SAUNDERS MANUAL OF CLINICAL LABORATORY SCIENCE

SAUNDERS MANUAL OF CLINICAL LABORATORY SCIENCE

Edited by

Craig A. Lehmann, PhD, CC(NRCC)

Associate Dean, School of Health Technology
and Management
Associate Professor/Chair, Division of
Diagnostic and Therapeutic Sciences
Health Sciences Center
State University of New York at Stony Brook
Stony Brook, New York

W.B. SAUNDERS COMPANY
A Division of Harcourt Brace & Company
Philadelphia London Toronto Montreal Sydney Tokyo

W.B. SAUNDERS COMPANY
A Division of Harcourt Brace & Company

The Curtis Center
Independence Square West
Philadelphia, Pennsylvania 19106

Library of Congress Cataloging-in-Publication Data

Saunders manual of clinical laboratory science / [edited by] Craig A. Lehmann.—1st ed.

p.   cm.

ISBN 0–7216–2185–6

1. Diagnosis, Laboratory—Handbooks, manuals, etc.   I. Lehmann, Craig A.
   [DNLM: 1. Diagnosis, Laboratory—laboratory manuals.   2. Chemistry, Clinical—laboratory manuals.   3. Microbiology—laboratory manuals.
   QY 25 S257 1998]

RB38.2.S28   1998   616.07′56—dc21

DNLM/DLC   97-27842

Saunders Manual of Clinical Laboratory Science   ISBN 0–7216–2185–6

Printed in the United States of America

Last digit is the print number: 9   8   7   6   5   4   3   2   1

CONTRIBUTORS

Robert J. Borley, MS, MT(ASCP)SBB

Associate Technical Director, University Hospital and Medical Center, State University of New York at Stony Brook, Stony Brook, New York

Compatibility Testing

Candace Breen, BS, MLT(ASCP)

Clinical Instructor, School of Health Technology and Management, Division of Diagnostic and Therapeutic Sciences, Department of Clinical Laboratory Sciences, Health Sciences Center, State University of New York at Stony Brook, Stony Brook, New York

Rheumatic and Autoimmune Diseases; Immunodeficiency; Lymphoproliferative Diseases; Immunology of Infectious Diseases; Transplantation Immunology

Elizabeth Cascone, BS, MT(ASCP)SBB

Training, Education and Quality Assurance Coordinator, University Hospital and Medical Center, State University of New York at Stony Brook, Stony Brook, New York

Basic Concepts of Immunohepatology; Compatibility Testing; Antibody Identification; Component Therapy; Quality Assurance

Donna D. Castellone, MS, MT(ASCP)SH

Clinical Assistant Professor, State University of New York at Stony Brook, Stony Brook; Technical Specialist, Department of Clinical Hematology, The New York Hospital–Cornell Medical Center, New York, New York

The Mechanism of Blood Coagulation; Evaluation of Bleeding Disorders; Evaluation of Thrombosis

Stuart Chaskes, MS, M(ASCP)

Associate Professor, State University of New York at Farmingdale, Farmingdale, New York

Virology

Stanley D. Cooper, PhD, FCACB

Partner, Triple G Corporation, Markham, Ontario, Canada

Laboratory Information Systems

Vincent Della Speranza, MS, HTL(ASCP), MT

Associate Technical Director for Anatomic Pathology, Chairman, Department of Laboratories Safety Committee, University Hospital and Medical Center, Stony Brook, New York

Safety Issues for the Clinical Laboratory

Karen M. Escolas, MS, MT(ASCP)

Chairperson and Assistant Professor, Medical Laboratory Technology Department, State University of New York at Farmingdale, Farmingdale, New York

Liver Function; Electrolytes and Water Balance; Renal Function and Nitrogen Balance; Blood Gases and Acid Base Balance; Mineral Metabolism; Endocrinology

Kathleen Finnegan, MS, MT(ASCP)SH

Clinical Assistant Professor, School of Health Technology and Management, Division of Diagnostic and Therapeutic Sciences, Department of Clinical Laboratory Sciences, Health Sciences Center, State University of New York at Stony Brook, Stony Brook, New York

Blood Collection and Anticoagulants; Routine Urinalysis; Routine Analysis of Body Fluids; Hematopoiesis; Erythrocyte Disorders; Leukocyte Disorders

Deborah Firestone, MA, MT(ASCP)SBB

Chair, Clinical Laboratory Sciences Program, and Clinical Assistant Professor, School of Health Technology and Management, Division of Diagnostic and Therapeutic Sciences, Department of Clinical Laboratory Sciences, Health Sciences Center, State University of New York at Stony Brook, Stony Brook, New York

Component Therapy; Transfusion Reactions

Marc Golightly, BS, PhD

Associate Professor, School of Medicine, Department of Pathology; Head of Clinical Immunology, University Hospital, State University of New York at Stony Brook, Stony Brook, New York

Rheumatic and Autoimmune Diseases; Immunodeficiency; Lymphoproliferative Diseases; Immunology of Infectious Diseases; Transplantation Immunology

Mary Hotaling, MS, MT(ASCP)DLM

Clinical Assistant Professor, School of Health Technology and Management, Division of Diagnostic and Therapeutic Sciences, Department of Clinical Laboratory Sciences, Health Sciences Center, State University of New York at Stony Brook, Stony Brook, New York

Amino Acids and Proteins; Carbohydrates; Enzymes; Cardiac Function

Bruce T. Kube, BS, MT(ASCP)H

Teaching Hospital Clinical Laboratory Technologist I, University Medical Center, State University of New York at Stony Brook, Stony Brook, New York

Erythrocyte Disorders; Hematology Procedures

Carolyn Kube, BS, MT(ASCP)

Medical Technologist, Clinical Laboratory, University Hospital Medical Center at Stony Brook, State University of New York at Stony Brook, Stony Brook, New York

Immunology of Infectious Diseases

Joseph T. Lanman, PhD (FACMG)

Assistant Professor of Clinical Pathology, Head of Cytogenetics, State University of New York at Stony Brook, Stony Brook, New York

Cytogenetics

Craig A. Lehmann, PhD, CC(NRCC)

Associate Dean, School of Health Technology and Management, Associate Professor/Chair, Division of Diagnostic and Therapeutic Sciences, Health Sciences Center, State University of New York at Stony Brook, Stony Brook, New York

Lipids and Lipoproteins; Pancreas and Gastrointestinal Function; Nutrition Assessment, Vitamins, and Trace Elements; Tumor Markers; Laboratory Mathematics

Alan M. Leiken, PhD

Chair and Associate Professor, Department of Health Care Policy and Management, Associate Dean for Graduate Studies, School of Health Technology and Management, State University of New York at Stony Brook, Stony Brook, New York

Laboratory Statistics

Ronald Malowitz, PhD, MT(ASCP)

Clinical Associate Professor, School of Health Technology and Management, Division of Diagnostic and Therapeutic Sciences, Department of Clinical Laboratory Science, Health Sciences Center; Assistant Head, Microbiology Laboratory, University Hospital, State University of New York at Stony Brook, Stony Brook, New York

Quality Control in the Clinical Microbiology Laboratory; Handling and Processing Specimens for Bacteriology, Mycology, and Parasitology; Clinical Parasitology; Clinical Mycology

Maria Reitano, PhD

Clinical Associate Professor, School of Health Technology and Management, Division of Diagnostic and Therapeutic Sciences, Department of Clinical Laboratory Sciences, Health Sciences Center, State University of New York at Stony Brook, Stony Brook, New York

Quality Control in the Clinical Microbiology Laboratory; Handling and Processing Specimens for Bacteriology, Mycology, and Parasitology; Clinical Bacteriology

Thomas R. Sexton, PhD

Associate Professor and Director, Harriman School for Management and Policy, State University of New York at Stony Brook, Stony Brook, New York

Laboratory Statistics

Vivien A. Soo, MS, MT(ASCP)

Section Supervisor, Special Chemistry/Toxicology, University Hospital, State University of New York at Stony Brook, Stony Brook, New York

Therapeutic Drug Monitoring; Clinical Toxicology

Eric D. Spitzer, MD, PhD

Associate Professor, Department of Pathology; Chief of Clinical Microbiology Laboratory, University Hospital, State University of New York at Stony Brook, Stony Brook, New York

Molecular Diagnostics

Silvia G. Spitzer, PhD

Research Assistant Professor, Department of Pathology; Head, Molecular Genetics Laboratory, University Hospital, State University of New York at Stony Brook, Stony Brook, New York

Molecular Diagnostics

FOREWORD

The decade of the 1990s will be remembered as one of significant and far-reaching changes in the field of health care—specifically medical care. Even as people were lamenting the "failure" of the President's health reform proposals, changes were taking place and the system was, in fact, being reformed, prodded by market forces rather than government-initiated reforms. Few changes in modern times have been so dramatic as those occurring in the biomedical sciences and the delivery of medical services. It is not easy to predict the configuration of the system when it reaches its equilibrium point, but it is safe to say that the changes occurring in the organization and financing of health care will have a material impact on all components of the health workforce. There are meaningful discussions taking place in the United States concerning the need to rationalize the supply of physicians as well as the demand for physicians' services. These conversations have been broadened to include yet another question: how many and what mix of health personnel does the nation need? Most policy makers have concluded that the United States has an oversupply of physicians, characterized by a large surplus of specialists and a relative shortage of primary care physicians. Incentives have been put in place to encourage academic medical centers to reverse this trend.

As we begin to address the supply of physicians and other health professionals, we note that the traditional professional roles and scopes of practice need to change along with the educational and training curricula that have traditionally served to carve out narrow, definitive scopes of practice, irrespective of the training of the professional. In the case of clinical laboratory scientists, the need for change is apparent, as the structure, management, and financing of the diagnostic services world are as confined as the rest of the health care system. As we move from a preponderance of in-hospital care to outpatient care in a variety of settings, we begin to observe new demands for professional autonomy, higher levels of competence, professional confidence, and a redefinition of the professional base of clinical laboratory scientists to more accurately reflect the increasing complexities of the job. As the system shifts from cost-based reimbursement to capitated payments and managed care, we are requiring that health professionals, at all levels, "do more with less." What this means is that professionals must broaden their professional horizons, retrain themselves, and move away from the intense specialization that was once associated with the field to a more generic and broad-based—a generalist—approach to clinical laboratory practice. This manual addresses the new configurations of the clinical laboratory operation and the need for students not only to perform tests, but to apply laboratory data to patient care.

Most industrialized nations are confronting the political and economic issues associated with financing health care. Policy makers, payers, and consumers are interested in ways of containing health care costs while achieving greater efficiencies. In almost every nation there are ongoing discussions about the future of medicine and health services in the context of aging populations, rapid technologic change, and growing consumer expectations. In the United States, the pressures for change—philosophical and organizational—have reached a crescendo, and health professionals are gearing up for the inevitable shifts, not only in their own professional milieus, but in the structure and management of the larger system. Both payers and policy makers have an increasing influence over medical decisions by the application of managed care controls. This stringent approach to cost containment and utilization management alters the way physicians and clinical laboratory scientists view the nature and frequency of laboratory tests and procedures. This has demanded new approaches to diagnosis and a new level of analytical skill in the laboratory.

In addition, many believe that the traditional infectious diseases have been controlled, if not totally eliminated. The more recent issues have to do with genetic re-engineering, organ transplantation, contraception, pain management, and rehabilitation from chronic degenerative diseases. The advances in biomedicine, taken together with those broader changes brought about by public health measures such as improvement in air, food, and water quality, signal that a profound change in human life has occurred. It has transformed the way that we think about disease, illness, and death. And certainly these events have changed the way in which we traditionally organize and deliver services. The clinical laboratory scientist has a role to play in all of these, especially in educating students for the new roles that will emerge.

Clearly, the work environment of health professionals has changed. For physicians, there has been the impact of attempts at rationalizing the field of medical care by utilizing a supply side strategy that favors the creation of more primary care providers and fewer specialists. Physicians acknowledge the stresses associated with these changes and the need to minimize uncertainty in clinical decision making by applying available medical science and technology to clinical decisions. As a result, physicians rely heavily on clinical laboratory findings and on the skill and expertise of the clinical laboratory scientist to provide accurate and relevant information to aid in diagnosis and decision making. This interdependent relationship illustrates the strides that have been made in the field to foster interdisciplinary practice and teamwork.

Saunders Manual of Clinical Laboratory Science addresses important aspects of the professional knowledge base that form the foundation for clinical laboratory professionals at all levels. It deals with the significant changes that affect the traditional world of work for laboratory scientists. The manual does an excellent job of embedding the work of clinical laboratory scientists into the fabric of both medicine and public health. It suggests changes in the processes of clinical laboratory science, as well as in the structure and management of the clinical laboratory enterprise. It suggests the necessary knowledge base that clinical laboratory scientists require in order to work efficiently and effectively in the changing world, and offers lessons for educators attempting to modify the curriculum in clinical laboratory science programs. Indeed, there is a need for curriculum redesign, since the duties of laboratory professionals must change as the work place expectations change. There is every indication of a need for more knowledge on a variety of broader issues than those contained in the originally accepted knowledge base of clinical laboratory scientists.

It is a fact that characteristics of the knowledge base are the foundations for distinguishing professions from occupations. The contents of this manual suggest that laboratory professionals must have problem solving skills, critical thinking abilities, and the capacity to synthesize and apply abstract knowledge. Clearly, the demands of the profession require more than the conventional knowledge base, because in the future clinical laboratory scientists will have considerably more autonomy as they move from highly structured, institutional work sites to remote, outpatient facilities where point-of-care testing and transmittal of results are becoming the normal mode of operation.

There will be a need for a scientist who not only performs tests and procedures but who also has the ability to analyze results.

The rapid introduction of technology into the health field makes many new models possible. Communications technology has greatly enriched the capacity of the laboratorian to work independently while functioning as part of a team. The rapid incorporation of new instruments and testing modalities requires a professional who has the capacity to understand the inner workings of biomedical equipment. This edition of *Saunders Manual of Clinical Laboratory Science* not only updates the day-to-day practice of laboratory medicine from the viewpoint of medical technology, but also establishes the new demands that are operating on the clinical laboratory scientist. The material included in the manual is as important to the educator and the manager as it is to the scientist.

LORNA S. MCBARNETTE, PhD
Dean of the School of Health Technology and Management
Professor of Health Policy and Management
Health Sciences Center
State University of New York at Stony Brook
Stony Brook, New York

PREFACE

Health care for the past several years has been changing owing to decreased government budgets and managed care. These changes have had major impacts on clinical laboratories and their personnel. The implementation of the core laboratory has forced many laboratorians to become proficient in more than one area. The new technologies' ability to consolidate workstations and sometimes entire departments such as the radioimmunoassay have forced many laboratorians into other parts of the clinical laboratory. Because of these changes and others, laboratorians are being asked to function in new and/or multiple disciplines (e.g., hematology, chemistry, coagulation), thus requiring many clinical laboratory scientists to relearn past knowledge. The environment is also requiring that many new clinical laboratory scientists enter the field as generalists. As a result of the present environment and a void in the clinical laboratory science literature, the following text will offer the clinical laboratory student and scientist, as well as others, laboratory diagnostic information in a format that is concise and easy to access.

The text assumes a basic level of clinical laboratory knowledge. It is not in any way a replacement of the standard texts such as *Tietz Fundamentals of Clinical Chemistry* by Burtis and Ashwood, *Diagnostic Hematology* by Rodak, or *Textbook of Diagnostic Microbiology* by Mahon amd Manuselis, to name a few. The primary intent of the text is to serve as a comprehensive resource for clinical laboratory students as well as clinical laboratory scientists and health care practitioners. For clinical laboratory science students, it will serve as a review text for registry and other examinations. The text covers the entire field of clinical laboratory science from routine areas such as clinical chemistry, hematology, and bacteriology to the more specialty areas such as molecular biology and mycology. At the end of each chapter there is a bibliography that will serve as a resource for additional queries. The text offers special sections on laboratory information systems, statistics, laboratory math, and laboratory safety.

Each chapter begins with a brief introduction to the topic, followed by concise paragraphs, charts, algorithms, and illustrations. This format places the most relevant information for each topic at the reader's fingertips. Clinical laboratory science students will find this format conducive to studying, as they will not have to thumb through endless pages of text for an answer. Clinical laboratory scientists who are being crosstrained or moved to a new department will find this text an excellent resource to acquaint themselves with forgotten, unlearned, or new subjects dealing with the clinical laboratory. Clinical laboratory scientists, as well as practitioners, will be able to find answers quickly on patient preparation, sample storage, test methodologies, test interferences, basic theories, and test result interpretation. For many pathologies, diagnostic algorithms are presented for easy interpretation and diagnostic testing strategies. The chapter on laboratory information systems is unique in that it explains the theory as well as the relevance of each LIS input and output for both the laboratorian and the practitioner.

Like myself, all the associate and assistant editors are educators. All but one (Karen Escolas) are from the Department of Clinical Laboratory Sciences, SUNY at Stony Brook. Karen Escolas was with the department for many years, until just recently when she accepted a position as Chair of Medical Technology, SUNY at Farmingdale (an associate degree level program). Because of this, Karen has also added her expertise in meeting the needs for this level. This group of editors and authors are unique in that for years we have worked together in education and curricular design for the field of clinical laboratory sciences. All the other authors are practitioners and educators from the University Medical Center, SUNY at Stony Brook, and are involved in SUNY Stony Brook's Clinical Laboratory Sciences program.

Overall, I believe this group of educators/clinical laboratory scientists has put together a body of knowledge in a format that will assist clinical laboratory students, clinical laboratory scientists, and health care practitioners in their quest for answers in the field of clinical laboratory science.

CRAIG A. LEHMANN, PhD, CC(NRCC)

ACKNOWLEDGMENTS

This text is a product of dedication, endless labor, and love for the profession of clinical laboratory sciences by relatively a small group of individuals. I would like to thank my editorial group and the contributors who have given so much of their time and knowledge to this endeavor over the last 3 years. Their commitment to the profession and the education of its students is meritorious.

I would also like to thank the following colleagues who supplied knowledge and/or visual material for this text. Without their assistance, we could have never produced such a high quality text.

Jacqueline H. Carr, MS, MT(ASCP)SH, DLM, Department of Pathology and Laboratory Medicine, Division of Hematopathology, Indiana University Medical Center, Indianapolis, Indiana

Andrea Ishigami, MS, Department of Clinical Laboratory Sciences, School of Health Technology and Management, SUNY, Stony Brook, New York

David T. John, MSPH, PhD, Oklahoma State University, College of Osteopathic Medicine, Tulsa, Oklahoma

Connie R. Mahon, MS, MT(ASCP), School of Allied Health Sciences, Department of Clinical Laboratory Sciences, The University of Texas Health Science Center at San Antonio, San Antonio, Texas

Edward K. Markell, MD, PhD, University of California, San Francisco, and Stanford University, Palo Alto, California

Michael R. McGinnis, PhD, Department of Pathology, University of Texas Medical Branch, Galveston, Texas

Bernadette F. Rodak, MS, CLSpH(NCA), MT(ASCP)SH, Medical Technology Program, Indiana University, Indianapolis, Indiana

Marcella Liffick Stevens, MA, MS, CLS(NCA), MT(ASCP), Clinical Laboratory Science Program, Indiana State University, Terre Haute, Indiana

Anne Stiene-Martin, PhD, Division of Clinical Laboratory Science, University of Kentucky, Chandler Medical Center, Lexington, Kentucky

Barbara Panessa Warren, PhD, Department of Clinical Laboratory Sciences, School of Health Technology and Management, SUNY, Stony Brook, New York

Eugene Wienke, MD, Pathology Laboratory, Deaconess Hospital Systems—Central Campus, St. Louis, Missouri

Elizabeth A. Zeibig, MT(ASCP), Department of Clinical Laboratory Science, School of Allied Health Professions, St. Louis University Health Science Center, St. Louis, Missouri

Thanks to the Triple G Corporation for their commitment of time and resources to the LIS chapter: Lee Green, Gary Friedman, Stanley Cooper, John Fitzgibbon, Amyn Hilari, and Sharon Smith. For clerical services, I would like to thank Kelly Ann Felice and Catherine Horgan, Dean's office, and Phyllis Brenna, Department of Clinical Laboratory Sciences, SUNY at Stony Brook. Thanks to the Saunders family, who are a group of true professionals: Selma Kaszczuk, Senior Editor, a true leader who has a vision beyond the horizon; Scott Weaver, Developmental Editor, for his ability to leave no rock unturned and go the extra mile to seek perfection; Karen Fabiano, Marketing Manager, for her marketing skills; as well as Gene Harris for the book design, Sharon Iwanczuk for the illustrations, and David Harvey and Gretchen Becker for the copy editing.

A **special thanks** to my wife Susan and my sons Jason and Aaron for their love, support, and praise.

CRAIG A. LEHMANN, PhD, CC(NRCC)

CONTENTS

Chapter

1

BLOOD COLLECTION AND ANTICOAGULANTS

Kathleen Finnegan, MS, MT (ASCP) SH

Q U I C K   C O N T E N T S

INTRODUCTION

Properly collected specimens represent a very important step for the laboratory and laboratory testing. The laboratory results are only as good as the specimens received for testing. Blood specimens are obtained by phlebotomy. Phlebotomy is defined as an incision made into the vein. Phlebotomy can be performed by the procedure of venipuncture, which involves collecting blood by penetrating a vein with a needle with a collection apparatus or syringe. The second method for blood collection is by the skin or dermal puncture, which involves the collection of capillary blood after an incision is made in the skin with a lancet. Blood specimens for laboratory testing are needed for laboratory analysis to diagnose and monitor medical conditions.

TYPES OF BLOOD SPECIMENS

There are various types of blood specimens required for laboratory testing. The type of specimen required depends on the type of test and the department of the laboratory that does the testing.

Types of Blood Specimens

TYPES	DESCRIPTION	USE
Clotted Blood	No anticoagulant added	For separation, to use the serum portion
Serum	Clotted blood is allowed to stand for 20 min and then centrifuged. The upper portion is termed serum. Does not contain fibrinogen	Chemistry testing Serology testing Blood banking
Whole Blood	Obtained by having a tube containing an anticoagulant that prevents the blood from clotting. The tube contains cells and plasma. Important that the tube is mixed well	Can be used for testing in hematology cell counting. For separation to use the plasma portion
Plasma	Whole blood is centrifuged and the upper layer is termed plasma. Plasma contains fibrinogen.	Coagulation Plasma chemistries
Capillary Blood	A combination of venous, arterial blood, and tissue fluid obtained through a skin puncture	When a venipuncture cannot be performed on newborns and children, a heel stick or finger stick procedure is performed.
Buffy Coat	The middle layer between the plasma and red blood cells Contains white blood cells and platelets	Special stains Hematology studies

SPECIMEN HANDLING

The integrity of specimens for laboratory testing is very important. The integrity of the specimen can be compromised by the methods of collection or by mishandling of the specimen. It is important for proper technique and procedures to ensure quality specimens. Poor specimens mean poor laboratory testing.

Unacceptable Specimens

TYPE	DESCRIPTION	CONSIDERATIONS
Lipemic	A cloudy turbid appearance, presence of lipids, indicates a nonfasting specimen.	Interferes with colorimetric analysis in chemistry and hemoglobin in hematology
Hemolysis	Destruction of the red blood cells results in plasma or serum appearing red to pink. This is due to the release of hemoglobin. Caused by traumatic phlebotomy or intravascular disease	Affects potassium and enzyme testing
Partially Filled Tubes	For proper ratio of blood to anticoagulant, all tubes should be filled until the vacuum is exhausted.	Most important for coagulation testing
Specimen Contamination	Improper antiseptic cleaning of the site before performing venipuncture, or the leaving of povidone iodine on a skin puncture	Aseptic technique very important for blood cultures Iodine increases potassium and uric acid results in a skin puncture.

Specimen Handling Requirements

TYPE	DESCRIPTION	EXAMPLES
Fasting	Patient should not have anything to eat or drink with the exception of water for 8–12 hr.	Glucose testing Cholesterol Triglycerides
Timed	Specimens to be collected at a specific time. Need to be labeled with time specimen was drawn.	Cardiac panel
Peak	Collected when the highest serum concentration of a drug is anticipated. Drawn 15–30 min after administration.	Drug levels
Trough	Collected when the lowest serum concentration of a drug is expected, usually before the next dose.	Drug levels
Iced	Chilling the specimen to slow down the metabolic process that will continue after it is drawn. Should be placed in a crushed ice and water solution for even cooling.	Ammonia Blood gases Coagulation testing
Keep Warm	Keep the specimen at body temperature or close to 37°C with the use of an incubator.	Cold agglutinins
Protect from Light	The specimen should be wrapped in aluminum foil or a light inhibiting container should be used. Components break down when exposed to light, causing a decreased value.	Bilirubin Vitamin B_{12} Carotene
Legal/Forensic	Samples that may be used as evidence in legal proceedings. Chain of custody is essential. Documentation of specimen handling begins with patient identification and continues until testing is completed. Must include date, time, and identification of handler. Should be done in front of a witness.	DNA analysis Drug levels Alcohol level

SPECIMEN HANDLING

BLOOD COLLECTION EQUIPMENT

The methods for blood collection for venipuncture are the evacuated tube system, the syringe method, and/or the butterfly infusion set. Organization and knowledge of phlebotomy equipment is important for venipuncture. For capillary blood, the skin puncture is done with the use of a lancet of various sizes, depending on the amount of blood needed.

TYPE	DESCRIPTION	FUNCTION	IMPORTANT INFORMATION
Needles	Vary in size, length, and gauge (the diameter) Gauge varies from 16 to 25 g. The larger the gauge, the smaller the diameter of the needle. Length varies from 1 to 1.5 inch. Most commonly used is a 21 g by 1.5 inch needle	Designed for single draw or multidraws. They are attached to the evacuated system or there are needles that attach to the syringe. Depending on the size and the integrity of the vein, the size of the needle should be determined.	Sterile, disposable, and used only once. Manufacturers package needles individually and color code them for gauge. Never recap, break, or bend needles. Dispose of properly.

Continued ▶

► Continued **BLOOD COLLECTION EQUIPMENT**

TYPE	DESCRIPTION	FUNCTION	IMPORTANT INFORMATION
Needle Disposal Containers	A container with a biohazard label for all sharp objects. Usually made of a sturdy plastic with openings on the top for needle disposal.	All used needles are disposed of. To avoid needle sticks, use the device on the container for safe removal of the needles.	Needles should never be re-capped, bent, or broken. Safety caps for needles are now available.
Needle Holders	These are adapters or holders for the needles. They are made of a hard, rigid plastic. They can be color coded for the particular needle system being used.	Needles used with the evacuated system are designed to be screwed into the holder, which also holds the collection tubes.	Some are disposable; others are used again and can be cleaned with a disinfectant.
Collection Tubes	Evacuated tubes for collection contain a premeasured vacuum, additive or nonadditive. They range in size from 2 to 15 mL and are color coded depending on additive.	To be used with multisample needles and needle holder for collection of blood.	Vacuum is guaranteed by the manufacturer until the expiration date on each tube is passed. Always read the manufacturer's label on the tube for additive and level of fill.
Syringe	A single sample needle attached to a sterile disposable plastic barrel with plunger. Can be used with a variety of needle sizes and syringe size ranging from 2 to 50 mL.	Used for veins that are too fragile for the evacuated system. You can regulate the amount of pressure by how hard you pull on the plunger.	Blood needs to be transferred from the syringe into collection tubes. Use correct order of draw.
Butterfly	A 0.5–0.75 inch stainless needle connected to a 5–12 inch length tubing with plastic extensions or wings.	Used for difficult veins, hand veins, pediatrics and elderly patients.	Can be used on the end of a syringe or with an adapter added to a holder to use with the evacuated system.
Lancet	A sterile, single use, disposable, sharp-pointed instrument. Different sizes for different depths.	Used to penetrate the skin in a finger or heel puncture.	Should never exceed 2.4 mm in depth.
Micro Collection Tubes	Plastic tubes with a variety of anticoagulant and additives. They are color coded the same as the vacuum collection tubes. Hold 600 μL of blood.	For finger-stick and heel-stick blood collection	Tubes with anticoagulant contain beads to help with mixing. Should be mixed often; they tend to clot quickly.
Tourniquet	Latex strip 2–3 inches in diameter, which does not support bacterial growth. Plastic strip with a Velcro closing, easy to put on and release	Applied above the elbow to cause blood to pool in the area and to enlarge the veins, making them easier to locate and penetrate.	Should not be left on for longer than 1 min. The pressure from the tourniquet causes biologic analytes to leak out of the cells into the blood.

Continued ►

▶ Continued **BLOOD COLLECTION EQUIPMENT**

TYPE	DESCRIPTION	FUNCTION	IMPORTANT INFORMATION
Antiseptic Pad	70% isopropyl alcohol	To prevent sepsis, bacteriostatis, which prevents or inhibits bacterial growth. Use to clean the site before performing venipuncture.	Iodine is used for blood cultures and for alcohol levels.
Gauze Pads	A 2 × 2 sterile cotton square	Used for drying the site that has been cleaned and also is placed over the site after withdrawal of the needle.	Cotton balls tend to stick to the site upon removal and may initiate bleeding.
Bandages	Adhesive strip	Placed on the site after needle withdrawal for protection and to prevent bleeding.	Should not be used on infants under 2 years of age because of aspiration.
Gloves	Latex Vinyl Polyethylene	Used for universal protection for each patient.	A new pair of gloves must be worn for each patient.

Color-Coded Collection Tubes

Collection tubes are color coded for the type of specimen that will be obtained and type of laboratory testing that will be done. The tubes are color coded for the type of additive or nonadditive that the tube may or may not contain. Two types of stoppers (tube tops) are now available: rubber stoppers or a plastic shield that covers the rubber stopper (Hemogard). Most collection tubes have been universally color coded for easy use. Each laboratory may interchange the use of a particular tube for a particular test.

TIP   Always refer to the laboratory manual of each facility for correct tube and specimen collection.

Collection Tube Colors and Additives*

TYPE	ADDITIVE	ADDITIVE FUNCTION	CONSIDERATIONS	LABORATORY USE
Plain Red	None	Contains no anticoagulants and no additives.	Sterile with no additive best choice for blood banking. Clot formation takes 30 min.	Serum chemistries Serology Blood bank
Lavender	EDTA	Removes calcium to prevent clotting.	Should be well mixed; invert 6–8 times.	Whole blood hematology cell counting CBC

Continued ▶

▶ Continued **Collection Tube Colors and Additives***

TYPE	ADDITIVE	ADDITIVE FUNCTION	CONSIDERATIONS	LABORATORY USE
Light Blue	Sodium citrate 0.105 M or 0.129 M	Removes calcium to prevent clotting.	Tube should be full and mixed well. Blood to anticoagulant ratio is very important (9:1).	Coagulation studies PT APTT Factor assay
Green	Sodium heparin Lithium heparin Ammonium heparin	Inhibits thrombin formation to prevent clotting.	Be careful of the type of heparin that is being used for the type of testing.	Plasma chemistries
Gray	Sodium fluoride Potassium oxalate	Inhibits glycolysis. Removes calcium to prevent clotting.	Should not be used for other chemistries.	Glucose testing usually Glucose tolerance Alcohol levels
Yellow	Sodium polyethylene sulfonate (SPS)	Prevents blood from clotting and stabilizes bacterial growth.	Invert 8 times	Blood cultures
Royal Blue	None Sodium heparin EDTA	Contains no anticoagulant Anticoagulant	Chemically cleaned and the rubber stoppers contain low levels of metals.	Toxicology Trace metals
Red/Marbled	Gel separator/clot activator	Clot activators shorten the time for clot formation. The gel forms a barrier between cells and serum.	Tubes should be inverted 5 times to expose the blood to the activator. Centrifuged after clot formation is complete.	Most chemistry testing Not suitable for blood bank testing.
Light Green/ Marbled	Gel separator/lithium heparin	Heparin prevents clotting. Gel separator prevents cell contamination.		Potassium determinations
Yellow/ Marbled	Thrombin	Thrombin is a clot activator for faster clot formation, usually within 5 min.	Should be inverted 8 times	STAT chemistries
Black	Sodium citrate	Binds calcium	4:1 ratio of blood to anticoagulant	Westergren sedimentation rates
Brown	Sodium heparin	Inhibits thrombin formation.	Less than 0.1 μg/mL of lead	Lead determinations
Plain Pink	None	None		Used for blood banking

*See inside front cover for color photos of stoppers included within this chart.

Order of Draw

When multiple specimens are collected, the order in which the tubes are drawn can affect test results. As recommended by Becton-Dickinson, a tube manufacturer, the order of draw for a routine venipuncture is that sterile specimens are drawn first followed by plain red, light blue (sodium citrate), green (heparin), lavender (EDTA), clot activators, or clot separators; last is gray (oxalate/fluoride). The National Committee for Clinical Laboratory Standards (NCCLS) recommends the order of draw as blood cultures, non-additive or serum, coagulation, additive tubes.

If only coagulation studies are being drawn, a plain red top tube should be drawn first in view of the release of tissue thromboplastin from the skin puncture, which can interfere with coagulation testing.

> **TIP** A light blue tube should never be drawn first and should always be full and well mixed.

The order of draw changes for a syringe procedure. The order for tube fill from a syringe is first the sterile specimens, followed by coagulation studies, EDTA, heparin, or other anticoagulants, followed by plain red and serum separators.

For the skin puncture, the order of draw is a slide for a blood smear, EDTA, green, followed by red and gel separators last.

VENIPUNCTURE PROCEDURE

For a routine venipuncture, the choice of site involves three primary veins including the cephalic, the basilic, and the median cubital, which is located in the antecubital fossa at the bend of the elbow. The median cubital is the vein of choice because of easy access and because it is anchored better than the others (see below). A tourniquet is applied to increase stasis and to aid in vein selection. In selecting a vein, the tip of the index finger is used to palpate the vein. This will help determine the size, depth, and direction of the vein. After the vein is selected, the arm should be cleansed with 70% isopropyl alcohol. Let the alcohol dry and do not touch the site after this step. Then proceed with the venipuncture procedure.

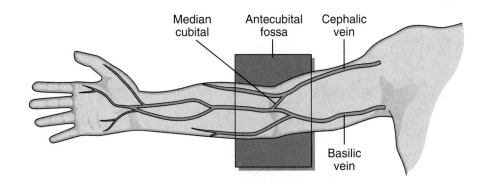

> **TIP** Never leave a tourniquet on a patient's arm for longer than 1 minute.

VENIPUNCTURE PROCEDURE

The most important step of venipuncture is patient identification and the proper labeling of all tubes. Patients should state and spell their full name, birth date, and identification number, which can be the social security number or number assigned to them by the hospital. All labeling should be performed at the bedside or before the patient leaves your side. Always label tubes after blood is drawn; never label tubes after you leave the patient. Labeling should also contain the date, the time of collection, and the phlebotomist's initials.

Venipuncture Steps

1. **Prepare paperwork.** Carefully look over requisitions slips. Note any special instructions.

2. **Identify the patient.** A crucial step. Always ask the patient to state and spell his or her full name and identification number.

3. **Verify diet restrictions.** A fasting or nonfasting specimen. Note any medication that may interfere with testing.

4. **Wash hands, put on gloves, and assemble equipment.** Always wash hands before and after attending to each patient. Universal Precautions state that a clean pair of gloves should be used for each patient. Organization is important.

5. **Reassure and position the patient.** Never tell a patient it will not hurt. A patient should be seated in a blood drawing chair or lying down. Never have them standing or seated on a high stool.

6. **Apply tourniquet.** The tourniquet is applied 3 to 4 inches above the intended site and should never be left in place for longer than 1 minute.

7. **Select venipuncture site.** Have the patient make a fist; this makes the veins more prominent. A vein has bounce or resilience. Never select a blue line. You must feel the vein.

8. **Cleanse the site.** Using 70% isopropyl alcohol, make a circular motion starting from the center and moving outward. Allow the site to dry. *Do not touch the site after cleaning!*

9. **Uncover needle and inspect.** Remove the cover from the needle and visually inspect the needle for imperfections or barbs. Do not touch the needle.

10. **Perform venipuncture.** Anchor the vein using your nondominant hand and use the thumb to pull the skin taut but not tight. Do not use the two finger method. Insert the needle into the skin with the bevel up at a 15 to 30 degree angle with a quick smooth motion.

11. **Fill tubes: order of draw.** Always fill tubes according to the order of draw. If the tube has an additive, mix well by inverting several times. Tubes will stop filling when the vacuum is exhausted.

12. **Release tourniquet.** The tourniquet should be released after the first tube is full. It should not be left on for more than 1 minute.

13. **Withdrawal and needle disposal.** After the last tube is filled, release it from the holder, remove the needle in one swift motion, and immediately apply pressure to the site. Hold in place until bleeding stops. It is not acceptable to have patients bend their arm up. Dispose of the needle immediately in the proper container. Never cut, bend, break, or recap needles.

⑭ **Label tubes.** All tubes should be labeled with the patient's full name, birth date, and/or identification number; the time; the date; and the phlebotomist's initials. Never label tubes prior to venipuncture.

⑮ **Apply bandage.** Check the patient's arm; if bleeding has stopped, apply a bandage. Never apply a bandage on a child under 2 years of age.

⑯ **Dispose of contaminated materials, thank the patient, remove gloves, and wash hands.** All contaminated material should be disposed of properly. Do not leave any blood drawing equipment in the patient's bed or room. Always remove gloves and wash hands after each patient.

⑰ **Transport the specimen to the laboratory.** The specimen should be transported in a timely fashion. Proper specimen handling and transport are important for the integrity of the specimen.

SKIN OR DERMAL PUNCTURE PROCEDURE

The skin puncture procedure is the obtaining of blood from either the finger or the heel of a patient. Microcollection by skin puncture follows the same steps used during venipuncture. Skin puncture is the method of choice for infants and children under the age of 2 years. In adults, skin puncture may be required because of inability to find a vein for the venipuncture procedure. Other reasons for the use of skin puncture for adults are burned or scarred patients, geriatric patients with fragile veins, patients receiving chemotherapy, and when only a small sample is needed, as in point of care testing.

The composition of blood collected from a skin or dermal puncture is different from that of blood drawn from a vein. The blood collected from the skin is a combination of venous, arterial, and interstitial fluid. It contains a higher amount of arterial blood, especially if the area has been warmed. It should always be noted on the laboratory slip when capillary blood is drawn for laboratory testing.

Heel Puncture Site

The heel is used in newborns and infants who have not started to walk. The acceptable area for the heel stick is the medial and lateral areas of the plantar surface (see below).

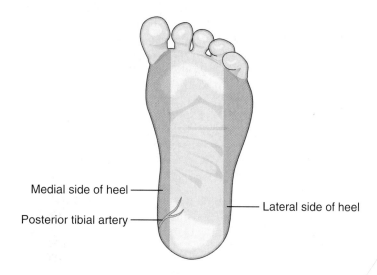

Medial side of heel ——

Posterior tibial artery ——

—— Lateral side of heel

SKIN OR DERMAL PUNCTURE PROCEDURE

The posterior curvature, the arch, or the toes are not acceptable for the collection of blood. If these areas are used for collection, damage to the nerves and tendons of the foot may be caused. There is also a risk of puncturing the bone. The heel puncture should never exceed 2.4 mm in depth.

Finger Puncture Site

The recommended site for the finger stick is the palmar surface of the distal phalanx of the ring or middle finger (see below). The puncture should be made in the central fleshy area of the finger. The puncture should be perpendicular to the fingerprint and not parallel to it. It is not recommended to use the index finger because of increased nerve endings, the little or fifth fingers because of their decreased tissue mass, and the thumb because it is sometimes callused. The finger stick puncture also should never exceed 2.4 mm in depth.

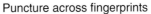

Puncture across fingerprints

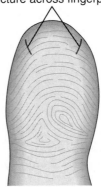

Performing the Skin Puncture

In performing a heel or finger stick procedure, the same basic steps of venipuncture apply. The heel or finger should be well supported by holding firmly. The area should not be excessively squeezed. You may want to warm or massage the area before performing the stick. Warming increases the blood flow and allows for better blood collection. Always wipe the first drop of blood away. This will prevent contamination of residual alcohol and the introduction of tissue fluid into the specimen. Specimens are obtained by capillary action. If using the microcontainer system that contains additives, tap the tube several times and invert six to eight times for complete mixing. Microsamples must be labeled with the full name of the patient, identification number, date, time, and phlebotomist's initials. If transporting the smaller tube in a large tube, both tubes should contain all labeling information.

SYRINGE PROCEDURE

The procedure and steps for the drawing of blood using a syringe are the same as for the evacuated tube method. A syringe consists of a plastic barrel and a plunger. The needle is attached on the end of the barrel. Pull on the syringe plunger to break the seal, and see that it moves freely. Make sure the plunger is pushed all the way into the syringe before you begin. Hold the syringe as you would a needle holder.

Syringe drawing is used for a patient who has fragile or weak veins that may collapse with the evacuated method. By using the syringe, you can control the pressure by pulling on the plunger and then allowing the syringe to fill slowly. When the syringe is full, the blood needs to be transferred into collection tubes. The needle should be replaced with a 18 gauge needle. Penetrate the stoppers of the collection tubes and allow the vacuum to draw in the blood. Never force blood into the tube. Use proper order of draw, label all tubes correctly, and dispose of syringe and needle into a sharps container.

BUTTERFLY PROCEDURE

The butterfly method can be used with the evacuated tube system or can be attached to a syringe. Butterfly or winged infusion sets are used for pediatric patients, or for patients who have small veins, especially in the hand.

Again, all venipuncture steps apply to the butterfly procedure. Remove the butterfly from the sealed package. Pull on the tubing gently to uncoil it. Attach the butterfly to a syringe. The butterfly can also be attached to a needle holder with an adapter (or with the use of an adapter for the needle holder). Using the wings, insert the needle at a 10 to 15 degree angle into the vein with the bevel up. Make sure the butterfly is secure at the site. Fill the collection tubes or syringe. When the procedure is complete, remove the butterfly and dispose of the needle and tubing into the sharps container with it still attached to the holder or syringe; then detach. Use extreme care with butterfly disposal.

COMPLICATIONS IN BLOOD COLLECTION

COMPLICATION	CAUSE	CORRECTIVE ACTION
Failure to Draw Blood	Inserting the needle too deep and going through the vein. Inserting the needle not deep enough, being above the vein. The bevel of the needle not facing up. Losing the vacuum of the collection tube.	Sometimes you can slowly pull back or withdraw the needle. Redirect the needle and go deeper; never probe. Need to begin again. Always check expiration dates of tubes and have extra tubes handy.
Fainting (Vasovagal Syncope)	Patient experiences dizziness during or after the venipuncture through an emotional stimuli such as fright or the sight of blood. There is a sudden decrease in blood pressure and a temporary loss of consciousness.	Protect the patient from falling, lower the patient's head between the knees. Alert the physician. If fainting occurs during the procedure, always remove the tourniquet and withdraw the needle. Have an ammonia inhalant ready.
Hematoma	Blood leaks from the vein into the surrounding tissue, resulting in a purple bruise.	Remove the tourniquet and withdraw the needle. Apply pressure until the site stops bleeding.
Edema	Swelling caused by an abnormal accumulation of fluid under the skin. Sometimes caused by the IV line.	Avoid the site. Specimens can be contaminated with excess tissue fluid.

COMPLICATIONS IN BLOOD COLLECTION

Continued ▶

▶ Continued **COMPLICATIONS IN BLOOD COLLECTION**

COMPLICATION	CAUSE	CORRECTIVE ACTION
Obesity	In the heavier patient, veins may not be accessible.	The use of a blood pressure cuff can make the veins more prominent. Do not probe blindly.
Intravenous (IV) Therapy	If an IV is running, blood should not be drawn from that arm.	Draw below the IV site or stop the infusion for 2 min, discard 5 mL of blood, and document that the specimen was drawn from the IV arm.
Hemoconcentration	An increase of analytes in the blood due to a shift in water balance. The tourniquet or prolonged massaging can cause this increase.	The tourniquet should not remain on any longer than 1 min.
Hemolysis	The damaging or breakdown of red blood cells with the release of hemoglobin into the specimen.	Use a correct gauge needle for blood collection, practice good technique, mix gently, and make sure alcohol is dry before performing blood collection.
Scarred or Sclerosed Veins	After repeated venipunctures, the wall of the vein develops scar tissue; or veins may have been damaged by chemotherapy.	Should be avoided. Try to use an alternative site. If not possible, avoid inserting the needle through the vein.
Seizures	Can be from a preexisting condition or an adverse response to the needle stick.	The tourniquet is removed immediately and the needle is withdrawn. Do not restrain the convulsing patient except to prevent self-injury. Alert the physician.
Mastectomy	The removal of a breast whereby the patient may have had the lymph nodes removed. These patients are susceptible to infections.	Never draw blood from the same side as the mastectomy. Never apply a tourniquet to this site. Use an alternate site.
Vomiting	Ejection of stomach contents usually brought on by the thought or sight of blood, in response to an adverse reaction to blood collection.	Have the patient take deep breaths. Place a cold compress on the patient's head and make him or her comfortable. Alert the physician.
Allergies	Reactions to the antiseptic or the adhesive bandages.	Do not use alcohol, use iodine. Use a hypoallergenic tape.
Rolling Veins	When veins tend to move away from the needle.	To avoid rolling, a firm pressure to anchor the vein is applied until the needle is inserted.
Collapsing Veins	Small veins or veins with thin walls. The pressure from the vacuum in the tubes causes a sucking action and prevents the blood from flowing into the tube.	Use a syringe or a butterfly with a small gauge needle where the pressure can be controlled in the drawing.

QUALITY ASSURANCE IN SPECIMEN COLLECTION

Quality assurance (QA) guarantees quality care by providing reliable and accurate laboratory testing in a timely manner. The quality of laboratory testing is very dependent on the quality of specimens received. A specimen of low quality can produce inaccurate and potentially dangerous results. Many aspects of venipuncture can affect specimen collection. Failure to properly identify the patient is one of the most serious mistakes. To avoid this error, always identify your patient before beginning any venipuncture procedure. Patient preparation, technique, and collection priorities are all part of quality assurance. Always check your equipment for defects, cracks, and expiration dates. Proper specimen handling includes the use of the proper collection tube, tubes that are correctly filled and inverted for thorough mixing, the use of correct order of draw, and specimens transported back to the laboratory in a timely manner.

Causes for Specimen Rejection

1. Unlabeled or improperly labeled tubes.
2. Hemolyzed specimen.
3. Lipemic specimen.
4. Discrepancies between requisition form and labeled tube.
5. Clots in an anticoagulated tube.
6. Wrong tube drawn for a particular test.
7. Insufficient amount of blood in collection tube.
8. Outdated equipment and collection tubes.
9. Poor specimen handling (exposed to light).
10. Specimen collected at the wrong time (drug level).
11. Specimen contamination.

In summary, the types of specimens rejected, the number of specimens recollected, the number of collection attempts, the number of duplicate draws, and the incidence of untimeliness and patient complaints are indicators for the need for a quality assurance program.

QUALITY ASSURANCE IN SPECIMEN COLLECTION

BIBLIOGRAPHY

Gauger C: Specimen collection. In Lotspeich C, ed: Clinical Hematology. Philadelphia, JB Lippincott, 1992, pp 10–19.

Garza D, Bean-McBride K: Phlebotomy Handbook, 4th ed. Stamford, CT, Appleton & Lange, 1996.

McCall R, Tankersley CM: Phlebotomy Essentials. Philadelphia, JB Lippincott, 1993.

Mullins C: Specimen collection. In Rodak B, ed: Diagnostic Hematology. Philadelphia, WB Saunders, 1995, pp 7–19.

St. Hill H: Topics in Phlebotomy Workshop, American Society for Clinical Pathologists, Associate Member Section, Philadelphia, 1995.

Strasinger SK, Di Lorenzo MA: Phlebotomy Workbook for the Multiskilled and Healthcare Professional. Philadelphia, FA Davis, 1996.

I

CLINICAL CHEMISTRY

Chapter 2

AMINO ACIDS AND PROTEINS

Mary Hotaling, MS, MT (ASCP) DLM

Q U I C K   C O N T E N T S

AMINO ACIDS

INTRODUCTION

Structure

Each α-amino acid is configured as an L optical isomer and contains at least one amino group (—NH$_2$), one carboxyl group (—COOH) bonded to the α-carbon (carbon next to the carboxylic acid group), and one R group:

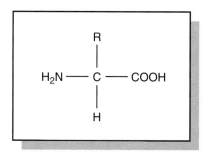

Amino acids are amphoteric and, depending on the pH of the solution, some exist primarily as anions (basic amino acids) and some exist primarily as cations (acidic amino acids). The differing acid base and solubility properties among the various amino acids allow separation by electrophoresis and chromatography methods, while the characteristic chemical properties of the R group permit identification and quantitation by photometric methods.

METABOLISM

The body requires 20 different α-amino acids to synthesize necessary proteins. Humans cannot synthesize about one half of the 20 necessary amino acids in quantities sufficient for normal growth and maintenance. These nutritionally "essential" amino acids and other amino acids are derived from dietary proteins. Proteolytic enzymes in the gastrointestinal tract, such as trypsin and pepsin, catabolize dietary proteins into their constituent amino acids. Dietary amino acids are absorbed from the intestine into the portal circulation and become part of the amino acid pool.

The amino acid pool also includes endogenously synthesized amino acids and those released during normal protein turnover. The amino acid pool is primarily used for endogenous protein synthesis, and is also used as an energy source and in the formation of nonprotein nitrogen compounds, such as creatine, purines, and pyrimidines. Blood amino acids are filtered through the glomerulus and are actively reabsorbed by the renal tubules.

PATIENT PREPARATION, SPECIMEN COLLECTION AND STORAGE

AMINO ACID TEST	PATIENT PREPARATION	SPECIMEN COLLECTION	SPECIMEN STORAGE	COMMENT
Whole Blood Amino Acid Screening Test (Guthrie Test)	6-8 hr fast is preferred Avoid use of drugs known to cause interference, i.e., certain antibiotics* Patient should be >24 hr old and have adequate protein intake for ≥48 hr prior to test	Collect whole blood on standardized filter paper Avoid hemolysis	10 days at 30°C 60 days at 4°C	Positive test should be verified by amino acid quantitation or identification method
Urine Amino Acid Screening Test	As above, except fast is not necessary	Random urine collection	Freeze at −20°C if testing is delayed for more than a few hours	Positive test should be verified by amino acid quantitation or identification method
Plasma Amino Acid Quantitative Test	Normal diet 2–3 days prior to test As above for Guthrie test	Heparinized plasma, collect on ice, deliver to laboratory immediately Avoid hemolysis	Immediately separate plasma from cells Freeze plasma within 1 hr of collection Stable for 1 wk at −20°C	Collect blood and urine samples simultaneously to help differentiate renal from overflow, and no-threshold aminoaciduria types
Urine Amino Acid Quantitative Test	As above, except fast is not necessary (unless blood is also collected)	24 hr urine collection is preferred Refrigerate or preserve with thymol or organic solvent during collection	Freeze at −20°C if testing is delayed for more than a few hours	As above

*See Tietz for list of specific interfering drugs.

REFERENCE RANGES

Plasma amino acid levels display diurnal variation, with lowest levels in the morning and highest in the midafternoon. Amino acid reference values are age dependent. Normal urine usually has five prominent amino acids: alanine, glutamine, glycine, histidine, and serine. Pediatric urine may also contain β-aminoisobutyric acid, phosphoethanolamine, glutamic acid, lysine, taurine, and threonine. Amino acid testing results should be evaluated with caution.

Amino Acid Reference Ranges

AMINO ACID	PLASMA AMINO ACID (μmol/L)		URINE AMINO ACID (μmol/L)	
	Children (3–16 yr)	Adults (>16 yr)	Children (3–16 yr)	Adults (>16 yr)
Alanine	200–450	230–510	65–190	160–690
Alpha-amino-*N*-butyric acid	8–37	15–41	7–25	0–28
Arginine	44–120	45–130	10–25	13–64
Asparagine	8–37	24–79	15–40	34–100
Aspartic acid	0–26	0–6	10–26	14–89
Beta-alanine	0–49	0–29	0–42	0–93
Citrulline	16–32	16–55	0–13	0–11
Cystine	19–47	30–65	11–53	28–115
Glutamic acid	32–140	18–98	13–22	27–105
Glutamine	420–730	390–650	150–400	300–1,040
Glycine	110–240	170–330	195–855	750–2,400
Histidine	68–120	26–120	46–725	500–1,500
Hydroxyproline	0–5	Not measured	Not measured	Not measured
Isoleucine	37–140	42–100	3–15	4–23
Leucine	70–170	66–170	9–23	20–77
Lysine	120–290	150–220	19–140	32–290
Methionine	13–30	16–30	7–20	5–30
3-Methylhistidine	0–52	0–64	42–1345	64–320
Ornithine	44–90	27–80	3–16	5–70
Phenylalanine	26–86	41–68	20–61	36–90
Phosphoethanolamine	0–12	0–55	24–66	17–95
Proline	130–290	110–360	Not measured	Not measured
Serine	93–150	56–140	93–210	200–695
Taurine	11–120	45–130	62–970	267–1,290
Threonine	67–150	92–240	25–100	80–320
Tyrosine	26–110	45–74	30–83	38–145
Valine	160–350	150–310	17–37	19–74

DIAGNOSTIC TESTS AND METHODOLOGIES

Diagnosis

Aminoacidurias must be diagnosed and treated as early as possible to prevent permanent damage such as mental retardation or early death. Diagnosis is chiefly dependent on laboratory testing, since many of these disorders produce nonspecific symptoms in affected newborns and infants and in older children (see symptom table below).

SYMPTOMS OF AMINO ACID DISORDERS OF METABOLISM

NEWBORN	INFANTS AND OLDER CHILDREN
Failure to thrive, poor feeding Neurologic disorder, i.e., seizures, irritability, lethargy Vomiting, diarrhea, dehydration Hepatomegaly Metabolic acidosis, increased anion gap Hyperglycemia, hypoglycemia Neutropenia, thrombocytopenia	Mental retardation Seizures Development delay (mental, physical, motor) Hematologic disorders, anemias CNS defects, speech, behavior problems Hepatomegaly, splenomegaly Renal calculi, defects Blindness Recurrent infections, fever of unknown origin

LABORATORY EVALUATION OF AMINOACIDURIAS

Laboratory testing for aminoaciduria is a component of routine neonatal screening, diagnosis of a symptomatic infant or child, and routine follow-up of treatment for aminoaciduria. In these applications, laboratory analyses are used to detect amino acids and metabolites in urine, blood, and body fluids. The level of testing includes screening, quantitation, and identification methods (see four tables below). Prenatal diagnosis of aminoaciduria may be requested in cases in which there is a positive family history, or if the mother is a known carrier. Currently, this testing requires identification of the specific enzyme defect through measurement of enzyme activity of patient skin fibroblast culture. A method of identifying the presence of the genetic defect causing the primary aminoaciduria by direct DNA analysis is under development.

Amino Acid Screening Tests

In general, urine specimen is more useful than plasma for amino acid screening purposes. However, urine may not be effective in very early neonatal detection of phenylketonuria (PKU) and maple syrup urine disease (MSUD). If these are suspected, use plasma.

Amino Acid Screening Tests

METHOD/PRINCIPLE	DIAGNOSTIC UTILITY/COMMENT
Two-Dimensional TLC Amino acids are allowed to migrate along one solvent front, then the chromatogram is rotated 90° and allowed to migrate with a second solvent front.	Preferred amino acid screening method, can generally separate and detect all significant amino acids in blood, urine, other body fluids. Semiquantitative

Continued ▶

▶ Continued *Amino Acid Screening Tests*

METHOD/PRINCIPLE	DIAGNOSTIC UTILITY/COMMENT
Guthrie Microbiological Test Bacterial spores and a competitive growth inhibitor are incorporated into the agar medium. Patient whole blood is spotted onto a standard sized filter paper disk and placed on the media. In the presence of increased amounts of the amino acid of interest, growth inhibition is overcome and zones of bacterial growth are observed.	Useful for routine neonatal screening Semiquantitative Growth inhibitor is varied according to amino acid of interest. Some antibiotics interfere with interpretation of the zone of inhibition (false negative).
Colorimetric Spot Tests Several colorimetric urine spot tests are available.	Used for screening, to supplement other test information, i.e. spot checking TLC results See table below for individual tests. Qualitative
TLC, thin layer chromatography.	

Colorimetric Urine Spot Amino Acid Tests

METHOD/PRINCIPLE	AMINOACIDURIA(S) ASSOCIATED WITH POSITIVE TEST	OTHER URINE FINDINGS/ TEST LIMITATIONS
Cyanide/Nitroprusside In alkaline medium, free sulfhydryl groups react with nitroprusside to produce a red color.	Cystinuria Cystinosis Homocystinuria	Cystinuria, homocystinuria may have a sulfurous odor. Cystinuria, cystinosis also may have cystine crystals in urine. Test cannot differentiate between cystine and homocystine.
Ferric Chloride Ferric chloride produces various colors (green-blue-gray) with aromatic hydroxyl groups.	PKU (dark blue-green) Tyrosinuria (green) Alkaptonuria (blue) MSUD (gray-blue)	Phenistix is a commercial dipstick version and is more specific. Alkaptonuria and MSUD may be negative with Phenistix. Salicylates and phenothiazines interfere, producing purple and purple-brown colors, respectively.
2,4-Dinitrophenylhydrazine 2,4-Dinitrophenylhydrazine produces yellow-white precipitate of hydrazones when it reacts with aliphatic or aromatic α-keto acids.	PKU Tyrosinemia MSUD	PKU urine has a characteristic mousy, musty odor. MSUD urine has a characteristic maple syrup odor.
α-Nitroso-β-Naphthol (ANBN) Nitrosonaphthol in the presence of nitrite reacts with certain parasubstituted phenols to produce an orange-red color	Tyrosinemia	Tyrosinemia urine has a dark brown color and may have tyrosine crystals.
PKU, phenylketonuria; MSUD, maple syrup urine disease.		

Amino Acid Quantitative Tests

METHOD/PRINCIPLE	DIAGNOSTIC UTILITY/COMMENT
Chromatography HPLC, ion-exchange, GLC	HPLC is the method of choice to confirm a positive screening test and is also used to monitor therapy. Sample purification may be required in HPLC to remove interfering substances. If identification is uncertain, use GC-MS identification (see below).
HPLC, high performance (pressure) liquid chromatography; GLC, gas liquid chromatography.	

Amino Acid Identification Test

METHOD/PRINCIPLE	DIAGNOSTIC UTILITY/COMMENT
Gas chromatography-mass spectroscopy (GC-MS)	Exact determination of unknown amino acid or metabolite when needed, i.e., diagnosis of equivocal data by other methods Not commonly requested, since quantitation methods are generally sufficient for diagnosis

EVALUATING TEST RESULTS

Aminoacidopathies

Disorders of amino acid metabolism (aminoacidopathies) generally result in abnormal urine amino acid patterns (aminoaciduria). The etiology of aminoaciduria may be primary or secondary, and the types may be classified as overflow, no-threshold, or renal.

Types of Aminoacidurias

AMINOACIDURIA TYPE	DEFECT	PLASMA AMINO ACID PATTERN	URINE AMINO ACID PATTERN
Overflow	Plasma level of one or more amino acids exceeds the renal threshold, and excess amino acid(s) spill(s) into the urine.	↑	↑
No-threshold	Owing to an inborn error of metabolism, excessive amounts of one or more amino acid are present in the urine, but plasma levels remain essentially normal because all the amino acid is excreted.	Normal or Sl ↑	↑
Renal	Plasma amino acid levels are essentially normal, but the renal tubular reabsorption system has congenital or acquired defects resulting in excessive amino acid excretion in the urine.	Normal or ↓	↑

Primary Aminoaciduria

Primary aminoaciduria is rare, genetically determined, and generally inherited in an autosomal recessive manner. These inborn errors of amino acid metabolism involve two main mechanisms: an enzyme deficiency or defect in enzyme activity in a specific amino acid metabolic pathway, or a defect in a specific renal tubular amino acid reabsorption mechanism. With an interruption in normal metabolism, the primary substrate accumulates or is diverted into an alternative, but ineffective pathway. Clinical symptoms, such as mental retardation, may result when essential products of the normal pathway are not formed at all or are formed in decreased amounts, or when the products of an alternate pathway accumulate and become toxic. There are more than 50 primary aminoacidurias. Selected aminoacidurias and their respective attributes are outlined in the table on the following three pages.

Primary Overflow and Renal Aminoacidurias

	PRIMARY OVERFLOW AMINOACIDURIAS					
Aminoaciduria	Enzyme Disorder/Other Defect	Plasma Metabolite	Urine Metabolite	Population Frequency	Clinical Symptoms	Treatment/Comment
Phenylketonuria (PKU)	Phenylalanine hydroxylase (PH) (absent)	Phenylalanine	Phenylalanine and metabolites: phenylpyruvate, phenylacetate, o-hydroxyphenylacetate	1:10,000 (most common type)	Mental retardation, seizures, eczema	Mandated neonatal screening test. May be treated with dietary restriction of phenylalanine. Several PKU variants exist.
Tyrosinemia Type I (Tyrosinosis)	Fumarylacetoacetate (FAA) hydrolase (absent)	Tyrosine Methionine	Tyrosine and metabolites: p-hydroxyphenyl lactic acid (PHPLA), p-hydroxyphenyl pyruvic acid (PHPPA), p-hydroxyphenyl acetic acid (PHPAA)	1:100,000	Hepatic cirrhosis, renal damage (Fanconi's syndrome)	May be treated with dietary restriction of phenylalanine, tyrosine, methionine.
Tyrosinemia Type II	Tyrosine aminotransferase (absent)	Tyrosine	Tyrosine and metabolites	Rare	Eye and skin lesions, mental retardation	May be treated with dietary restriction of phenylalanine, tyrosine.
Alkaptonuria	Homogentisic acid oxidase (absent)	Homogentisic acid	Homogentisic acid	1:250,000	Dark urine on exposure to air. May not be diagnosed until middle age with development of connective tissue pigmentation (ochronosis) and arthritic changes.	Currently, no treatment available

Continued ▶

EVALUATING TEST RESULTS

▲ Continued *Primary Overflow and Renal Aminoacidurias*

Aminoaciduria	Enzyme Disorder/Other Defect	Plasma Metabolite	Urine Metabolite	Population Frequency	Clinical Symptoms	Treatment/Comment
PRIMARY OVERFLOW AMINOACIDURIAS						
Homocystinuria	Cystathionine β-synthase (absent or deficient)	Homocystine Methionine	Homocystine Methionine	1:200,000	Ocular, skeletal, vascular effects, frequently mental retardation	Pyridoxine administration is effective for responsive form. Unresponsive form may be treated with methionine restricted diet.
Maple Syrup Urine Disease (MSUD)	Branched chain keto acid decarboxylase (deficient)	Leucine Isoleucine Alloisoleucine Valine Corresponding keto acids	Maple syrup odor: Leucine Isoleucine Alloisoleucine Valine Corresponding keto acids	1:250,000	Metabolic acidosis CNS symptoms May have mental retardation, respiratory failure	Mandated neonatal screening test in some states. Dietary restriction of leucine, isoleucine, and valine.
PRIMARY RENAL AMINOACIDURIAS						
Cystinuria, Classic Form	Defect of amino acid reabsorption at renal tubules causing ↑ urinary excretion of amino acids	N/A	Cystine Lysine Ornithine Arginine	1:13,000 (most common type)	Cystine renal calculi and urinary crystals	High fluid intake and urine alkalinization, penicillamine to avoid renal calculi

Continued ▲

▶ Continued *Primary Overflow and Renal Aminoacidurias*

PRIMARY RENAL AMINOACIDURIAS

Aminoaciduria	Enzyme Disorder/Other Defect	Plasma Metabolite	Urine Metabolite	Population Frequency	Clinical Symptoms	Treatment/Comment
Hartnup's Disease	Defect of amino acid reabsorption at renal tubules causing ↑ urinary excretion of amino acids	N/A	All neutral amino acids: Alanine, threonine, glutamine, serine, asparagine, valine, leucine, isoleucine, phenylalanine, tyrosine, tryptophan, histidine, citrulline	1:18,000	May be symptomless unless there is nicotinamide deficiency manifesting in pellagra-like symptoms including dermatitis, neurologic and psychiatric symptoms	Treat with nicotinamide administration.

Secondary Aminoaciduria

Secondary aminoaciduria is the result of disease of an active site of amino acid metabolism, such as the liver; generalized renal tubular dysfunction; or protein-energy malnutrition. Secondary aminoacidurias affect many amino acids simultaneously, and the defects may be overflow or renal types.

OVERFLOW	RENAL

Acute viral hepatitis
Acetaminophen hepatotoxicity
	PHYSIOLOGIC:
	Premature newborns during the first week of life
	Pregnancy
	
	PATHOLOGIC:
	Due to progressive proximal renal tubule dysfunction
	▮ Acquired forms:
	  Starvation
	  Heavy metal poisoning
	  Acute tubular necrosis
	
	▮ Inherited forms:
	  Fanconi's syndrome
	  Wilson's disease
	  Galactosemia

PROTEINS

INTRODUCTION

Proteins are complex macromolecules composed of more than 40 amino acids linked by peptide bonds. Proteins are found in all cells and body fluids, with the plasma alone containing more than 100 different species. The plasma proteins serve a large array of important functions and exist in a variety of shapes, sizes, and structures.

Protein Functions

Transport: lipids, metals, vitamins, toxic substances
Antibodies
Buffers
Coagulation factors
Regulation of metabolism
Catalysis of metabolic reactions
Hormones
Chromosomes
Plasma oncotic pressure
Nutrients

PROTEIN STRUCTURE (SHAPE) DETERMINANTS

STRUCTURE	ASPECT	BOND TYPE
Primary	Amino acid sequence, number, type	Peptide
Secondary	Twisted shape of the primary structure due to rotation of bonds. Shape may be α-helix (most common globular protein shape), pleated sheet, or random coil.	Hydrogen bonds within the same or different peptide chains within the same molecule
Tertiary	Three-dimensional structure that forms when the amino acid chain folds back on itself	Relatively weak interactions of amino acid R groups, which include disulfide linkages, and noncovalent attraction, i.e., hydrogen bonds, electrostatic, hydrophobic, and van der Waals forces
Quaternary	≥ 2 polypeptide chains joined to form a functional protein molecule, i.e., dimer, trimer, tetramer. Single chain proteins do not have this structural component.	Noncovalent attraction (as above for tertiary)

PROTEINS—INTRODUCTION

Structure

Proteins are composed of up to 20 different primary L-α-amino acids in characteristic combinations, numbers, and sequences determined by genetic code. The amino acids are covalently linked in a head to tail manner through peptide bonds. Peptide bonding is illustrated by the formation of a dipeptide below:

Peptide bond

At the amino acid's N-terminal end, there is a free amino group, which can form a peptide bond (through the removal of a water molecule) with another amino acid's C-terminal end, where there is a free carboxyl group.

DENATURATION

When the secondary, tertiary, or quaternary structure of a protein is disrupted, the protein may lose its "native" or original biologic character, i.e., immunogenicity or enzyme activity. In the clinical laboratory, important sources of denaturation of protein based specimens and reagents include exposure to heat, pH changes, solvents, and mechanical forces (i.e., repeated freeze/thaw cycles, and vigorous mixing).

Classification

Proteins are generally classified as either simple or conjugated. Simple proteins contain only amino acids and may be globular or fibrous. The globular proteins are the most commonly measured by the clinical laboratory and include most plasma proteins, hemoglobin, and enzymes. Conjugated proteins consist of apoprotein (amino acids) and prosthetic (non–amino acid) portions. Conjugated proteins are named for the prosthetic group, since they lend certain attributes to the protein: i.e., the lipoprotein prosthetic group is lipid and apoprotein is amino acids.

METABOLISM

Almost all plasma proteins are synthesized in the liver, except for the immunoglobulins, which are produced by the plasma cells of the immune system. Proteins are mainly catabolized in the liver to their constituent amino acids, which are deaminated, producing ammonia and keto acids. Ammonia is converted by the liver via the urea cycle to urea, which is then excreted into the urine. Keto acids are oxidized via the citric acid cycle and converted to glucose or fat.

Protein Catabolism

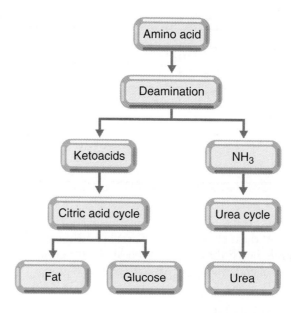

Nitrogen Balance

Although the rate of protein turnover varies widely between the individual proteins, there is an overall balance between protein anabolism (synthesis) and catabolism. This equilibrium is referred to as *nitrogen balance*. A "negative" nitrogen balance occurs when protein catabolism or loss exceeds synthesis; a "positive" nitrogen balance occurs when protein synthesis exceeds catabolism.

PATIENT PREPARATION, SPECIMEN COLLECTION AND STORAGE, REFERENCE RANGE

Patient Preparation

No special patient preparation is required for protein analysis. However, patient position, i.e., ambulatory vs. recumbent, affects the reference range for serum total protein and albumin (see table below) and may affect urine total protein values in certain patients having orthostatic proteinuria (see "Renal and Nonrenal Proteinurias" on p 36).

Specimen Storage

Specimen storage requirements for protein analyses are identical regardless of test or specimen type: 4°C <72 hours, or freeze at −20°C for up to 6 months. Centrifuge urine, cerebrospinal fluid (CSF), and body fluid specimens before analysis to remove particulate matter.

Specimen Collection, Reference Range

TEST	SPECIMEN	SPECIMEN COLLECTION	REFERENCE RANGE (g/dL)	COMMENTS
Total Protein and Albumin	*Serum*	Avoid prolonged application of tourniquet, which causes hemoconcentration, leading to spurious increase of all plasma proteins.	TOTAL PROTEIN Ambulatory: 6.4–8.3 Recumbent: 6.0–7.8 ALBUMIN 3.5–5.0	Avoid hemolysis, lipemia. Both total protein and albumin are decreased by about 0.3 g/dL in recumbent patients.
	Urine (24 hr)	No preservatives; refrigerate specimen at 4°C during collection.	TOTAL PROTEIN 1–14 mg/dL 50–80 mg/day ALBUMIN 1–14 mg/dL 50–80 mg/day	Strenuous exercise increases urine total protein <250 mg/dL and albumin is also increased.
	CSF	Lumbar puncture is most common site.	TOTAL PROTEIN 15–40 mg/dL ALBUMIN 10–30 mg/dL	Avoid traumatic tap, which invalidates protein results even when blood is occult.
	Body Fluid	—	TOTAL PROTEIN Transudate <2.0 mg/dL Exudate >2.0 mg/dL	Avoid traumatic collection, which invalidates protein results even when blood is occult.

Continued ▶

▶ Continued **Specimen Collection, Reference Range**

TEST	SPECIMEN	SPECIMEN COLLECTION	REFERENCE RANGE (g/dL)	COMMENTS
Protein Electrophoresis	*Serum*	Avoid prolonged application of tourniquet, which causes hemoconcentration, leading to spurious increase of all plasma proteins.	For cellulose acetate method: Albumin: 3.5–5.0 Alpha-1: 0.1–0.3 Alpha-2: 0.6–1.0 Beta: 0.7–1.1 Gamma: 0.8–1.6	Avoid hemolysis, lipemia.
	Urine	24 hr urine collection Simultaneously collect urine and serum specimens for protein electrophoresis.	Normal urine contains a trace of protein, mainly albumin.	Requires sample preconcentration or sensitive dye, i.e., CBB, owing to normally low protein content.
	CSF	Lumbar puncture is most common site. Simultaneously collect serum and CSF specimens and run in parallel.	Prealbumin, albumin, transferrin are normal major constituents.	HRE techniques generally used with sample preconcentration or sensitive dye, i.e., CBB for detection of oligoclonal bands in MS.
Specific Protein	*Serum*	As above for serum total protein	See "Characteristics and Clinical Significance of Selected Plasma Proteins" on page 41.	Avoid hemolysis, lipemia

HRE, high resolution electrophoresis; CBB, Coomassie brilliant blue; MS, multiple sclerosis.

DIAGNOSTIC TESTS AND METHODOLOGIES

Laboratory Evaluation of Proteins

Diseases and nutritional disorders often alter the expected amounts and relative proportions of the plasma proteins. The clinical laboratory evaluation of plasma proteins is performed using three general methods:

1. Quantitation of total protein and albumin by routine chemical methods
2. Semiquantitation of serum and other body fluid proteins by routine and/or special electrophoresis techniques, i.e., immunoelectrophoresis (IEP).
3. Quantitation of normal and abnormal specific proteins by immunoassay methods, i.e., nephelometry, turbidity, and radial immunodiffusion (RID)

Total Protein Methods

Method/Principle	Interferences	Comment
SERUM		
Biuret In alkaline medium, violet colored chelate forms between cupric ions and peptide bonds.	Hemolysis Lipemia	Requires ≥2 peptide bonds. Routine method.
Refractometry Measures refractive index	Hemolysis Icterus Lipemia Excessive nonprotein solids, i.e., electrolytes, urea, glucose	Rapid method requires very small volume. Temperature dependent; some refractometers have a built-in temperature compensation device.
Kjeldahl Acid digestion of protein with measurement of total nitrogen.	Ammonia contamination	Reference method, not used routinely. Total protein calculated based on assumed 16% nitrogen content of proteins.
URINE AND CSF		
Turbidimetric/Nephelometric Protein denaturing agent precipitates proteins with trichloroacetic acid (TCA), sulfosalicylic acid (SSA), or benzethonium chlorides (BZC).	Each denaturing agent suffers at varying degrees from the problem that all plasma proteins do not react equally. BZC and TCA are least affected.	Use calibrators that contain mixture of proteins similar to proteins in sample to be analyzed for dye binding and precipitation methods.
Dye Binding Pyrogallol red, Coomassie brilliant blue (CBB)	Proteins do not give the same response (affinity and/or binding capacity vary).	As above

Albumin Methods

METHOD/PRINCIPLE	SPECIMEN	COMMENT
Dye Binding Binding increases the absorbance of the dye proportionately to the concentration.	Serum	Routine method Bromocresol green dye (BCG)—most common Bromocresol purple dye (BCP)—more precise
Nephelometry	Serum Urine CSF	Method of choice for urine and CSF
Protein Electrophoresis Protein separation based on electric charge. Albumin migrates fastest toward the anode (⊕) at pH 8.6 in routine electrophoresis methods.	Serum Urine CSF	Normally the largest plasma protein fraction (40%–60%), normally present in urine and CSF

DIAGNOSTIC TESTS AND METHODOLOGIES

Protein Electrophoresis Methods

ROUTINE ELECTROPHORESIS METHODS

In practice, most routine protein electrophoresis is performed using a commercially integrated electrophoresis apparatus (power supply, sample applicators, chamber) and kit material and reagents (stain, fixative, clearant [if necessary]) from a single supplier for consistent protein separation patterns.

HIGH RESOLUTION ELECTROPHORESIS METHODS

High resolution electrophoresis techniques, such as polyacrylamide gel electrophoresis (PAGE) and two-dimensional electrophoresis (2-DE), are not often performed in the clinical laboratory but are generally performed by research laboratories.

Specific Protein Methods

Specific proteins are measured by immunochemical methods, i.e., nephelometry, immunodiffusion, or immunoassays such as immunoelectrophoresis (IEP) and immunofixation (IFE). Refer to Section II, "Immunology," for discussion of these methods.

EVALUATING TEST RESULTS

Protein analysis provides information regarding nutritional status and the presence of severe disease states involving the liver, kidney, and bone marrow. Protein fractionation, i.e., electrophoresis and quantitation by specific protein assays, yields far more clinically useful data.

Total Protein

Total protein concentration of various specimens yields vastly different clinical information and therefore has distinct diagnostic utility, as can be seen in the table below:

DIAGNOSTIC UTILITY OF TOTAL PROTEIN

TOTAL PROTEIN SPECIMEN TYPE	DIAGNOSTIC UTILITY
Serum	Provides general information regarding nutritional status and the presence of severe disease states involving the liver, kidney, and bone marrow.
Urine	Evaluation of glomerular integrity, renal tubular function, presence of overflow of abnormal plasma protein
CSF	Evaluation of blood-brain barrier integrity, ↑ CNS protein synthesis, CNS infection
Body Fluid	Provides data to distinguish transudate from exudate.
CSF, cerebrospinal fluid; CNS, central nervous system.	

SERUM

Serum total protein is composed of albumin and globulins in an A/G ratio of about 1.6:1.0. A change in serum total protein is generally caused by a change in plasma water volume or a change in concentration of one or more of the plasma proteins. For example, albumin is in such high levels of total protein (40%–60%) that a change in this single protein commonly influences total protein values.

Alterations of Serum Total Protein

HYPERPROTEINEMIA	HYPOPROTEINEMIA
Dehydration Monoclonal or polyclonal gammopathies	↑ Protein loss ▌ Nephotic syndrome, blood loss, burns ↑ Protein catabolism ▌ Inflammation ▌ Malignancy ↓ Protein synthesis ▌ Liver disease ▌ ↓ Amino acid intake

URINE TOTAL PROTEIN

Urine is formed by ultrafiltration of plasma across the glomerulus. Plasma proteins with a molecular weight greater than 40,000 are almost entirely retained in the plasma, while lower molecular weight proteins easily enter the glomerular ultrafiltrate, and are actively reabsorbed from the ultrafiltrate and catabolized by the proximal tubules. Normally, total protein excreted in urine consists of about one half albumin and one half Tamm-Horsfall protein.

Proteinuria

Proteinuria is often detected initially by urine dipstick screening methods. These methods are more sensitive to albumin than other plasma proteins. This sensitivity to albumin makes this test an excellent screening method for glomerular proteinuria, but it is unsatisfactory for tubular proteinuria. A 24 hour urine total protein assay is commonly performed to confirm and quantitate positive urine protein screening results. Tubular proteinuria is better detected and the degree of glomerular selectivity better determined by correlating the results of concurrent serum and urine protein assays, such as protein electrophoresis or immunoelectrophoresis.

Renal and Nonrenal Proteinurias

TYPE OF PROTEINURIA		DEFECT	DISEASES	PROTEIN FOUND IN URINE	COMMENT
R E N A L	**Glomerular**	↑ Glomerular permeability	Glomerulonephritis	Low MW protein (mainly albumin) to start with, then increasing MW as proteinuria becomes nonselective	Most common and severe type. Usually detected by urine dipstick test. End-stage renal disease has decreasing proteinuria as renal failure occurs.
	Tubular	Defective reabsorption at proximal tubules	Nephrotoxicity Metabolic disturbances Chronic pyelonephritis	Low MW protein	Screening test is beta-microglobulin quantitation. Usually not detected by urine dipstick test (not enough albumin).
N O N R E N A L	**Overload**	Overflow of abnormal protein from plasma	Multiple myeloma Hemolytic disease	Low MW abnormal proteins: Bence Jones protein, hemoglobin, myoglobin	Precipitation of these proteins in the kidney may lead to renal disease.
	Physiological "Nonpathologic"	↑ Glomerular permeability	Functional: heavy exercise, fever, pregnancy Orthostatic proteinuria	Low MW protein (mainly albumin)	Orthostatic "postural" proteinuria occurs when the patient is in the upright position. When the patient is in the recumbent position, the proteinuria resolves.
	Postrenal	Protein produced in urinary tract	Inflammation Malignancy	WBCs and malignant cells	Absence of urinary casts and RBCs is good indication that the proteinuria is nonrenal.

MW, molecular weight; WBCs, white blood cells; RBCs, red blood cells.

CSF TOTAL PROTEIN

More than 80% of CSF protein content is formed by ultrafiltration of the plasma across the blood-brain barrier. Twenty percent of central nervous system (CNS) protein is synthesized locally by the choroid plexus of the ventricles of the brain. Since CSF is mainly an ultrafiltrate, low molecular weight plasma proteins normally predominate and include prealbumin, albumin, and transferrin.

Increased CSF total protein concentration may be further evaluated by measurement of CSF albumin and/or CSF immunoglobulin G (IgG). Albumin is used as a protein marker of blood-brain barrier permeability, since it is not produced to any significant amount by the CNS. In multiple sclerosis, increased amounts of myelin basic protein (MBP) is produced by demyelination of the nerve axon sheath. Increased amounts of IgG are also synthesized within the CNS by B lymphocytes, which infiltrate demyelinating nerve sheath lesions. This produces an increased $IgG_{CSF}:IgG_{serum}$ ratio and the appearance of oligoclonal IgG bands on CSF electrophoresis. These abnormal CSF protein results should be correlated with clinical findings, since similar CSF results may be found in chronic meningoencephalitis and in Guillain-Barré syndrome.

Alterations of CSF Total Protein

CNS DEFECT	CONDITIONS	EVALUATION METHOD
↑ **Blood-Brain Barrier Permeability**	↑ Intracranial pressure ■ Brain tumor ■ Intracerebral hemorrhage/trauma Inflammation ■ Meningitis (especially high in bacterial meningitis) ■ Encephalitis Obstruction of CSF circulation ■ Tumor above puncture site	CSF/serum albumin index: $Albumin_{CSF}$ (mg/dL)/$Albumin_{SER}$ (g/dL) Evaluates the integrity of blood-brain barrier: <9 = intact 9–14 = slight impairment 30–100 = severe impairment >100 = complete breakdown
↑ **CNS Synthesis (IgG)**	Demyelinating CNS diseases ■ Multiple sclerosis Chronic CNS inflammatory diseases ■ Guillain-Barré syndrome ■ Chronic meningoencephalitis Neoplasia	CSF-serum IgG-albumin Index: IgG_{CSF} (mg/dL) $\times$ $albumin_{SER}$ (g/dL)/$Albumin_{CSF}$ (mg/dL) $\times$ IgG_{SER} (g/dL) Increased index (>0.70) indicates ↑ CNS synthesis

TOTAL PROTEIN IN OTHER BODY FLUIDS

Body fluids are arbitrarily designated according to total protein concentration:

FLUID TYPE	TOTAL PROTEIN CONCENTRATION	DEFECT
Transudate	<3 mg/dL	Reflects changes in filtering membrane permeability
Exudate	>3 mg/dL	Usually the result of infection or malignancy and may contain WBCs or malignant cells

See "Routine Analysis of Body Fluids," Chap. 34, for further discussion.

Albumin

SERUM

Since albumin makes up 40% to 60% of the serum total protein concentration, many of the causes of altered serum total protein levels also result in altered serum albumin levels (or vice versa). For more information regarding serum albumin, see "Characteristics and Clinical Significance of Selected Plasma Proteins" on page 41.

Alterations of Serum Albumin

HYPERALBUMINEMIA	HYPOALBUMINEMIA
Dehydration	↑ Albumin loss
	∎ Nephrotic syndrome, blood loss, burns
	↑ Albumin catabolism
	∎ Inflammation
	∎ Malignancy
	↓ Albumin synthesis
	∎ Liver disease
	∎ ↓ Amino acid intake
	Altered albumin distribution into extravascular compartment
	∎ Ascites fluid

URINE AND CSF ALBUMIN

Urine albumin is used as a protein marker of glomerular permeability, while CSF albumin is used as a marker of blood-brain barrier permeability. For further discussion of these assays, refer to "Urine Total Protein" on page 35 and "CSF Total Protein" on page 36.

Serum Protein Electrophoresis (SPE)

Routine SPE is a zonal electrophoresis method that separates serum proteins into five major fractions (bands) based on their electric charge properties. Routine methods include cellulose acetate electrophoresis (CAE) and agarose gel electrophoresis (AGE) performed at pH 8.6. The electrophoretogram result gives relative increases and decreases of expected fractions and provides clues to the presence of abnormal proteins. Some disorders display a characteristic protein electrophoresis pattern. Any abnormality of electrophoresis pattern can be investigated by immunochemical methods, which can determine individual protein concentration.

COMMON ELECTROPHORESIS PATTERNS

Many of the individual proteins have relatively very low concentrations and cannot be determined by electrophoresis pattern changes: e.g., ceruloplasmin (CER) is overshadowed by proteins of higher concentration, such as α_2-macroglobulin (AMG). However, some diseases have characteristic patterns. Probably the most striking clinically significant finding on an electrophoresis pattern is monoclonal gammopathy, which demonstrates a spike from anywhere in the alpha$_2$ to the gamma region.

COMMON SPE PATTERN	COMMENTS
Normal SPE pattern (normal pattern is dotted) 	Used to compare with the patient's pattern to detect changes in peak slope or shape.
Hypogammaglobulinemia 	In this case, the gamma region is almost absent. If severe, it is called agammaglobulinemia.
Monoclonal gammopathy 	Marked, single spike in gamma region Caused by multiple myeloma, heavy chain disease, or Waldenström's macroglobulinemia. These diseases are indistinguishable on SPE; further laboratory testing by immunoelectrophoresis (IEP) or immunofixation (IF) is needed to identify abnormal immunoglobulins.

Continued ▶

EVALUATING TEST RESULTS

▶ Continued

COMMON SPE PATTERN	COMMENTS
Nephrotic syndrome 	$\downarrow$ in most serum proteins $\uparrow\uparrow$ A$_2$ fraction Nephrotic syndrome generally results in a loss of most of the proteins except α_2 -macroglobulin because it is a very large protein.
Active hepatocellular damage (cirrhosis) 	$\uparrow\uparrow$ IgA "Beta-gamma bridging," or fusion of the beta and gamma regions, is very characteristic for cirrhosis. Pattern suggests $\uparrow\uparrow$ IgA, which migrates in the valley between beta and gamma.

Characteristics and Clinical Significance of Selected Plasma Proteins

SPE REGION	PROTEIN	MW (kD)	FUNCTION	ACUTE PHASE REACTANT? (APR) ⊕ OR ⊖	CLINICAL SIGNIFICANCE/COMMENTS
Prealbumin	*Prealbumin*	55	Transport protein: T3, T4	⊖	Band appears on high resolution electrophoresis methods. Indicator of nutritional status or liver dysfunction due to very short half-life (12 hr). ↓ in malnutrition, inflammation, liver cirrhosis.
	Retinol Binding Protein (RBP)	21	Transport protein: retinol (vitamin A)	⊖	
Albumin	*Albumin*	66	Transport protein, maintains oncotic pressure, source of endogenous amino acids	⊖	Indicator of nutritional status or liver dysfunction; also a sensitive marker for glomerular and blood-brain barrier integrity. ↓ in malnutrition, nephrotic syndrome, inflammation, liver cirrhosis, and many other nonspecific disorders. ↓ may result in edema and decreased albumin transport function, i.e., unexpected drug toxicity.
α_1	α_1-*Antitrypsin (AAT)*	53	Antiprotease, prevents tissue breakdown by neutrophil proteases released during inflammation	⊕	Makes up 90% of α_1 region. Congenital decrease may cause early onset emphysema or infantile hepatitis, leading to cirrhosis.
	α_1-*Acid Glycoprotein*	44	APR, exact function unknown	⊕	Stains very weakly in SPE owing to ↑ carbohydrate content.
	α_1-*Lipoprotein (HDL)*	200	Transports lipids	—	Stains very weakly in SPE owing to ↑ lipid content.
	α_1-*Fetoprotein (AFP)*	76	Principal fetal protein; no known adult function	—	Fetal ↑ may indicate neural tube defect. Adult ↑ may indicate hepatocellular tumor

Continued ▶

EVALUATING TEST RESULTS

► Continued **Characteristics and Clinical Significance of Selected Plasma Proteins**

SPE REGION	PROTEIN	MW (kD)	FUNCTION	ACUTE PHASE REACTANT? (APR) ⊕ OR ⊖	CLINICAL SIGNIFICANCE/COMMENTS
α_2	*Haptoglobin (HAP)*	85–1000	Binds and transports free hemoglobin	⊕	Monitor APR and hemolytic processes: ↓ in intravascular hemolysis, ↑ inflammation (APR), nephrotic syndrome, burns due to high molecular weight
	α_2-Macroglobulin (AMG)	800	Unknown	—	One of the largest plasma proteins. Dramatic ↑ in nephrotic syndrome.
	Ceruloplasmin (CER)	160	Involved in copper metabolism	⊕	↓ in Wilson's disease ↑ in copper toxicity
β_1	*Transferrin (TFR)*	77	Transports iron	⊖	↑ iron deficiency anemia (correlates with TIBC) ↓ inflammation (negative APR)
	Hemopexin (HPX)	57	Binds circulating heme	—	↓ Hemolytic processes
	β-Lipoprotein (Apoprotein B)	~3000	Transports lipids	—	See "Lipids and Lipoproteins," Chapter 4.
	C_4	206	Immune system factor	⊕	May only be found on electrophoresis when fresh serum is used.
β_2	*Fibrinogen*	340	Coagulation factor	⊕	Artifact on SPE when plasma specimen is used instead of serum.
	C_3	180	Immune system factor	⊕	May only be found on electrophoresis when fresh serum is used.
	β_2-Microglobulin (BMG)	11.8	Unknown, found on cell surfaces of nucleated cells, particularly WBCs and tumor cells	⊕	Indicator of renal tubular function, especially useful for detection of kidney transplant rejection. Also useful as a tumor marker to monitor B cell tumors.

Continued ►

► Continued **Characteristics and Clinical Significance of Selected Plasma Proteins**

SPE REGION	PROTEIN	MW (kD)	FUNCTION	ACUTE PHASE REACTANT? (APR) ⊕ OR ⊖	CLINICAL SIGNIFICANCE/COMMENTS
γ	*C-Reactive Protein (CRP)*	~120	Immune function	⊕⊕	Migrates in the beta-gamma region. Nonspecific, but most sensitive acute phase reactant. ↑ in inflammation, and used to monitor inflammatory processes.
	IgG	160	Immune function, most abundant immunoglobulin	⊕	Monoclonal ↑ B cell tumors, i.e., myelomas
	IgA	170	Immune function, found mainly in secretions	⊕	Monoclonal ↑ Liver cirrhosis
	IgM	9000	Immune function, early response	⊕	Monoclonal ↑ Waldenström's macroglobulinemia

TIBC, total iron binding capacity.

BIBLIOGRAPHY

Beetham R, Cattell WR: Proteinuria: pathophysiology, significance, and recommendations for measurement in clinical practice. Ann Clin Biochem 30:425–434, 1993.

Bishop ML: Clinical Chemistry: Principles, Procedures, Correlations, 3rd ed. Philadelphia, JB Lippincott, 1996.

Burtis CA, Ashwood ER: Tietz Fundamentals of Clinical Chemistry, 4th ed. Philadelphia, WB Saunders, 1996.

Burtis CA, Ashwood ER: Tietz Textbook of Clinical Chemistry, 2nd ed. Philadelphia, WB Saunders, 1994.

Deodhar SD: C-reactive protein: the best laboratory indicator available for monitoring disease activity. Cleve Clin J Med 56:126–130, 1989.

Guthrie R, Susi A: A simple phenylalanine method for detecting phenylketonuria in large populations of newborn infants. Pediatrics 32:338–343, 1963.

Kaplan LA, Pesce AJ: Clinical Chemistry: Theory, Analysis, Correlation, 3rd ed. St. Louis, Mosby–Year Book, 1996.

Putnam FW: The Plasma Proteins, 2nd ed, Vol 1. New York, Academic Press, 1975.

Scriver CR, et al: The Metabolic Basis of Inherited Disease, 7th ed. New York, McGraw-Hill, 1995.

Snider GL: Pulmonary disease in alpha₁-antitrypsin deficiency. Ann Intern Med 111:957–959, 1989.

Tietz NW, ed: Clinical Guide to Laboratory Tests, 3rd ed. Philadelphia, WB Saunders, 1995.

Woo SLC: Prenatal diagnosis and carrier detection of classic phenylketonuria by gene analysis. Pediatrics 74:412–423, 1984.

Chapter **3**

CARBOHYDRATES

Mary Hotaling, MS, MT (ASCP) DLM

Q U I C K C O N T E N T S

INTRODUCTION

Glucose is the primary energy source for the human body. Glucose is derived from the diet, through the digestion of dietary carbohydrates; from body stores (glycogen); and from the endogenous synthesis of glucose from noncarbohydrate sources (amino acids, glycerol, lactate). The blood glucose level is held within a fairly constant range by regulatory hormones and metabolic processes.

Disorders of carbohydrate metabolism may result in either hyperglycemia or hypoglycemia. The most frequently occurring hyperglycemic disorder is diabetes mellitus. Hypoglycemia is much less frequently encountered. Patients with diabetes mellitus, especially those requiring insulin therapy, need close monitoring of blood glucose to maintain "normal" glucose levels. Interest in maintaining nearly normal blood glucose levels has gained popularity in recent years because the latest clinical studies indicate that this factor may reduce the frequency and severity of specific complications associated with diabetes mellitus. These microvascular and neurologic complications include retinopathy leading to blindness, renal failure, neuropathy, and atherosclerosis.

METABOLISM

Metabolism of dietary carbohydrates begins in the mouth, where salivary amylase hydrolyzes starch to form the disaccharide maltose and intermediate products (dextrins). Pancreatic amylase completes digestion of the intermediate products to produce maltose. In the intestinal mucosa, maltose and any ingested disaccharides (lactose, sucrose) are hydrolyzed by enzymes to form monosaccharides: glucose, galactose, fructose. The monosaccharides are absorbed into the bloodstream and transported to the liver via the portal circulation. Liver enzymes convert the nonglucose monosaccharides to glucose, after which the glucose is reacted with adenosine triphosphate (ATP), forming glucose-6-phosphate dehydrogenase (G6PD). Further glucose metabolism proceeds according to the body's requirements and may follow three possible pathways: immediate energy production (to ATP) by complete conversion to CO_2 and water; storage as glycogen in the liver or as triglyceride in adipose tissue; or conversion to keto acids, amino acids, or protein.

Glucose Metabolism Processes

GLUCOSE METABOLISM PROCESSES	SUBSTRATE	PRODUCT	GLUCOSE METABOLISM USE
Glycolysis (Anaerobic) Anaerobic conversion of glucose to pyruvate or lactate	Glucose	Pyruvate/ lactate + ATP	Energy production (2 ATP)
Glycogenesis Process of glycogen formation from glucose	Glucose	Glycogen	Storage of glucose as glycogen in liver and muscle
Glycogenolysis Breakdown of glycogen to form glucose	Glycogen	Glucose	Release of glucose from glycogen for energy (muscle) or increase of blood glucose (liver) to maintain homeostasis
Gluconeogenesis Formation of glucose from noncarbohydrate sources (proteins, lipids)	Amino acids Lactate Glycerol	Glucose	Increase of blood glucose (liver) when glycogen stores are depleted
TCA (Tricarboxylic Acid) Cycle and Electron Transport System Aerobic phase of glucose metabolism within the mitochondria of the cell	Pyruvate → acetyl CoA	ATP	Energy production (24 ATP, 12 per acetyl CoA molecule)
Hexose Monophosphate Pathway (HMP) Alternate pathway for glucose oxidation	Glucose	NADPH	Energy source for many anabolic reactions and glycolysis in RBCs, since they lack mitochondria

NADPH, reduced form of nicotinamide adenine dinucleotide phosphate; RBCs, red blood cells.

Regulation of Glucose Metabolism

The blood glucose level is regulated by complex interactions of many metabolic pathways, which are controlled by a number of hormones that move glucose into and out of the blood. These hormones include insulin, which decreases blood glucose, and the counterregulatory hormones (glucagon, cortisol, epinephrine, and growth hormone), which increase blood glucose levels.

ACTION OF MAJOR HORMONES REGULATING BLOOD GLUCOSE CONCENTRATION

HORMONE	EFFECT ON BLOOD GLUCOSE CONCENTRATION	SITE OF ORIGIN	ACTION
Insulin	↓	β cells of pancreas	Increases cell membrane permeability to glucose, stimulates glycogenesis
Glucagon	↑	α cells of pancreas	Principal hormone to ↑ blood glucose; stimulates liver glycogenolysis, gluconeogenesis
Epinephrine	↑	Adrenal medulla	Stimulates glycogenolysis; immediate glucose production, and a back-up for glucagon
Growth Hormone ACTH	↑	Anterior pituitary	Insulin antagonist; inhibits glucose uptake by the cells; also stimulates liver glycogenolysis
Cortisol	↑	Adrenal cortex	Stimulates gluconeogenesis, and insulin antagonist

PATIENT PREPARATION, SPECIMEN COLLECTION AND STORAGE, REFERENCE RANGE

Glucose Tests

SERUM/PLASMA				
Test	Patient Preparation	Specimen Collection	Specimen Storage	Reference Range (mg/dL)
FBG (fasting blood glucose, formerly FBS)	6–8 hr fast	SERUM: Separate from cells within 30 min PLASMA: Commonly collected using Na fluoride preservative/anticoagulant	SERUM: 25°C for 8 hr 4°C for 72 hr PLASMA: When preserved with Na fluoride or iodoacetate, 25°C for 24 hr	Adult: 70–105 Adult >60: 80–115 Neonate: 30–60 Glucose is physiologically higher in arterial than in venous blood.

Continued ▶

▶ Continued **Glucose Tests**

		SERUM/PLASMA		
Test	**Patient Preparation**	**Specimen Collection**	**Specimen Storage**	**Reference Range (mg/dL)**
2-hr PP (postprandial)	Patient eats breakfast or lunch containing carbohydrates, or a glucose solution (75 g) is administered by mouth.	Collect plasma/serum 2-hr postprandially.	Same as FBG	<120
Oral GTT (glucose tolerance test)	Patient receives 150 g carbohydrate diet for 3 days prior to test. 10–16 hr fast is required prior to test. 75 g glucose load is administered by mouth.	Collect plasma/serum at timed intervals: Fasting, then every 30 min for 2 hr after glucose load is administered.	Same as FBG	Fasting: 70–105 30 min: 110–170 60 min: 120–170 90 min: 100–140 120 min: 70–120
		A 5 hr GTT is occasionally requested to diagnose postprandial hypoglycemia.	Same as FBG	Many factors influence OGTT results; unless they are grossly abnormal, the test should be repeated to confirm.
		Urine samples for glucose and/or ketones may be collected simultaneously with the blood if desired.	Same as FBG	
Intravenous GTT (glucose tolerance test)	As above for OGTT, except glucose dose is 25 g/100 mL IV solution administered within 1–2 min.	Fasting, then allow administered glucose to reach equilibrium at about 15 min. Collect specimens at 5 min intervals for 30–45 min.	Same as FBG	Blood glucose decreases exponentially (K) when $K = 70/t_{1/2}$ and $t_{1/2}$ = half-life of glucose clearance.
		This is one method; timing varies appreciably among various sources.	Same as FBG	$(K = 1.4\%–2.0\%)$ IV glucose administration eliminates factors related to GI tract glucose absorption.

Continued ▶

▶ Continued **Glucose Tests**

SERUM/PLASMA				
Test	**Patient Preparation**	**Specimen Collection**	**Specimen Storage**	**Reference Range (mg/dl)**
1-hr PP Gestational Diabetes Screen	Perform screening at 24–28 wk of gestation. Administer 50 g glucose load by mouth; fasting not required.	Collect specimen 1 hr postprandially.	Same as FBG	>140 mg/dL requires full OGTT work-up using 100 g glucose load and collecting specimens at fasting, and at 1 hr intervals for 3 hr
OTHER BODY FLUIDS				
Whole Blood (capillary)	Fasting specimen requires 6–8 hr fast.	Collect from finger stick or earlobe without excessive squeezing.	Avoid fluoride preservative.	<100 Whole blood glucose results are ≈10%–15% lower than simultaneously collected plasma/serum values.
Urine (24 hr, quantitative)	—	Collect in dark container, keep on ice.	Preserve with 5 mL glacial acetic acid.	<0.5 g/day 1–15 mg/dL
Urine (random, qualitative, semiquantitative)	—	—	Analyze immediately or store at 2°–4°C if testing is delayed.	Negative Diabetics may have a decreased renal threshold
CSF	—	Blood glucose may be obtained 30–60 min prior to lumbar puncture CSF for correlation.	Analyze CSF immediately. Store at −20°C.	40–70 Changes in blood glucose are reflected in CSF after 1–3 hr.

PATIENT PREP/SPECIMEN COLLECTION/STORAGE/REFERENCE RANGE

Other Carbohydrate Metabolism Tests

TEST	PATIENT PREPARATION	SPECIMEN COLLECTION	SPECIMEN STORAGE	REFERENCE RANGE
Ketones	—	Serum or urine Avoid hemolysis in serum.	Store tightly covered at 4°C for 5 days	Negative
Insulin	Fasting	Serum	Freeze at −20°C for 3 mo	6–24 μU/mL
C Peptide	Fasting	Serum	Freeze at −70°C for 3 mo	0.78–1.89 ng/mL
Glycated Hemoglobin	—	Whole blood EDTA anticoagulant is preferred Prepare washed RBCs or hemolysate.	Whole blood 4°C for 5 days Hemolysate 4°C for 4–7 days −70°C for 30 days	Reference range is method dependent. Affinity or column chromatography = 5.3%–7.5% of total hemoglobin.

DIAGNOSTIC TESTS AND METHODOLOGIES

Diagnostic Tests

A variety of glucose and other carbohydrate metabolism tests are available to diagnose and monitor different states of altered carbohydrate metabolism. The clinical utility of these tests may be the diagnosis of hyperglycemia or hypoglycemia, or the tests may be used to monitor efficacy of treatment and compliance with therapeutic regimens within the short or long term.

GLUCOSE AND GLUCOSE LOADING TESTS

SERUM/PLASMA	
Test	**Clinical Utility/Comment**
FBG (fasting blood glucose, formerly FBS)	Detect disorders of carbohydrate metabolism, mainly to diagnose diabetes mellitus (DM) and to monitor DM therapy. Other tests (5-hr OGTT) are generally more useful for diagnosis of hypoglycemia.
2-hr PP (postprandial)	Simple glucose loading test; result generally evaluated in conjunction with FBG to screen for or monitor therapy of DM.
Oral GTT (glucose tolerance test)	Glucose loading test, most sensitive test to detect DM, conducted at 7–9 AM, usually lasting 2–3 hr. 5 hr OGTT, or preferably 5 hr meal tolerance test, is used to detect postprandial hypoglycemia. Abnormal results should be verified by repeat testing unless results are initially grossly abnormal.
Intravenous GTT (glucose tolerance test)	As above for OGTT; used if the patient cannot tolerate oral glucose or when a defect in gastrointestinal glucose absorption is suspected.
1-hr PP Gestational Diabetes Screen	Simple glucose loading test, used to detect gestational diabetes at 24–28 wk of gestation. Increased results should be confirmed by OGTT.

Continued ▶

▶ Continued **GLUCOSE AND GLUCOSE LOADING TESTS**

WHOLE BLOOD AND BODY FLUIDS	
Whole Blood	Most commonly, patient (or an individual performing point of care testing) measures the glucose level using a glucose meter. Results are used to modify insulin dosage therapy and must not be used to *diagnose* DM.
Urine	Screen for hyperglycemia that exceeds the renal threshold (>160–180 mg/dL), no longer recommended to monitor DM therapy.
CSF	Detect increased glucose usage by the CNS, i.e., presence of WBCs, or microorganisms within the CNS.

CNS, central nervous system; WBCs, white blood cells.

OTHER CARBOHYDRATE METABOLISM TESTS

TEST	CLINICAL UTILITY/COMMENT
Ketones	Indicator of altered carbohydrate metabolism resulting in excessive fat and protein utilization (gluconeogenesis). Helpful in differentiating between diabetic coma and insulin shock.
Insulin	Useful for the evaluation of fasting hypoglycemic patients and establishing diagnosis of insulinoma.
C Peptide	Useful as an indicator of surreptitious injection of insulin resulting in factitious fasting hypoglycemia. Also aids in the detection of endogenous insulin secretion in the presence of anti-insulin antibodies.
Glycated Hemoglobin	Index of long-term plasma glucose control (2-3 mo period), indicating compliance and efficacy of DM therapy.
Fructosamine	Index of long-term plasma glucose control (2–3 wk period), indicating compliance and efficacy of DM therapy; glycated hemoglobin measurement is currently preferred.
Reducing Substances	Used in conjunction with a negative glucose specific assay to detect reducing sugars (other than glucose) in the urine of newborns and infants for screening of inherited disorders of carbohydrate metabolism.

DIAGNOSTIC TESTS AND METHODOLOGIES

Methodologies

GLUCOSE METHODS

METHOD/PRINCIPLE	INTERFERENCE/COMMENT
Glucose Hexokinase (HK)–Coupled Enzyme Reaction Glucose + ATP $\xrightarrow{\text{HK}}$ glucose-6-phosphate (G6P) + ADP G6P + NADP$^+$ $\xrightarrow{\text{GPD}}$ 6-phosphogluconate + NADPH Measure indicator reaction (NADP$^+$ → NADPH) as absorbance increases at 340 nm (UV)	Reference method and most frequently performed automated method; virtually no interferences.
Glucose Oxidase (GO)–O_2 Consumption Glucose + O_2 $\xrightarrow{\text{GO}}$ gluconic acid + H_2O_2 O_2 consumption is measured by O_2 electrode	Less common than HK method, but still frequently used, especially for glucose meter testing; accurate and precise method; virtually no interferences.
Glucose Oxidase (GO)–Coupled Enzyme Reaction (Trinder) Glucose + O_2 $\xrightarrow{\text{GO}}$ gluconic acid + H_2O_2 H_2O_2 + reduced dye (colorless) $\xrightarrow{\text{Peroxidase}}$ oxidized dye (colored) Measure photometric indicator reaction (colorless dye → colored dye)	Frequently used for urine and whole blood glucose rapid reagent strip testing. Also used for automated methods for serum/plasma. Initial glucose oxidase reaction is specific for glucose, but the indicator reaction is subject to interference by substances oxidized by H_2O_2 (uric acid, bilirubin, ascorbic acid).
Glucose Meter (Self-Monitoring and Point of Care Testing) Reflectance meter measures the glucose oxidase–Trinder coupled enzyme reaction occurring on a reagent strip Glucose + O_2 $\xrightarrow{\text{GO}}$ gluconic acid + H_2O_2 H_2O_2 + reduced dye (colorless) $\xrightarrow{\text{Peroxidase}}$ oxidized dye (colored) Measure photometric indicator reaction (colorless dye → colored dye) Popular instruments include: Accu-Chek (Boehringer-Mannheim) Glucometer (Ames)	Frequently used for capillary whole blood glucose testing. Glucose meters utilizing the glucose oxidase–Trinder coupled enzyme reaction have the same interferences as discussed above. Very low or very high results are unreliable and must be verified by another method. Commonly, errors arise from improper sample collection. See "Specimen Collection" on page 49. Adequate training and adherence to manufacturer's procedures are essential to achieve reliable and reproducible results.

OTHER CARBOHYDRATE METABOLISM TEST METHODS

METHOD/PRINCIPLE	INTERFERENCE/COMMENT
Ketones, Semiquantitative Method for Urine or Serum Nitroprusside reaction Acetoacetic acid and acetone form a purple color with nitroprusside under alkaline conditions.	Serum specimens must be performed using the tablet form of the reagent (Acetest tablets); the reagent impregnated strip or tablet may be used for urine specimens. β-Hydroxybutyric acid does not react, while the test is 10–20 times more sensitive to acetoacetic acid than acetone.
Insulin Immunoassay Radioimmunoassay (RIA) method is still frequently performed; IEMA and MEIA are also frequently used	Interferences include exogenously administered insulin and circulating insulin antibodies.
C Peptide Immunoassay RIA	Cross-reactivity with proinsulin can significantly interfere with the assay.
Glycated Hemoglobin (Hemoglobin A$_1$ or GHb) Separation from nonglycated Hgb is based on charge, chemical reactivity, or structure. Most common methods include affinity and ion exchange chromatography, spectrophotometry, electrophoresis, and immunoassay. Affinity chromatography is the recommended routine method and measures all glycated hemoglobins.	Reduced in vivo RBC survival rates result in falsely decreased levels, as in hemolytic anemias. Hemoglobinopathies, the presence of labile Hb A$_{1c}$ (pre-Hb A$_{1c}$), and nonglucose adducts of hemoglobin interfere with the methods, except for affinity chromatography and colorimetric thiobarbituric acid methods. The colorimetric method has interference with free glucose and must be removed. Ion exchange methods, including HPLC (the reference method), are sensitive to variation in pH and temperature. The presence of Hgb F results in falsely ↑ values. Lipemia interferes only with the column method. Electrophoresis methods are falsely ↑ in the presence of Hgb F and labile intermediates.
Hemoglobin A$_{1c}$ Ion exchange chromatography (HPLC and column chromatography methods). Separation of Hgb fractions based on characteristic charge differences.	Ion exchange methods, including HPLC (the reference method), are sensitive to variation in pH and temperature. The presence of Hgb F results in falsely ↑ values. Lipemia interferes only with the column method.
Isoelectric Focusing (IEF) Separation of Hgb fractions based on characteristic isoelectric points.	IEF methods produce falsely elevated results in the presence of Hgb F.
Reducing Substances Benedict's (copper reduction) Based on the ability of glucose and other reducing sugars to reduce cupric ion (Cu^{2+}) to cuprous ion (Cu^+).	Semiquantitative test for glucose and total reducing substances in urine, nonspecific for reducir 1 sugars.

IEMA, immunoenzymetric assay; MEIA, microparticle enzyme immunoassay.

DIAGNOSTIC TESTS AND METHODOLOGIES

DIABETES MELLITUS

Diabetes mellitus is a group of hyperglycemic disorders caused by insulin deficiency or resistance at the tissues. Glucose utilization is impaired because the deficiency of insulin action hinders glucose entry into the cells. As a result, blood glucose levels rise, and when levels exceed the renal threshold, glucose is excreted into the urine (glycosuria). If severe hyperglycemia is left uncontrolled, some patients, particularly type I diabetics, may develop acute life-threatening complications such as diabetic ketoacidosis (DKA). Type II diabetics tend to develop another life-threatening complication, hyperosmolar coma.

Diabetes Mellitus Types and Characteristics

TYPE	ONSET	PATHOGENESIS	SYMPTOMS	THERAPY/COMMENT
Type I, IDDM (insulin dependent diabetes mellitus) 5%–10% prevalence	Juvenile ($\leq$ 20 yr old)	Insulin deficiency due to autoimmune destruction of pancreatic β cells	Symptoms appear abruptly and include polyuria, polydipsia, rapid weight loss, ketosis.	Patient is dependent on exogenous insulin administration to sustain life and prevent DKA.
Type II, NIDDM (non–insulin dependent diabetes mellitus) $\approx$90% prevalence	Adult ($\geq$20 yr old, usually after 40)	Insulin resistance and/or decreased insulin amounts	Minimal symptoms; obesity is commonly associated with NIDDM; generally no ketosis.	Patient may be controlled by diet, exercise, or oral hypoglycemic agents or may require insulin administration.
GDM $\approx$3% of pregnancies prevalence	Pregnancy, usually resolves after delivery	Insulin resistance	May be asymptomatic. Family and/or reproductive history is sometimes helpful.	Patient may be controlled by diet or oral hypoglycemic agents or may require insulin administration. Universal screening is recommended at 24–28 wk of gestation. Patients with positive history or symptoms may be screened earlier.

Other Causes of Hyperglycemia, "Secondary Diabetes"

$\uparrow$ Glucocorticosteroids
Acute stress, including acute myocardial infarction, cerebrovascular accident
Anti-insulin antibodies
Drug-induced pancreatic islet cell destruction

HYPOGLYCEMIA

In hypoglycemia, plasma glucose levels are usually less than 50 mg/dL, but there is no universal agreement concerning exact diagnostic values. A transient hypoglycemia may normally occur about 2 hours after an oral glucose load. Hypoglycemia occasionally occurs in the absence of disease and may also be asymptomatic.

Hypoglycemia Types and Characteristics

SYMPTOM CLASSIFICATION	GLUCOSE LEVEL AND RATE OF DECREASE	SYMPTOMS
Adrenergic Activation of sympathetic nervous system, which releases epinephrine	Rapid Glucose level may or may not remain within reference range	Sweating, weakness, shakiness, lightheadedness, rapid pulse, hunger, nausea
Neuroglycopenia Depriving the brain of glucose causes CNS dysfunction	Gradual Glucose level of <20–30 mg/dL	Headache, confusion, seizures, coma. May be asymptomatic until the CNS is impaired. Repeated or extended episodes may result in irreversible CNS damage.

EVALUATING TEST RESULTS

Hyperglycemia

DIABETES MELLITUS CLASSIFICATION

Glucose tolerance testing is widely accepted for the diagnosis of diabetes mellitus and detects lesser degrees of impaired glucose tolerance (IGT). Criteria developed by the National Diabetes Data Group (NDDG) is widely used in the United States and is outlined below (all results in mg/dL units):

Adult, Nonpregnant (NDDG Diagnostic Criteria for Glucose Tolerance Testing)

CLASSIFICATION (75 g GLUCOSE LOAD)	FASTING GLUCOSE	POSTPRANDIAL GLUCOSE (½ HR, 1 HR, 1½ HR)	2 HR GLUCOSE	COMMENT
"Normal"	<115	<200	<140	Must meet all three criteria.
IGT	<140	≥200	140–199	Must meet all three criteria.
Diabetes Mellitus	≥140 or meets postprandial glucose and 2 hr glucose criteria	≥200	≥200	Can stop at fasting specimen if ≥140 on two separate occasions or if one increased glucose level is accompanied by classic symptoms of diabetes mellitus.
Nondiagnostic	Other results not fitting the above criteria			

Adult, Pregnant (O'Sullivan Criteria for Gestational Diabetes)

CLASSIFICATION	FASTING GLUCOSE	POSTPRANDIAL GLUCOSE	COMMENT
"Normal"	≤105	1 hr ≤ 190 2 hr ≤ 165 3 hr ≤ 145	3 hr OGTT is recommended for gestational diabetes diagnosis.
Gestational Diabetes Screening Test (50 g glucose load)	Not recommended, since just missing one meal may lead to ketosis.	1 hr >140	Positive screening, refer for routine OGTT using 100 g glucose load (criteria below).
Gestational Diabetes (100 g glucose load)	>105	1 hr >190 2 hr >165 3 hr >145	At least two values must meet the criteria.

DIABETIC KETOACIDOSIS

In DKA, carbohydrate metabolism pathways are severely compromised and/or overwhelmed. The carbohydrate metabolism derangements include inhibition of glycolysis, while glycogenolysis and gluconeogenesis are stimulated. Besides hyperglycemia, laboratory findings for a patient with acute DKA reflect a complex array of acid base and electrolyte disturbances.

Typical Laboratory Findings in Diabetic Ketoacidosis

ANALYTE	TYPICAL FINDINGS	MECHANISM/COMMENT
Glucose	300–500 mg/dL	Glucose usually remains within this range provided that renal function is maintained.
Ketones	Positive	Excessive ketoacids: acetone, β-hydroxybutyric acid, acetoacetic acid are produced during gluconeogenesis, mainly by increased fatty acid oxidation to acetyl CoA.
Blood Gases	Metabolic acidosis: pH ↓ Bicarbonate ↓↓ After compensation: Bicarbonate ↓↓ Pco_2 ↓↓	Bicarbonate and Pco_2 are usually decreased owing to metabolic acidosis compensation mechanism of Kussmaul breathing (deep respirations) to "blow-off" CO_2 to remove excess hydrogen ions.
Electrolytes	Na^+ ↓ K^+ ↑ Total CO_2 ↓ Anion gap ↑	Hyperkalemia is due to movement of cellular K^+ into the extracellular fluids, including the blood. K^+ must be monitored closely, since there is hyperkalemia even though total body K^+ is frequently ↓.
Osmolality	Moderately ↑	Moderate ↑ osmolality reflects ↑ plasma glucose levels, since plasma Na^+ is commonly ↓.

Hypoglycemia

The initial step in diagnosing adult hypoglycemia is to determine whether it is the reactive or fasting type. Rule out fasting hypoglycemia before making a diagnosis of postprandial hypoglycemia. Diagnosis should be based on Whipple's triad criteria: low blood glucose, accompanied by typical symptoms, which are resolved by glucose administration.

HYPOGLYCEMIA CLASSIFICATION

CLASSIFICATION	CAUSES	LABORATORY DIAGNOSIS	COMMENT
"Postprandial" (reactive)	May occur in patients with gastrointestinal surgery or mild diabetes. Usually benign and may be considered a variant of normal physiology.	GLUCOSE: Obtain blood specimen when patient is symptomatic; if not possible, perform 5 hr meal tolerance test. Plasma glucose within the reference range with the presence of symptoms is strongly suggestive that hypoglycemia is not the diagnosis.	5 hr meal tolerance test is preferred to 5 hr OGTT.
Postabsorptive (fasting) Loss of glycemic control during a fast	Drugs, e.g., insulin or oral hypoglycemic agents, administered in excess and ethanol abuse are most common. Other causes are rare but usually serious underlying organic disease, e.g., insulinomas, liver dysfunction, sepsis, depleted glycogen stores, ↓ glucocorticoids.	INSULIN AND C PEPTIDE: ↑ Insulin with normal or ↓ C peptide → excessive exogenous insulin administration ↑ Insulin with ↑ C peptide → insulinoma GLUCOSE: Obtain blood specimen after prolonged fast (up to 48 hr). Hypoglycemia is usually detectable within 12 hr.	5 hr OGTT is not appropriate testing for suspected fasting hypoglycemia.
Neonatal	Prematurity Maternal diabetes or toxemia, which are usually transient	GLUCOSE: Full term <30 mg/dL Premature <20 mg/dL	Neonates are less sensitive to hypoglycemia and may be asymptomatic even at very low glucose levels.
Early Infancy	Inborn errors of carbohydrate metabolism, e.g., von Gierke's disease (type I). For discussion, refer to Burtis and Ashwood: Tietz Textbook of Clinical Chemistry.		

EVALUATING TEST RESULTS

BIBLIOGRAPHY

American Diabetes Association position statement: Urine glucose and ketone determinations. Diabetes Care 14:39–40, 1991.

American Diabetes Association position statement: Standards of medical care for patients with diabetes mellitus. Diabetes Care 14:10–13, 1991.

American Diabetes Association position statement: Prevention of type I diabetes mellitus. Diabetes Care 14:14–15, 1991.

Bishop ML: Clinical Chemistry: Principles, Procedures, Correlations, 3rd ed. Philadelphia, JB Lippincott, 1996.

Burtis CA, Ashwood ER: Tietz Fundamentals of Clinical Chemistry, 4th ed. Philadelphia, WB Saunders, 1996.

Burtis CA, Ashwood ER: Tietz Textbook of Clinical Chemistry, 2nd ed. Philadelphia, WB Saunders, 1994.

Fajans SS, Floyd JC Jr: Fasting hypoglycemia in adults. N Engl J Med 294:766–772, 1976.

Gerich JE: Glucose counterregulation and its impact on diabetes mellitus. Diabetes 37:1608–1617, 1988.

Haymond MW: Hypoglycemia in infants and children. Endocrinol Metab Clin North Am 18:211–252, 1989.

Hofelt FD: Reactive hypoglycemia. Endocrinol Metab Clin North Am 18:185–201, 1989.

Kaplan LA, Pesce AJ: Clinical Chemistry: Theory, Analysis, Correlation, 3rd ed. St. Louis, Mosby–Year Book, 1996.

Lev-Ran A, Anderson RW: The diagnosis of postprandial hypoglycemia. Diabetes 30:996–999, 1981.

Nathan D: Intensive diabetes treatment and complications in IDDM. The Diabetes Control and Complications Trial Research Group. N Engl J Med 329:977–986, 1993.

National Diabetes Data Group: Classification and diagnosis of diabetes mellitus and other categories of glucose intolerance. Diabetes 28:1039–1057, 1979.

National Diabetes Data Group: Report of the expert committee on glucosylated hemoglobin. Diabetes Care 7:602–606, 1984.

O'Sullivan JB, Mahaw CM: Criteria for the oral glucose tolerance test in pregnancy. Diabetes 13:278–285, 1964.

Super DM, et al: Diagnosis of gestational diabetes in early pregnancy. Diabetes Care 14:288–294, 1991.

Tietz NW, ed: Clinical Guide to Laboratory Tests, 3rd ed. Philadelphia, WB Saunders, 1995.

Chapter

4

LIPIDS AND LIPOPROTEINS

Craig A. Lehmann, PhD, CC(NRCC)

Q U I C K   C O N T E N T S

INTRODUCTION

The term *lipid* represents a large group of compounds that are virtually insoluble in water. This group can be separated into four primary groups: cholesterol and its esters, glycerol esters (triglycerides being the most abundant), fatty acids, and phospholipids. Among these, cholesterol and triglycerides are the two most prominent lipids found in serum. The association of cholesterol and/or triglycerides with coronary heart disease, arteriosclerosis, hepatic disease, diabetes, hyperlipoproteinemia, and pancreatitis explains the large number of tests on these substances requested by health practitioners. The remaining lipids provide valuable diagnostic information for many primary and secondary disorders. However, requests for such tests as apolipoproteins are significantly less common than those for cholesterol and triglycerides and in many cases are considered to be esoteric and not routine.

Cholesterol

Almost all of endogenous cholesterol is synthesized by the liver and gut and exists in two forms, free cholesterol and esterified cholesterol. Approximately 75% to 85% of the total cholesterol is present in the esterified form. Cholesterol is a major constituent of cellular membranes and serves as a metabolic precursor for other steroids (e.g., sex hormones). Cholesterol can also be derived from dietary sources such as meat, eggs, butter, and plants. Cholesterol derived from dietary sources needs to be mixed with fatty acids, conjugated bile acids, phospholipids, and monoacylglycerides in order to be absorbed. From 30% to 60% of dietary cholesterol intake is actually absorbed. Once cholesterol is absorbed into the mucosal cell, it becomes part of a very large micelle called a *chylomicron*. This chylomicron consists of a variety of lipids other than cholesterol, including triglycerides, phospholipids, and apolipoproteins. The chylomicrons that are produced enter the lymphatics and are eventually discharged into the thoracic duct and finally on to systemic venous circulation (see "Lipoprotein Metabolism" on p 62).

Dietary cholesterol seems to influence endogenous levels by only 10% to 20%, primarily because dietary cholesterol inhibits hepatic production and therefore keeps plasma cholesterol levels fairly constant. This deviation from the true value is small enough for nonfasting samples to offer pertinent information in screening for hypercholesterolemia. When an individual's true cholesterol level is assessed, especially in the case of diagnosing hypercholesterolemia, a number of 12 to 14 hour fasting samples are required (see Patient Preparation, Specimen Collection and Storage, Reference Range on p 65).

Glycerol Esters

Of the dietary glycerol esters, triglycerides are the most abundant and encompass 95% of all fat stored in the body's adipose tissue. Their fundamental function is to furnish energy for the cell. Dietary triglycerides come from a variety of sources such as plants, animals, and fish. In the presence of lipases and bile acids in the duodenum and proximal ileum, triglycerides are hydrolyzed into monoglycerides, glycerol, and fatty acids. Upon absorption, like cholesterol, triglycerides are resynthesized and form chylomicrons. Unlike cholesterol, concentrations of plasma triglycerides are very much affected by dietary factors, and therefore patients need to fast for 12 or more hours (see Patient Preparation, Specimen Collection and Storage, Reference Range on p 65).

Among the glycerol esters are a group referred to as phosphoglycerides. These are different in that they contain phosphatidic acid. Some important members are phosphatidyl ethanolamine, phosphatidyl choline (lecithin), and phosphatidyl serine.

Fatty Acids

Most fatty acids, with the exception of linoleic acid, can be synthesized by humans. The unsaturated fatty acid linoleic is considered an essential fatty acid for good health and must be acquired through dietary sources (vegetable oils). Fatty acids that are relevant to nutrition and metabolism are those that contain even carbon numbers and are long chain. In the metabolic process the two most important fatty acids are palmitic acid and stearic acid.

The formation of acetyl coenzyme A (acetyl CoA) is a byproduct of excessive mobilization of fatty acids and is diverted to an alternate pathway that produces ketone bodies. Ketone bodies become present in both starvation and severe uncontrolled diabetes mellitus. The actual quantitation of fatty acids is generally not requested by health practitioners unless impaired absorption or metabolism is suspected.

Apolipoproteins

Apolipoproteins are the hydrophilic components of lipoproteins. Lipids such as cholesterol and triglycerides are hydrophobic and need to be placed in water soluble micellar structures in order to be transported in plasma. At present there are five major apolipoproteins (Apo A, B, C, D, E) along with their subgroups.

The two most requested apolipoproteins are Apo A and B. Apo A-I and A-II are one of the major components of high density lipoprotein (HDL). Each of these proteins is also present in chylomicrons and enters circulation via this route. They are synthesized both in the liver and intestine. Apo A-I plays a major role in the reverse transport of cholesterol as Apo A-I activates the needed enzyme lecithin-cholesterol acyltransferase (LCAT), which esterifies cholesterol. Interestingly, there seems to be a correlation between Apo A-I and HDL concentrations. Apo A-II, on the other hand, inhibits LCAT. Apo B exists in two forms: B-100 and B-48. Apo B-100 is associated with low density lipoprotein (LDL) and very low density lipoprotein (VLDL), is synthesized in the liver, and is responsible for the transport of endogenous cholesterol. Apo B-48 is synthesized in the intestine and is responsible for transporting exogenous lipid. The half-lives of these two apoproteins are significantly different. Apo B-100 has a half-life of days while Apo B-48 has a half-life of hours. Very little to no Apo B-48 is found in normal fasting patients. Since most patients fast for lipid testing, the actual assay really only evaluates Apo B-100.

It should be noted that apolipoprotein assays have only a confined clinical value owing to the inability to standardize testing procedures.

INTRODUCTION

LIPOPROTEIN METABOLISM

Exogenous Metabolism

Dietary intake of fat

Upon entering the small intestine the pancreatic enzyme lipase begins to break down fats to fatty acids, glycerol, and monoglycerides, and with the help of bile salts these are absorbed by the intestinal mucosa.

The lipids are then resynthesized into what are known as chylomicrons and are passed into circulation via the thoracic duct.

Circulating chylomicrons interact with lipoprotein lipase, which hydrolyzes triglycerides to fatty acids, monoglycerides, and glycerol. The byproducts are absorbed by cells for energy and/or reassembled back into triglycerides for future energy.

The portion of the chylomicron that is not broken down is referred to as the remnant. This remnant is quickly removed from circulation via the liver.

Endogenous Metabolism

Endogenous lipoprotein synthesis starts at the liver. The liver begins with the production of the very low density lipoprotein (VLDL), a lipoprotein rich in triglycerides. VLDLs are acted upon by lipoprotein lipase in the same manner as chylomicrons. The remnant that remains is now referred to as the intermediate density lipoprotein (IDL).

IDLs are continually acted upon by lipoprotein lipase with the end product being low density lipoproteins (LDLs). LDLs are rich in cholesterol. LDLs are catabolized in both the liver and peripheral tissue.

The creation of nascent high density lipoprotein (HDL) comes from two sources, the liver and intestine. It appears that the primary purpose of HDLs is to reduce the amount of stored cholesterol.

*LCAT = lecithin cholesterol
acetyl transferase

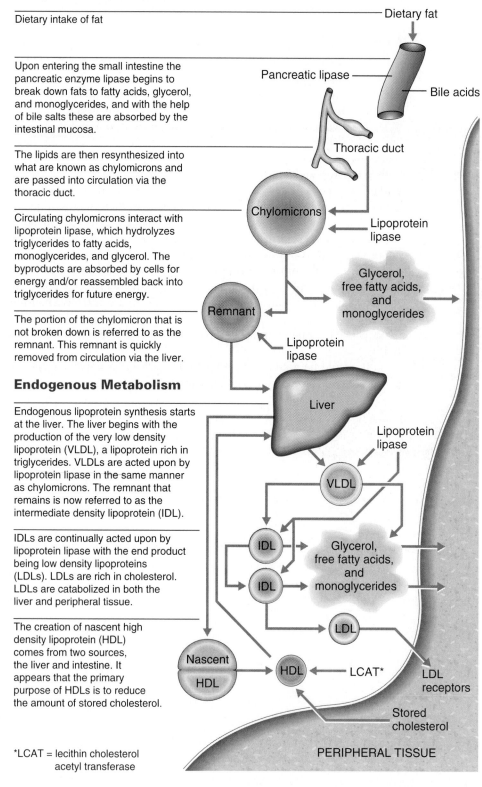

Dietary fat

Pancreatic lipase

Bile acids

Thoracic duct

Chylomicrons

Lipoprotein lipase

Glycerol, free fatty acids, and monoglycerides

Remnant

Lipoprotein lipase

Liver

Lipoprotein lipase

VLDL

IDL

IDL

Glycerol, free fatty acids, and monoglycerides

LDL

Nascent HDL

HDL

LCAT*

LDL receptors

Stored cholesterol

PERIPHERAL TISSUE

LIPOPROTEINS

As previously discussed, the primary lipids found in blood are triglycerides and cholesterol. Neither of these lipids is soluble in a aqueous environment, and therefore both require the assistance of other lipids and proteins for transportation. These soluble macromolecular complexes (lipoproteins) are composed of varying concentrations of cholesterol, triglycerides, phospholipids, and apoproteins. These lipoproteins can be separated into distinct classifications: chylomicrons, VLDL, LDL, and HDL.

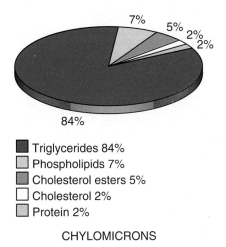

7% 5% 2% 2%

84%

■ Triglycerides 84%
□ Phospholipids 7%
▨ Cholesterol esters 5%
□ Cholesterol 2%
▨ Protein 2%

CHYLOMICRONS

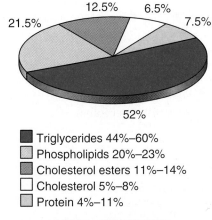

12.5% 6.5% 7.5%

21.5%

52%

■ Triglycerides 44%–60%
□ Phospholipids 20%–23%
▨ Cholesterol esters 11%–14%
□ Cholesterol 5%–8%
▨ Protein 4%–11%

VERY LOW DENSITY
LIPOPROTEINS

CHYLOMICRONS. Chylomicrons are the primary lipoproteins responsible for the transportation of fat from the diet (exogenous). Triglycerides are the predominant lipid component of this lipoprotein. Chylomicrons also contain cholesterol, cholesterol esters, phospholipids, proteins, and apoproteins but at a much smaller concentration. The most prevalent apoproteins found in this lipoprotein are Apo AI, AII, B48, and C. Once the chylomicrons enter the circulation, they are acted upon by lipoprotein lipases (LPLs). LPL hydrolyzes the triglycerides to glycerol, monoglycerol, and free fatty acids, which are either utilized for cellular energy or resynthesized for storage. The byproduct of this interaction with LPL is referred to as the remnant. Remnants are removed from circulation rapidly via the liver.

VERY LOW DENSITY LIPOPROTEINS. VLDLs are a product of endogenous lipoprotein synthesis in the liver. While triglyceride is still the dominant lipid of this lipoprotein, there is a significant increase of cholesterol, cholesterol esters, phospholipids, and protein. The apolipoprotein make-up of this lipoprotein also changes, as Apo C, B-100, and E become the most prevalent. In the circulation Apo C activates the release of lipoprotein lipase, which once again hydrolyzes triglycerides to glycerol, monoglycerol, and free fatty acids. Because of this, the concentration of its constituents will vary. This action results in the formation of an intermediate density lipoprotein (IDL).

LIPOPROTEIN METABOLISM

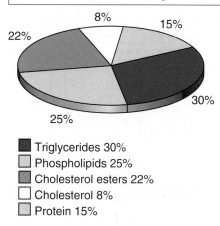

- Triglycerides 30%
- Phospholipids 25%
- Cholesterol esters 22%
- Cholesterol 8%
- Protein 15%

INTERMEDIATE DENSITY
LIPOPROTEINS

INTERMEDIATE DENSITY LIPOPROTEINS. This lipoprotein now contains almost equal amounts of cholesterol, triglycerides, and phospholipids. The dominant apolipoprotein in this lipoprotein is clearly Apo B-100, making up 50% to 70% with Apo E and C following. This intermediate lipoprotein is further catabolized to LDL with the aid of Apo E.

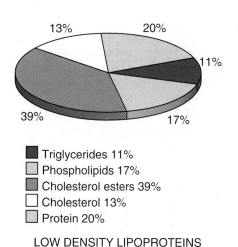

- Triglycerides 11%
- Phospholipids 17%
- Cholesterol esters 39%
- Cholesterol 13%
- Protein 20%

LOW DENSITY LIPOPROTEINS

LOW DENSITY LIPOPROTEINS. Of all the lipoproteins, LDL has the highest percentage of cholesterol (>50%). This lipoprotein now has one dominant apolipoprotein, Apo B-100 (98%), with traces of Apo C and E. Apo B-100 enables the lipoprotein to bind to specific sites at peripheral tissue and liver. At the Apo B receptor sites the LDL is degraded and incorporated. Once in the cell, the degradation of Apo B to amino acids takes place. At the same time, esterified cholesterol is being hydrolyzed to free cholesterol. The free cholesterol concentration plays a role in regulating cellular cholesterol synthesis, which includes repressing 3-hydroxy-3-methylglutaryl-coenzyme A (HMG-CoA), activating acyl CoA:cholesterol acyltransferase (ACAT) action, and modifying LDL receptors.

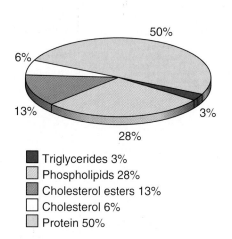

- Triglycerides 3%
- Phospholipids 28%
- Cholesterol esters 13%
- Cholesterol 6%
- Protein 50%

HIGH DENSITY LIPOPROTEINS

HIGH DENSITY LIPOPROTEINS. Proportionally, HDLs contain very few triglycerides. They contain a high percentage of protein, phospholipids, and cholesterol. The dominant apoprotein is A-I (67%) followed by A-II, C, and E. The origination of this lipoprotein is at the liver and intestine. It is released in the form of a nascent and can later assume the typical spherical form by absorbing lipids. This process is very much dependent on the enzyme LCAT. Absorption of lipids take place at peripheral sites and/or other lipids. HDL transports cholesterol back to the liver, in which it serves as a precursor for bile acids and/or part of VLDL composition.

PATIENT PREPARATION, SPECIMEN COLLECTION AND STORAGE, REFERENCE RANGE

LIPID TEST	PATIENT PREPARATION	SPECIMEN COLLECTION	SPECIMEN STORAGE	REFERENCE RANGE
Total Cholesterol	Nonfasting is acceptable for screening, otherwise 12-14 hr fast	Serum or plasma (EDTA) or heparin with separation from cells within 2 hr	4°C 5-7 days. −20°C 90 days	Age dependent Males, 114-265 mg/dL Females, 112-280 mg/dL Coronary risk adults: Low <200 mg/dL Moderate 200-240 mg/dL High >240 mg/dL
HDL Cholesterol	12 hr or more fast	Serum or plasma (EDTA)	4°C 4 days	Age dependent Males 38-67 mg/dL Females 36-92 mg/dL
LDL Cholesterol	12 hr or more fast	Serum or plasma (EDTA)	4°C 3 days	Age dependent Male 63-210 mg/dL Females 68-224 mg/dL Coronary risk adults: Low <130 mg/dL Moderate 130-159 mg/dL High >160 mg/dL
RATIO Total Cholesterol/ HDL Cholesterol	Same as total cholesterol and HDL cholesterol	Same as total cholesterol and HDL cholesterol	Same as total cholesterol and HDL cholesterol	Coronary risk Average: Male 5.0 Female 4.4 2× average: Male 9.6 Female 7.1 3× average: Male 23.4 Female 11.0
Triglycerides	12 hr or more fast	Serum or plasma (EDTA or heparin) separation from cells within 2 hr	4°C 7 days −20°C 90 days	Age dependent Males 30-327 mg/dL Females 35-262 mg/dL Triglyceridemic rank: Average <200 mg/dL Borderline 200-500 mg/dL High (pancreatitis) >1000 mg/dL
Apolipoproteins:				Age and method dependent EIA method ref. range
A-I	12 hr or more fast	Serum or plasma (EDTA)	4°C 4 days −20°C 180 days	Males 104-150 mg/dL Females 121-173 mg/dL
A-II	12 hr or more fast	Serum or plasma (EDTA)	4°C 7 days −20°C 3 yr	Males 50-72 mg/dL Females 58-78 mg/dL
B	12 hr or more fast	Serum or plasma (EDTA)		Males 73-127 mg/dL Females 69-115 mg/dL

Continued ▶

▶ Continued **PATIENT PREPARATION, SPECIMEN COLLECTION AND STORAGE, REFERENCE RANGE**

LIPID TEST	PATIENT PREPARATION	SPECIMEN COLLECTION	SPECIMEN STORAGE	REFERENCE RANGE
Ratio Apo A-1/Apo B	Same as Apo A-1 and Apo B	Same as Apo A-1 and Apo B	Same as Apo A-1 and Apo B	Coronary risk: Average risk 1.4 Increased risk <1.1
Free Fatty Acids	12 hr fast	Plasma (heparin or EDTA)	Storage not recommended	Adults 8-25 mg/dL Children <31 mg/dL
Lipoproteins	12 or more hr fast	Serum or plasma (EDTA)	4°C	See phenotyping chart, p 72

DIAGNOSTIC TESTS AND METHODOLOGIES

TEST	METHOD	INTERFERENCE	COMMENTS
Total Cholesterol	Direct enzymatic that measures either O_2 or H_2O_2 production	Interference will occur from samples that are turbid, lipemic, or hemolyzed or demonstrate increased bilirubin.	Samples with cholesterol values >500 mg/dl need to be diluted. Bilirubin does not interfere with methods that measure O_2 electrochemically. Plasma sample results should be multiplied by 1.03.
High Density Lipoprotein Cholesterol HDL-C	Precipitating reagents such as divalent cations, along with sulfate polysaccharides or sodium phosphotungstate, are used to create a insoluble complex of all lipoproteins except HDLs. The same direct enzymatic method used for total cholesterol must be used for HDL cholesterol.	Procedures that use Mn^{2+} with a phosphate buffer will increase results. Liquid EDTA will produce false low values. Procedure has same interferences as total cholesterol.	Mn^{2+} interference can be eliminated by reconstituting reagent in a EDTA solution or using a method that does not use a phosphate buffer.
Low Density Lipoprotein Cholesterol LDL-C	LDL-cholesterol = total cholesterol − $\dfrac{\text{(HDL-cholesterol} + \text{Triglycerides)}}{5}$	Same as total cholesterol	Triglyceride values should be under 400 mg/dL.
Low Density Lipoprotein Cholesterol (Direct)	Immunoseparation-latex beads coated with affinity purified goat polyclonal antisera	None	Patient does not have to be fasting

Continued ▶

► Continued **DIAGNOSTIC TESTS AND METHODOLOGIES**

TEST	METHOD	INTERFERENCE	COMMENTS
Apoproteins	Radial immunodiffusion (RID)	CVs range from 8% to 15%	2-3 days to complete
	Electroimmunoassay	CVs for A-I & B range from 6% to 10% CVs for A-II, C-II, and E range from 10% to 15%	Faster than RID
	Enzyme linked immunoassay	CVs under 10%	Good precision
	Immunonephelometry and turbidimetric immunoassay	Pretreatment required because of triglyceride interference	Method of choice for Apo A-I and B for kits and is applicable to automation
Triglycerides	Methods measure free glycerol by a variety of coupled enzymes.	Collection tubes that have lubricated stoppers should not be used. Free glycerol can cause increased values. However, sample blanks can correct error.	If plasma samples are used, multiply test results by 1.03.
Lipoproteins	Ultracentrifugation	None	Reference method; expensive instrumentation requires high technical skills.
	Electrophoresis	Cellulose acetate methods may be unable to identify chylomicrons that migrate with VLDL.	Labor intensive and requires high technical skills

CVs, coefficients of variation.

ASSESSMENT OF LIPIDS

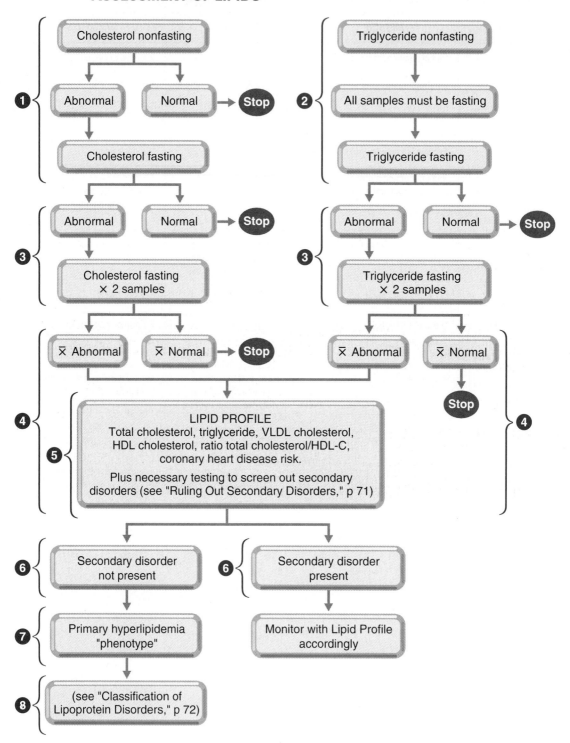

①
Cholesterol nonfasting
→ Abnormal / Normal → Stop
Abnormal → Cholesterol fasting

②
Triglyceride nonfasting
→ All samples must be fasting
→ Triglyceride fasting

③
Abnormal / Normal → Stop
Abnormal → Cholesterol fasting × 2 samples

③
Abnormal / Normal → Stop
Abnormal → Triglyceride fasting × 2 samples

④
x̄ Abnormal / x̄ Normal → Stop

④
x̄ Abnormal / x̄ Normal → Stop

⑤
LIPID PROFILE
Total cholesterol, triglyceride, VLDL cholesterol, HDL cholesterol, ratio total cholesterol/HDL-C, coronary heart disease risk.

Plus necessary testing to screen out secondary disorders (see "Ruling Out Secondary Disorders," p 71)

⑥
Secondary disorder not present

⑥
Secondary disorder present

⑦
Primary hyperlipidemia "phenotype"

Monitor with Lipid Profile accordingly

⑧
(see "Classification of Lipoprotein Disorders," p 72)

1 Nonfasting cholesterol assays are satisfactory as a screening test. If results are > 200 mg/dL, a 12 hour fasting sample should be evaluated.

2 Triglyceride assays must come from patients who have fasted for at least 12 hours.

3 If a fasting sample results in abnormal cholesterol and/or triglyceride (cholesterol > 200 mg/dL; triglycerides: males > 160 mg/dL, females > 135 mg/dL), two additional samples should be assayed over the next 6 to 8 weeks.

4 If the average of all three assays for any given lipid are abnormal, a lipid profile should be performed.

5 Tests found in lipid profiles vary with each laboratory and can contain some or all that are present in the following lipid profile. The most common lipid profile contains total cholesterol, HDL cholesterol, LDL cholesterol (calculated), and triglycerides.

6 At the same time as or shortly after the lipid profile, the clinician should be encouraged to consider a possible secondary disorder (see "Ruling Out Secondary Disorders," p 71) and should order the appropriate test or tests to rule out such a condition.

7 If there is no secondary condition and hyperlipidemia is considered to be the primary disorder, one should consider classifying the phenotype (see "Classification of Lipoprotein Disorders," p 72).

8 As seen, Fredrickson-Levy classification can be made with cholesterol, triglyceride, LDL cholesterol, HDL cholesterol, and a plasma 4°C test. By placing the plasma in a 4°C refrigerator for 16 hours, an observation can be made as to turbidity and/or the appearance of a creamy layer at the top of the sample. For the most part, this information is sufficient for classifying a phenotype. However, if apolipoprotein assays are available, they can help distinguish the underlying causes. For example: phenotype 1 can be caused by either LDL deficiency or Apo C-II deficiency. This is also applicable for performing lipoprotein electrophoresis, as the procedure can present a broad beta band found in phenotype III.

ASSESSMENT OF LIPIDS

DIAGNOSING HYPERTRIGLYCERIDEMIA

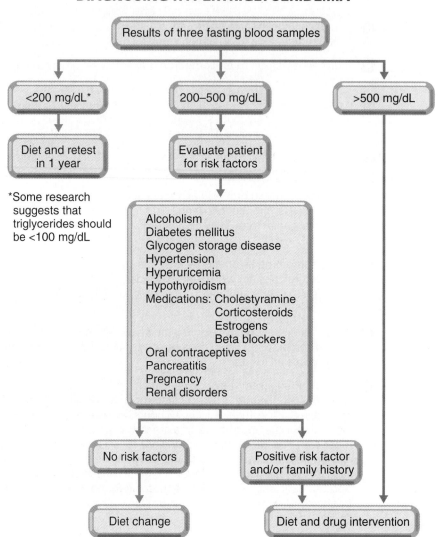

Results of three fasting blood samples

<200 mg/dL*

200–500 mg/dL

>500 mg/dL

Diet and retest
in 1 year

Evaluate patient
for risk factors

*Some research
suggests that
triglycerides should
be <100 mg/dL

Alcoholism
Diabetes mellitus
Glycogen storage disease
Hypertension
Hyperuricemia
Hypothyroidism
Medications: Cholestyramine
Corticosteroids
Estrogens
Beta blockers
Oral contraceptives
Pancreatitis
Pregnancy
Renal disorders

No risk factors

Positive risk factor
and/or family history

Diet change

Diet and drug intervention

RULING OUT SECONDARY DISORDERS

SECONDARY DISORDERS	DIAGNOSTIC TESTS	LIPID EFFECT	LIPOPROTEIN EFFECT
Alcoholism	Gamma glutamyl transferase	↑Triglycerides	↑Chylomicrons ↑VLDL
Chronic Renal Disease	Creatinine, urea nitrogen, K	↑Triglycerides ↑Cholesterol	↑Chylomicrons ↑VLDL ↑LDL
Chronic Anemia	CBC, vitamin B_{12}/folate	↓Cholesterol	↓LDL
Diabetes Mellitus	Glucose	Triglycerides	↑Chylomicrons ↑VLDL ↑HDL
Diet	Triglycerides, cholesterol	↑Triglycerides ↑Cholesterol	↑Chylomicrons ↑VLDL ↑HDL
Malnutrition	Prealbumin, albumin, transferrin, retinol binding protein	↓Cholesterol	↓LDL ↓HDL
Liver Disease	LDH, ALK-PHOS, AST, ALT	↑Cholesterol	↑LDL ↓HDL
Hypothyroidism	Thyroid stimulating hormone	↑Triglycerides ↑Cholesterol	↑Chylomicrons ↑VLDL ↑LDL
Pancreatitis	Amylase, lipase	↑Triglycerides	↑Chylomicrons ↑VLDL ↑LDL
Pregnancy	Beta-hCG	↑Triglycerides	↑Chylomicrons ↑VLDL ↑LDL
Nephrotic Syndrome	Urine protein	↑Cholesterol	↑VLDL ↑LDL
Beta Blockers	Platelet function	↑Triglycerides ↑Cholesterol	↑Chylomicrons ↑VLDL ↑LDL
Estrogens	Estradiol	↑Triglycerides ↑Cholesterol	↑Chylomicrons ↑VLDL ↑LDL ↑HDL
Androgens	Testosterone, 17-ketosteroids	↑Cholesterol	↑LDL
Progestogens	Progesterone	↑Triglycerides ↑Cholesterol	↑Chylomicrons ↑VLDL ↑LDL
Glycogen Storage Disease	Specific to disease	Triglycerides	Chylomicrons ↑VLDL
Storage Disease (Gaucher's, Niemann-Pick)	Specific enzyme	↑Triglycerides	↑Chylomicrons ↑VLDL
Anorexia Nervosa	Albumin, transferrin, retinol binding protein	↑Cholesterol	↑LDL

ALK-PHOS, alkaline phosphatase; ALT, alanine aminotransferase; AST, aspartate aminotransferase; CVs, coefficients of variation; LDH, lactate dehydrogenase.

FREDRICKSON-LEVY CLASSIFICATION OF LIPOPROTEIN DISORDERS

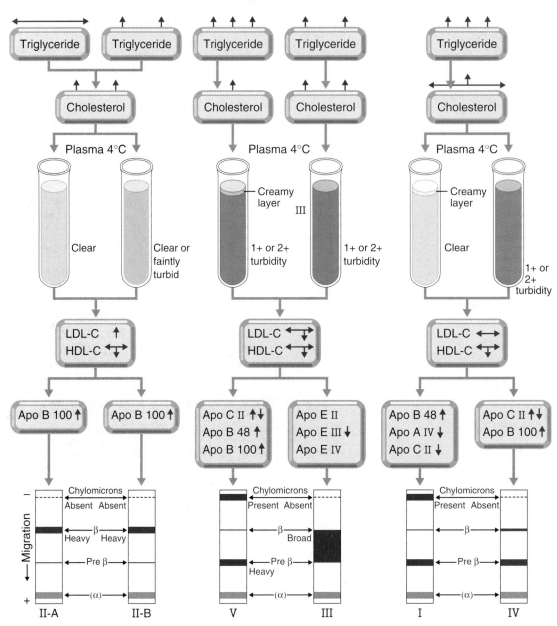

LIPID INTERPRETATION FOR CORONARY HEART DISEASE

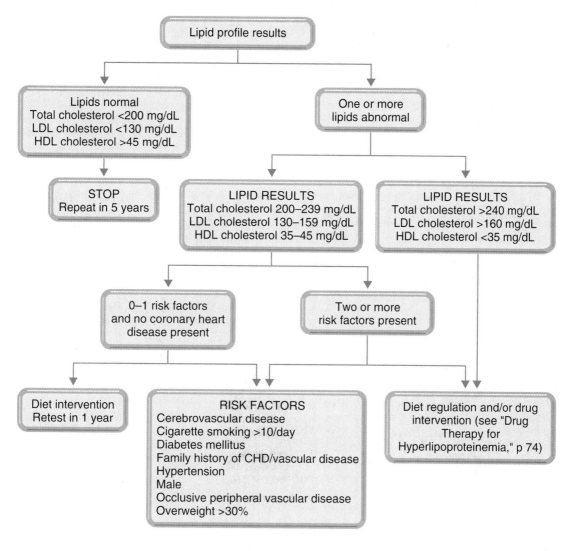

DRUG THERAPY FOR HYPERLIPOPROTEINEMIA

DRUG	PHENOTYPE	EFFECT	ADVERSE EFFECT	LABORATORY MONITORING
Nicotinic Acid (Niacin) Mechanism for lipid reduction unknown	II III IV	↓Triglyceride ↓VLDL cholesterol ↓LDL cholesterol ↑HDL cholesterol	Hepatic Peptic ulcers	HDL cholesterol, Liver function tests, glucose, triglyceride, LDL cholesterol, uric acid
Cholestyramine and Colestipol Anion exchange resin that binds intestinal bile acids	IIa	↓LDL cholesterol	Constipation Nausea Hypoprothrombinemia (<vitamin K)	Cholesterol, triglyceride, prothrombin time, LDL cholesterol, HDL cholesterol
Clofibrate Mechanism not yet clear	III IV	↓Triglyceride ↓VLDL cholesterol ↓LDL cholesterol ↑HDL cholesterol	Myositis Hepatic Gastrointestinal Many additional effects	HDL cholesterol, cholesterol, triglyceride, liver function tests, complete blood count, protein, creatine kinase
Gemfibrozil Mechanism not clear; research has demonstrated that the drug inhibits peripheral lipolysis and decreases hepatic extraction of free fatty acids.	IIa IIb III IV V	↓VLDL cholesterol ↓HDL cholesterol ↑LDL cholesterol	Myositis Hepatic Many additional effects	Cholesterol, triglyceride, K levels, complete blood count, HDL cholesterol, LDL cholesterol, liver function tests
Probucol Increased rate of fractional catabolism of LDL also inhibits cholesterol synthesis	II	↓LDL cholesterol ↓HDL cholesterol	Hepatic Diarrhea Nausea	Cholesterol, triglyceride, HDL cholesterol, liver function tests, glucose, urea nitrogen, uric acid, LDL cholesterol
Fluvastatin Sodium HMG-CoA reductase inhibitors	IIa IIb	↓Total cholesterol ↓LDL cholesterol	Digestive	Liver function tests, CK, total cholesterol, LDL cholesterol
Lovastatin HMG-CoA reductase inhibitor	IIa IIb	↓Total cholesterol ↓LDL cholesterol	Central nervous system Gastrointestinal Hypersensitivity ↑Creatine kinase, aspartate aminotransferase, alanine aminotransferase	CK, AST, total cholesterol, LDL cholesterol, VLDL cholesterol

ALT, alanine aminotransferase; AST, aspartate aminotransferase; CK, creatine kinase.

BIBLIOGRAPHY

Badimon JJ, Fuster V, Badimon L: Role of high density lipoproteins in the regression of athero-sclerosis (review). Circulation 86(6 Suppl):III86-94, 1992.

Barrett-Connor EL: Testosterone and risk factors of cardiovascular disease in men (review). Diabet Metab 21(3):156–161, 1995.

Beisiegel U, Ameis D, Will H, Greten H: [Hypertriglyceridemia and arteriosclerosis. Physiology and pathophysiology of chylomicron catabolism] (review) [German]. Internist 36(4):357–361, 1995.

Burchfiel CM, Laws A, Benfante R, et al: Combined effects of HDL cholesterol, triglyceride, and total cholesterol concentrations on 18-year risk of atherosclerotic disease. Circulation 92(6):1430–1436, 1995.

Burtis CA, Ashwood ER: Tietz Fundamentals of Clinical Chemistry, 4th ed. Philadelphia, WB Saunders, 1996.

Corti MC, Guralnik JM, Salive ME, et al: HDL cholesterol predicts coronary heart disease mortality in older persons [see comments]. JAMA 274(7):539–544, 1995.

Davies MJ, Woolf N, Rowles P, Richardson PD: Lipid and cellular constituents of unstable human aortic plaques. Basic Res Cardiol 89(Suppl 1):33–39, 1994.

Denke MA: Review of human studies evaluating individual dietary responsiveness in patients with hypercholesterolemia (review). Am J Clin Nutr 62(2):471S–477S, 1995.

Denke MA, Winker MA: Cholesterol and coronary heart disease in older adults. No easy answers (editorial; comment). JAMA 247(7):575–577, 1995.

Fukuyo Y, Kobayashi Y: [New approach for lipids and its clinical significance. Part II. Remnant like particles of cholesterol] (review) [Japanese]. Nippon Ika Daigaku Zasshi 61(5):506–509, 1994.

Ginsberg HN: Low HDL cholesterol: what are the prospects of increasing it? (editorial). *Ann Med* 27(3):283–284, 1995.

Howanitz JH: Laboratory Medicine Test Selection and Interpretation. New York, Churchill Livingstone, 1991.

Jialal I, Hirany SV, Devaraj S, Sherwood TA: Comparison of an immunoprecipitation method for direct measurement of LDL-cholesterol with beta-quantification (ultracentrifugation). Am J Clin Pathol 104(1):76–81, 1995.

Khosla P, Hayes KC: Dietary trans-fatty acids and lipoprotein cholesterol (letter). Am J Clin Nutr 629(40):843–844, 1995.

Kitagawa S, Yamaguchi Y, Kunitomo M, et al: Impairment of endothelium dependent relaxation in aorta from rats with arteriosclerosis induced by excess vitamin D and high cholesterol diet. Jpn J Pharmacol 59(3):339–347, 1992.

Lane DM, McConathy WJ, Laughlin LO, et al: Selective removal of plasma low density lipoprotein with the HELP system: biweekly versus weekly therapy. Atherosclerosis 114(2):203–211, 1995.

Lawn RM: Lipoprotein(a) in heart disease. Sci Am 266(6):54–60, 1992.

Lupatelli G, Siepi D, Pasqualini L, et al: Lipoprotein(a) in peripheral arterial occlusive disease. Vasa 23(4):321–324, 1994.

Masse J: Effect of interleukin-3 on lipoprotein(a) and lipoprotein cholesterol levels (letter). Am J Cardiol 76(10):747, 1995.

Mize CE, Uauy R, Kramer R, et al: Lipoprotein cholesterol responses in healthy infants fed defined diets from ages 1 to 12 months: comparison of diets predominant in oleic acid versus linoleic acid, with parallel observations in infants fed a human milk-based diet. J Lipid Res 36(6):1178–1187, 1995.

McClatchery KD: Clinical Laboratory Medicine. Baltimore, Williams & Wilkins, 1994.

Nawrocky JW, Weiss SR, Davidson MH, et al: Reduction of LDL cholesterol by 25% to 60% in patients with primary hypercholesterolemia by atorvastatin, a new HMG-CoA reductase inhibitor. Arterioscl Thromb Vasc Biol 15(5):678–682, 1995.

Nofer JR, Von Ecardstein A, Wielbusch H, et al: Screening for naturally occurring apolipoprotein A-I variants: apo A-I (delta K107) is associated with low HDL-cholesterol levels in men but not in women. Hum Genet 96(2):177–182, 1995.

Otto C, Richter WO: Hemostatic factors and the risk of myocardial infarction (letter, comment). N Engl J Med 333(6):389–390, 1995.

Patch W, Gotto AM Jr: High density lipoprotein cholesterol, plasma triglyceride, and coronary heart disease: pathophysiology and management (review). Adv Pharmacol 32:375–426, 1995.

DRUG THERAPY FOR HYPERLIPOPROTEINEMIA

Perova NV, Oganov RG, Williams DH, et al: Association of high-density-lipoprotein cholesterol with mortality and other risk factors for major chronic noncommunicable diseases in samples of US and Russian men. Ann Epidemiol 5(3):179–185, 1995.

Purnell JQ, Marcovina SM, Hokanson JE, et al: Levels of lipoprotein(a), apolipoprotein B, and lipoprotein cholesterol distribution in IDDM. Results from follow-up in the Diabetes Control and Complications Trial. Diabetes 44(10):1218–1226, 1995.

Rindone JP, Achacoso R, Bledsoe R: Effect of lovastatin administered every other day on serum low-density lipoprotein cholesterol > 160 mg/dl. Am J Cardiol 76(4):312–313, 1995.

Sachinidis A, Ko Y, Vetter W, Vetter H: [Action of intrinsic low density lipoprotein in the vascular wall. Significance for the pathogenesis of essential hypertension and arteriosclerosis] (review) [German]. Med Klin 89(12):662–667, 1994.

Sacks FM, Gibson CM, Rosner B, et al: The influence of pretreatment low density lipoprotein cholesterol concentrations on the effect of hypocholesterolemic therapy on coronary atherosclerosis in angiographic trials. Harvard Atherosclerosis Reversibility Project Research Group (review). Am J Cardiol 76(9):78C–85C, 1995.

Schaefer EJ, Lichtenstein AH, Lamon-Fava S, et al: Efficacy of National Cholesterol Education Program Step 2 diet in normolipidemic and hypercholesterolemic middle-aged and elderly men and women. Arterioscl Thromb Vasc Biol 15(8):1079–1085, 1995.

Shi Y, Nardone D, Hernandez-Martinez A, et al: Fibrinolytic activity after vessel wall injury. J Am Coll Cardiol 19(2):441–443, 1992.

Sugiuchi H, Uji Y, Irie T, et al: Direct measurement of high-density lipoprotein cholesterol in serum with polyethylene glycol–modified enzymes and sulfated alpha-cyclodextrin. Clin Chem 41(5):717–723, 1995.

Uesugi S, Yamaguchi I: [Significance of clinical examination concerning arteriosclerosis] [Japanese]. Rinsho Byori 43(2):101–103, 1995.

Vecera R, Chmela Z, Hrebicek J, Skottova N: Unsaturated fatty acids incorporated in HDL in hypo- and hyperalphalipoproteinemia—relation to the HDL-cholesterol level. Acta Univ Palacki Olomuc Fac Med 137:35–38, 1994.

Wilder LB, Bachorik PS, Finney CA, et al: The effect of fasting status on the determination of low-density and high-density lipoprotein cholesterol. Am J Med 99(4):374–377, 1995.

Zhu BQ, Sun YP, Sievers RE, et al: Effects of etidronate and lovastatin on the regression of atherosclerosis in cholesterol fed rabbits. Cardiology 85(6):370–377, 1994.

Chapter *5*

ENZYMES

Mary Hotaling, MS, MT (ASCP) DLM

Q U I C K   C O N T E N T S

INTRODUCTION

This chapter presents the more general aspects of clinical enzymology. Additional information regarding the specific organ systems such as the liver, gastrointestinal, cardiac, and prostate (carcinoma) may be found in their respective chapters.

Alterations of plasma enzyme levels are used to assist in disease detection, differential diagnosis, and monitoring efficacy of treatment. Differential diagnosis is most possible when a pattern of plasma enzyme elevation is established and compared with the known distribution of enzymes and isoenzymes among the various tissues. With this information, the location and nature of the pathologic tissue changes may be identified.

Plasma Enzyme Characteristics

Enzymes are important biologic catalysts that enable metabolic processes to proceed rapidly enough to maintain life. Enzymes are produced intracellularly, and most perform their catalytic function within the cytosol and/or mitochondrion. Intracellular enzyme levels are extremely high compared with the plasma. Some enzymes, mainly the digestive variety, are secreted and function within the extracellular fluids. In health, characteristic amounts of intracellular enzymes enter the plasma mainly as a result of leakage from the cells during normal cell turnover.

Factors Influencing Increased Plasma Enzyme Levels

Plasma enzyme levels can become elevated by a number of factors increasing the rate of enzyme entry into the circulation. When tissues are subjected to stress, injury, or necrosis, they release increased amounts of certain enzymes (native to that tissue) into the circulation. Because of a significant concentration gradient between intracellular and extracellular enzyme levels, even a relatively small change in plasma enzyme levels can be a sensitive indicator of such a pathologic process. These factors and mechanisms, along with common examples, are briefly described in the table below:

FACTOR	MECHANISM	EXAMPLE
↑ Enzyme leakage from cells	Cell stress, through injury, through necrosis Results in varying degrees of loss of cell membrane integrity (which increases cell membrane permeability) through complete cell necrosis.	AMI results in hypoxia, leading to cardiac cell death and subsequent necrosis. Cardiac enzymes, e.g., CK, LD, AST, are released over time from the damaged tissue.
↑ Enzyme production	Enzyme induction Increased rate of intracellular enzyme production	■ Drug administration, e.g., ↑ GGT production with antiepileptics such as phenytoin ■ Ethanol intake
	Proliferation of a cell type producing a specific enzyme	Proliferation of PAP-producing cells in prostatic carcinoma

AMI, acute myocardial infarction; CK, creatine kinase; LD, lactic dehydrogenase; AST, aspartate aminotransferase; GGT, gamma-glutamyltransferase; PAP, prostatic acid phosphatase.

Enzyme Clearance

Consideration of enzyme clearance rate or half-life in the circulation is most valuable when assessing acute conditions elevating plasma enzyme levels. With the exception of the smallest enzyme molecule, amylase, the healthy kidney is not a major enzyme clearance route out of the circulation. The major enzyme clearance route is believed to be the reticuloendothelial system via receptor mediated endocytosis.

PATIENT PREPARATION, SPECIMEN COLLECTION AND STORAGE REQUIREMENTS, REFERENCE RANGES

Specimen Collection

Serum is the specimen of choice. Heparinized plasma is sometimes acceptable, but EDTA or oxalate plasma specimens should not be used because they generally cause extensive enzyme activity inhibition.

Reference Ranges

Reference ranges may vary significantly among assay methods, such as enzymatic versus immunoassay. Even among the various enzymatic assays, different reference ranges may be obtained because reagent systems often contain different types and/or concentrations of substrates, cofactors, and buffers (to adjust pH). Reference ranges may also vary as a result of different reaction temperature conditions.

Patient Preparation, Specimen Storage Requirements, Reference Ranges for Enzyme and Isoenzyme Assays

TEST	PATIENT PREPARATION	SPECIMEN STORAGE	REFERENCE RANGE (U/L) AT 37°C
Alanine Aminotransferase (ALT)	None	0°–4°C for 1–3 days Frozen for longer periods Best to assay on day of collection because no storage temperature is entirely satisfactory.	M: 10–40 F: 10–28 Range for optimized reagent system containing the cofactor pyridoxal phosphate
Alkaline Phosphatase (ALP)	None	0°–4°C for 2–3 days −25°C for 30 days Thawed specimens may ↑ ALP activity by up to 30%	F > 15 yr: 25–100 M > 20 yr: 25–100 F 1–12 yr: <350 M 1–12 yr: <350 M 12–14 yr: <500
Alkaline Phosphatase (ALP) Isoenzymes	Fasting	Analyze immediately or store at 4°C	% Inactivation, 56°C, 16 min Bone (50%–70%) Liver (90%–100%) Intestinal (50%–60%) Placental (0%) Regan (0%)
Amylase (AMS)	SERUM: None URINE: Collect 1–24 hr timed specimen.	SERUM: RT for 7 days 4°C for 30 days URINE: Adjust to alkaline pH before storage. Storage same as serum.	Maltotetraose substrate SERUM: 27–131 URINE: 1–17 U/hr

Continued ▶

► Continued **Patient Preparation, Specimen Storage Requirements, Reference Ranges for Enzyme and Isoenzyme Assays**

TEST	PATIENT PREPARATION	SPECIMEN STORAGE	REFERENCE RANGE (U/L) AT 37°C
Amylase (AMS) Isoenzymes	None	Best when analyzed immediately or store as for AMS.	P type (30%–55%) S type (45%–70%) Ranges are method dependent.
Aspartate Aminotransferase (AST)	None	RT for 24 hr 4°C for 28 days −20°C for at least 1 yr	M: 15–40 F: 13–35 Range for optimized reagent system containing the cofactor pyridoxal phosphate.
Cholinesterase (SChE) (Pseudocholinesterase) SChE should not be confused with acetylcholinesterase	None	RT for 6 hr 4°C for 7 days −70°C for 6 mo	Colorimetric: 4.9–11.9 U/mL Butylthiocholine: 7–19 U/mL
Creatine Kinase (CK)	Avoid excessive physical activity.	RT for 4–8 hr 4°C for 1–2 days −20°C for 30 days	M: 38–174 F: 26–140 African-Americans have higher levels than non–African-Americans.
Creatine Kinase (CK) Isoenzymes	Avoid excessive physical activity.	RT for 4–8 hr 4°C for 1–2 days −20°C for 30 days Preserve for CK-BB analysis with 2-ME and EDTA, protect from light, and keep tightly stoppered.	Electrophoresis method: CK-BB (CK-1) (0% or trace) CK-MB (CK-2) ($<$4%–6%) CK-MM (CK-3) ($>$94%–96%) Immunoassay CK-MB$_{mass}$: $<$10 μg/L (method dependent)
γ-Glutamyltransferase (GGT)	None	4°C for 30 days −20°C for 1 yr	M: 10–35 F: 8–25
Lactate Dehydrogenase (LD)	None	Serum *or* heparinized plasma Separate from cells and analyze ASAP. RT only, *do not* refrigerate or freeze.	Lactate → pyruvate: 140–280 Pyruvate → lactate: 208–378

Continued ►

▶ Continued **Patient Preparation, Specimen Storage Requirements,**
Reference Ranges for Enzyme and Isoenzyme Assays

TEST	PATIENT PREPARATION	SPECIMEN STORAGE	REFERENCE RANGE (U/L) AT 37°C
Lactate Dehydrogenase (LD) Isoenzymes	None	RT only; LD-5 is least stable fraction.	Cellulose acetate electrophoresis method: LD-1 (18%–33%) LD-2 (28%–40%) LD-3 (18%–30%) LD-4 (6%–16%) LD-5 (2%–13%) Isoenzyme patterns cannot be reliably interpreted without clinical data. Immunoassay LD-1 (immunoinhibition) <40% (method dependent).
Lipase (LPS)	None	RT for several days 4° is optimal	Triolein substrate: <200 Olive oil substrate: <160
Prostatic Acid Phosphatase (PAP)	Collect serum specimen *before* any prostate manipulation.	Immunoassay methods: 2°–8°C for 24 hr ≤−20°C for ≥24 hr Enzyme methods (i.e. tartrate): Separate serum from cells and analyze immediately. If testing is delayed, acidify serum to a pH of 5.4–6.2 with citrate buffer or acetic acid. Store acidified serum at 4°C or −20°C	Immunoassay: <2.5 ng/mL Tartrate inhibition: 0–0.6 U/L
Prostate Specific Antigen (PSA)	Collect serum specimen *before* any prostate manipulation.	2°–8°C for 2 wk ≤−20°C for longer periods	<4.0 ng/mL PSA values ↑ with age

F, female; M, male; RT, room temperature; 2-ME, 2-mercaptoethanol; EDTA, ethylenediaminetetraacetate.

DIAGNOSTIC ENZYMOLOGY AND METHODOLOGIES
Diagnostic Enzymology
ENZYME PANELS

Although single enzyme results are sometimes helpful in diagnosis, the use of enzyme panels consisting of more than one enzyme (or isoenzyme) provides greater diagnostic sensitivity and specificity in disease detection. Results of enzyme panels revealing a "pattern" of enzyme elevation is especially useful for differentiating various disorders. The clinically important enzymes are listed below by common name with the principal tissue source(s) and clinical application.

CLINICALLY SIGNIFICANT ENZYMES

ENZYME	PRINCIPAL TISSUE SOURCE(S)	PRINCIPAL CLINICAL APPLICATIONS
Acid Phosphatase (ACP)	See Prostatic Acid Phosphatase (PAP)	
Alanine Aminotransferase (ALT)	Liver, kidney	Hepatic parenchymal diseases, not usually ↑ in renal diseases
Alkaline Phosphatase (ALP)	Liver, bone, placenta	Bone diseases, hepatobiliary disease
Alkaline Phosphatase (ALP) Isoenzymes Liver Bone Intestinal Placental Regan	Tissue specific sources Liver Bone Intestine Placenta Regan—some neoplasia	Identify likely tissue source causing ↑ ALP levels; especially to differentiate bone from liver diseases.
Amylase (AMS)	Pancreas, salivary glands	Pancreatic diseases
Amylase (AMS) Isoenzymes P types S types	P types: pancreas S types: e.g., salivary glands, ovaries, lung	Identify likely tissue source causing ↑ AMS levels, especially to rule out pancreatic source in postoperative ↑ AMS.
Aspartate Aminotransferase (AST)	Liver, skeletal, and cardiac muscle	Acute myocardial infarction (AMI), hepatic parenchymal diseases, skeletal muscle diseases.
Cholinesterase (SChE) (Pseudocholinesterase)	Liver	Insecticide poisoning (organophosphorus), suxamethonium sensitivity, rarely used for hepatic parenchymal diseases.
Creatine Kinase (CK)	Skeletal and cardiac muscle, brain	AMI, skeletal muscle diseases.
Creatine Kinase (CK) Isoenzymes CK-BB (CK-1) CK-MB (CK-2) CK-MM (CK-3)	CK-BB: brain CK-MB: cardiac, skeletal muscle CK-MM: skeletal, cardiac muscle	Identify likely tissue source causing ↑ CK levels, especially to rule out AMI. CK-MB isoenzyme quantitation is used for this purpose.

Continued ▶

► Continued **CLINICALLY SIGNIFICANT ENZYMES**

ENZYME	PRINCIPAL TISSUE SOURCE(S)	PRINCIPAL CLINICAL APPLICATIONS
γ-Glutamyltransferase (GGT)	Liver	Hepatobiliary disease, alcoholism
Lactate Dehydrogenase (LD)	Cardiac muscle, liver, skeletal muscle, RBCs	AMI, hemolysis, hepatic parenchymal diseases
Lactate Dehydrogenase (LD) Isoenzymes LD-1 (HHHH) LD-2 (HHHM) LD-3 (HHMM) LD-4 (HMMM) LD-5 (MMMM)	LD-1: cardiac muscle, RBCs, kidney LD-2: cardiac muscle, kidney, RBCs LD-3: spleen, kidney, lungs, RBCs LD-4: spleen, lungs, kidney LD-5: liver, skeletal muscle	Identify likely tissue source causing ↑ LD levels, especially to rule out AMI LD-1 isoenzyme quantitation is used for this purpose.
Lipase (LPS)	Pancreas	Pancreatic diseases
Prostate Specific Antigen (PSA)	Prostate	Prostatic carcinoma
Prostatic Acid Phosphatase (PAP)	Prostate	Prostate carcinoma

Enzyme Methodologies

GENERAL ENZYME REACTIONS

Enzymes function as biochemical catalysts by reducing the activation energy required to energize the substrate so that the reaction proceeds at an accelerated rate at normal body temperature. In the simple enzymatic reaction for one substrate and one product listed below:

$$E + S \rightleftharpoons ES \rightarrow E + P$$

the enzyme *(E)* reversibly binds with its substrate *(S)*, forming the enzyme-substrate complex *(ES)*. The ES complex decomposes to enzyme [E] and product [P] without the enzyme being altered by the overall reaction.

FACTORS INFLUENCING ENZYME ACTIVITY

Some enzymes require cofactors, such as coenzymes, for the proper formation of the ES complex to achieve maximal enzyme activity. Enzyme activity is also altered by the reaction pH and temperature because these conditions affect the enzyme's three-dimensional conformation. Beyond certain pH and temperature limits, the protein is denatured and the enzyme is inactivated. Enzymes may bind to molecules other than the substrate that may reduce or enhance catalytic activity. These substances are called inhibitors and activators, respectively.

DIAGNOSTIC ENZYMOLOGY AND METHODOLOGIES

MEASUREMENT OF ENZYME ACTIVITY

Under appropriate reaction conditions, enzyme activity is directly proportional to enzyme concentration. Enzyme activity is commonly monitored by measuring the quantity of the (1) product formed, (2) substrate depleted, or (3) coenzyme converted. Some of these reactions yield a colored end product, while many more methods take advantage of the ultraviolet (UV) absorbance properties of the coenzymes NAD^+ (or $NADP^+$) as they are converted to NADH (or NADPH) (reduced form) or vice versa. The absorbance at 340 nm increases significantly as NAD^+ (or $NADP^+$) is converted to NADH (or NADPH).

COUPLED ENZYME REACTIONS

An enzyme reaction that does not utilize NAD^+ or NADH as a coenzyme and does not form a convenient colored end product can be *coupled* to one or more enzymatic reactions. Coupled enzyme reactions terminate in a final indicator reaction that produces a convenient end product for reliable measurement of enzyme activity. An example couple enzyme reaction for the assay of creatine kinase (CK) is outlined in the table below:

Coupled Enzyme Reaction Steps

REACTION STEP	CREATINE KINASE (CK) COUPLED ENZYME REACTION METHOD
Primary Reaction step catalyzed by the enzyme whose activity is to be determined	Creatine phosphate + ADP $\xrightarrow[Mg^{++}]{CK}$ creatine + ATP ▪ CK is the enzyme being determined. ▪ Mg^{++} is a required cofactor.
Auxiliary One or more subsequent reaction steps catalyzed by auxiliary enzymes (except for Indicator reaction)	ATP + glucose $\xrightarrow{HK}$ glucose-6-phosphate + ADP ▪ The product ATP from the primary reaction is reacted with glucose and the auxiliary enzyme hexokinase (HK), forming glucose-6-phosphate (G6P)
Indicator Final reaction step producing a product whose absorbance is measured as a colored end product or UV measurable product, i.e., $NAD^+ \leftrightarrow NADH$	G6P + $NADPH^+$ $\xrightarrow{GPD}$ 6-phosphogluconate + NADPH ▪ Measure indicator reaction ($NADP^+ \rightarrow NADPH$) as absorbance increases at 340 nm (UV).

ENZYME METHODOLOGIES

TEST	METHOD	SPECIMEN INTERFERENCE	PHYSIOLOGIC INTERFERENCE	COMMENT
Alanine aminotransferase (ALT)	Coupled enzyme reaction Substrate: L-alanine Indicator reaction: Conversion of NADH → NAD$^+$ is monitored 340 nm.	Avoid hemolysis, RBC contains ↑ AST and ALT.	Many drugs are hepatotoxic and also may cause cholestasis; many also ↑ ALT transiently without necessarily indicating hepatotoxicity.	Pyridoxal phosphate is added to most modern reagent systems.
Alkaline Phosphatase (ALP)	Photometric enzyme reaction Substrate: 4-nitrophenyl phosphate (4-NPP) Indicator reaction: Production of yellow colored 4-nitrophenol (4-NP) is monitored 405 nm.	Avoid EDTA and oxalate anticoagulants, which ↓ ALP activity.	Many drugs are hepatotoxic and many also ↑ ALP transiently without necessarily indicating hepatotoxicity.	
Amylase (AMS)	Coupled enzyme reaction 1. Substrate: maltotetraose or maltopentaose Indicator reaction: Conversion of NAD$^+$ → NADH is monitored 340 nm. 2. Substrate: 4-NP-glucoside Indicator reaction: Production of free, yellow colored 4-nitrophenol (4-NP) is monitored 405 nm.	Avoid contamination with saliva. Lipemia, anticoagulants EDTA, fluoride, citrate ↓ AMS.	Renal insufficiency may falsely ↑. Presence of macroamylase ↑ serum AMS and is accompanied by normal or ↓ urine AMS.	
Aspartate aminotransferase (AST)	Coupled enzyme reaction Substrate: L-aspartate Indicator reaction: Conversion of NADH → NAD$^+$ is monitored 340 nm.	Avoid hemolysis; RBC contains ↑ AST and ALT.	Many drugs are hepatotoxic and also may cause cholestasis; many also ↑ AST transiently without necessarily indicating hepatotoxicity.	Pyridoxal phosphate is added to most modern reagent systems.

Continued ▶

DIAGNOSTIC ENZYMOLOGY AND METHODOLOGIES

E METHODOLOGIES

METHOD	SPECIMEN INTERFERENCE	PHYSIOLOGIC INTERFERENCE	COMMENT
Photometric enzyme reaction Substrate: butylthiocholine Indicator reaction: Hydrolyzed substrate reacts with colorless DTNB → colored 5-MNBA is monitored 410 nm.	Avoid hemolysis, citrate, fluoride anticoagulants.	↓ in genetic SChE variants.	
Creatine Kinase (CK) Coupled enzyme reaction Substrate: phosphocreatine Indicator reaction: Conversion of $NAD^+ \rightarrow NADH$ is monitored 340 nm.	Gross hemolysis. RBC contains adenylate kinase, causing positive interference.	Physical activity, skeletal muscle damage	Reagent system utilizes thiol compound, i.e., NAC (n-acetyl cysteine) for reactivation of CK activity.
γ-Glutamyltransferase (GGT) Photometric enzyme reaction Substrate: L-γ-glutamyl-*p*-nitroanilide or L-γ-glutamyl-3-carboxy-nitroanilide Indicator reaction: Production of *p*-nitroaniline (yellow) or 5-amino-2-nitrobenzoate is monitored 405 nm or 410 nm, respectively.	Heparin interference is variable depending on method.	None known	
Lactate Dehydrogenase (LD) Photometric enzyme reaction Lactate → pyruvate (L→P) Substrate: lactate Indicator reaction: Conversion of $NAD^+ \rightarrow NADH$ is monitored 340 nm.	Avoid hemolysis. RBCs contain very high LD concentration.	In vivo hemolysis	Although P → L is theoretically preferred method, L → P is commonly used in US because of ↑ linearity.

Continued ▶

▶ Continued **ENZYME METHODOLOGIES**

TEST	METHOD	SPECIMEN INTERFERENCE	PHYSIOLOGIC INTERFERENCE	COMMENT
Lipase (LPS)	Turbidimetric enzyme reaction Substrate: olive oil or triolein Indicator reaction: ↓ turbidity is monitored as LPS hydrolyzes the turbid substrate fat emulsion.		Heparin administration releases lipoprotein lipase and hepatic lipase, resulting in falsely ↑ serum lipase by some nonoptimized methods.	Optimized assays contain bile salts and colipase for optimal pancreatic lipase activity.
Prostatic Acid Phosphatase (PAP)	■ Immunoassay RIA, IRMA, MEIA ■ Photometric enzyme reaction Differential substrate: α-naphthyl phosphate or thymolphthalein monophosphate Indicator reaction: Production of yellow colored 4-nitrophenol (4-NP) is monitored **405 nm.** ■ Chemical inhibition (tartrate) — photometric enzyme reaction Substrate: 4-nitrophenyl phosphate (4-NPP) at acid pH Indicator reaction: As above for differential substrates	■ None known for immunoassay methods ■ For enzyme methods, avoid moderate hemolysis, separate from RBCs immediately. If testing is delayed, acidify serum specimen.	Prostate manipulation, benign prostatic hypertrophy (BPH)	Tartrate inhibits PAP fraction of total ACP. Calculate difference between: (total ACP activity) — (ACP activity after tartrate inhibition) = PAP. Immunoassay methods are more specific for PAP than either enzyme method.
Prostate Specific Antigen (PSA)	Immunoassay RIA, IRMA, IEMA	None known	Prostate manipulation, benign prostatic hypertrophy (BPH)	

IRMA, immunoradiometric assay; MEIA, microparticle enzyme immunoassay; RIA, radioimmunoassay; IEMA, immunoenzymetric assay.

DIAGNOSTIC ISOENZYMES AND METHODOLOGIES

Diagnostic Isoenzymes

Many enzymes exist in multiple molecular forms called isoenzymes. Although these isoenzyme forms are molecularly distinct from one another, they perform the same or similar catalytic reactions. Enzymes are measured as total enzyme activity or as distinct isoenzymes by several methods outlined in the table below. Isoenzyme measurement is especially important in the differential diagnosis of elevated enzyme levels because they are entirely or partially derived from discrete tissue sources. Isoenzyme data are used to detect the affected tissue or organ causing elevated enzyme levels.

Isoenzyme Methodologies

ISOENZYME(S)	METHOD	SPECIMEN INTERFERENCE	PHYSIOLOGIC INTERFERENCE	COMMENT
Alkaline Phosphatase (ALP) Isoenzymes: Bone Liver Intestinal Placental Regan	▪ Heat inactivation at 56°C for 10 min ▪ Electrophoresis ▪ Selective Inhibition Urea and phenyl-alanine	Fasting specimen is most appropriate since eating may ↑ intestinal ALP in some individuals of blood types O or B.	Placental and Regan isoenzymes have similar pattern in heat and electrophoresis methods. Placental ALP is produced during pregnancy, especially in third trimester. Regan isoenzyme is found to be associated with neoplastic disorders.	Heat inactivation method is routinely performed and reported as % heat stable. This method is best used to estimate bone or liver source of ↑ ALP.
Amylase (AMS) Isoenzymes: P types S types	▪ Electrophoresis ▪ Isoelectric focusing ▪ Selective Inhibition AMS (S type) Wheat germ ▪ Immunoassay	Specimen storage may result in aberrant isoenzyme bands on electrophoresis and isoelectric focusing methods.	Ovarian and bronchial tumors produce AMS similar to S type. Macroamylase is an S type AMS bound to immunoglobulin.	Results and number of P type and S type isoenzymes recovered are very method dependent.
Creatine Kinase Isoenzymes: CK-BB (CK-1) CK-MB (CK-2) CK-MM (CK-3)	▪ Electrophoresis Activity of all isoenzymes ▪ CK-MB *activity* Immunoinhibition ▪ CK-MB *mass* Immunoassay ELISA, IRMA	None known for immunoassay For immunoinhibition methods: hemolysis produces positive interference.	Electrophoresis Macro-CK can be misidentified as CK-MB band. Immunoinhibition methods cannot distinguish between CK-BB and CK-MB activity.	Immunoinhibition results are generally confirmed with a CK-MB mass assay.

Continued ▶

▶ Continued **Isoenzyme Methodologies**

ISOENZYME(S)	METHOD	SPECIMEN INTERFERENCE	PHYSIOLOGIC INTERFERENCE	COMMENT
LD Isoenzymes: LD-1 LD-2 LD-3 LD-4 LD-5	▮ Electrophoresis Activity of all isoenzymes	LD-5 is least stable isoenzyme. Avoid hemolysis, may grossly ↑ LD-1 band.	In vivo hemolysis may grossly ↑ LD-1 and LD-2 bands. Presence of LD bound to Ig A or IgG can produce variable results, including ↑ or ↓ fractions or distorted electrophoresis patterns.	
	▮ LD-1 immunoassay ▮ Immunoinhibition ▮ Chemical inhibition 1,6 hexanediol or sodium perchlorate	Avoid hemolysis, may grossly ↑ LD-1.		LD-1 immunoassay and Inhibition methods only measure LD-1.

CARCINOMA

Plasma levels of several enzymes and some of their isoenzymes may be increased in malignant conditions such as carcinoma. Some enzymes may be used as tumor markers to assist in the diagnosis and monitoring of some types of malignancies. However, practical utilization of enzymes as tumor markers is limited because specificity is generally inadequate to identify distinct types of malignancies and their location. Elevated plasma enzyme levels, suspected to be a result of a malignancy, may be further evaluated by clinical laboratory methods by correlation with other, more specific types of tumor markers, such as oncofetal antigens, hormones, steroid receptors, specific proteins, monoclonal immunoglobulins, immunophenotyping, or DNA analysis. Some enzymes and their respective clinical carcinoma applications are outlined in the table below. Refer to the section on tumor markers for further discussion.

DIAGNOSTIC ISOENZYMES AND METHODOLOGIES

Clinically Useful Enzyme and Isoenzyme Tumor Markers

ENZYME/ISOENZYME	PRINCIPAL TISSUE SOURCE(S)	TUMOR MARKER APPLICATIONS
Alkaline Phosphatase (ALP)	Liver Bone Placenta	Primary and metastatic liver, bone malignancies, hematologic diseases, i.e. leukemia, lymphoma
Amylase (AMS)	Pancreas, salivary glands	Some lung and ovarian tumors
Creatine Kinase Isoenzyme (CK-BB)	Brain, smooth muscle, many other minor sources including lung, bladder, prostate, uterus, liver, gut, breast.	Many types of malignancies, particularly prostate, lung (small cell) carcinoma, and bladder and GI tract malignancies
Lactate Dehydrogenase (LD)	Cardiac muscle, liver, skeletal muscle, RBCs	Many types of primary and metastatic carcinomas; see specific LD Isoenzymes
Lactate Dehydrogenase (LD) Isoenzymes	Cardiac muscle, liver, skeletal muscle, RBCs	LD-1: germ cell tumors, LD-3: leukemias, LD-5: breast, lung, stomach, colon tumors
Neuron Specific Enolase (NSE)	Neurons, neuroendocrine cells	Neuroendocrine system malignancies, such as lung (small cell), neuroblastoma, carcinoid, and pancreatic islet cells
Prostatic Acid Phosphatase (PAP)	Prostate	Prostatic carcinoma. Not recommended for screening purposes since it is usually not significantly ↑ until tumor is metastasized. PSA is preferred marker.
Prostate Specific Antigen (PSA)	Prostate	Prostatic carcinoma detection, monitoring, and staging. Should be used in conjunction with digital rectal examination for screening men over 50 yr of age. Most useful for monitoring therapy and tumor recurrance since PSA may not be significantly ↑ until tumor is grown out of prostate capsule.

EVALUATING TEST RESULTS

In this section, diagnostic information is grouped into two tables. The first table, "Clinically Significant Causes of Altered Enzyme Levels," provides general data by listing the often numerous disorders that either increase or decrease plasma enzyme levels. The second table, "Clinically Significant Enzymes by Tissue," provides much more specific data and can be used when a particular tissue or organ system injury is suspected.

Clinically Significant Causes of Altered Enzyme Levels

ENZYME	INCREASED		DECREASED
Acid Phosphatase	See Prostatic Acid Phosphatase (PAP)		
Alanine Aminotransferase (ALT)	HEPATIC PARENCHYMAL DISEASES: Viral hepatitis Toxic hepatitis Reye's syndrome Obstructive jaundice (cholestasis) Cirrhosis (variable)	OTHERS: Heart failure or acute myocardial infarction (AMI) with hepatic congestion Infectious mononucleosis Muscular dystrophy	Not clinically significant
Alkaline Phosphatase (ALP)	BONE DISEASES: Paget's disease Bone tumors Osteomalacia and rickets Bone fractures (physiologic increase) HEPATOBILIARY DISEASES: Obstructive jaundice (cholestasis) Viral hepatitis Hepatic malignancy Alcoholic cirrhosis	OTHERS: Hyperparathyroidism Pregnancy (physiologic increase, especially in 3rd trimester) Malabsorption (sprue) Other malignancies	Not clinically significant
Amylase (AMS)	PANCREATIC: Acute pancreatitis Chronic pancreatitis (may be variable) Pancreatic cyst or pseudocyst SALIVARY GLANDS: Parotitis Mumps	OTHERS: Intestinal obstruction Ectopic pregnancy Diabetic ketoacidosis Biliary tract disease Macroamylasemia Malignancies, i.e., some ovarian, lung tumors	Pancreatic insufficiency
Aspartate Aminotransferase (AST)	CARDIAC MUSCLE DISEASES: Acute myocardial infarction Heart failure with or without hepatic congestion Pericarditis Myocarditis SKELETAL MUSCLE DISEASES: Muscular dystrophy Muscle trauma	HEPATIC PARENCHYMAL DISEASES: Viral hepatitis Toxic hepatitis Reye's syndrome Infectious mononucleosis Obstructive jaundice (cholestasis) Cirrhosis (variable) OTHERS: Acute pancreatitis	Uremia

Continued ▶

► Continued **Clinically Significant Causes of Altered Enzyme Levels**

ENZYME	INCREASED		DECREASED
Cholinesterase (SChE) (Pseudo-cholinesterase)	Not clinically significant but occurs in: Hyperlipoproteinemia (type IV) Obesity Nephrosis Breast cancer		HEPATIC PARENCHY-MAL DISEASES: Rarely used for diagnosis since ↓ SChE generally parallels serum albumin levels) Hepatitis Cirrhosis Malignancy OTHERS: Insecticide poisoning (organophosphorus) Genetic variants displaying suxamethonium sensitivity
Creatine Kinase (CK)	CARDIAC MUSCLE DISEASES: Acute myocardial infarction Myocarditis Cardiac catheterization, angioplasty Cardiac surgery Congestive heart failure Tachycardia BRAIN AND CNS DISEASES: Cerebrovascular accident (CVA) Cerebral ischemia	SKELETAL MUSCLE DISEASES: Muscular dystrophy, (especially early stage Duchenne's) and female carriers Muscle trauma Excessive exercise Malignant hypothermia Myopathic disorders, i.e., rhabdomyolysis, myocarditis, alcoholism OTHERS: Reye's syndrome Hypothyroidism Malignancies, i.e., prostate, bladder, GI tract	Not clinically significant but occurs in: Hyperthyroidism Decreased muscle mass
γ-Glutamyltransferase (GGT)	LIVER: Obstructive jaundice (cholestasis) Cirrhosis Tumors Infectious mononucleosis Hepatotoxicity, i.e., acetaminophen toxicity	OTHERS: Alcohol abuse Antiepileptic drug administration	Not clinically significant

Continued ►

▶ Continued **Clinically Significant Causes of Altered Enzyme Levels**

ENZYME	INCREASED		DECREASED
Lactate Dehydrogenase (LD)	CARDIAC MUSCLE DISEASES: Acute myocardial infarction Congestive heart failure (CHF) Myocarditis SKELETAL MUSCLE DISEASES: Muscular dystrophies Muscle trauma Excessive physical activity	HEPATIC PARENCHYMAL DISEASES: Viral hepatitis Infectious mononucleosis Cirrhosis Obstructive jaundice (cholestasis) OTHERS: Megaloblastic and pernicious anemias Shock or circulatory failure Malignancies Renal diseases of many types	Not clinically significant
Lipase (LPS)	PANCREATIC: Pancreatitis Pancreatic cyst or pseudocyst	OTHERS: Obstructive jaundice (cholestasis) Peritonitis Intestinal obstruction, infarct	Pancreatic insufficiency
Prostate Specific Antigen (PSA)	PROSTATE: Prostate carcinoma Benign prostatic hypertrophy (BPH) After prostate manipulation, including surgery, catheterization, digital massage, biopsy		Not clinically significant
Prostatic Acid Phosphatase (PAP)	PROSTATE: Prostate carcinoma (especially metastatic) Benign prostate hypertrophy After prostate manipulation, including surgery, catheterization, digital massage, biopsy (Rarely) Prostatitis Prostate infarct		Not clinically significant

EVALUATING TEST RESULTS

Clinically Significant Enzymes by Tissue

The table below provides the "diagnostic window" that may be used to further confirm or rule out the selected acute disorder.

"DIAGNOSTIC WINDOW"

In some acute conditions, certain enzymes may display a "diagnostic window," which is the expected time frame of the enzyme's initial rise, its peak, and return to normal in the blood. It is important to evaluate these enzyme test results sequentially, over a designated period, when either establishing or ruling out these disorders. Along with knowledge of the primary tissue sources and "diagnostic window," plasma enzyme results should be correlated with other analytes and clinical findings for final diagnosis.

Clinically Significant Enzymes by Tissue

PANCREATIC			
Enzyme	**Principal Source**	**"Diagnostic Window" of Selected Acute Disorders**	**Comment**
Amylase (AMS)	Pancreas, salivary glands	Acute pancreatitis Rise: 2–12 hr Peak: 12–72 hr Normal: 3–4 days	Renal insufficiency may falsely ↑ serum AMS.
Lipase (LPS)	Pancreas	Acute pancreatitis Rise: 4–8 hr Peak: 24 hr Normal: 8–14 days	LPS is more specific and sensitive than AMS for pancreatic disorders.
CARDIAC			
Aspartate Aminotransferase (AST)	Liver, skeletal, and cardiac muscle	Acute myocardial infarction (AMI) Rise: 6–8 hr Peak: 18–24 hr Normal: 4–5 days	See "Cardiac Function," Chapter 6 for further discussion of AMI, CK isoenzymes, and LD isoenzymes.
Creatine Kinase (CK)	Skeletal and cardiac muscle, brain	AMI Rise: 6–8 hr Peak: 24–36 hr Normal: 3–4 days	
Lactate Dehydrogenase (LD)	Cardiac muscle, liver, skeletal muscle, RBCs	AMI Rise: 8–12 hr Peak: 24–48 hr Normal: 7–12 days	

Continued ▶

▶ Continued **Clinically Significant Enzymes by Tissue**

	PROSTATE		
Enzyme	**Principal Source**	**"Diagnostic Window" of Selected Acute Disorders**	**Comment**
Prostate Specific Antigen (PSA)	Prostate Prostate carcinoma cells produce more PSA than normal prostate cells.	Prostate carcinoma No acute diagnostic window because PSA may not be significantly ↑ until tumor is grown out of prostate capsule.	Currently, most sensitive prostate carcinoma marker When used in conjunction with digital rectal examination, PSA may be used to screen men over 50 yr of age for prostatic carcinoma. Most useful for monitoring therapy and tumor recurrence
Prostatic Acid Phosphatase (PAP)	Prostate, RBCs	Prostate carcinoma Generally not significantly ↑ until tumor is metastasized.	Prostate carcinoma, but PSA is a more appropriate marker to detect *early stage* prostate carcinoma and to monitor therapy and tumor recurrence than PAP.
	LIVER		
Aspartate Aminotransferase (AST)	Liver, skeletal and cardiac muscle	Acute viral hepatitis Rise: before onset of jaundice Peak: 7–12 days after onset of jaundice Normal: 3–4 wk after onset of jaundice	Characteristically, ALT ≥ AST levels in viral hepatitis
Alanine Aminotransferase (ALT)	Liver, kidney	Acute viral hepatitis Rise: before onset of jaundice Peak: 7–12 days after onset of jaundice Normal: 3–4 wk after onset of jaundice	Characteristically, ALT ≥ AST levels in viral hepatitis. Not usually ↑ in renal diseases
Alkaline Phosphatase (ALP)	Hepatobiliary, bone, placenta	Acute hepatobiliary obstruction Rise: immediately Normal: soon after obstruction is resolved	ALP "diagnostic window" parallels GGT in hepatobiliary obstruction.

EVALUATING TEST RESULTS

Continued ▶

▶ Continued **Clinically Significant Enzymes by Tissue**

LIVER			
Enzyme	**Principal Source**	**"Diagnostic Window" of Selected Acute Disorders**	**Comment**
Cholinesterase (SChE) (Pseudocholinesterase)	Liver	No defined diagnostic window for insecticide poisoning or hepatic diseases. However, in acute cases, ChE levels ↓, then return to normal shortly after recovery, and may be used to monitor recovery.	Unlike other plasma enzymes, ↓ SChE is clinically significant, instead of elevation. To detect atypical SCheE variants, total SCheE assay results may be correlated with ChE enzyme inhibition (i.e., dibucaine) assay results.
γ-Glutamyltransferase (GGT)	Liver, kidney	Acute hepatobiliary obstruction Rise: immediately Normal: soon after obstruction is resolved	Most sensitive enzyme in liver diseases Not usually elevated in renal disease ↑ GGT > ↑ ALP in hepatobiliary obstruction
Lactate Dehydrogenase (LD)	Cardiac muscle, liver, skeletal muscle, RBCs	No defined "diagnostic window" for hepatic diseases	LD-5 isoenzyme is elevated in many hepatic diseases, but this fraction is also elevated in skeletal muscle disorders.

BIBLIOGRAPHY

Akoun GM, et al: Serum neuron-specific enolase. A marker for disease extent and response to therapy for small-cell lung cancer. Chest 87:39–43, 1985.

Bhayana V, Henderson AR: Biochemical markers of myocardial damage. Clin Biochem 28:1–29, 1995.

Bishop ML: Clinical Chemistry: Principles, Procedures, Correlations, 3rd ed. Philadelphia, JB Lippincott, 1996.

Black HR, et al: Racial differences in serum creatine kinase levels. Am J Med 81:479–487, 1986.

Bruns DE, et al: Lactate dehydrogenase isoenzyme-1: changes during the first day after acute myocardial infarction. Clin Chem 27:1821–1823, 1981.

Burtis CA, Ashwood ER: Tietz Fundamentals of Clinical Chemistry, 4th ed. Philadelphia, WB Saunders, 1996.

Burtis CA, Ashwood ER: Tietz Textbook of Clinical Chemistry, 3rd ed. Philadelphia, WB Saunders, 1995.

Catalona WJ, et al: Comparison of digital rectal examination and serum prostate specific antigen in the early detection of prostate cancer: results of a multicenter clinical trial of 6630 men. J Urol 151:1283–1290, 1994.

Evans RT: Cholinesterase phenotyping: clinical aspects and laboratory application. Crit Rev Clin Lab Sci 23:35–64, 1986.

Galen RS: The enzyme diagnosis of myocardial infarction. Hum Pathol 6:141–155, 1975.

Kaplan LA, Pesce AJ: Clinical Chemistry: Theory, Analysis, Correlation, 3rd ed. St. Louis, Mosby–Year Book, 1996.

Moss DW: Alkaline phosphatase isoenzymes. Clin Chem 28:2007–2016, 1982.

Panteghini M, Pagani F: Diagnostic value of measuring pancreatic lipase and the P3 isoform of the pancreatic amylase isoenzyme in serum of hospitalized hyperamylasemic patients. Clin Chem 35:417–421, 1989.

Tietz NW, ed: Clinical Guide to Laboratory Tests, 3rd ed. Philadelphia, WB Saunders, 1995.

Tietz NW, et al: Laboratory tests in the differential diagnosis of hyperamylasemia. Clin Chem 32:301–307, 1986.

Wilkinson JH: The Principles and Practice of Diagnostic Enzymology. Chicago: Year Book, 1976.

EVALUATING TEST RESULTS

Chapter **6**

CARDIAC FUNCTION

Mary Hotaling, MS, MT (ASCP) DLM

Q U I C K   C O N T E N T S

INTRODUCTION

Heart Structure and Function

The heart is a muscular organ composed of cardiac muscle cells. The heart structure consists of four chambers: two atria and two ventricles. The atria collect blood from the systemic circulation and pump it into the ventricles. The right ventricle pumps blood to the lungs (pulmonary artery) for reoxygenation and release of carbon dioxide. The left ventricle pumps blood to the heart itself (coronary circulation) and the systemic circulation (aorta artery).

Metabolism

Cardiac muscle (myocardial) cells are quite metabolically active and require a continuous supply of oxygenated blood. The coronary circulation furnishes the heart with oxygenated blood, and the muscle protein myoglobin optimizes uptake of the oxygen presented. High metabolic activity of myocardial tissue makes it particularly susceptible to ischemia, which may result in reversible or irreversible myocardial tissue damage. Cell damage is generally reversible if reperfusion (restoration of blood flow) occurs within 15 to 20 minutes of the ischemic event. After this time, irreversible cell damage is signaled when the integrity of the cell membrane is no longer sustained. Intracellular enzymes and soluble proteins are released through the damaged cell membranes into the surrounding tissues and subsequently are carried into the circulation.

Myocardial Ischemia

Myocardial ischemia is most often caused by coronary atherosclerosis. Less commonly, ischemia is caused by inflammation of the coronary arteries, thrombosis, or coronary vasospasm. The three patterns of ischemic heart disease (IHD) include chronic IHD, angina pectoris (AP): stable and unstable forms, and acute myocardial infarction (AMI). The above disorders are listed from lowest to highest risk of morbidity and mortality and represent a continuum based on the degree and distribution of coronary insufficiency.

Evaluation of Acute Myocardial Infarction (AMI)

Early and accurate AMI diagnosis is of the utmost clinical importance to minimize the mass of infarcted tissue and prevent death due to arrhythmia. Administration of reperfusion therapy (i.e., thrombolytics or percutaneous transluminal coronary angioplasty [PCTA]) within 4 to 6 hours after the infarction is essential for the most positive clinical outcome.

AMI DIAGNOSTIC CRITERIA

The classic World Health Organization (WHO) diagnosis of AMI is based on the presence of two of the three following criteria: history of characteristic chest pain; electrocardiographic (ECG) changes (pathologic Q waves, ST segment and T wave changes); and a typical pattern of serum cardiac enzyme rise, peak, and return to reference range. It is known that the WHO diagnosis method has limitations in early AMI diagnosis because some of these findings are frequently absent or not easily recognized. For example, a history of chest pain is often a diagnostic dilemma, because cardiac and noncardiac conditions, e.g., musculoskeletal pain and indigestion, can produce chest pain. Each year in the United States, about 6 million patients with chest pain are admitted to hospital emergency departments to rule in or rule out AMI; approximately 20% of these patients have AMI, while 80% do not.

Recently, new rule in/rule out AMI triage strategies have been developed that combine the most sensitive and specific diagnostic tests to better accomplish the goal of early and accurate diagnosis (see "Current Cardiac Marker Testing and Triaging Strategies for Suspected Acute Myocardial Infarction," p 105). Beside better clinical outcomes, it is expected that these chest pain triage strategies will help contain costs by more efficiently utilizing health care resources and simultaneously reducing the danger of discharging a high risk patient.

CARDIAC FUNCTION TESTS: ECG AND CARDIAC IMAGING

Important cardiac function tests include the electrocardiogram (ECG) and myocardial imaging techniques. An ECG is noninvasive and records the electrical impulses throughout the heart. This technique is useful in cardiac arrhythmia assessment and is relatively specific for the diagnosis of AMI. However, on initial presentation of chest pain caused by AMI, diagnostic sensitivity has been reported to be as low as 50%.

Cardiac imaging techniques, such as scintigraphy, monitor myocardial tissue uptake of a radiotracer, technetium-99m pyrophosphate, to detect infarcted areas from 18 to 24 hours after the infarction. Although this test is relatively sensitive (as high as 84%) for transmural ("Q wave") infarctions, it has been found to lack sensitivity (as low as 32%) in nontransmural ("non–Q wave") infarctions. These cardiac function tests are clearly inadequate in their efficacy to diagnose early AMI. Because of these limitations, the clinical laboratory's ability to measure biochemical cardiac markers is an integral component of the differential diagnosis of AMI.

PATIENT PREPARATION, SPECIMEN COLLECTION AND STORAGE, REFERENCE RANGE

Patient Preparation

No special patient preparation is required. Excessive physical activity should be avoided prior to creatine kinase (CK) total enzyme, CK isoenzyme, and myoglobin testing.

Specimen Collection

SPECIMEN

Serum is the specimen of choice, but heparinized plasma is also generally acceptable. There is also a rapid cardiac troponin T method available that uses venous whole blood.

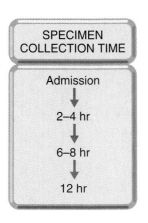

SPECIMEN
COLLECTION TIME

Admission
↓
2–4 hr
↓
6–8 hr
↓
12 hr

COLLECTION TIME

Accurate clinical interpretation of cardiac marker values in AMI rule in/rule out diagnosis requires that serial specimens be collected at appropriate time intervals. Serial measurements, as opposed to single sample values, are most effective. The current recommendations to rule out AMI suggest that samples be drawn on admission, at 2 to 4 hours, at 6 to 8 hours, and at 12 hours.

Specimen Storage Requirements and Reference Ranges

TEST	SPECIMEN STORAGE	REFERENCE RANGE
Creatine Kinase (CK), Total Activity	RT for 4–8 hr 4°C for 1–2 days −20°C for 30 days	M: 38–174U/L F: 26–140U/L African-Americans have higher levels than non–African-Americans.
Creatine Kinase (CK) Isoenzymes, CK-MB Isoenzyme with Relative Index (RI)	RT for 4–8 hr 4°C for 1–2 days −20°C for 30 days	Immunoassay CK-MB$_{mass}$: <10 μg/L (method dependent) CK-MB$_{mass}$ RI: <6% (method dependent) Electrophoresis method: CK-BB (CK-1) (0% or trace) CK-MB (CK-2) (<4%–6%) CK-MM (CK-3) (>94%–96%)
Creatine Kinase-MB Isoforms (CK-MB Isoforms) and CK-MB$_2$/CK-MB$_1$ Isoform Ratio	2°–8°C up to 5 days −20°C for several weeks	0.5–1.0 U/L (both isoforms) <1.5 Isoform ratio
Myoglobin (Mb)	2°–8°C up to 7 days	<100 μg/L
Cardiac Troponin I (cTnl)	−80°C for several weeks	<3.1 μg/L (nonparametric, 95% interval)
Cardiac Troponin T (cTnT)	Serum 2°–8°C 24 hr −20°C up to 3 mo	0.0–0.1 μg/L
	Whole blood (venous) 25°C for 8 hr (do not refrigerate)	0.0–0.1 μg/L

RT, room temperature.

DIAGNOSTIC TESTS AND METHODOLOGIES

Diagnostic Tests

CARDIAC ENZYMES

Routine measurement of serum enzymes and isoenzymes (creatine kinase [CK], lactic dehydrogenase [LD], and aspartate aminotransferase [AST]) have been utilized for more than a decade as a major determinant by which AMI is diagnosed. The application of these enzymes for AMI diagnosis (except for total CK and CK-MB isoenzyme) is less common today because of relatively poor cardiac specificity and sensitivity. Refer to Chapter 5 for further discussion of these enzymes.

CURRENT CARDIAC MARKERS

Biochemical cardiac markers currently include total CK, CK-MB isoenzyme, CK-MB isoforms, and the muscle proteins myoglobin and troponin. These markers demonstrate excellent sensitivity to rule in or rule out AMI. Each cardiac marker has its own characteristics, particularly its "diagnostic window." The "diagnostic window" is the expected time frame of the cardiac marker's initial rise, its peak, and its return to normal in the blood. Very early markers of AMI are myoglobin and CK-MB isoforms. Both of these markers are detectable as early as ½ hour after the infarction. Early markers include CK-MB isoenzyme and the cardiac troponins. The cardiac troponins T and I are also later markers of AMI because they remain elevated for >14 and >5 days, respectively. It is important to evaluate these test results sequentially, over a designated period, when either establishing or ruling out these disorders.

Typical Cardiac Marker Diagnostic Window Curves and Serum Levels, Post AMI

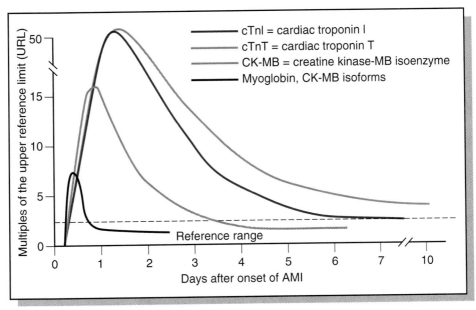

Current Cardiac Marker Characteristics and Clinical Utility

MARKER	TISSUE SOURCE	PHYSIOLOGIC FUNCTION	"DIAGNOSTIC WINDOW"	CLINICAL UTILITY
Creatine Kinase (CK), Total Activity	Skeletal muscle Cardiac muscle Brain and other tissues	Rephosphorylation of ADP, forming ATP in muscle contraction	Rise: 6–8 hr Peak: 24–36 hr Normal: 3–4 days	Limited diagnostic value since it is increased in various disease states CK isoenzyme analysis is more useful for diagnosis.

Continued ▶

► Continued **Current Cardiac Marker Characteristics and Clinical Utility**

MARKER	TISSUE SOURCE	PHYSIOLOGIC FUNCTION	"DIAGNOSTIC WINDOW"	CLINICAL UTILITY
CK-MB Isoenzyme, Mass	Cardiac muscle Skeletal muscle to a much lesser extent	Same as above	Rise: 4–6 hr Peak: 12–24 hr Normal: >48 hr	Mass assay of CK-MB isoenzyme is the current "gold standard" for early diagnosis of AMI.
CK-MB Isoforms and Isoforms Ratio	Same as above	Same as above	Rise: 2–6 hr Peak: 6–12 hr Normal: 24–36 hr	Early marker of AMI, more specific than myoglobin
Myoglobin (Mb)	Cardiac muscle Skeletal muscle	Oxygen binding protein	Rise: 2–3 hr Peak: 6–9 hr Normal: 24–36 hr	Nonspecific early marker to rule in/rule out AMI
Cardiac Troponin I (cTnI)	Cardiac muscle	Muscle contraction regulatory protein; bound to tropomyosin and actin	Rise: 4–8 hr Peak: 14–18 hr Normal: 5–9 days	Highly specific for myocardial injury Useful for patients with atypical symptoms or those who delay seeking medical attention Potential to diagnose AMI in patients who also have concomitant skeletal muscle trauma/disease Potential usage to risk stratify angina patients
Cardiac Troponin T (cTnT)	Cardiac muscle; regenerating skeletal muscle	Same as above	Rise: 4–8 hr Peak: 14–18 hr Normal: >14 day	As above for cTnI

**Current Cardiac Marker Testing and Triaging Strategies
for Suspected Acute Myocardial Infarction**

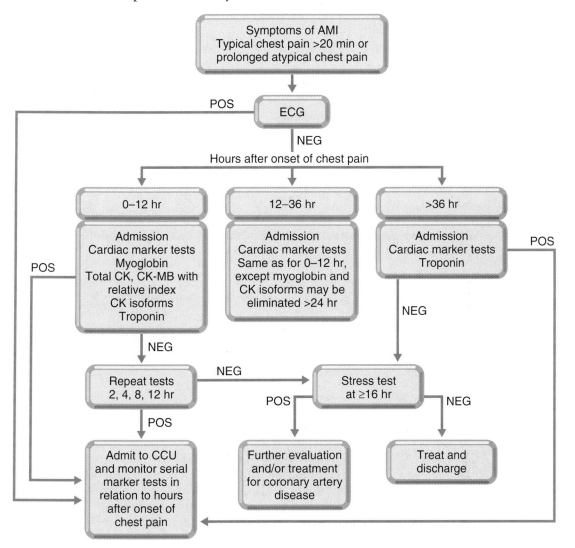

Creatine Kinase (CK)

CK is a cytoplasmic and mitochondrial enzyme that catalyzes the reversible phosphory-lation of creatine by ATP for striated muscle cell contraction. Total CK is measured in the diagnosis and treatment of AMI and skeletal muscle diseases such as Duchenne type progressive muscular dystrophy. CK is usually dramatically higher in skeletal muscle in-jury than in cardiac injury because the absolute amount of CK in skeletal muscle is 5 to 10 times that of cardiac tissue. Total CK values evaluated alone have limited diagnostic utility, since the enzyme is increased in various diseases. Measurement of the CK isoen-zyme distribution is vastly more useful for diagnosis, especially for AMI.

CK Isoenzymes

CK is composed of two subunits (M = muscle, B = brain), forming three different isoenzymes: CK-BB (CK-1), CK-MB (CK-2), and CK-MM (CK-3). The isoenzymes are numbered on the basis of relative electrophoretic mobility, with the most anodal fraction (CK-BB) having the lowest number (CK-1), as can be seen in the figure below:

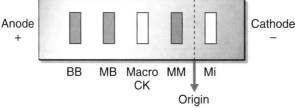

CK isoenzyme determination is more useful than total CK for diagnosis because different tissues consist of known proportions of isoenzymes:

Relative Proportion of CK Isoenzymes in "Normal Serum" and Major Tissue Sources

SERUM	SKELETAL MUSCLE	CARDIAC MUSCLE	BRAIN
0 trace BB	0 trace BB	0% BB	97% BB
<6% MB	1% MB	20% MB	3% MB
>94% MM	99% MM	80% MM	0% MM

CREATINE KINASE-MB ISOENZYME (CK-MB). CK-MB isoenzyme measured by mass assay methods is the current "gold standard" biochemical marker of AMI. CK-MB determinations that display the typical "diagnostic window" (expected time of rise, peak, and subsequent fall to within the reference range) are highly diagnostic for AMI. CK-MB values must be interpreted with caution, since there is overlap between cardiac and skeletal muscle tissue sources of the isoenzyme.

Relative Index (RI). Relative index (RI) relates the CK-MB isoenzyme mass concentration to the total CK activity. The RI is a tool to evaluate increased total CK activity. It should not be used to interpret total CK values within the reference range or CK-MB mass values of <10 μg/L. The RI is calculated as follows:

$$\text{RI } (\%) = \frac{\text{CK-MB } (\mu g/L)}{\text{Total CK } (U/L)} \times 100$$

Increased serum CK-MB level with an RI of >6% of total CK is usually indicative of cardiac damage, especially AMI. Increased serum CK-MB level with an RI of <6% of total CK is usually indicative of skeletal muscle damage. The RI need not be calculated for a percentage CK-MB value obtained by electrophoresis methods, since this value is already directly related to the total CK activity.

ATYPICAL CK ISOENZYMES. Atypical CK isoenzymes are generally two types: macro-CK and mitochondrial CK (CK-Mt). Atypical CK isoenzymes may be distinguished from each other and the three typical CK isoenzymes by their unique electrophoretic properties (see "CK Isoenzyme Migration Pattern" on p 106). The presence of atypical CK forms is not directly correlated to any specific disease state.

Macro-CK. Macro-CK is composed of immunoglobin (usually IgG) bound to CK-BB and most frequently occurs in women over the age of 50. Accurate identification of macro-CK on electrophoresis is critical because of the band's proximity to the expected position of the CK-MB band. Misidentification of a macro-CK band as a CK-MB band may result in the reporting of a false positive biochemical marker for AMI. Observing the macro-CK band on electrophoresis may also be helpful in troubleshooting certain CK-MB assays, e.g., immunoinhibition methods. (See "Methodologies" on p 109.)

Mitochondrial CK (CK-Mi). Mitochondrial CK (CK-Mi) exists in both dimeric and oligomeric forms, bound to the outer surface of the inner mitochondrial membranes. CK-Mi is not present in "normal serum" but may occur occasionally in severe illnesses, resulting in extensive cell membrane and mitochondria breakdown, e.g., malignant tumors.

CK ISOFORMS (ISOENZYME SUBTYPES). Although CK-MB has proved to be the current "gold standard" for AMI detection, CK-MB and CK-MM isoform assays have been developed to further improve the sensitivity of the biochemical diagnosis of AMI. There are at least two isoforms of the CK-MB isoenzyme and at least three isoforms of the CK-MM isoenzyme. Isoforms are produced in the bloodstream in a time dependent manner by sequential and irreversible cleavage of lysine residues from the CK-M subunit(s) by the enzyme lysine carboxypeptidase.

The CK-MB isoforms are more specific to cardiac tissue injury than CK-MM isoforms, since CK-MB itself is more specific than CK-MM to cardiac tissue. Normally, serum $CK-MB_2$ and $CK-MB_1$ levels are approximately equal, producing an $CK-MB_2:CK-MB_1$ ratio of about 1.0. However, after AMI, $CK-MB_2$ rapidly rises above $CK-MB_1$, producing an increased $CK-MB_2:CK-MB_1$ ratio, which is reported to be a highly sensitive and specific indicator of early stage AMI. The sensitivity of the CK-MB isoform ratio in detecting early AMI is second only to myoglobin, while possessing a good degree of cardiac specificity (albeit not absolute) that myoglobin lacks.

Troponin (Tn)

The troponin protein complex is located on the thin filament of striated muscle (both cardiac and skeletal). The physiologic role of the troponin complex is regulation of calcium mediated muscle contraction, via its interaction with actin and myosin. The troponin complex consists of three subunit proteins: T (TnT), I (TnI), and C (TnC). Troponin T (TnT) is the tropomyosin binding subunit that binds the troponin complex to tropomyosin along actin (thin filament). Troponin I (TnI) is the myosin ATPase inhibiting subunit blocking myosin (thick filament) movement in the absence of calcium. Troponin C (TnC) is the calcium binding subunit. The troponin subunits exist as three immunochemically unique isoforms that are distributed in a muscle tissue specific manner: cardiac muscle, slow twitch striated muscle, and fast twitch striated muscle. Troponin C lacks cardiac specificity and will not be discussed further.

Serial measurements of cardiac troponin T (cTnT) and cardiac troponin I (cTnI) are used in the diagnosis of AMI because they are highly specific for myocardial damage,

DIAGNOSTIC TESTS AND METHODOLOGIES

and because troponins are not usually detectable in the normal population by available methods. Cardiac troponins may be most helpful in the diagnosis of AMI in patients with concomitant skeletal muscle injury, because there is often considerable controversy concerning whether increases in CK-MB are due to skeletal muscle or cardiac injury, especially when the CK-MB Relative Index is borderline.

The initial rise of the cardiac troponins in AMI at least parallels that of CK-MB (and may occur as early as 3 hours after AMI) and remains elevated up to 5 to 9 days for cTnI and up to 14 days for cTnT. This lengthy "diagnostic window" can be both an advantage and a disadvantage. The advantage lies in diagnosing patients who delay in presentation because of denial or atypical symptoms. An example of a disadvantage includes diagnosing a current AMI patient with reinfarction, since elevations remain so long. In this case, myoglobin, CK-MB isoenzyme, and CK isoforms should be measured, since these markers return to within the reference range more quickly than the cardiac troponins.

Risk Stratification

Recent studies have reported that increased cardiac troponin levels may predict poor outcomes in some patients with unstable angina. In risk stratification, unstable angina patients (presenting with normal CK-MB levels along with increased cardiac troponin levels), are placed in an increased risk category. These patients with unstable angina have a significantly increased (40%) likelihood of short term complications such as death or AMI. These patients also have long term outcomes similar to those patients diagnosed with AMI. Patients identified as high risk may be treated more aggressively (e.g., cardiac catheterization), while patients deemed to be low risk can be managed conservatively in less expensive chest pain evaluation units or medical telemetry beds pending further testing and discharge.

Myoglobin (Mb)

Myoglobin is a cytoplasmic oxygen binding heme protein present in striated muscle cells (skeletal and cardiac). It is rapidly released into the blood circulation after muscle injury, making it a sensitive marker for early rule in/rule out AMI in the absence of concomitant skeletal muscle trauma or renal failure. The negative predictive value of myoglobin in the early detection of AMI may be its greatest utility in evaluating acute chest pain, especially early after symptom onset. Myoglobin is reported to have high clinical sensitivity and specificity when specimens are collected serially every 1 to 2 hours during the first 2 to 10 hours after infarction. Myoglobin has a relatively wide reference range, but recent studies indicate that myoglobin levels that double within 1 to 2 hours are highly suggestive of AMI, even when the second level remains within the reference range.

Carbonic Anhydrase III

Carbonic anhydrase III is a small (28 kDa) cytoplasmic protein mainly present in skeletal muscle, with only trace amounts found in cardiac muscle. It displays a similar rise and fall pattern as myoglobin in AMI. It is proposed that elevated myoglobin levels due to skeletal muscle injury may be differentiated from AMI by determining the myoglobin:carbonic anhydrase III ratio. Assays for carbonic anhydrase III are under development.

Methodologies

TEST	METHOD	SPECIMEN INTERFERENCE	PHYSIOLOGIC INTERFERENCE	COMMENT
Creatine Kinase (CK), Total Activity	Coupled enzymatic reaction. Production of NADPH is monitored as an increase in absorbance at 340 nm.	Gross hemolysis. RBCs contain adenylate kinase, which causes positive interference.	Physical activity, skeletal muscle damage	Reagent system utilizes thiol compound, i.e., NAC (n-acetyl cysteine), for restoration of CK activity.
CK-MB Isoenzyme, Mass	Immunoassay ELISA, IRMA Monoclonal antibody is bound to solid support and binds CK-MB. Second labeled antibody forms antibody-CK-MB-antibody sandwich complex.	No interferences	Skeletal muscle damage	Most frequently used CK-MB method. Current "gold standard" to confirm AMI diagnosis.
CK-MB, Isoenzyme Activity	Immunoinhibition Anti-CK-M inactivates the M subunit of CK-MM and CK-MB. Residual B subunit enzyme activity is measured as above for total CK. This result is multiplied by 2 to calculate CK-MB activity.	Same as total CK above	Presence of CK-BB or macro-CK. Method cannot distinguish between BB and MB activity.	Generally used as a rapid screening method, to be confirmed with a CK-MB mass assay.
	Electrophoresis At pH 8.6, CK isoenzymes migrate as follows: $\leftarrow$ $\oplus$ CK-BB, CK-MB, CK-MM $\ominus$ Bands are visualized by incubating gels with CK substrate and measuring reaction via fluorescence or by coupling with dye, e.g., tetranitrozolium blue.	None reported	End stage renal dialysis patient serum may contain a fluorescent compound that migrates near the area where CK-BB is expected. This causes errors only in the fluorescence visualization method.	Helpful when atypical CK forms are suspected. High voltage electrophoresis methods have improved testing turnaround time.
CK-MB Isoforms and Ratio	Electrophoresis $CK-MB_1$ isoform migrates most anodally, since a positively charged lysine is removed, making it more negatively charged than $CK-MB_2$. $\leftarrow$ $\oplus$ $CK-MB_1$ $CK-MB_2$ $\ominus$ Bands are visualized by incubating gels with CK substrate and measuring reaction via fluorescence or by coupling with dye, e.g., tetranitrozolium blue.	None reported	Skeletal muscle damage, other conditions, e.g., urosepsis, congestive heart failure, pulmonary edema.	High voltage electrophoresis is the current method of choice. Not a routine assay in most laboratories, since it requires relatively long assay time, specialized training, and equipment.

DIAGNOSTIC TESTS AND METHODOLOGIES

Continued ▶

► Continued **Methodologies**

TEST	METHOD	SPECIMEN INTERFERENCE	PHYSIOLOGIC INTERFERENCE	COMMENT
Myoglobin (Mb)	Immunoassay Turbidimetry/nephelometry ELISA Monoclonal antibody is bound to solid support and binds myoglobin. Second labeled antibody forms antibody-myoglobin-antibody sandwich complex.	Hemolysis, icterus, and lipemia interference is method dependent.	Skeletal muscle damage, renal disease	Increases due to skeletal muscle damage may be differentiated from AMI by determining myoglobin:carbonic anhydrase III ratio. Routine carbonic anhydrase III assay is under development.
Cardiac Troponin I (cTnI)	Immunoassay ELISA Monoclonal antibody is bound to solid support and binds troponin I. Second labeled antibody forms antibody-troponin I-antibody sandwich complex.	None reported	None reported	May also be used to risk stratify patients with unstable angina. Assay recently FDA approved; interferences may be discovered as the assay is utilized.
Cardiac Troponin T (cTnT)	Immunoassay ELISA Monoclonal antibody is bound to solid support and binds troponin T. Second labeled antibody forms antibody-troponin T-antibody sandwich complex.	Hemolysis causes positive interference.	Unstable angina, chronically stressed skeletal muscle may produce cardiac form of troponin T; probably due to regenerating muscle. Also found in chronic renal disease.	May also be used to risk stratify patients with unstable angina.

ELISA, enzyme linked immunoabsorbent assay; IRMA, immunoradiometric assay.

BIBLIOGRAPHY

Adams JE, et al: Comparable detection of acute myocardial infarction by creatine kinase MB isoenzyme and cardiac troponin I. Clin Chem 40:1291–1295, 1994.

Adams JE, et al: Cardiac troponin I: a marker with high specificity for cardiac injury. Circulation 88:101–106, 1993.

Apple FS: Acute myocardial infarction and coronary reperfusion: serum cardiac markers for the 1990s. Am J Clin Pathol 97:217–226, 1992.

Bhayana V, Henderson AR: Biochemical markers of myocardial damage. Clin Biochem 28:1–29, 1995.

Bishop ML: Clinical Chemistry: Principles, Procedures, Correlations, 3rd ed. Philadelphia, JB Lippincott, 1996.

Brogan GX, et al: Evaluation of a new rapid quantitative immunoassay for serum myoglobin versus CK-MB for ruling out acute myocardial infarction in the emergency department. Ann Emerg Med 24:665–671, 1994.

Burtis CA, Ashwood ER: Tietz Fundamentals of Clinical Chemistry, 4th ed. Philadelphia, WB Saunders, 1996.

Burtis CA, Ashwood ER: Tietz Textbook of Clinical Chemistry, 2nd ed. Philadelphia, WB Saunders, 1994.

Gibler WB, et al: Early detection of acute myocardial infarction in patients presenting with chest pain and non-diagnostic ECGs: serial CK-MB sampling in the emergency department. Ann Emerg Med 19:1359–1366, 1990.

Jesse RL, Wu AH: Triaging the chest pain patient (insert). Clin Lab News 22(7), 1996.

Kaplan LA, Pesce AJ: Clinical Chemistry: Theory, Analysis, Correlation, 3rd ed. St. Louis, Mosby–Year Book, 1996.

Mair J, et al: Equivalent early sensitivities of myoglobin, creatine kinase MB mass, creatine kinase isoform ratios, and cardiac troponins I and T for acute myocardial infarction. Clin Chem 41:1266–1272, 1995.

Mercer DW: A historical background in cardiac markers. Med Lab Obs 28:45–51, 1996.

Montague C, Kircher T: Myoglobin in the early evaluation of acute chest pain. Am J Clin Pathol 104:472–476, 1995.

Newby LK, et al: Biochemical markers in suspected acute myocardial infarction: the need for early assessment (editorial). Clin Chem 41:1263–1265, 1995.

Puleo PR, et al: Early detection of acute myocardial infarction based on assay for subforms of creatine kinase-MB. Circulation 82:759–764, 1990.

Statland BE: Signals from the injured heart: the role of cardiac markers in managing patients with acute coronary syndrome. Med Lab Obs 28:42–44, 1996.

Tietz NW, ed: Clinical Guide to Laboratory Tests, 3rd ed. Philadelphia, WB Saunders, 1995.

Tucker JF, et al: Value of serial myoglobin levels in the early diagnosis of patients admitted for acute myocardial infarction. Ann Emerg Med 24:704–708, 1994.

Vaidya HC: Myoglobin. Lab Med 23:306–310, 1992.

Vuori J, et al: Myoglobin/carbonic anhydrase II ratio: highly specific and sensitive early indicator for myocardial damage in acute myocardial infarction. Clin Chem 42:107–108, 1996.

Wu AHB, Azar R: Prognostic value of cardiac troponin I in chest pain patients (letter). Clin Chem 42:651–652, 1996.

DIAGNOSTIC TESTS AND METHODOLOGIES

Chapter **7**

LIVER FUNCTION

Karen M. Escolas, MS, MT(ASCP)

QUICK CONTENTS

INTRODUCTION

The liver is a large organ with 80% of its volume taken up by hepatocytes, the cells that carry out the metabolic functions of the liver. These cells are capable of regeneration and response to an increased metabolic demand through their reserve capabilities, which are able to compensate for destruction of up to 80% of the hepatocytes. Most of the endogenous energy sources for the body are produced by the hepatocytes in the liver. Chemical materials received, processed, and stored by the liver include amino acids, carbohydrates, fatty acids, cholesterol, and vitamins. Many proteins are synthesized in the liver, including albumin, α and β globulins, clotting factors, and transport proteins. The liver synthesizes bile acids from cholesterol for secretion into the intestine to facilitate further dietary fat absorption. The liver is also responsible for detoxification of potentially toxic substances such as drugs or metabolic products and for regulation of hormone levels through metabolism of the hormones themselves. In response to hormonal and neural signals, the liver regulates the blood glucose level.

    Liver function tests are those clinical tests that indicate hepatic structure, cell integrity, and function. Most commonly measured are substances released from damaged tissue, such as enzymes found in hepatocytes, and substances metabolized or produced by the liver, such as proteins and bilirubin. Liver function tests are used to screen for liver function abnormalities, document the presence of an abnormality, identify the type and site of liver injury, and monitor the progress of patients diagnosed with liver disease.

PATIENT PREPARATION, SPECIMEN COLLECTION AND STORAGE, AND REFERENCE RANGE

TEST	PATIENT PREPARATION	SPECIMEN COLLECTION	SPECIMEN STORAGE	REFERENCE RANGE
Conjugated (Direct) Bilirubin	AM fasting specimen preferred (avoids lipemia)	SERUM OR HEPARINIZED PLASMA: No hemolysis or lipemia	SERUM/PLASMA: Protect from exposure to light (bilirubin is photooxidized, causing unconjugated form to react with Diazo reagents as well as conjugated form). Store at low temperature (minimizes photooxidation). Stable 3 days at 1°–6°C, 3 mo at −70°C (when in dark).	SERUM/PLASMA: <0.2 mg/dL
		URINE: Fresh random specimen preferred.	URINE: Protect from light (to avoid oxidation). Stable 1 day at 1°–4°C	URINE: Negative
Total Bilirubin	See Conjugated Bilirubin	See Conjugated Bilirubin Does not apply to urine	See Conjugated Bilirubin Does not apply to urine	Serum/plasma: <1.5 mg/dL
Urobilinogen	No preparation necessary.	URINE: Fresh random acceptable (may be false negative as majority is excreted 2–3 hr postprandially.) 2–3 hr postprandially preferred (after the noon meal for best results)	Stable at 2°–8°C in dark for less than 24 hr (unstable in light at room temperature)	<1 mg/dL
Bile Acids	Fasting specimen preferred	Serum	Stable 6 mo at 4°C in absence of bacterial contamination	0.3–2.3 μg/mL

Continued ▶

► Continued **PATIENT PREPARATION, SPECIMEN COLLECTION AND STORAGE, AND REFERENCE RANGE**

TEST	PATIENT PREPARATION	SPECIMEN COLLECTION	SPECIMEN STORAGE	REFERENCE RANGE
Ammonia	AM fasting specimen preferred No smoking by patient after 12 midnight or in vicinity of specimen collection and testing No fist clenching	PLASMA: EDTA or heparin (no ammonium heparin) Good venipuncture technique No hemolysis	PLASMA: Keep on ice in anaerobic conditions (results will become falsely elevated, as nitrogenous compounds are metabolized if aerobic). Analyze ASAP.	PLASMA: 19–60 μg/dL
		URINE: 24 hr preferred Avoid contamination with bacteria or ammonia.	URINE: Store at 4°–8°C. Analyze without delay.	URINE: 140–1500 mg/day

DIAGNOSTIC TESTS AND METHODOLOGIES

TEST	METHOD	INTERFERENCE	COMMENTS
Conjugated (Direct) Bilirubin (Blood)	Diazo reaction (diazo reagent reacts directly with conjugated bilirubin, forming a colored product that is measured photometrically).	Hemolysis (falsely decreased results due to high absorbance of the blank) Lipemia (falsely increased results due to high absorbance of turbidity)	Most widely used routine method
	High performance liquid chromatography		Reference method for all forms of bilirubin
Total Bilirubin (Blood)	Diazo reaction (accelerator added for unconjugated form to react with diazo reagent: Jendrassik-Grof = caffeine; Evelyn-Malloy = alcohol).	See Conjugated Bilirubin	Most widely used routine method
	High pressure liquid chromatography		Reference method for all forms of bilirubin

Continued ►

▶ Continued **DIAGNOSTIC TESTS AND METHODOLOGIES**

TEST	METHOD	INTERFERENCE	COMMENTS
Conjugated (Direct) Bilirubin (Urine)	Direct spectrophotometric (bilirubin pigment in serum measured directly at 450 nm)	Serum pigments in adults such as carotene also have absorbance in the same range.	Applicable only to neonatal patients
	Dipstick (bilirubin reacts with dry diazo reagent on the reaction pad, causing a color change).	False positive results with medications that produce red urine (e.g., phenazopyridine) Large quantities of ascorbic acid or nitrite lower the detection limit.	Highly specific Most widely used routine method
	Ictotest (bilirubin remains on the surface of the testing mat while all other constituents are washed into mat—diazo added to surface of mat reacts with bilirubin).	Any interference may be washed off the reaction surface.	Increased sensitivity Used for confirmation and quantitation of positive dipstick result
Urobilinogen (Urine)	Dipstick (urobilinogen reacts with Ehrlich's reagent [*p*-dimethylaminobenzaldehyde] on the reaction pad, causing a color change).	False negative result occurs when nitrites are present. False positive result occurs when other Ehrlich's reactive compounds are present (e.g., porphobilinogen, indican, *p*-aminosalicylic acid, sulfonamides).	Most widely used routine method Detects normal or elevated levels; does not detect low or absent levels Other Ehrlich's reacting compounds are elevated proportionally to urobilinogen; thus, elevation may be interpreted as elevated urobilinogen.
Urobilinogen (Fecal)	Same as urine reaction after pretreatment (aqueous fecal extract treated with alkaline ferrous hydroxide to convert urobilin to urobilinogen)		

Continued ▶

▶ Continued **DIAGNOSTIC TESTS AND METHODOLOGIES**

TEST	METHOD	INTERFERENCE	COMMENTS
Bile Acids	Gas-liquid chromatography		Requires deconjugation, which is time consuming and tedious
	High performance liquid chromatography		Current detectors have limited sensitivity.
	Enzymatic with fluorescent or chemiluminescent measurement of NADH		Increased sensitivity
			May separate bile acids first through thin layer chromatography to measure each individually
	Immunoassay (radioimmunoassay or enzyme-linked immunosorbent assay)		Simple procedure
			Good sensitivity and specificity
Ammonia	*Two-stage* (requires initial separation of ammonia and ammonium)	FALSE ELEVATIONS IN ALL METHODS:	Requires labor-intensive and specific equipment
	One-stage (direct measurement of ammonia): Enzymatic (kinetic measurement as NADPH converted to NADP) Ion-selective electrodes	1. Smoking by patient or phlebotomist 2. Laboratory atmosphere 3. Poor venipuncture (probing for vein, use of heparin lock, transfer from syringe to evacuated tube, partially filled tube allowing air to enter) 4. Metabolism of nitrogenous constituents (prevented by keeping on ice, separating from cells, and performing assay ASAP)	Fast, no specific equipment, readily automated

DIAGNOSTIC TESTS AND METHODOLOGIES

EVALUATING TEST RESULTS

Indicators of Hepatic Excretory Function

INDICATOR	ANALYTES MEASURED	NORMAL FINDINGS	FINDINGS WITH LIVER DISEASE
Bilirubin	Total bilirubin Conjugated bilirubin	Low blood levels Negative urine levels	UNCONJUGATED HYPERBILIRUBINEMIA: Overproduction in hemolytic processes Impaired uptake by liver in Gilbert's disease Defective conjugation ■ Crigler-Najjar syndrome ■ Physiologic jaundice of the newborn CONJUGATED HYPERBILIRUBINEMIA: Reduced excretion by liver and biliary tract ■ Hepatobiliary obstruction (gallstone or tumor) ■ Dubin-Johnson or Rotor's syndrome HYPERBILIRUBINEMIA (BOTH CONJUGATED AND UNCONJUGATED FORMS): Liver disease *Note:* Urine bilirubin and urobilinogen will both be elevated in conjugated hyperbilirubinemia
Bile Acids	Primary and secondary bile acids	Low blood levels	DECREASED LEVELS: Loss of functioning hepatocytes ■ Hepatitis ■ Cirrhosis ELEVATED LEVELS: Regurgitation from hepatocytes ■ Biliary obstruction ■ Hepatocellular disease
Xenobiotic Dyes	Bromsulphthalein Indocyanine green	Less than 5% retained 45 min after infusion	INCREASED RETENTION: Hepatocellular disease Biliary obstruction disease Space filling lesions (tumors)

BILIRUBIN METABOLISM

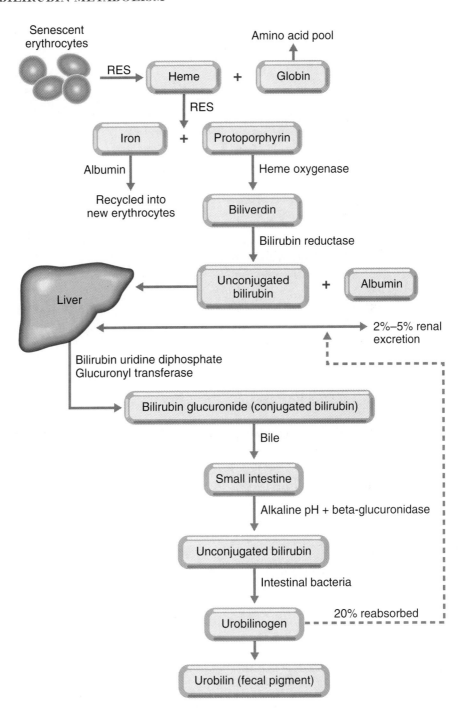

BILE ACID METABOLISM

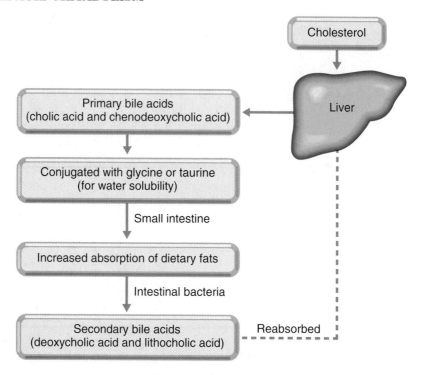

Indicators of Hepatic Synthetic Function

INDICATOR	NORMAL PRODUCTION	FINDINGS WITH LIVER DISEASE
Plasma Proteins	All plasma proteins except hemoglobin and the immunoglobulins are produced by the hepatocytes.	DECREASED PLASMA PROTEINS: Hepatic disease with decreased production of albumin, α_1-antitrypsin, fibrinogen, ceruloplasmin, haptoglobin, transferrin, and coagulation proteins ELEVATED PLASMA PROTEINS: Hepatic injury or inflammation with increased production of acute phase reactants (haptoglobin, prealbumin, α_1-antitrypsin, C-reactive protein, and ceruloplasmin) *Note:* Extensive liver damage must occur before a significant change in protein levels is detectable.
Lipids and Lipoproteins	Synthesis of cholesterol, triglycerides, and phospholipids Packaging of low density lipoprotein (LDL) and very low density lipoprotein (VLDL)	ACUTE LIVER DISEASE: Hypertriglyceridemia OBSTRUCTIVE LIVER DISEASE: Elevated cholesterol and phospholipids Presence of lipoprotein X
Urea	Conversion of amino acids to ammonia, which is then converted to urea	LOSS OF HEPATIC SYNTHETIC ABILITY: Decreased blood and urine levels of urea Elevated blood levels of amino acids and ammonia

Indicators of Hepatic Metabolic Function

INDICATOR	NORMAL METABOLISM	FINDINGS WITH LIVER DISEASE	COMMENTS
Ammonia	Conversion of amino acids to ammonia, which is then converted to urea	LOSS OF HEPATIC SYNTHETIC ABILITY: Decreased blood and urine levels of urea Elevated blood levels of amino acids and ammonia	Accumulation of ammonia is toxic to the central nervous system.
Carbohydrates	Dietary glucose used for energy through glycolysis or stored as glycogen. When glucose is needed, glycogen is broken down and glucose is produced from amino acids and fatty acids through gluconeogenesis.	Nonspecific and uninformative for diagnosis of liver disease because of variation due to dietary status, hormonal control, and pancreatic function	Not used to assess liver function

Indicators Released from Damaged Hepatocytes

ENZYME	LOCATION IN HEPATOCYTE	HALF-LIFE IN BLOOD	TISSUE SOURCES	CLINICAL SIGNIFICANCE
Alanine Transaminase (ALT)	Cytosolic and mitochondrial forms	47 hr	Many tissues, highest concentration in liver	Specific for liver Released when there is hepatocellular damage or necrosis Elevated higher than AST
Aspartate Transaminase (AST)	Cytosolic and mitochondrial forms	17 hr	Equal levels in liver and skeletal and cardiac muscle	Nonspecific for liver Released when there is hepatocellular damage or necrosis
Alkaline Phosphatase (ALP)	Membrane associated	10 days	In cell membranes of many tissues, highest activity in liver, bone, intestine, kidney, and placenta	Nonspecific for liver Elevated owing to enhanced synthesis in liver disease Highest elevation (10 × ULN) with extrahepatobiliary obstruction Lesser elevations (2–3 × ULN) with intrahepatobiliary obstruction
Gamma-Glutamyl-Transferase (GGT)	Membrane associated	4 days	Sources include liver, renal, and prostatic tissues	Elevated owing to enhanced synthesis in liver disease Elevated earlier than other enzymes Also elevated owing to increased mitochondrial production with ingestion of alcohol, barbiturates, tricyclic antidepressants, and anticonvulsants
Lactate Dehydrogenase (LD)	Cytosolic	Several days	Found in many tissues; isoenzymes 4 and 5 originate in liver	Total LD activity is nonspecific for liver disease. Valuable only if liver is the only organ involved in the disease Isoenzyme analysis is more specific for liver disease.
5′ Nucleotidase (5′NT)	Microsomal and membrane associated	Several days	Found in a wide variety of tissues, most specifically liver tissue	Elevated owing to enhanced synthesis in liver disease No elevation with ingestion of drugs or alcohol Not routinely used owing to lack of available methods

ULN, upper limits of normal.

SUMMARY OF FINDINGS WITH LIVER DISEASE

DISEASE	ANALYTE ALTERATIONS		COMMENTS
Acute Viral Hepatitis (A-E, CMV, EBV)*	AST/ALT	10–100 × ULN	Rise early (prior to bilirubin)
	Total bilirubin (conjugated and unconjugated)	5–20 mg/dL (icteric phase) Normal–slightly elevated (anicteric phase)	Elevated at 2–8 wk post infection
	ALP	2 × ULN	5 × ULN if intrahepatic cholestasis present
	GGT	5 × ULN	10 × ULN if intrahepatic cholestasis present
Chronic Hepatitis*	ALT/AST	Slight persistent elevation	*Note:* Usually associated with persistent hepatitis B viral infection.
	Total bilirubin	Slight persistent elevation	
Alcoholic Liver Disease	GGT	2–3 × ULN	Returns to normal with abstinence unless liver is damaged
	ALT/AST	Mild elevation	AST may be more elevated if concurrent alcoholic myopathy
	Albumin	Decreased	Due to decreased nutritional status
	Globulins	Elevated	Due to decreased nutritional status
	Lipids	Elevated	Due to decreased nutritional status
Cirrhosis	AST/ALT, LD	Slight elevation	Due to liver cell injury
	ALP, GGT, total bilirubin	Mild elevation	Indicates cholestasis
	Albumin, cholesterol	Decreased	Due to loss of synthetic ability
	Prothrombin time	Prolonged	Due to loss of synthetic ability
Primary Biliary Cirrhosis	Total and conjugated bilirubin	Elevated	Due to progressive destruction of intrahepatic bile ducts Occurrence in females 9× that in males, predominantly in middle age
	ALP	2–10 × ULN	
	AST/ALT	Moderately elevated	
Hepatic Tumors	LD GGT ALP	2–10 × ULN Up to 20 × ULN Elevated	Liver function altered when tissue is compressed by tumor mass Ratio of metastatic tumors to primary liver tumors is 20:1. Presence of elevated α-fetoprotein level used as a tumor marker

Continued ▶

SUMMARY OF FINDINGS WITH LIVER DISEASE

▶ Continued **SUMMARY OF FINDINGS WITH LIVER DISEASE**

DISEASE	ANALYTE ALTERATIONS		COMMENTS
Cholestasis (Intra-hepatic or Extra-hepatic)	GGT, ALP	Markedly elevated	*Note:* May be either intrahepatic or extrahepatic in nature.
	ALT/AST	Slightly elevated	
	Bilirubin	Elevated, mostly conju-gated form	

*Refer to Chapter 21, "Immunology of Infectious Diseases," for serologic findings associated with hepatitis.

BIBLIOGRAPHY

Anderson SC, Cockayne S: Clinical Chemistry: Concepts and Applications. Philadelphia, WB Saunders, 1993.

Bishop M, Duben-Engelkirk JL, Fody EP: Clinical Chemistry: Principles, Procedures, Correlations, 3rd ed. Philadelphia, JB Lippincott, 1996.

Burtis CA, Ashwood ER: Tietz Fundamentals of Clinical Chemistry, 4th ed. Philadelphia, WB Saunders, 1996.

Doumas BT, Wu TW: The measurement of bilirubin fractions in serum. Crit Rev Clin Lab Sci 28:415–446, 1991.

French SW: Biochemistry of alcoholic liver disease. Crit Rev Clin Lab Sci 29:83–115, 1992.

Henry JB: Clinical Diagnosis and Management by Laboratory Methods, 19th ed. Philadelphia, WB Saunders, 1996.

Kaplan L, Pesce AJ: Clinical Chemistry: Theory, Analysis, Correlation, 3rd ed. St. Louis, Mosby–Year Book, 1996.

Marshall WJ: Clinical Chemistry, 3rd ed. St. Louis, Mosby–Year Book, 1995.

Tietz NW, ed: Clinical Guide to Laboratory Tests, 3rd ed. Philadelphia, WB Saunders, 1995.

Tygstrup N: Assessment of liver function: Principle and practice. J Gastroenterol Hepatol, 5:468–682, 1990.

Chapter 8

PANCREAS AND GASTROINTESTINAL FUNCTION

Craig A. Lehmann, PhD, CC(NRCC)

Q U I C K   C O N T E N T S

INTRODUCTION

The pancreas serves as both an endocrine and an exocrine gland. Its endocrine function is to synthesize hormones such as glycogen, insulin, and gastrin. Endocrine functions originate from a group of cells called islets, which are located in an area known as the islets of Langerhans. There are 1 to 2 million islets and they make up about 1% out of 100 g of pancreatic tissue. The islet cells contain beta, alpha, and delta cells, which are responsible for the production of the above-named hormones. The islet cells are surrounded by acinar cells, which are responsible for the production of exocrine digestive enzymes. Among these enzymes, amylase and lipase have been used extensively to evaluate pancreatic functions.

Endocrine Functions from the Islets of Langerhans

CELL	PRODUCTION	ACTION	OUTCOME
Alpha Cells	Glucagon	↑ Glycogenolysis ↑ Gluconeogenesis	↑ Glucose ↑ Glucose
Beta Cells	Preinsulin → insulin	↑ Glucose uptake	↓ Glucose
Delta Cells	Gastrin	↑ Digestion	↑ Gastric acid

Exocrine Functions from the Acinar Cells

CELL	PRODUCTION	ENZYMES	DIGESTIVE STIMULATION
Acinar Cells	Enzymes and proteolytic enzyme precursors	↑ Trypsin ↑ α-Amylase ↑ Cholesterol esterase ↑ Phospholipase A ↑ Lipase	↑ Protein ↑ Starch ↑ Cholesterol esters ↑ Phospholipids ↑ Triglycerides

PANCREATIC AND GASTROINTESTINAL DISEASES

The pancreas is the primary provider of the enzyme amylase for the body. However, there are other sources that produce this enzyme (e.g., parotid salivary glands). Because of this, laboratories are often required to identify the source of the enzyme's elevation. This is accomplished by identifying the isoenzymes of amylase (pancreatic and salivary). Amylase is responsible for hydrolyzing internal α-1,4 starch linkages. The most predominant pathology associated with pancreatic exocrine function is pancreatitis. Pancreatitis can be separated into two primary categories: acute and chronic.

Acute Pancreatitis

Acute pancreatitis can be caused by a variety of conditions, including obstruction (gallstones), toxins (alcohol), hyperlipidemias, and trauma. In some hyperlipidemias, serum amylase levels may appear to be normal. However, urine amylase will still demonstrate an increase. The condition can present in two forms: acute edematous or hemorrhagic. The hemorrhagic form is the most serious and is responsible for most acute pancreatitis fatalities. While it is extremely difficult, if not impossible, to distinguish between the two forms, most cases (80%) are the less severe acute edematous form.

Chronic Pancreatitis

Chronic pancreatitis presents with inflammation of the pancreatic tissue and is difficult to diagnose. Because of this, in addition to laboratory tests, a variety of techniques such as radiology are used to help make a diagnosis. Other pancreatic laboratory tests used to diagnose pancreatitis are urine amylase, serum lipase, and trypsin tests. Most serum lipase is produced in the pancreas and remains elevated longer than amylase. As, like lipase, trypsin is produced in the pancreas, the test is more specific than total amylase testing. It should be noted that some pathologies demonstrate subnormal urine and serum levels of amylase.

Pancreatic Exocrine

Pancreatic exocrine function tests are used in the diagnosis of other pathologies also, e.g., malabsorption and cystic fibrosis. Tests such as β-carotene and vitamin B_{12} tests are among the many absorption processes evaluated by the laboratory. Cystic fibrosis is an inherited defect causing malabsorption and chronic pulmonary disease involving sweat glands, pancreas, and lungs. While the increase in sweat chloride is the dominant diagnostic test, 90% of the patients present with pancreatic endocrine dysfunction.

Pancreatic Endocrine

Among all the pancreatic endocrine disorders, diabetes (type 1 insulin dependent) is the most prevalent. Strong evidence supports the theory that insulin dependent diabetes is an autoimmune disorder. Other endocrine disorders include Zollinger-Ellison syndrome, a condition caused by duodenal or pancreatic endocrine tumors leading to a increase in gastrin production. Most gastrin production is from the antral G cells, with the remainder from the small intestine and pancreas. Because of this, gastric and gastrin analysis are useful in diagnosing Zollinger-Ellison and other gastric disorders. Multiple endocrine neoplasia syndrome caused by hyperplasia or tumors in two or more endocrine glands also results in increased gastrin due to gastrinoma. Islet tumors that originate in the A cell produce high levels of glucagon (>500 pg/mL). Most of these tumors are malignant. Glucagon secreting neoplasms of the islet cells of the pancreas present glucagon levels greater than 100 pg/mL. The condition is usually malignant and well established before a diagnosis can be made. Adenocarcinoma of the pancreas is difficult to diagnose as it presents no early signs or symptoms, thus accounting for at least 5% of all cancer fatalities in the United States. Other conditions such as malnutrition, ulcers, pyloric obstruction, and cancer can be evaluated by gastrointestinal function tests, which are discussed later in this chapter.

PATIENT PREPARATION, SPECIMEN COLLECTION AND STORAGE, REFERENCE RANGE

TEST NAME	PATIENT PREPARATION	SPECIMEN COLLECTION	SPECIMEN STORAGE	REFERENCE RANGE
Amylase Serum	No special preparation	Serum or heparinized sample	Stable at room temperature for a few days; for months, store at 4°C	Method specific: starch based method: Roche 450–2000 dye U/L
Amylase Urine	No special preparation	Urine random or timed	Store at 4°C; amylase unstable in acidic urine	Method specific: starch based method: Roche 40–330 dye U/hr
Amylase Isoenzymes	No special preparation	Same as serum and urine amylase	Same as serum and urine amylase	Method specific: 45%–70% S type

Continued ▶

► Continued **PATIENT PREPARATION, SPECIMEN COLLECTION AND STORAGE, REFERENCE RANGE**

TEST NAME	PATIENT PREPARATION	SPECIMEN COLLECTION	SPECIMEN STORAGE	REFERENCE RANGE
Amylase/Creatinine Clearance Ratio	Timed urine collection not necessary; 2–4 hr collection acceptable	Same as serum and urine amylase	Same as serum and urine amylase	2%–5% clearance
Lipase	No special preparation	Serum	Room temperature for a couple of days, longer if refrigerated	<200 U/L triolene; <160 U/L olive oil
Trypsin	No special preparation	Serum or plasma acceptable; no citrate or oxalate	Store 4°C or −20°C	25± 5.3 μg/L
β-Carotene	Overnight fast	Serum	Separated from cells. Store frozen prior to analysis. Protect from light.	20–40 μg/dL; high performance liquid chromatography (HPLC)
Vitamin B$_{12}$ Absorption	Overnight fast	Serum, plasma (EDTA), no heparin, urine, or feces; urine the most widely used	Protect from light. 4 hr 2°–8°C. −20°C for increased periods.	8% in urine of 0.5 μg B$_{12}$; oral dose in a 24 hr urine
Glucagon	No special preparation	Plasma (EDTA)	Store frozen prior to analysis. Stable up to 74 days at −20° C	Adults 20–100 pg/mL
Gastrin	Fasting 12 hours or more	Serum	Store frozen prior to analysis	Up to 100 pg/mL
Tripeptide Hydrolysis Test	Overnight fast. Restrict non-essential medication for 24 hours	Urine is collected for 6 hours in EDTA tubes.	Urine should be centrifuged and keep frozen until analyzed	Para-aminobenzoic acid excreted 48%–72%
Fecal Fat	Normal fat diet 50–150 g/day for several days	Stool is collected for 3 days.	Store at 4°C	Fecal fat 5–10 g% indicate malabsorption. Values >10 g% suggest maldigestion.
14C-Triolein Breath	Overnight fast	Breath is collected in a trapping solution.	14CO2 is measured hourly for 6 hr.	Peak of 3.4% of dose per hr
D-Xylose Absorption	Overnight fast and begin with an empty bladder	Serum and urine	Store at 4°C	5 g dose, 2 hr serum level >20 mg/dL, 5 hr urine >1.2 g
Sweat Chloride	No special preparation	Skin surface	Collection of at least 100 mg of sweat	5–35 mmol/L

DIAGNOSTIC TESTS AND METHODOLOGIES

TEST	METHOD	INTERFERENCE	COMMENTS
Amylase Serum	Saccharogenic: measurement of reducing materials		Saccharogenic methods are generally not used any longer.
	Chromogenic: dye-labeled substrates that are attacked at the 1,4 bonds by serum amylase producing dye fragments. Some methods use fluorescein labeled amylopectin as the substrate.	Certain drugs can produce increased amylase values.	Infants for the first year of life have below normal values.
	Defined substrates: maltopentaose and maltotetraose		Both methods under controlled conditions produce good results.
Amylase Urine	See serum method	See serum method	See serum method
Amylase Isoenzymes Types P and S	Ion exchange technique		
	Electrophoresis	Storage can change isoenzyme patterns.	All methods separating pancreatic and salivary amylase produce reliable results.
	Selective inhibition (wheat germ inhibitor) or immunoassay		Wheat germ accuracy declines when pancreatic isoenzymes are present in <10% or >90%.
Amylase/Creatinine Clearance Ratio	Amylase: see serum method		
	Creatinine: Jaffe reaction	Hemolysis will increase creatinine results. If urine preservative is needed, use only thymol or toluene.	Caution should be taken when interpreting results, as amylase creatinine clearance ratio lacks specificity.
Lipase	Titrimetric	Titrimetric: enzyme reaction not linear; also lacks specificity for pancreatic lipase	Bacterial contamination contributes to lipase activity.
	Turbidimetric	Turbidimetric: possible negative results from patients with rheumatoid factor	Kinetic titrimetric is used as reference method.
	Spectrophotometric and fluorometric		Kodak Ektachem uses spectrophotometric reaction rate.
	Immunoassay sandwich technique		Good sensitivity and specificity. Availability and use of such methods are still limited.

Continued ▶

▶ Continued **DIAGNOSTIC TESTS AND METHODOLOGIES**

TEST	METHOD	INTERFERENCE	COMMENTS
Trypsin	Immunoreactive trypsin serum radioimmunoassay (RIA)		Rises parallel with serum amylase. As with amylase, renal failure must be ruled out. The method appears to have no greater sensitivity than other pancreatic diagnostic tests. Because of the methodology (RIA), tests are usually batched, thereby restricting its use as a STAT test. Test offers the possibility of a screen for cystic fibrosis
β-carotene	HPLC	β-Carotene levels are inversely proportional to the number of cigarettes smoked per day.	For malabsorption diagnosis, a single assay is not as diagnostic as an absorption test.
Vitamin B$_{12}$	Competitive protein binding	Certain foods can increase results.	Laboratory should determine its own reference range. Absorption test affords the opportunity to distinguish between pernicious anemia and malabsorption.
Gastrin	Double antibody radioimmunoassay	Gastrin immunoreactivity decreases with refrigeration storage time.	CG-34 is the dominant structure of gastrin, but the standard is G-17. Because of this, all results should be reported as G-17.
Tripeptide Hydrolysis	Ability of intraluminal chymotrysin to hydrolyze oral synthetic peptide bentiromide. Spectrophotometric measurement of PABA.	Sulfonamides, thiazides, furosemide, acetaminophen, chloramphenicol.	The patient must have adequate renal function and gastrointestinal absorptivity.
Fecal Fat	Quantitation of fat in stool	Patient compliance is difficult.	When steatorrhea is suspected, a 3 day collection is recommended.

Continued ▶

▶ Continued **DIAGNOSTIC TESTS AND METHODOLOGIES**

TEST	METHOD	INTERFERENCE	COMMENTS
^{14}C-Triolein Breath	^{14}C-labeled triglyceride is hydrolyzed by pancreatic lipase in the bowel. Free fatty acids are absorbed and metabolized.	Secondary conditions can influence results.	The test offers a good alternative to fecal fat measurements.
D-Xylose Absorption	Quantitation of D-xylose in serum and urine. Xylose is dehydrated to furfural, which reacts with *p*-bromoalinine and is measured at 520 nm.	Diuretics, anti-inflammatory drugs, antibiotics, dehydration, edema, and ascites can produce false positive results.	Reference ranges for elderly and others differ.
Sweat Chloride	Sweat is collected on paper after stimulation with pilocarpin and low electric current. Chloride is washed off and measured by coulometric-amperometric titration or ion selective electrode (ISE).	Skin must be cleaned properly or increased results will occur. Patients in hot climates need to have electrolytes measured to rule out salt depletion.	Avoid contamination of testing site.

DIAGNOSING ACUTE AND CHRONIC PANCREATITIS

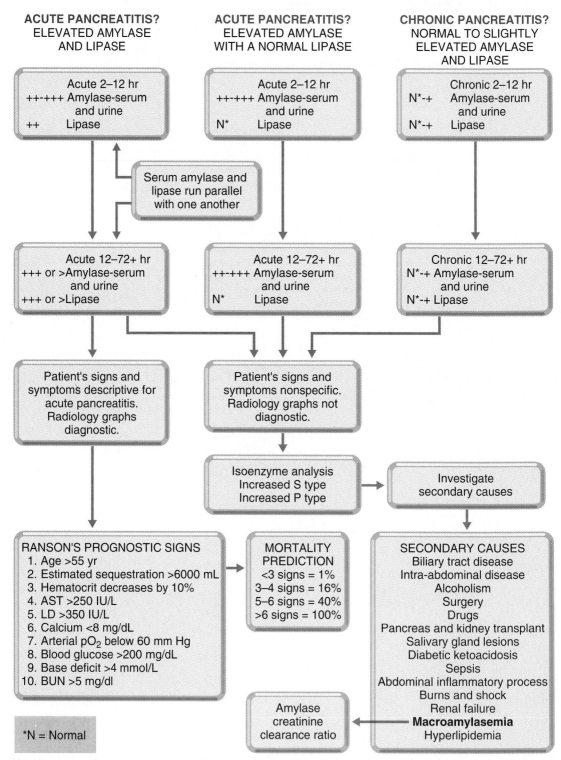

ACUTE PANCREATITIS?
ELEVATED AMYLASE
AND LIPASE

ACUTE PANCREATITIS?
ELEVATED AMYLASE
WITH A NORMAL LIPASE

CHRONIC PANCREATITIS?
NORMAL TO SLIGHTLY
ELEVATED AMYLASE
AND LIPASE

Acute 2–12 hr
++-+++ Amylase-serum
and urine
++ Lipase

Acute 2–12 hr
++-+++ Amylase-serum
and urine
N* Lipase

Chronic 2–12 hr
N*-+ Amylase-serum
and urine
N*-+ Lipase

Serum amylase and
lipase run parallel
with one another

Acute 12–72+ hr
+++ or >Amylase-serum
and urine
+++ or >Lipase

Acute 12–72+ hr
++-+++ Amylase-serum
and urine
N* Lipase

Chronic 12–72+ hr
N*-+ Amylase-serum
and urine
N*-+ Lipase

Patient's signs and
symptoms descriptive for
acute pancreatitis.
Radiology graphs
diagnostic.

Patient's signs and
symptoms nonspecific.
Radiology graphs not
diagnostic.

Isoenzyme analysis
Increased S type
Increased P type

Investigate
secondary causes

RANSON'S PROGNOSTIC SIGNS
1. Age >55 yr
2. Estimated sequestration >6000 mL
3. Hematocrit decreases by 10%
4. AST >250 IU/L
5. LD >350 IU/L
6. Calcium <8 mg/dL
7. Arterial pO$_2$ below 60 mm Hg
8. Blood glucose >200 mg/dL
9. Base deficit >4 mmol/L
10. BUN >5 mg/dl

MORTALITY
PREDICTION
<3 signs = 1%
3–4 signs = 16%
5–6 signs = 40%
>6 signs = 100%

SECONDARY CAUSES
Biliary tract disease
Intra-abdominal disease
Alcoholism
Surgery
Drugs
Pancreas and kidney transplant
Salivary gland lesions
Diabetic ketoacidosis
Sepsis
Abdominal inflammatory process
Burns and shock
Renal failure
Macroamylasemia
Hyperlipidemia

Amylase
creatinine
clearance ratio

*N = Normal

The above chart in no way represents all variations of amylase and lipase in acute and chronic pancreatitis
(i.e., acute pancreatitis in hyperlipidemia, see p 126).

TESTING FOR MALABSORPTION AND CYSTIC FIBROSIS

TESTING FOR MALABSORPTION	
Tripeptide Hydrolysis Test	Decreased para-aminobenzoic acid results suggest pancreatic insufficiency.
Fecal Fat	Values 5–10 g% suggest malabsorption. Values > 10 g% suggest maldigestion.
^{14}C-Triolein Breath	Decreased $^{14}CO_2$ in expired air suggests fat malabsorption.
D-Xylose Absorption	Values below reference ranges suggest little to no absorption capacity of the proximal small bowel mucosa.
Vitamin B_{12} Malabsorption	Patients who excrete <7% are suspected to have pernicious anemia.
β-Carotene	Decreased levels are seen in patients with malabsorption and/or malnutrition.
TESTING FOR CYSTIC FIBROSIS	
Sweat Chloride	Increased levels are diagnostic of cystic fibrosis.

GASTRIC ANALYSIS

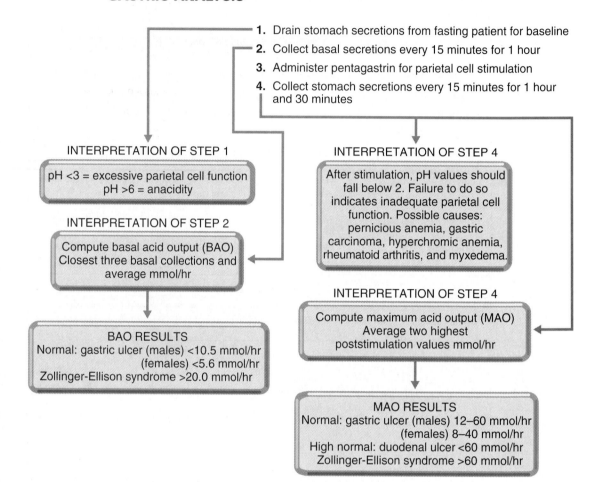

1. Drain stomach secretions from fasting patient for baseline
2. Collect basal secretions every 15 minutes for 1 hour
3. Administer pentagastrin for parietal cell stimulation
4. Collect stomach secretions every 15 minutes for 1 hour and 30 minutes

INTERPRETATION OF STEP 1

pH <3 = excessive parietal cell function
pH >6 = anacidity

INTERPRETATION OF STEP 2

Compute basal acid output (BAO)
Closest three basal collections and
average mmol/hr

BAO RESULTS
Normal: gastric ulcer (males) <10.5 mmol/hr
(females) <5.6 mmol/hr
Zollinger-Ellison syndrome >20.0 mmol/hr

INTERPRETATION OF STEP 4

After stimulation, pH values should
fall below 2. Failure to do so
indicates inadequate parietal cell
function. Possible causes:
pernicious anemia, gastric
carcinoma, hyperchromic anemia,
rheumatoid arthritis, and myxedema.

INTERPRETATION OF STEP 4

Compute maximum acid output (MAO)
Average two highest
poststimulation values mmol/hr

MAO RESULTS
Normal: gastric ulcer (males) 12–60 mmol/hr
(females) 8–40 mmol/hr
High normal: duodenal ulcer <60 mmol/hr
Zollinger-Ellison syndrome >60 mmol/hr

INTERPRETATION OF GASTRIN ANALYSIS

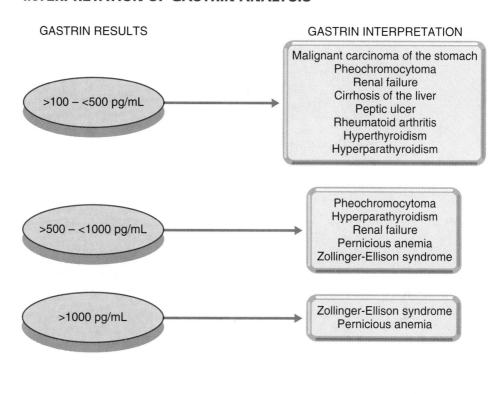

GASTRIN RESULTS

GASTRIN INTERPRETATION

>100 – <500 pg/mL

Malignant carcinoma of the stomach
Pheochromocytoma
Renal failure
Cirrhosis of the liver
Peptic ulcer
Rheumatoid arthritis
Hyperthyroidism
Hyperparathyroidism

>500 – <1000 pg/mL

Pheochromocytoma
Hyperparathyroidism
Renal failure
Pernicious anemia
Zollinger-Ellison syndrome

>1000 pg/mL

Zollinger-Ellison syndrome
Pernicious anemia

BIBLIOGRAPHY

Bank S, Chow KW: Diagnostic tests in chronic pancreatitis (review). Gastroenterologist 2(3):224–232, 1994.

Banks PA, Carr-Locke DL, Slivka A, et al: Urinary trypsinogen activation peptides (TAP) are not increased in mild ERCP-induced pancreatitis. Pancreas 12(3):294–297, 1996.

Burtis CA, Ashwood ER: Tietz Fundamentals of Clinical Chemistry, 4th ed. Philadelphia, WB Saunders, 1996.

Chen CC, Wang SS, Chao Y, et al: Serum pancreas-specific protein in acute pancreatitis. Its clinical utility in comparison with serum amylase. Scand J Gastroenterol 29(1):87–90, 1994.

Corsetti JP, Cox C, Schulz TJ, Arvan DA: Combined serum amylase and lipase determinations of diagnosis of suspected acute pancreatitis. Clin Chem 39(12):2495–2499, 1993.

Dominguez-Munoz JE, Pieramico O, Buchler M, Malfertheiner P: Ratios of different serum pancreatic enzymes in the diagnosis and staging of chronic pancreatitis. Digestion 54(4):231–236, 1993.

Dorner K, Schulze S: In vivo interference of heparin bolus injection with photometric continuous lipase determination. Eur J Clin Chem Clin Biochem 34(4):363–364, 1996.

Dressler C, Franke KP, Herzig M: [Acute pancreatitis—what are the diagnostically and prognostically relevant chemical laboratory parameters?] [German]. Anaesthesiol Reanim 19(3):67–72, 1994.

Dugernier T, Laterre PF, Reynaert M: [Prognosis and intensive care of severe acute pancreatitis] (review) [French]. Rev Praticien 46(6):696–703, 1996.

El-Omar EM, Penman ID, Ardill JE, et al: *Helicobacter pylori* infection and abnormalities of acid secretion in patients with duodenal ulcer disease. Gastroenterology 109(3):681–691, 1995.

Gumaste VV, Roditis N, Mehta D, Dave PB: Serum lipase levels in nonpancreatic abdominal pain versus acute pancreatitis. Am J Gastroenterol 88(12):2051–2055, 1993.

Howantiz JH, Howantiz PJ: Laboratory Medicine: Test Selection and Interpretation. New York, Churchill Livingstone, 1991.

INTERPRETATION OF GASTRIN ANALYSIS

Kaplan LA, Pesce AJ: Clinical Chemistry: Theory, Analysis and Correlation, 2nd ed. St. Louis, CV Mosby, 1989.

Lankisch PG, Droge M, Becher R: Pulmonary infiltrations. Sign of severe acute pancreatitis. Int J Pancreatol 19(2):113–115, 1996.

Lankisch PG, Petersen M, Gottesleben F: High, not low, amylase and lipase levels indicate severe acute pancreatitis. Z Gastroenterol 32(4):213–215, 1994.

Lowe AW, Luthen RE, Wong SM, Grendell JH: The level of the zymogen granule protein GP2 is elevated in a rat model for acute pancreatitis. Gastroenterology 107(6):1819–1827, 1994.

McClatchery KD: Clinical Laboratory Medicine. Baltimore, MD, Williams & Wilkins, 1994.

Nakae Y, Hayakawa T, Kondo T, et al: Serum alpha-2-macroglobulin-trypsin complex and early recognition of severe acute pancreatitis after endoscopic retrograde pancreatography. J Gastroenterol Hepatol 9(3):272–276, 1994.

Orebaugh SL: Normal amylase levels in the presentation of acute pancreatitis. Am J Emerg Med 12(1):21–24, 1994.

Paredes Cotore JP, Bustamante Montalvo M, Fernandez Rodriguez E, et al: [Prognosis of acute pancreatitis: Ranson or Apache II?] [Spanish]. Rev Esp Enferm Dig 87(2):121–126, 1995.

Sibert A: [Imaging of pancreatitis] [French]. Rev Praticien 46(6):689–695, 1996.

Tenner S, Dubner H, Steinberg W: Predicting gallstone pancreatitis with laboratory parameters: a meta-analysis. Am J Gastroenterol 89(10):1863–1866, 1994.

Tietz NW: Clinical Guide to Laboratory Tests. Philadelphia, WB Saunders, 1995.

Turcotte GE, Nadeau L, Forest JC, et al: A new rapid immunoinhibition pancreatic amylase assay: diagnostic value for pancreatitis. Clin Biochem 27(2):133–139, 1994.

Chapter *9*

ELECTROLYTES AND WATER BALANCE

Karen M. Escolas, MS, MT (ASCP)

Q U I C K   C O N T E N T S

INTRODUCTION

Electrolytes are defined as substances whose molecules dissociate into ions when in solution. The major electrolytes found in the human body are positively charged cations (sodium, potassium, calcium, and magnesium) or negatively charged anions (chloride, bicarbonate, phosphate, sulfate, proteins, and a variety of organic acids such as lactate). To maintain electroneutrality within the body system, the total concentration of the cations must equal that of the anions. The overall functions of electrolytes in the body include maintenance of osmotic pressure and water distribution, maintenance of proper pH, regulation of proper function of heart and other muscles, involvement in oxidation-reduction (electron transfer) reactions, and service as cofactors to a variety of enzymatic reactions. The electrolyte profile run routinely in clinical laboratories includes assessment of the most abundant electrolytes: sodium, potassium, chloride, and bicarbonate. This profile is one of the most important tests performed in the clinical laboratory, as alterations of the electrolyte levels may be the cause or consequence of a variety of disorders. Calcium, magnesium, and phosphate are covered in Chapter 12, "Mineral Metabolism"; the proteins are covered in Chapter 2, "Amino Acids and Proteins."

ROUTINE ELECTROLYTE PROFILE

ELECTROLYTE	REGULATION	FUNCTION	COMMENTS
Sodium (Na$^+$) Major extracellular cation	RENAL: 100% filtered at glomerulus 70% reabsorbed in proximal tubule 25% reabsorbed in loop of Henle More reabsorbed in distal tubule when aldosterone is present	Maintenance of water distribution Maintenance of osmotic pressure in plasma	The ratio of plasma Na$^+$ to osmolality is 0.43:0.50. An increase in osmotically active substances will result in a decreased ratio.
Potassium (K$^+$) Major intracellular cation	RENAL: Secreted in distal tubule at a rate dependent on: ▮ Level of K$^+$ intake ▮ Availability of Na$^+$ for reabsorption ▮ Balance of H$^+$ and K$^+$ ▮ Ability of cells to secrete H$^+$ ▮ Acid base status ▮ Presence of aldosterone to stimulate secretion ▮ Tubular flow rate	Important to cellular metabolism Necessary for neuromuscular function, particularly of cardiac tissue	K$^+$ moves into cells in response to increased glucose and insulin levels.
Chloride (Cl$^-$) Major extracellular anion	RENAL: Filtered at glomerulus Passively reabsorbed at proximal tubule Further reabsorbed in loop of Henle	Maintenance of water balance and osmotic pressure in conjunction with sodium	Chloride shift = Cl$^-$ move into cells in exchange for bicarbonate produced in cells Plasma level closely linked to sodium level except in acid base disorders
Bicarbonate (HCO$_3^-$) Major component of total carbon dioxide in plasma	RENAL: Filtration and reabsorption regulated in response to acid base status of body	Maintenance of acid base balance	Further discussed in Chapter 11, "Blood Gases and Acid Base Balance"

ANION GAP

The anion gap is the mathematical approximation of the difference between the concentration of unmeasured cations and unmeasured anions in serum. Thus, the anion gap will detect altered concentrations of ions other than those measured in the routine electrolyte panel (Na$^+$, K$^+$, Cl$^-$, HCO$_3^-$), such as calcium, magnesium, phosphate, sulfate, proteins, and various organic acids. Electroneutrality must be maintained in the body; therefore, the number of positively charged ions will equal the number of negatively charged ions at all times and the anion gap will always be zero. For this reason, the anion gap determined during an electrolyte panel is merely an analytical term and not an actual physiologic finding. The following two equations may be used to calculate the anion gap:

$$([Na^+] + [K^+]) - ([Cl^-] + [HCO_3^-]) \qquad \text{Reference range} = 10\text{–}20$$

$$([Na^+]) - ([Cl^-] + [HCO_3^-]) \qquad \text{Reference range} = 8\text{–}16$$

Elevated or decreased anion gap results not only may be used to indicate true alterations in electrolyte levels, but also may be used as a means of quality control in performing electrolyte results. If anion gaps are either elevated or decreased for several patients consecutively, this indicates that a problem exists in the instrument on which the electrolyte levels are being measured.

WATER BALANCE

In health, the water content accounts for 50% to 60% of body weight in males and 45% to 55% of body weight in females. Approximately two thirds of the water is found in intracellular fluid and the remaining one third in the extracellular fluid. The plasma content accounts for 8% of the extracellular water. Water levels are maintained through a balance between intake through food, fluids, and metabolism; and excretion through gastrointestinal fluids, sweat at skin surfaces, respiration, and urine. Water is freely permeable throughout the body, depending on the osmotic contents of each compartment, the major osmotic particles being the electrolytes. Normally, the various compartments are isotonic, thereby maintaining water levels in both the intracellular and extracellular spaces. The primary exception is in the renal compartments where the osmotic content is varied to regulate the amount of water that is excreted or retained in response to the body water content. In response to a decreased body water content, the hypothalamus stimulates the thirst mechanism and the production of antidiuretic hormone (ADH or vasopressin) by the posterior pituitary gland. ADH is responsible for increasing the permeability of the collecting ducts in the kidney to allow for increased reabsorption of water. The renin-angiotensin-aldosterone hormonal system also affects water content through regulation of blood pressure and sodium and potassium levels.

OSMOLALITY

The water content of extracellular fluid is assessed by determining the osmolality of the plasma. Osmolality is defined as the number of moles of particles dissolved in solution and is expressed as milliosmoles per kilogram water (mOsm/kg H_2O). Osmolality is measured using one of the colligative properties: those properties of a solution related only to the number of particles rather than to the nature of the particles. Dissolved particles will affect the colligative properties in the following ways: depression of the vapor pressure and freezing point, and elevation of the boiling point and osmotic pressure. Plasma osmolality is maintained within an extremely tight range through the hormonal regulation of renal water excretion. The main contributors to the osmolality of plasma are sodium, chloride, urea, and glucose. As a result, osmolality may be estimated using the following equation:

$$([Na^+] \times 2) + \frac{[\text{urea}]}{2.8} + \frac{[\text{glucose}]}{18}$$

ROUTINE ELECTROLYTE PROFILE

OSMOLAL GAP

The mathematical difference between the measured and calculated osmolality is the osmolal gap. The presence of osmotically active particles other than the main contributors is detected through determination of the osmolal gap. The reference range is 0 to 6 in the absence of any abnormal osmotic contributors.

PATIENT PREPARATION, SPECIMEN COLLECTION AND STORAGE, REFERENCE RANGE

TEST	PATIENT PREPARATION	SPECIMEN COLLECTION	SPECIMEN STORAGE	REFERENCE RANGE
Sodium (Na^+)	Nonfasting is acceptable.	Serum, heparinized plasma, or whole blood (*not* sodium heparin) Timed urine, feces (liquid), or GI fluids (filtered)	Severe hemolysis has a dilutional effect on blood levels. No preservative is required for urine. Serum, plasma, and urine are stable for 1 wk at room temperature or 1°–4°C, 1 yr frozen.	SERUM/PLASMA: 135–145 mmol/L URINE: 40–220 mmol/day
Potassium (K^+)	Nonfasting is acceptable. Prolonged tourniquet application or repeated clenching of the fist during venipuncture will falsely elevate values. High platelet or white blood cell counts will produce elevated values.	Same specimens as sodium EDTA cannot be used (contains K^+)	Any degree of hemolysis will falsely elevate levels. Serum/plasma is separated from cells within 3 hr to prevent leakage of K^+ from red blood cells. Same sample stability as sodium	SERUM: 3.5–5.0 mmol/L PLASMA: Slightly lower owing to release of K^+ from platelets during clot formation with serum URINE: 25–125 mmol/day
Chloride (Cl^-)	Fasting specimen is required except in emergencies (level decreases following meals).	Serum, heparinized plasma/whole blood, 24 hr urine, sweat	Separate from cells promptly, as change of pH will alter distribution of chloride. Hemolysis should be avoided. Same sample stability as sodium	SERUM/PLASMA: 98–109 mmol/L URINE: 110–250 mEq/day SWEAT: 5–35 mEq/L

Continued ▶

► Continued **PATIENT PREPARATION, SPECIMEN COLLECTION AND STORAGE, REFERENCE RANGE**

TEST	PATIENT PREPARATION	SPECIMEN COLLECTION	SPECIMEN STORAGE	REFERENCE RANGE
Bicarbonate (HCO_3^-) or Total CO_2 (tCO_2)	Nonfasting is acceptable.	Serum or heparinized plasma	Maintain anaerobic conditions until separated from cells; decreases 6 mmol/hr after becomes aerobic. Stable for several days if separated, tightly capped, and refrigerated	SERUM/PLASMA: 22–29 mmol/L
Osmolality	Nonfasting is acceptable.	Serum or heparinized plasma	Serum must be removed from cells as soon as possible; stable 3 hr at room temperature, 3 days at 1°–4°C.	SERUM: 275–300 mOsm/kg H_2O
		Urine (24 hr specimen preferred, random acceptable)	Urine must be centrifuged to remove cellular debris; stable 24 hr at 1°–4°C.	URINE: Random: 50–1200 mOsm/kg H_2O 24 hr: 300–900 mOsm/kg H_2O

DIAGNOSTIC TESTS AND METHODOLOGIES

TEST	METHOD	INTERFERENCE	COMMENTS
Sodium	Atomic absorption spectroscopy	ALL METHODS: Increased lipids (turbidity) cause falsely decreased Na^+ values in indirect methods (those requiring dilution) owing to Na^+ content confined to water portion of sample not being properly diluted—may be corrected by ultracentrifugation. Increased protein levels due to a paraprotein may cause falsely elevated Na^+ levels in direct methods (those not requiring dilution of sample) owing to positive charge of protein or viscosity of sample.	Reference method
	Flame emission spectroscopy		Rarely used
	Ion selective electrodes (glass electrode selective for sodium)		Most commonly used
	Spectrophotometric/colorimetric		Currently in development

Continued ►

► Continued **DIAGNOSTIC TESTS AND METHODOLOGIES**

TEST	METHOD	INTERFERENCE	COMMENTS
Potassium	Same methods as sodium Ion selective electrode (liquid membrane with Valinomycin selective for potassium)	Potassium levels are not affected by lipids or protein owing to the larger proportional reference range in comparison with sodium levels.	Same as sodium Most commonly used method
Chloride (Blood or Urine)	Colorimetry (chloride reacts with mercury thiocyanate to form red colored complex). Coulometric-amperometric titration (chloride precipitates with silver generated at electrode). Ion selective electrodes (solid-state electrode with silver chloride membrane) Mercurimetric titration (Schales & Schales method using mercury to titrate chloride to a colored end point)	Bilirubin, hemoglobin, and lipemia cause false elevations. ALL METHODS: Other halides cause falsely elevated Cl⁻ levels (e.g., bromide, which is present in many drug compounds).	Constant temperature necessary for accurate results Limited to plasma, serum, and CSF ranges Reference method Most commonly used Difficult to detect end point of titration
Chloride (Sweat)	Pilocarpine iontophoresis (pilocarpine induces sweating when driven into the skin through iontophoresis—sweat collected is measured using one of the above methods).	Gloves must be worn by technologist at all stages to avoid contamination with sweat.	Used as screening test for cystic fibrosis
Bicarbonate	P_{CO_2} electrode after treatment with acid buffer to convert all forms to CO_2 gas Enzymatic after treatment with alkaline to convert all forms to bicarbonate Ion selective electrode (refer to Chapter 11, "Blood Gases and Acid Base Balance")		Reference method, rarely used for routine measurement Commonly used routine method Commonly used routine method

Continued ►

▶ Continued **DIAGNOSTIC TESTS AND METHODOLOGIES**

TEST	METHOD	INTERFERENCE	COMMENTS
Osmolality	Freezing point (FP) depression: measures the degree to which the FP of the sample differs from that of water (each osmole of particles depresses the FP by 1.86°C).	Requires a large sample volume.	Most commonly used Precision = ±2 mOsm/kg H_2O
	Vapor pressure depression: measures the degree to which the vapor pressure of the sample differs from that of water by measuring the dew point of the sample.	Does not detect volatile substances that may contribute to the osmolality (ethanol, methanol, ethylene glycol).	Requires smaller sample; thus, preferable for neonatal testing Less precise, more variation in results

EVALUATING TEST RESULTS

Causes of Electrolyte Alterations

ALTERATION	CAUSES	
Hypernatremia	DEHYDRATION (water loss greater than sodium loss): Profuse sweating Prolonged hyperpnea Vomiting Diarrhea Polyuria Decreased ADH secretion or activity Osmotic diuresis	ABSOLUTE SODIUM EXCESS: Saline solution administration Hyperaldosteronism Hyperadrenocorticism (Cushing's disease) Associated with hypercalcemia and hypokalemia: ▮ Liver disease ▮ Cardiac failure ▮ Pregnancy ▮ Burns
Hyponatremia	DEPLETIONAL (absolute loss of sodium from the body): Excessive sweating Prolonged vomiting Persistent diarrhea Salt losing enteropathies (salt loss greater than water loss) Renal loss of sodium: ▮ Inappropriate diuretic use ▮ Aldosterone deficiency (Addison's disease) ▮ Severe polyuria ▮ Metabolic acidosis (sodium coexcreted with anions) ▮ Osmotic diuresis ▮ Renal tubular acidosis (RTA)	DILUTIONAL (decrease in sodium relative to increase in body water): Excessive water retention Edema Chronic cardiac failure (due to formation of ascites) Uncontrolled diabetes mellitus Hepatic cirrhosis Nephrotic syndrome Malnutrition Syndrome of inappropriate ADH secretion (SIADH)

Continued ▶

▶ Continued **Causes of Electrolyte Alterations**

ALTERATION	CAUSES	
Hyperkalemia	ABSOLUTE INCREASE IN TOTAL BODY POTASSIUM: Overtreatment with K^+-rich fluids (especially with decreased renal function) Tumor lysis syndrome Salt losing congenital adrenal hyperplasia Administration of diuretics (those that block K^+ secretion) Decreased excretion of potassium in urine: ▪ Renal failure ▪ Acidosis ▪ Adrenocortical insufficiency	SHIFT OF INTRACELLULAR POTASSIUM TO EXTRACELLULAR FLUID: Dehydration Shock with tissue hypoxia Diabetic ketoacidosis Massive intravascular hemolysis severe burns Violent muscular activity (as with epileptic seizures) Thrombocytosis Leukocytosis
Hypokalemia	DECREASED INTAKE OF POTASSIUM: Chronic starvation Postoperative therapy with fluids low in potassium REDISTRIBUTION OF POTASSIUM FROM EXTRACELLULAR TO INTRACELLULAR FLUID: Insulin therapy of diabetes mellitus (K^+ and water into cells with glucose) Alkalosis (K^+ into cells as H^+ moves out of cells)	INCREASED LOSS OF POTASSIUM FROM BODY: Gastrointestinal ▪ Vomiting ▪ Diarrhea ▪ Intestinal fistulas Renal ▪ RTA ▪ Hyperaldosteronism ▪ Diuretic therapies (those that promote K^+ secretion)
Hyperchloremia	Dehydration Renal tubular acidosis Acute renal failure Diabetes insipidus Adrenocortical hyperfunction Metabolic acidosis with prolonged diarrhea and loss of bicarbonate Salicylate intoxication Respiratory alkalosis Increased dietary intake Excessive saline administration Primary hyperparathyroidism	
Hypochloremia	Salt losing nephritis Metabolic acidosis (competes with increased organic acid production) Prolonged vomiting (loss of gastric HCl) Persistent gastric secretion Metabolic alkalosis (replaced by bicarbonate) Hyperaldosteronism Bromide intoxication Cerebral salt wasting after head injury SIADH Expansion of extracellular fluid volume	

Causes of Alterations of Osmolality

ALTERATION	CAUSES		
Hyperosmolality	NORMAL OSMOLAL GAP: Dehydration Hyperglycemia without ketoacidosis Hypernatremia Azotemia Diabetes insipidus	MODERATELY ELEVATED OSMOLAL GAP (UP TO 10): Ketoacidosis Renal acidosis Lactic acidosis	MARKEDLY ELEVATED OSMOLAL GAP (GREATER THAN 10): Poisoning (both the parent compound and the metabolites contribute to the osmolality). ▐ Ethanol ▐ Methanol ▐ Isopropanol ▐ Ethylene glycol ▐ Diethyl ether ▐ Paraldehyde ▐ Trichloroethane ▐ Salicylate
Hypo-osmolality	A decreased plasma osmolality will be found only in the presence of hyponatremia. Therefore, any pathologic condition resulting in hyponatremia will also result in hypo-osmolality.		

BIBLIOGRAPHY

Anderson SC, Cockayne S: Clinical Chemistry: Concepts and Applications. Philadelphia, WB Saunders, 1993.

Badrick T, Hickman PE: The anion gap—a reappraisal. Am J Clin Pathol 98:249, 1992.

Bishop M, Duben-Engelkirk JL, Fody EP: Clinical Chemistry: Principles, Procedures, Correlations, 3rd ed. Philadelphia, JB Lippincott, 1996.

Burtis CA, Ashwood ER: Tietz Fundamentals of Clinical Chemistry, 4th ed. Philadelphia, WB Saunders, 1996.

Dennis VW: Investigations of renal function. In Wyngaarden JB, Smith LH Jr, Bennett JC, eds: Cecil Textbook of Medicine, 19th ed. Philadelphia, WB Saunders, 1992, p 492.

DeVita MV, Michelis MF: Perturbations in sodium balance: hyponatremia and hypernatremia. Clin Lab Med 13:135, 1993.

Dinovo EC, Sansone P, Lee DBN: Changes in the reference range of the serum anion gap. Clin Chem 38:935, 1992.

Henry JB: Clinical Diagnosis and Management by Laboratory Methods, 19th ed. Philadelphia, WB Saunders, 1996.

Kamel SK, Ethier JH, Richardson RMA, et al: Urine electrolytes and osmolality: when and how to use them. Am J Nephrol 10:89, 1990.

Kaplan L, Pesce AJ: Clinical Chemistry: Theory, Analysis, Correlation, 3rd ed. St. Louis, Mosby–Year Book, 1996.

Latta K, Hisano S, Chan JCM: Perturbations in potassium balance. Clin Lab Med 13:149, 1993.

Maas AHJ: IFCC reference methods and materials for measurement of pH, gases, and electrolytes in blood. Scand J Clin Lab Invest 53(Suppl 214):83, 1993.

Marshall WJ: Clinical Chemistry, 3rd ed. St. Louis, Mosby–Year Book, 1995.

Narins RG, ed: Maxwell and Kleeman's Clinical Disorders of Fluid and Electrolyte Metabolism, 5th ed. New York, McGraw-Hill, 1994, p 886.

Southgate JH, Collins JS, Short SM: Comparison of colorimetric potassium method with flame photometry and ion-selective electrodes. Ann Clin Biochem 28:412, 1991.

Tietz NW, ed: Clinical Guide to Laboratory Tests, 3rd ed. Philadelphia, WB Saunders, 1995.

EVALUATING TEST RESULTS

Chapter *10*

RENAL FUNCTION AND NITROGEN BALANCE

Karen M. Escolas, MS, MT (ASCP)

QUICK CONTENTS

INTRODUCTION

The kidney is responsible for three areas of function: excretory, regulatory, and endocrine.

Excretion

Excretory function involves removal of waste products of metabolism (urea, creatinine, uric acid, amino acids) and inorganic substances ingested in the diet (sodium, potassium, chloride, calcium, phosphate, magnesium, sulfate, bicarbonate). The kidney is also the site of excretion of many foreign chemicals, such as heavy metals, and certain drugs, such as antibiotics.

Regulation

Regulatory function involves homeostatic control through reabsorption and secretion processes that establish the equilibrium of water and electrolytes in all body fluid compartments. As part of this homeostatic regulation, the kidney balances the acid and base levels in the body, thereby maintaining the proper body pH. The kidney also serves as a regulator of protein levels by conserving the concentration of protein when urine is formed.

Endocrine

The endocrine function of the kidney includes both primary and secondary activity in the control of hormone production. The kidney has primary control through the production of the following hormones: renin, which regulates blood pressure in conjunction with angiotensin; 1,25-$(OH)_2D_3$ or calcitriol, which regulates mineral homeostasis by controlling the deposit and removal of calcium and phosphate from bone structure; and erythropoietin, which regulates the production of red blood cells by the bone marrow. The kidney serves as a secondary site of endocrine function by degrading the following hormones: insulin, which is responsible for the uptake and use of glucose by tissue cells; and aldosterone, which controls the renal regulation of sodium and potassium plasma levels.

URINE FORMATION

Much of the kidney's function is tied to the process of urine formation by the nephrons through the steps of filtration, reabsorption, secretion, and excretion. These events are carried out through interaction between the nephron and the surrounding vasculature of the kidney, thereby producing urine through removal of components from the plasma (see figure on next page). Each kidney contains one-half million nephrons that carry out the function of urine formation. Therefore, impairment of kidney function is not detectable until up to 80% of the nephrons have been destroyed.

BOWMAN'S CAPSULE:
Hollow structure that collects the glomerular ultrafiltrate, which resembles plasma without the large molecular weight molecules such as proteins

GLOMERULUS:
Tuft of capillaries with semipermeable basement membrane through which small molecular weight molecules are freely filtered

DISTAL CONVOLUTED TUBULE:
• Reabsorption of small amounts of Na^+, Cl^-, and water in response to ADH and aldosterone
• K^+ secreted in response to aldosterone
• H^+, ammonia, urea, and uric acid secreted and bicarbonate reabsorbed

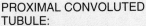

PROXIMAL CONVOLUTED TUBULE:
• 65% of ultrafiltrate is reabsorbed including water, salt, glucose, amino acids, low molecular weight proteins, urea, uric acid, bicarbonate, phosphate, chloride, potassium, magnesium, and calcium
• Some H^+ and ammonia secreted

COLLECTING DUCT:
• ADH controls water reabsorption
• Aldosterone regulates NaCl reabsorption
• K^+, H^+, and ammonia reabsorbed
• Urine formed is carried to ureter and then bladder for excretion

LOOP OF HENLE:
• Selectively permeable to Na, urea, and water
• Responsible for conservation of water through movement of salt and water in the countercurrent mechanism:
  Descending loop = highly permeable to water but not salt; urine becomes concentrated as water into vasculature
  Ascending loop = impermeable to water but actively reabsorbs salt, decreasing the concentration of the urine

URINE FORMATION

PATIENT PREPARATION, SPECIMEN COLLECTION AND STORAGE, REFERENCE RANGE

TEST	PATIENT PREPARATION	SPECIMEN COLLECTION	SPECIMEN STORAGE	REFERENCE RANGE
Urea	Nonfasting specimen is acceptable. Increased with high protein diet Males have higher level than females. Reference level higher with age	SERUM PLASMA (for indirect methods: fluoride and citrate anticoagulants inhibit urease, and ammonium heparin causes falsely elevated results). Serum or plasma must be nonhemolyzed. URINE: 24 hr specimen	SERUM/PLASMA: Stable 24 hr at 22°C Stable several days at 4°–8°C (prevents bacterial conversion of urea to ammonia) Stable 2–3 mo frozen URINE: Stable 4 days at 4°–8°C pH must be adjusted to 4. Preserve with thymol to prevent bacterial growth and conversion of urea to ammonia.	SERUM/PLASMA: Urea: 5–39 mg/dL BUN: 7–18 mg/dL Convert urea to BUN: Urea × (28/60) = BUN Convert BUN to urea: BUN × (60/28) = urea (where BUN and urea are both in mg/dL and 28 g of nitrogen is in each 60 g urea molecule) URINE: Urea: 17–20 g/day
Creatinine	Nonfasting specimen is acceptable. Varies with age, gender, and lean body mass. Severe exercise and high meat diet elevates level.	SERUM/PLASMA (heparin or fluoride anticoagulant) Hemolysis of specimen releases chromagens that falsely elevate results. Lipemic and icteric specimens also have erroneously high results. URINE: 24 hr specimen	Stable 7 days at 4°C if Jaffe reaction used for assay Separate from cells ASAP if enzymatic method used for assay, because of ammonia production upon standing.	SERUM/PLASMA: M: 0.9–1.5 mg/dL F: 0.7–1.3 mg/dL URINE: M: 14–26 mg/kg/day F: 11–20 mg/kg/day

Continued ▶

▶ Continued **PATIENT PREPARATION, SPECIMEN COLLECTION AND STORAGE, REFERENCE RANGE**

TEST	PATIENT PREPARATION	SPECIMEN COLLECTION	SPECIMEN STORAGE	REFERENCE RANGE
Uric Acid	Nonfasting specimen is acceptable. Severe exercise elevates levels.	SERUM OR PLASMA EDTA and fluoride cause positive interference with the uricase method. URINE: 24 hr specimen	SERUM/PLASMA: Stable 3–5 days at 2°–6°C Stable 6 mo at −20°C URINE: Preserve with NaOH (10 mL per 24 hr collection) Stable for 3 days at 22°–25°C in the absence of bacterial growth	SERUM/PLASMA: M: 3.6–7.7 mg/dL F: 2.5–6.8 mg/dL URINE: 250–750 mg/24 hr

DIAGNOSTIC TESTS AND METHODOLOGIES

TEST	METHOD	INTERFERENCE	COMMENTS
Urea	INDIRECT METHOD: Step 1: urease hydrolyzes urea. Step 2: quantitate ammonium ion.	Ammonia in the sample causes positive interference (not suitable for urine samples unless pretreated to remove ammonia).	
	Enzymatic assay of NH_3	Best done kinetically, as other enzymes (e.g., LD) compete for NADH in the reaction.	Most frequently used
	pH indicator dye		Very common in dry chemistry
	Conductimetric assay (electrode selective for ammonia)		Frequency of use is increasing.
	DIRECT METHOD: Fearon reaction (diacetyl condenses with urea, forming a colored complex).	Sulfa drugs cause positive interference. No interference by ammonia	Rarely used owing to caustic chemical nature of diacetyl

Continued ▶

PATIENT PREP/SPECIMEN COLLECTION/STORAGE/REFERENCE RANGE

► Continued **DIAGNOSTIC TESTS AND METHODOLOGIES**

TEST	METHOD	INTERFERENCE	COMMENTS
Creatinine	Jaffe reaction: creatinine and picrate form a red-orange complex.	Chromagens react with picrate: protein, glucose, ascorbic acid, uric acid, guanidine, acetone, cephalosporins, acetoacetate, pyruvate—overestimation by 20%.	Kinetic assay improves the specificity (bilirubin still causes negative interference and ketoacids still cause elevated values).
	Enzymatic: creatinine aminohydrolase converts creatinine to creatine, and indicator added.	Avoid ammonium heparin anticoagulant: falsely elevates.	Better specificity
	High performance liquid chromatography	No interference	Reference method owing to high accuracy, specificity, and precision
Uric Acid	Phosphotungstic acid (PTA) reduced by uric acid, forming a blue color reaction	Protein and lipids cause turbidity and quench absorbance. Other substances reduce PTA, causing falsely elevated results: glucose, ascorbic acid, acetaminophen, caffeine, theophylline, and the amino acids glutathione, ergothionine, and cysteine released from RBC.	Infrequently used Protein must be removed from specimen prior to reaction with PTA. Method modifications have not improved the positive interference of other reducing substances.
	Uricase oxidizes uric acid, forming allantoin, carbon dioxide, and hydrogen peroxide, which is then quantitated.	Very little interference Protein removal not required	Most commonly used method Increased specificity

EVALUATING TEST RESULTS

Tests of Renal Function

RENAL CLEARANCE AND GLOMERULAR FILTRATION RATE (GFR)

Measurement of the clearance of a substance by the kidney approximates the patient's GFR. Clearance is defined as the quantity of blood cleared of a substance per unit time and depends on the plasma concentration of the substance and the excretion rate of the kidney, which reflects the GFR and the renal plasma flow. The substance used to estimate the clearance must be filtered exclusively by the glomeruli and not reabsorbed, secreted, synthesized, or degraded in other parts of the nephron. Clearance tests are the best laboratory tests currently available to detect mild to moderate glomerular damage. The general formula for calculation of the renal clearance is

$$C_s = \frac{(U_s \times V)}{P_s}$$

where:　C_s = clearance of the substance, reported in mL/min
　　　　U_s = urine concentration of the substance
　　　　V = total volume of urine collected per unit time, typically 24 hr
　　　　P_s = plasma concentration of the substance

Summary of Clearance Tests

TEST	DESCRIPTION	COMMENTS
Urea Clearance	Urea is an endogenous substance that may be used to estimate GFR by measuring both the serum and urine levels followed by use of the clearance formula.	Urea is not a reliable substance for use in determining GFR, as many other factors influence the levels of urea in serum and urine other than renal function. Urea is also reabsorbed and secreted in areas of the nephron other than the glomerulus.
Creatinine Clearance	Creatinine is an endogenous substance that may be measured in both serum and urine followed by use of the clearance formula, with the following adjustment made for the patient's body surface area: $$C_s = \frac{(U_s \times V)}{P_s} \times \frac{1.73}{A}$$ where: 1.73 = the body surface area of an average individual in mm^2 A = the body surface area of the patient in mm^2 (may be obtained using a standardized nomogram)	Most commonly used clearance test owing to convenience of endogenous substance and routine methods available for measurement. Creatinine levels in plasma have very little daily variation and the molecule is freely filtered, with a relatively small amount secreted in the tubules. Overestimates GFR by 7% owing to error inherent in creatinine measurement: Jaffe reaction overestimates creatinine as a result of interference by other chromagens. When GFR falls below 10 mL/min, the test becomes less accurate. In the presence of high plasma proteins, creatinine secretion is increased, leading to a marked overestimation of GFR.
Inulin Clearance	Inulin is an exogenous substance that may be measured in both serum and urine followed by use of the clearance formula.	Inulin is freely filtered by the glomeruli with no additional reabsorption or secretion in the nephron, resulting in increased precision over the creatinine clearance, making this the reference method for estimation of GFR. The necessity to administer inulin to the patient intravenously, and the technical difficulty of inulin analysis in the laboratory, limit its usefulness in routine determinations of GFR.
Para-Aminohippurate (PAH) Clearance	Measurement of the clearance of the exogenous substance PAH from the blood estimates the rate of renal blood flow.	PAH has a high extraction rate from the blood as it is both filtered and secreted by the kidney. In normal conditions, the PAH clearance is determined to be 580–600 mL/min. PAH clearance is limited by its unreliability in the presence of renal disease, as it is an accurate assessment only if the kidney is functioning properly.

EVALUATING TEST RESULTS

ASSESSMENT OF GLOMERULAR PERMEABILITY

Under normal conditions, macromolecules such as proteins are not allowed to be filtered at the glomerulus. Therefore, measurement of protein levels in urine provides an indication of the integrity of the glomerular basement membrane. Measurement may be made using a protein dipstick, microalbumin assay, or total protein assay or protein electrophoresis on a 24 hour urine specimen.

Tubular Function Tests

A variety of tests are available to assess the ability of the tubules to reabsorb and secrete substances during formation of the urine.

Summary of Tubular Function Tests

TEST	DESCRIPTION	COMMENTS
Phenolsulfon-phthalein (PSP)	PSP is an exogenous substance used to assess tubular secretory function. It is injected into the patient, and the amount secreted into the urine is tested at 15 min intervals. The results of the PSP test reflect the renal plasma flow and the tubular secretory function.	94% of PSP is secreted with very little filtered by the glomeruli, because the substance binds to albumin in the blood. When the kidney is functioning normally, 25%–50% of the injected PSP should be secreted in the first 15 min, with an additional 10%–15% secreted in the next 15 min.
Beta$_2$-Microglobulin	This protein is present on all nucleated cells and is filtered but not normally reabsorbed in the kidney. The measurement of serum and urine levels thus serves as a sensitive indicator of renal excretory function.	When reabsorption is diminished owing to tubular damage, elevations in urine beta$_2$-microglobulin will be found. This test is useful in the diagnosis of renal allograft rejection, cyclosporine nephrotoxicity, and cytomegalovirus infection.

Continued ▶

► Continued **Summary of Tubular Function Tests**

TEST	DESCRIPTION	COMMENTS
Concentration Tests: Osmolality and Specific Gravity	OSMOLALITY: Measures the number of particles present per unit of solution, expressed as milliosmoles per kilogram water (mOsm/kg H_2O). Ranges from 50–1200 mOsm/kg H_2O, depending on the patient's hydration. Improved clinical utility when serum osmolality is measured simultaneously and serum:urine ratio is determined. The ratio should be between 1:1 and 1:3 when the concentrating ability of the kidney is intact. SPECIFIC GRAVITY: Test is included in the routine urinalysis. Reference range is 1.003–1.035, depending on the state of patient hydration. When the concentrating ability of the kidney is impaired, the urine becomes isosthenuric, having the same specific gravity as the original ultrafiltrate: 1.007–1.010.	The concentrating ability of the kidney requires adequate GFR, renal plasma flow, tubular mass, and healthy renal tubular cells to pump salt against the concentration gradient. Impairment of this ability leads to nocturia and polyuria. Testing the concentrating ability of the kidney is one of the most sensitive means of evaluating renal function.

NONPROTEIN NITROGENOUS COMPOUNDS

The nonprotein nitrogenous compounds include all compounds containing nitrogen except protein. The kidney is the main elimination route of most of these compounds; thus, measurement of the serum concentration is a test of renal function status. Urea constitutes 45% of the total nonprotein nitrogens in serum; amino acids and uric acid are 20% each, creatinine is 5%, creatine is 1%–2%, and ammonia is 0.2%.

Summary of Nonprotein Nitrogenous Compounds

COMPOUND	SOURCE	RENAL HANDLING	CLINICAL SIGNIFICANCE
Urea	Product of protein metabolism: hepatic enzymes convert ammonia from amino acids to urea.	Freely filtered without reabsorption or secretion Up to 50% of filtered urea may passively diffuse back into plasma.	Elevated with renal disease Also affected by nonrenal factors: ❚ Water status ❚ Dietary protein ❚ Protein catabolism ❚ Muscle wasting

Continued ▶

ASSESSMENT OF GLOMERULAR PERMEABILITY

▶ Continued **Summary of Nonprotein Nitrogenous Compounds**

COMPOUND	SOURCE	RENAL HANDLING	CLINICAL SIGNIFICANCE
Creatinine	The amino acids arginine, methionine, and glycine are converted to creatine in the kidney, liver, and pancreas. Creatine is converted to the high energy compound phosphocreatine in muscle and brain tissue. 1%–2% of creatine is spontaneously converted to creatinine daily.	Freely filtered, very little secreted, and none reabsorbed	Elevated with renal disease although not a sensitive index (not elevated until up to 50% of renal function is lost) Creatinine clearance is a more sensitive index. Amount of creatinine produced is dependent upon the muscle mass of the patient; therefore, varies with age and gender.
Uric Acid	Product of degradation of dietary and endogenous purines by the liver	100% filtered at glomerulus 98% reabsorbed in proximal tubule Reabsorption and secretion in distal tubule results in 6%–12% excreted in urine.	Elevated with renal disease Also influenced by liver function and turnover rate of nucleated cells

BUN/Creatinine Ratio

Comparison of the BUN and creatinine levels is a better indicator of the source of elevations of either substance than the substance value alone. In health, the ratio should be between 10:1 and 20:1.

ALTERATION	CAUSES	COMMENTS
Decreased Ratio	Acute tubular necrosis Low protein intake Severe diarrhea and/or vomiting Starvation Severe liver disease Renal dialysis (urea dialyzes better than creatinine and is removed from plasma at a higher rate)	Less common than an increased ratio
Increased Ratio with Normal Creatinine Level	Dehydration High protein diet Increased protein catabolism Muscle wasting Reabsorption of blood proteins after gastrointestinal hemorrhage Treatment with cortisol Decreased perfusion of kidneys (congestive heart failure, shock, hemorrhage)	Usually 20:1–30:1 as urea is cleared at a lower rate than creatinine Referred to as prerenal azotemia

Continued ▶

► Continued **BUN/Creatinine Ratio**

ALTERATION	CAUSES	COMMENTS
Increased Ratio with Elevated Creatinine Level	Obstruction of urine flow due to: ■ Nephrolithiasis ■ Prostatism ■ Tumors of genitourinary tract ■ Severe infection	Most commonly found with postrenal azotemia May be found when prerenal azotemia is superimposed on renal disease.
Normal Ratio with Elevated Urea and Creatinine Levels	End stage renal disease Acute renal failure Glomerular disease (acute nephritic syndrome, rapidly progressing glomerulonephritis, chronic glomerulonephritis, nephrotic syndrome) Tubular disease (acute pyelonephritis)	Typically found with renal diseases

Summary of Uric Acid Alterations

ALTERATION	DESCRIPTION	CAUSES
Hyperuricemia	Plasma uric acid level >7 mg/dL in men and >6 mg/dL in women May lead to gout in which the urates precipitate in joints, causing arthritic symptoms and in the kidney, causing urate crystals in the urine that may lead to stone formation.	Overproduction due to enzyme deficiency Renal disease Increased breakdown of nucleated cells (as in malignancy) Low doses of salicylates
Hypouricemia	Plasma uric acid level <2 mg/dL	Secondary to severe hepatocellular disease, defective renal tubular reabsorption, or overtreatment of hyperuricemia with drugs High doses of salicylates Use of thiazide diuretics

NONPROTEIN NITROGENOUS COMPOUNDS

BIBLIOGRAPHY

Anderson SC, Cockayne S: Clinical Chemistry: Concepts and Applications. Philadelphia, WB Saunders, 1993.

Bishop M, Duben-Engelkirk JL, Fody EP: Clinical Chemistry: Principles, Procedures, Correlations, 3rd ed. Philadelphia, JB Lippincott, 1996.

Burtis CA, Ashwood ER: Tietz Fundamentals of Clinical Chemistry, 4th ed. Philadelphia, WB Saunders, 1996.

Chonko AM, Grantham JJ: Disorders of urate metabolism and excretion. In Brenner BM, Rector FC, eds: The Kidney, 4th ed. Philadelphia, WB Saunders, 1991.

Cohen EP, Lehmann J Jr: The role of the laboratory in evaluation of kidney function. Clin Chem 37:785, 1991.

Davis BB, Zenser TV: Evaluation of renal concentrating and diluting ability. Clin Lab Med 13:131, 1993.

Duarte CG, Preuss HG: Assessment of renal function—glomerular and tubular. Clin Lab Med 13:33, 1993.

Garcia PJ, Mateos FA: Clinical and biochemical aspects of uric acid overproduction. Pharm World Sci 16:40, 1994.

Geyer SJ: Urinalysis and urinary sediment in patients with renal disease. Clin Lab Med 13:30, 1993.

Henry JB: Clinical Diagnosis and Management by Laboratory Methods, 19th ed. Philadelphia, WB Saunders, 1996.

Kaplan L, Pesce AJ: Clinical Chemistry: Theory, Analysis, Correlation, 3rd ed. St. Louis, Mosby–Year Book, 1996.

Levey AS, Madaio MP, Perrone RD: Laboratory assessment of renal disease: clearance, urinalysis, and renal biopsy. In Brenner BM, Rector RC Jr, eds: The Kidney, 4th ed, Vol 1. Philadelphia, WB Saunders, 1991, p 919.

Madias NE, Perrone RD: Acid-base disorders in association with renal disease. In Schrier RW, Gottschalk CW, eds: Disease of the Kidney. Boston, Little, Brown, 1993.

Marshall WJ: Clinical Chemistry, 3rd ed. St. Louis, Mosby–Year Book, 1995.

Orsonneau J, Massoubre C, Cabanes M, Lustenberger P: Simple and sensitive determination of urea in serum and urine. Clin Chem 38:619, 1992.

Perrone RD, Madias NE, Levey AS: Serum creatinine as an index of renal function: new insights into old concepts. Clin Chem 38:1933, 1992.

Rajs G, Mayer M: Oxidation markedly reduces bilirubin interference in the Jaffe creatinine assay, Clin Chem 38:2411, 1992.

Rosano TG, Ambrose RT, Wu AHB, et al: Candidate reference method for determining creatinine in serum: method development and interlaboratory validation. Clin Chem 36:1951, 1990.

Sugita O, Uchiyama K, Yamada T, et al: Reference values of serum and urine creatinine, and of creatinine clearance by a new enzymatic method. Ann Clin Biochem 29:523, 1992.

Tietz NW, ed: Clinical Guide to Laboratory Tests, 3rd ed. Philadelphia, WB Saunders, 1995.

Weber JA, van Zanten AP: Interferences in current methods for measurement of creatinine. Clin Chem 37:965, 1991.

Chapter **11**

BLOOD GASES AND ACID BASE BALANCE

Karen M. Escolas, MS, MT (ASCP)

Q U I C K   C O N T E N T S

INTRODUCTION

Blood Gases

The process of respiration supplies oxygen to tissues and removes the carbon dioxide produced by cellular metabolic activity. External respiration takes place at the alveolar surface in the lung where oxygen in the air is exchanged with carbon dioxide in the blood. Internal respiration takes place at the body tissues where oxygen in the blood is delivered to the cells and carbon dioxide is transferred from the cells to the blood for disposal.

Regulation of respiration is carried out through neurochemical mediation. The medullary respiratory center of the brain stem is capable of altering the rate and depth of respiration. Central chemoreceptors at the medulla oblongata and peripheral chemoreceptors in the carotid bodies and aortic bodies regulate the medullary respiratory center. The peripheral chemoreceptors are stimulated by either a decreased oxygen or an increased carbon dioxide level, while the central chemoreceptors respond only to an increased carbon dioxide level.

The exchange of gases is dependent on the partial pressure gradients at the surfaces of the cells involved in the exchange. For example, at the alveolar surface, the partial pressure of oxygen in the air is greater than that in the blood; therefore, oxygen moves into the blood. Hemoglobin in the red blood cell is responsible for transportation of oxygen and carbon dioxide through the circulatory system. The oxygen saturation refers to the amount of hemoglobin that is saturated with oxygen at the time of sampling.

Acid Base Control

The body normally maintains the arterial blood pH within a very strict range of 7.35 to 7.45. This is accomplished through the buffering capacity of the interaction of the bicarbonate system, hemoglobin, phosphate, and proteins.

Metabolic processes produce 15 to 20 mol of hydrogen ions in the body each day. The body is capable of functioning with plasma levels between 36 and 44 nmol/L of hydrogen ions. Deviations from this hydrogen ion concentration cause changes in the rates of chemical reactions in cells and metabolic processes in the body. At concentrations greater than 44 nmol/L, consciousness is altered, leading to eventual coma and death. At concentrations below 36 nmol/L, symptoms of neuromuscular irritability and tetany are evident, followed by loss of consciousness and eventual death.

The respiratory system controls the body pH through removal of the waste product carbon dioxide, a component of the bicarbonate system. The chemical reactions of the bicarbonate system are as follows:

$$H_2O + CO_2 \leftrightarrow H_2CO_3 \leftrightarrow H^+ + HCO_3^-$$

In the tissues, hemoglobin picks up a portion of the cellular carbon dioxide forming carbaminohemoglobin. The remainder of the carbon dioxide combines with water to form carbonic acid, which dissociates to form hydrogen ions and bicarbonate ions. The hydrogen ions will bind to deoxygenated hemoglobin and the bicarbonate will move out of the cell in exchange for chloride moving into the cell, referred to as the chloride shift. At the lungs, the hydrogen ions bound to deoxygenated hemoglobin are released when oxygen binds the hemoglobin. The hydrogen ions then bind to bicarbonate ions to form carbonic acid, which then forms water and carbon dioxide that is expired into the air.

The renal system controls the pH by altering the rates of reabsorption, secretion, and excretion. The kidney is able to increase either the excretion or reabsorption of hydrogen ions in exchange for sodium and potassium ions to maintain electroneutrality. The rate of bicarbonate reabsorption may also be altered in response to the pH as bicarbonate acts as a base in the carbonic acid system. Bicarbonate is exchanged for other anions such as chloride and phosphate to maintain electroneutrality. The kidney is also capable of increasing or decreasing the rate of ammonia (NH_3) formation to either excrete excess hydrogen ions as ammonium ions (NH_4^+) in acidosis or conserve hydrogen ions in alkalosis.

The ability of both the respiratory and renal systems to react to acid base disturbances by attempting to restore the pH to a normal level is termed *compensation*. The respiratory system is capable of immediate compensatory response, while the renal system may take several days to reach a detectable level of compensation.

Henderson-Hasselbalch Equation

Defined as the log expression of the ionization constant equation of a weak acid, the Henderson-Hasselbalch equation is used to express mathematically the pH that is obtained as the components of the buffer system become altered:

$$pH = pK_a + \log \frac{[HCO_3^-]}{[H_2CO_3]}$$

The pK_a of the bicarbonate system is 6.1 and the carbonic acid concentration may be expressed as the partial pressure of carbon dioxide (PCO_2) multiplied by the solubility coefficient or alpha factor (0.03). As a result, the pH is equal to the pK$_a$ added to the log of the ratio of bicarbonate to carbon dioxide. In the normal pH range of 7.35 to 7.45, this ratio should be approximately 20:1. As the bicarbonate level rises or lowers, the pH will rise or lower in direct proportion. Conversely, as PCO$_2$ rises or lowers, pH will be altered in inverse proportion.

PATIENT PREPARATION, SPECIMEN COLLECTION AND STORAGE, REFERENCE RANGE

TEST	PATIENT PREPARATION	SPECIMEN COLLECTION	SPECIMEN STORAGE	REFERENCE RANGE
Arterial or Venous Blood Gases	Avoid patient pain and anxiety, which may cause hyperventilation (results in decreased carbon dioxide and increased pH results). Must be timed as appropriate to any respiratory treatment. No finger flexing or clenched fist (lowers PO$_2$ and increases acid metabolites). PCO$_2$ values become decreased in sitting or standing position (in comparison with supine position).	Whole blood is required. ARTERIAL: Syringe and needle, no tourniquet, no pull on plunger VENOUS: Needle and syringe or heparinized evacuated tube completely filled, drawn few seconds after tourniquet applied Drawn anaerobically (air exposure causes increased pH, decreased carbon dioxide, and increased oxygen unless patient is on oxygen therapy). Liquid heparin is the only suitable anticoagulant in the proper amount (low levels result in clot formation, high levels increase carbon dioxide and decrease pH and cause dilutional error). Glass collection device better than plastic (glass remains gastight for 2 hr while plastic is not gastight—oxygen and carbon dioxide blood levels shift to match atmospheric levels).	Stored anaerobically (see Collection) Analyze ASAP (glycolysis causes decreased pH, increased carbon dioxide, and decreased oxygen levels upon standing). If testing delayed more than 5 min, store in ice water slush for up to 30 min (slows the process of glycolysis).	PO$_2$: 80–108 mm Hg (dependent on altitude) PCO$_2$ (adult): Males: 35–48 mm Hg Females: 32–45 mm Hg pH: Arterial: 7.35–7.45 Venous: 7.32–7.43 O$_2$ SATURATION: 94%–98% (decreases with age) HCO$_3$: 22–26 mmol/L

Continued ▶

▶ Continued **PATIENT PREPARATION, SPECIMEN COLLECTION AND STORAGE, REFERENCE RANGE**

TEST	PATIENT PREPARATION	SPECIMEN COLLECTION	SPECIMEN STORAGE	REFERENCE RANGE
Capillary Blood Gases	Same precautions as arterial and venous collection. Used primarily for neonatal testing. Warm site to 45°C before collection. Wipe away the first drop of blood.	Same precautions as arterial and venous collection Use capillary tube coated with heparin and insert a metal flea to mix after collection.		

DIAGNOSTIC TESTS AND METHODOLOGIES

TEST	METHOD	INTERFERENCE	COMMENTS
Pco_2	Electrochemistry (a Teflon or silicone gas permeable membrane allows CO_2 to enter the tip of the electrode, and an internal hydrogen ion sensitive electrode measures the change in pH as the CO_2 enters the electrode and interacts with the interior buffer).		Levels increase with increased temperature; therefore, the value measured may be temperature corrected for increased accuracy.
PO_2	Polarography (a polypropylene membrane allows oxygen into the electrode—oxygen reacts with the cathode generating current that is measured).	Anesthetics may cause slight false elevations. Must be calibrated to appropriate range. Sensitive to temperature of instrument for accurate results. High WBC counts result in false decreases as WBCs use oxygen for glycolysis when specimen is not handled properly.	Must be temperature corrected if 1°C difference from 37°C.
pH	Ion selective electrode (glass tip sensitive to hydrogen ions)	Protein, lipid, and platelet deposits on the glass tip cause erratic response.	May be temperature corrected for accuracy.

EVALUATING TEST RESULTS

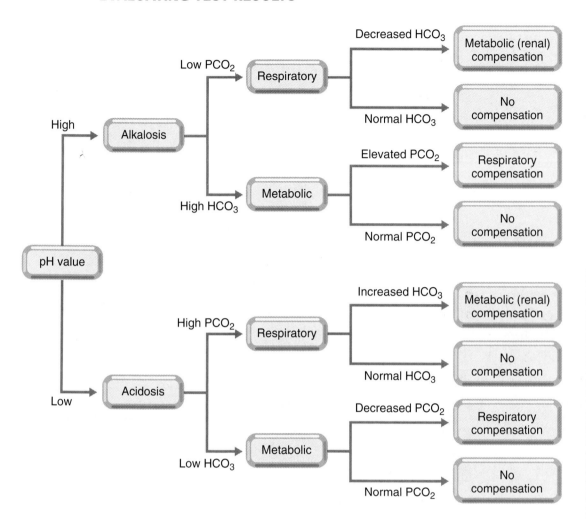

Change of Analyte in Disease

ANALYTE	MEASUREMENT	CLINICAL SIGNIFICANCE	COMMENTS
Partial Pressure of Oxygen (PO$_2$)	Clark oxygen electrode used to measure arterial blood gas level	ELEVATED: Angiomas of the brain DECREASED: Hypoxemia Decreased cardiac output Carbon monoxide exposure Anesthesia Near drowning Decreased alveolar gas exchange (as in respiratory distress syndrome) Ventilation/perfusion inequalities (as in bronchitis, asthma, emphysema, pneumonia, obstruction of airway) Alveolar hypoventilation (as in suffocation, submersion, respiratory center depression by drugs or head injury)	Elevated levels also occur when the patient is breathing oxygen enriched air or is undergoing strenuous exercise. Levels of <40 mm Hg indicate severe hypoxemia. Levels of <20 mm Hg frequently result in death.
P$_{50}$ Oxygen	The PO$_2$ at half saturation of hemoglobin as measured spectrophotometrically in whole blood	ELEVATED: Oxygen dissociation curve shifted to right (hemoglobin has decreased affinity for oxygen): ■ Hyperthermia ■ Acidosis ■ Hypercapnia ■ Increased 2,3-DPG DECREASED: Oxygen dissociation curve shifted to the left (hemoglobin has increased affinity for oxygen): ■ Hypothermia ■ Acute alkalosis ■ Hypocapnia ■ Decreased 2,3-DPG ■ Preeclampsia	Measurement of the affinity of hemoglobin for oxygen is an indicator of the delivery rate of oxygen to tissues. Temperature, pH, 2,3-DPG level, and type of hemoglobin influence the P$_{50}$ value. Elevated levels occur during uncomplicated pregnancy.
Oxygen Saturation (SO$_2$)	Arterial whole blood oxygen saturation is estimated using the following calculation: $$SO_2 = \frac{O_2Hb}{(O_2Hb + HHb)} \times 100\%$$	NORMAL VALUES: 94%–98% saturation DECREASED: Hypoxemia Anemia (low level of RBC and/or hemoglobin) Abnormal hemoglobins	SO$_2$, in conjunction with P$_{50}$ value, indicates the availability of oxygen to the tissues.

Continued ▶

▶ Continued **Change of Analyte in Disease**

ANALYTE	MEASUREMENT	CLINICAL SIGNIFICANCE	COMMENTS
Partial Pressure of Carbon Dioxide (P_{CO_2})	Determined in whole arterial blood by potentiometric method	ELEVATED: Respiratory acidosis Compensation for metabolic alkalosis DECREASED: Respiratory alkalosis Compensation for metabolic acidosis	Levels >80 mm Hg may result in death.
pH	Measured in arterial whole blood sample by potentiometry	ELEVATED: Metabolic alkalosis Respiratory alkalosis DECREASED: Metabolic acidosis Respiratory acidosis	Must be maintained between 6.80 and 7.80 for compatibility with life.
Bicarbonate	Calculated by the following formula (Henderson-Hasselbalch equation): $$pH = pK_a + \frac{[HCO_3]}{0.03(P_{CO_2})}$$	ELEVATED: Metabolic alkalosis Compensated respiratory acidosis DECREASED: Metabolic acidosis Compensated respiratory alkalosis	Nomograms are also available for determination of bicarbonate value.
Base Excess	Determined from a nomogram or computed in blood gas instruments.	POSITIVE BASE EXCESS (excess bicarbonate): Metabolic alkalosis Acute respiratory alkalosis NEGATIVE BASE EXCESS (deficit of bicarbonate or base deficit): Metabolic acidosis Acute respiratory acidosis	Represents base concentration of whole blood upon titration with strong acid to pH 7.4 at P_{CO_2} of 40 mm Hg at 37°C. Allows estimation of milliliters of sodium bicarbonate or ammonium chloride that should be administered to correct the patient's pH when an acid base disturbance is diagnosed.

EVALUATING TEST RESULTS

DISORDERS OF ACID BASE BALANCE

DISORDER	DEFINITION	COMPENSATION	CAUSES
Metabolic Acidosis	An absolute bicarbonate deficit resulting in decreased pH and bicarbonate and a base deficit	Pco_2 becomes decreased owing to respiratory compensation, and urine becomes acidic with normal renal function as hydrogen ions are excreted and bicarbonate ions are re-absorbed.	Increased production of acid: ■ Ketoacidosis (diabetes, starvation) ■ Lactic acidosis (hypoxia) Decreased excretion of hydrogen ions ■ Renal failure ■ Renal tubular acidosis ■ Fanconi's syndrome ■ Addison's disease Accumulation of acid metabolites: ■ Late salicylate poisoning Increased loss of alkaline body fluids ■ Intestinal (diarrhea)
Metabolic Alkalosis	An absolute bicarbonate excess that results in increased pH and bicarbonate level and a base excess	Pco_2 becomes increased with respiratory compensation, and urine becomes alkaline with normal renal function owing to decreased excretion of hydrogen ions and re-absorption of bicarbonate.	Excessive $NaHCO_3$ infusion Citrate (as with blood transfusions) Antacids Prolonged vomiting (due to loss of HCl) Potassium depletion (K^+ and H^+ exchanged at cells and distal tubules) Prolonged use of diuretics
Respiratory Acidosis	An absolute carbon dioxide excess that results in decreased pH and increased Pco_2 and a base deficit	Bicarbonate becomes increased with normal renal function owing to increased excretion of hydrogen ions and reabsorption of bicarbonate.	Emphysema Pneumonia Rebreathing air (as in a paper bag) Airway obstruction (as in choking) Pulmonary edema Drugs that depress the respiratory control center in the brain (e.g., barbiturates) Congestive heart failure
Respiratory Alkalosis	An absolute carbon dioxide deficit that results in increased pH and decreased Pco_2 and a base excess	Renal compensatory mechanisms are too slow to adjust pH before the patient loses consciousness and proper breathing rate is restored.	Hyperventilation Early salicylate poisoning Anxiety Head injury that results in stimulation of the control center in the brain Excessive artificial ventilation

BIBLIOGRAPHY

Anderson SC, Cockayne S: Clinical Chemistry: Concepts and Applications. Philadelphia, WB Saunders, 1993.

Arieff Al, Defronzo RA: Fluid, Electrolyte and Acid-Base Disorders, 2nd ed., New York, Churchill Livingstone, 1995.

Bishop M, Duben-Engelkirk JL, Fody EP: Clinical Chemistry: Principles, Procedures, Correlations, 3rd ed., Philadelphia, JB Lippincott, 1996.

Burnett RW, Covington AK, Fogh-Anderson N, et al: Recommendations on whole blood sampling, transport, and storage for simultaneous determination of pH, blood gases, and electrolytes. J Int Fed Clin Chem 6:115, 1994.

Burtis CA, Ashwood ER: Tietz Fundamentals of Clinical Chemistry, 4th ed. Philadelphia, WB Saunders, 1996.

Ehrmeyer S, et al: Definitions of quantities and conventions related to blood pH and gas analysis (C12-T2). Villanova, PA, National Committee for Clinical Laboratory Standards, 1991.

Ehrmeyer S, et al: Fractional oxyhemoglobin, oxygen content and saturation, and related quantities in blood: terminology, measurement, and reporting (C-25T). Villanova, PA, National Committee for Clinical Laboratory Standards, 1992.

Ehrmeyer S, et al: Performance characteristics for devices measuring PO_2 and PCO_2 in blood sample (C21-A). Villanova, PA, National Committee for Clinical Laboratory Standards, 1992.

Ehrmeyer S, et al: Blood gas pre-analytical considerations: specimen collection, calibration, and controls (C27-A). Villanova, PA, National Committee for Clinical Laboratory Standards, 1993.

Haber RJ: A practical approach to acid-base disorders. West J Med 155:146, 1991.

Henry JB: Clinical Diagnosis and Management by Laboratory Methods, 19th ed. Philadelphia, WB Saunders, 1996.

Kaplan L, Pesce AJ: Clinical Chemistry: Theory, Analysis, Correlation, 3rd ed. St. Louis, Mosby–Year Book, 1996.

Maas AHJ: IFCC reference methods for measurement of pH, gases, and electrolytes in blood. Scand J Clin Lab Invest 53:83, 1993.

Mahoney JJ, et al: Changes in oxygen measurements when whole blood is stored in iced plastic or glass syringes. Clin Chem 37:1244, 1991.

Marshall WJ: Clinical Chemistry, 3rd ed. St. Louis, Mosby–Year Book, 1995.

Miller-Plathe O, Heyduck S: Stability of blood gases, electrolytes, and hemoglobin in heparinized whole blood samples: influence of the type of syringe. Eur J Clin Chem Biochem 30:349, 1992.

Preuss HG: Fundamentals of clinical acid-base evaluation. Clin Lab Med 13:103, 1993.

Roberts GH: Acid-base balance and arterial blood gases: an instructional text. Clin Lab Sci 3:171, 1990.

Rosenberg E, Price N: Diffusion of CO_2 and O_2 through the walls of plastic syringes. Clin Chem 37:1244, 1991.

Scanlon CL, Spearman CD, Sheldon R: Egan's Fundamentals of Respiratory Care, 6th ed. St. Louis, Mosby–Year Book, 1995.

Tietz NW, ed: Clinical Guide to Laboratory Tests, 3rd ed. Philadelphia, WB Saunders, 1995.

Chapter **12**

MINERAL METABOLISM

Karen M. Escolas, MS, MT (ASCP)

QUICK CONTENTS

INTRODUCTION

The metabolism of the body minerals calcium, phosphate, and magnesium is intricately tied to the process of skeletal homeostasis. Bone is made of organic collagen and inorganic deposits of calcium phosphate called hydroxyapatite. A small portion of the bone structure is occupied by osteoblasts, the cells that undertake the process of synthesizing bone matrix referred to as deposition or formation, and osteoclasts, the cells that demineralize and digest bone matrix in the process of resorption. The remainder of the bone structure is a calcified matrix of collagen, consisting of the amino acids proline and hydroxyproline; noncollagen protein, primarily osteocalcin; and glycosaminoglycans containing ground substance in which hydroxyapatite crystals are embedded. The process of bone modeling or skeletal homeostasis is a balance between the formation and resorption processes that is also reliant upon the functions of intestinal absorption and renal clearance to maintain mineral levels in the body. This homeostatic process is regulated primarily by the calcitropic hormones parathyroid hormone (PTH or parathyrin), $1,25\text{-}(OH)_2\text{-vitamin } D_3$ (calcitriol), and calcitonin. Assessment of mineral and skeletal homeostasis is accomplished through evaluation of the following chemical markers: total and free (ionized) calcium, phosphate, magnesium, PTH, vitamin D metabolites, calcitonin, PTH related protein (PTHrP), markers of bone formation including osteocalcin and alkaline phosphatase (ALP), and markers of bone resorption such as pyridinoline crosslinks.

SUMMARY OF THE MAJOR MINERALS

MINERAL	BODY SOURCES	HANDLING	FUNCTION	COMMENTS
Calcium	99% in bone structure Plasma forms: ▪ 50% free or ionized (active) ▪ 40% bound to protein ▪ 10% complexed with anions	Absorption in intestine influenced by vitamin D Deposition on bone with excess excreted by kidney influenced by PTH	Maintenance of intracellular Ca^{++} Bone mineralization and structure Blood coagulation Maintenance of plasma membrane potential Muscle contraction Neurotransmission Cofactor in enzymatic reactions	Decreased Ca^{++} causes increased neuromuscular excitability and tetany. Elevated Ca^{++} causes decreased neuromuscular excitability and weakness. Protein-bound fraction is pH dependent: a higher pH will result in increased negative charge on protein and higher level of bound calcium (and thus lower ionized calcium).
Phosphorus	80%–85% bone structure 9% muscular tissue Remainder viscera and extracellular fluid	Absorption in intestine influenced by vitamin D Deposition on bone and excretion by kidney influenced by PTH	Contributor to structural support and regulation of phosphate pools Energy generation and storage (ATP or NADP) Phospholipid structure in cellular membranes Nucleic acids Phosphoproteins Enzyme systems Gene transcription Cell growth	
Magnesium	50%–60% skeletal Remainder intracellular fluid (muscle and other cells) 1% plasma ▪ 55% free or ionized form ▪ 30% protein bound ▪ 15% complexed with anions	Absorption in intestine Excretion by kidney	Cofactor for more than 300 enzymes Activator for many other enzymes Oxidative phosphorylation Glycolysis Cellular respiration Nucleotide metabolism Protein biosynthesis	Decreased Mg^{++} causes increased neuromuscular excitability and tetany. Increased Mg^{++} causes decreased neuromuscular excitability and weakness.

HORMONES THAT REGULATE MINERAL HOMEOSTASIS

HORMONE	PRODUCTION	FORMS	REGULATION OF SYNTHESIS	RECEPTORS	OVERALL EFFECTS
Parathyroid Hormone (PTH)	In chief cells of parathyroid gland: ■ PreproPTH produced ■ Pre and pro segments removed ■ PTH released into plasma	N-terminal fragment = active C-terminal fragment = inactive Intact PTH = active form	Inverse, negative feedback mechanism of Ca^{++} main regulator Inverse, negative feedback mechanism of calcitriol and extreme Mg^{++} levels Direct negative effect of phosphorus levels	Cell membranes of kidney and bone	Increased plasma levels of Ca^{++} and calcitriol Decreased plasma level of phosphorus Increased urine levels of calcium, phosphorus, and cyclic AMP
Vitamin D	1. Dietary vitamin D converted to provitamin D in small intestine 2. Provitamin D converted to vitamin D_3 through exposure of skin to sunlight 3. Vitamin D_3 hydroxylated to calcidiol in the liver 4. Kidney hydroxylates calcidiol to form calcitriol and 24,25-$(OH)_2$-vitamin D_3.	Provitamin D_3 = 7-dehydrocholesterol Vitamin D_3 = cholecalciferol Calcidiol = 25-hydroxyvitaminD_3 (main storage form) Calcitriol = 1,25-$(OH)_2$-vitaminD_3 (active form) 24,25-$(OH)_2$-vitaminD_3 = waste product	Stimulated by increased levels of plasma PTH and decreased levels of phosphorus Indirect stimulation by decreased Ca^{++} through PTH action	Cells of bone and intestine	Increased plasma levels of calcium and phosphorus
Calcitonin	C cells of thyroid gland main site of production Also pituitary gland, gastrointestinal tract, and liver	Intact calcitonin	Directly stimulated by elevated Ca^{++} level	Osteoclasts in bone	Decreased plasma Ca^{++} level
PTH Related Protein (PTHrP)	Many tissues normally produce very small amounts. Tumors secrete large concentrations.	Intact PTHrP	Uncontrolled secretion by tumor cells	Same as PTH	Markedly elevated plasma Ca^{++} level

HORMONAL REGULATION OF MINERAL HOMEOSTASIS

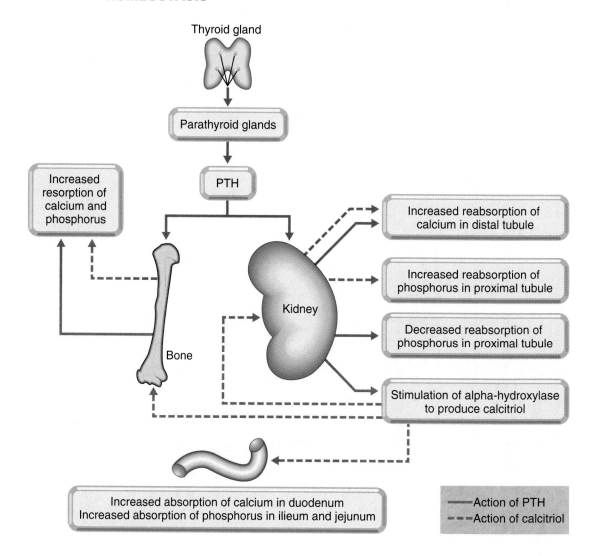

Thyroid gland

Parathyroid glands

PTH

Increased resorption of calcium and phosphorus

Bone

Kidney

Increased reabsorption of calcium in distal tubule

Increased reabsorption of phosphorus in proximal tubule

Decreased reabsorption of phosphorus in proximal tubule

Stimulation of alpha-hydroxylase to produce calcitriol

Increased absorption of calcium in duodenum
Increased absorption of phosphorus in ilieum and jejunum

—— Action of PTH
– – – Action of calcitriol

PATIENT PREPARATION, SPECIMEN COLLECTION AND STORAGE, REFERENCE RANGE

TEST	PATIENT PREPARATION	SPECIMEN COLLECTION	SPECIMEN STORAGE	REFERENCE RANGE
Ionized Calcium	Nonfasting specimen is acceptable. Stasis should be avoided.	Serum Heparinized plasma or whole blood (excess heparin lowers results by 3%–5%). Anticoagulants that chelate calcium cannot be used (citrate, oxalate, EDTA).	Stable 6 hr at 4°C (reduces glycolysis, which would alter pH and protein binding). Maintain anaerobic until tested (minimizes CO_2 loss, which would also alter pH).	4.65–5.28 mg/dL
Total Calcium	Fasting specimen is preferred. Venous stasis or erect posture elevate result by 0.6 mg/dL. Diurnal variation (higher in PM than in AM)	Serum Heparinized plasma (no chelating additives as with ionized calcium) Urine: 24 hr specimen	Stable 8 hr at 22°–25°C, days at 4°C, months if frozen Separate from RBC promptly to avoid RBC uptake of calcium. 10–20 mL 6M HCl added to 24 hr urine	SERUM/PLASMA: 8.0–10.5 mg/dL URINE: 100–300 mg/day
Inorganic Phosphate	Fasting AM specimen (diurnal variation causes elevated levels in PM and dietary intake influences level). Exercise causes increased levels. Transient lower level after meals due to change in pH and insulin action Avoid venous stasis.	Serum Heparinized plasma (other anticoagulants inhibit complex formation in assay). Hemolysis falsely elevates level by releasing phosphate esters from RBC. Urine: 24 hr specimen	Stable at 4°C for days, months when frozen Separate from cells ASAP to avoid leakage of phosphate from cells. Level will increase when stored at room temperature or 37°C. Urine specimen must be acidified with HCl to pH of 2–3 after collection; stable for 6 mo.	SERUM/PLASMA: 2.5–4.8 mg/dL URINE: 0.4–1.3 g/day

Continued ▶

▶ Continued **PATIENT PREPARATION, SPECIMEN COLLECTION AND STORAGE, REFERENCE RANGE**

TEST	PATIENT PREPARATION	SPECIMEN COLLECTION	SPECIMEN STORAGE	REFERENCE RANGE
Total Magnesium	Fasting specimen is preferred. Avoid venous stasis.	Serum or heparinized plasma (other anti-coagulants chelate magnesium). No hemolysis (Mg^{++} released from RBC) Urine: 24 hr specimen	Stable 4°C for several days, months frozen Separate from RBC ASAP to avoid leakage from cells. Urine acidified to pH of 1 with concentrated HCl (prevents precipitation)	SERUM/PLASMA: 1.5–2.6 mEq/L or 1.8–2.3 mg/dL URINE: 6.0–10.0 mEq/day
Free Magnesium	Fasting specimen is preferred.	Serum Heparinized plasma or whole blood	Same as total magnesium	1.0–1.5 mEq/L
PTH	Fasting AM specimen is preferred.	Serum or plasma (EDTA anticoagulant of choice)	Place on ice. Separate promptly in refrigerated centrifuge and store frozen if not assayed immediately.	C-TERMINAL: 50–330 pg/mL N-TERMINAL: 8–24 pg/mL INTACT MOLECULE: 10–65 pg/mL
Vitamin D (Calcitriol and Calcidiol)	Nonfasting specimen is acceptable.	Serum (for metabolites) Plasma (acceptable for extraction and chromatography methods)	Stable at 22°–25°C or 4°C, freeze if delayed assay Not sensitive to light exposure	CALCITRIOL: 16–65 pg/mL CALCIDIOL: 14–60 pg/mL
Calcitonin	Fasting specimen Males have higher levels than females. Levels higher in pregnant/lactating females and childhood/infancy	Serum or heparinized plasma	Freeze immediately at −20°C or lower.	SERUM: <150 pg/mL PLASMA: M: <19 pg/mL F: <14 pg/mL

Continued ▶

► Continued **PATIENT PREPARATION, SPECIMEN COLLECTION AND STORAGE, REFERENCE RANGE**

TEST	PATIENT PREPARATION	SPECIMEN COLLECTION	SPECIMEN STORAGE	REFERENCE RANGE
PTHrP	Nonfasting specimen is acceptable.	Serum or heparinized plasma Collect in tubes with protease inhibitors (e.g., aprotinin, leupeptin).	Chill ASAP in ice water and separate using refrigerated centrifuge. Freeze for prolonged storage. Separate from RBC promptly.	<1.5 pmol/L

DIAGNOSTIC TESTS AND METHODOLOGIES

TEST	METHOD	INTERFERENCE	COMMENTS
Ionized Calcium	Ion selective electrode	Protein build-up	Routine method
Total Calcium	Photometric assay (calcium binds dyes such as cresolphthalein, arsenazo III)	Biologic pigments cause false positive results (hemolysis, icterus, lipemia, paraproteins, magnesium).	Magnesium interference removed by 8-hydroxyquinoline Addition of potassium cyanide (KCN) stabilizes color, eliminates metal interference. Most commonly used routine method
	Atomic absorption spectroscopy	Protein (resolved through dilution) Phosphate (resolved through addition of lanthanum)	Highly sensitive and specific Reference method
	Isotope dilution-mass spectroscopy		Definitive method with which all other methods are compared
Inorganic Phosphate	Photometric assay (ammonium molybdate forms phosphomolybdate complex, which may be read in ultraviolet (UV) range or reduced to read in visible range)	Hemolysis, icterus, lipemia, mannitol, and fluoride interfere with chemical reaction. Anticoagulants other than heparin interfere with complex formation.	Phosphorus contamination on glassware must be avoided (common in detergent). Oldest but still most commonly used routine method

Continued ►

► Continued **DIAGNOSTIC TESTS AND METHODOLOGIES**

TEST	METHOD	INTERFERENCE	COMMENTS
Total Magnesium	Photometric assay (metal-lochromic indicators such as calmagite, formazan dye, methylthymol blue, and magon react with Mg).	Hemolysis, icterus, lipemia cause positive interference.	Addition of KCN eliminates metal interference. Addition of EGTA prevents interference by calcium. Commonly used for automated methods
	Atomic absorption spectroscopy		Reference method owing to greater precision and accuracy
Ionized Magnesium	Ion selective electrode		Not routinely measured at present time
PTH	Competitive RIA for C-terminal, N-terminal, or midregion	Heterogeneity of circulating PTH makes it difficult to determine accurate PTH levels.	Limited specificity and sensitivity
	Two-site labeled antibody for intact PTH		Improved clinical usefulness
Vitamin D	Separated by polarity owing to presence and number of hydroxyl groups		Measures both vitamin D_2 and D_3 forms
Calcidiol,	Requires extraction from protein carriers, purification to separate interferents, and quantitation by competitive protein binding assay, RIA, or UV absorption		Calcidiol good indicator of vitamin D status
Calcitriol			Calcitriol good indicator of active form status
Calcitonin	RIA	Gross lipemia and hemolysis may interfere with reaction.	Wide range of sensitivity and specificity
	IRMA		Improved sensitivity and specificity
PTHrP	RIA		Wide range of sensitivity and specificity
	IRMA		More sensitive and specific
			Newer development

EVALUATING TEST RESULTS

Summary of Causes of Mineral Alterations

ALTERATION	DEFINITION	CAUSES	COMMENTS
Hypercalcemia	Plasma level >10.5 mg/dL	MALIGNANCY: Skeletal metastases Humoral hypercalcemia of malignancy (PTHrP) Hematologic Coexisting hyperparathyroidism Multiple myeloma ENDOCRINE DISORDERS: Primary hyperparathyroidism Acute adrenal insufficiency (Addison's disease) Hyperthyroidism Withdrawal of steroids MISCELLANEOUS: Vitamin D overdose Thiazide diuretics Milk-alkali syndrome Sarcoidosis and other granulomatous diseases Renal failure	Typically accompanied by muscle weakness and disorientation Approximately 90% of cases are the result of either hyperparathyroidism or hypercalcemia of malignancy.
Hypocalcemia	Plasma calcium level <8.5 mg/dL	Hypoalbuminemia Chronic renal failure Hypomagnesemia Vitamin D deficiency Hypoparathyroidism (lack of PTH) Pseudohypoparathyroidism (lack of response to PTH)	Typically accompanied by tetany The most common cause is hypoalbuminemia, in which the ionized fraction may actually be normal while the total calcium level is decreased owing to a low percentage of calcium bound to albumin. The following formula may be used to correct the total calcium result: Corrected calcium = (measured calcium − albumin [g/dL]) +4

Continued ▶

▶ Continued **Summary of Causes of Mineral Alterations**

ALTERATION	DEFINITION	CAUSES	COMMENTS
Hyperphosphatemia	Plasma level >4.7 mg/dL	**INCREASED RENAL REAB-SORPTION:** Hypoparathyroidism Pseudohypoparathyroidism Hyperthyroidism Hypogonadism Excess vitamin D Growth hormone excess **MASSIVE CELL DESTRUCTION:** Cytotoxic therapy Tissue injuries such as: ▪ Crushing injuries ▪ Hyperthermia ▪ Hypoxia **INCREASED BODY LOAD:** Blood transfusion Hyperalimentation High-phosphorus laxatives High-phosphorus enemas	The most common cause is renal failure.
Hypophosphatemia	Plasma level <2.4 mg/dL	Decreased intestinal absorption Increased renal excretion (as in hyperparathyroidism) Impaired renal reabsorption Intracellular shift due to insulin action (as during recovery phase of diabetic ketoacidosis with administration of insulin or glucose therapy)	
Hypermagnesemia	Plasma level >2.5 mEq/L	Dehydration Renal insufficiency (may result in significantly elevated levels) Uncontrolled diabetes mellitus Adrenocortical insufficiency Addison's disease Tissue trauma Hypothyroidism	Significant hypermagnesemia is an uncommon occurrence. Extremely high concentrations cause respiratory paralysis and cardiac arrest.
Hypomagnesemia	Plasma level <1.0 mEq/L	Malabsorption, malnutrition, fistulas Alcoholism (chronic) Cirrhosis Diuretic therapy Renal tubular disorders (level elevated in advanced stages) Chronic mineralocorticoid excess Hypoparathyroidism	Typically accompanied by tetany, agitation, delirium, muscle weakness, and cardiac arrhythmias Often found in conjunction with hypocalcemia, hypophosphatemia, and hypokalemia

BIBLIOGRAPHY

Altura BT, Altura BM: Measurement of ionized magnesium in whole blood, plasma and serum with a new ion-selective electrode in healthy and diseased human subjects. Magnes Trace Elem 10:90, 1992.

Anderson SC, Cockayne S: Clinical Chemistry: Concepts and Applications. Philadelphia, WB Saunders, 1993.

Aurbach GD, Marx SJ, Speigel AM: Parathyroid hormone, calcitonin, and the calciferols. In Wilson JD, Foster DW, eds: Williams Textbook of Endocrinology, 8th ed. Philadelphia, WB Saunders, 1992, pp 1397–1476.

Bilezikian JP: Calcium and bone metabolism. In Becker KL, ed: Principles and Practice of Endocrinology and Metabolism. Philadelphia, JB Lippincott, 1990, pp 398–569.

Birkeland KI, Gallefoss F, Olsson S, et al: Primary hyperparathyroidism or hypercalcemia of malignancy? Scand J Clin Lab Invest 52:347, 1992.

Bishop M, Duben-Engelkirk JL, Fody EP: Clinical Chemistry: Principles, Procedures, Correlations, 3rd ed. Philadelphia, JB Lippincott, 1996.

Body JJ: Calcitonin: from the determination of circulating levels in various physiological and pathological conditions to the demonstration of lymphocyte receptors. Horm Res 39:166, 1993.

Broadus AE, Stewart AF: Parathyroid hormone–related protein: structure, processing and physiologic actions. In Bilezikian JP, ed: The Parathyroids. New York, Raven Press, 1994.

Burtis CA, Ashwood ER: Tietz Fundamentals of Clinical Chemistry, 4th ed. Philadelphia, WB Saunders, 1996.

Burtis WJ: Parathyroid hormone related protein: structure, function, and measurement. Clin Chem 38:2171, 1992.

Cadeau BJ, MacKay JS: Serum calcium: review of methods. ASCP Check Sample, Vol 4, No. 8, PTS 92-1 (PTS-59), American Society of Clinical Pathologists, 1992.

Delmas PD: Biochemical markers of bone turnover. J Bone Miner Res 8(Suppl 2):S549, 1993.

DeLuca HF: New concepts of vitamin D functions. Ann N Y Acad Sci 669:59, 1992.

Elin RJ: Laboratory tests for the assessment of magnesium status in humans. Magnes Trace Elem 10:172, 1992.

Endres DB, Rude RK: Mineral and bone metabolism. In Burtis CA, Ashwood ER, eds: Tietz Textbook of Clinical Chemistry, 2nd ed. Philadelphia, WB Saunders, 1994, pp 1887–1973.

Forman DT, Lorenzo L: Ionized calcium: its significance and clinical usefulness. Ann Clin Lab Sci 21:297, 1991.

Henry JB: Clinical Diagnosis and Management by Laboratory Methods, 19th ed. Philadelphia, WB Saunders, 1996.

Holick MF, Adams JS: Vitamin D metabolism and biological function. In Avioli LV, Krane SM, eds: Metabolic Bone Disease and Clinically Related Disorders, 2nd ed. Philadelphia, WB Saunders, 1990, pp 155–195.

Igbal SJ: Vitamin D metabolism and the clinical aspects of measuring metabolites. Ann Clin Biochem 31:109, 1994.

Kao CP, Grnat CS, Klee GG, et al: Clinical performance of parathyroid hormone immunometric assays. Mayo Clin Proc 67:637, 1992.

Kaplan L, Pesce AJ: Clinical Chemistry: Theory, Analysis, Correlation, 3rd ed. St. Louis, Mosby–Year Book, 1996.

Lafferty FW: Differential diagnosis of hypercalcemia. J Bone Miner Res 6:S51, 1991.

Marshall WJ: Clinical Chemistry, 3rd ed. St. Louis, Mosby–Year Book, 1995.

Martin BJ, McGregor CW: Measurement of serum magnesium: effect of delay in separation from erythrocytes. Clin Chem 32:564, 1986.

Scott MG: Inorganic phosphorus: review of methods. ASCP Check Sample, Vol 8, No. 5, PTS 92-5 (PTS-63), American Society of Clinical Pathologists, 1992.

Segre GV, Potts JT Jr: Differential diagnosis of hypercalcemia: methods and clinical applications of parathyroid assays. In DeGroot LJ, ed: Endocrinology, 2nd ed, Vol 2. Philadelphia, WB Saunders, 1989, pp 984–1001.

Tietz NW, ed: Clinical Guide to Laboratory Tests, 3rd ed. Philadelphia, WB Saunders, 1995.

Wysolmerski JJ, Broadus AE: Hypercalcemia of malignancy: the central role of parathyroid hormone–related protein. Annu Rev Med 45:189, 1994.

Chapter

13

ENDOCRINOLOGY

Karen M. Escolas, MS, MT (ASCP)

Q U I C K   C O N T E N T S

HYPOTHALAMUS AND PITUITARY FUNCTION

INTRODUCTION

The hypothalamus and pituitary glands are located in close proximity at the base of the brain. The two glands share direct circulatory connection, which allows for the control of pituitary hormone production by the hypothalamus in response to brain stimulation. Hypothalamic hormones are neuropeptides that either stimulate or inhibit release of corresponding pituitary hormones. The levels of pituitary hormones produced in turn control the hypothalamic production of hormones through a feedback mechanism.

The pituitary gland is composed of two lobes: the anterior lobe or adenohypophysis, composed primarily of glandular tissue, and the posterior lobe or neurohypophysis, composed primarily of neural tissue. The anterior lobe produces trophic hormones that regulate virtually all other endocrine functions, the secretion of which is controlled by the hypothalamus. The posterior lobe stores hormones produced in the hypothalamus, releasing them in response to stimulation by the hypothalamus.

HORMONES OF THE HYPOTHALAMUS

HORMONE	REGULATION	PHYSIOLOGIC ACTION
Corticotropin Releasing Hormone (CRH)	Regulated through negative feedback by pituitary ACTH and adrenal cortisol	A corticotrope that stimulates production and secretion of ACTH by the anterior pituitary gland
Thyrotropin Releasing Hormone (TRH)	Regulated through negative feedback by pituitary TSH and thyroid hormones	A thyrotrope that stimulates production and secretion of TSH and prolactin by the anterior pituitary gland
Growth Hormone Releasing Hormone (GHRH or Somatocrinin)	Regulated through negative feedback by pituitary GH	A somatotrope that stimulates production and secretion of GH by the anterior pituitary gland
Growth Hormone Inhibiting Hormone (GHIH or Somatostatin)	Regulated through positive feedback by pituitary GH	Inhibits production and secretion of GH and TSH by the anterior pituitary gland
Gonadotropin Releasing Hormone (GnRH)	Regulated through negative feedback by pituitary FSH and LH	A gonadotrope that stimulates production and secretion of FSH and LH by the anterior pituitary gland
Prolactin Inhibiting Factor (PIF)	Regulated through positive feedback by pituitary prolactin, TSH, FSH, LH, and GH	Postulated to be dopamine, a neurotransmitter that inhibits the production and secretion of prolactin, TSH, FSH, LH, and GH by the anterior pituitary gland

HORMONES OF THE ANTERIOR PITUITARY GLAND (ADENOHYPOPHYSIS)

HORMONE	REGULATION	PHYSIOLOGIC ACTION
Adrenocorticotropic Hormone (ACTH)	CRH of the hypothalamus causes secretion in response to biorhythms of the brain with circadian variation.	Stimulates secretion of cortisol by the adrenal gland Causes sedation, increased pain threshold, autonomic regulation of respiration, blood pressure, and heart rate
Thyroid Stimulating Hormone (TSH) or Thyrotropin	TRH of the hypothalamus causes secretion in response to low levels of thyroid hormones in the blood.	Stimulates secretion of the thyroid hormones T_3 and T_4 by the thyroid gland
Growth Hormone (GH)	GHRH and GHIH of the hypothalamus regulate the release of GH in response to exercise; physiologic and emotional stress; hypoglycemia; amino acid, testosterone, and estrogen levels.	Promotes growth in soft tissue, cartilage, and bone Stimulates protein synthesis, fat and carbohydrate metabolism Changes electrolyte metabolism: elevates phosphorus and intestinal absorption of calcium, and decreases renal excretion of sodium and potassium Opposes insulin action in chronic disease by increasing glucose levels In acute disease, decreases glucose levels.
Prolactin (PRL)	TRH and PIF (dopamine) from the hypothalamus regulate prolactin levels. Levels are increased in fetal pituitary glands and during pregnancy. Release of PRL is stimulated by suckling and suppressed by stress.	The primary role of PRL is initiation and maintenance of lactation. PRL induces ductal growth, development of the lobular alveolar system, and synthesis of milk production. PRL controls osmolality, fat and carbohydrate metabolism, calcium and vitamin D metabolism, fetal lung development, and steroidogenesis in the ovary and testis.
Follicle Stimulating Hormone (FSH)	GnRH from the hypothalamus regulates FSH secretion by the pituitary gland.	FSH controls the functional activity of the gonads. FEMALES: Stimulates growth of ovarian follicles In presence of LH, promotes secretion of estrogen by maturing follicles MALES: Stimulates spermatogenesis

Continued ▶

▶ Continued **HORMONES OF THE ANTERIOR PITUITARY GLAND (ADENOHYPOPHYSIS)**

HORMONE	REGULATION	PHYSIOLOGIC ACTION
Luteinizing Hormone (LH)	GnRH from the hypothalamus regulates LH secretion by the pituitary gland.	LH controls the functional activity of the gonads. FEMALES: Causes release of ovum from the follicles ripened by FSH Transforms the follicle into a corpus luteum that secretes progesterone MALES: Produces testosterone by Leydig cells of the testes

HORMONES OF THE POSTERIOR PITUITARY GLAND (NEUROHYPOPHYSIS)

HORMONE	REGULATION	PHYSIOLOGIC ACTION
Antidiuretic Hormone (ADH) or Arginine Vasopressin	Stimulated by increased osmolality, plasma volume depletion, pain, stress, sleep, exercise, and chemical agents (opiates, catecholamines, angiotensin II, prostaglandins, anesthetics, nicotine, and barbiturates) Inhibited by increased plasma volume, decreased osmolality, alcohol, glucocorticoids, and phenytoin	Maintains water homeostasis (both blood osmolality and plasma volume) by increasing water reabsorption in the distal tubules and collecting ducts of the kidney, which increases the urine concentration. Also stimulates vasoconstriction to increase blood pressure.
Oxytocin	Primarily stimulated by suckling and stretch receptors of the uterus, which is enhanced by estrogen Emotional stress and psychogenic factors (e.g., fear) inhibit the release.	FEMALES (only known action): Stimulates uterine contractions during labor Stimulates the letdown reflex in mammary glands, constricting mammary ducts to release milk May be used to induce labor

PATIENT PREPARATION, SPECIMEN COLLECTION AND HANDLING, REFERENCE RANGE

TEST	PATIENT PREPARATION	SPECIMEN COLLECTION	SPECIMEN HANDLING	REFERENCE RANGE
ACTH	Exhibits diurnal variation (highest 6–8 AM, lowest 9–10 PM → with normal sleep cycle) Stressful venipuncture elevates levels.	Collected in prechilled plastic tubes with EDTA or heparin. ACTH is very labile, requires antiprotease in the collection vial.	Place immediately on ice, centrifuge at 4°C, and store at −20°C within 15 min of collection. Aprotonin (500 kU/mL) added for long term storage	8 AM: <120 pg/mL 4–8 PM: <85 pg/mL *Note:* Highest at birth, decreases until reaches adult level
TSH	Refer to "Thyroid Function" section.			
GH	Patient should be fasting and at complete rest for 30 min before collection. Spikes occur 3 hr after meals, stress, or exercise and 90 min after onset of sleep, peaking during deepest sleep.	Serum is preferred; refrigerate immediately. EDTA plasma results in lower values with some methods.	Stable at 2°–8°C for 8 hr Specimen frozen for longer periods of storage	ADULT MALES: 0–4 ng/mL ADULT FEMALES: 0–18 ng/mL *Note:* Highest levels in childhood
PRL	Collect 3–4 hr after awakened; will be increased during sleep and peak in early morning hours. Avoid emotional stress, exercise, ambulation, and protein ingestion, all of which increase the level.	Fresh, nonhemolyzed serum is preferred.	Stable at 4°C for 24 hr Specimen frozen for longer periods of storage	*Nonpregnant women, men, and children:* 5–20 ng/mL PREGNANCY: 1st trimester = <80 ng/mL 2nd trimester = <169 ng/mL 3rd trimester = <400 ng/mL

Continued ▶

▶ Continued **PATIENT PREPARATION, SPECIMEN COLLECTION AND HANDLING, REFERENCE RANGE**

TEST	PATIENT PREPARATION	SPECIMEN COLLECTION	SPECIMEN HANDLING	REFERENCE RANGE
FSH and LH	Exhibit episodic, circadian, and cyclic variations → best to use serial blood tests or timed urine collections. Time of menstrual cycle must be noted in women to allow proper interpretation of results.	Serum, plasma, and urine are acceptable.	Stable 8 days at room temperature, 2 wk at 4°C Specimen frozen at −20°C for longer periods of storage	FSH: 5–20 mIU/mL LH: 5–25 mIU/mL
ADH and Oxytocin	ADH samples should be measured in conjunction with osmolality, as ADH varies with osmolality.	Plasma collected in prechilled tubes containing EDTA Random urine samples	Separate immediately in refrigerated centrifuge and store frozen at −20°C. No preservatives necessary for urine Levels deteriorate with prolonged storage	ADH: 2–8 pg/mL OXYTOCIN: 1–5 pg/mL

DIAGNOSTIC TESTS AND METHODOLOGIES

TEST	METHOD	INTERFERENCE	COMMENTS
ACTH	Immunoassays: RIA (competitive binding)	Insensitive and nonspecific: measures intact ACTH, precursor molecules, and ACTH fragments	Sensitivity may be improved by concentrating the specimens Recommended for ectopic sources of ACTH → tumors may secrete fragments rather than intact ACTH.
	IRMA	May be too specific to recognize all associated forms → measures intact ACTH only	Low detection limit (1–4 pg/mL) More sensitive and precise
TSH	Refer to "Thyroid Function" section.		
GH	Immunoassays: RIA (competitive binding)		Sensitivity = 0.5–1.0 ng/mL
	IRMA		Sensitivity = 0.1–0.5 ng/mL
PRL	Immunoassays: RIA (competitive binding)		
	IRMA	May not recognize some forms	Lower detection limit (0.2–1.0 ng/mL) Improved precision (coefficient of variation <8%) Superior specificity
FSH	Immunoassay: RIA	Less than 1% cross-reactivity with LH, TSH, and hCG or with free alpha or beta chains	
LH	Immunoassays: RIA	10%–25% cross-reactivity with hCG	Invalid test in pregnancy or when hCG secreting tumors are present
	IRMA	Eliminates cross-reactivity	Lower detection limits (0.2 IU/L) Better precision
ADH and Oxytocin	Immunoassay: RIA	Blood assays require preliminary extraction to isolate the hormones.	Not routinely used owing to lack of sensitivity and specificity

EVALUATING TEST RESULTS

Tests of Hypothalamic/Pituitary Function

TEST	PROCEDURE	INTERPRETATION	COMMENTS
GnRH Test	GnRH administered IV. Serum collected prior to dose for baseline followed by sampling at 30, 60, 90, and 120 min after dose for measurement of FSH and LH levels.	NORMAL RESPONSE: LH peak 3–10 × baseline FSH peak 1.5–3 × baseline Pituitary disease = absent or lesser response Hypothalamic disease = normal or lesser response	FSH and LH secreted in a pulsatile manner; therefore, necessary to determine baseline level using serial samples.
GH Stimulation Test (after arginine)	Arginine HCl administered IV. Serum drawn prior to dose for baseline followed by sampling at 30, 60, and 90 min after dose for determination of GH level.	NORMAL RESPONSE: Baseline = <5 ng/mL Peak = >10 ng/mL No response = hypopituitarism	No response may be seen if the baseline level is >5 ng/mL. Because 20% of healthy patients may not respond to arginine, a negative response must be confirmed with other tests.
GH Stimulation Test (after glucagon and propranolol)	Propranolol administered orally at 7 AM to patient fasting since 12 AM, followed by IM injection of glucagon at 9 AM. Serum tested for baseline at 7 AM, at 9 AM before glucagon, and again at 11 AM and 12 PM.	NORMAL RESPONSE: Peak = >10 ng/mL No response or inadequate response = hypopituitarism	Other stimulation tests are preferred since glucagon is not a potent stimulus.
GH Stimulation Test (after insulin)	Insulin administered IV. Serum tested at 30, 60, and 90 min after dose.	NORMAL RESPONSE: GH peak = >10 ng/mL Cortisol peak = >7 ng/dL No response or inadequate response = hypothalamic or pituitary dysfunction	Blood glucose must fall below 40 mg/dL within 1 hr after insulin dose, or a second injection should be administered. Patient placed at risk owing to the level of hypoglycemia induced by the test.
GH Stimulation Test (after L-dopa)	L-Dopa given orally after overnight fast. Serum collected prior to dose for baseline followed by sampling at 30, 60, 90, and 120 min after dose while patient at rest for GH determination.	NORMAL RESPONSE: Peak = >10 ng/dL No response = hypopituitarism	20% of healthy patients may not respond to L-dopa; therefore, all negative responses should be confirmed with other tests.

Continued ▶

▶ Continued **EVALUATING TEST RESULTS**

Tests of Hypothalamic/Pituitary Function

TEST	PROCEDURE	INTERPRETATION	COMMENTS
GH Stimulation Test (after exercise)	Patient exercises for 20 min after which specimen is drawn immediately and tested for GH level.	NORMAL RESPONSE: >6 ng/dL No response = hypopituitarism	The patient must be physically able to undergo strenuous exercise in order to complete this test.
GH Stimulation Test (after CRH)	A CRH injection is given to the patient followed by measurement of the blood level of GH.	NORMAL RESPONSE: GH level elevated compared with baseline No response = hypopituitarism	GH stimulation test with the lowest risk factors for the patient
GH Suppression Test (after glucose)	Glucose taken orally after overnight fast. Serum collected prior to dose for baseline followed by sampling at 60 and 120 min after dose for GH determination.	NORMAL RESPONSE: GH <2 ng/mL or undetectable No or incomplete suppression = gigantism or acromegaly	GH level may actually increase after glucose dose in patients with acromegaly.
TRH/TSH Stimulation Tests	Refer to "Thyroid Function" section.		
Overnight Water Deprivation Test	Water withheld from patient for 8 hr during which blood and urine samples are collected and tested for osmolality.	NORMAL RESPONSE: Serum osmolality within reference range Urine osmolality high, indicating concentrated urine RESPONSE IN ADH DEFICIENCY: Serum osmolality elevated Urine osmolality low, indicating diluted urine	Indirectly measures ADH content through renal response to water deprivation Valid only if the patient has normal renal function
ADH Stimulation Test	Exogenous ADH administered to evaluate patient's response through urine output and osmolality.	NORMAL RESPONSE: Decreased urine output Increased urine osmolality NEPHROGENIC DIABETES INSIPIDUS: No response NEUROGENIC DIABETES INSIPIDUS: >10% increase in urine osmolality	Used to differentiate the cause of diabetes insipidus

CHANGE OF ANALYTE IN DISEASE

ANALYTE	CLINICAL SIGNIFICANCE	COMMENTS
ACTH	ELEVATIONS: Addison's disease Congenital adrenal hyperplasia (CAH) Pituitary-dependent Cushing's disease Ectopic ACTH-producing tumors DECREASES: Secondary adrenocortical insufficiency Adrenal carcinoma Adrenal adenoma Hypopituitarism	Elevations also occur in response to the physiologic conditions of pregnancy and stress, and during different phases of the menstrual cycle.
TSH	Refer to "Thyroid Function" section.	
GH	ELEVATIONS: Pituitary adenomas Acromegaly in adults (overgrowth of skeleton and soft tissues) Pituitary gigantism (GH excess before long bone growth is complete) DECREASES: Congenital or acquired deficiency Idiopathic or pituitary damage Isolated or with other pituitary hormone fluctuations	Excesses and deficiencies of GH rarely occur.
Prolactin	ELEVATIONS: Pituitary adenomas (30% of cases) Acromegaly Hypotension Chronic renal failure DECREASES: No disease correlation	HYPERPROLACTINEMIA RESULTS IN: Alteration of fertility in females: ▪ Anovulation with or without menstrual irregularity ▪ Amenorrhea and galactorrhea Alteration of fertility in males: ▪ Oligospermia with or without impotence
FSH	Refer to "Gonadal Function" section.	
LH	Refer to "Gonadal Function" section.	
ADH	ELEVATIONS: Syndrome of inappropriate ADH secretion (SIADH) caused by: ▪ Malignancy ▪ Disease of central nervous system ▪ Pulmonary disorders ▪ Side effect of drug therapies DECREASES: Hypothalamic or neurogenic diabetes insipidus (deficient ADH production) Nephrogenic diabetes insipidus (deficient ADH action on the kidney) Psychogenic or primary polydipsia (excessive water intake)	FINDINGS WITH SIADH: Decreased urine volume Increased urine sodium and osmolality Increased plasma volume Decreased plasma sodium and osmolality FINDINGS WITH DIABETES INSIPIDUS: Polyuria (>2.5 L/day urine output) Increased urine volume Decreased urine osmolality
Oxytocin	No known disease correlation exists.	Most active in pregnant women

THYROID FUNCTION

INTRODUCTION

The thyroid gland is a two-lobed endocrine gland located in the anterior region of the throat. Two types of cells are responsible for the production of hormones by the thyroid gland: parafollicular and follicular cells. The parafollicular cells, also referred to as C cells, produce the hormone calcitonin, which is involved in the regulation of calcium levels in the blood (see Chapter 12, "Mineral Metabolism"). The follicular cells secrete the active hormones T_4 (thyroxine or 3,5,3′,5′-L-tetraiodothyronine) and T_3 (triiodothyronine or 3,5,3′-L-triodothyronine), as well as smaller amounts of the inactive compound reverse T_3 (rT_3 or 3,3′,5′-L-triodothyronine) and the T_3/T_4 precursors MIT (monoiodotyrosine) and DIT (diodotyrosine). The production of thyroid hormones is regulated by the secretion of TSH (thyroid stimulating hormone) from the pituitary gland, which in turn is controlled by TRH (thyrotropin releasing hormone) from the hypothalamus. TSH causes an increase in the number of follicles in the thyroid gland and in the uptake of the iodide required for hormone production. The transportation of iodide to the thyroid gland is the rate-limiting step in the production process. Once iodide reaches the thyroid, it is oxidized, allowing for combination with the tyrosine residues in the thyroglobulin molecule, thus forming MIT and DIT, which are coupled to form T_3 and T_4. The thyroid gland secretes approximately 7 μg of T_3 daily along with 80 to 100 μg of T_4, 30% to 50% of which will be converted to T_3 and rT_3 once released. The actual circulating level of T_3 is 22 to 47 μg, 80% to 85% of which results from the deiodination of T_4 in peripheral tissue, particularly the liver and kidney, after release from the thyroid gland. More than 99% of the circulating thyroid hormones are bound to the carrier proteins TBG (thyroxine binding globulin), TBPA (thyroxine binding prealbumin), and albumin, resulting in a large, stable reservoir of inactive hormone. Because the levels of binding proteins fluctuate greatly, the total hormone levels in euthyroid individuals will have a wide reference range. The remainder of the circulating hormone, less than 0.1%, is in the free or active form. The activity of T_3 is three to five times more potent than that of T_4. The thyroid hormones exert their effects by binding to receptors and undergoing a degradation process in which they become deiodinated. Their functions include control of energy expenditure; regulation of growth, development, and sexual maturation; and stimulation of heart rate and contraction, protein synthesis and carbohydrate metabolism, synthesis and degradation of cholesterol and triglyceride, and enhanced sensitivity of beta-adrenergic receptors to catecholamines.

CHANGE OF ANALYTE IN DISEASE

Hypothalamic-Pituitary-Thyroid Axis

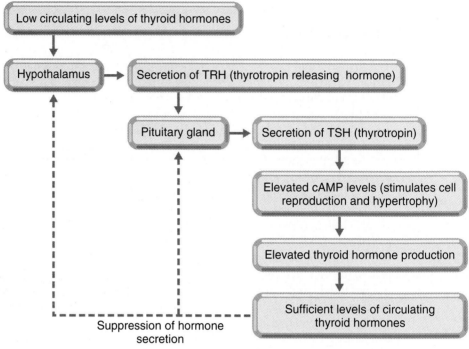

SUMMARY OF THYROID DISEASE

DISEASE	DEFINITION	CAUSES	SYMPTOMS
Hyperthyroidism	Excessive production of thyroid hormones	Graves' disease (most common) Toxic multinodular goiter Solitary toxic adenoma Exogenous iodine and iodine containing drugs Excessive T_3/T_4 ingestion Ectopic thyroid tissue Pituitary tumor	Thyrotoxicosis causes decreased weight with normal appetite, fatigue, heart palpitations, goiter, eyelid retraction, oligomenorrhea, diarrhea, angina, sweating, heat intolerance, tremors, and muscle weakness. Thyroid storm is a rare medical crisis characterized by hyperpyrexia, dehydration, and cardiac failure.
Hypothyroidism	Inadequate production of thyroid hormones	>90% of cases caused by: Atrophic hypothyroidism (most common) Autoimmune hypothyroidism (Hashimoto's thyroiditis) Post surgery, radioactive iodine therapy, or antithyroid drug therapy Congenital hypothyroidism Secondary hypothyroidism (pituitary disease, TSH deficiency) Tertiary hypothyroidism (hypothalamus disease, TRH deficiency)	Myxedema syndrome is characterized by dry skin, coarse features, and subcutaneous swelling. Accompanying symptoms include lethargy, tiredness, cold intolerance, hoarseness, and weight gain. Myxedema coma is a complication with high mortality characterized by stupor and hypothermia.

PATIENT PREPARATION, SPECIMEN COLLECTION AND STORAGE, REFERENCE RANGE

TEST	PATIENT PREPARATION	SPECIMEN COLLECTION	SPECIMEN STORAGE	REFERENCE RANGE
TSH	Exhibits diurnal variation: 2–4 AM = highest levels 5–6 PM = lowest levels	Serum preferable Plasma acceptable depending on method used No hemolysis or lipemia	Stable 5–7 days at 2°–8°C, 1 mo if frozen Best to freeze if testing delayed for 24 hr	0.5–5.75 MIU/L *Note:* Varies with method and reference population, increases after age 55
T_4	Nonfasting specimen is acceptable.	Serum Plasma (heparin or EDTA) No hemolysis or lipemia Centrifuge turbid samples before testing	Stable 7–14 days at room temperature or 2°–8°C, 1 mo if frozen Cannot be repeatedly frozen and thawed	4.6–11 μg/dL (higher in premenopausal women owing to estrogen) *Note:* Varies considerably owing to fluctuations in TBG levels, higher during pregnancy
T_3	Same as T_4	Same as T_4	Same as T_4	70–204 ng/dL *Note:* Decreases after age 50

DIAGNOSTIC TESTS AND METHODOLOGIES

TEST	METHOD	INTERFERENCE	COMMENTS
TSH	IMMUNOASSAY: RIA—competitive binding using antibody to alpha subunit of TSH	Antibodies used cross-react with LH, FSH, and hCG (refer to "Pituitary Function" section)	First generation test → detection limit = 1–2 mU/L Limited sensitivity—only capable of detecting elevated levels of TSH Limited specificity due to cross-reactivity with other hormones
	Immunometric—sandwich assay using multiple antibodies to beta subunit of TSH	High dose hook effect occurs with IRMA methods (at very high levels patient results are underestimated → solved by dilution)	Second generation test → detection limit = 0.1–0.2 mU/L Improved sensitivity—wider measurement range capable of detecting suppressed levels as well as elevated levels Improved specificity—no cross-reactivity with other hormones Better turnaround time
	Chemiluminescence and Time Resolved Fluorescence		Third and fourth generation tests → detection limit = 0.01–0.02 mU/L Even greater sensitivity
T$_4$	IMMUNOASSAY: Isotopic: RIA—competitive binding		Heterogeneous assay—requires separation of bound antibody from free during testing
	Nonisotopic: Enzyme-multiplied immunoassay technique/ fluorescence polarization immunoassay (EMIT/FPIA)		Homogeneous assay—no separation step required
T$_3$	Same as T$_4$		

EVALUATING TEST RESULTS

Tests of Thyroid Function

TEST	PROCEDURE	INTERPRETATION	CLINICAL USE
Thyroid Uptake of Iodine	The amount of labeled iodine that is present in the thyroid is measured after administration of a specific dose.	Normal uptake is 8%–30% after 24 hr. Uptake is increased (>55% after 24 hr) in Graves' disease and other causes of hyperthyroidism. Uptake is decreased (0%–1% after 24 hr) in hypothyroidism and also in a few hyperthyroid conditions.	Reflects the functional status of the thyroid gland for synthesis and secretion of thyroid hormones.
TRH Stimulation Test	TRH is administered intravenously and the subsequent levels of TSH and T_3/T_4 are measured.	Normal → the TSH, T_3, and T_4 levels increase. Normal, but delayed → tertiary hypothyroidism (TRH production is deficient). Low TSH production → blunted response associated with pituitary dysfunction (secondary hypothyroidism). High TSH production with no T_3/T_4 response → indicates primary hypothyroidism.	A normal result rules out the diagnosis of hyperthyroidism. May be used to diagnose subclinical hyperthyroidism and evaluate patients with ophthalmopathy without overt hyperthyroidism. Most useful in diagnosis of secondary and tertiary hypothyroidism. Rarely needed with better TSH tests available.
TSH Stimulation Test	A labeled dose of iodine is administered to the patient and the baseline uptake is determined. Bovine TSH is then administered along with another dose of labeled iodine and the uptake is again evaluated. For best results, the results are monitored for 3 consecutive days.	Normal response → uptake after TSH administration should be 1.5 times that of the baseline; T_4 levels should also be increased. Primary hypothyroidism → no response Secondary or tertiary hypothyroidism → increased uptake and T_4	Differentiates primary hypothyroidism from secondary and tertiary hypothyroidism. Replaced by TRH stimulation test and TSH quantitative assays.
T_3/T_4 Suppression Test	Uptake of a labeled dose of iodine is determined before and after administration of T_3/T_4 for 7–10 days. Images of the thyroid are taken to determine areas of the gland that are unresponsive to the change in TSH.	Normal → T_3/T_4 suppress the production of TSH; uptake is reduced 30%–50%. Overactive thyroid (hyperthyroidism) → will not respond and hormone levels will remain elevated, including TSH.	T_4 suppression test is better tolerated by most patients. Normal result rules out hypothyroidism and subclinical Graves' disease. Clinical utility is limited → replaced by TSH and TRH stimulation tests.

CHANGE OF ANALYTE IN DISEASE

ANALYTE	MEASUREMENT	CLINICAL SIGNIFICANCE	COMMENTS
Total Serum T_4	Serum levels are routinely measured by immunoassay when TSH is altered.	Elevated when the synthesis, release, or binding protein capacity is increased Elevations most frequently seen with hyperthyroidism Also elevated in subacute thyroiditis, Hashimoto's thyroiditis, and after radiation therapy Decreased in hypothyroidism	An increase in thyroxine binding globulin (TBG) will result in an elevated total serum T_4. A decrease in TBG will result in a decreased total serum T_4. The FT_4I should be reported.
Total Serum T_3	Serum levels may be measured by immunoassay.	Elevated proportionately to T_4 in hyperthyroidism and other causes Decreased in hypothyroidism In 5% of individuals, T_3 elevated while T_4 normal → T_3 thyrotoxicosis	Not routinely measured except to monitor treatment of T_3 thyrotoxicosis. Fluctuates with TBG levels, same as T_4.
Resin Uptake Test (RT_3U or RT_4U)	The available binding sites on binding protein (esp. TBG) are estimated by mixing the patient sample with labeled hormone. The amount of labeled hormone that does not bind is removed by adding a resin and measured as inversely proportional to the binding sites available.	Hyperthyroidism → the serum level of thyroid hormones is high; thus, few or no binding sites are available and the uptake result is elevated. With increased TBG levels, more labeled hormone is able to bind and the uptake result is decreased. With decreased TBG levels, less labeled hormone is able to bind and the uptake result is increased.	Drugs such as salicylates, phenytoin, furosemide, and fenclofenac compete with the hormone for binding sites on TBG, thus resulting in an increased resin uptake with concurrent decreased total hormone levels and normal free hormone levels. Replaced by the THBR value.
Free Thyroxine Hormone Index (FT_4I)	The free T_4 in blood may be calculated using the following formula: FT_4I = (total T_4 × %T_4 uptake in patient serum)/%T_4 uptake in reference serum *or* FT_4I = (total T_4 × THBR)	Decreased binding protein without thyroid disease → decreased total T_4 with elevated T_4 uptake result → normal FT_4I estimate Hypothyroidism → decreased T_4 level with elevated T_4 uptake result → decreased FT_4I estimate Hyperthyroidism → increased T_4 level with decreased T_4 uptake result → increased FT_4I estimate	The same estimate may be used for the free T_3 hormone index (FT_3I) → only necessary in the case of T_3 thyrotoxicosis.

Continued ▶

► Continued **CHANGE OF ANALYTE IN DISEASE**

ANALYTE	MEASUREMENT	CLINICAL SIGNIFICANCE	COMMENTS
Thyroid Hormone Binding Ratio (THBR)	Uptake test is performed and the following calculation made: $$\frac{\% \; T_4 \text{ uptake (patient)}}{\% \; T_4 \text{ uptake (reference)}}$$	Normal ratio should be 1. Increased ratio indicates hyperthyroidism or low TBG levels. Decreased ratio indicates hypothyroidism or high TBG levels.	If the T_4 level is increased or decreased in proportion to the THBR → the primary alteration is of thyroid function. If the T_4 level is increased or decreased inversely to the THBR → the primary alteration is of the TBG level.
Free T_4 (FT_4) and Free T_3 (FT_3)	Analytical methods available to measure serum levels directly	Parallel the alterations in total hormone levels in hyperthyroidism and hypothyroidism	Not clinically useful to measure directly owing to the quality of current methods. Advantage over total serum levels → not influenced by fluctuating TBG levels.
Thyroxine Binding Globulin (TBG)	Serum levels measured by immunoassay	Elevated TBG → elevated total hormone levels with or without hyperthyroidism Decreased TBG → decreased total hormone levels Normal adult level → 3–42 ng/mL	Quantitative alterations result in change in TBG concentration. Qualitative alterations result in change in TBG ability to bind thyroid hormones
Thyroid Stimulating Hormone (TSH)	Serum levels routinely measured by immunoassay	Primary hypothyroidism → elevated TSH Secondary or tertiary hypothyroidism → normal or decreased TSH Hyperthyroidism → low or undetectable TSH level	The TRH stimulation test is needed to differentiate between secondary and tertiary hypothyroidism. TSH secretion is inhibited by glucocorticoids (e.g., dopamine, somatostatin).
Thyroglobulin (Tg)	Serum levels measured by immunoassay	Elevated in thyroid carcinoma and hyperthyroidism Decreased in thyrotoxicosis factitia	Lack of sensitivity and specificity combined with inability to measure Tg when Tg antibodies are present limit the usefulness of Tg measurement.

CHANGE OF ANALYTE IN DISEASE

Continued ►

▶ Continued **CHANGE OF ANALYTE IN DISEASE**

ANALYTE	MEASUREMENT	CLINICAL SIGNIFICANCE	COMMENTS
Thyroglobulin Antibodies	Serum levels measured by ELISA or IRMA immunoassays	PRESENT IN: 85% Hashimoto's thyroiditis (highest levels) 30% Graves' disease 45% thyroid carcinoma 95% idiopathic myxedema 50% pernicious anemia (low levels) 30% systemic lupus erythematosus 10% normal (low levels)	Normal level does not rule out Hashimoto's thyroiditis (microsomal antibodies are a more sensitive indicator).

LABORATORY FINDINGS WITH DISEASE

DISEASE	LABORATORY	TREATMENT
Hyperthyroidism	Elevated T_3, T_4 levels Decreased TSH levels	Antithyroid drugs → may lead to remission but relapse can occur as much as many years later. Radioactive iodine and surgery → may lead to hypothyroidism in 35% of cases. Beta-adrenergic blocking drugs → relieve the symptoms but do not cure.
Hypothyroidism	Decreased levels of thyroid hormones Primary → elevated TSH levels Secondary or tertiary → decreased TSH levels	Replacement therapy → T_3, T_4 T_3 is preferred for treatment owing to short half-life, which allows for quicker adjustment of therapeutic levels.

DIAGNOSIS OF HYPOTHYROIDISM

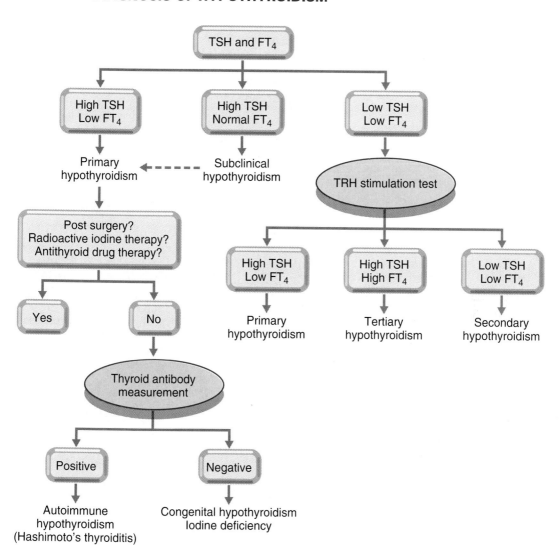

DIAGNOSIS OF HYPERTHYROIDISM

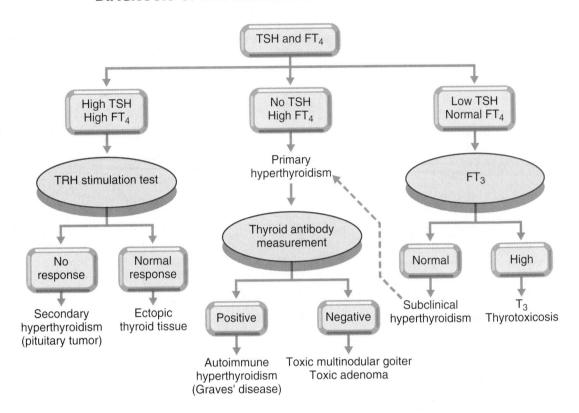

ADRENAL FUNCTION

INTRODUCTION

The adrenal glands are pyramid shaped endocrine glands located at the upper pole of each kidney. Each adrenal gland is composed of a gray inner medulla and a yellow outer cortex. The chromaffin cells in the medulla produce the catecholamine hormones epinephrine, norepinephrine, and dopamine. The cortex produces steroid hormones within its three layers: the outer layer or zona glomerulosa produces mineralocorticoids; the middle layer (zona fasciculata) and the inner layer (zona reticularis) produce glucocorticoids and androgens.

Catecholamines

The catecholamines consist of a catechol or dihydroxybenzene ring with an amine attached. Norepinephrine and dopamine are primary amines and epinephrine is a secondary amine. The main sites of catecholamine production are the brain, chromaffin cells of the adrenal medulla, and sympathetic neurons. The adrenal medulla produces the greatest quantity of epinephrine and the sympathetic neurons produce the greatest quantity of norepinephrine.

Production of catecholamines begins with tyrosine as the hormonal precursor. The hydroxylation of tyrosine is the rate-limiting step of catecholamine production in the sympathetic neurons and the adrenal medulla. Levels of norepinephrine and epinephrine inhibit this hydroxylation step through a negative feedback mechanism. The product of tyrosine hydroxylation is dihydroxyphenylalanine (DOPA), which is further converted to dopamine in many tissues. Dopamine levels build up in the granulated vesicles of the sympathetic nerve endings and chromaffin granules of the adrenal medulla. Within these storage granules dopamine is converted to norepinephrine. In the adrenal medulla, the norepinephrine is converted to epinephrine in response to cortisol levels. Stimulation by the nervous system causes the release of stored catecholamines from the storage granules in response to hypotension, hypoxia, exposure to cold, muscular exertion, pain, and emotional disturbance. The catecholamines bind to alpha- and beta-adrenergic receptors in tissues throughout the body.

CATECHOLAMINE RECEPTORS

RECEPTOR TYPE	CATECHOLAMINE SPECIFICITY	EFFECTS OF BINDING
α-Adrenergic	Norepinephrine Epinephrine	Vasoconstriction Decreased insulin secretion, increased glycolysis (elevates blood glucose) Sweating Piloerection (hairs stand on end)
β-Adrenergic	Epinephrine	Vasodilation Stimulates insulin release Increases heart contractions Relaxes smooth muscle of intestinal tract Bronchodilation Stimulates renin release (increases sodium reabsorption) Increases lipolysis

The catecholamines are transported in the blood bound to protein with a short half-life of 2 minutes. The enzyme catechol-O-methyltransferase (COMT) in the liver, kidney, and erythrocytes forms metanephrine and normetanephrine from epinephrine and norepinephrine. The kidneys excrete 20% of the metanephrine and normetanephrine in either the free or the conjugated form. Most of the metabolites are further deaminated by monoamine oxidase (MAO), and most is oxidized to vanillylmandelic acid (VMA) with lesser amounts reduced to methoxyhydroxyphenylglycol (MHPG), both of which are then excreted by the kidney. Urinary measurement of VMA reflects the total production of norepinephrine and epinephrine in the body. The final metabolite of dopamine is homovanillic acid (HVA).

ADRENAL FUNCTION—INTRODUCTION

SUMMARY OF CATECHOLAMINE-SECRETING TUMORS

TUMOR TYPE	DESCRIPTION	SYMPTOMS	INCIDENCE
Pheochromocytoma	Benign or malignant tumor in autonomic nervous system and adrenal medulla, resulting in high blood levels of epinephrine, norepinephrine, or both catecholamines	Sustained hypertension Weight loss Sweating spells Headache Palpitations Anxiety Heat intolerance Tremors Increased basal metabolic rate	Rare, life-threatening tumors are curable with surgery. Adults → 90% in adrenal medulla, most benign Children → more commonly malignant
Neuroblastoma	Malignant tumor that grows rapidly and metastasizes, resulting in high blood levels of all catecholamines	Hypertension Sweating Tachycardia Headaches	One of the most common malignant tumors in pediatric patients

Corticosteroids

The adrenal cortex produces the corticosteroids in response to levels of adrenocorticotropic hormone (ACTH) secreted by the pituitary gland and levels of angiotensin I and II in the renin-angiotensin system. The rate-limiting step of corticosteroid production is the conversion of cholesterol to pregnenolone. The source of the cholesterol is either synthesis within the adrenal cortex or transport to the adrenal cortex after synthesis into low density lipoprotein (LDL) in the liver. The corticosteroids are transported bound to albumin and corticosteroid binding globulin (CBG). The major corticosteroids produced by the adrenal cortex are cortisol, aldosterone, and a group of androgens.

SUMMARY OF CORTICOSTEROIDS

HORMONE	DESCRIPTION	EFFECTS	REGULATION
Cortisol	Glucocorticoid hormone is secreted at rate of 10–30 mg/day that influences carbohydrate metabolism through increasing gluconeogenesis and decreasing glucose utilization. The result is an elevation of the plasma glucose level.	Inhibits amino acid uptake Increases protein breakdown Inhibits protein synthesis Increases lipid breakdown Amino acids and fatty acids used for gluconeogenesis Increases red blood cell and neutrophil production, decreases production of other white blood cells Suppresses inflammatory and immune responses	Refer to diagram of hypothalamus-pituitary-adrenal axis. Cortisol produced within a few minutes of ACTH release

Continued ▶

▶ Continued **SUMMARY OF CORTICOSTEROIDS**

HORMONE	DESCRIPTION	EFFECTS	REGULATION
Aldosterone	Mineralocorticoid hormone is secreted at rate of 150–200 μg/day that regulates the salt content and extracellular fluid level.	Conservation of sodium and secretion of potassium in the distal convoluted tubule Water moves with sodium	Produced predominantly in response to the renin-angiotensin system. Elevated potassium level stimulates production, decreased level inhibits production. ACTH stimulates production of aldosterone.
Androgens	Dehydroepiandrosterone (DHEA) Androstenedione Testosterone (major source in females) Dihydrotestosterone (DHT)	Effect sexual function (refer to Gonadal Endocrinology section).	Regulated by ACTH and secreted in parallel to cortisol

Hypothalamus-Pituitary-Adrenal Axis

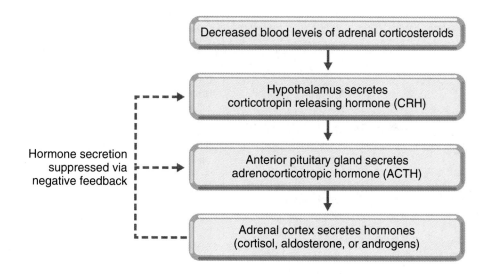

ADRENAL FUNCTION—INTRODUCTION

DISEASES OF THE ADRENAL CORTEX

DISEASE	DESCRIPTION	CAUSES	SYMPTOMS
Primary Adrenal Insufficiency (Addison's Disease)	Relatively rare deficiency of all adrenal steroids	Results from progressive destruction of adrenals by local disease or systemic disorder 70% caused by autoimmune adrenalitis with circulating adrenal antibodies OTHER CAUSES: Tuberculosis Adrenalectomy Adrenal hemorrhage Congenital primary hypoaldosteronism	Gradual onset of fatigue, weakness, weight loss, gastrointestinal disturbances, postprandial hypoglycemia Leads to dehydration, hypotension, hyponatremia, and hyperkalemia Hyperpigmentation caused by high levels of ACTH
Secondary or Tertiary Adrenal Insufficiency	Secondary is a deficiency of ACTH. Tertiary is a deficiency of CRH.	Secondary is caused by pituitary insufficiency. Tertiary is caused by hypothalamic insufficiency.	Similar to those seen in primary adrenal insufficiency with less severe hypotension and without the hyperpigmentation caused by high levels of ACTH
Corticosteroid Excess (Cushing's Syndrome)	Hyperadrenalism with production of excess cortisol	Most common cause is exogenous glucocorticoid therapy (iatrogenic origin). OTHER CAUSES: 60% pituitary tumors 20% ectopic ACTH-producing tumors (lung, thymic, or pancreatic cancer) 20% adrenal adenoma and carcinoma	Clinical presentation of truncal obesity, hypertension, hypokalemia, metabolic alkalosis, carbohydrate intolerance, disturbance of reproductive function, and neuropsychotic symptoms
Adult Adrenogenital Syndrome	Adrenal hyperplasia caused by elevated ACTH	Adrenal adenoma and carcinoma major causes	Results in masculinization in females owing to the high levels of androgens produced
Congenital Adrenal Hyperplasia	Blockage of the pathway that produces cortisol from cholesterol, either partial or complete	Caused by a congenital absence or deficiency of the enzymes necessary to the cortisol production pathway 95% caused by deficiency of 21-hydroxylase	Results in virilization Partial block has varied clinical manifestations → may be compensated by increased secretion of ACTH by pituitary to restore cortisol levels. Complete block is incompatible with life.

Continued ▶

▶ Continued **DISEASES OF THE ADRENAL CORTEX**

DISEASE	DESCRIPTION	CAUSES	SYMPTOMS
Primary Hyperaldosteronism or Conn's Syndrome	Characterized by hypertension and hypokalemia resulting from hypersecretion of aldosterone	70% caused by aldosterone-producing adrenal adenoma (APA) 30% caused by idiopathic adrenal hyperplasia (IAH) May also occur secondary to renal lesions in which high levels of renin are produced	Major feature is hypertension caused by retention of sodium and water accompanied by loss of potassium. Also impaired glucose tolerance due to the effect of low potassium on insulin release. OTHER SYMPTOMS: Muscle weakness Fatigue Polyuria (esp. nocturnal) Polydipsia

PATIENT PREPARATION, SPECIMEN COLLECTION AND STORAGE, REFERENCE RANGE

TEST	PATIENT PREPARATION	SPECIMEN COLLECTION	SPECIMEN STORAGE	REFERENCE RANGE
Catecholamines (Epinephrine, Norepinephrine, Dopamine)	Diurnal variation → higher in AM than in PM Posture essential as levels are 2–3 times higher when patient is upright → best to have patient rest 30 min in recumbent position prior to collection. No eating, drinking coffee or tea, or using tobacco for 4 hours prior to collection. Venipuncture may cause elevated levels → best to use indwelling catheter.	Plasma: heparin or EDTA *Note:* Add antioxidants such as glutathione or metabisulfate. Urine: 24 hr collection with 10–20 mL 6M HCl, refrigerated during collection	Plasma: Transport on ice, centrifuge at 4°C within 30 min, separate, and freeze until tested. Both plasma and urine are stable 8 mo at −70°C.	PLASMA: Epinephrine = <50 pg/mL Norepinephrine = 110–410 pg/mL Dopamine = <87 pg/mL URINE: Epinephrine = 0–20 μg/day Norepinephrine = 15–80 μg/day Dopamine = 65–400 μg/day

Continued ▶

► Continued **PATIENT PREPARATION, SPECIMEN COLLECTION AND STORAGE, REFERENCE RANGE**

TEST	PATIENT PREPARATION	SPECIMEN COLLECTION	SPECIMEN STORAGE	REFERENCE RANGE
Metanephrine and Normetanephrine		24 hr urine with 10–20 mL 6M HCl. Random urine acidified to pH of 1–3	Stable several weeks at 1°–4°C, frozen indefinitely	Metanephrine = 74–297 μg/day Normetanephrine = 105–354 μg/day
VMA	No intake of chocolate, coffee, bananas, foods with vanilla, citrus fruits, drugs (aspirin, antihypertensives) as all cause false elevations with some methods.	Urine: 24 hr recommended with 10–20 mL 6M HCl as stabilizer, refrigerated during collection	Stable 2 wk at 1°–4°C, may be frozen indefinitely	2.1–7.6 mg/day *Note:* The reference range is dependent on the method used to measure VMA.
HVA	See VMA.	Urine: 24 hr specimen preserved with 20 mL 6M HCl and refrigerated during collection	Stable 2 wk at 1°–4°C, may be frozen indefinitely Adjust pH to 3–4 with 6M HCl.	1.4–8.8 mg/day
Cortisol	Highest level at 8 AM, >50% reduction at 8 PM (based on a normal sleep-wake cycle) Elevated by stress, glucocorticoid administration, pregnancy, depression, hypoglycemia, and hypertension	Serum Heparinized plasma Urine: 24 hr specimen preserved with boric acid	Stable 2 days at 2°–8°C Must be frozen for long term storage	SERUM/PLASMA (TOTAL CORTISOL): 5–20 μg/dL URINE (FREE CORTISOL): 20–90 μg/day *Note:* Cortisol levels are lowest in children, increasing over time to adult levels.
Aldosterone	Patient must be upright for 2 hr prior to collection. AM levels are higher than PM levels.	Plasma (heparin, EDTA, or citrate) Serum Urine: 24 hr specimen preserved with boric acid and refrigerated during collection	Frozen in airtight container at −20°C for up to 2 yr Urine: pH adjusted with 50% acetic acid to 2–4, frozen at −20°C	Recumbent: 50–150 ng/L Upright: 150–300 ng/L *Note:* Highest levels in neonates, decreasing over time to adult levels.
Androgens	Refer to "Gonadal Function" section.			

DIAGNOSTIC TESTS AND METHODOLOGIES

TEST	METHOD	INTERFERENCE	COMMENTS
Catecholamines (Epinephrine, Norepinephrine, Dopamine)	HPLC: Preliminary extraction and concentration of plasma Different column and detector types may be used.		Limited ability to obtain good precision owing to technical difficulty of the procedure
Urinary Metanephrine and Normetanephrine	HPLC—fractionated: Preliminary extraction Column and phases vary.		HPLC has better sensitivity and specificity.
	Colorimetric—total: Pisano method	Colorimetric method more prone to interference by chromagenic substances	Colorimetric method does not distinguish metanephrine from normetanephrine.
Urinary VMA	Preliminary extraction Spectrophotometric or chromatographic quantitation	HPLC has fewest interferences.	HPLC has best sensitivity, accuracy, reproducibility, and speed of analysis.
Urinary HVA	Spectrophotometric and chromatographic methods	HPLC has fewest interferences.	HPLC has excellent sensitivity and better specificity.
Cortisol	HPLC/GC-MS	Requires preanalytical extraction of cortisol	Not routine because labor intensive and relatively slow HPLC more specific for urine
	Immunoassay—RIA	No initial extraction needed *Note:* Urine requires extraction of metabolites regardless of method.	Method of choice for routine measurement
Aldosterone	Immunoassay—RIA	Cross-reacts with other steroids and thus requires separation by extraction if other steroids present in high levels.	Simple and reliable
Androgens	Refer to "Gonadal Function" section.		

PATIENT PREP/SPECIMEN COLLECTION/STORAGE/REFERENCE RANGE

EVALUATING TEST RESULTS

Tests of Adrenal Function

TEST	PROCEDURE	INTERPRETATION	CLINICAL USE
Low Dose Dexamethasone Suppression Test	Dexamethasone administered over 2 day period (0.5 mg every 6 hr = equivalent to 4× normal adrenal output) Serum and 24 hr urine collected on second day and tested for free cortisol level	Normal → 50% of normal cortisol output suppressed: Urine = <18 µg/L AM serum = <50 µg/L Cushing's disease → no significant suppression, cortisol levels remain elevated.	Used for diagnosis of Cushing's disease A 20 µg/kg/day dose should be used for children and obese patients.
High Dose Dexamethasone Suppression Test	Dexamethasone administered over 2 day period (2 mg every 6 hr) Response tested by measuring serum cortisol or 24 hr urine free cortisol.	Normal → same as low dose test Cushing's disease due to pituitary tumor → >50% suppression of cortisol and ACTH due to continued responsiveness of pituitary tumor to high levels of cortisol Cushing's disease due to adrenal carcinoma, adenoma, or ectopic ACTH source → no suppression of response	Used to determine cause of Cushing's disease
Overnight Dexamethasone Suppression Test	A single dose is administered at 11 PM. The level of cortisol in the blood is measured in a sample drawn at 8 AM the next morning.	Normal response: AM cortisol <5 µg/dL Cushing's disease response: AM cortisol <10 µg/dL	Used as a screening test only; results must be confirmed with other tests.
Metyrapone Stimulation Test	Metyrapone administered to inhibit 11-hydroxylase and cortisol synthesis. Response detected by measurement of blood 11-deoxycortisol or urine 17-hydroxycorticosteroids → measure baseline at 8 AM, give 750 mg metyrapone every 4 hr for 24 hr and repeat measurement.	Normal → cortisol drops and ACTH, 11-deoxycortisol, and 17-hydroxycorticosteroid levels elevated No response → Cushing's disease with pituitary source and hypopituitarism	Used to detect cause of Cushing's disease Not routinely used, although may be better than high dose dexamethasone suppression test

Continued ▶

▶ Continued **Tests of Adrenal Function**

TEST	PROCEDURE	INTERPRETATION	CLINICAL USE
Furosemide Stimulation Test, Rapid	Furosemide dose given orally after overnight fast after 1 week of normal diet without medications. Plasma renin levels are measured prior to dose and 5 hr after dose while patient is in upright position.	Normal response: Renin level rises 1–6 ng/mL/hr Exaggerated response: Renin dependent hypertension, pheochromocytoma No response: Hypertension from mineralocorticoid excess (primary aldosteronism)	Test used for screening purposes on an outpatient basis
ACTH Stimulation Test (after insulin—Insulin Tolerance Test)	Serum drawn at 0, 30, 60, and 90 min after insulin injection. Cortisol level should rise 30 min after maximum fall in blood glucose.	Normal response: Insulin-induced hypoglycemia causes ACTH secretion by pituitary gland, which elevates blood cortisol level. No response or lesser response: Hypothalamic lesions or pituitary ACTH deficiency	Assesses hypothalamus-pituitary-adrenal axis. Should be used only if the adrenal gland responds to ACTH.
ACTH Stimulation Test (Prolonged Infusion)	Cosyntropin dose administered IV for 8 hr on 3 days. Serum is tested for cortisol and/or urine is tested for 17-ketogenic steroids (17-KGS).	Normal response: Peak blood cortisol response 2–5 fold rise in 17-KGS No or inadequate response: Primary adrenal insufficiency (Addison's disease) Delayed but normal response: Secondary adrenal insufficiency (hypopituitarism) No cortisol change with rise in 17-KGS: Congenital adrenal hyperplasia due to 21-hydroxylase and 17-hydroxylase deficiency	Not useful in differential diagnosis of Cushing's disease

EVALUATING TEST RESULTS

Continued ▶

▶ Continued **Tests of Adrenal Function**

TEST	PROCEDURE	INTERPRETATION	CLINICAL USE
ACTH Stimulation Test (Rapid)	Cosyntropin dose administered IV after overnight fast. Serum tested at 0, 30, and 60 min after injection to detect peak cortisol level.	Normal response: Cortisol peak greater than 20 μg/dL Subnormal response: Decreased adrenal reserve and primary adrenal insufficiency (Addison's disease or adrenal failure), secondary to pituitary disease or supplemental steroid medications	Screening test only Normal response rules out primary and secondary adrenal insufficiency. Prolonged ACTH stimulation test and plasma ACTH measurement needed to distinguish primary from secondary insufficiency.
Aldosterone Stimulation Test (after sodium restriction)	Sodium restricted from patient's diet until urine sodium level <5–6 mmol/12 hr, then plasma renin level determined after patient upright for 2 hr and 24 hr urine collected for aldosterone, creatinine and sodium measurements.	Normal response: Renin level becomes increased Slight or no response: Primary aldosteronism	May be combined with aldosterone suppression test (after saline administration) for best evaluation of adrenal aldosterone production.
Aldosterone Suppression Test (after saline administration)	After 2 hr in upright position, 2 L normal saline is administered to recumbent patient. Plasma specimens are tested for aldosterone level before and after saline dose.	Normal response: Aldosterone <5 ng/dL No response (aldosterone remains >10 ng/dL): Primary aldosteronism	Useful for diagnosis of primary aldosteronism
Captopril Stimulation Test	Captopril dose administered orally after overnight fast with patient seated during the test. Plasma specimen collected before and 2 hr after dose is given.	Normal response: Aldosterone <15 ng/dL No response (aldosterone level remains high): Primary aldosteronism	Best discrimination provided by aldosterone:plasma renin activity ratio: Ratio >50 in primary aldosteronism Ratio <50 in essential hypertension
Clonidine Suppression Test	Clonidine administered orally after overnight fast. Plasma specimen collected 3 hr later to measure norepinephrine level.	Normal response: Norepinephrine level within reference range Exaggerated response: Pheochromocytoma	False negative results may occur with pheochromocytoma owing to intermittent secretion of catecholamines.

Continued ▶

► Continued **Tests of Adrenal Function**

TEST	PROCEDURE	INTERPRETATION	CLINICAL USE
CRH Stimulation Test	Administration of 100 µg CRH should cause elevated ACTH release. Blood cortisol level measured at 5, 15, 30, 60, and 120 min post dose and compared with baseline measurement.	Normal → 2–4 fold increase of ACTH and cortisol levels Cushing's disease → ACTH secreting tumors retain CRH receptors and ACTH/cortisol levels rise. Other causes → no response	90% diagnostic accuracy for Cushing's disease, which is only marginally better than the high dose dexamethasone suppression test

CHANGE OF ANALYTE IN DISEASE

ANALYTE	MEASUREMENT	CLINICAL SIGNIFICANCE	COMMENTS
Aldosterone	Blood level measured by RIA	ELEVATED: Primary aldosteronism (Conn's syndrome) Pseudoprimary aldosteronism Secondary aldosteronism DECREASED WITHOUT HYPERTENSION: Addison's disease Isolated aldosterone deficiency Syndrome of hypoaldosteronism due to renin deficiency DECREASED WITH HYPERTENSION: Excess secretion of deoxycorticosterone, corticosterone, and 18-hydroxydeoxycorticosterone Turner's syndrome Diabetes mellitus Acute alcohol intoxication	Overlap exists in test results between normal patients and those with aldosterone insufficiency

EVALUATING TEST RESULTS

Continued ►

▶ Continued **CHANGE OF ANALYTE IN DISEASE**

ANALYTE	MEASUREMENT	CLINICAL SIGNIFICANCE	COMMENTS
Catecholamines (Fractionated)	Measurement in plasma or urine by HPLC	ELEVATED: Pheochromocytoma (norepinephrine greater than epinephrine) Pheochromocytoma in adrenal medulla (epinephrine greater than norepinephrine) Neuroblastoma Myocardial infarction Stress Hypotension Diabetic acidosis DECREASED: Autonomic neuropathy (e.g., Parkinson's disease)	Exercise, stress, smoking, and pain cause elevations. Levels are lower during the night. Determination of homovanillic acid, vanillylmandelic acid, and metanephrines in urine should be used to confirm the diagnosis of pheochromocytoma.
Cortisol	Measurement in urine or blood by RIA or HPLC	ELEVATED: Cushing's syndrome Adrenal adenoma Carcinoma Late pregnancy Stress Obesity EXTREME ELEVATIONS: Ectopic ACTH syndrome DECREASED: Addison's disease Congenital adrenal hyperplasia Hypopituitarism	Most sensitive and specific test for screening for Cushing's syndrome. Diurnal variation may be absent in Cushing's syndrome.
17-Hydroxycorticosteroids	Colorimetric assay of a 24 hr urine specimen preserved with boric acid	NORMAL: 2–10 mg/day excreted ELEVATED: Cushing's syndrome Stress Obesity Pregnancy Severe hypertension Acromegaly Hydrocortisone treatment DECREASED: Addison's disease Congenital adrenal hyperplasia Hypopituitarism Hypotension Dexamethasone treatment	Any acute illness may cause increased excretion. Test has been replaced by plasma and urine cortisol assays.

Continued ▶

▶ Continued **CHANGE OF ANALYTE IN DISEASE**

ANALYTE	MEASUREMENT	CLINICAL SIGNIFICANCE	COMMENTS
17-Ketosteroids/17-Ketogenic Steroids (17-KS/17-KGS)	Colorimetric assay of a 24 hr urine specimen preserved with boric acid	ELEVATED: Cushing's disease Ectopic ACTH-producing tumors Congenital adrenal hyperplasia DECREASED: Addison's disease Hypopituitarism Generalized wasting disease	Assays for specific plasma and urine steroids have replaced this test.

LABORATORY FINDINGS WITH DISEASE

DISEASE	LABORATORY	TREATMENT
Primary Adrenal Insufficiency (Addison's Disease)	ELEVATED BLOOD LEVELS OF: ACTH Potassium Calcium Urea nitrogen DECREASED BLOOD LEVELS OF: Cortisol Glucose Sodium	Administration of cortisol replacement therapy
Secondary or Tertiary Adrenal Insufficiency	Both ACTH and cortisol decreased. Differentiated from primary causes by ACTH stimulation test.	Administration of cortisol replacement therapy
Corticosteroid Excess (Cushing's Syndrome)	ELEVATED: Cortisol Glucose Sodium DECREASED: Potassium ACTH LEVEL: Elevated when pituitary origin Decreased when adrenal origin The high dose dexamethasone test is used to differentiate between pituitary and adrenal causes.	Alteration of exogenous glucocorticoid therapy when of iatrogenic origin Resection of tissue when of carcinogenic origin

CHANGE OF ANALYTE IN DISEASE

Continued ▶

▶ Continued **LABORATORY FINDINGS WITH DISEASE**

DISEASE	LABORATORY	TREATMENT
Adult Adrenogenital Syndrome	ELEVATED: Blood DHEA Urine 17-ketosteroids Blood ACTH DECREASED BLOOD LEVELS OF: Cortisol	Adrenalectomy to remove carcinogenic tissue
Congenital Adrenal Hyperplasia (CAH)	ELEVATED BLOOD LEVELS OF: ACTH Androgen levels DECREASED BLOOD LEVELS OF: Cortisol Aldosterone	Administration of exogenous cortisol and aldosterone
Primary Hyperaldosteronism (Conn's Syndrome)	ELEVATED LEVELS OF: Blood and urine aldosterone Blood sodium DECREASED BLOOD LEVELS OF: Potassium Renin No response in aldosterone suppression tests In hyperaldosteronism secondary to renal lesions, the blood renin level will be elevated.	Surgical removal of the adrenal tumor when present Treatment with a diuretic that antagonizes aldosterone activity when cause is idiopathic or while patient awaits surgery

Continued ▶

GONADAL FUNCTION

INTRODUCTION

The female and male sex steroids are synthesized in the ovaries, testes, and adrenal glands (refer to "Adrenal Function" section). The precursor of all steroids is acetate, which is derived from cholesterol. The rate limiting step of steroid production is the conversion of cholesterol to pregnenolone. The source of the cholesterol is either through synthesis at the site of steroid production or from circulating low density lipoprotein (LDL) synthesized in the liver. Production of the hormones is controlled through a feedback mechanism with the hypothalamus-pituitary axis. The hypothalamus secretes gonadotropin releasing hormone (GnRH) in pulses every 2 minutes. At the anterior pituitary gland, GnRH stimulates the release of follicle stimulating hormone (FSH) and leuteinizing hormone (LH). (Refer to "Hypothalamus and Pituitary Function" section).

Androgens

The androgens are produced in the male testes and in lesser amounts in the adrenal glands of both males and females. In the testes, the Leydig cells contain enzymes for synthesis of the androgens. LH receptors in the Leydig cells bind LH, stimulating the generation of cyclic AMP and other messengers that result in secretion of the androgens. FSH binds receptors in the Sertoli cells of the testes, which stimulates production of androgen binding protein (ABP) and initiates spermatogenesis. High levels of androgens, particularly testosterone, inhibit the production of hypothalamic and pituitary hormones through negative feedback.

HYPOTHALAMUS-PITUITARY-TESTICULAR AXIS

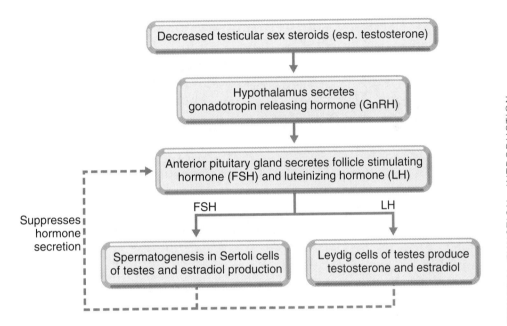

The major androgen produced by the testes is testosterone, which is also produced in minor amounts in the adrenal glands. Testosterone is produced from pregnenolone by two pathways in the testes:

1. pregnenolone → 17-hydroxypregnenolone → DHEA → androstenediol → testosterone
2. pregnenolone → progesterone → 17-hydroxyprogesterone → androstenedione → testosterone

The testosterone produced is not stored in the testes but is immediately released into the blood, where the free form carries out the hormonal actions. In males, testosterone is responsible for embryonic differentiation of male traits, male secondary sexual development at puberty, and maintenance of libido and potency in the adult male. In females, the androgens serve as precursors for the estrogens.

Estrogens and Progesterone

In females, the ovaries produce the ova, releasing one every 28 to 30 days, and secrete the female sex hormones progesterone, from the granulosa cells of the corpus luteum, and estrogens, from the thecal cells. FSH binds to receptors in the ovary, stimulating conversion of androgens to estrogens. The estrogens produced regulate the secretion of FSH and LH by the pituitary gland through feedback mechanisms. Estradiol and progesterone both inhibit the secretion of FSH, and progesterone also inhibits the secretion of LH through negative feedback. Estradiol stimulates the secretion of LH through positive feedback. The female sex hormones are responsible for development and maintenance of the female sex organs and secondary sex characteristics. They also regulate the menstrual cycle and pregnancy. The estrogens are produced mainly by the ovarian follicles, corpus luteum, and placenta, with minute amounts secreted by the adrenal glands and testes. Estradiol is the most potent estrogen, almost all of which originates in the ovaries. The adrenal cortex in both sexes and the testes in males are also a minor source of progesterone, as well as the placenta during pregnancy.

HYPOTHALAMUS-PITUITARY-OVARIAN AXIS

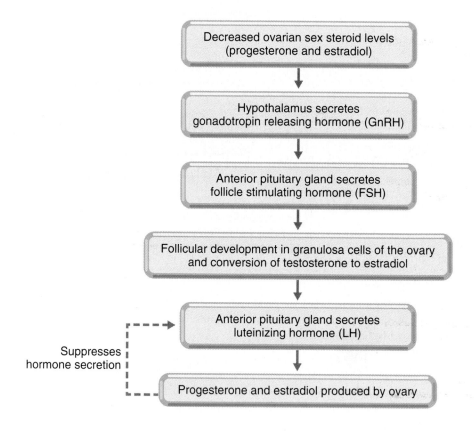

OVARIAN PHASES OF THE MENSTRUAL CYCLE

OVARIAN PHASE	MAJOR EVENTS	HORMONE LEVELS	CORRESPONDING UTERINE PHASES
Early Follicular Phase	Several follicles develop. Corpus luteum is nonfunctioning.	FSH elevated to stimulate follicular growth and increase estrogen secretion LH, estradiol, and progesterone levels low	Menstruation begins because follicles do not secrete enough estrogen to support endometrium. During pregnancy, the fertilized egg implants in the uterus, preventing menstruation.
Late Follicular Phase	Continued development of the follicle in preparation for release of the ovum.	FSH levels drop as estradiol levels increase. LH level increases. Estradiol peaks at days 7–8 of cycle.	Proliferative phase of uterine development → elevated estradiol stimulates reconstruction of endometrium, blood vessels, and secretory gland of uterus.
Midcycle Phase	Final maturation and rupture of ovum at ovulation (day 14) occurs 16–24 hr after the LH peak.	Estradiol level drops, LH level peaks, and estradiol level rises again.	Continuation of the proliferative phase of uterine development in preparation for implantation of ovum
Luteal Phase	Corpus luteum forms from ruptured follicle.	FSH drops as estradiol rises. 3 days after ovulation progesterone rises, causing LH to drop. Progesterone peaks 8–9 days after LH peak (day 23–25 of cycle). Estradiol and progesterone elevated, LH and FSH decreased. Low FSH causes regression of corpus luteum and lowering of estradiol and progesterone levels. FSH rises again, starting the cycle over.	Secretory phase of endometrium in which uterine glands secrete substances

SUMMARY OF MAJOR SEX STEROIDS

HORMONE	BIOCHEMISTRY	METABOLITES	TRANSPORT
Testosterone	Metabolized from the weak gonadal androgens (androstenedione and DHEA) and adrenal androgens (DHEA, DHEA-S, androstenadione, androstenediol) Converted to androstanolone, androstanediol, and dihydrotestosterone (DHT) in the prostate gland and other peripheral tissues DHT is the most potent androgen.	In the liver, the main metabolites of testosterone are androsterone and DHT, which are further metabolized to androstenedione and etiocholanelone. Metabolites are excreted by the kidneys. Main metabolites of adrenal, testicular, and ovarian hormones are 17-ketosteroids: ▪ Males: one third from testosterone from testes, two thirds from adrenal steroids ▪ Females: almost all from adrenal steroids	Testosterone and DHT in plasma exist as either free or bound form: ▪ Males: 2%–3% free, 60%–65% bound to sex hormone binding globulin (SHBG), remainder bound to albumin. ▪ Females: 1% free, 80% bound to SHBG, 19% bound to albumin.
Estrogens	Testosterone rapidly converted to estradiol, the most potent estrogen. Estradiol is the main estrogen produced and secreted by the ovary (100–300 μg/day). 1% of secreted androstenedione is converted to estrone in peripheral tissue (100–200 μg/day).	Estradiol and estrone are converted to estriol and conjugated with glucuronic acid or sulfuric acid by the liver in preparation for renal excretion.	ESTRADIOL: 2%–3% free, remainder bound to SHBG and albumin ESTRONE: Almost exclusively bound to albumin
Progesterone	Synthesis same as in adrenal cortex; cholesterol converted to pregnenolone then progesterone under control of LH and FSH.	Progesterone is converted to pregnanediol and conjugated with glucuronic acid by the liver in preparation for renal excretion.	PROGESTERONE: 2%–10% free, remainder bound to corticosteroid binding globulin (CBG)

SUMMARY OF PATHOLOGIC CONDITIONS

DISEASE	DEFINITION	CAUSES	SYMPTOMS
Primary Ovarian Hypofunction	Functional or developmental dysfunction of the ovary resulting in low levels of steroids and elevated gonadotropins	FUNCTIONAL CAUSES: Premature ovarian failure Resistant ovary syndrome Ovarian tumors DEVELOPMENTAL CAUSES: Gonadal agenesis Turners syndrome 17-Alpha-hydroxylase deficiency NORMAL PHYSIOLOGIC OCCURRENCE: Menopause	PREPUBERTAL: Delayed or absent menarche (primary amenorrhea) POSTPUBERTAL: Secondary amenorrhea
Secondary or Tertiary Ovarian Hypofunction	Low levels of steroids due to pituitary (secondary) or hypothalamic (tertiary) disturbance	Pituitary trauma most common secondary cause (Injury, surgery) as well as tumors and necrosis from postpartum hemorrhage Emotional stress or physical illness as well as anorexia nervosa may cause hypothalamic hyposecretion.	Amenorrhea, as with primary ovarian hypofunction.
Primary Ovarian Hyperfunction	High estrogen occurring before puberty in 5% of cases, during reproductive years in 55% of cases, and after menopause in 40% of cases	Main cause is estrogen secreting tumors such as granulosa and thecal cell tumors.	BEFORE PUBERTY: Precocious puberty Intermittent uterine bleeding DURING REPRODUCTIVE YEARS: Irregular uterine bleeding Amenorrhea AFTER MENOPAUSE: Uterine bleeding
Secondary Ovarian Hyperfunction	Hypersecretion of FSH/LH from pituitary gland resulting in high levels of estrogen	Caused by hyperfunction of the pituitary gland or hypothalamus	Sexual precocity

Continued ▶

SUMMARY OF PATHOLOGIC CONDITIONS

▶ Continued **SUMMARY OF PATHOLOGIC CONDITIONS**

DISEASE	DEFINITION	CAUSES	SYMPTOMS
Primary Testicular Hypogonadism	Low levels of androgens accompanied by high levels of gonadotropins	PREPUBERTAL: Developmental abnormalities POSTPUBERTAL: Testicular infection Trauma Irradiation Tumor (replacing testicular parenchyma) Surgical or accidental castration	PREPUBERTAL: Persistent infantile genitalia Barely palpable prostate Poor secondary sexual development Lack of normal secondary sex characteristics Eunuchoid characteristics POSTPUBERTAL: Decreased beard growth Thinning body hair Prostate atrophy Decreased sexual desire and performance Genitalia decreased in size
Secondary Testicular Hypogonadism	Failure of the pituitary gland to produce LH/FSH and subsequent lack of androgen production	Usually due to pituitary failure; may be due to hypothalamic failure to produce GnRH	As seen with primary testicular hypogonadism
Primary Testicular Hypergonadism	Excessive production of testicular androgens	Caused by testicular tumor (e.g., Leydig cell or interstitial cell carcinoma)	CHILDREN: Precocious puberty ADULT MALES: Little change
Secondary Testicular Hypergonadism	Hypersecretion of gonadotropins by the pituitary gland with subsequent elevation of blood androgens	Caused by hyperfunction of pituitary gland or hypothalamus	As seen with primary testicular hypergonadism

PATIENT PREPARATION, SPECIMEN COLLECTION AND STORAGE, REFERENCE RANGE

TEST	PATIENT PREPARATION	SPECIMEN COLLECTION	SPECIMEN STORAGE	REFERENCE RANGE
Total Testosterone	MALES: Increased during puberty Levels high in AM for adults and 25% lower in evening (13 hr after AM maximum) FEMALES: Lower values with increase 1–2 days midcycle Elevated after exercise. Decreased after glucose load; slow progressive decrease after age 50	Serum Heparinized plasma Urine: 24 hr specimen	Separate from cells within 6 hr, otherwise levels become falsely elevated. Stable 1 wk at 1°–4°C, 6 mo at –20°C.	SERUM/PLASMA: Males: 280–1100 ng/dL Females: 15–70 ng/dL URINE: Males: 50–135 µg/day Females: 2–12 µg/day *Note:* Vary with age and sex
Free and Weakly Bound (Albumin) Testosterone (Bioavailable Testosterone)	See "Total Testosterone"	Serum	Stable 2 days at 1°–4°C or 2 mo at –20°C	Males: 66–417 ng/dL Females: 0.6–5.0 ng/dL
Free Testosterone	See "Total Testosterone."	Serum	Stable 2 days at 1°–4°C or 2 mo at –20°C	Males: 50–210 pg/mL Females: 1–8.5 pg/mL

Continued ▶

▶ Continued **PATIENT PREPARATION, SPECIMEN COLLECTION AND STORAGE, REFERENCE RANGE**

TEST	PATIENT PREPARATION	SPECIMEN COLLECTION	SPECIMEN STORAGE	REFERENCE RANGE
DHEA	Circadian variation similar to cortisol (highest levels in AM)	Serum Heparinized or EDTA plasma Urine: 24 hr specimen	SERUM: Store in glass tubes at 1°–4°C for 2 days. Stable frozen at −20°C for up to 2 mo URINE: Preserve with boric acid and refrigerate until tested.	SERUM: Males: 180–1250 ng/dL Females: 130–980 ng/dL *Note:* Highest levels occur in adults. URINE: Males: <3.1 mg/day Females: <1.5 mg/day
DHEA-S	No variation	Serum or EDTA plasma	Same as DHEA	Males: 125–619 μg/dL Females: 29–781 μg/dL *Note:* Increases to age 30 then declines.
17-Ketosteroids (17-KS)		24 hr urine		Males: 9–22 mg/24 hr Females: 6–15 mg/24 hr

Continued ▶

▲ Continued **PATIENT PREPARATION, SPECIMEN COLLECTION AND STORAGE, REFERENCE RANGE**

TEST	PATIENT PREPARATION	SPECIMEN COLLECTION	SPECIMEN STORAGE	REFERENCE RANGE
Estradiol	FEMALES: Increases progressively through-out puberty Peaks at midcycle and luteal phases Exhibits diurnal variation → best to draw samples at specific time of day	Freshly drawn nonhemolyzed serum preferred Plasma Urine: 24 hr specimen preserved with boric acid	Stable 2 days at 1°–4°C in glass tubes Stable at −20°C for up to 2 mo.	SERUM: Males: 10–50 pg/mL Females: Early follicular = 20–150 pg/mL Late follicular = 40–350 pg/mL Midcycle = 150–750 pg/mL Luteal = 30–450 pg/mL Postmenopausal = less than 20 pg/mL URINE: Males: 1–4 µg/g creat. Females: Follicular = 1–13 µg/g creat. Midcycle = 4–20 µg/g creat. Luteal = 1–17 µg/g creat.
Estrogen		Serum Urine: 24 hr specimen preserved with boric acid and refrigerated during collection	Serum must be frozen immedi-ately after collection.	SERUM: Males: 20–80 pg/mL Females: Follicular = 60–200 pg/mL Luteal = 160–400 pg/mL Postmenopausal = <130 pg/mL URINE: Males: 4–23 µg/g creat. Females: Follicular = 7–65 µg/g creat. Midcycle = 32–104 µg/g creat. Luteal = 8–135 µg/g creat.

Continued ▲

► Continued **PATIENT PREPARATION, SPECIMEN COLLECTION AND STORAGE, REFERENCE RANGE**

TEST	PATIENT PREPARATION	SPECIMEN COLLECTION	SPECIMEN STORAGE	REFERENCE RANGE
Progesterone	FEMALES (NONPREGNANT): Reference value depends on phase of cycle (elevated during luteal, maximal level 5–10 days after LH peak at midcycle). FEMALES (PREGNANT): Gradual elevation between weeks 5–40 (up to 10–40 times normal level)	Serum Heparinized or EDTA plasma	Stable 7 days at 2°–8°C Stable up to 3 mo at −20°C	Males: 0.12–0.3 ng/mL Females: DURING MENSTRUAL CYCLE: Follicular phase = <1 ng/mL Luteal phase = 5–20 ng/mL DURING PREGNANCY: 1st trimester = 20–50 ng/mL 2nd trimester = 50–100 ng/mL 3rd trimester = 100–400 ng/mL

DIAGNOSTIC TESTS AND METHODOLOGIES

TEST	METHOD	INTERFERENCE	COMMENTS
Total Testosterone	Immunoassay: RIA–2 step	Other steroids and drugs removed by chromatography or solvent extraction	Method of choice Most widely used routine measurement
	Nonisotopic	Cross-reacts with DHT	In development Cross-reaction a problem only when DHT is elevated
Free and Weakly Bound Testosterone	Labeled testosterone added to sample and allowed to bind SHBG precipitated out by ammonium sulfate Supernatant tested for testosterone.	Does not depend upon alterations in SHBG levels in blood	Measures all testosterone but that bound to SHBG Useful indicator of androgen activity
Free Testosterone	RIA–competitive binding assay: Add labeled testosterone to compete with unlabeled testosterone → ratio estimates the level of free testosterone.	Problems due to tracer impurity and separation methods	Problems best solved by ultrafiltration used for separation
DHEA/DHEA-S	Immunoassay: RIA	DHEA requires extraction owing to low levels found in blood. DHEA-S does not require extraction.	Assay has replaced the measurement of urinary 17-ketosteroids.
17-Ketosteroids	Photometric: Color reaction of 17-ketosteroids with m-dinitrobenzene in alcoholic KOH.		Replaced by plasma DHEA-S measurement
Estradiol (Both Free and Bound)	Immunoassay Direct (no extraction) RIA or enzymatic	SHBG and albumin compete with the antibody to bind estradiol.	A large excess of DHT displaces the binding proteins from the antibody. Sensitive, reliable, and practical method

Continued ▶

DIAGNOSTIC TESTS AND METHODOLOGIES

► Continued **DIAGNOSTIC TESTS AND METHODOLOGIES**

TEST	METHOD	INTERFERENCE	COMMENTS
Urinary Estrogens	Kober spectrophotometric reaction Requires extensive extraction	Urinary contaminants interfere with color development.	
	Immunoassay: RIA		Increased specificity with preliminary chromatography
	Nonisotopic		Replaced by more specific serum estradiol measurement
Progesterone	GC-MS		Reference method
	Immunoassay-direct RIA		Routine method of choice
			Simple, rapid, precise, accurate
	Nonisotopic		

EVALUATING TEST RESULTS

Tests of Gonadal Function

TEST	PROCEDURE	INTERPRETATION	CLINICAL USE
Clomiphene (Clomid) Stimulation Test	Clomid is administered orally for 7 days. On day 8, serum is collected and the LH/FSH levels are compared with those at baseline.	NORMAL RESPONSE: LH/FSH increased as Clomid blocks the feedback mechanism to the hypothalamus, resulting in increased secretion of GnRH. NO RESPONSE: Hypothalamic or pituitary dysfunction, prepubertal state, anorexia nervosa, and post menopause	Owing to the pulsatile nature of LH/FSH secretion, three samples should be drawn 20 min apart to determine the baseline and response levels of LH/FSH.

CHANGE OF ANALYTE IN DISEASE

ANALYTE	MEASUREMENT	CLINICAL SIGNIFICANCE	COMMENTS
Corticosteroid Binding Globulin (CBG or Transcortin)	Serum levels measured by RIA	ELEVATED: Ovarian hyperfunction Estrogen therapy Pregnancy Chronic active hepatitis Anticonvulsant drug treatment DECREASED: Ovarian hypofunction Fetal death Septic shock Inflammation Chronic liver disease Hypertension Nephrosis	Synthesized in the liver; binds cortisol, progesterone, and testosterone. Concentration is sensitive to exogenous estrogen in dose-response manner.
Sex Hormone Binding Globulin (SHBG)	Serum levels measured by RIA	ELEVATED: Elevated estrogens Hypertension Liver cirrhosis DECREASED: Elevated androgens Hypotension Glucocorticoids Malnutrition and malabsorption Protein losing states Obesity (esp. in females)	Binds both testosterone and estradiol, although has a greater affinity for testosterone.
Estradiol	Serum or urine levels measured by immunoassay	ELEVATED: Feminization in children Estrogen producing tumors (ovarian, adrenal, testicular) Gynecomastia Hepatic cirrhosis Hypertension DECREASED: Primary and secondary hypogonadism (ovarian failure)	Most active endogenous estrogen Higher levels occur during pregnancy. Used to evaluate menstrual and fertility problems in women Most useful in assessment of ovarian function
Estriol	Immunoassay method used to measure free or total levels in blood, urine or amniotic fluid	ELEVATED: When delivery is imminent DECREASED: High risk pregnancy (diabetes, preeclampsia, intrauterine fetal death, anencephalic fetus, malnutrition)	Predominant estrogen present during pregnancy Serial measurements collected at same time of day are best for evaluation of fetal integrity.

Continued ▶

CHANGE OF ANALYTE IN DISEASE

► Continued **CHANGE OF ANALYTE IN DISEASE**

ANALYTE	MEASUREMENT	CLINICAL SIGNIFICANCE	COMMENTS
Estradiol Receptor Protein	Immunochemical or immunocytochemical measurement of protein in tissue samples	POSITIVE (PROTEIN PRESENT): Better prognosis for survival after breast cancer Indicates that the cancer will respond to estrogen therapy	Primary use for identification of patients with breast cancer who will respond to estrogen therapy
Total Estrogens	Serum and urine levels measured by immunoassay	ELEVATED: Ovarian tumors producing estrogen Granulosa and thecal cell tumors Testicular tumors Hyperplasia of adrenal cortex DECREASED: Ovarian agenesis Primary ovarian malfunction Hypopituitarism Hypofunction of adrenal cortex Menopause GnRH deficiency Anorexia nervosa Psychogenic stress	Used to identify gonadal hypofunction and hormonally active tumors Used to evaluate ovulation and oocyte recovery in in vitro fertilization
Testosterone	Blood levels measured by RIA	ELEVATED: Testicular tumors Ovarian masculinizing tumors DECREASED: Hypogonadism	Total testosterone levels are greatly influenced by SHBG levels.
Progesterone	Blood levels measured by immunoassay	ELEVATED: Congenital adrenal hyperplasia due to 21-hydroxylase, 17-hydroxylase, and 11-hydroxylase deficiency Lipoid ovarian tumor Theca lutein cyst Molar pregnancy Chorioepithelioma of ovary DECREASED: Threatened abortion Primary or secondary hypogonadism Short luteal phase syndrome	Used primarily to evaluate fertility in females through detection of ovulation Interpretation must be made in reference to the menstrual cycle.

Continued ►

▶ Continued **CHANGE OF ANALYTE IN DISEASE**

ANALYTE	MEASUREMENT	CLINICAL SIGNIFICANCE	COMMENTS
FSH	Blood and urine levels measured by immunoassay	ELEVATED: Primary gonadal failure Klinefelter's syndrome Castration Alcoholism Menopause Gonadotropin secreting pituitary hormones DECREASED: Anterior pituitary hypofunction Hypothalamic disorders Pregnancy Anorexia nervosa Polycystic ovary disease	Episodic, circadian, and cyclic nature of pituitary gonadotropin secretion requires multiple samplings for appropriate interpretation of results.
LH	Serum levels measured by immunoassay	ELEVATED: Primary gonadal dysfunction Polycystic ovary syndrome Post menopause Pituitary adenoma DECREASED: Pituitary or hypothalamic impairment Anorexia nervosa Severe stress Malnutrition Severe illness	See FSH comments.
Androstenedione	Blood, amniotic fluid, and saliva levels measured by RIA.	ELEVATED: Polycystic ovary disease Hirsutism Congenital adrenal hyperplasia Cushing's syndrome Ectopic ACTH-producing tumors Hyperplasia of ovarian stroma or ovarian tumor DECREASED: Adrenal or ovarian failure	Produced in both adrenals and gonads Useful to evaluate and manage androgen disorders Used to monitor congenital adrenal hyperplasia treatment with glucocorticoids

Continued ▶

CHANGE OF ANALYTE IN DISEASE

▶ Continued **CHANGE OF ANALYTE IN DISEASE**

ANALYTE	MEASUREMENT	CLINICAL SIGNIFICANCE	COMMENTS
DHEA	Serum levels measured by RIA	ELEVATED: Adrenogenital syndrome due to deficiency of beta-dehydrogenase, 21-hydroxylase, and 11-hydroxylase Hirsutism Polycystic ovary disease Cushing's syndrome Ectopic ACTH producing tumors DECREASED: Decreases with age Hyperlipidemia Psychosis Psoriasis Pregnancy	Valuable in assessment of delayed puberty
DHEA-S	Serum levels measured by RIA	ELEVATED: Female hirsutism Congenital adrenal hyperplasia Adrenal cortex tumors Cushing's syndrome Ectopic ACTH producing tumors Polycystic ovary disease DECREASED: Primary or secondary adrenal insufficiency	Replaced the urinary measurement of 17-ketosteroids to estimate adrenal androgen production

BIBLIOGRAPHY

Hypothalamus and Pituitary Function

Anderson SC, Cockayne S: Clinical Chemistry: Concepts and Applications. Philadelphia, WB Saunders, 1993.

Bishop M, Duben-Engelkirk JL, Fody EP: Clinical Chemistry: Principles, Procedures, Correlations, 3rd ed. Philadelphia, JB Lippincott, 1996.

Burtis CA, Ashwood ER: Tietz Fundamentals of Clinical Chemistry, 4th ed. Philadelphia, WB Saunders, 1996.

Challinor SM, Winters SJ, Amico JA: Patterns of oxytocin concentrations in the peripheral blood of healthy women and men: effect of the menstrual cycle and short-term fasting. Endocrinol Res 20:117, 1994.

Chevenne D, Beau N, Leger J, et al: Variability of serum human growth hormone levels in different commercial assays: specificity of growth hormone–releasing hormone stimulation. Horm Res 40:168, 1993.

Claybaugh JR, Uyehara CFT: Metabolism of neurohypophysial hormones. Ann N Y Acad Sci 689:250, 1993.

Cuneo RC, Salomon F, McGauley GA, Sonksen PH: The growth hormone deficiency syndrome. Clin Endocrinol 37:387, 1992.

Finding JW, Tyrrell JB: Anterior pituitary gland. In Greenspan F, ed: Basic and Clinical Endocrinology. Norwalk, CT, Appleton & Lange, 1991, pp 79–132.

Hartman ML, Veldhuis JD, Thorner MO: Normal control of growth hormone secretion. Horm Res 40:37, 1993.

Henry JB: Clinical Diagnosis and Management by Laboratory Methods, 19th ed. Philadelphia, WB Saunders, 1996.

Holtzman EJ, Ausiello DA: Nephrogenic diabetes insipidus: causes revealed. Hosp Pract 29:89, 1994.

Jenkins D, Stewart PM: Advances in medial therapy for pituitary disease: treating patients with growth hormone excess and deficiency. J Clin Pharm Ther 18:155, 1993.

Kaplan L, Pesce AJ: Clinical Chemistry: Theory, Analysis, Correlation, 3rd ed. St. Louis, Mosby–Year Book, 1996.

Kovacs L, Robertson GL: Syndrome of inappropriate antidiuresis. Endocrinol Metab Clin North Am 21:859, 1992.

Loriaux DL, Nieman L: Corticotropin-releasing hormone testing in pituitary disease. Endocrinol Metab Clin North Am 20:363, 1991.

Marshall WJ: Clinical Chemistry, 3rd ed. St. Louis, Mosby–Year Book, 1995.

Mauri M, Pico AM, Alfayate R, et al: Usefulness of urinary growth hormone (GH) measurement for evaluating endogenous GH secretion in acromegaly. Horm Res 39:13, 1993.

Melby JD: Diagnosis of hyperaldosteronism. Endocrinol Metab Clin North Am 20:247, 1991.

Ober K: Diabetes insipidus. Crit Care Clin 7:109, 1991.

Ramsay DF: Posterior pituitary gland. In Greenspan F, ed: Basic and Clinical Endocrinology. Norwalk, CT, Appleton & Lange, 1991, pp 177–187.

Reeves WB, Andreoli TE. The posterior pituitary and water metabolism. In Wilson JD, Foster DW, eds: Williams Textbook of Endocrinology, 8th ed. Philadelphia, WB Saunders, 1992, pp 311–356.

Rudd B: Growth, growth hormone and the somatomedins: an historical perspective and current concepts. Ann Clin Biochem 28:542, 1991.

Smith C, Norman M: Prolactin and growth hormone: molecular heterogeneity and measurement in serum. Ann Clin Biochem 27:542, 1990.

Thorner MO, Vance ML, Horvath E, Kovacs K: The anterior pituitary. In Wilson JD, Foster DW, eds: Williams Textbook of Endocrinology, 8th ed. Philadelphia, WB Saunders, 1992, pp 221–310.

Tietz NW, ed: Clinical Guide to Laboratory Tests, 3rd ed. Philadelphia, WB Saunders, 1995.

Thyroid Function

American Thyroid Association. Optimal use of blood tests for assessment of thyroid function. JAMA 269:2736, 1993.

Anderson SC, Cockayne S: Clinical Chemistry: Concepts and Applications. Philadelphia, WB Saunders, 1993.

Bayer MF: Effective laboratory evaluation of thyroid status. Med Clin North Am 75:1, 1991.

Becks GP, Burrow GN: Thyroid disease and pregnancy. Med Clin North Am 75:121, 1991.

Bishop M, Duben-Engelkirk JL, Fody EP: Clinical Chemistry: Principles, Procedures, Correlations, 3rd ed. Philadelphia, JB Lippincott, 1996.

Bristow A, Gaines-Das R, Buttress N: The international standard for thyroxine binding globulin. Clin Endocrinol 38:361, 1993.

Burtis CA, Ashwood ER: Tietz Fundamentals of Clinical Chemistry, 4th ed. Philadelphia, WB Saunders, 1996.

Cavalieri RR: The effects of nonthyroid disease and drugs on thyroid function tests. Med Clin North Am 75:27, 1991.

Demers LM: The influence of nonthyroidal factors on thyroid function. Lab Med 24:495, 1994.

Ekins R: Analytic measurements of free thyroxine. Clin Lab Med 13:599, 1993.

Faix JD, Rosen HN, Velazquez FR: Indirect estimates of thyroid hormone–binding proteins to calculate free thyroxine index: comparison of nonisotopic methods that use labeled thyroxine ("t-uptake"). Clin Chem 41:41, 1995.

Hay ID, Bayer MF, Kaplan MK, et al: American Thyroid Association assessment of current free thyroid hormone and thyrotropin measurement and guidelines for future clinical assays. Clin Chem 37:2002, 1991.

Hay ID, Klee GG: Linking medical needs and performance goals: clinical and laboratory perspectives on thyroid disease. Clin Chem 39:1519, 1993.

Helfand M, Schmitter J: Screening for thyroid dysfunction: which test is best? JAMA 270:2297, 1993.

Henry JB: Clinical Diagnosis and Management by Laboratory Methods, 19th ed. Philadelphia, WB Saunders, 1996.

Kaplan L, Pesce AJ: Clinical Chemistry: Theory, Analysis, Correlation, 3rd ed. St. Louis, Mosby–Year Book, 1996.

Kaye TB: Thyroid function tests. Application of newer methods. Postgrad Med 94:81, 1993.

Klee GG, ed: Pathophysiology of thyroid disease. Clin Lab Med 13:531, 1993.

Klee GG, Hay ID: Role of thyrotropin measurements in the diagnosis and management of thyroid disease. Clin Lab Med 13:673, 1993.

Larsen PR, Ingbar SH: The thyroid gland. In Wilson JH, Foster DW, eds: Williams Textbook of Endocrinology, 8th ed. Philadelphia, WB Saunders, 1992, pp 357–487.

Lechan RM: Update on thyrotropin-releasing hormone. Thyroid Today XVI (1), 1993.

Liewendahl K: Assessment of thyroid status by laboratory methods: developments and perspectives. Scan J Clin Lab Invest (Suppl) 201:83, 1990.

Liewendahl K: Thyroid function tests: performance and limitations of current methodologies. Scand J Clin Lab Invest 52:435, 1992.

Marshall WJ: Clinical Chemistry, 3rd ed. St. Louis, Mosby–Year Book, 1995.

Martinez M, Derksen D, Kapsner P: Making sense of hypothyroidism. Postgrad Med 93:135, 1993.

Meek JC: Tests of thyroid function: update in the diagnosis and management of thyroid disease. Comp Ther 16:20, 1990.

Nicoloff JT, Spencer CA: The use and misuse of sensitive thyrotropin assays. J Clin Endocrinol Metab 71:553, 1990.

Spencer CA, Schwarzbein D, Guttler RB, et al: Thyrotropin (TSH)-releasing hormone stimulation test responses employing third and fourth generation TSH assays. J Clin Endocrinol Metab 76:494, 1993.

Surks MI: Guidelines for thyroid testing. Lab Med 24:270, 1994.

Surks MI, Chopra IJ, Mariash CN, et al: American Thyroid Association guidelines for use of laboratory tests in thyroid disorders. JAMA 263:1529, 1989.

Taylor CS, Brandt DR: Developments in thyroid-stimulating hormone testing: the pursuit of improved sensitivity. Lab Med 24:337, 1994.

Tietz NW, ed: Clinical Guide to Laboratory Tests, 3rd ed. Philadelphia, WB Saunders, 1995.

Volpe BO: Thyroid Function and Disease. Philadelphia, WB Saunders, 1990.

Wartofsky L, Ingbar SH: Diseases of the thyroid. In Wilson JD, Braunwald E, Isselbacher KJ, et al, eds: Harrison's Principles of Internal Medicine, 12th ed. New York, McGraw-Hill, 1991.

Whitley RJ, Meikle AW, Watts NB: Endocrinology. In Burtis CA, Ashwood ER, eds: Tietz Textbook of Clinical Chemistry, 2nd ed. Philadelphia, WB Saunders, 1994.

Adrenal Function

Anderson SC, Cockayne S: Clinical Chemistry: Concepts and Applications. Philadelphia, WB Saunders, 1993.

Biglieri EG, Kater CE: Mineralocorticoids. In Greenspan FS, Forsham PH, eds: Basic and Clinical Endocrinology. East Norwalk, CT, Appleton & Lange, 1992.

Bishop M, Duben-Engelkirk JL, Fody EP: Clinical Chemistry: Principles, Procedures, Correlations, 3rd ed. Philadelphia, JB Lippincott, 1996.

Blumenfeld JD, Sealey JE, Schlussel Y, et al: Diagnosis and treatment of primary hyperaldosteronism. Ann Intern Med 121:877, 1994.

Bravo EL: Primary aldosteronism. Endocrinol Metab Clin North Am 23:271, 1994.

Burtis CA, Ashwood ER: Tietz Fundamentals of Clinical Chemistry, 4th ed. Philadelphia, WB Saunders, 1996.

Candito M, Albertini M, Politano S, et al: Plasma catecholamine levels in children. J Chromatogr 617:304, 1993.

Candito M, Thyss A, Albertini M, et al: Methylated catecholamine metabolites for the diagnosis of neuroblastoma. Med Pediatr Oncol 20:215, 1992.

Cryer PE: Pheochromocytoma. West J Med 156:399, 1992.

Davenport J, Kellerman C, Reiss D, et al: Addison's disease. Am Fam Physician 43:1338, 1991.

Findling J: Cushing's syndrome—an etiological work-up. Hosp Pract 27:107, 1992.

Gerlo EA, Sevens C: Urinary and plasma catecholamines and urinary catecholamine metabolites in pheochromocytoma: diagnostic value in 19 cases. Clin Chem 40:250, 1994.

Grua JR, Nelson DH: ACTH producing pituitary tumors. Endocrinol Metab Clin North Am 20:319, 1991.

Henry JB: Clinical Diagnosis and Management by Laboratory Methods, 19th ed. Philadelphia, WB Saunders, 1996.

Kaplan L, Pesce AJ: Clinical Chemistry: Theory, Analysis, Correlation, 3rd ed. St. Louis, Mosby–Year Book, 1996.

Karet FE, Brown MJ: Phaeochromocytoma: diagnosis and management. Postgrad Med J 70:326, 1994.

Kaye TB, Crapo L: The Cushing syndrome: an update on diagnostic tests. Ann Intern Med 112:434, 1990.

Marshall WJ: Clinical Chemistry, 3rd ed. St. Louis, Mosby–Year Book, 1995.

Meikle AW, Daynes RA, Araneo BA: Adrenal androgen secretion and biologic effects. Endocrinol Metab Clin North Am 20:381, 1991.

Melby J: Diagnosis of hyperaldosteronism. Endocrinol Metab Clin North Am 20:247, 1991.

Orth DN: Cushing's syndrome. N Engl J Med 332:791, 1995.

Orth DN: Differential diagnosis of Cushing's syndrome. N Engl J Med 325:957, 1991.

Parker LN: Control of adrenal androgen secretions. Endocrinol Metab Clin 20:401, 1991.

Peplinski GR, Norton JA: The predictive value of diagnostic tests for pheochromocytoma. Surgery 116:1101, 1994.

Ram CVS, Fierro-Carrion GA: Pheochromocytoma. Semin Nephrol 15:126, 1995.

Rosano TG, Swift TA, Hayes LW: Advances in catecholamine and metabolite measurements for diagnosis of pheochromocytoma. Clin Chem 37:1854, 1991.

Ross GA, Newbould EC, Thomas J, et al: Plasma and 24-hour urinary catecholamine concentrations in normal and patient populations. Ann Clin Biochem 30:38, 1993.

Snow K, Jiang N, Kao PC, et al: Biochemical evolution of adrenal dysfunction: the laboratory perspective. Mayo Clin Proc 67:1055, 1992.

Tietz NW, ed: Clinical Guide to Laboratory Tests, 3rd ed. Philadelphia, WB Saunders, 1995.

Werbel SS, Ober KP: Pheochromocytoma. Update on diagnosis, localization, and management. Med Clin North Am 79:131, 1995.

Gonadal Function

Adashi EY: The ovarian cycle. In Yen SSC, Jaffe RB, eds: Reproductive Endocrinology. Philadelphia, WB Saunders, 1992, pp 181–237.

Anderson SC, Cockayne S: Clinical Chemistry: Concepts and Applications. Philadelphia, WB Saunders, 1993.

Bishop M, Duben-Engelkirk JL, Fody EP: Clinical Chemistry: Principles, Procedures, Correlations, 3rd ed. Philadelphia, JB Lippincott, 1996.

Braunstein GD: Testes. In Greenspan FS, ed: Basic and Clinical Endocrinology. Norwalk, CT, Appleton & Lange, 1991.

Burtis CA, Ashwood ER: Tietz Fundamentals of Clinical Chemistry, 4th ed. Philadelphia, WB Saunders, 1996.

Carr BR: Disorders of the ovary and female reproductive tract. In Wilson JD, Foster DW, eds: Williams Textbook of Endocrinology, 8th ed. Philadelphia, WB Saunders, 1992, pp 733–798.

Catt KJ, Dufau ML: Gonadotropic hormone biosynthesis, secretion, receptors, and actions. In Yen SSC, Jaffe RB, eds: Reproductive Endocrinology, Physiology, Pathophysiology and Clinical Management. Philadelphia, WB Saunders, 1991, pp 105–155.

Goldfien A, Monroe SE: Ovaries. In Greenspan FS: Basic and Clinical Endocrinology. Norwalk, CT, Appleton & Lange, 1991.

Griffin JE, Wilson JD: Disorders of the testes and male reproductive tract. In Wilson JD, Foster DW, eds: Williams Textbook of Endocrinology, 8th ed. Philadelphia, WB Saunders, 1992, pp 799–852.

Henry JB: Clinical Diagnosis and Management by Laboratory Methods, 19th ed. Philadelphia, WB Saunders, 1996.

Hylka VW, DiZerega GS: Reproductive hormones and their mechanism of action. In Mishell DR, Davajan V, Lobo RA, eds: Infertility, Contraception, and Reproductive Endocrinology. Boston, Blackwell Scientific Publications, 1991.

Kaplan L, Pesce AJ: Clinical Chemistry: Theory, Analysis, Correlation, 3rd ed. St. Louis, Mosby–Year Book, 1996.

Lobo RA, Kletzky OA: Dynamics of hormone testing. In Mishell DR, Davajan V, Lobo RA, eds: Infertility, Contraception, and Reproductive Endocrinology. Boston, Blackwell Scientific Publications, 1991.

Marshall WJ: Clinical Chemistry, 3rd ed. St. Louis, Mosby–Year Book, 1995.

Mooradian AP, Morley JE, Korenman SG: Biological action of androgens. Endocrinol Rev 8:1, 1987.

Rojanasakul A, Udomsubpayakul U, Chinsomboon S: Chemiluminescence immunoassay versus radioimmunoassay for the measurement of reproductive hormones. Int J Gynecol Obstet 45:141, 1994.

Selby C: Sex hormone–binding globulin: origin, function and clinical significance. Ann Clin Biochem 27:532, 1990.

Tietz NW, ed: Clinical Guide to Laboratory Tests, 3rd ed. Philadelphia, WB Saunders, 1995.

Veldhuis JD: The hypothalamic-pituitary-testicular axis. In Yen SSC, Jaffe RB, eds: Reproductive Endocrinology. Philadelphia, WB Saunders, 1992, pp 409–460.

Yen SSC: The human menstrual cycle: neuroendocrine regulation. In Yen SSC, Jaffe RB, eds: Reproductive Endocrinology. Philadelphia, WB Saunders, 1992, pp 273–308.

Chapter **14**

THERAPEUTIC DRUG MONITORING

Vivien A. Soo, MS, MT (ASCP)

Q U I C K   C O N T E N T S

INTRODUCTION

Therapeutic drug level monitoring is one of the fastest growing areas in many laboratories since the mid-1970s. This came about as a result of the introduction of new analytical technologies into the clinical laboratory. Most notable is the development of immunoassay methodologies and the introduction of the high throughput immunoassay automated analyzers. As a result, drug level monitoring that used to require hours of labor intensive analysis has become available to clinicians on a routine basis to aid in optimization of drug therapy in the management of their patients.

The role of the laboratory scientist is to provide clinicians with reliable analytical as well as clinically relevant results. To ensure the quality of the results generated, the laboratory scientist must have a knowledge of the basic principles of pharmacokinetics as they relate to monitoring some of the most commonly monitored drugs, and a thorough understanding of the methods used to measure these drug levels. This chapter will discuss some of the basic principles of therapeutic drug monitoring of some of the most commonly monitored drugs as well as their analytical methodologies.

PHARMACOKINETICS

Pharmacokinetics is the study of drug disposition within the body. This includes the absorption, distribution, metabolism, and elimination of the drug.

Disposition of Drug in the Body

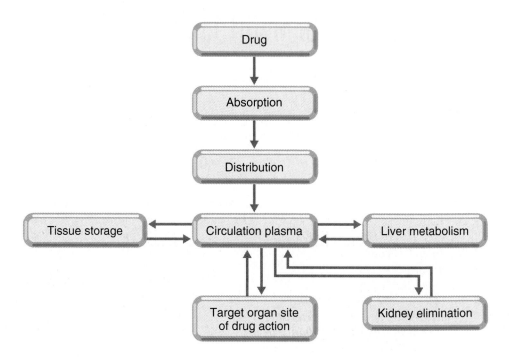

ABSORPTION

For the drug to exert its pharmacologic effects, it must be absorbed and distributed to its target organ or tissue. The rate of drug absorption is dependent on two major factors:

Route of Administration

Generally, parenteral administration, especially by the intravenous route, elicits the most rapid effect by bypassing the gastrointestinal tract. Drugs taken orally may be convenient for the patient, but their rate of absorption may vary widely depending on the type of drug formulation (sustained release), the rate of gastric emptying, and the pH of the absorption site.

Physiochemical Characteristics

For the drug to reach its target organ, it must cross cell membranes. Only the nonionized form of the drug molecule can diffuse across cell membranes. The pKa value of the drug therefore determines the rate of absorption of the drug at the absorption site. (pKa value is the pH at which 50% of the drug is ionized and 50% is in the nonionized form.) Another drug characteristic that determines how well it is absorbed is its solubility in lipids. All biologic membranes are composed of lipid molecules, which act as a barrier. The more lipid soluble the drug, the more easily it crosses the biologic membranes to reach its target organ.

DISTRIBUTION

After the drug absorption phase, the drug enters into the circulatory system to reach its site of action. The rate of drug distribution to various tissues and organs depends on several factors:

Blood Perfusion

A well perfused organ such as the liver and the lungs will receive drugs at a higher rate than a poorly vascular organ such as fat tissues.

Volume of Distribution

Each drug has its characteristic volume of distribution. This can be estimated by dividing the drug dosage by the plasma concentration of the drug.

$$VD = \frac{\text{Amount of drug in the body}}{\text{Concentration of drug in plasma}}$$

Drugs with a small volume of distribution (e.g., gentamicin) generally remain in the plasma, while drugs with a high volume of distribution (e.g., digoxin) will remain in the tissue. Drugs that are highly lipid soluble and readily pass through most biologic barriers will exhibit a very large volume of distribution.

Protein Binding

Some drugs are bound to plasma proteins for their transport. Only the free drugs can cross the cell membrane to exert their pharmacologic effects. As free drugs leave the plasma, bound drugs are displaced from their binding protein. The plasma concentration of the some of the highly protein bound drugs such as phenytoin and valproic acid may be affected by changes in the availability of these plasma proteins. Some disease states can increase or decrease plasma protein concentrations, resulting in decreased or increased concentration of free drugs. Since most therapeutic drug monitoring methods measure total drug concentration (bound + free drugs), free drug level monitoring is recommended for these highly protein bound drugs in patients whose disease state may have altered the protein binding capacity of these proteins.

DRUG METABOLISM

After the drugs have reached their site of action and exerted their pharmacologic effects, they either are eliminated from the body in the unchanged form via the kidneys or are metabolized in the liver to more water soluble metabolites to enable them to be eliminated by the kidneys or in the bile. Drug metabolism occurs mainly in the liver, involving liver enzymes. These biochemical processes are broadly divided into two general classes, nonsynthetic and synthetic. In some cases, some of these processes are genetically determined.

Nonsynthetic Reactions

A functional group, including oxidation, hydroxylation, reduction, and hydrolysis reactions, is added to the parent drug. These reactions all render the parent drug compound more water soluble.

Synthetic Reactions

These combine the parent drug molecule with a conjugating agent such as glucuronic acid or any compound that contain functional groups such as carboxyl, amino, hydroxyl, or sulfhydryl groups. After the parent drugs are conjugated to these functional groups, they become more polar and water soluble.

Genetic Factors

The rate of drug metabolism may be genetically determined. It is well known that the rate of metabolism of procainamide to its active metabolite is genetically determined. Procainamide is metabolized to *N*-acetylprocainamide by the liver enzyme *N*-acetyltransferase. In some patients, the activity of this enzyme is slower or faster than the normal population as predetermined by their genetic make-up. Measurement of both the parent and the active metabolite is therefore recommended.

DRUG ELIMINATION

Drug elimination involves several organs. Highly water soluble drugs such as the aminoglycosides are eliminated unchanged in the urine via the kidneys. Most drugs are metabolized in the liver and eliminated through renal excretion. The rate of drug elimination is determined by the following factors:

Renal Blood Flow and Glomerular Filtration Rate

These determine the amount of drug or drug metabolites to be cleared from the body. Patients with renal disease may not be able to clear the drug compounds efficiently, which results in accumulation of a toxic level of the drug.

Urine pH

Acid urine favors the reabsorption of acidic drugs, because at that pH most of the drugs are in the nonionized forms, allowing them to diffuse across tubular cell plasma membranes. Conversely, alkaline pH favors the reabsorption of basic drugs. The elimination of acid drugs such as aspirin may be facilitated by alkalinization of the urine pH, and vice versa for the elimination of basic drugs.

Half-Life

Each drug has its characteristic elimination half-life, which is defined as the time it takes for the serum drug concentration to decrease by one half.

SPECIMEN COLLECTION

Sampling Time

To obtain clinically relevant therapeutic drug levels, proper specimen collection time is important. Some of the general principles that apply to sampling time are as follows:

POSTDISTRIBUTION SAMPLING

After a single dose, sampling should be done after the distribution phase. Sampling before the postdistribution phase will result in misleadingly elevated blood levels, even though the tissue level is adequate. This is particularly important in monitoring drugs that have a prolonged distribution phase, such as digoxin.

STEADY STATE

For drugs given orally, sampling should be done when they have reached steady state. At steady state, the quantity of drug entering and leaving the body is in equilibrium. It takes approximately five to seven half-lives.

CONSTANT INFUSION

For drugs given in a constant infusion, sampling can be taken at any time.

PEAK AND TROUGH LEVELS

Peak drug level represents the highest drug concentration in a dosing interval. It should be obtained shortly after a dose is given. Trough drug level is the lowest drug concentration within a dosing interval. It is obtained just before the administration of the next dose. Low peak drug levels are usually associated with subtherapeutic dosing, while elevated trough drug levels are usually associated with a toxic concentration of the drug. Drugs that require both peak and trough levels are the aminglycoside antibiotics and vancomycin.

Sample Types

SERUM

Serum is the specimen of choice for most therapeutic drug monitoring. Plasma may be used, depending on the type of anticoagulants used. Some anticoagulants may interfere with some immunoassay methodologies.

WHOLE BLOOD

Whole blood is the specimen of choice for immunosuppressive drugs such as cyclosporine and tacrolimus (FK-506).

SPECIMEN COLLECTION

MOST COMMONLY MONITORED DRUGS

Antiepileptic Drugs: Characteristics, Therapeutic and Toxic Values

DRUG	INDICATIONS	HALF-LIFE (HR)	% PROTEIN BOUND	VD (L/KG)	ELIMINATION	THERAPEUTIC RANGES (μG/ML)	CRITICAL VALUE/TOXICITY (μG/ML)	ANALYTICAL METHODS
Carbamazepine	Grand mal seizures	10–30	67–87	0.8–1.0	Hepatic	4–12	>20 Hypotension, tachycardia	EIA, FPIA, HPLC, GC
Free Carbamazepine						1–3		FPIA
Ethosuximide	Petit mal seizures	40–60	Negligible	0.62	Hepatic	40–100	>200 Anorexia, diarrhea, aplastic anemia	EIA, FPIA, HPLC, GC
Phenobarbital	Effective for all seizures except petit mal	50–120	50	0.7–1.0	Hepatic	15–40	>60 CNS sedation	EIA, FPIA, HPLC, GC
Primidone	Similar to phenobarbital	6–10	0–20	0.6	Hepatic; 15%–20% metabolized to phenobarbital	5–12	>24 CNS sedation due to phenobarbital effect	EIA, FPIA, HPLC, GC
Phenytoin	Effective for most seizures except petit mal	20–40	88–92	0.7	Hepatic; zero order kinetics	10–20	>40 Nystagmus, ataxia, tremor, lethargy	EIA, FPIA, HPLC, GC
Free Phenytoin						1–2		FPIA

Continued ▶

▶ Continued **Antiepileptic Drugs: Characteristics, Therapeutic and Toxic Values**

DRUG	INDICATIONS	HALF-LIFE (HR)	% PROTEIN BOUND	VD (L/KG)	ELIMINATION	THERAPEUTIC RANGES (μG/ML)	CRITICAL VALUE/TOXICITY (μG/ML)	ANALYTICAL METHODS
Valproic Acid	Effective for general and partial seizures	8–15	90–95	0.2	Hepatic	50–100	>200 CNS depression, thrombocytopenia, liver dysfunction	EIA, FPIA, HPLC, GC
Free Valproic Acid						5–15		FPIA

Cardioactive Drugs: Characteristics, Therapeutic and Critical Values

DRUG	INDICATIONS	HALF-LIFE (HR)	% PROTEIN BOUND	VD (L/KG)	ELIMINATION	THERAPEUTIC RANGES (µG/ML)	CRITICAL VALUE/TOXICITY (µG/ML)	ANALYTICAL METHODS
Digoxin	Antiarrhythmic treatment for congestive heart failure	30–50	25	500–600	Hepatic and renal	0.5–2.0 ng/mL Interacts with quinidine to cause digoxin level to increase two- to threefold	>2.5 ng/ml Nausea, confusion, arrhythmia, and vasoconstriction	EIA, FPIA, HPLC
Disopyramide	Antiarrhythmic, effective for ventricular tachycardia	6–8	20–40	0.45–0.7	Hepatic and renal	3–5	>7 Congestive heart failure, anticholinergic effects (dry mouth, urinary retention, constipation)	EIA, FPIA, HPLC, GC
Lidocaine	Drug of choice to treat ventricular arrhythmias due to myocardial infarction or cardiac manipulation	1.5	40–80	130	Hepatic	1.5–5.0	>9 Nausea, confusion, arrhythmias, vasoconstriction	EIA, FPIA, HPLC, GC
Procainamide NAPA	Wide spectrum antiarrhythmic for both ventricular and atrial tachycardia; active metabolite *N*-acetylprocainamide (NAPA)	3.5 6–11	15	2.4	Hepatic and renal; genetic variation in rate of procainamide metabolism—fast and slow acetylators	4–10 Procainamide + NAPA 10–30	>12 Nausea, confusion, vomiting, arrhythmia, lupus syndrome	EIA, FPIA, HPLC, GC

Continued ▶

▲ Continued **Cardioactive Drugs: Characteristics, Therapeutic and Critical Values**

DRUG	INDICATIONS	HALF-LIFE (HR)	% PROTEIN BOUND	VD (L/KG)	ELIMINATION	THERAPEUTIC RANGES (μG/ML)	CRITICAL VALUE/TOXICITY (μG/ML)	ANALYTICAL METHODS
Quinidine	One of the earliest natural agents extracted from tree bark to treat atrial fibrillation	6–7	80–90	3.0	Hepatic; reduces digoxin clearance, thereby increasing serum digoxin level	2–5	>10 Nausea, vomiting, arrhythmias	EIA, FPIA, HPLC

Antibiotic and Bronchodilator Drugs: Characteristics, Therapeutic and Critical Values

DRUG	INDICATIONS	HALF-LIFE (HR)	% PROTEIN BOUND	VD (L/KG)	ELIMINATION	THERAPEUTIC RANGES (μ/ML)		CRITICAL VALUE/TOXICITY (μG/ML)		ANALYTICAL METHODS
Antibiotics										
Amikacin Gentamicin Tobramycin	Aminoglycoside antibiotics against gram negative bacterial infections	2–3	<10 <30 10	0.25	Renal	*Trough* 4–8 0.5–1.5 0.5–1.5	*Peak* 20–30 6–10 6–10	*Trough* >10 >3.0 >3.0 Nephrotoxicity and ototoxicity	*Peak* >50 >15 >15	EIA, FPIA, HPLC, GC
Vancomycin	Antibiotic agent against gram positive bacterial infections	5–6	55	0.4	Renal	*Trough* 5–10	*Peak* 30–40	*Trough* >20 Nephrotoxicity and ototoxicity	*Peak* >60	EIA, FPIA, HPLC, GC
Bronchodilators										
Theophylline	Bronchodilator to relieve symptoms of asthma attacks	4–16	50	0.5	Hepatic and renal; zero order kinetics	10–20		30 GI distress, CNS tremors, and arrhythmia		EIA, FPIA, HPLC, GC
Caffeine	Active metabolite of theophylline, used to treat neonatal apnea	Adult 4 Neonate 30–300	35	0.6	Hepatic and renal	Neonate 8–20		Neonate >50 CNS and skeletal muscle stimulation		EIA, HPLC, GC

Tricyclic Antidepressants, Methotrexate, and Cyclosporin A: Characteristics, Therapeutic and Critical Values

DRUG	INDICATIONS	HALF-LIFE (HRS)	% PROTEIN BOUND	VD (L/KG)	ELIMINATION	THERAPEUTIC RANGES (NG/ML)	CRITICAL VALUE/TOXICITY (NG/ML)	ANALYTICAL METHODS
Tricyclic Antidepressants								
Amitriptyline (Nortriptyline)	Drugs used to control mental depressions, often associated with intentional and unintentional overdose. Drugs are metabolized to secondary active metabolites shown in parentheses.	16–20 / 25–35	95 / 92	14 / 18	Hepatic / Hepatic	100–250	>500	EIA, FPIA, HPLC, GC
Nortriptyline		15–20	95	23	Hepatic	50–150	>300	
Imipramine (Desipramine)		15–20	90	34	Hepatic	150–250	>500	
Desipramine		8–36	70–90		Hepatic	100–300	>500	
Doxepin (Desmethyldoxepin)						*Dox. + metabolite* 100–300	>300 Anticholinergic effects, blurred vision, hypotension	
Antineoplastic								
Methotrexate	Antimetabolite used to treat acute leukemia in children and other solid tumors. High dose treatment requires "rescue" dose of Leucovorin to protect normal tissues from the lethal effects of the drug.	2	50	0.18	Renal	Dose dependent	>5.0 µmol Nephrotoxicity, nausea, vomiting, thrombocytopenia	EIA, FPIA, HPLC
Immunosuppressive								
Cyclosporin A	Immunosuppressive drug that interferes with the activities of T cells; given to organ transplant patients to suppress organ rejection.	6–15	93	1.22	Hepatic	Organ dependent	>300 Reduced renal function, hypomagnesemia, hypertension	EIA, FPIA, HPLC

THERAPEUTIC DRUG MONITORING METHODS

The most commonly used methods for the measurements of serum drug levels are enzyme immunoassay (EIA) and fluorescent polarization immunoassay (FPIA). These have essentially replaced the radioimmunoassays that were widely used in the 1970s. Other methods still in use include high performance liquid chromatography (HPLC) and gas chromatography (GC). Generally, these are used as reference methods or when measurement of both the parent drugs and their metabolites is required.

Indications for Therapeutic Drug Monitoring

Since there are so many drugs in use today, it is not practical to monitor all of them. The following lists some of the situations in which drug level monitoring would benefit patient management.

- Therapeutic drug level is useful only if the drug concentration in the blood correlates with predictable clinical response in the patients.
- Drugs with narrow therapeutic to toxic ranges may require monitoring to prevent toxicity.
- Drugs that exhibit zero order elimination kinetics (saturation kinetics) may require monitoring to prevent drug overdose. For these drugs, a small increment in drug dose may result in disproportionate increase in serum drug level to toxic concentration.
- Drug level monitoring is necessary in patients who have altered drug disposition owing to age, disease state, or other physiologic conditions.
- When multiple drugs are administered concomitant to each other, drug monitoring of their levels is necessary to avoid toxicity due to drug interaction.
- Patient compliance can best be assessed by periodic drug level monitoring.

Common Problems Encountered in Therapeutic Drug Monitoring

To provide clinicians with clinically relevant serum drug levels, laboratory scientists must not only have a good understanding of the pharmacokinetics of the drugs, but also know the limitations of the analytical methods and the potential interferences from endogenous as well as exogenous substances.

See chart on page 248.

Comparison of Therapeutic Drug Monitoring Methodologies

METHOD	PRINCIPLE	SAMPLE PREP.	REAGENT COST	MULTIPLE DRUGS	TURNAROUND TIME (MIN)	TECH. SKILL
Enzyme Immunoassays EMIT, CEDIA	Competitive binding of enzyme labeled drugs with drugs in the patient for limited antibody binding sites. Enzyme activity is blocked when the enzyme labeled drug is bound to the antibody. The amount of enzyme activity is directly proportional to the drug concentration in the patient.	None	High	Single drug	8–15	Medium
Fluorescent Polarization Immunoassays ABBOTT, ROCHE	Competitive binding of fluorescein labeled drugs with drugs in the patient. Labeled drugs, when bound to the antibody, will rotate more slowly than labeled drugs that are free. As a result, they will react to an incident beam of polarized light differently. Bound labeled drug will cause emitted light to remain polarized; free labeled drug will cause reduced polarization of emitted light. Drug concentration is indirectly proportional to the rate of polarization.	None	High	Single drug	8–15	Medium
High Performance Liquid Chromatography (HPLC)	Physical separation of a mixture of compounds based on their differential affinity for the solid stationary and the liquid mobile phase. The sample is introduced to the column under high pressure liquid flow. The analytes are separated by size, polarity, or degree of ionization. The separated analytes are detected by a UV detector at selected wavelengths and converted to electrical signals in the form of peaks whose peak heights are proportional to the concentration of the analytes present in the sample. HPLC is the reference method for the measurement of many therapeutic drug monitoring drugs.	Yes Sample extraction	Low	Multiple drugs and metabolites	45–90	High
Gas Chromatography (GC)	Physical separation of a mixture of compounds based on the differential distribution between the stationary and the gas phase. The sample is vaporized under high temperature. The carrier inert gas (mobile) phase then moves the vaporized sample through a column (stationary) phase where separation takes place. The separated analytes are detected by a flame-ionization detector, electron capture, or a nitrogen-phosphorus detector. The signal produced is proportional to the concentration of the analyte and is then electronically converted into a series of printed peaks.	Yes Sample extraction	Low	Multiple drugs and metabolites	45–90	High

THERAPEUTIC DRUG MONITORING METHODS

Common Problems Encountered in Therapeutic Drug Monitoring

TEST	PROBLEM	PROBABLE CAUSE	SOLUTION
Digoxin	Toxic digoxin level	Overdosed Sampling before distribution phase Cross-reactivity with digoxin-like immunoactive substances (DLIAs) Drug interaction with quinidine	Administer Digibind. Sample 9–10 hr after dosing (after distribution phase). Use HPLC methods. Measure when patient is not on quinidine/reduce digoxin dosage.
Antibiotics	Peak and trough level discrepancies	Mislabelling peak and trough Incorrect sampling times	Verify sampling time. Educate staff.
Phenytoin Valproic Acid Carbamazepine	Toxic drug level	Drug interaction. These highly protein bound drugs compete for limited binding proteins, resulting in increased level of free drugs.	Measure free drug.
		Interaction with endogenous substances: i.e., bilirubin competes for binding proteins.	Measure free drug.
		Renal disease will decrease protein binding to phenytoin, thereby increasing free drug level.	Measure free drug.
Amikacin Tobramycin	Toxic drug level	Drug cross-reactivity	Measure when patient is no longer on the cross-reacting drug. These drugs are not normally coadministered.

BIBLIOGRAPHY

Baselt RC, Cravey RH: Disposition of Toxic Drugs and Chemicals in Man, 3rd ed. Chicago, Year Book, 1990.

Burtis CA, Ashwood ER: Textbook of Clinical Chemistry, 2nd ed. Philadelphia, WB Saunders, 1994.

Goldfrank LR, Floenbaum NE, Lewin NA, et al: Goldfrank's Toxicologic Emergencies, 5th ed. Norwalk, CT, Appleton & Lange, 1994.

Goodman AG, Goodman LS, Gilman A: The Pharmacologic Basis of Therapeutics, 6th ed. New York, Macmillan, 1990.

Halsted CH, Halsted JA: The Laboratory in Clinical Medicine, 2nd ed. Philadelphia, WB Saunders, 1981.

Kaplan LA, Pesce AJ: Clinical Chemistry, 2nd ed. St. Louis, CV Mosby, 1987.

Ochs HR, Bodem G, Greenblatt DS: Impairment of digoxin clearance by coadministration of quinidine. J Clin Pharmacol 21:396, 1981.

Perucea E: Free level monitoring of antiepileptic drugs: clinical usefulness and case studies. Clin Pharmacokinet; 9(Suppl 1):71, 1984.

Pesce AJ, Kaplan LA: Methods in Clinical Chemistry. St. Louis, CV Mosby, 1987.

Tilton RC, Balows A, Hohnadel DC, Reiss RF: Clinical Laboratory Medicine. St. Louis, Mosby–Year Book, 1992.

Ward KM, Lehmann CA, Leikan AM: Clinical Laboratory Instrumentation and Automation: Principles, Applications and Selection. Philadelphia, WB Saunders, 1994.

Chapter # 15

CLINICAL TOXICOLOGY

Vivien A. Soo, MS, MT (ASCP)

Q U I C K   C O N T E N T S

INTRODUCTION

Clinical toxicology is the detection and measurement of drugs in human biologic fluids to aid clinicians in the diagnosis and treatment of patients who overdose on drugs or who are abusive drug users. Some of these agents are common over the counter drugs. Others are controlled drugs that have the potential to be highly addictive and abusive.

The use of illicit drugs has been on the rise in recent years and has become a national problem. Many employers have required workplace drug testing on their employees. Many psychiatric emergency rooms routinely perform screening for drugs of abuse in their patients. The role of the clinical toxicology laboratory is to perform accurate drug testing to identify and confirm the presence of drugs, and to rule out negative drug use by performing preliminary screening tests. This chapter will discuss some of the commonly encountered drugs, their characteristics, and their assay methodologies.

MOST ABUSED SUBSTANCES

Ethanol

Ethanol is commonly referred to as "alcohol." It is a two carbon aliphatic alcohol and is the most commonly abused substance in the United States. It is physically addicting. In New York State, a person with a blood alcohol level of 100 mg/dL or greater is considered intoxicated. Alcohol is associated with 50% of traffic fatalities. For the average adult person, one ounce of whiskey, a glass of wine, or a 12 ounce bottle of beer will raise blood alcohol approximately 25 mg/dL.

METABOLISM

Ninety percent of the ethanol ingested is eliminated by enzymatic oxidation in the liver. At high blood concentration, ethanol may be detected in the breath as the lungs become involved with the excretion of ethanol.

$$\text{ethanol} \xrightarrow{\text{ADH}} \text{acetaldehyde} \xrightarrow{\text{ALDH}} \text{acetate}$$

ADH alcohol dehydrogenase
ALDH aldehyde dehydrogenase

TOXICITY

BLOOD ALCOHOL CONCENTRATION (MG/DL)	CLINICAL MANIFESTATIONS
100–200	Emotional instability, loss of critical judgment
200–300	Confusion, disorientation, impaired balance
300–400	Stupor, inability to stand or walk
>500	Coma, depressed circulation and respiration
>2000	Death from respiratory paralysis

Other Common Alcohols

CHARACTERISTICS, SIGNS, AND SYMPTOMS OF TOXICITY. In addition to ethanol, other alcohols such as methanol, isopropanol, and ethylene glycol are sometimes ingested accidentally or intentionally.

SUBSTANCE	METABOLITES	ACIDOSIS	KETOSIS	CLINICAL MANIFESTATIONS
Ethanol	Acetaldehyde	+	+	Alcoholic ketoacidosis
Ethylene Glycol	Oxalic acid Glycolic acid	+ +	−	Renal failure, calcium oxalate crystals
Isopropanol	Acetone	−	+ +	Hemorrhagic tracheobronchitis, gastritis
Methanol	Formaldehyde Formic acid	+ +	−	Blindness

+, presence and degree of symptoms; −, absence of symptoms.

DETECTION METHODS

Enzyme Assay

Blood ethanol level can be measured accurately by enzyme assays. The enzyme is alcohol dehydrogenase, which is specific for ethanol and does not react with other alcohols. In this assay, NAD is reduced to NADH by the enzyme, and the change in absorbance is measured at 340 nm. The method is easily adaptable to automated instrumentation.

Gas Chromatography (GC)

Gas chromatographic analysis of blood alcohols is the reference method. It allows for simultaneous measurement of other alcohols such as methanol and isopropanol. However, this procedure requires a high degree of technical skills, and the instrumentation is expensive.

COMMON OVER THE COUNTER DRUGS

Acetaminophen (Tylenol) and acetylsalicylate (aspirin) are two of the over the counter drugs most frequently cited as the causative agents for accidental overdose.

Acetaminophen (Tylenol)

Acetaminophen is one of the most commonly used over the counter analgesics.

MOST ABUSED SUBSTANCES

METABOLISM

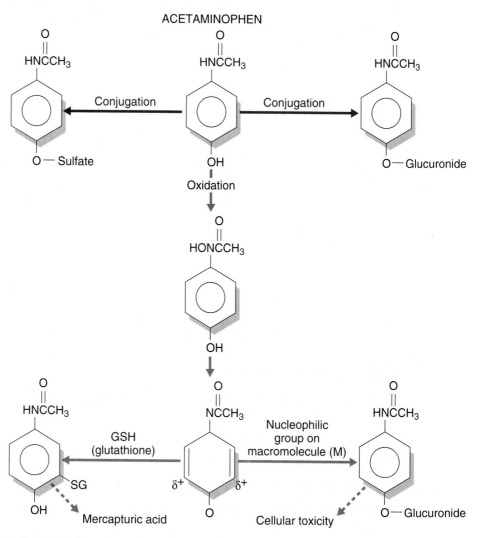

Modified from Mitchell JR, Nelson SD, Thorgeirsson SS, et al: Metabolic activation: biochemical basis for many drug induced liver injuries. In Popper H, Schaffner F, eds: Progress in Liver Disease, Vol 5. New York, Grune & Stratton, 1976, p 259.

Relationship Between Plasma Concentration of Acetaminophen, Time of Ingestion, and Likelihood of Toxicity

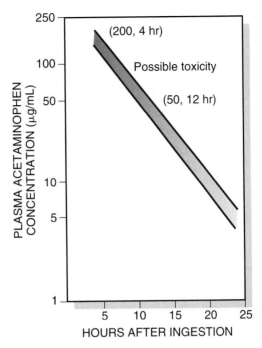

Modified from McNeil Consumer Products Company. Management of acetaminophen overdose with *N*-acetylcysteine. Fort Washington, Pa, McNeilab, Inc., 1980.

Acetaminophen is mainly metabolized in the liver, where it is oxidized and conjugated with sulfate and glucuronic acid. At normal therapeutic dosage, these metabolites will be eliminated in the urine by the kidneys. A small amount of the drug will be metabolized by the cytochrome P-450 system in the liver to a highly reactive metabolite that, under normal conditions, will be inactivated and eliminated by binding to glutathione in the liver. However, in an overdose situation, the normal metabolic pathways are saturated and the glutathione levels become depleted. As a result, the reactive metabolites bind with cellular macromolecules such as DNA, RNA, and proteins in the cytosol to cause liver necrosis. This process may continue for days before the patient exhibits any signs of liver dysfunction. Therefore, if acetaminophen overdose is suspected, it is important to obtain information on the approximate time of ingestion and to check serial plasma acetaminophen levels to assess the risk of liver damage.

ANTIDOTE

N-Acetylcysteine (Mucomyst) is a specific antidote for acetaminophen overdose. It acts as a precursor for glutathione, replenishing reduced glutathione stores. It is most effective if given 8 to 24 hours after ingestion.

COMMON OVER THE COUNTER DRUGS

REFERENCE RANGES

THERAPEUTIC	TOXIC
5–20 μg/mL	>50 μg/mL 12 hr after ingestion >200 μg/mL 4 hr after ingestion

Acetylsalicylic Acid (Aspirin)

Acetylsalicylic acid (aspirin) is the most widely used analgesic, antipyretic, and anti-inflammatory nonprescription drug in the world.

METABOLISM

Acetylsalicylic acid is hydrolyzed to salicylic acid by esterases in the blood as well as in the liver. Salicylic acid is the active analgesic and is rapidly absorbed in the stomach. It is metabolized to salicyluric acid and glucuronides. It has a half-life of 3 hours. It is highly protein bound. Therefore, disease states that affect protein binding will increase or decrease drug levels.

TOXICITY

Toxic symptoms include respiratory alkalosis followed by metabolic acidosis, fever, and coma at levels greater than 600 μg/mL.

ANTIDOTE

Alkalinization of the urine by intravenous administration of sodium bicarbonate may increase the amount of the ionized form of the salicylic acid and prevent its reabsorption in the kidneys.

REFERENCE RANGES

THERAPEUTIC	TOXIC
15–30 mg/dL	>100 mg/mL

Methods for the Analysis of Acetaminophen and Salicylate

DRUG	METHOD	PRINCIPLE	USAGE
		Urine	
Acetaminophen	Spot test	Acetaminophen + *o*-cresol ⟶ indophenol blue	Qualitative Urine screen
Salicylate	Spot test	Salicylate + ferric nitrate ⟶ colored complex	Qualitative Urine screen

Continued ▶

BARBITURATES

Characteristics

Barbiturates are all derivatives of barbituric acid, which has no central depressant activities. They are categorized into four groups based on their elimination half-lives (long acting, intermediate acting, short acting and ultrashort acting). The shorter-acting barbiturates are more lipid soluble, are more protein bound, and have a higher pKa. Pharmacologic effects of these shorter acting barbiturates have a more rapid onset and a shorter duration.

Clinical Manifestations

Symptoms of barbiturate intoxication include ataxia, lethargy, nystagmus, headaches, and confusion. As dosage increases, users may become comatose. Deaths are due to respiratory arrest and cardiovascular collapse.

BENZODIAZEPINES

Characteristics

Benzodiazepines are among the most widely prescribed drugs in the world. They are also the most frequent causes of acute overdose. Some benzodiazepines are metabolized in the liver by demethylation and hydroxylation to active intermediates. Diazepam is demethylated to N-desmethyldiazepam (Nordazepam), which is converted to oxazepam, conjugated with glucuronide, and excreted. Others, such as oxazepam, lorazepam, and temazepam, are metabolized to inactive metabolites by conjugation with glucuronide in the liver, and excreted.

Clinical Manifestations

Toxic doses of benzodiazepines cause progressive loss of consciousness, and at higher dosages deep coma and death.

Narcotics/Analgesics

Narcotic/analgesic is a term used to describe any natural or synthetic drug that has morphine-like pharmacologic actions. These include heroin, morphine, codeine, methadone, and propoxyphene.

HEROIN

Characteristics

Heroin is a semisynthetic derivative of opium, which is an extract of the seed of the poppy plant. It is highly addictive. Heroin has a very short half-life. It is quickly converted to the active 6-monoacetylmorphine (6-MM) in the liver and other tissues, with a half-life of less than 10 minutes. 6-MM is then slowly metabolized to morphine, which is then conjugated to glucuronide or excreted unchanged. Consequently, only morphine and morphine conjugates are found in the urine of heroin users.

DRUGS OF ABUSE IN URINE (DAU)

Clinical Manifestations

Patients who overdose on heroin suffer from pulmonary complications such as pulmonary edema and respiratory depression. Hypotension and bradycardia are some of the cardiovascular complications. CNS depression may lead to coma and death.

MORPHINE/CODEINE

Characteristics

Both morphine and codeine are natural opium derivatives with potent analgesic activities. Codeine is found in many over the counter analgesic medications. Both drugs are rapidly absorbed and distributed. Morphine is conjugated to glucuronide in the liver. Codeine is extensively metabolized to norcodeine, and at least 10% is transformed to morphine. These agents are in turn conjugated with glucuronide and eliminated in the urine. Both heroin and codeine users have morphine in their urine.

Clinical Manifestations

Morphine and codeine overdoses produce clinical manifestations similar to those in heroin users. Pinpoint pupils, respiratory depression, and coma are common symptoms.

METHADONE

Characteristics

Methadone is a synthetic narcotic analgesic with pharmacologic properties similar to those of morphine. However, the development of tolerance to methadone is slower than that to morphine. It is used to treat chronic heroin users. Methadone, like other narcotic analgesics, is well absorbed and distributed to various tissue compartments. It is metabolized in the liver to normethadone and excreted in the urine.

Clinical Manifestations

Toxic side effects from methadone overdose are similar to those caused by morphine.

PROPOXYPHENE

Characteristics

Propoxyphene is a synthetic narcotic analgesic. It is used for the management of mild to moderate pain when aspirin is not effective. It is well absorbed. It is metabolized in the liver to norpropoxyphene and eliminated in the urine.

Clinical Manifestations

Propoxyphene intoxication is accompanied by respiratory and CNS depression. Other symptoms include confusion, hallucinations, and convulsions.

DIAGNOSTIC TESTS AND METHODOLOGIES FOR DRUGS OF ABUSE IN URINE

Screening Tests

These are qualitative tests designed to rule out the absence of drug. They must be sensitive and specific enough to detect classes of drugs of abuse in urine. Both federal and some state agencies have established cut-off concentrations for each drug to divide specimens into negatives and positives. The methodology is easily automated and provides a relatively fast turnaround time of less than 1 hour. Methods include spot tests and immunoassays.

SPOT TESTS

These are colorimetric, end point qualitative assays for group specific drugs in the urine. They indicate presumptive presence or absence of the drug. They must be confirmed.

ADVANTAGES. Low cost and no instrumentation required.

DISADVANTAGES. Lack sensitivity and specificity.

IMMUNOASSAYS

$$AB + Drug + Drug^\circ \rightleftarrows AB\text{-}Drug + AB\text{-}Drug^\circ + Drug^\circ$$
$$\text{(bound)} \qquad\qquad \text{(free)}$$

AB	antibody
Drug	drug in sample
Drug°	labeled drug
AB-Drug°	bound drug in sample
AB-Drug°	bound labeled drug
Drug°	free labeled drug

Heterogeneous. Immunoassays that require physical separation of the bound drug from the free drug, e.g., RIA.

Homogeneous. Immunoassays that do not require physical separation of the bound drug from the free drug, e.g., EMIT and FPIA.

Immunoassays used in the toxicology laboratory are enzyme immunoassay (EIA), fluorescent polarization immunoassay (FPIA) kinetic interaction of microparticle (KIM), and cloned enzyme donor immunoassay (CEDIA). These are sensitive and group specific assays that can easily be adapted to high throughput automated analyzers.

ADVANTAGES. Sensitive and easily adaptable to high throughput analyzers.

DISADVANTAGES. High reagent/instrument costs; some drugs of abuse in urine (DAU) immunoassays are drug class specific, e.g., amphetamine/methamphetamine, opiates, and benzodiazepines. At high serum concentrations, many over the counter cold medications, diet pills, and sleep aids or even food substances may cause potential cross-reactivity, producing false positive results.

Interferences in Immunoassays

Signal Interferences

Urine from patients who have ingested aspirin may contain an aspirin metabolite that will cause a reduction in signal of the EMIT DAU assay, a potential for a false negative result.

Cross-Reactivity

Drugs with similar chemical structures may cross-react with the antibody in the assay to cause a false positive result.

ASSAY	CROSS-REACTING SUBSTANCES
Amphetamine/Methamphetamine	Pseudoephedrine/ephedrine (decongestant)
	Phentermine (anorectic)
	Phenylpropanolamine (decongestant)
Opiates (Morphine)	Codeine (analgesic/cold medication)
	Hydrocodone, hydromorphone, and oxycodone (narcotic analgesics)
	Poppy seeds
Propoxyphene	Diphenhydramine (antihistamine)

Types of Immunoassays

ENZYME MULTIPLIED IMMUNOASSAY TEST (EMIT)

$$AG + AB \longrightarrow AG\text{-}AB + AB + AG\text{-}ENZ$$

$$NAD \smile NADH$$
$$AG\text{-}AB + AG\text{-}ENZ\text{-}AB + AG\text{-}ENZ$$
$$G6P \frown 6\text{-}GLUCONATE$$

AG	unlabeled drug
AG-ENZ	drug labeled with enzyme G6PD
AB	specific antibody

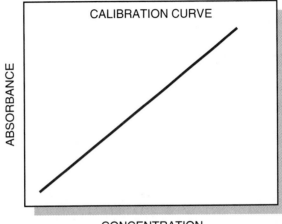

CALIBRATION CURVE

ABSORBANCE

CONCENTRATION

Drug concentration is directly
proportional to rate of absorbance

DIAGNOSTIC TESTS AND METHODOLOGIES FOR DRUGS OF ABUSE IN URINE

CLONED ENZYME DONOR IMMUNOASSAY (CEDIA)

Cloned enzyme donor immunoassay is a novel enzyme immunoassay. It uses recombinant DNA technology to produce a donor enzyme unit and an enzyme receptor unit. When these two units are combined, they form an active enzyme molecule beta-galactosidase, which reacts with the substrate galactopyranoside to form a colored product that can be measured spectrophotometrically.

This technology has been applied to therapeutic drug monitoring as well as drugs of abuse testing. For drug analysis, drug in the patient sample competes with the drug labeled with the donor enzyme for limited antibody binding sites. When drug concentration is high, most of the antibody molecules are bound to the drug molecules in the patient sample, leaving most of the drugs labeled with the donor enzyme unit to combine with the enzyme acceptor unit to form the active enzyme molecule beta-galactosidase. The amount of enzyme activity is directly proportional to the drug concentration in the patient sample.

$$\text{Drug} + \text{Drug-ED} + \text{AB} + \text{EA} \longrightarrow \text{Drug-AB} + \text{Drug-ED-AB} + \text{Drug-ED-EA}$$

$$\underline{\text{SUBSTRATE}}\Bigg/$$

$$\underline{\text{COLORED PRODUCT}}$$

A	absorbance (nm)
AB	antibody
ED	enzyme donor
EA	enzyme acceptor
Drug-ED	drug conjugated to enzyme donor unit
Drug-AB	drug bound to antibody
Drug-ED-EA	drug conjugated to active enzyme molecule

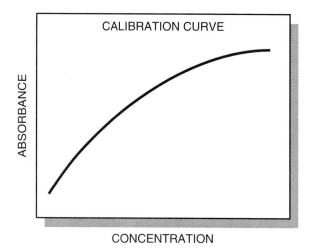

CALIBRATION CURVE

ABSORBANCE

CONCENTRATION

Drug concentration is directly
proportional to rate of absorbance

FLUORESCENCE POLARIZATION IMMUNOASSAY (FPIA)

$$AG + AB + AG^* \longrightarrow AGAB + AG^*AB + AG^*$$

large molecules	small molecules
rotate slowly	rotate rapidly
↓	↓
emitted light	emitted light
remains polarized	polarization reduced

AG   unlabeled drug
AG*   drug labeled with fluorescein
AB   specific antibody

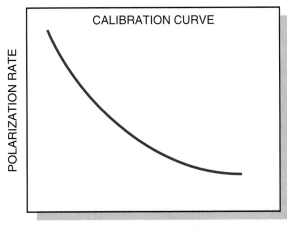

CALIBRATION CURVE

POLARIZATION RATE

CONCENTRATION

Drug concentration is indirectly
proportional to rate of polarization

DIAGNOSTIC TESTS AND METHODOLOGIES FOR DRUGS OF ABUSE IN URINE

KINETIC INTERACTION OF MICROPARTICLE IN SOLUTION (KIM)

The kinetic interaction of microparticle immunoassay is an example of a turbidimetric immunoassay that is based on the light scattering property of an antibody bound drug molecule conjugated to a microparticle. Drug molecule in the patient competes with drug conjugated to microparticles for limited antibody sites. When there is low drug concentration in the sample, most of the drug conjugated to microparticles will bind with antibody molecules to form lattices that are large enough to scatter light. When this happens, light transmission through the reaction solution is blocked, resulting in increased absorbance. The drug concentration in the sample is inversely related to the absorbance of the reaction mixture.

$$\text{Drug} + \text{Drug-M} + \text{AB} \longrightarrow \text{Drug-AB} + \text{Drug-M-AB} + \text{Drug-M}$$
$$\downarrow$$

Lattice formation blocks light transmission, resulting in increased absorbance.

A	absorbance (nm)
AB	antibody
Drug-M	drug conjugated to microparticle
Drug-AB	drug bound to antibody
Drug-M-AB	drug microparticle, and antibody complex

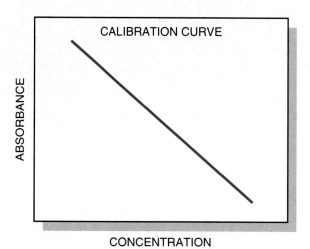

Drug concentration is inversely related to absorbance value

Confirmatory Tests

These are analytical procedures used to confirm the positive urine drug screen and to positively identify the specific drug or metabolite. These procedures should employ techniques or chemical principles different from those used in the initial screening procedure.

THIN LAYER CHROMATOGRAPHY (TLC)

This is a chromatographic method in which a mobile phase moves by capillary action across a thin layer of stationary phase (usually silica gel base material) bonded onto a glass plate or fiberglass sheet. When a mixture of drugs is applied to the plate and developed with the mobile phase, the drugs move across the plate at different rates, depending on their solubility, the pKa values, and the capacity of the hydrogen bonding. The distance the drugs travel from the origin relative to the distance the solvent front has traveled is referred to as the Rf value. Identification of the drug is based on its Rf value and its differential reaction with various chemical agents. Some drugs, such as amphetamine, have characteristic fluorescence under ultraviolet (UV) light.

ADVANTAGES. Low reagent cost; no instrument required; multiple drug analysis.

DISADVANTAGES. Lacks sensitivity; requires high level of technical skills.

HIGH PERFORMANCE LIQUID CHROMATOGRAPHY (HPLC)

HPLC is used as screening as well as a confirmation method. It consists of an autosampler where the sample is introduced to the column. The column consists of a stationary phase and the mobile phase (liquid). Drugs in the sample are separated by size, polarity, or the degree of ionization, depending on the type of stationary phase materials used. The separated analytes are detected by a UV detector at selected wavelengths.

ADVANTAGES. High sensitivity and specificity; ability to detect and quantify several drugs and their metabolite in the same run.

DISADVANTAGES. High instrument cost; sample extraction required; high level of technical skills; slow turnaround time.

GAS CHROMATOGRAPHY (GC)

GC is the method of choice for measuring volatile agents such as ethanol, methanol, isopropanol, and ethylene glycol. Samples are introduced to the injector port where they are vaporized under high temperature. The carrier inert gas (mobile phase) carries the vaporized sample through a column (stationary phase) where separation takes place. Separation of the analytes is highly temperature dependent. The analyte with the higher boiling point will be retained on the stationary phase longer than another compound with a lower boiling point (lower partition coefficient). To control the temperature of the separation, the column is placed in a temperature controlled oven. The separated analytes are detected by flame ionization detector (FID), electron capture detector (ECD), or nitrogen phosphorus detector (NPD). The signal produced is proportional to the concentration of the analyte and is then electronically converted into a series of printed peaks.

ADVANTAGES. High sensitivity and specificity; simultaneous measurement of multiple drugs and their metabolites.

DISADVANTAGES. High instrumentation cost; high technical skills; samples require pretreatment; some may require derivatization.

DIAGNOSTIC TEST AND METHODOLOGIES FOR DRUGS OF ABUSE IN URINE

GAS CHROMATOGRAPHY–MASS SPECTROMETRY (GC-MS)

The use of MS as a detector on a GC provides the ultimate tool for the analysis of drugs. Identification of unknowns can be based on computer matching of the unknown mass spectrum with those of known drugs in the MS library. Both quantitative and qualitative analysis can be performed.

ADVANTAGES. High sensitivity and specificity; ability to identify unknown drugs if they are in the MS library.

DISADVANTAGES. High instrumentation cost; high technical skills requiring special training; require sample pretreatment and derivatization procedure to optimize drug recovery and identification.

SENSITIVITY, SPECIFICITY, AND CUT-OFF CONCENTRATION

SENSITIVITY. The minimal concentration of a drug or metabolites that can be detected; expressed in ng/mL of undiluted urine.

SPECIFICITY. The degree to which a test can discriminate among closely related drugs, metabolites, and naturally occurring substances.

CUT-OFF CONCENTRATION. A drug concentration at which point a drug test is considered positive or negative. If the drug level is equal to or above the cut-off concentration, it is considered positive. If the drug concentration is below the cut-off, the test is considered negative.

MOST COMMONLY ABUSED DRUGS: CHARACTERISTICS AND DETECTION METHODS

CLASS	DRUG	PKA	HALF-LIFE (HR)	PRIMARY METABOLITES	METHOD OF DETECTION
Stimulants	Amphetamine	9.8	4–24	Benzoic acid *p*-Hydroxyamphetamine *p*-Hydroxynorephedrine	CEDIA, EIA, KIM, FPIA, TLC GCMS
	Methamphetamine	9.9	9–24	Amphetamine 4-Hydroxymetamphetamine 4-Hydroxyamphetamine	CEDIA, EIA, KIM, FPIA, TLC GCMS
	Cocaine	8.7	2–4	Benzoylecgonine	CEDIA, EIA, KIM, FPIA, TLC HPLC, GCMS
Hallucinogens	Phencyclidine	8.5	7–16	*N,N*-diethyl-1-phenylcyclohexylamine PCDE	CEDIA, EIA, KIM, FPIA, TLC GCMS
	Delta-9-THC	10.6	14–38	8-β-Hydroxy 9-THC 11-Hydroxy 9-THC 11-Nor-9-THC-9-carboxylic acid	CEDIA, EIA, KIM, FPIA, TLC GCMS
Hypnotics/Sedatives	Pentobarbital	7.9	15–48	3-Hydroxypentobarbital *N*-Hydroxypentobarbital	CEDIA, EIA, KIM, FPIA, TLC GCMS, HPLC
Barbiturates	Amobarbital	7.9	12–16	3-Hydroxyamobarbital *N*-Glucosyl amobarbital	CEDIA, EIA, KIM, FPIA, TLC GCMS, HPLC
	Secobarbital	7.9	15–40	3-Hydroxysecobarbital, secodiol	CEDIA, EIA, KIM, FPIA, TLC GCMS, HPLC
	Butalbital	7.6	30–40	5-(2,3-dihydroxypropyl-5-isobutylbarbituric acid, glucuronide conjugates	CEDIA, EIA, KIM, FPIA, TLC GCMS, HPLC
	Phenobarbital	7.2	48–120	*N*-Glucosyl phenobarbital *p*-Hydroxyphenobarbital Glucuronide conjugates	CEDIA, EIA, KIM, FPIA, TLC GCMS, HPLC

Continued ▶

COMMONLY ABUSED DRUGS: CHARACTERISTICS/DETECTION METHODS

▶ Continued **MOST COMMONLY ABUSED DRUGS: CHARACTERISTICS AND DETECTION METHODS**

CLASS	DRUG	PKA	HALF-LIFE (HR)	PRIMARY METABOLITES	METHOD OF DETECTION
Benzodiazepines	Alprazolam	2.4	7–13	α-Hydroxyalprazolam 4-hydroxyalprazolam Glucuronide conjugates	CEDIA, EIA, KIM, FPIA, TLC GCMS, HPLC
	Chlordiazepoxide	4.8	6–27	Norchlordiazepoxide Oxazepam, nordazepam Glucuronide conjugates	CEDIA, EIA, KIM, FPIA, TLC GCMS, HPLC
	Diazepam	3.4	20–50	Nordazepam, oxazepam Glucuronide conjugates	CEDIA, EIA, KIM, FPIA, TLC GCMS, HPLC
	Flurazepam	1.9/8.2	2–3	N-Desalkylflurazepam N-Hydroxyethylflurazepam	CEDIA, EIA, KIM, FPIA, TLC GCMS, HPLC
	Lorazepam	1.3/11.5	9–16	Glucuronide conjugates	CEDIA, EIA, KIM, FPIA, TLC GCMS, HPLC
Narcotics/Analgesics	Heroin	7.6	1–1.5	6-Acetylmorphine Morphine glucuronide	CEDIA, EIA, KIM, FPIA, TLC, GCMS
	Codeine	8.2	2–4	Morphine, norcodeine	CEDIA, EIA, KIM, FPIA, TLC GCMS, HPLC
	Morphine	8.1	2–4	Morphine glucuronide Normorphine Codeine	CEDIA, EIA, KIM, FPIA, TLC GCMS, HPLC
	Methadone	8.2	15–60	Normethadol	CEDIA, EIA, KIM, FPIA, TLC GCMS, HPLC
	Propoxyphene	6.3	8–24	Norpropoxyphene	CEDIA, EIA, TLC, GCMS

CEDIA, cloned enzyme donor immunoassay; TLC, thin-layer chromatography; KIM, kinetic interaction of microparticle; EIA, enzyme immunoassay; GC-MS, gas chromatography–mass spectroscopy; FPIA, fluorescence polarization immunoassay; HPLC, high performance liquid chromatography.

DRUGS OF ABUSE: METHODS AND DETECTION LIMITS

DRUG	SCREENING METHOD	DETECTION LIMITS (NG/ML)	CONFIRMATION METHOD	DETECTION LIMITS (NG/ML)	SAMHSA† (NG/ML)
Stimulants					
Amphetamine/ Methamphetamine	EIA, FPIA KIM	1000	TLC GCMS	1000 250	500
Benzoylecgonine (Cocaine)	EIA, FPIA KIM	300	TLC GCMS	300 100	150
Hallucinogens					
Cannabinoids (11-NOR-9-THC-9COOH)	EIA, FPIA KIM	50	TLC GCMS	100 10	15
Phencyclidine (PCP)	EIA, FPIA KIM	25	TLC GCMS	100 10	25
Sedatives					
Barbiturates (seco., amo., pento., butalb.)	EIA, FPIA KIM	300	TLC GCMS	1000 250	
Benzodiazepines (oxazepam, nor-diazepam)	EIA, FPIA KIM	300	TLC GCMS	500* 300	
Narcotics/Analgesics					
Methadone	EIA, FPIA KIM	300	TLC GCMS	500 100	
Opiates (morphine, codeine)	EIA, FPIA KIM	300-Morphine	TLC GCMS	300 250	300-Morphine 300-Codeine
Propoxyphene	EIA GCMS	300 300	TLC	500	

*Detection of aminobenzophenones as hydrolysis products of most benzodiazepine metabolites.
†Substance Abuse and Mental Health Service Administration.

COMPARISON OF DAU ANALYTICAL METHODS

METHOD	SAMPLE EXTRACTION	INSTRUMENTATION	SENSITIVITY (NG/ML)	TAT (MIN)	MULTIPLE DRUGS	TECHNICAL SKILLS
TLC	Yes	No	100–1000	60	Yes	High
GC	Yes	Yes	50–100	60	Yes	High
GCMS	Yes	Yes	10–100	60	Yes	High
HPLC	Yes	Yes	50–100	60	Yes	High
EIA	No	Yes	25–1000	2–5	No	Moderate
FPIA	No	Yes	25–1000	2–5	No	Moderate
Spot Test	No	No	1–2 ug/ml	5–10	Yes	Low

TAT, turnaround time; HPLC, high performance liquid chromatography; TLC, thin layer chromatography; EIA, enzyme immunoassay; GC, gas chromatography; FPIA, fluorescent polarization immunoassay; GC-MS, gas chromatography–mass spectrometry.

MISCELLANEOUS POISONOUS SUBSTANCES

CARBON MONOXIDE

Characteristics

Carbon monoxide (CO) is an odorless, colorless, tasteless gas. It is a byproduct of incomplete combustion of organic materials. Sources include automobile exhausts, improperly maintained heating systems, and improperly ventilated coal and gas stoves.

Clinical Manifestations

Carbon monoxide has high affinity for hemoglobin (210 times that of oxygen). In the blood, CO binds to hemoglobin to form carboxyhemoglobin (HbCO). Under normal conditions, carboxyhemoglobin constitutes only a small fraction of the total hemoglobin (<0.5%). At higher levels, the following toxic symptoms may occur as a direct result of hypoxia:

HBCO CONCENTRATION (%)	SYMPTOMS
10–20	Headache
20–30	Severe headache accompanied by syncope and confusion
30–40	Nausea, vomiting, weakness, and dizziness accompanying severe headache
40–50	Tachycardia and tachypnea
>50	Coma
>70	Death

Specimen Requirement

Whole blood using heparin or EDTA as anticoagulant. Specimen must be thoroughly mixed before assay.

Detection Methods

Measurement of carboxyhemoglobin at its characteristic wavelength at 535 and 570.9 nm can easily be performed using a spectrophotometer.

CYANIDE

Characteristics

Cyanides are used in various chemical and electroplating industries. They may be found in household products such as silver polish, insecticides, and rodenticides. Some fruit seeds such as apricot seeds also contain cyanides. They react with cytochrome oxidase to block cellular respiration, producing cytotoxic hypoxia. This action is rapid. There is no known pharmacologic use for cyanide. Most deaths from cyanide poisoning are due to accidental exposure, suicide, or genocide.

Clinical Manifestations

Cyanide ions are readily absorbed. Part of the absorbed cyanide is excreted unchanged by the lungs, giving off the characteristic cyanide odor (oil of bitter almond). The larger portion of the cyanide ions is transformed by the enzyme sulfurtransferase to thiocyanate ions, which are relatively harmless. During acute poisoning, this pathway is saturated. Cyanide ions react with the cytochrome oxidase system in the mitochondria to form cyanomethemoglobin. Methemoglobin competes with cyanide ion for the cytochrome oxidase. This forms the basis for the treatment of cyanide poisoning.

Antidote

Sodium nitrite is the best agent to use for the formation of methemoglobin. Methemoglobin displaces cyanide ions and restores normal cellular respiration. The administration of thiosulfate allows the cyanide ions to form the thiocyanate ions, which can be safely eliminated.

MISCELLANEOUS POISONOUS SUBSTANCES

FORENSIC URINE DRUG TESTING

Forensic drug testing differs from clinical toxicology drug testing in the following areas:

- Forensic drug testing laboratories must meet state and/or federal licensure or certification requirements, including passing on-site inspections.
- Forensic drug testing laboratories require special laboratory facilities with limited access.
- Forensic laboratories should have protocols that protect the confidentiality of all laboratory records, including limiting computer access to authorized personnel.
- Chain of custody of specimens must be well documented.
- Both initial screening and confirmatory testing must be performed at the same laboratory site.
- Forensic drug testing results must be definitive and are both scientifically and legally defensible in a court of law.
- Rapid turnaround time for result reporting is not required for a forensic laboratory, whereas it is very important in a clinical laboratory for the management of patient care.

BIBLIOGRAPHY

Baselt RC, Cravey RH: Disposition of Toxic Drugs and Chemicals in Man, 3rd ed. Chicago, Year Book, 1990.

Burtis CA, Ashwood ER: Textbook of Clinical Chemistry, 2nd ed. Philadelphia, WB Saunders, 1994.

Department of Health and Human Services: Mandatory Guidelines for Federal Workplace Drug Testing Programs. Fed Regist 59:29908, 1991.

Done AK: Salicylate intoxication: significance of measurement of salicylate in blood in cases of acute ingestion. Pediatrics 26:800, 1960.

Epidemiologic Data System (AEDS)—National Institute on Alcohol Abuse and Alcoholism: US Alcohol Epidemiologic Data Reference Manual, vol 3, 3rd ed. Rockville, MD, U.S. Department of Health and Human Services, 1991.

Goldfrank LR, Flomenbaum NE, Lewin NA, et al: Toxicologic Emergencies, 5th ed. Norwalk, CT, Appleton & Lange, 1994.

Goodman AG, Goodman LS, Gilman A: The Pharmacologic Basis of Therapeutics, 6th ed. New York, Macmillan, 1990.

Gossel TA, Bricker JD: Principles of Clinical Toxicology, 2nd ed. New York, Raven Press, 1990.

Haddad LM, Winchester JF, Shannon MW: Clinical Management of Poisoning and Drug Overdose, 3rd ed. Philadelphia, WB Saunders, 1998.

Moffat AC: Clarke's Isolation and Identification of Drugs in Pharmaceuticals, Body Fluids and Post-mortem Materials, 2nd ed. London, Pharmaceutical Press, 1986.

Pesce AJ, Kaplan LA: Methods in Clinical Chemistry. St. Louis, CV Mosby, 1987.

Chapter *16*

NUTRITION ASSESSMENT, VITAMINS, AND TRACE ELEMENTS

Craig A. Lehmann, PhD, CC(NRCC)

Q U I C K   C O N T E N T S

INTRODUCTION

Interest in nutrition over the years has increased for a variety of reasons. The public is far better educated about the effects food has on its health; cholesterol and its relationship to coronary heart disease is a good example. Clinicians are also more aware of how the nutritional status of patients can affect their health as well as their recovery ability. This is particularly true of individuals in hospitals and nursing homes.

The body requires a number of essential nutrients such as water, carbohydrates, amino acids, fatty acids, vitamins, minerals, and trace elements for its metabolism. Nutrients can be placed into two primary groups: macronutrients and micronutrients. The body requires more than 1 g a day of each of the macronutrients. Carbohydrates, proteins, and fats are the primary macronutrients. Macronutrients are generally used for energy. Micronutrients are those nutrients that are needed in concentrations of milligrams or less. Vitamins, minerals, and trace elements would be considered micronutrients.

Nutritional Deficiencies

Nutritional deficiencies can involve many nutrients or just one. Such deficiencies can occur in a short time or can be chronic and not immediately obvious. There are three stages in which the body responds to nutritional deficiency. The first stage is when the body receives insufficient intake of a nutrient or nutrients; it then relies on its reserves, provided that they have not already been depleted. Stage 2 is when the body's concentrations of these nutrients or their metabolites begin to fall and can be detected in the serum and urine. Generally, the patient is asymptomatic in stage two. In stage 3 the patient is almost always symptomatic, as at this point all fat stores have been depleted and protein is being utilized as the source of energy.

Eating Disorders

There are two well known eating disorders associated with nutritional deficiencies: anorexia nervosa and bulimia. Anorexia nervosa is a disorder in which patients virtually starve themselves. Individuals see themselves as overweight and restrict their nutritional intake and/or inflict self-induced vomiting. It is more prevalent in teenagers and more common in females than in males. Bulimia patients indulge in binge eating and/or consume large quantities of food, which is followed by self-induced vomiting in order not to gain weight. Acute malnutrition is also seen in many cancer patients. This malnutrition can be a result of the cancer itself or of the treatment (e.g., radiation therapy). Protein-calorie malnutrition (PCM) is seen in many third world countries and leads to the state of starvation. Of the PCMs, kwashiorkor and marasmus are the two most common. Kwashiorkor is a syndrome in which there is adequate caloric intake (from carbohydrates) yet severe protein deficiency. Marasmus occurs when the diet is deficient not only in protein but also in carbohydrates.

Chronic Conditions

There are many malnutrition conditions that are chronic in nature. Individuals who have improper diets either by choice (high carbohydrate/low protein diets) or because of secondary conditions (drug addicts, alcoholics) are good examples of chronic malnutrition. Anthropometric measurements have been useful in monitoring patients' nutritional status. Body weight is a good indicator of nutritional condition; it can be used as a reference point or can be compared against standard reference tables. Skinfold thickness is a good indicator of body fat, as subcutaneous fat decreases with malnutrition. Changes in muscle mass can be assessed by midarm circumference measurement (MAC). Muscle mass can also be assessed by creatinine/height index and/or 3-methylhistidine excretion. While these tests are useful, they must be carefully interpreted. The combination of anthropometric tests along with a number of biochemical tests can begin to provide a better understanding of an individual's nutritional condition.

Biochemical Markers

Plasma proteins are the most popular of the biochemical markers, since they can help provide an assessment of a patient's nutritional condition. Proteins such as albumin, transferrin, transthyretin (prealbumin), and retinol binding protein have been used to assess nutritional status as well as monitor nutritional therapy. In addition to protein, mineral, and hematologic assays, vitamin and trace element analyses are also becoming part of nutritional evaluations, as they too can provide information about nutritional status.

Vitamins

Vitamins are essential for good health and can be separated into two groups, fat soluble (A, D, E, and K) and water soluble (C and B complex). The body can be deprived of vitamins either directly (diet) or indirectly (patients who have fat absorption problems demonstrate decreases in fat soluble vitamins).

Trace Elements

Trace elements are found in very small concentrations in tissue but play a vital role in human metabolism. The absence or decrease in such elements may produce functional impairment. Trace elements have so far been shown to play major roles in amplification of action, specificity, homeostasis, and interactions. Many trace elements are essential nutrients. Trace elements are stored in various parts of the body; because of this, the most pertinent body fluid must be selected for its analysis.

PATIENT PREPARATION, SPECIMEN COLLECTION AND STORAGE, REFERENCE RANGE

TEST	PATIENT PREPARATION	SPECIMEN COLLECTION	SPECIMEN STORAGE	REFERENCE RANGE
Albumin	Fasting	Serum	4°C up to 72 hr; −20°C up to 6 mo	Child 3.8–5.4 g/dL Adult 3.4–4.8 g/dL
		Urine	Urine 4°C for long periods; freeze −20°C	24 hr urine: adult 1–14 mg/dL
Transferrin	Fasting	Serum	4°C up to 72 hr; −20°C up to 6 mo	Serum: adult 200–400 mg/dL
		Urine	Urine: adjust pH to 7.0; freeze −20°C up to 1 yr	24 hr urine 0.68/d
Transthyretin (Prealbumin)	Fasting	Serum	4°C up to 72 hr; −20°C up to 6 mo	Serum: adult 16–35 mg/dL
		Urine	Urine: adjust pH to 7.0; freeze −20°C up to 1 yr	24 hr urine: 0.017–0.047 mg/d
Retinol Binding Protein	Fasting	Serum Plasma: EDTA, heparin, or citrate	4°C up to 72 hr; −20°C up to 6 mo	Adult 2.6–7.6 mg/dL
Triglycerides	12 or more hr fast	Serum	4°C—7 days; −20°C 90 days	Adult recommended ranges: Male 40–160 mg/dL Female 35–135 mg/dL (age dependent, see Lipid chapter)
Vitamin A	Fasting	Serum Plasma (heparin)	4 wk at 4°C; 2 yr frozen at −20°C; protect from light	Child 30–65 μg/dL Adult 30–80 μg/dL

Continued ▶

► Continued **PATIENT PREPARATION, SPECIMEN COLLECTION AND STORAGE, REFERENCE RANGE**

TEST	PATIENT PREPARATION	SPECIMEN COLLECTION	SPECIMEN STORAGE	REFERENCE RANGE
Vitamin D	Fasting	Serum Plasma (heparin)	Stable at room temperature for 72 hr and at −20°C for longer storage periods	25-(OH)D: Child 2–8 ng/mL Adult 8–45 ng/mL 1,25(OH)2D: Child 19–70 pg/mL Adult 15–40 pg/mL
Vitamin E	Fasting	Serum Plasma (heparin)	4°C for 4 wk and for longer periods at −20°C	5.0–18 μg/mL
Vitamin K	Fasting	Serum Plasma	−20°C up to 3 mo	0.13–1.19 ng/mL
Thiamine B$_1$	Fasting	Serum	<1 yr at −20°C	0.75–1.30 IU/g Hgb
Riboflavin B$_2$	Fasting	Urine 24 hr Serum Plasma (EDTA) Erythrocytes	Urine: −4°C Serum or plasma: −20°C Erythrocytes: −20°C; protect from light	24 hr urine >100 μg/d Serum 4–24 μg/dL Erythrocytes 10–50 μg/dL
Vitamin B$_6$	Fasting	Serum Plasma (EDTA, heparin, Na citrate)	10 days at −50°C	5–30 ng/mL
Niacin		24 hr urine in 1% HCl		2.4–6.4 mg/d
Vitamin B$_{12}$	Fasting	Serum	24 hr at 8°C; 8 wk at −0°C; protect from light	200–835 pg/mL
Pantothenic Acid B$_3$		Serum Whole blood (Na citrate) Urine 24 hr in chlorobenzene		0.2–1.8 μg/mL Urine 1–15 mg/d
Vitamin C (Ascorbic Acid)		Plasma (oxalate, heparin, or EDTA) Whole blood Leukocyte levels Urine	3 hr at 4°C; deproteinized sample stable for 2 mo at −20°C; leukocyte assay immediately	Plasma >0.30 mg/dl Whole blood >0.50 mg/dL Leukocyte >15 μg/dL Urine: Adult 8–27 mg/24 hr Child 35–54 mg/24hr
Iron	Morning specimen	Serum Urine: adjust pH to 1	No hemolysis	Child 50–120 μg/dL Adult: Female 50–170 μg/dL Male 65–170 μg/dL

Continued ►

► Continued **PATIENT PREPARATION, SPECIMEN COLLECTION AND STORAGE, REFERENCE RANGE**

TEST	PATIENT PREPARATION	SPECIMEN COLLECTION	SPECIMEN STORAGE	REFERENCE RANGE
Zinc	Fasting morning specimen	Serum/plasma Urine 24 hr: adjust pH to 2.0 Erythrocytes Hair	Separate from cells before 45 min	Serum/plasma: 70–120 μg/dL Urine 150–1200 μg/d Erythrocytes 10–16 μg/mL Hair 124–320 μg/g day wt
Copper		Serum Plasma Erythrocytes Urine 24 hr: adjust pH to 2	Separate from cells immediately	Adult: Male 70–140 μg/dL Female 80–155 μg/dL Plasma: Male 56–111 μg/dL Female 69–169 μg/dL Erthrocytes 90–150 μg/dL Urine 3–35 μg/d
Magnesium	Fasting	Serum Erythrocytes Urine 24 hr: adjust pH to 1.0	Stable for several days at 4°C	Adult 1.6–2.6 mEq/L Erythrocytes 3.3–5.3 mEq/L Urine 6.0–10 mEq/L
Manganese		Whole blood Serum Plasma (no sodium heparin) Urine Erythrocytes	Stable at room temperature for 7 days	Whole blood 10.9 + 0.6 μg/L Plasma 0.9 + 0.1 μg/L Serum 0.59 + 0.16 μg/L Urine 0.5–9.8 μg/L Erythrocytes: Male 1.4 + 0.03 μg/dL Female 1.7 + 0.06 μg/dL
Selenium		Whole blood (EDTA or heparin) Serum Urine 24 hr Erythrocytes Hair		Whole blood 58–234 μg/dL Serum 46–143 μg/dL Urine 7–160 μg/L Erythrocytes 75–240 μg/kg Hair 0.2–1.4 μg/g day wt
Molybdenum		Serum Plasma (citrate) Whole blood Urine Hair		Serum 0.1–3.0 μg/L Plasma 36–82 μg/L Whole blood 0.8–3.3 μg/L Urine 8–34 μg/L Hair 20–490 μg/kg day wt

DIAGNOSTIC TESTS AND METHODOLOGIES

TEST	METHOD	INTERFERENCE	COMMENTS
Albumin	Binding with anionic dyes brom-cresol green or purple Immunochemical methods RID and nephelometry Electrophoresis	Lipemic samples will interfere. Samples should be ultracentrifuged if lipemia is suspected.	Posture, age, and hemo-concentration will alter results. Half-life 15–21 days
Transferrin	Nephelometry and RID	Transferrin can be estimated from total iron binding capacity value. This method can provide a false increase of transferrin by as much as 20%.	Half-life 8 days
Transthyretin (Prealbumin)	Nephelometry and RID		Half-life 2 days
Retinol Binding Protein	Nephelometry and RID		Zinc deficiencies will decrease RBP. Half-life 10 hr
Triglycerides	Methods measure free glycerol by a variety of coupled enzymes (see lipid chapter).	Collection tubes that have lubricated stoppers should not be used. Free glycerol can cause increased values. However, sample can correct error.	If plasma samples are used, multiply test results by 1.03.
Vitamin A	Neeld-Pearson method: trifluoroacetic HPLC	Neeld-Pearson method sensitive to light	HPLC is the method of choice.
Vitamin D	RIA or ultraviolet detection	Almost all methods use a 3 step procedure: extraction—HPLC, separation, detection.	Methods that detect multiple metabolites should not be used.
Vitamin E	Emmeric-Engel color reaction Fluorimetric HPLC separates α-tocopherol and its five oxidation products with ultraviolet (UV) detection RBC hemolysis test with H_2O_2	Medications interfere with fluorimetry.	HPLC is the preferred method. The stability of the RBC membranes should be measured, as it is an excellent indicator of vitamin E status.
Vitamin K	After extraction and separation methods that react vitamin K with acidic phenylhydrazine, 2,6-dichloroindophenol and active methylene compounds have been utilized. Vitamin K can also be assessed using prothrombin time.		
Thiamine B_1	HPLC with UV detection Measuring transketolase in whole blood or erythrocytes.		

Continued ▶

▶ Continued **DIAGNOSTIC TESTS AND METHODOLOGIES**

TEST	METHOD	INTERFERENCE	COMMENTS
Riboflavin B_2	Urinary determinations from fasting, timed, or 24 hr samples are performed either by HPLC separation with fluorimetric detection or direct fluorimetric measurement. A more common method is one that assays flavin adenine dinucleotide dependent glutathione reductase activity of lysed erythrocytes from a small amount of heparinized venous blood.	Factors such as physical activity, stress, temperature, and some therapeutic drugs can make borderline interpretations difficult.	Sensitivity can be improved with a load return test.
Vitamin B_6	Urinary determinations from 24 hr samples: microbiologic using *Saccaromyces uvarum,* which measures free B_6; plasma levels are measured by enzymatic, radiometric, and HPLC methods. Tryptophan load test most common test for vitamin B_6 nutrient.	Factors influencing tryptophan load test are protein intake, exercise, lean body mass, and circadian rhythm. Pregnant women and women taking oral contraceptives can also demonstrate excessively high values.	Hematologic assays are helpful; normocytic, microcytic, or sideroblastic anemia possible.
Niacin	Measurements of $N(1)$-methylnicotinamide and $N(1)$-methyl-3-carboxamide-6-pyridone are the two most widely used methods. HPLC is the method of choice for determining pyridone to methylnicotinamide ratios.	$N(1)$-Methylnicotinamide increases during pregnancy.	
Vitamin B_{12}/ Folate	Microbiologic, competitive protein binding, and immunometric methods are presently being utilized for the measurement of B_{12}/folate. Competitive protein binding methods: folate competes with 125-I labeled folate for binding sites on β-lactoglobulin binder and B_{12} competes with Co-labeled cobalamin for binding sites on the intrinsic factor.		Reference ranges vary and are method dependent. Laboratories should establish their own reference range.
Pantothenic Acid	Microbiologic and RIA present methods used		

Continued ▶

► Continued **DIAGNOSTIC TESTS AND METHODOLOGIES**

TEST	METHOD	INTERFERENCE	COMMENTS
Vitamin C (Ascorbic Acid)	Most methods rely on the reductive properties of ascorbic acid. The reduction of 2,4-dinitrophenylhydrazine to hydrazone and the reduction of 2,4-dichlorophenol-indophenol to its colorless form are two good examples. A fluorimetric method along with a method that utilizes L-ascorbate oxidase to oxidize ascorbic acid to dehydroascorbic acid, coupled to the production of ferrous ions, has demonstrated excellent sensitivity and specificity.		Urine is not as reliable as serum or leukocyte values in the evaluation of ascorbic acid nutriture.
Iron	Serum iron, iron binding capacity, and transferrin saturation are based on the principle that when the pH is decreased in serum, iron is released from transferrin. Fe^{3+} is reduced to Fe^{2+} and complexes with either bathophenanthroline or ferrozine. Unsaturated iron binding capacity and total iron binding capacity is accomplished by saturating transferrin binding sites with excess Fe^{3+}. Ferritin can be performed by several methods, IRMA and ELISA being the most prevalent.	Samples that demonstrate high levels of hemolysis should be avoided. Contamination of reagents and glassware should be avoided.	Immunoassays are available for serum transferrin.
Zinc	Flame or electrothermal atomic absorption spectroscopy are the desired methods.	Contamination of sample, (e.g., by water, reagents) can present false elevations.	Plasma and serum concentrations are not valid in the presence of hypoalbuminemia.
Copper	Flame or electrothermal atomic absorption spectroscopy are the methods of choice. Methods detecting ceruloplasmin can be either photometric or "immuno" methods. Photometric methods utilize a oxidase reaction with dimethyl-*p*-phenylenediamine. "Immuno" methods consist of immunonephelometry, radial immunodiffusion, and immunoelectrophoresis.	Environmental contamination can increase values.	An acid washed polypropylene bottle should be used for urine.
Manganese	Furnace atomic absorption spectroscopy (AAS) is the method of choice.	Environmental contamination must be avoided.	Urine levels are usually very low.

Continued ►

▶ Continued **DIAGNOSTIC TESTS AND METHODOLOGIES**

TEST	METHOD	INTERFERENCE	COMMENTS
Selenium	Spectrofluorimetry and flameless AAS are the methods of choice.		
Molybdenum	AAS methods have been used for this trace element, but none were acceptable.		This trace element has no present clinical significance, except for the diagnosis of inborn error.

TESTS FOR MONITORING AND EVALUATING NUTRITIONAL STATUS AND DIAGNOSIS OF SELECTED CONDITIONS

TEST AND PRIMARY FUNCTION	CLINICAL SIGNIFICANCE
Albumin Vascular colloidal pressure and transports many compounds	Decreases in malnutrition Half-life 15–21 days Affected by fluid retention
Transferrin Transports iron	Low in malnutrition Half-life 8 days
Transthyretin (Prealbumin) Stabilizes and prevents retinol binding protein from glumerular filtration. Plays a significant role in vitamin A metabolism.	Low in malnutrition, reflects hepatic protein synthesis Half-life 2 days
Retinol Binding Protein Transports vitamin A	Low in malnutrition Half-life 10 hr
Triglycerides Energy storage and metabolic energy	Assessment of hypertriglyceridemia in peripheral parental nutrition
Prognostic Nutritional Index (PNI) Albumin, transferrin, triceps skinfold thickness, and delayed hypersensitivity reaction: $PNI(\%) = 158 - 16.6\ (ALB) - 0.2\ (TRF)$ $\quad - 0.78\ (TSF) - 5.8\ (DHR)$	Assessment of patient's surgical risk and selection criteria for preoperative nutrition support: PNI <40% Low Risk 40–49% Intermediate Risk >50% High RIsk
Vitamin A Involved in vision	Decreased levels of vitamin A in liver stores are seen in chronic infection, fever, hepatic disease, and many disorders that involve lipid metabolism. Vitamin A absorption test is recommended for assessment of intestinal absorption.
Vitamin D Skeletal growth and calcium needs	Decreased levels are found in malabsorption, rheumatoid arthritis, nephrotic syndrome, usage of anticonvulsants (e.g., phenytoin), renal osteodystrophy, rickets, hypoparathyroidism, and decreased dietary intake or decreased sunlight.

Continued ▶

► Continued **TESTS FOR MONITORING AND EVALUATING NUTRITIONAL STATUS AND DIAGNOSIS OF SELECTED CONDITIONS**

TEST AND PRIMARY FUNCTION	CLINICAL SIGNIFICANCE
Vitamin E Antioxidant for unsaturated fatty acyl moieties	Decreased values are seen in fat absorption disorders, abetalipoproteinemia, and malabsorption. Toxicity can occur from increased intake of vitamin (e.g., anticoagulant therapy).
Vitamin K Required for the synthesis of clotting factors II, VII, IX, and X	Decreased values are observed in newborns who have hemorrhaged. Mothers who have been receiving vitamin K antagonists place their newborn at high risk of having decreased vitamin K. Decreased values in adults are seen in chronic fat malabsorption and obstructive jaundice. Decreased vitamin K leads to impairment in the synthesis of VII, IX, X, and prothrombin. Gut sterilization with antibiotics.
Thiamine B$_1$ Involved in the aldehyde transfers of alpha keto acids.	Alcohol abuse is one of the leading causes of thiamine deficiency. Decreases are also seen in diabetes, cancer, and dialysis patients. A number of inborn errors respond to thiamine therapy.
Riboflavin B$_2$ Involved in oxidation and reduction reactions	Decreased values are generally associated with decreases of other water soluble vitamins.
Vitamin B$_6$ Involved in many reactions (metabolism of proteins, carbohydrates, lipids, and amino acids)	Vitamin B$_6$ dependency syndromes Drugs such as isoniazid, D-cycloserine, and penicillamine
Nicotinamide NAD and NADP dependent enzymes are required in (NAD) catabolic and (NADP) biosynthetic reactions.	Pellagra (diets of predominantly corn). This condition can also be caused by Hartnup's disease or carcinoid syndrome.
Vitamin B$_{12}$ Involved in the synthesis of methionine and conversion of methylmalonic to succinic acid	Vitamin B$_{12}$, unsaturated B$_{12}$ binding capacity (UBBC), and total B$_{12}$ binding capacity (TBBC) are the tests used to evaluate this vitamin. Decreased conditions in all three tests are seen in pernicious anemia. Increases in all three are seen in liver disease, polycythemia vera, myelofibrosis, chronic myelocytic leukemia, and acute myelocytic leukemia. Leukocytosis and late pregnancy present increased UBBC and TBBC with decreased vitamin B$_{12}$. Decreases in B$_{12}$ are seen in inadequate dietary intake and malabsorption syndromes (e.g., celiac disease. The most common cause is the defective production of intrinsic factor.
Pantothenic Acid B$_3$ A primary component of acyl thiol esters of CoA	Because of the abundance of pantothenic acid in food, decreases are not seen.
Vitamin C (Ascorbic Acid) Cofactor for protocollagen hydroxylase	Inefficient intake of vitamin C leads to scurvy. Some populations have demonstrated deficiencies in vitamin C: smokers; alcoholics; individuals under stress; and patients with rheumatic fever, tuberculosis, and acute and chronic inflammatory conditions.

Continued ►

▶ Continued **TESTS FOR MONITORING AND EVALUATING NUTRITIONAL STATUS AND DIAGNOSIS OF SELECTED CONDITIONS**

TEST AND PRIMARY FUNCTION	CLINICAL SIGNIFICANCE
Iron Required in a variety of processes such as cellular oxidation mechanisms and transport of oxygen to tissues	Diurnal variation demonstrates normal values in the early part of the day, decreasing midafternoon and decreasing to its lowest level by midnight. Decreased values are observed in menstrual cycle, pregnancy, acute and chronic inflammation, myocardial infarction, malignancy, kwashiorkor, and iron deficiency. Increased values are seen in hepatitis, oral contraceptive usage, and increased ingestion.
Zinc Plays a role in protein synthesis	Nutritional deficiency demonstrates decreased levels in serum, urine, and erythrocytes. Hepatic cirrhosis demonstrates a decrease in serum, an increase in urine, and a normal concentration in erythrocytes. Other decreases in serum levels are seen in pregnancy, sickle cell anemia, chronic renal failure, carcinoma of the lung, myocardial infarction, and oral contraceptive usage. Increases just in urine are seen in nephrosis, chronic infection, and hepatic porphyria.
Copper Required for hemoglobin synthesis	Deficiency is seen in kwashiorkor, marasmus, malabsorption syndromes, malnutrition, malabsorption, and premature infants. Hereditary disorders such as kinky hair disease and Wilson's disease demonstrate decreased values of ceruloplasmin. Increases are seen in Addison's disease, hypopituitarism, infection, lymphomas, liver disease, pregnancy, and testosterone therapy.
Magnesium Cofactor for many enzymes as well as an allosteric activator for enzyme systems	Decreases have been observed in chronic alcoholism, malnutrition, lactation, malabsorption, acute pancreatitis, hypothyroidism, and aldosteronism. Increases have been observed in dehydration, diabetic acidosis, and Addison's disease.
Manganese Involved in metalloenzymes	Increased urine levels have been observed in acute hepatitis, myocardial infarctions, and rheumatoid arthritis. Low tissue values have been observed in children with maple syrup disease and phenylketonuria.
Selenium Plays a role in the metabolism of enzymes	Decreased values have been reported in gastrointestinal cancer and protein-calorie malnutrition (PCM).
Molybdenum Involved in metalloenzymes (xanthine, aldehyde, and sulfite oxidases)	Presently there is no need to perform molybdenum assays. The only condition associated with this trace element is the inborn error of molybdenum metabolism.

TESTS FOR MONITORING AND EVALUATING NUTRITIONAL STATUS

BIBLIOGRAPHY

Bailey KV, Ferro-Luzzi A: Use of body mass index of adults in assessing individual and community nutritional status. Bull World Health Organ 73:673–680, 1995.

Barrocas A, White JV, Gomez C, Smithwick L: Assessing health status in the elderly: the nutrition screening initiative. J Health Care Poor Underserved 7:210–218, 1996.

Burtis CA, Ashwood ER: Tietz Fundamentals of Clinical Chemistry, 4th ed. Philadelphia, WB Saunders, 1996.

Chapman KM, Ham JO, Pearlman RA: Longitudinal assessment of the nutritional status of elderly veterans. J Geront A Biol Sci Med Sci 51:B261–269, 1996.

Conwell Y: Nutrition. Crisis 16:56–58, 1995.

Cotton E, Zinober B, Jessop J: A nutritional assessment tool for older patients. Prof Nurse 11:609–610, 621, 1996.

Davis C, Stables I: Audit of nutrition screening in patients with acute illness. Nurs Times 92:35–37, 1996.

Fisher GG, Opper FH: An interdisciplinary nutrition support team improves quality of care in a teaching hospital. J Am Diet Assoc 96:176–178, 1996.

Howanitz JH, Howanitz PJ: Laboratory Medicine: Test Selection and Interpretation. New York, Churchill Livingstone, 1991.

Hsu LK, Lee S: Is weight phobia always necessary for diagnosis of anorexia nervosa? (review). Am J Psychiatry 150:1466–1471, 1993.

Kaplan LA, Pesce AJ: Clinical Chemistry: Theory, Analysis and Correlation, 2nd ed. St. Louis, CV Mosby, 1989.

Peterson AE, Maryniuk MD: Using a nutrition assessment to determine a nutrition prescription (review). Diabetes Educator 22:205–206, 209–210, 1996.

Phang PT, Aeberhardt LE: Effect of nutritional support on routine nutrition assessment parameters and body composition in intensive care unit patients. Can J Surg 39:212–219, 1996.

Rault JP, Adam F, Simon F: Limits of PINI (prognostic nutritional and inflammatory index) in the evaluation of nutritional status in children [French]. Med Trop 55:343–346, 1995.

Tietz NW: Clinical Guide to Laboratory Tests, 3rd ed. Philadelphia, WB Saunders, 1995.

Verity S: Nutrition and its importance to intensive care patients (review). Intens Crit Care Nurs 12:71–78, 1996.

Watson R: Nutrition in elderly people (review). Elderly Care 7:23–27, 28–29, 1995.

17

TUMOR MARKERS

Craig A. Lehmann, PhD, CC(NRCC)

Q U I C K   C O N T E N T S

INTRODUCTION

The role of the clinical laboratory in screening, diagnosing, and monitoring neoplasia has increased over the years, but not without controversy. Many of the present tumor markers do not clearly delineate between benign and malignant cells. Because of this, their use, especially in screening, is limited. The low sensitivity and specificity of tumor markers have for the most part required physicians to use a combination of markers as well as other diagnostic tools (e.g., biophysical methods) to enhance their accuracy and aid in their decision process. The costs associated with screening for neoplasia have also been raised. The economic costs of screening for early detection have been demonstrated to not always be cost effective. One example is the screening for cervical cancer with Papanicolaou (Pap) testing. In women who had screenings every 3 years, the incidence of cancer was reduced by 90.8% compared with women who were screened annually in whom the incidence decreased by 93.5%. Because of the costs associated with testing every year, recommendations are that Pap testing be performed every 1 to 3 years based on the presence of risk factors (e.g., sexual history).

Etiology

Cancer is a long term multistage genetic process. The first stage is when the DNA is damaged by some form of carcinogen (e.g., smoking, radiation, chemicals, virus). At some later time, additional damage occurs that eventually leads to chromosome breakdown and rearrangement. This process produces a new phenotype that loses control over the process of mitosis. The process of mitosis continues and ultimately produces malignant tumor cells. Eventually, there is a production of a growing mutant cell that expresses oncogenes. Oncogenes are genes capable of inducing or maintaining transformation of cells. The metastatic phenotype is the supreme stage in the advancement of cancer cells. The mutational events that lead to the metastatic phenotype produce cells that leave the tumor. These cells are now capable of entering the interstitial stroma, and can invade the walls of blood vessels and enter circulation. Once in circulation, these cells eventually spread to other organs.

Classification of Tumor Markers

Tumor markers come from a variety of groups: enzymes, glycoproteins, hormones and hormone-like substances, hormone receptors, oncogenes, and oncogene receptors. The list of tumor markers that arise from this list is quite extensive. However, because of the low sensitivity and specificity of most tumor markers, the Food and Drug Administration (FDA) has approved only a few assay kits as tumor markers. The FDA approved list of tumor markers includes alpha-fetoprotein, carcinoembryonic antigen, estrogen receptors, ovarian CA (CA 125), progesterone receptor, prostate specific antigen (PSA), and soluble interleukin-2 (IL-2) receptor.

Tumor markers may not be ideal for screening purposes but have been very effective in tumor staging, monitoring, detecting the recurrence of cancer, and monitoring therapeutic response. In April 1995 the FDA reclassified serum tumor markers used in monitoring cancer patients from class III into class II. This will increase the availability of tumor markers in monitoring tumors to the public. This is a clear sign that the use of tumor markers to aid physicians in diagnosing, treating, and monitoring cancer patients will most likely continue to grow. The use of genetic markers in evaluating chromosomal changes could very well help in the early detection of cancer. Oncogenes and suppresser genes have already begun to demonstrate their value in hematologic and solid tumor malignancies.

PATIENT PREPARATION, SPECIMEN COLLECTION AND STORAGE, REFERENCE RANGE

TEST	PATIENT PREPARATION	SPECIMEN COLLECTION	SPECIMEN STORAGE	REFERENCE RANGE
Alpha-fetoprotein (AFP)	—	Serum	2°–8°C up to 24 hr >24 hr −20°C	<15 µg/L
Cancer Antigen (CA) 15-3	—	Serum or plasma (citrate)	<5 days 2°–8°C >5 days −20°C	<30 U/mL
CA 19-9	—	Serum	2°–8°C up to 24 hr >24 hr −20°C	<70 U/mL
CA 50	—	Serum	2°–8°C up to 24 hr >24 hr −20°C	<17 U/mL
CA 72-4	—	Serum	2°–8°C up to 24 hr >24 hr −20°C	<4.0 ng/mL
CA 125	—	Serum	2°–8°C up to 24 hr >24 hr −20°C	<35 U/mL

Continued ▶

▶ Continued **PATIENT PREPARATION, SPECIMEN COLLECTION AND STORAGE, REFERENCE RANGE**

TEST	PATIENT PREPARATION	SPECIMEN COLLECTION	SPECIMEN STORAGE	REFERENCE RANGE
CA 549	—	Serum	2°–8°C up to 24 hr >24 hr −20°C	<15.5 U/mL
Carcinoembryonic Antigen (CEA)	—	Serum	2°–8°C up to 24 hr >24 hr −20°C	<5.0 ng/L
Calcitonin	Fasting	Serum or plasma (heparin)	Freeze immediately at −20°C	Serum: adult <150 pg/mL Plasma: adult Male <19 pg/mL Female <14 pg/mL
Human Chorionic Gonadotropin (hCG)	—	Serum	2°–8°C <7 days >7 days −20°C	<2 ng/mL
Progesterone Receptors	—	0.1–1.0 g of tissue	Store in liquid nitrogen within 30 min	negative <6 fmol/mg borderline 6–10 fmol/mg positive >10 fmol/mg
Estrogen Receptors	—	Serum	Freeze immediately at −20°C	Male 20–80 pg/mL Female: Luteal phase 160–200 pg/mL Postmenopausal <130 pg/mL
Progesterone	—	Serum	4 days at 4°C 3 mo −20°C	Male 13–97 ng/dL Female: Luteal phase 200–2500 ng/dL
Alkaline Phosphatase	—	Serum	<3 days 4°C 1 mo −25°C	Method specific; AACC, IFCC ref. method 37°C 20–50 yr Male 53–128 U/L Female 42–98 U/L >60 yr Male 56–155 U/L Female 43–160 U/L
Creatine Kinase CK-BB	—	Serum	4°C <2 days >2 days −20°C	Absent or trace
Lactic Dehyrogenase and Its Isoenzymes	—	Serum or plasma (heparin) Serum only for isoenzymes	Remove from clot and store at room temperature	Total LDH 120–280 U/L
Prostate Specific Antigen (PSA)	—	Serum	<14 days 2°–8°C >14 days −20°C	Males 80% <4.0 μg/L

DIAGNOSTIC TESTS AND METHODOLOGIES

TEST	METHOD	INTERFERENCE	COMMENTS
Alpha-fetoprotein (AFP)	Immunoassay	Turbid samples need to be clarified	
Cancer antigen (CA) 15-3	Immunoradiometric assay	None reported	Use in conjunction with CEA.
CA 19-9	Immunoradiometric assay	None reported	
CA 50	Immunoradiometric assay	None reported	
CA 72-4	Immunoradiometric assay	None reported	
CA 125	Immunoassay Immunoradiometric assay	Human antimouse antibody	Avoid gross hemolysis, jaundice, and lipemic samples.
CA 549	Immunoradiometric assay	None reported	Results correlates with those found using CA 15-3.
Carcinoembryonic antigen (CEA)	Enzyme immunoassay and radioimmunoassay	Turbid samples should be avoided or cleared	
Calcitonin	Radioimmunoassay	Epinephrine, estrogen, oral contraceptives. Also avoid gross hemolysis and lipemic samples.	Ranges vary with method.
Human Chorionic Gonadotropin (hCG)	Immunometric assay, immunoassay		Methods that measure both subunits (intact and free beta-hCG) should be used for tumor markers.
Progesterone Receptors	Cytochemical, immunocytochemical, and immunochemical		Cytochemical is subject to individual interpretations.
Estrogen Receptors	Radioimmunoassay	Oral contraceptives, estrogen therapy, digoxin	
Progesterone	Radioimmunoassay	Oral contraceptives, ampicillin	
Alkaline Phosphatase	Enzymatic: phenyl phosphate, 4-NPP, AMP, DEA	Numerous hepatotoxic drugs, ascorbic acid, oral contraceptives, estrogen, clofibrate	Isoenzymes can offer greater specificity.
Creatinine kinase CK-BB	Immunochemical, electrophoresis, ion exchange	Electrophoresis method has interference from albumin in chronic hemodialysis patients.	

Continued ▶

▶ Continued **DIAGNOSTIC TESTS AND METHODOLOGIES**

TEST	METHOD	INTERFERENCE	COMMENTS
Lactic Dehydrogenase (LD) and Its Isoenzymes	Pyruvate to lactate or lactate to pyruvate; Isoenzymes: electrophoresis, immunoinhibition and chemical inhibition	Hemolysis and numerous drugs	LD-1 is increased in germ cell tumors.
Prostate Specific Antigen (PSA)	Radioimmunoassay, immunoradiometric assay, and immunoenzymatic assay	Finasteride	Screening with PSA for prostatic cancer is recommended only for men >50 yr.

CLINICAL SIGNIFICANCE

TEST	CLINICAL SIGNIFICANCE
Alpha-fetoprotein is an oncofetal glycoprotein and is synthesized by heptoma cells.	Hepatocellular carcinoma Testicular germ cell tumors (nonseminoma) Pancreatic carcinoma Gastric carcinoma
CA-15-3 is a glycoprotein mucin.	Breast carcinoma Pancreatic cancer Lung cancer Colorectal cancer Ovarian cancer Liver cancer
CA-19-9 is a carbohydrate antigen and occurs in serum (mucin) and in tissue (monosialogangliosides).	Abdominal carcinoma Pancreatic cancer Lung cancer Gastric cancer Hepatobiliary cancer Colorectal cancer
CA-50 has a sialylated Lewis A determinant.	Gastrointestinal cancer Pancreatic cancer
CA-72-4 TAG is a mucin-like, human adenocarcinoma associated antigen.	Gastric carcinoma monitoring Ovarian carcinoma
CA-125 is a serum carbohydrate antigen and is a glycoprotein antigen.	Ovarian and endometrial cancer monitoring Elevated also in lung, breast, and gastrointestinal carcinoma
C-549 is an acidic glycoprotein.	Monitoring breast cancer Ovarian cancer Prostate cancer Lung cancer

CLINICAL SIGNIFICANCE

Continued ▶

▶ Continued **CLINICAL SIGNIFICANCE**

TEST	CLINICAL SIGNIFICANCE
CEA in a glycoprotein present in colonic adenocarcinoma and fetal gut.	FDA approved for colorectal cancer Also used in the management of breast, gastrointestinal, colorectal, and lung cancer
Calcitonin is a circulating peptide hormone produced by the perifollicular C cells of the thyroid gland.	Thyroid medullary carcinoma Bronchogenic carcinoma Skeletal metastases
hCG is a glycoprotein hormone with two dissimilar subunits, alpha and beta, with a half life <20 hr	Monitoring nonseminomatous germ cell testicular tumors Trophoblastic tumors
Progesterone receptors in tumor tissue	Ovarian cancer The presence of progesterone and estrogen receptors in a tumor indicates that the patient will respond well to endocrine therapy.
Estrogen receptors in tumor tissue	Breast cancer: treatment and prognosis
Progesterone total in serum	Lipoid ovarian tumor
Alkaline phosphatase in serum	Liver and bone leukemia, carcinoma
Creatinine kinase CK-BB in serum	Prostate and lung (small cell) carcinoma
Lactate dehydrogenase in serum	Elevated in many carcinomas as well as in patients with metastatic carcinoma
Prostate specific antigen is a seminal plasma protein (gamma-seminoprotein)	Monitoring and staging of prostate cancer

TUMOR MARKERS IN DIAGNOSING, MONITORING, STAGING, AND DETECTING THE RECURRENCE OF CANCER

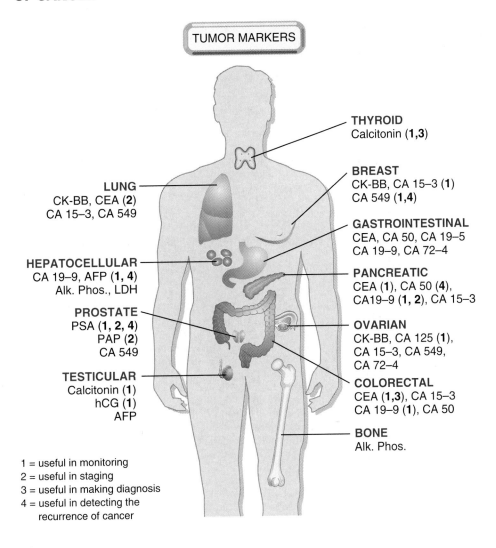

TUMOR MARKERS

THYROID
Calcitonin (**1,3**)

BREAST
CK-BB, CA 15–3 (**1**)
CA 549 (**1,4**)

GASTROINTESTINAL
CEA, CA 50, CA 19–5
CA 19–9, CA 72–4

PANCREATIC
CEA (**1**), CA 50 (**4**),
CA19–9 (**1, 2**), CA 15–3

OVARIAN
CK-BB, CA 125 (**1**),
CA 15–3, CA 549,
CA 72–4

COLORECTAL
CEA (**1,3**), CA 15–3
CA 19–9 (**1**), CA 50

BONE
Alk. Phos.

LUNG
CK-BB, CEA (**2**)
CA 15–3, CA 549

HEPATOCELLULAR
CA 19–9, AFP (**1, 4**)
Alk. Phos., LDH

PROSTATE
PSA (**1, 2, 4**)
PAP (**2**)
CA 549

TESTICULAR
Calcitonin (**1**)
hCG (**1**)
AFP

1 = useful in monitoring
2 = useful in staging
3 = useful in making diagnosis
4 = useful in detecting the
    recurrence of cancer

BIBLIOGRAPHY

Anonymous: Biology, Biochemistry and Clinical Usefulness of Tumor Markers. 23rd Meeting of the International Society for Oncodevelopmental Biology and Medicine, September 10–13, 1995, Montreal, Canada. Abstracts: Tumor Biol 17 suppl 1:1–85, 1996.

Bosl GJ, Chaganti RS: The use of tumor markers in germ cell malignancies (review). Hematol Oncol Clin North Am 8:573–587, 1994.

Burtis CA, Ashwood ER: Tietz Fundamentals of Clinical Chemistry, 4th ed. Philadelphia, WB Saunders, 1996.

Giai M, Roagna R, Ponzone R, et al: TPS and CA 15.3 serum values as a guide for treating and monitoring breast cancer patients. Anticancer Res 16:875–881, 1996.

Gion M, Mione R, Barioli P, Dittadi R: Dynamic use of tumor markers, rationale—clinical applications and pitfalls (review). Anticancer Res 16:2279–2284, 1996.

Hayes DF: Serum (circulating) tumor markers for breast cancer (review). Recent Results Cancer Res 140:101–113, 1996.

Howanitz PJ, Howanitz JH: Laboratory Medicine: Test Selection and Interpretation. New York, Churchill Livingstone, 1991.

Huncharek M, Muscat J: Serum prostate-specific antigen as a predictor of staging abdominal/pelvic computed tomography in newly diagnosed prostate cancer. Abdom Imaging 21:364–367, 1996.

Kaplan LA, Pesce AJ: Clinical Chemistry: Theory, Analysis and Correlation, 2nd ed. St. Louis, CV Mosby, 1989.

Kato H: Gynecologic malignancies (review) [Japanese]. Nippon Rinsho 54:1637–1641, 1996.

Lee WJ, Park YT, Choi JS, et al: Solid and papillary neoplasms of the pancreas. Yonsei Med J 37:131–141, 1996.

Massidda B, Ionta MT, Foddi MR, et al: Usefulness of pyridinium crosslinks and CA 15-3 as markers in metastatic bone breast carcinoma. Anticancer Res 16:2221–2223, 1996.

Masukagami T, Akimoto S, Akakura K, et al: Prognostic factors in stage D2 prostate cancer: results of univariate and multivariate analyses [Japanese]. Hinyokika Kiyo 42:269–274, 1996.

McClatchery KD: Clinical Laboratory Medicine. Baltimore, Williams & Wilkins, 1994.

Miralles RM: Pelvic masses and endoscopic surgery: diagnosis (review). Eur J Obstet Gynecol Reprod Biol 65:75–79, 1996.

Motoo Y, Watanabe H, Sawabu N: Sensitivity and specificity of tumor markers in cancer diagnosis (review) [Japanese]. Nippon Rinsho 54:1587–1591, 1996.

Plebani M, De Paoli M, Roveroni G, et al: Serum tumor markers in colorectal cancer staging, grading, and follow-up. J Surg Oncol 62:239–244, 1996.

Plebani M, Giacomini A, Beghi L, et al: Serum tumor markers in monitoring patients: interpretation of results using analytical and biological variation. Anticancer Res 16:2249–2252, 1996.

Posner MR, Mayer RJ: The use of serologic tumor markers in gastrointestinal malignancies (review). Hematol Oncol Clin North Am 8:533–553, 1994.

Roviello F, Garosi L, Marrelli D, et al: Preoperative serum levels of CEA and CA 19-9 in patients with gastric cancer [Italian]. Minerva Chir 51:133–139, 1996.

Schuurman JJ, Bong SB, Einarsson R: Determination of serum tumor markers TPS and CA 15-3 during monitoring of treatment in metastatic breast cancer patients. Anticancer Res 16:2169–2172, 1996.

Schwartz PE, Chambers JT, Taylor KJ: Early detection and screening for ovarian cancer (review). J Cell Biochem (suppl) 23:233–237, 1995.

Sixteenth Annual Arnold O. Beckman Conference in Clinical Chemistry: Clinical laboratory testing in cancer patient diagnosis and management. Clin Chem 39/11 (B) 1993.

Suresh MR: Classification of tumor markers (review). Anticancer Res 16:2273–2277, 1996.

Takami H, Kodaira S: Tumor markers: neoplasms in digestive organs (review) [Japanese]. Nippon Rinsho 54:1616–1620, 1996.

Tamakoshi K, Kikkawa F, Shibata K, et al: Clinical value of CA125, CA19-9, CEA, CA72-4, and TPA in borderline ovarian tumor. Gynecol Oncol 62:67–72, 1996.

Tietz NW: Clinical Guide to Laboratory Tests, 3rd ed. Philadelphia, WB Saunders, 1995.

Villena V, Lopez-Encuentra A, Echave-Sustaeta J, et al: Diagnostic value of CA 72-4, carcinoembryonic antigen, CA 19-9 assay in pleural fluid. A study of 207 patients. Cancer 78:736–740, 1996.

von Kleist S, Hesse Y, Kananeeh H: Comparative evaluation of four tumor markers, CA 242, CA 19-9, TPA and CEA in carcinomas of the colon. Anticancer Res 16:2325–2331, 1996.

Watanabe N: Organ specificity of tumor markers and its application for clinical diagnosis (review) [Japanese]. Nippon Rinsho 54:1592–1596, 1996.

Section

II

IMMUNOLOGY

Chapter **18**

RHEUMATIC AND AUTOIMMUNE DISEASES

Candace Breen, BS, MLT (ASCP)

Marc Golightly, PhD

QUICK CONTENTS

INTRODUCTION

The rheumatic and autoimmune diseases can generally be classified into two groups. The first group are systemic diseases, which includes the major autoimmune disorders such as systemic lupus erythematosus (SLE), Sjögren's syndrome, progressive systemic sclerosis, rheumatoid arthritis, and mixed connective tissue disease. The second group are those that are organ or tissue directed. Examples of this type are autoimmune thyroid disease, myasthenia gravis, and certain skin diseases such as bullous pemphigoid. This section is concerned with the systemic diseases, but it should be realized that these diseases often fail to fit squarely into these categorizing groups, and many have characteristics common to both.

SYSTEMIC DISEASES

CLINICAL MANIFESTATIONS: SYSTEMIC

The clinical manifestations of both groups usually reflect the organ system(s) or tissue(s) involved. The disease manifestations between and within individuals are highly variable and may range in severity from being extremely mild to severe and protracted leading to death. Since the specific clinical manifestations of the autoimmune diseases are so variable and complex, a detailed treatment of this topic is beyond the scope of this chapter; the interested reader is referred to the appropriate clinical text. While the pathogenic mechanism of the autoimmune diseases is complex and variable, they share the commonality of antibodies being produced to modified or unmodified structures on cell surfaces, autoantigen-autoantibody immune complexes, or autoreactive cytotoxic cells as the mechanisms by which autoimmune damage seems to occur.

LABORATORY DIAGNOSIS: SYSTEMIC

The laboratory diagnosis of rheumatic and autoimmune diseases centers on detection of the autoantibody being produced in the disease process. Whether it is an inciting autoantibody or an antibody produced as a result of the tissue insult and subsequent release of autoantigens yielding a break in B-cell tolerance, or both, is not clear.

ANA Positivity with Connective Tissue Disease

CONNECTIVE TISSUE DISEASE	PERCENT POSITIVE ANA TEST
Systemic Lupus Erythmatosus	90–100
Sjögren's Syndrome	85
Scleroderma	88
Rheumatoid Arthritis	55
Juvenile Arthritis	22
Mixed Connective Tissue Disease	100

Antinuclear Antibodies (ANA)

The detection of antinuclear antibodies (ANA) has been one of the major laboratory screening tests for detection of systemic rheumatic diseases since the early 1960s (see "ANA Positivity with Connective Tissue Disease" above). Since the substrate in the ANA test is the whole cell, including the intact nucleus with most of the cellular antigens present, many different autoantibodies can be detected and screened for by this method. The major ANA antigens of interest are the following nuclear macromolecules:

1. DNA (both double and single stranded)
2. DNP (deoxyribonucleoprotein)
3. Histones

4. Extractable nuclear antigens (ENA)
   Nuclear proteins
   RNA-protein conjugates

ANA PATTERN RECOGNITION. Autoantibodies to these antigens are evidenced by the ANA pattern of staining that occurs in the nucleus or cytoplasm of the cell. While the ANA pattern recognition gives clues to the disease involved, it is not terribly specific for an individual antigen (with a few exceptions—see "Antigens Associated with Autoimmune Disease" below). Therefore, when a positive ANA is reported, further testing should be performed to determine the antigen that is reacting with the autoantibody. More than one autoantibody may be present in an autoimmune disease, and this often translates to more than one ANA pattern in a particular sample. This should be reported when found, as it may be significant to the disease process or prognosis.

ANTIGENS ASSOCIATED WITH AUTOIMMUNE DISEASE

AUTOANTIBODY/ANTIGENS RECOGNIZED	ANA PATTERN	DISEASE ASSOCIATION	COMMONLY USED CLINICAL TEST
Double and Single Stranded IF DNA	Homogeneous/rim	SLE and low level in other rheumatic disease	ELISA, *Crithidia luciliae*
Histones	Homogeneous/rim	Drug induced lupus, SLE	ELISA, treated ANA
Deoxynucleoprotein	Homogeneous/rim	Drug induced lupus, SLE	ELISA, LE Prep (seldom used)
Smith (SM)	Speckled	Diagnostic of SLE	ELISA, ID, WB
Nuclear RNP	Speckled	High titer: mixed connective tissue disorder/SLE	ELISA, ID, WB
SS-A (Ro)	Speckled or negative (low titer)	Sjögren's syndrome, SLE	ELISA, ID, WB
SS-B (La)	Speckled	Sjögren's syndrome	ELISA, ID, WB
ScL-70	Atypical speckled	Diagnostic of scleroderma	ID, WB
Centromere	Centromere	CREST variant of scleroderma	ANA, W.B.
RNA Polymerase I	Nucleolar	Scleroderma: high prevalence	ANA, WB
Fibrillarin	Nucleolar	Scleroderma	ANA, WB
DNA Topoisomerase I	Nucleolar	Scleroderma	ID
Mitotic Spindle Apparatus	MSA	Carpal tunnel syndrome, SLE	ANA
Jo-1	Cytoplasmic nucleolus	Polymyositis	ID
Pm-ScL	Cytoplasmic nucleolus	Polymyositis	IF

ANA, antinuclear antibodies; ELISA, enzyme linked immunosorbent assay; ID, immunodiffusion; IF, immunofluorescence fixation; LE Prep, lupus erythematosus preparation; WB, Western blot.

LABORATORY DIAGNOSIS: SYSTEMIC

ANA PATTERN TITERS. Following the disease course by ANA titer has been suggested by some, but because of the multiple reactivities that can occur in the ANA, this is not always accurate. Following the specific autoantibody titer is usually more productive and may be a better prognostic indicator. Elucidating the ANA specific reactivities is discussed below. It should be noted that autoantibodies are not unique to autoimmune diseases. Any disease process in which cellular injury or alteration is included in the pathogenesis has the potential to stimulate autoantibody production. This includes, but is not limited to, various infectious, neoplastic, and liver diseases. Any of these diseases could potentially be in the differential diagnosis and may not be excluded by a positive ANA result. Fortunately, the ANA titer in these cases is usually less than those caused by connective tissue diseases.

Specific Autoantigens and Extractable Nuclear Antigens

The specific antigenic reactivity of an autoantibody causing a positive ANA should be determined in a reflexive manner, as there are many possibilities, and to test all would represent an unwarranted health care expense. The methods used to determine the specific autoantibody reactivity are EIAs, immunodiffusion assays, countercurrent electrophoresis, and (recently) immunoblot. The first two methods are those used by most laboratories. The most common autoantibodies/antigens are listed on p 297 along with the ANA pattern that occurs when the antibody is present. "Clinically Suspect Autoimmune Disease," p 299, presents an algorithm for further testing when a significant ANA titer is found. At the present time, antibodies to native DNA and the extractable nuclear antigens (SM, RNP, SS-A, SS-B) are the most common secondary tests performed. Occasionally, anti-ScL-70 and Jo-1 tests are performed but usually not before the others. Many of these antibody-antigen systems are being further defined. For example, there are several subunits to Sm and the RNP antigens, and the antibodies that are specific to each of these subunits can be determined by Western or immunoblot techniques. There appears to be clinical significance to the pattern of subunit reactivity, but further clinical and laboratory studies are required before their use in the routine clinical laboratory becomes justified and common. The test methodology/parameters and reference ranges are listed under "Diagnostic Tests and Methodologies" and "Immunologic Autoimmune Assays," pp 302 and 304.

CLINICALLY SUSPECT AUTOIMMUNE DISEASE

Rheumatoid Factor

Rheumatoid factor is traditionally thought of as the hallmark test for rheumatoid arthritis. However, it also occurs in SLE (30%), in Sjögren's syndrome (90%), and occasionally in scleroderma and polymyositis. Like the ANA, rheumatoid factor can occur in some nonautoimmune diseases also (e.g., chronic active hepatitis, sarcoidosis, chronic infectious diseases, neoplasia, syphilis). Furthermore, rheumatoid factor has been reported to occur with increasing prevalence in the elderly in the absence of disease.

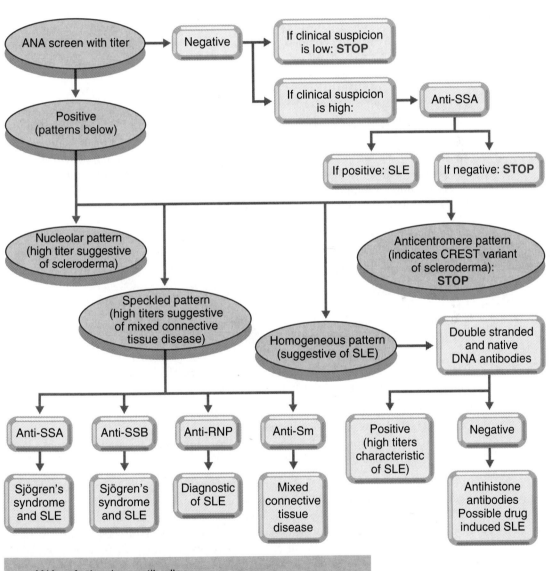

LABORATORY DIAGNOSIS: SYSTEMIC

ANA = Antinuclear antibodies

CREST = Calcinosis cutis, Raynaud's phenomenon, esophageal dysmotility, sclerodactyly, and telangiectasia syndrome

SLE = Systemic lupus erythematosus

Rheumatoid factor is monomeric and pentameric IgM that has reactivity to IgG. However, IgA and IgG rheumatoid factors also exist. When complexed with IgG, rheumatoid factor may accumulate in the various tissues (such as the synovium), activate complement, and cause intense inflammatory reactions and tissue damage and in some cases vascular damage. The most common methods for rheumatoid factor are latex agglutination assays and nephelometry.

Nonspecific Tests

Other nonspecific tests such as CBC and sedimentation rate are often performed. Most autoimmune patients exhibit normochromic, normocytic anemia. The sedimentation rate is usually elevated during active disease, indicating the inflammatory process. Complement levels (CH50, C3, C4) often give an indication of disease activity, as this is related to antigen-antibody complexes consuming complement and/or reduced complement formation.

TREATMENT: SYSTEMIC

Treatment of the various autoimmune diseases is highly individual but is basically anti-inflammatory and/or immunosuppressive in nature. It ranges from little or no treatment to severe immunosuppressive and cytotoxic regimens (e.g., systemic corticosteroids, methotrexate, alkylating agents, purine analogs).

ORGAN SPECIFIC AUTOIMMUNE DISEASES

CLINICAL MANIFESTATIONS: ORGAN SPECIFIC

Organ specific autoimmune diseases occur in most major organ systems. These include, but are not limited to, endocrine, hematologic, cardiac and vascular, gastrointestinal, liver, kidney, skin, lung, and brain disorders. See "Organ Specific Antigens and Antibodies," p 301. When a specific organ system is the target of an autoimmune antibody, several possible clinical outcomes can occur as a result:

1. Organ failure or malfunction can result from tissue damage similar to that which occurs in systemic autoimmune diseases.
2. Cellular receptors or ligands on the target organ may be stimulated or blocked if the autoantibody is directed against them.

If the receptors are stimulated, the autoantibody behaves like the target organ's natural ligand without the appropriate downregulating mechanisms. This results in clinical manifestations characteristic of overstimulation of the organ. On the other hand, the autoantibody may block the receptor without triggering it or may be directed at the receptor's natural ligand. This results in clinical manifestations characteristic of understimulation of the organ.

Organ Specific Antigens and Antibodies

AUTOANTIBODY/ANTIGEN RECOGNIZED	ORGAN SPECIFIC PRIMARY DISEASE ASSOCIATION	SENSITIVITY	SPECIFICITY	COMMONLY USED TESTS
Thyroglobulin	*Hashimoto's Thyroiditis*	40%–70%	Moderate	IFA, EIA
	Graves' Disease	20%–40%	Low	IFA, EIA
Microsomal Antigen (Thyroid Peroxidase)	*Hashimoto's Thyroiditis*	80%–95%	High	IFA, EIA
	Graves' Disease	50%–80%	Low	IFA, EIA
Thyroid Stimulating Immunoglobulin (TSI)	*Graves' Disease*	50%–90%	High	Bioassay
	Hashimoto's Thyroiditis	10%–20%	Low	Bioassay
Thyroid Binding Inhibitory Immunoglobulin (TBII)	*Graves' Disease*	50%–80%	High	Bioassay
	Hashimoto's Thyroiditis	5%–10%	Low	Bioassay
Anti–Islet Cell Antibodies	*Insulin Dependent Diabetes Mellitus*	35%–80%	High	IFA (not prognostic of development)
Anti–Smooth Muscle Antibodies	*Autoimmune Chronic Active Hepatitis*	40%–70%	Good	IFA, EIA
Antimitochondrial Antibodies	*Primary Biliary Cirrhosis*	50%	Low	IFA, EIA
	Primary Biliary Cirrhosis	>90%	In high titer, High	IFA, EIA
Anti–Acetylcholine Receptor Antibodies	*Myasthenia Gravis*	80%–95%	High	HA, RIA
Antistriated Cardiac Muscle	*Autoimmune Myocarditis*		In high titer, High	IFA
Antiepidermis Antibodies	*Pemphigus Vulgaris*	80%–90%	Moderate	IIF
Anti–Skin Basement Membrane Region Antigens	*Bullous Pemphigoid*	70%	High	IIF
Antigastric Parietal Cell	*Pernicious Anemia*	>90%	Low	IIF, CF
	Atrophic Gastritis	60%	Low	IIF, CF

LABORATORY DIAGNOSIS: ORGAN SPECIFIC

The presence of organ specific autoantibodies can be important in helping to establish the diagnosis (see "Organ Specific Antigens and Antibodies" above). Their presence has also been utilized in monitoring these patients. However, there are problems when examining autoantibodies using complex bioassays (such as used to examine hormone receptor binding), as these are not standardized and may demonstrate considerable variation in sensitivity. Determinations of autoantibodies to poorly defined antigens are also problematic, since the antigens used in the assays often vary. Finally, even in the well established and defined tests, caution must be used in the interpretation of positive results, since the presence of these specific autoantibodies does not always correlate with a specific disease or disease activity. The tests, methodologies, and reference ranges are listed at the end of this chapter.

TREATMENT: ORGAN SPECIFIC

The treatment varies considerably but is generally directed at replacement therapy if an organ hormone is lacking, or alternatively suppressing the production of hormone through various inhibitors if overproduction is the problem. In addition, controlling the autoimmune process through immune suppression can be effective provided that the autoantibody is involved in the pathogenesis (which is not always the case).

DIAGNOSTIC TESTS AND METHODOLOGIES

TEST	METHOD	INTERFERENCE	COMMENTS
Antinuclear Antibody (ANA)	IFA	None found	Patterns seen included, but not limited to, speckled, homogeneous, nucleolar, and peripheral rim. High titers of homogeneous pattern are indicative of systemic lupus erythematus (SLE).
Anti Acetylcholine Receptor	AChR-binding antibody assay- RIA	Interference can occur with muscle relaxant drugs. They can cause false positive results with succinylcholine or snake venom.	Binding assay is increased with myasthenia gravis.
	AChR-modulating antibody assay- RIA		Modulating and blocking assays should be done after negative results with binding assay for patients with high clinical suspicion of myasthenia gravis.
	AChR-blocking antibody assay- RIA		Assay diagnostic for myasthenia gravis and is useful in managing patients' response to immunosuppressive therapy.
Anti–Extractable Nuclear Antigen Antibodies (ENA),	EIA/ID, WB	None found	
Anti-SS-A (Ro)			SS-A(Ro) antibodies are present in about 35% of patients with SLE and about 60% of patients with primary Sjögren's syndrome.
Anti-SS-B (La)	EIA/ID, WB		SS-B (La) antibodies are present in about 60% of patients with vasculitis.

Continued ▶

► Continued **DIAGNOSTIC TESTS AND METHODOLOGIES**

TEST	METHOD	INTERFERENCE	COMMENTS
Anti-Smith (Sm)	EIA/ID, WB		Sm antibodies are found in about 30% of patients with SLE.
Antinuclear RNP	EIA/ID, WB		RNP antibodies are found in many patients with mixed connective tissue disease (MCTD) and about 35% of SLE patients.
Anti-DNA	EIA	None found	Antibodies to native DNA are of considerable importance in diagnosis and management of patients with SLE.
Antigastric Parietal Cells	IIF	None found	These antibodies can be found in 90% or more of patients with pernicious anemia. Antibodies can also be found in conditions such as chronic thyroiditis and gastric ulcer.
Antihistones Antibodies	EIA	None found	Assay detects antihistone antibodies encountered in drug induced and idiopathic SLE. Assay is used to discriminate a positive ANA (homogeneous pattern).
Anti–Islet Cell Antibodies	FA	None found	Detection of antibodies is found in about 35%–80% of patients with newly diagnosed insulin dependent diabetes mellitus (IDDM).
Anti-Jo-1	ID	None found	Anti-Jo-1 antibodies are found in about 35% of patients with polymyositis.
Antimitochondrial Antibodies	EIA, IFA	None found	Demonstration of antimitochondrial antibodies alone does not confirm diagnosis of primary biliary cirrhosis (PBC). Assay may be useful in distinguishing between extrahepatic biliary obstruction, where antibodies are rarely seen, and PBC.
Anti–Skin Basement Membrane Region Antigens	IIF	None found	Antibodies found with bullous pemphigoid. Assay usually done in research laboratories.
Antistriated Cardiac Muscle	IFA		Assay usually done in research laboratories. Non-specific fluorescent staining can be caused by heterophile autoantibodies.
Anti–Smooth Muscle Antibodies	IFA, EIA	None found	Titers of smooth muscle autoantibodies are found in 50% of patients with autoimmune and chronic active hepatitis. Low positive titers are seen in viral hepatitis, primary biliary cirrhosis, and infectious mononucleosis. The antibody is generally not seen in SLE.
Antithyroglobulin	IFA, EIA	None found	5% to 10% of the normal population may demonstrate low positive titers. High positive titers ($>$1:25,600) strongly suggest Hashimoto's disease. This assay is routinely done with antimicrosomal antibody assay. A normal thyroglobulin antibody titer does not rule out Hashimoto's thyroiditis.

Continued ►

► Continued **DIAGNOSTIC TESTS AND METHODOLOGIES**

TEST	METHOD	INTERFERENCE	COMMENTS
Antimicrosomal Antigen (Thyroid Peroxidase)	ISA, IFA	None found	Antibodies are associated with patients with either Graves' disease or Hashimoto's thyroiditis, with titer correlating strongly with active clinical disease.
Thyroid Stimulating Immunoglobulin (TSI)	Bioassay	None found	This assay is ordered when TBII is positive. Antibodies are associated with hyperthyroidism in Graves' disease.
Thyroid Binding Inhibitory Immunoglobulin (TBII)	Bioassay	None found	Assay recommended test for initial evaluation of TSH receptor antibodies.

IFA, fluorescent tagged antibody reacts with antigen. Antigen-antibody complex visible as microscopic fluorescence by ultraviolet light; IIF, a double antibody immunofluorescence technique; EIA, use of a conjugated enzyme to a known antigen or antibody for quantification of antigen or antibody; ID, detects reaction of antigen and antibody by precipitation reaction; Bioassay, a category of techniques involving in vivo cell lines; WB, Western blot technique detects specific proteins within a complex after separation by gel electrophoresis.

IMMUNOLOGIC AUTOIMMUNE ASSAYS

TEST	SPECIMEN	STORAGE	REFERENCE RANGES*
Antiacetylcholine Receptor			
Binding Assay-RIA	Serum	Freeze −20°C 12 mo	<0.03 nmol/L
Modulating Antibody-RIA	Serum	Freeze −20°C 12 mo	Negative
Blocking Antibody-RIA	Serum	Freeze −20°C 12 mo	<20% inhibition of $I\alpha$-bungarotoxin
Antinuclear Antibody (ANA), IFA	Serum	Freeze −20°C 12 mo	Negative
Anti-nDNA-ELISA	Serum	Freeze −20°C 12 mo	>250 U/L
Anti-nDNA-*Crithidia luciliae*-RIA	Serum		<1:10
Anti-ENA, Antibodies Against Acidic Nuclear Ribonucleoproteins			
Anti-SS-A (Ro)-ELISA/ID, WB	Serum	Freeze −20°C 12 mo	Negative
Anti-SS-B (La)-ELISA/ID, WB	Serum	Freeze −20°C 12 mo	Negative
Anti-Smith (Sm)-ELISA/ID, WB	Serum	Freeze −20°C 12 mo	Negative

Continued ►

► Continued **IMMUNOLOGIC AUTOIMMUNE ASSAYS**

TEST	SPECIMEN	STORAGE	REFERENCE RANGES*
Anti-Nuclear RNP-ELISA/ID, WB	Serum	Freeze −20°C 12 mo	Negative
Antiepidermal Antibodies IIF	Serum	Freeze −20°C 12 mo	Negative
Antigastric Parietal Cell IIF, CF	Serum	Freeze −20°C 12 mo	Negative
Antihistones-ELISA	Serum	Freeze −20°C 12 mo	Negative
Anti–Islet Cell Antibodies-IFA	Serum	Freeze −20°C 12 mo	Negative
Anti-Jo Antibodies-ELISA	Serum	Freeze −20°C 12 mo	Negative
Anti-Mitochondrial Antibodies-IFA, ELISA	Serum	Freeze −20°C 12 mo	EIA—Negative IFA—Titer <20
Anti–Basement Membrane Region Antigens-ELISA	Serum	Freeze −20°C 12 mo	Negative
Antistriated Cardiac Muscle	Serum	Freeze −20°C 12 mo	Negative
Antithyroglobulin-IFA	Serum-freeze −20 degrees immediately	Freeze −20°C 12 mo	Negative
Antimicrosomal Antigen (Thyroid Peroxidase)-IFA, ELISA	Serum	Freeze −20°C 12 mo	IFA—Nondetectable ELISA—Negative
Anti–Thyroid Stimulating Immunoglobulin (TSI)-Bioassay	Serum	4°C 24 hr	Bioassay—<130% of basal activity EIA—Negative
Anti–Thyroid Binding Inhibitory Immunoglobulin (TBII)-Bioassay	Serum	Freeze −20°C 12 mo	<10% inhibition
Anti–Smooth Muscle Antibodies-ELISA, IFA	Serum	Freeze −20°C 12 mo	Negative or None Detected

IMMUNOLOGIC AUTOIMMUNE ASSAYS

BIBLIOGRAPHY

Bach JF: Organ-specific autoimmunity. Immunol Today 16(7):353–355, 1995.

Callegari PE, Williams WV: Laboratory tests for rheumatic diseases. When are they useful? Postgrad Med 97(4):65–68, 71–74, 1995.

Coutinho A, Kazatchkine MD, Avrameas S: Natural autoantibodies. Curr Opin Immunol 7(6):812–818, 1995.

Lefkowith JB, Gilkeson GS: Nephritogenic autoantibodies in lupus: current concepts and continuing controversies. Arthritis Rheum 39(6):894–903, 1996.

Radic MZ, Weigert M: Origins of anti-DNA antibodies and their implications for B-cell tolerance. Ann NY Acad Sci 764:384–396, 1995.

Schnabel A, Hauschild S, Gross WL: Anti-neutrophil cytoplasmic antibodies in generalized autoimmune diseases. Int Arch Allergy Immunol 109(3):201–206, 1996.

Spronk PE, Limburg PC, Kallenberg CG: Serological markers of disease activity in systemic lupus erythematosus. Lupus 4(2):86–94, 1995.

Steinman L: Escape from "horror autotoxicus": pathogenesis and treatment of autoimmune disease. Cell 80(1):7–10, 1995.

Stites D, Terr AI, Parslow TG: Basic and Clinical Immunology, 8th ed. Norwalk, CT, Appleton & Lange, 1994.

van Venrooij WJ, Pruijn GJ: Ribonucleoprotein complexes as autoantigens. Curr Opin Immunol 7(6):819–824, 1995.

von Muhlen CA, Tan EM: Autoantibodies in the diagnosis of systemic rheumatic diseases. Semin Arthritis Rheum 24(5):323–358, 1995.

Chapter *19*

IMMUNODEFICIENCY

Candace Breen, BS, MLT (ASCP)

Marc Golightly, PhD

Q U I C K   C O N T E N T S

INTRODUCTION

Clinical Manifestations: General

The immune system is organized with the cell mediated, humoral, phagocytic, and complement cascade systems all linked together by a network of regulatory and synergistic interactions in a highly complex fashion. Owing to this extreme complexity, there are a tremendous number of possibilities for defects. The clinical presentation of suspected immunodeficient patients may point to the type of immune dysfunction present. However, since all arms of the immune system are inter-related, a defect in one arm often affects the function of the others, resulting in clinical symptoms more encompassing than expected. Depending on the extent of deficiency, the clinical manifestations may range from no notable clinical symptoms to severe illness and/or death. Patients with a defective cell mediated immunity are more susceptible to infection by fungal, protozoan, and viral organisms (notably chronic skin, pneumonia, and mucous membrane infections). A history of recurrent bacterial infections, particularly bacterial pneumonia and otitis media, suggests a humoral immune defect. Phagocytic and complement deficiencies are suggested by skin and systemic infections with pyogenic bacteria.

PRIMARY IMMUNODEFICIENCIES. Immunodeficiencies are classified into two groups: primary and secondary. Primary immunodeficiencies are those deficiencies that are inherent in the immune system itself and are often caused by congenital genetic defects. However, they may be acquired and can occur in ages from infancy to adulthood. A large number of primary immunodeficiencies are known, but they are uncommon except for selective immunoglobulin deficiency.

SECONDARY IMMUNODEFICIENCIES. These deficiencies are much more common. They are usually transient in nature and are secondary to a variety of diseases and disorders (infection, malignancy, autoimmune diseases, protein losing states, immunosuppressive therapy, and many others). These immunodeficiencies usually resolve when the primary disorder is successfully treated. Secondary immunodeficiencies will not be discussed further, with the exception of human immunodeficiency virus (HIV), which has its own section. However, the association of secondary immunodeficiencies with the various primary diseases and disorders (and vice versa) is important for supportive and diagnostic purposes.

Diagnosis: General

A discussion of all the specific immunodeficiencies is beyond the scope of this book, but this section will examine some of the general approaches to laboratory evaluation and diagnosis of suspected immunodeficiencies. The subsequent section will then discuss some of the more common ones as examples.

EVALUATION OF IMMUNODEFICIENCY

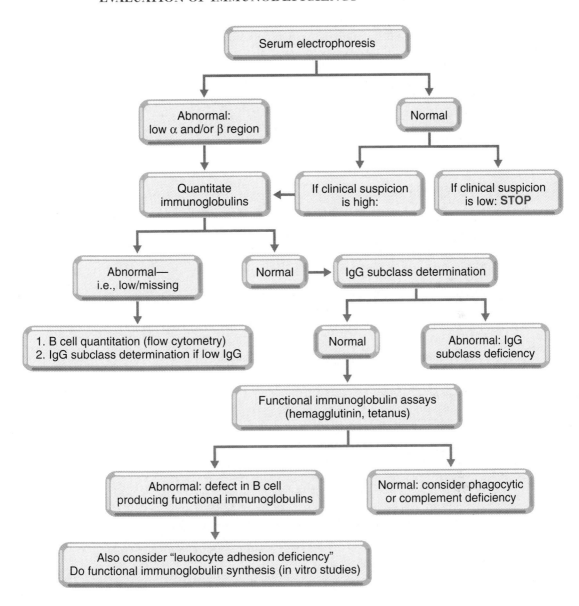

INTRODUCTION-DIAGNOSIS: GENERAL

HISTORY

As mentioned, the patient's medical history may provide valuable clues as to which arm or arms of the immune system are involved in the suspected immunodeficiency (see "Evaluation of Immunodeficiency" above.). Recurrent infections, their type, and complications after vaccination with live viral vaccines should be noted. In addition to these considerations, some immunodeficiencies are associated with autoimmune diseases, malignancies, and certain neurologic abnormalities. Since many are genetic, the family history should be questioned. The physical evaluation may also provide evidence of immunodeficiency. This might include evidence of past or present severe and/or chronic infections via scars from skin infections/abscesses/viral infections, and pulmonary involvement. The physical presence of lymphoid tissue should also be determined.

LABORATORY DIAGNOSIS

A single screening test for most primary immunodeficiencies does not exist, and laboratory tests to assess the immune system both quantitatively and functionally tend to be quite extensive. In today's environment, the simple and inexpensive quantitative tests should be run first, followed by the functional tests if necessary (see list below). The specifics and requirements of the immunologic tests used to examine the individual arms of the immune system are listed in tables at the end of this chapter.

Assessment of Immunodeficiencies

Humoral Immunity

Basic assessment:

1. White blood cell (WBC) count with differential
2. Serum immunoelectrophoresis
3. Immunoglobulin determination (quantitation IgG, IgA, IgM)

Secondary assessment:

1. B cell quantitation (flow cytometry)
2. IgG subclass determination
3. Functional immunoglobulin assays: Hemagglutinin titers
   Tetanus/Pneumovac titer
4. Immunoglobulin synthesis (in vitro studies)

Cellular Immunity

Basic assessment:

1. WBC count with differential
2. T cell quantitations (flow cytometry) (CD3, CD4, CD8)

Secondary assessment:

1. Skin tests
2. Monocellular proliferation studies (mitogen/antigen blastogenesis test)

Phagocytic Immunity

Basic assessment:

1. WBC count with differential

Secondary assessment:

1. Oxidative burst test: NBT, chemiluminescence
2. Chemotactic response (migration tests)
3. Cell adhesion molecules (flow cytometry) (CD11a, CD18)

Complement Immunity

Basic assessment:

1. Total functional complement (CH50)
2. C3 and C4 quantitation

Secondary assessment:

1. Functional and quantitations of individual components (C1q, C2)

HUMORAL ASSESSMENT. Laboratory evaluation of the humoral immune system should start with serum electrophoresis, followed by the quantitation of the immunoglobulin levels, specifically IgG, IgA, and IgM if indicated. IgG subclass determinations may be performed but only if subclass deficiency is strongly suspected. Occasionally, the evaluation proceeds to the functional level when quantitative levels are normal or slightly low and inability to mount a specific response is suspected. Functional immunoglobulin may be assessed by determining isohemagglutination titers (mostly IgM) and the Shick test or tetanus toxoid titers (mostly IgG) in appropriately immunized individuals. These tests expose most humoral defects. Once a defect has been found, it can be further characterized by highly specialized laboratories, if required. This may include B cell quantitations and cell surface antigenic expression as well as in vitro immunoglobulin synthesis studies.

CELLULAR ASSESSMENT. Laboratory evaluation of cell mediated immunity (T cells) should start with a simple determination of the absolute lymphocyte count (WBC with differential). Counts consistently below 1200/mm^3 may indicate a T cell deficiency (most of the peripheral blood lymphocytes are T cells). If the clinical suspicion of a cellular defect is high, T cell quantitation may be helpful even in the presence of normal lymphocyte counts, since there may be an imbalance in the various regulatory T cell subsets (i.e., helper cells vs. cytotoxic cells) without this being evident in the absolute numbers. This is especially true in HIV. If T cell numbers are normal and a cellular defect is still in the differential diagnosis, functional studies such as in vivo skin tests (delayed hypersensitivity) or in vitro mitogen and antigen blastogenesis assays can be performed. Skin testing is inexpensive and good for the overall assessment of cellular immunocompetence, but does have several restrictions:

1. In the first years of life, skin testing is of limited value, since the patient has had little or no previous exposure to the recall test antigens.
2. It depends on patient compliance (i.e., a follow-up examination at a specified time interval is required). The in vitro blastogenesis test examines the ability of purified patient mononuclear cells to respond and proliferate to a variety of stimuli. This is more expensive and usually available only in large reference laboratories, but it does not suffer from the above restrictions.

PHAGOCYTIC ASSESSMENT. In the evaluation of the phagocytic system, a WBC count with a differential quantifying the number of neutrophils should be the starting point and generally will have already been performed. A new group of leukocyte deficiencies has recently been described in which the cell adhesion molecules found on the cell surface are missing or reduced. This causes the leukocytes to interact improperly in the immune response. Many of these adhesion molecules have commercially available monoclonal antibodies directed against them (CD11a, CD18) and can be quantitated by flow cytometry (see Lymphoproliferative Diseases, Chapter 20). Functional tests of the various phagocytic cell activities exist but are often performed only in the major institutions and reference laboratories. One of the oldest of these tests is the nitroblue tetrazolium (NBT) dye reduction test, which ultimately indicates the ability of the polymorphonuclear cells to produce the hydrogen peroxide and oxygen radicals necessary for intracellular killing. Other tests that often use some of the newer technologies to assess various phagocytic cell functions are chemiluminescence, quantitative intracellular in vitro killing curves, and migration tests (chemotactic and nonchemotactic).

INTRODUCTION-DIAGNOSIS: GENERAL

COMPLEMENT ASSESSMENT. Clinically apparent complement abnormalities and deficiencies can usually be detected in the laboratory by functional hemolytic complement assays for both the classic and alternative pathways. When a decrease in one of these assays is found, the individual components of the complement system should then be quantified to determine the exact deficient component. Occasionally, absolute levels are normal but the protein is nonfunctional. In these cases, functional assays may be performed on the individual components. Of the eight components of the classic complement cascade, only C3 and C4 are readily available in most hospital laboratories. While primary C3 and C4 deficiencies are extremely rare, significant decreases are associated with many secondary immunodeficiencies, including various autoimmune diseases.

Laboratory Assessment Practicalities

There are no simple screening tests for most primary immunodeficiencies, but many of the basic tests required to start the work-up evaluation are readily available. These patients with suspected immunodeficiency are then usually referred to the larger institutions where the more sophisticated tests are available for the final laboratory diagnosis.

COMBINED B AND T CELL IMMUNODEFICIENCIES

Severe Combined Immunodeficiency

CLINICAL MANIFESTATIONS. The immunodeficiencies of this type are variable in their severity and cause. The survival rates of these patients are also highly variable, ranging from under 1 year of age to adulthood. The symptoms usually begin in early infancy and include susceptibility to a wide range of bacterial, fungal, protozoal, and viral infections. These deficiencies have associations with enzyme deficiencies, genetic components, short limbed dwarfism, and thymoma. Severe combined immunodeficiency (SCID) is the most severe of this class of immunodeficiency. As the name implies, it is characterized by a severe defect of both B and T cell arms. Lymphoid tissue is scarce and there is a depression in the numbers and/or functions of T and B cells. SCID is extremely serious and life threatening, and these patients usually die within the first 1 or 2 years of life, often before the diagnosis can be made. During the first few months of life, patients are usually protected from bacterial infections and some viral infections by maternal IgG transferred in utero. However, these children fail to thrive; suffer from chronic diarrhea; and become susceptible to a wide range of microbial infections, usually of the skin and respiratory and gastrointestinal tracts. Death from progressive viremia is almost always the outcome to vaccination with live attenuated vaccines. For the same reason, because of the risk of graft vs. host reactions, transfusions with non-irradiated blood should never be given to an infant suspected of having SCID or any other immunodeficiency.

LABORATORY DIAGNOSIS. As mentioned above, lymphoid tissue is scarce, and x-ray tests have been used with some success to determine this. In addition, this deficiency should be reflected in the WBC with differential. There is a depression in the numbers and/or functions of T and B cells, which can be determined by flow cytometry and mitogen/antigen stimulation studies, respectively. Immunoglobulin determinations should be made if B cells are present, to examine the functionality of B cells in terms of immunoglobulin production. SCID is a collection of disorders, and therefore varying degrees of abnormalities are expected in the laboratory.

TREATMENT. SCID has been treated by bone marrow transplantation, fetal liver transplantation, and fetal thymus transplantation, with varying success.

Wiskott-Aldrich Syndrome (Immunodeficiency with Thrombocytopenia and Eczema)

CLINICAL MANIFESTATIONS. Wiskott-Aldrich syndrome (WAS) is an X-linked inherited genetic disease that involves both T and B cells. It is characterized by severe thrombocytopenia, often with bleeding; recurrent infections with a broad spectrum of microbial organisms; and eczema. The recurrent infections, as in most congenital immunodeficiencies, do not generally begin before 6 months of age owing to the presence of maternal antibodies. However, the thrombocytopenia usually begins at birth, and by the end of the first year eczema is evident and is commonly infectious. There is an increasing prevalence of pneumonias, meningitis, and septicemia, and survival rarely exceeds the first decade of life. Most immunodeficiencies exhibit an increase in the frequency of lymphoreticular malignancies; for WAS patients, it occurs in 30%.

LABORATORY DIAGNOSIS. In contrast to SCID, B cells are present in normal numbers, but their responses to polysaccharide antigens are abnormal and reduced. The response to polysaccharides is primarily IgM; therefore the serum levels of IgM are usually decreased. Serum IgA and IgE are frequently elevated, possibly as a compensatory mechanism. The cellular responses are also deficient, with normal mitogen response and little or no antigen response. It should be noted that the T cell immunity may deteriorate both quantitatively and functionally with increasing age.

TREATMENT. Increased immunoglobulin catabolism, regulatory cell failure, and defective T cell membranes have all been implicated in the pathogenesis of WAS. Bone marrow transplantation has been performed to treat these patients.

Hereditary Ataxia-Telangiectasia with Immunodeficiency

CLINICAL MANIFESTATIONS. This is primarily an autosomal recessive neurologic disorder, but it also severely affects the immune, vascular, and endocrine systems. It is characterized by ataxia (incoordination), telangiectasia of the eye (lesions caused by dilated venules), and recurrent sinopulmonary infections. The ataxia begins in infancy; the telangiectasia occurs later. The neurologic and immunologic functions progressively deteriorate with age. The infections usually begin early in the first decade, but when they begin before the ataxia-telangiectasia, it is difficult to distinguish them from other combined immunodeficiencies with abnormal immunoglobulin production and selective IgA deficiency. Death usually occurs from chronic respiratory infection or lymphoreticular malignancy during the second or third decade of life.

LABORATORY DIAGNOSIS. T and B cells are variably affected. The B cell numbers are relatively normal to slightly increased, while the levels of serum and secretory IgA are absent or decreased. IgE deficiencies have also been noted. The T cells may be reduced in numbers, frequency, and functional ability.

TREATMENT. While the pathogenesis of this disorder is still not clearly defined, a specific immunologic defect is unlikely. A genetic defect that affects DNA repair, and possibly chromosomal translocations involving breakpoints in the T cell receptor gene, have been postulated. Fetal thymus transplantation and intravenous gammaglobulin have been used.

COMBINED B AND T CELL IMMUNODEFICIENCIES

Other Combined T and B Cell Immunodeficiencies

The above immunodeficiencies are the major disorders that have been traditionally classified as primary combined immunodeficiencies. There are other disorders of T and B cells with varying degrees of severity that apparently cannot be classified into any of the groups discussed above. As our ability to elucidate the defects in these disorders increases, the distinction between combined, T cell, and B cell deficiencies will change. For example, laboratory tests have now shown certain "B cell deficiencies" to actually be the result of defective T cell regulation.

HUMORAL IMMUNODEFICIENCIES (B CELL AND ANTIBODY IMMUNODEFICIENCIES)

Characteristic of most primary immunodeficiencies, B cell and antibody deficiencies exhibit a variable range of defects and symptoms. The result is a range from an absence of all immunoglobulin classes to a selective deficiency of an immunoglobulin subclass, and a clinical range from severe recurrent infections to no clinical presentation. The age of onset is also variable and usually depends on the severity of the antibody deficiency. These patients generally do very well after the institution of proper therapy (usually gamma globulin). The pathogenesis of these defects involves several mechanisms that range from inherent B cell abnormalities at the various stages of B cell maturation to misregulation by T cells and improper response to cytokines. Most of the laboratory diagnoses for the detection of B cell deficiencies can be performed by tertiary care hospital laboratories and are represented in the flow diagram on p 315.

Humoral Assessment

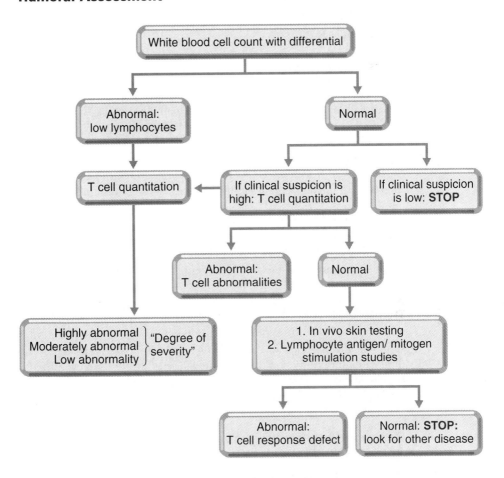

X-Linked Infantile Agammaglobulinemia (Bruton's Agammaglobulinemia)

CLINICAL MANIFESTATIONS. X-linked infantile agammaglobulinemia is the most severe B cell deficiency. It is characterized by a lack of circulating B cells and plasma cells. Pre-B cells are present in the bone marrow and peripheral blood but are not functionally competent and do not secrete immunoglobulin. The deficiency is genetically inherited in an X-linked recessive fashion and occurs in approximately 1 in 100,000. Like most childhood immunodeficiencies, the patient is usually not symptomatic in the first months of life owing to the passive transfer of maternal antibodies. As these antibodies are catabolized, recurrent/excessive pyogenic bacterial infections (commonly sinusitis, dermatitis, pneumonia, otitis media, sepsis, and meningitis) by streptococci, staphylococci, and *Haemophilus influenzae* become evident. These patients usually handle the common viral diseases of childhood without sequelae.

LABORATORY DIAGNOSIS. Early diagnosis and treatment are extremely important to the successful long term maintenance of these patients. The laboratory diagnosis may start with serum electrophoresis when the gamma globulins are severely depressed or absent. Subsequent immunoglobulin quantitations reveal levels that are drastically reduced; typically, IgG is less than 100mg/dl, and IgA and IgM are less than 1% of normal. T cells are generally normal in both quantitation and function.

TREATMENT. The treatment for most B cell deficiencies is intravenous gamma globulins coupled with appropriate antibiotic therapy for infections that do occur. Patients respond quickly to antibiotic therapy, which unfortunately may delay early diagnosis.

Transient Hypogammaglobulinemia of Infancy

CLINICAL MANIFESTATIONS. Infants with transient hypogammaglobulinemia exhibit a delayed production of IgG (occasionally IgM and IgA as well) by up to 2 years of age. This is in contrast to normal infants who begins to synthesize IgM at birth, IgA within 3 weeks, and IgG by 6 to 8 weeks. Like infants with other B cell deficiencies, these infants are also prone to recurrent respiratory tract and skin infections. However, the severity of infections is less than in X-linked infantile agammaglobulinemia. These infections gradually decrease as the patient's delayed immunoglobulin synthesis begins.

LABORATORY DIAGNOSIS. These infants do have circulating B cells, in contrast to the situation in X-linked infantile agammaglobulinemia. Most patients with transient hypogammaglobulinemia lack only IgG, and this helps in the differentiation. Occasionally, IgA and IgM are also absent, which complicates the diagnosis. Cellular immunity is intact.

TREATMENT. It has been postulated that a passive transfer of a maternal anti-IgG (GM) antibody could suppress the production of IgG in the infant, or a transient deficiency in the number and/or function of the T helper cells required for proper immunoglobulin production could be the cause of this deficiency. Although this condition is generally less severe than X-linked hypogammaglobulinemia, some patients present with the same severity and type of infections and therefore should be treated similarly.

Common Variable Immunodeficiency (Primary Acquired Agammaglobulinemia)

CLINICAL MANIFESTATIONS. Common variable immunodeficiency (CVI) is a heterogeneous population of disorders with similar features. The clinical presentation is similar to that of X-linked agammaglobulinemia, but this disorder may occur at any age (although usually between 15 and 35 years of age). There is also a higher than normal incidence of collagen vascular disease and malignancy in these patients. While there is no definitive inheritance pattern, there does seem to be a high incidence of immunologic abnormalities in the patient's family members.

LABORATORY DIAGNOSIS. Most CVI patients have circulating B cells, and the immunoglobulin levels are slightly better than in X-linked agammaglobulinemia. Serum electrophoresis should show a marked decrease in gamma globulins. Quantitative immunoglobulins are substantially decreased, with the total immunoglobulin levels not uncommonly less than 300 mg/dl. A significant number of these patients demonstrate quantitative and functional abnormalities in T cells, which may worsen in time.

TREATMENT. The pathogenesis is variable, since this is a collection of similar type disorders. B cell defects, enzymatic abnormalities, increased activated cytotoxic T cells, and decreased helper T cells have all been reported in the pathogenesis. The treatment is virtually the same as for X-linked agammaglobulinemia, but the long term prognosis of treated patients is good.

Selective Immunoglobulin Deficiencies (Including Subclass Deficiency)

CLINICAL MANIFESTATIONS. Selective immunoglobulin deficiency involves the lack of only one immunoglobulin class or subclass, while the rest are present in normal or even increased concentrations. The most common of all primary immunodeficiencies is selective IgA deficiency, occurring in approximately 1 in 600 individuals. However, it is becoming apparent that the incidence of IgG subclass deficiency is much higher than previously thought. The clinical presentations range from recurrent sinopulmonary infections and sepsis to asymptomatic presentation (most selective IgA deficient and many IgG subclass deficient patients are asymptomatic). When IgG subclass deficiencies present clinically, some correlations, such as IgG2 with encapsulated bacteria and IgG1 with features common to severe hypogammaglobulinemia, have been noted. However, these correlations do not always occur because of host compensation. In fact, it has been demonstrated that both levels and specific antibody response of the nondeficient subclasses may be increased over normal in an apparent compensatory mechanism. This has been demonstrated to occur in IgA deficiency also, in which IgG subclass or IgM specific antibodies and/or levels are increased.

LABORATORY DIAGNOSIS. Normal numbers of circulating B cells are present. IgA deficiency is easy to diagnose in the laboratory (i.e., lack of IgA). However, IgG subclass deficiency is much more difficult, since subclass deficiency can occur in the face of normal total IgG concentrations or even hypergammaglobulinemia. Furthermore, selective IgG subclass deficiency or combined IgG subclass deficiency may occur with an associated immunoglobulin isotype deficiency. Complicating this further is the fact that the actual subclass testing has a history of problems and inaccuracies. Fortunately, in many cases, subclass determinations add little or nothing to the diagnosis or to how the patient will be managed, and may represent unnecessary testing.

TREATMENT. Treatments vary from no gamma globulin in IgA deficiencies to gamma globulins in some of the other class and subclass deficiencies. The pathogenesis is not always known. In IgG2 and IgG4 subclass deficiency, the defect may not be in the B cell itself but rather may be the end result of a defect in T cell, T cell–B cell interactions, or lymphokine production (interferon gamma and transforming growth factor [TGF]-beta). On the other hand, those deficiencies inherent in the B cell seem to be due to homozygous deletion of immunoglobulin heavy chain constant region genes. In many pediatric cases, the mechanism appears to be a transient immaturity or block of the immune system.

T CELL IMMUNODEFICIENCIES

T cell immunodeficiencies almost always secondarily affect the humoral immune system owing to the dependency of B cells on the regulatory T cells to mount a proper antibody response. However, in select cases, T cell deficiencies can occur with normal to near normal antibody production. These individuals suffer from severe recurrent infections with opportunistic fungal, viral, and protozoal organisms, while having a relatively normal response to bacteria. The laboratory assessment is represented below.

HUMORAL IMMUNODEFICIENCIES

Cellular Assessment

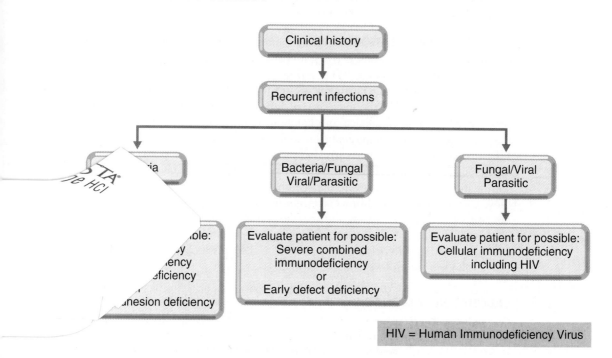

HIV = Human Immunodeficiency Virus

Thymic Hypoplasia (DiGeorge's Syndrome)

CLINICAL MANIFESTATIONS. DiGeorge's syndrome is a congenital malformation of the third and fourth pharyngeal pouches that occurs early in gestation. At birth there are multiple anomalies, including abnormal facial structures, congenital heart defects, hypoparathyroidism, and a reduced or absent thymus. The cellular immune defect varies with the severity of the thymic abnormality. In these infants the congenital heart defects and hypocalcemia require immediate attention and bring the patient to presentation. These immediately life threatening defects must be corrected before the cellular defect can be addressed.

LABORATORY DIAGNOSIS. Depending on the severity and other factors, the cellular immunity, if left untreated, may spontaneously recover or deteriorate further. The lymphocyte counts, the percentage of T cells, and the response to mitogens are all usually decreased. On the other hand, B cell percentages may actually be increased with somewhat normal function. Since most of the immunoglobulin will be of maternal origin at the time when these infants present, immunoglobulin quantitations are not helpful.

TREATMENT. There are reported cases of thymic hypoplasia in infants of alcoholic mothers, but the cause of this congenital defect is generally not known; it does not appear to be inherited. Successful reconstitution of the T cell immunity has been accomplished with fetal thymus transplants, resulting in long term survival.

Chronic Mucocutaneous Candidiasis

CLINICAL MANIFESTATIONS. This is a relatively restricted T cell immunodeficiency characterized by a selective inability to mount a cellular immune response against *Candida albicans* and related fungi. Other cellular function remains intact and these patients can generally mount a response against viral, protozoal, bacterial, and other fungal organisms. Clinically, the infections range from a very mild involvement of a single fingernail to a severe infection of the mucous membranes and skin. These patients do relatively well and life threatening infections are not common. As in most immunodeficiencies, there are several forms of this deficiency, including association or no association with endocrine abnormalities, and early or late onsets. Autosomal recessive inheritance is postulated in view of the reported familial pattern of occurrences.

LABORATORY DIAGNOSIS. The B cell numbers and immunoglobulin levels are normal. The lymphocyte count is generally normal. Skin tests and blastogenesis assays are the best diagnostic tools. The patients are not responsive to *Candida,* but the response to other antigens and mitogens is usually normal.

TREATMENT. Treatment is directed at the infections, using antifungal agents. Immunostimulatory techniques have been tried with limited success. The pathogenesis of this disorder is unclear.

PHAGOCYTIC DEFICIENCIES

CLINICAL MANIFESTATIONS. Primary phagocytic dysfunctions all result in the inability of the phagocytic cell to kill microorganisms for various reasons. Usually this is due to an enzymatic defect or deficiency in the oxidative burst cycle. The most common of these is chronic granulomatous disease, which occurs in several genetic forms and generally affects children during the first 2 years of life. The clinical manifestations of these disorders range from recurrent mild bacterial infections to severe systemic fatal infections. The patients generally do not have viral or protozoal infections. Our knowledge of the cellular interactions at the molecular level has led to the description of another phagocytic disorder that results from abnormalities of leukocyte adhesion molecules that are required for normal immune interactions. These leukocyte adhesion defects also affect T cells. As might be expected, the clinical manifestations of these defects potentially can be broader in scope.

LABORATORY DIAGNOSIS. For most phagocytic deficiencies the T and B cell systems are intact. The tests performed to elucidate these deficiencies are generally highly specialized (NBT dye reduction test, chemiluminescence, quantitative intracellular in vitro killing curves, and migration tests [chemotactic and nonchemotactic]) and not available in routine hospital laboratories.

TREATMENT. Aggressive antibiotic treatment for the infecting organism(s) is required. Some interferon gamma therapy has been reported to increase the respiratory burst of monocytes and neutrophils.

T CELL IMMUNODEFICIENCIES

DIAGNOSTIC TESTS AND METHODOLOGIES

TEST	METHODOLOGY	INTERFERENCE	COMMENTS	UTILITY
Serum Electrophoresis	Electrophoresis	Hemolyzed, precipitous, or chylous specimens should not be used	For presumptive diagnosis of hypogammaglobulinemia. Decreases in only IgA or IgM immunoglobulins are difficult to detect by this method since they represent a small fraction of the total.	General B cell function
Immunoglobulin Quantitation (IgG, IgA, IgM)	Nephelometry, single radial immunodiffusion (SRID), turbidimetry	Lipemic, precipitous, or hemolyzed specimens should not be used	Nephelometry is the method of choice.	General B cell function
B Cell Quantitation	Flow cytometry, CD19, CD20, CD21, surface and/or cytoplasmic immunoglobulin	Factors affecting viability: extremes of temperature	IgG, IgA, IgM, and IgD bearing cells of peripheral blood B lymphocytes	B cell quantitation
IgG Subclasses (IgG1, IgG2, IgG3, IgG4)	Radial immunodiffusion (RID)	Lipemic, precipitous, or hemolyzed specimens should not be used	IgG subclass deficiencies often occur with Ig isotype deficiency. IgG2 determinations may be problematic and subclass testing is not well standardized.	General B cell function
	Nephelometry	Same		
	Enzyme linked immunoassay	Same		
Isohemagglutinin Titers Tetanus/Pneumococcal Antibody Titers	Microhemagglutination assay	Hemolyzed specimens should not be used	Isohemagglutinin assays measure functional IgM. Tetanus assays measure functional IgG.	Specific B cell and immunoglobulin function (in vivo)
Immunoglobulin Synthesis (In Vitro Studies)	In vitro antibody production in cell culture assayed using radioactive isotope	Factors affecting viability: extremes of temperature	Highly specialized test. Reference/research labs only.	Specific B cell and immunoglobulin function (in vitro)
T Cell Quantitation	Flow cytometry, CD3, CD1, CD2	Extremes of temperature after results. Transport at room temperature.	Quantitates immature and mature T cells.	T cell quantitation

Continued ▶

▶ Continued **DIAGNOSTIC TESTS AND METHODOLOGIES**

TEST	METHODOLOGY	INTERFERENCE	COMMENTS	UTILITY
T Cell Subsets **CD3/CD4** **CD3/CD8**	Flow cytometry, CD3, CD4, CD8	Extremes of temperature alter results. Transport at room temperature.	Determines the total number of T cells in addition to CD4 (helper), CD8 (suppresser) number and ratio.	T cell subset quantitation
Delayed Hypersensitivity Skin Test (DHST)	Intradermal injection antigens used: *C. albicans*, mumps, tetanus, diphtheria, staphylococci lysate, streptokinase-streptodornase, *Trichophyton*, and histoplasmin, among others Multitest: 7-antigen disk pressed onto skin	False-negative delayed reactions can occur if preceded by a strong immediate reaction to site of injection. Expired, contaminated, or heat exposed antigens can cause inaccurate testing.	A positive test reaction indicates that the patient's cellular responses are intact. Clinical history of exposure must be used for proper interpretation.	T cell function
T Cell Proliferation Assays: *Lymphocyte*				T cell function
Mitogen Stimulation	Radioactive isotope	Factors negatively affecting lymphocyte viability (temperature extremes).	Very labor intensive and expensive. Mitogens should be positive, while the clinical history of exposure must be used for proper interpretation of antigen studies.	
Antigen Stimulus	Radioactive isotope	Same		
Oxidative Burst Tests By: *Nitroblue Tetrazolium (NBT)*	Dye reduction	Same as above	Useful means of assessing metabolic integrity of phagocytosing neutrophils.	Phagocytic function

Continued ▶

DIAGNOSTIC TESTS AND METHODOLOGIES

► Continued **DIAGNOSTIC TESTS AND METHODOLOGIES**

TEST	METHODOLOGY	INTERFERENCE	COMMENTS	UTILITY
Flow Cytometry	Flow cytometry, fluorescent reduced products	Same	Lack of response is indicative of chronic granulomatous disease (CGD) and myeloperoxidase deficiency.	Flow cytometry can detect carrier states.
Detection of Cell Adhesion Molecules	Flow cytometry, CD11a, CD18	Factors affecting viability: extremes of temperature	Deficiencies seen in leukocyte adhesion (integrin) disorders.	Leukocyte function
Chemotactics	Migration assay through agar or filter pores	Factors negatively affecting lymphocyte viability (temperature extremes). Interference caused by anti-inflammatory agents, corticosteroids, and chemotherapeutic agents.	Measures chemotactive ability of any purified cell population. There is a profound defect, with no cell migration seen in patients with primary chemotactic deficiency states.	Phagocytic function
CH50	Hemolytic assay	Specimens not immediately frozen will be falsely decreased. Hemolyzed specimens should not be used.	CH50 should detect deficiencies that are inborn and acquired. Individual component assays should follow up decreased CH50 results.	Complement component quantitation
C3 and C4 Quantitation	Nephelometry, RID	Interference occurs with hemolyzed and lipemic specimens.	Nephelometry is method of choice.	Complement component quantitation

SPECIMEN COLLECTION AND STORAGE, REFERENCE RANGE

TEST	SPECIMEN COLLECTION	SPECIMEN STORAGE	REFERENCE RANGE*
Serum Electrophoresis	Serum	−20°C 6 mo −70°C indefinitely	Age dependent Adult: g/dL Total protein: 6.3–7.9 Albumin: 3.1–4.3 Alpha$_1$ globulin: 0.1–0.3 Alpha$_2$ globulin: 0.6–1.0 Beta globulin: 0.7–1.4 Gamma globulin: 0.7–1.6
B Cell Quantitation CD19, CD20, CD21	Whole blood (heparinized or EDTA). Transport at room temperature.	Do not refrigerate or freeze. CDC recommends specimen be assayed within 8 hr.	Age dependent Adult CD19: 5%–20%
Immunoglobulin Quantitations IgG, IgA, IgM	Serum	−20°C 6 mo −70°C indefinitely	Age dependent Adult mg/dL IgG 650–1600 IgA 40–350 IgM 050–300
IgG Subclasses IgG1, IgG2, IgG3, IgG4	Serum	−20°C 6 mo −70°C indefinitely	Age dependent Adult mg/dL IgG1 456–893 IgG2 189–527 IgG3 17–100 IgG4 7–74
Isohemagglutinin Titers Tetanus/Pneumovac titer	Serum	−20°C 6 mo −70°C indefinitely	ABO typing-positive as appropriate. Tetanus/Pneumovac titer depends on exposure.
T Cell Quantitation CD1, CD2, CD3	Whole blood (heparinized or EDTA). Transport at room temperature.	Do not refrigerate or freeze. CDC recommends specimen be assayed within 8 hr.	Age dependent Adult CD1 * CD2 74%–90% CD3 68%–88%
T Cell Subsets CD3/CD4 CD3/CD8	Whole blood (heparinized or EDTA). Transport at room temperature.	Do not refrigerate or freeze. CDC recommends specimen be assayed within 8 hr.	Age dependent Adult CD3 68%–88% CD4 38%–60% CD8 21%–41%
Delayed Hypersensitivity Skin Tests (DHST)	Obtain all in vitro test samples prior to DHST.	NA	Skin reaction after exposure to known immunized antigen
T Cell Proliferation Assays: Mitogen Stimulation Antigen Stimulation	Whole blood (heparinized). Specimen to be assayed within 24 hr. Transport at room temperature.	Specimen should be assayed within 24 hr. Do not refrigerate, do not freeze.	Positive mitogen test = normal; negative test = deficiency. Antigen test results depend on exposure.
Oxidative Burst Tests: Flow Cytometry Nitroblue Tetrazolium	Whole blood (heparinized or EDTA)	Specimen should be assayed within 4 hr. Do not refrigerate, do not freeze.	Positive test = normal; negative test = deficiency. Some tests can detect carrier.

Continued ▶

▶ Continued **SPECIMEN COLLECTION AND STORAGE, REFERENCE RANGE**

TEST	SPECIMEN COLLECTION	SPECIMEN STORAGE	REFERENCE RANGE*
Cell Adhesion Molecules CD11a, CD18	Whole blood (heparinized or EDTA). Transport at room temperature.	Do not refrigerate or freeze. CDC recommends specimens be assayed within 8 hr.	*See note
Chemotaxis	Whole blood (heparinized)	Do not refrigerate or freeze. Specimens should be assayed within 4 hr.	Laboratory established ranges must be used.
Total Functional Complement Assay (CH50)	Serum. Allow specimen to clot at room temperature. Assay or freeze immediately.	−70°C	Age dependent Adult 95–151 units
C3 Quantitation	Serum or plasma (EDTA)	4°C short term −20°C long term	Age dependent Adult 76–142 mg/dL
C4 Quantitation	Serum or plasma (EDTA)	4°C short term −20°C long term	Age dependent Adult 5–40 mg/dL
C1q, C2 Quantitation	Serum or plasma (EDTA)	4°C short term −20°C long term	Age dependent Adult C1q 6.5 ± 0.7 C2 2.8 ± 0.6

*Quantitation values are dependent on kit manufacturer and geographical location.

BIBLIOGRAPHY

Aucouturier P, Lacombe C, Preud'homme JL: Serum IgG subclass level determination: methodological difficulties and practical aspects. Ann Biol Clin 52(1):53–56, 1994.

Conley ME: Primary immunodeficiencies: a flurry of new genes. Immunology Today 16(7):313–315, 1995.

Epstein MM, Gruskay F: Selective deficiency in pneumococcal antibody response in children with recurrent infections. Ann Allergy Asthma Immunol 75(2):125–131, 1995.

Inoue R, Kondo N, Kobayashi Y, et al: IgG2 deficiency associated with defects in production of interferon-gamma; comparison with common variable immunodeficiency. Scand J Immunol 41(2):130–134, 1995.

Kappes DJ, Alarcon B, Regueiro JR: T lymphocyte receptor deficiencies. Curr Opin Immunol 7(4):441–447, 1995.

Muller F, Aukrust P, Nilssen DE, Froland SS: Reduced serum level of transforming growth factor-beta in patients with IgA deficiency. Clin Immunol Immunopathol 76(2):203–208, 1995.

Oxelius VA, Carlsson AM, Hammarstrom L, et al: Linkage of IgA deficiency to Gm allotypes; the influence of Gm allotypes on IgA-IgG subclass deficiency. Clin Exp Immunol 99:211–215, 1995.

Rose N, de Marco EC, Fahey JL, et al: Manual of Clinical Laboratory Immunology, 4th ed. Washington, DC, American Society for Microbiology, 1992.

Rosen FS, Cooper MD, Wedgwood RJ: The primary immunodeficiencies. N Engl J Med 333(7):431–440, 1995.

Sigal L, Ron Y: Immunology and Inflammation. New York, McGraw-Hill, 1994.

Tietz NW: Clinical Guide to Laboratory Tests, 3rd ed. Philadelphia, WB Saunders, 1995.

Wahn U: Evaluation of the child with suspected primary immunodeficiency. Pediatr Allergy Immunol 6(2):71–79, 1995.

Chapter # 20

LYMPHOPROLIFERATIVE DISEASES

Candace Breen, BS, MLT(ASCP)
Marc Golightly, PhD

Q U I C K   C O N T E N T S

INTRODUCTION

The role of immunology in the diagnosis, prognosis, and treatment of cancer has increased tremendously since the mid-1980s. This has stemmed from our increased knowledge of the immune system and its function as well as by technologic advances using immunology as a tool. This section does not discuss the clinical manifestations of the various leukemias and lymphomas (covered in Chapter 37) but concentrates on the use of immunologic methods for diagnostic and prognostic adjuncts to standard histologic methodology.

LABORATORY DIAGNOSIS: GENERAL

The most significant advancement in clinical immunology for the diagnosis of leukemia and lymphomas in the 1970's was the discovery of monoclonal antibody technology and flow cytometry.

COMMONLY USED MONOCLONAL ANTIBODIES FOR CD ANTIGENS

CD ANTIGEN	DISTRIBUTION	FUNCTION
CD 1a	Thymus, dendritic cells	MHC class I–like molecule,
CD 1b,c	Cyto-B cells	
CD2	Pan T cells, thymocytes, NK cells	CD 58 (LFA-3); can activate T cells
CD2 R	Activated T cells	Activation dependent epitope
CD3	T cells, thymocytes	Associated with T cell–Ag receptor
CD4	Helper T cells, monocytes, macrophages	Coreceptor for MHC class II/HIV-I and HIV-2 receptor
CD5	T cells, B cell subset	Binds to CD72
CD6	Thymocytes, T cells, B cell CLL	
CD7	Most T cells, NK cells, eosinophils, thymocytes	Marker for T cell ALL and pluripotential stem cell leukemias
CD8	T cell and NK cell subsets, cytotoxic T cells	Coreceptor for MHC class I molecules
CD9	Pre-B cells, eosinophils, monocytes, platelets	
CD10	Pre-B cells, pre-T cells, PMNs	Metalloproteinase, pre-B cell ALL marker
CD11a	Monocytes, macrophages, lymphocytes, granulocytes	Alpha$_1$ subunit of integrin LFA-1 binds CD54 (ICAM-1) or ICAM-2.
CD11b	NK cells, neutrophils, monocytes	Alpha$_M$ subunit of integrin CR3, receptor for complement C3bi
CD11c	NK cells, neutrophils, monocytes	Alpha-X subunit of integrin CR4
CD12	Monocytes, granulocytes, platelets	
CD13	Monocytes, granulocytes	Aminopeptidase N
CD14	Monocytes, granulocytes	LPS and LPS binding protein receptor
CD15	Neutrophils, monocytes, eosinophils	Recognizes lacto-N-fucopentose III
CD16	Neutrophils, macrophages, NK cells	Low affinity Fc receptor, Fc gamma RIII, marker for NK cells
CD18	Leukocytes	Integrin beta subunit, associates with CD11
CD19	B cells	Coreceptor for B cells, CD21, CD81 association
CD20	B cells	Possible regulating B cell activation role
CD23	B cells, macrophages, eosinophils	Low affinity receptor for IgE, ligand for CD21
CD24	B cells, granulocytes	Possible heat stable antigen
CD25	T and B subsets, activated T cells	Low affinity IL-2 receptor

Continued ▶

▶ Continued **COMMONLY USED MONOCLONAL ANTIBODIES FOR CD ANTIGENS**

CD ANTIGEN	DISTRIBUTION	FUNCTION
CD26	Activated T and B cells	Dipeptidylpeptidase IV
CD28	T cell subsets	Receptor for costimulation of T cells, binding CD80 and B7-2
CD29	Leukocytes, platelets	Integrin b1 subunit, binds with CD49
CD30	Activated B and T cells	
CD33	Monocytes, myeloid cells	
CD34	Progenitor cells	Ligand for L-selectin
CD35	B cells, monocytes, neutrophils	Complement receptor for fragment C3b
CD38	Activated lymphocytes, plasma cells	
CD39	Activated T, B cells, NK cells	
CD40	B lymphocytes	
CD43	T cells, activated B cells	Ligand for CD54 (ICAM)
CD44	Leukocytes, erythrocytes	Hyaluronate receptor, mediates adhesion of leukocytes
CD45	All leukocytes	Protein tyrosine phosphatase, multiple isoforms of extracellular domain result from alternative RNA splicing.
CD45RA	Most T, B, NK cells	Isoforms of CD45, with A exon
CD45RB	Most T, B, NK cells	Isoforms of CD45, with B exon
CD45RO	Activated memory T, NK cells	Isoform of CD 45, without any A, B, and C exons, CD22 associated
CD49b	Platelets, monocytes, activated T cells	Alpha$_2$ integrin, binds collagen
CD49d	T and B lymphocytes, monocytes	Alpha$_4$ integrin, binds VCAM-1
CD54	Activated lymphocytes, macrophages	Integrin receptor for rhinoviruses; ICAM 1 binds CD11a/CD18
CD56	NK cells	Isoform of NCAM
CD58	Leukocytes	Ligand for CD2
CD64	Monocytes, macrophages	High affinity Fc receptor for IgG
CD71	Activated macrophages, lymphocytes	Transferrin receptor
CD72	B cells	Ligand for CD5
CD73	B cell subsets, T cell subsets	Ecto-5'-nucleotidase

Only selected markers are listed. HIV, human immunodificiency virus; PMN, polymorphonuclear cells; EBV, Epstein-Barr virus; IL-2, interleukin-2; ICAM, intercellular adhesion molecules; NCAM, neural cell adhesion molecules; MHC, major histocompatibility complex; ALL, acute lymphocytic leukemia; CLL, chronic lymphocytic leukemia; LFA-1, leucocyte function-associated antigen; VCAM, vascular cell-adhesion molecule; LPS, lipopolysaccharide.

LABORATORY DIAGNOSIS: GENERAL

Monoclonal Antibodies

There are now over 100 well characterized monoclonal antibodies available for clinical/investigational use (see "Commonly Used Monoclonal Antibodies for CD Antigens," p 326). These monoclonal antibodies recognize various specific epitopes or antigens (e.g., T cell receptor, surface immunoglobulin, various B cell epitopes, Fc receptors) and are given a "Cluster Designation" number (CD) to indicate the antibody's reactivity and to standardize the nomenclature. Various combinations of these antibodies are used as phenotypic markers in flow cytometry.

Flow Cytometry

Flow cytometry yields information regarding the biophysical and biochemical nature of a cell via analysis of light scatter and fluorescence signals from the cells labeled with various combinations of fluorescent monoclonal antibodies. Common analytes examined by flow cytometry are as follows:

- Surface and cytoplasmic antigens
- DNA content
- RNA content
- Enzyme studies
- DNA probe studies

The clinical arenas that flow cytometry is currently finding general utility for are listed below:

- Oncology
- Immunoregulatory and immunodeficiency diseases
    HIV diagnosis and monitoring
    Non-HIV immunodeficiencies
- Autoimmune disease (ANCAs, B27 typing, platelet antibodies)
- Reactive/inflammatory diseases

In the area of oncology, flow cytometry is used in the diagnosis as an adjunct or secondary procedure to traditional methods. It is also now being used to monitor for residual disease after treatment and to assess bone marrow harvesting and transplantation. New investigations suggest that it will be useful in the clinical determination of apoptosis (programmed cell death), which in turn may lead to new drug therapies and anticancer sensitivity determinations. This chapter is restricted to the discussion of the use of flow cytometry in the diagnosis of leukemias and lymphomas.

INSTRUMENTATION AND THEORY OF OPERATION

The flow cytometer has three component systems:

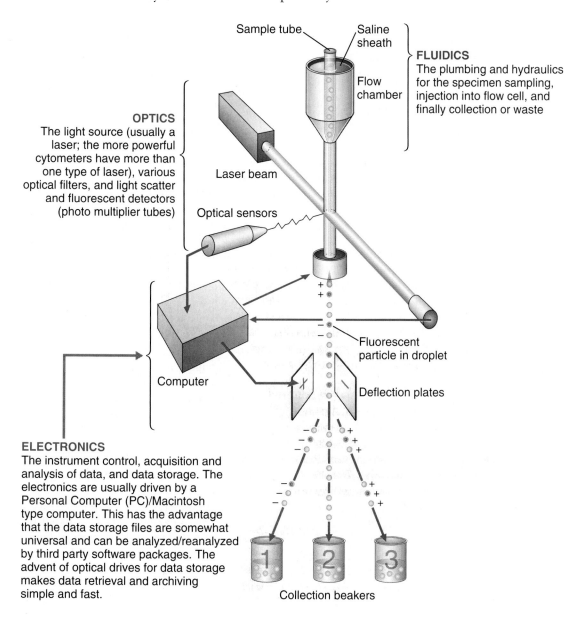

OPTICS
The light source (usually a laser; the more powerful cytometers have more than one type of laser), various optical filters, and light scatter and fluorescent detectors (photo multiplier tubes)

FLUIDICS
The plumbing and hydraulics for the specimen sampling, injection into flow cell, and finally collection or waste

Sample tube

Saline sheath

Flow chamber

Laser beam

Optical sensors

Computer

Fluorescent particle in droplet

Deflection plates

ELECTRONICS
The instrument control, acquisition and analysis of data, and data storage. The electronics are usually driven by a Personal Computer (PC)/Macintosh type computer. This has the advantage that the data storage files are somewhat universal and can be analyzed/reanalyzed by third party software packages. The advent of optical drives for data storage makes data retrieval and archiving simple and fast.

Collection beakers

ADVANTAGES

One of the main advantages to flow cytometry over histology is the quantitative ability (both in absolute numbers and fluorescent intensity), sensitivity, and shear statistical brute force. The cytometer is capable of analyzing over 10,000 cells in seconds, so that very rare cells can be analyzed with statistical significance.

DISADVANTAGES

The main disadvantages of the cytometer is that it is an expensive technology, and the architecture of the tissue is lost (see specimen preparation section below). It is often important to examine the cells in the content of the surrounding tissue. Therefore, flow cytometry should not be viewed as a replacement to standard histologic and immunohistologic procedures, but as a secondary procedure to be called upon when the diagnosis by traditional means is questionable or difficult.

BASIC PREPARATORY OPERATIONS

The type of samples that can be analyzed by flow cytometry include any specimen that can be manipulated into a single cell suspension. These include, but are not limited to, peripheral blood, bone marrow, lymph nodes, spleen, solid tumors, fine needle aspirates, and paraffin embedded tissue. The single cell suspension can then be labeled with an appropriate panel of monoclonal antibodies designed for the diagnosis being considered. The labeling procedure itself is very simple and basically no different from any direct fluorescent antibody test procedure. In fact, when blood is being examined, there are ways to label the whole blood without any purification procedures being required.

ANALYSIS

Light Scatter. The analysis of data from the cytometer first includes an analysis of the light scattering properties of the cells. When the laser beam hits the cell, light is scattered in the 90 degree direction (90LS) and also deflected at a low forward angle (FALS [forward angle light scatter]) direction. It has long been known that 90 degree light scatter gives an indication of the internal cellular complexity and hence is related to the density of the cell. The more 90LS, the higher is the density of the cell. On the other hand, FALS is related to the size of the cell: the higher the FALS, the larger is the cell. When both of these light scattering parameters are examined, a very characteristic pattern emerges for the different cell types. Mature lymphocytes, monocytes, and granulocytes can be easily identified by 90LS and FALS characteristics. Likewise, abnormal-sized and/or dense cells can often be identified and distinguished from normal populations on this basis.

Fluorescence. Once the population(s) to be examined is/are identified by light scattering properties, the analysis of the fluorescent properties (via fluorescent labeled monoclonal antibody markers) of the cells in question can be examined. This is usually performed on a gated population. This means that only fluorescent data are reported on the cells that have the light scattering properties that the operator of the instrument has identified. In most clinical cytometry laboratories, at least two or three markers can be examined on a single cell at the same time. This is done using two to three different colors of labeled monoclonal antibodies. Although multiple color analysis can represent a savings in labor/reagent costs, the main advantage of this type of analysis lies in the clinical diagnostic arena. The presence of several specific markers on the same cell is extremely important and often critical to the diagnosis. For example, CD5 (marker for T cells and a small subpopulation of B cells) and CD19 (marker for B cells), when run together in dual color, are a diagnostic combination for chronic lymphocytic leukemia (CLL). CLL cells are almost always B cells at the stage of maturity that marks with CD5. When a large number of cells are present that express both CD5 and CD19 together, the diagnosis of CLL can be made. Fluorescent data should be examined for the following:

1. Absolute number and percentage of cells that are positive.
2. Fluorescent intensity, which is related to the antigen density of the marker being investigated. The fluorescent intensity (antigen density) is important for further defining the maturational stages and phenotype of the cells in question.

DNA ANALYSIS

In addition to the examination of the various structures and antigens on and in the cell via monoclonal antibodies, flow cytometry can also be used to examine the DNA content of the cell. This is performed using various fluorescent dyes (e.g., propidium iodine) that stoichiometrically bind to the cellular DNA. When analyzed in the cytometer, the specimen's fluorescent intensity is directly correlated to the amount of DNA present. Like the fluorescent antibody labeling, this procedure is also simple. However, the analysis requires the use of complicated mathematical modeling programs. Recently, these have become more user friendly, but they still require a fairly sophisticated mathematical and technical knowledge to appropriately analyze and troubleshoot this testing. The determination of the DNA content/ploidy analysis to identify whether a tumor has an abnormal amount of DNA present (from as little as 5% to 10% above normal to three to four times normal) has gained clinical diagnostic utility. This type of analysis has been reported to have prognostic and diagnostic significance depending on the tumor type. The most common types of tumors for which DNA content/ploidy analysis has been used are:

- Breast
- Prostate
- Bladder
- Fetal tissue
- Lymphoid

For other tumors, the significance and validity in terms of cost effectiveness are still being established, but as the procedure and analysis are refined, the utility may become more widespread.

A modification of this technology has also been used for cell cycle analysis (the percentage of cells in each of the phases of mitosis). However, at present the demand for this type of analysis has not been great, since reports in the literature have found that cell cycle analysis by flow cytometry does not offer any great advantage over the more traditional methods for determining the prognosis of a given tumor.

LABORATORY DIAGNOSIS: SPECIFIC

Diagnostic Antibody Panel Selection

"Common Markers/Panels Used for Lymphoproliferative Studies in Flow Cytometry" on p 334 presents some general monoclonal antibody panels that may be used in the diagnosis of various leukemia and lymphomas. However, these panels are only a guide, and it is generally better if the panels are customized to the individual patient. This can be done in consultation with the pathologist and/or hematologist. During customization, the history, presentation, histology, and hematology results should be taken into account. These panels may be trimmed or expanded, depending on the certainty of the consultative information. For monitoring and follow-up studies after initial diagnosis and phenotyping, the panel is often dramatically reduced to only the monoclonal antibodies that were positive or significant.

Diagnostic Antibody Panel Theory

The choice of antibody panel is based on the fact that most leukemias and lymphomas are a proliferation of a single lymphoid cell, and consequently all the cells exhibit the same phenotypic characteristics. In addition, they have the maturational characteristics of the cell from which they arose. The figures below demonstrate ontogeny of the various lymphoid and myeloid lineages and the specific antigenic (CD) characteristic of each maturational stage of normal development:

CELLULAR ANTIGENS OF MYELOID AND MONOCYTIC CELLS

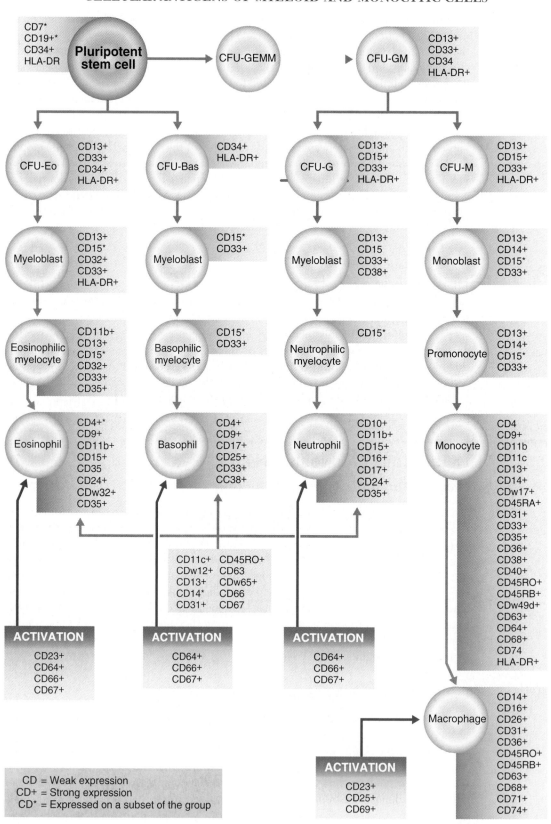

CELLULAR ANTIGENS OF LYMPHOID CELLS

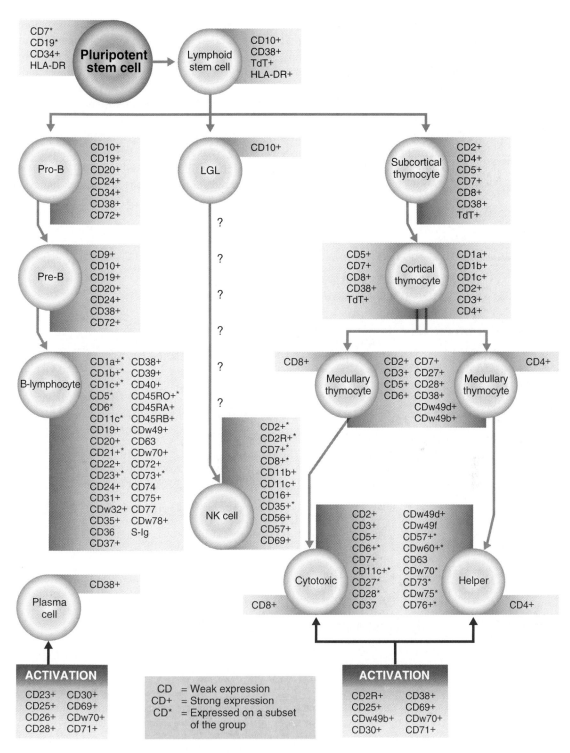

The various leukemia/lymphomas can then be identified by proper selection of a monoclonal antibody panel that recognizes a particular cell at a particular stage of maturation (See "Common Markers/Panels Used for Lymphoproliferative Studies in Flow Cytometry," p 334). It should be clear that correct consultative input is essential to the proper selection of antibody panel. Without this input, or if one does not have a high regard for its accuracy, the antibody panel should be expanded to account for this uncertainty. In addition, the specimen type should be considered. It is easy to acquire more peripheral blood if the antibody panel was too limited. However, another lymph node or bone marrow specimen is usually not a pleasant or possible option. One alternative is to sterile culture the left-over specimen for immediate future use if the initial panel yields inconclusive results. Most of the other leukemias and lymphomas are variations of the panels in "Common Markers/Panels Used for Lymphoproliferative Studies in Flow Cytometry" below, depending on the expected maturity of the cells to be tested. Ideally, flow cytometry studies should be ordered only after the pathologist receives a preliminary reading to determine whether flow cytometry is required. Therefore, the material received for flow cytometry should not be automatically processed as a first order test unless there is information already known to indicate it is needed. The biopsy material can be processed into a single cell suspension and cultured for 24 hours until flow cytometry is deemed necessary or not.

COMMON MARKERS/PANELS USED FOR LYMPHOPROLIFERATIVE STUDIES IN FLOW CYTOMETRY

DISEASE	ANTIBODY COMBINATIONS	INTERPRETATION AND PATTERN
Chronic Lymphocytic Leukemia (CLL) and Prolymphocytic Leukemia	CD3 with CD23	CD3 negative and CD23 positive
	CD5 with CD20	Dual staining CD5 positive and CD20 positive: characteristic of CLL and well differentiated lymphocytic lymphoma (WDLL)
	CD19 with kappa CD19 with lambda	CD19 positive with one light chain expressed in low intensity. Occasionally light chains are not detected.
	CD45 with CD14	CD45 brightly expressed and CD14 negative
	(Antiglycophorin added to bone marrows)	To determine erythroid component to the specimen
Hair Cell Leukemia (HCL)	CD3 with CD23	CD3 negative and CD23 negative
	CD11c with CD22	Brightly expressed CD11c and CD22, unlike CLL
	CD20 with CD5	CD20 positive and CD5 negative (occasionally weak expression of CD5)
	CD19 with kappa CD19 with lambda	CD19 positive with one monoclonal light chain expressed
	CD103 with CD25	CD103 is highly specific for HCL, and CD25 is usually expressed. Hairy cell variants may be negative for these two markers.
	CD21 with HLA-DR	CD21 negative and DR positive

Continued ▶

► Continued **COMMON MARKERS/PANELS USED FOR LYMPHOPROLIFERATIVE STUDIES IN FLOW CYTOMETRY**

DISEASE	ANTIBODY COMBINATIONS	INTERPRETATION AND PATTERN
B cell Acute Lymphocytic Leukemia (ALL)	CD45 with CD14	CD45 brightly expressed and CD14 negative
	(Antiglycophorin added to bone marrows)	To determine erythroid component to the specimen
	Others (which may be run PCA-1 and CD10)	PCA-1 the early plasma cell antigen is reported to be positive in HCL, and CD10 (Calla) is weakly expressed in 26% of cases.
	CD3 with HLA-DR	CD3 (T cell receptor) negative and DR positive
	CD5 with CD20	CD5 negative and CD20 variably positive (low intensity/negative on precursor B cell ALL, positive on more mature B cell ALL)
	CD19 with kappa CD19 with lambda	CD19 positive (stem cell is negative) and surface Ig negative (a mature B cell ALL may have surface immunoglobulin).
	CD34 with CD38	CD34 positive ALL correlates with good prognosis in pediatric patients and poor prognosis in adults. CD38 is positive from stem cell to pre-B.
	TdT with CD10	TdT and CD10 (Calla) positive in common ALL and pre-B ALL. CD10 positivity is associated with favorable complete treatment response and disease free survival.
	TdT with CD33	CD33 negative
Myeloma Plasmacytoid Leukemia/Lymphoma	CD45 with CD14	CD45 dimly expressed and CD14 negative
	(Antiglycophorin added to bone marrows)	To determine erythroid component to the specimen
	CD3 with HLA-DR	CD3 negative. Most are DR negative, although some early plasmacytoid cells may be DR positive
	CD5 with CD20	CD5 and CD20 negative
	CD19 with kappa CD19 with lambda	CD19 and surface Ig negative. Occasionally surface Ig is positive. Cytoplasmic Ig positive.
	CD45 with CD38	CD45 negative or low intensity. CD38 is positive.
	CD40 with CD56	Usually CD40 positive. CD56 has been reported to be positive on myeloma cells but negative on normal plasma cells.
	CD10	CD10 positivity indicates poor prognosis.

Continued ►

► Continued **COMMON MARKERS/PANELS USED FOR LYMPHOPROLIFERATIVE STUDIES IN FLOW CYTOMETRY**

DISEASE	ANTIBODY COMBINATIONS	INTERPRETATION AND PATTERN
T Cell Acute Lymphoblastic Leukemia (ALL)	PCA-1	PCA-1 positive
	CD45 with CD14	CD14 negative
	CD1 with CD3	CD1 positivity associated with longer disease free survival in adult T cell ALL. CD3 is negative in 99% (exception is mature medullary thymocyte T cell ALL).
	CD2 with CD25	CD2 variably expressed and CD25 negative
	CD38 with CD7	CD38 and CD7 are positive
	CD4 with CD8	CD4 and CD8 variably expressed depending on maturity: dual expression is common
	CD5 with CD20	CD5 positive except for prothymocyte stage T cell ALL. CD20 negative.
	CD45 with CD14	CD45 positive and CD14 negative
	HLA-DR with CD34	DR positive T cell ALL associated with a worse prognosis. CD34 in pediatric patients associated with CNS involvement and poor prognosis, and predicts myeloid expression.
	TdT with CD10	TdT is positive. CD10 positive T cell ALL associated with prolonged disease free survival.
	CD19 and kappa	Negative
	CD19 and lambda	Negative
	(Antiglycophorin added to bone marrows)	To determine erythroid component to the specimen
Postthymic T Cell Leukemia/Lymphoma **Peripheral T Cell Leukemia** **Sézary's Syndrome** **Adult T Cell Leukemia**	CD1 with CD3	CD1 negative, CD3 positive. *Note:* Peripheral T cell lymphomas lack ≥1 pan-T cell antigen (CD3, 2, 5, or 7) 75% of the time.
	CD2 with CD25	CD2 positive. CD25 positive in adult T cell leukemias and some peripheral T cell lymphomas.
	CD7 with CD5	CD5 positive; CD7 positive except in adult T cell leukemia
	CD4 with CD8	Variable expression
	CD19 with kappa	Negative
	CD19 with lambda	Negative

Continued ►

▶ Continued **COMMON MARKERS/PANELS USED FOR LYMPHOPROLIFERATIVE STUDIES IN FLOW CYTOMETRY**

DISEASE	ANTIBODY COMBINATIONS	INTERPRETATION AND PATTERN
	CD45 with CD14	CD45 positive and CD14 negative
	TdT with CD10	Negative
	(Antiglycophorin added to bone marrows)	To determine erythroid component to the specimen
T γ Proliferative Disease (NK-like T cell Leukemia) NK-like T Cell Lymphoma NK Cell Leukemia	CD2 with CD57	NK-like T cell lymphoma tends to be CD56 positive, CD57 negative and is usually clinically aggressive. NK cell leukemias tend to be CD56 and/or CD16 positive, CD57 negative and are usually clinically aggressive. Tγ proliferative disease is CD56 negative, CD57 positive and exhibits a chronic indolent course. CD2 is usually positive for all, but there are variants.
	CD3 with CD56, CD16	Surface CD3 is positive in Tγ proliferative disease and NK-like T cell lymphoma. CD3 is negative in NK cell leukemia. For CD56 and CD57, see above.
	CD11b with CD11c	Usually positive
	CD4 with CD8	Usually CD8 positive, CD4 negative. However, dual staining and CD4 positivity has been reported.
	CD19	Negative
	CD45 with CD14	CD45 positive and CD14 negative
Acute Myelogenous Leukemia (AML)	CD11c with CD11b	CD11c positive on mature myeloid cells. CD11b positive on myelomonocytic cells, eosinophilic myelocytes, eosinophils, and neutrophils. Differentiated AML usually expresses mature markers.
	CD13 with CD15	Poorly differentiated AML usually lacks CD15, CD11c, CD11b.
	CD33 with TdT	CD33 in the absence of CD34, DR, and/or CD13 suggests immature acute basophilic or mast cell leukemia. TdT is often expressed in low intensity in poorly differentiated AML.
	CD14 with CD45	Low intensity CD45. CD14 on early promonocytes to mature monocytes. High expression of CD14 and CD11b predicts poor outcome.
	CD3 with CD7	CD3 negative. Some immature AML expresses CD7.
	CD19 with kappa	CD19 occasionally expressed on some primitive AML

Continued ▶

▶ Continued **COMMON MARKERS/PANELS USED FOR LYMPHOPROLIFERATIVE STUDIES IN FLOW CYTOMETRY**

DISEASE	ANTIBODY COMBINATIONS	INTERPRETATION AND PATTERN
	CD19 with lambda	Surface Ig negative
	CD34 with HLA-DR	Poorly differentiated AML often expresses CD34. High intensity CD34 has worse prognosis. CD34 coexpressed with DR has worse prognosis than CD34 alone.
	CD10 with TdT	CD10 is present on neutrophils.
	(Antiglycophorin added to bone marrows)	To determine erythroid component to the specimen

BIBLIOGRAPHY

Bauer KD, Duque RE, Shankey TV: Clinical Flow Cytometry, Principles and Application. Baltimore, Williams & Wilkins, 1993.

Foa R: Interleukin 2 in the management of acute leukaemia. Br J Haematol 92(1):1–8, 1996.

Freedman AS: Cell surface antigens in leukemias and lymphomas. Cancer Invest 14(3):252–276, 1996.

Jaffe E: Classification of natural killer (NK) cell and NK-like T cell malignancies. Blood 87:1207–1210, 1996.

Keren DF: Flow Cytometry in Clinical Diagnosis. Chicago, American Society of Clinical Pathologists, 1989.

Oshimi K: Lymphoproliferative disorders of natural killer cells. Int J Hematol 63(4):279–290, 1996.

Paietta E: Immunobiology of acute leukemia. In Wiernik P, ed: Neoplastic Diseases of the Blood, 3rd ed. New York, Churchill Livingstone, 1996.

Paietta E, Andersen J, Wiernik PH: A new approach to analyzing the utility of immunophenotyping for predicting clinical outcome in acute leukemia. Eastern Cooperative Oncology Group. Leukemia 10(1):1–4, 1996.

Sachs L: The control of hematopoiesis and leukemia: from basic biology to the clinic. Proc Nat Acad Sci USA 93(10):4742–4749, 1996.

Shapiro H: Practical Flow Cytometry, 3rd ed. New York, Wiley-Liss, 1995.

Tabbara IA: Allogeneic bone marrow transplantation: acute and late complications. Anticancer Res 16(2):1019–1026, 1996.

Wiernik PH: Leukemias and myeloma. Cancer Chemoth Biol Response Modif 16:347–375, 1996.

Chapter

21

IMMUNOLOGY OF INFECTIOUS DISEASES

Candace Breen, BS, MLT (ASCP)
Carolyn Kube, BS, MT (ASCP)
Marc Golightly, PhD

Q U I C K   C O N T E N T S

INTRODUCTION

In many infectious diseases, culture, isolation, and identification of the organism are the "gold standard" laboratory diagnostic indication of infection. Unfortunately, isolation, culture, and identification may not always be feasible because of the time involved, because the procedure may have a low yield, or because a fairly invasive procedure may be necessary depending on the specimen required (e.g., skin biopsy). Therefore, indirect evidence is often the only practical choice. (The most common diagnostic methods and the specimen requirements for the infectious diseases discussed in this chapter are given in "Specimen Collection, Storage and Reference Range" on p 366 and "Diagnostic Tests and Methodologies" on p 370.

The most important recommendation that can be made in the use and interpretation of serologic diagnostic tests for infectious diseases is to integrate the clinical symptoms, history, and other laboratory data with the serologic results. This applies not only to the actual interpretation of the test result but also to the ordering of the test (i.e., testing only those patients for whom there is a valid or good suspicion that they were exposed or infected). The importance of this has been demonstrated by predictive value calculations. When tests are ordered without regard for clinical presentation and history (i.e., used as a screen despite the lack of appropriate symptoms and/or risk factors), the predictive value (that a positive test actually indicates the presence of the disease) is extremely low. However, the positive predictive value is very high when the clinical data are used and only patients with a good clinical history for the disease are tested. Therefore, inappropriate testing of patients (shotgun approach) should be strongly avoided because positive results are virtually meaningless under these conditions and may lead to unneeded and potentially harmful therapy.

IMMUNOLOGIC INFECTIOUS DISEASE TESTS (BACTERIAL)

Spirochetal Infections

Spirochetes are bacteria belonging to the order Spirochaetales. These include two families: Spirochaetaceae and Leptospiraceae. The three most clinically important spirochetes are *Treponema*, *Borrelia*, and *Leptospira*. These spirochetes are motile, gram negative bacteria with a tightly helical shape that ranges from 10 to 50 μm in length. They have an enclosed flagellum that is responsible for their corkscrew movement. Although they are gram negative, silver stains or direct visualization with darkfield examination is needed to demonstrate the organisms for clinical diagnosis. There are several diseases caused by these bacteria. These include, but are not limited to, Lyme disease, syphilis, and leptospirosis. Not only are the causative organisms similar, but often so are the clinical manifestations. Therefore it is important to know the subtle differences and similarities in both the clinical and the laboratory diagnostic tests. This knowledge is invaluable in explaining the patterns of laboratory test results obtained and coming to the correct diagnosis.

SYPHILIS

Syphilis is a sexually transmitted diseases caused by the spirochete *Treponema pallidum.* Syphilis was known as early as the late 1400s and is thought to be the cause of the "great pox" epidemic in 15th and 16th century Europe. In the urban areas, over 10% of the population in the United States and Europe had serologic evidence of exposure by the 19th century. With the advent of antibiotics in the 1940s the incidence of this disease dropped. However, in the late 1980s and the 1990s the incidence of syphilis in the United States has increased again because of the increased use of crack cocaine and increased prevalence of human immunodeficiency virus (HIV) infection. Therefore, the laboratory diagnosis of syphilis continues to be and is becoming more important to today's clinicians as the clinical diagnosis is now often complicated by other confounding diseases as discussed later.

Clinical Manifestations

Syphilis, like other spirochetal disease, has several recognizable clinical stages.

PRIMARY STAGE. The first, or primary, stage begins 3 to 6 weeks after infection. This stage is characterized by a chancre, a usually painless ulcer, that resolves with or without treatment in 2 to 8 weeks. It is this stage that, as in other spirochetal diseases, may be overlooked because of the occasional absence of the characteristic lesions or the presence of atypical forms. Darkfield examination of lesions is diagnostic for this stage.

SECONDARY STAGE. Secondary syphilis usually follows the primary stage by 2 to 24 weeks and may last 2 to 6 weeks, even if untreated. The symptoms are highly variable and can include fever, malaise, skin rash, and weight loss. Central nervous system (CNS) involvement may occur in up to 40% of the patients and is a severe complication when HIV coinfection occurs. The immunologic tests are the best method for laboratory diagnosis at this stage. Spontaneous subsidence of the secondary phase then occurs and is followed by a latent phase lasting several years.

TERTIARY STAGE. The first lesions of the tertiary stage are usually seen from 3 to 10 years after the primary stage. These are soft granulomatous lesions called *gummas*. The tertiary stage can be asymptomatic or can include CNS involvement, deafness, blindness, cardiovascular disease, and insanity.

TECHNICAL NOTE   The typical nontreponemal screening tests may be negative at this stage.

If negative rapid plasma reagin (RPR)–Venereal Disease Research Laboratory (VDRL) tests are obtained, the treponemal confirmatory tests should be considered [fluorescent treponemal antibody absorption (FTA-ABS)–microhemagglutination assay–*Treponema pallidum* (MHA-TP)].

Congenital Syphilis. Congenital syphilis can also occur. It is transmitted with greater frequency in pregnant women with untreated early infections as opposed to those with latent stages of the disease. Congenital syphilis may cause stillbirth, or fetal death due to premature birth. During the first weeks of life congenital syphilis can be asymptomatic. In fact, the majority of cases of congenital syphilis are diagnosed in patients older than 10 years. In these patients the disease manifestations include CNS involvement, abnormal tooth formation (Hutchinson's teeth), and nerve deafness. Other manifestations include interstitial keratitis, skeletal lesions, and fissuring around the mouth.

Syphilis in HIV Infected Patients. There is a high incidence of HIV infection in people with syphilis. These coinfected patients tend to have high nontreponemal titers and take a greater time to revert to nonreactive levels after treatment. HIV infected patients have a high incidence of biologic false positive syphilis tests, possibly due to the hypergammaglobulinemia that can occur in HIV patients.

Laboratory Diagnosis of Syphilis

▎ *Darkfield examination* from accessible lesions of syptomatic, primary syphilis patients is the most immediate method of diagnosis. Specific monoclonal and polyclonal fluorescent antibodies can be used on biopsied lesions in a direct fluorescent assay to rule out the presence of nonpathogenic commensal spirochetes that are commonly mistaken for *T. pallidum*.

IMMUNOLOGIC INFECTIOUS DISEASE TESTS (BACTERIAL)

▪ *Nontreponemal tests* test for the presence of antibodies to phospholipids that occur in syphilis. These tests (RPR and VDRL) are used for screening patients because they are easy and cost effective. They should be used when patients are suspected of having syphilis and have atypical lesions or a negative darkfield microscopic examination. Quantitative RPR testing is primarily used in monitoring therapy of primary and secondary syphilis. However, tertiary syphilis patients revert to being nonreactive in these tests with or without treatment. Cerebrospinal fluid (CSF) can be tested by the VDRL method only. All reactive nontreponemal tests must be confirmed by treponemal testing to rule out false positives caused by infectious and noninfectious diseases and conditions (e.g., measles, mononucleosis, leptospirosis, malaria, autoimmune disorders, pregnancy, drug addiction, and old age).

▪ *Treponemal tests* (FTA-ABS and MHA-TP) are used to confirm reactive nontreponemal procedures. A positive FTA-ABS test almost always remains positive, so it is not recommended for monitoring therapy. This test should also be done if tertiary syphilis is suspected and a nonreactive RPR is obtained.

▪ *PCR testing* has been reported to be useful in detecting treponemal antigens but has not yet been perfected for routine clinical use.

Treatment for Syphilis

Penicillin is the drug of choice for all stages of syphilis.

LEPTOSPIROSIS

The *Leptospira* spirochete is tightly coiled and motile, measuring 6 to 20 μm long. The species of *Leptospira* that are generally recognized have many serotypes and subserotypes. *Leptospira biflexa* is a saprophyte, not often associated with human infection and usually found in fresh waters. *Leptospira interrogans* is pathogenic for humans and other mammals. The reservoirs for these bacteria are rodents and domestic animals; the bacteria are shed in the urine. The occurrence is worldwide with person to person transmission being rare. Farmers and those whose occupations involve dealing with livestock or working in sewers are at high risk. Recreational exposure is also possible (camping, swimming in ponds and rivers, and so forth).

Clinical Manifestations

Infection by *Leptospira* is by ingestion or passage through the skin or mucous membranes. Leptospirosis is usually "biphasic," causing chills, fever, and severe headaches lasting about 4 to 7 days. An interval of being asymptomatic, lasting 1 to 2 days, is followed by a serovar specific immunity phase when antibodies are produced. This phase lasts about 30 days and is generally characterized by uveitis, rash, aseptic meningitis, and hepatic and renal damage. At this time organisms are detected in urine but not in CSF or blood.

Laboratory Diagnosis

CULTURE. Isolation of the organisms from blood or CSF, when collected in the first 7 to 10 days of the illness, and urine collected after the first week of infection, is diagnostic for leptospirosis. Spinning hooked ends of the *Leptospira* allow easy identification with darkfield microscopy.

ANTIBODIES. Pooled bacterial antigens are used to detect agglutinating antibodies in the microagglutination test (MAT). The end point of the reaction is taken at the dilution for which 50% of the leptospiras are agglutinated. Antibodies can also be detected by enzyme immunoassay (EIA). Immunoblotting has demonstrated that patients produce IgM antibodies to leptospiral lipopolysaccharide and flagellin. Some patients can also produce IgG to a 65 kDa protein.

Treatment

Penicillin G is the treatment of choice. Ampicillin is recommended for severe disease, and doxycycline for preventing the disease in exposed persons. There are vaccines for some domestic livestock and pets, helping to reduce the prevalence of the disease.

LYME DISEASE

Lyme disease is caused by infection with the spirochete *Borrelia burgdorferi*. As previously noted, spirochetal diseases exhibit a wide range of presentations but are generally characterized by periods of clinical activity separated by periods of remission. When untreated, spirochetal diseases are generally of long duration. Being a spirochetosis, Lyme disease shares the general and some specific characteristics of diseases caused by other spirochetes (*Leptospira* spp., *Treponema* spp., and other *Borrelia* spp.).

Clinical Manifestations

Patients with Lyme disease can demonstrate early and late cutaneous; cardiac; peripheral and central nervous system; articular; and ocular manifestations. As in any other disease, the frequency of these manifestations as well as their severity can be variable. Only in 1990 did the Centers for Disease Control and Prevention (CDC) develop a case definition.

EARLY LYME DISEASE. The early clinical sign that is the hallmark of Lyme disease is erythema migrans (EM). EM is an enlarging lesion of the skin that can begin as a red macule at the site of the tick bite. This lesion can expand into either a uniform or an annular reddish plaque and can at times become vesicular. In a number of patients, EM lesions can be multiple. The presence of an EM in a patient epidemiologically at risk is usually sufficient to establish a diagnosis of Lyme disease. Unfortunately, EM does not occur in, or is not reported by, all patients with Lyme disease.

TECHNICAL NOTE The laboratory is not very helpful in establishing a diagnosis of Lyme disease during the initial cutaneous stage since antibodies are generally not present. This is probably the greatest problem associated with the diagnosis of Lyme disease.

LATE LYME DISEASE. The laboratory is of significant assistance to the clinician for patients who present with late manifestations of this disease but without a history of the pathognomonic lesion. Articular manifestations are possibly the best characterized of all the disseminated or late manifestations of Lyme disease.

Lyme Arthritis. The late arthritis seen in Lyme disease patients is oligoarticular, usually inflammatory, and predominantly affects the large joints, notably the knees. Both arthralgias and arthritis can become chronic in the late stage of Lyme disease. Patients with late Lyme disease are usually reactive in serologic assays. Unfortunately, arthralgias along with malaise, fatigue, and myalgias can also be part of the early musculoskeletal complaints of Lyme disease.

Cardiovascular Disease. Spirochetal diseases can also cause cardiovascular disease. Leptospirosis and syphilis cause prominent abnormalities in the heart and in the aorta; thus, it is not surprising that such manifestations (including conduction system abnormalities, arrhythmias, pericarditis, and myocarditis) may be part of the clinical spectrum of Lyme disease.

Neurologic Disease. The neurologic manifestations of Lyme disease can occur early as well as late and involve both the peripheral and central nervous systems. It should be noted that other spirochetoses produce neurologic manifestations and that in Lyme disease, as well as in syphilis, there appears to be an early invasion of the nervous system. The range of neurologic abnormalities is very large and can include cognitive impairment and psychiatric disease. Meningitis can often accompany seventh cranial nerve palsy, and late complications of progressive *Borrelia* encephalomyelitis can include encephalopathy and polyneuropathy. In some instances, the diagnosis of neuroborreliosis may be aided by the finding of specific antibodies in the CSF.

Laboratory Diagnosis

The clinical diagnosis of Lyme borreliosis can often be a severe problem for the clinician because of the often variable and vague clinical symptoms when there is a lack of definitive clinical hallmarks of Lyme disease. Because of these facts as well as patient pressure, the laboratory has often been used as the primary source for making the definitive diagnosis.

CULTURE. In many bacterial infections, the laboratory evidence is usually very powerful since culture followed by identification of the causative organism is usually diagnostic. Although culture in Lyme disease is better than that in syphilis (*T. pallidum* cannot be cultured in vitro), culturing *B. burgdorferi* is difficult because of (1) its fastidious in vitro growth characteristics, (2) its scarcity in easily obtained body fluids or tissues, or a combination of both. Therefore, culture, the usual "gold standard" for bacterial diagnosis and identification, is not a good diagnostic option for *B. burgdorferi*.

ANTIGEN DETECTION. Urine has been examined for excreted *B. burgdorferi* antigens; however, more work and clinical studies need to be performed in this area before this can be considered a diagnostic option as an indication of Lyme borreliosis.

POLYMERASE CHAIN REACTION. Polymerase chain reaction (PCR) has been used to detect DNA of pathogenic organisms. However, in the clinical setting there are still many questions to be answered and PCR has not yet been extensively used clinically. It has been demonstrated that the detection of spirochetal DNA does not necessarily prove the existence of viable culturable organisms. One of the most important considerations is what specimen should be used, since the spirochetemia is short lived in humans; blood is not optimal for this and other reasons. Recently, Goodman and colleagues demonstrated that PCR is three times more sensitive than culture in early Lyme disease and may be useful as a diagnostic indicator of disease dessemination. Urine, joint fluid, skin, and CSF have been used with success. However, without a Food and Drug Administration (FDA) approved diagnostic PCR kit, it is doubtful that the test will be performed by the average hospital or diagnostic laboratory for some time. Presently, PCR is performed by specialized referral laboratories.

ANTIBODY DETECTION. The detection of antibodies to *B. burgdorferi* is the most common method used to obtain laboratory evidence of past or present exposure to the organism. These assays include EIA, indirect immunofluorescence antibody (IFA), and the Western blot or immunoblot.

Indirect Immunofluorescence Assays. The IFA is commonly used in diagnostic laboratories for many infectious agents. However, because of the subjectivity problems normally encountered with this type of assay, it has usually been replaced by EIA when possible.

Advantages. The IFA is ideally suited for low volume testing, and no special equipment is required (except for a fluorescence microscope, which most laboratories have for other fluorescence procedures such as antinuclear antibody tests).

Disadvantages. The IFA may have false positives due to crossreacting other spirochetal illnesses. The problems inherent in all IFA assays seem to outweigh the positive aspects of the Lyme disease IFA, and it is not the method of choice.

Enzyme Immunoassay. The Lyme disease EIA is the method used by most diagnostic laboratories, and many studies have evaluated and examined both commercial and research variations of this technique.

Advantages. Many of the disadvantages of the IFA (subjectivity, not amenable to high volume testing, and so forth) are eliminated by the EIA. However, the EIA is by no means a gold standard for Lyme disease diagnosis, and the CDC now recommends that all Lyme disease serologic studies by confirmed by a Western blot.

Disadvantages. EIA kit variability from different manufacturers has generally been the result of a lack of sensitivity of the test in patients with early Lyme disease. No test kits (including IFA kits) were able to detect specific antibody in patients with early Lyme disease (i.e., EM apparent for less than 1 week). This is unfortunate since the clinical symptoms at this stage may be quite vague, as previously discussed. However, most likely this is before significant amounts of specific antibody have been produced, and this should not be viewed as kit failure. However, intermanufacturer variability becomes more evident when Lyme disease patients further along in the disease process (EM longer than 1 week but less than 3 weeks) are tested. In this group, positive results were obtained for 0 to less than 57% of the patients, depending on the manufacturer. Patients with late Lyme disease are more reliably identified. It must be remembered that when any test is inappropriately used as a screen in patients with a low disease probability, problems can occur, even with a low false positive rate. For Lyme disease, false positives have been reported in patients with mononucleosis, certain bacterial diseases, autoimmune disease, and other causes of polyclonal B cell stimulation.

Western Blot (Immunoblot). The Western blot or immunoblot has an extremely important role in the clinical diagnostic laboratory as one of the confirmatory tests for HIV following a positive EIA. The CDC/Association of State Territory Public Health Laboratory Directors (ASTPHLD) recommended that the Lyme disease immunoblot be used in a two tier system in much the same fashion as that for HIV. All samples judged equivocal or positive by EIA or IFA should be tested by immunoblotting. Unfortunately, because of the common and crossreacting bacterial antigens expressed by *B. burgdorferi* as well as the individuality of the humoral response, the Lyme disease immunoblot is much more complex than the HIV immunoblot. Therefore, it cannot be used with the same degree of confidence as HIV immunoblotting. It is apparent from the Western blot proficiency testing from the College of American Pathologists (CAP) that there is much variation in results and interpretation. The sensitivity and specificity of immunoblotting is not significantly better or worst than the EIA. It is anticipated that there will continue to be large variations in reported sensitivities and specificities until the final standardization in method and interpretation is worked out. The CDC/ASTPHLD working group on the standardization of Lyme disease testing has published guidelines for the interpretation of Lyme disease immunoblots. However, a patient's diagnosis is still primarily a clinical one, and the laboratory should be used as a secondary source for support for or against the diagnosis. Complicating the laboratory interpretation is that antibiotic treatment (especially early in the disease course) may abrogate or alter the immune response so that an early Lyme disease patient may never seroconvert to positive. In addition, the reactivity of sera from patients with other diseases (many of which are in the clinical differential diagnosis of Lyme disease) is often known to be due to organisms that express crossreactive antigens. Patients with various autoimmune diseases (rheumatoid arthritis, systemic lupus erythematosis, and systemic sclerosis), acute Epstein-Barr virus (EBV) infection, polyclonal increases in immunoglobulin (acquired immunodeficiency disease [AIDS]), Sicca syndrome, fever of unknown origin, and chronic nephritis have been known to give false positive results.

Conclusions About Antibody Detection Assays. Although much has been written regarding the problems with Lyme disease serologic tests, it should be realized that, in general, serologic tests (of any type) are seldom diagnostic for infection without the integration of clinical input and patient history with the serologic results. Even then, the possibility of diseases within the clinical differential that may cause false positive results for one reason or another must be considered.

> **TECHNICAL NOTE** Despite these limitations, meaningful results can be obtained from these tests if caution is used in their interpretation and the clinical symptomatology, history, and examination are integrated with the laboratory results.

Treatment

The treatment of Lyme disease varies with the severity and duration. Generally, treatment is with amoxyicillin or doxycycline for 3 weeks. Occasionally, intravenous antibiotics are given for severe and/or chronic cases.

Streptococcal Infections

Streptococci are gram positive, ovoid or spherical shaped cocci often seen in chains or pairs. There are three schemes of classification:

1. Hemolytic reactions
2. Serologic reactivity to carbohydrates (Lancefield groups)
3. Physiologic characteristics

CLINICAL MANIFESTATIONS

One important pathogen is group A beta-hemolytic *Streptococcus pyogenes*, which is responsible for acute rheumatic fever and poststreptococcal glomerulonephritis. This species is also frequently associated with pharyngitis and its resultant disorder, and impetigo. Bacteremia can lead to infections in the bones and joints. Other infections include sinusitis in adults, otitis media in children, and neonatal septicemia. Complications frequently develop in untreated patients.

LABORATORY DIAGNOSIS

In addition to culture, extracellular products and bacterial toxins of *S. pyogenes* are important to the serologic diagnosis of streptococcal disease. Antibodies produced in response to these substances are measured by the following tests. As with all infectious diseases, serologic diagnosis must be made in association with clinical presentation.

ANTIGEN. Fluorescent monoclonal antibodies can be used directly on smears made from swab specimens. A rapid antigen detection test for streptococcal pharyngitis can be performed directly from throat swabs with commercially available kits. These are highly specific but have a low sensitivity, and culture should follow any negative direct test.

ANTIBODY TESTS

▪ *Antistreptolysin O (ASO) test* measures the antibodies produced against the extracellular toxin streptolysin O in patients' serum. A fourfold rise in the titer of acute and convalescent specimens is diagnostically significant. The normal adult reference range is less than 160 Todd U/mL; however, this varies with age. Results of 500 to 5000 Todd U/mL suggests acute poststreptococcal glomerulonephritis (AGN), active rheumatic fever (RF), or acute poststreptococcal endocarditis. It should be noted that 15% of acute RF patients test negative. The ASO is also not reliable for diagnosing poststreptococcal AGN after skin infection. A more reliable test is the anti-DNase B test, which detects about two thirds of patients with recent streptococcal impetigo.

▪ *Anti-DNase B* detects antibodies to the DNase B antigen produced by all group A streptococci. The levels increase after the patient recovers from a group A streptococcal infection. Adult normal titers are considered less than 85 Todd U/mL; school age children, less than 170 Todd U/mL; and preschoolers less than 60 Todd U/mL. Results of greater than 120 Todd U/mL in adults and 240 Todd U/mL in children are seen in 80% of patients with acute RF and 75% with poststreptococcal AGN.

▪ *Streptozyme (antistreptococcal enzyme)* test is considered nonspecific because it detects antibodies to multiple exoenzymes of group A streptococci. It can determine recent and current streptococcal infection but not the type of streptococcal infection. The normal reference range is less than 100 streptozyme units.

TREATMENT

Penicillin and penicillin derivatives are usually effective in the treatment of group A streptococci. There are some drug resistant strains that require multiple drug therapy for effective treatment.

Staphylococcus aureus Infections

Staphylococci are gram positive, catalase positive spherical cocci. The species *Staphylococcus aureus* is pathogenic and can colonize the skin, mucous membranes, and gastrointestinal tract. *S. aureus* is frequently seen in hospitals, where hospital staff spread infection among staff and patients through hand contact. There are antibiotic resistant strains of *S. aureus* (i.e., methicillin resistant [MRSA]) that are increasing in frequency.

LABORATORY DIAGNOSIS

CULTURE. Culture of *S. aureus* can be done with a high degree of accuracy. See Chapter 31, p 591.

ANTIBODY. Teichoic acid is present on the cell wall of gram positive bacteria, especially *S. aureus*. Detection of anti–teichoic acid antibodies by immunodiffusion has been used in diagnosis of *S. aureus* infection but has limited utility. The normal titer reference range is less than or equal to 1:2 and also less than a fourfold rise in titer between acute and convalescent samples. Increased titers are present in patients with serious infections and can support the diagnosis of endocarditis when combined with positive blood cultures. It may be necessary to repeat the test after 1 to 2 weeks if initial tests are negative because of low antibody production. False positives can be caused by *Haemophilus influenzae* infection.

TREATMENT

There is a high degree of variability in the resistance to antimicrobial agents. This makes susceptibility testing of the utmost importance. With the high prevalence of MRSA, the drug of choice for hospital acquired infections is vancomycin.

SPECIFIC IMMUNOLOGIC INFECTIOUS DISEASE TESTS (FUNGAL)

Introduction

Fungal infectious diseases are called *mycoses*. Since fungi are eukaryotes, they are similar to mammalian cells and contain a nucleus. Because of these similarities, treatment is more difficult than that of bacterial infections. The treatment for mycoses is amphotericin B and other antifungal azoles that act on the primary sterol of the fungi, ergosterol.

Except in the compromised host, relatively few fungi are pathogenic. Those immunocompromised patients often have invasive disease. Fungal diseases may be categorized as superficial, subcutaneous, and systemic invasive, depending on where the mycoses occurs. Mycoses are usually acquired by inhalation of specialized forms (conidia and spores), usually from the soil. Reproduction takes place in the form of yeasts, or spherules and endospores. They are then referred to as *dimorphic fungi* or *filamentous* (mycelial or hyphal).

Medically important fungi having immunologic based diagnostic tests are discussed in this chapter. It is important to note that generally, only positive serologic tests with significant titers are of value in indicating fungal diseases. When there is clinical suspicion and the titers are lower than what is considered significant, several explanations should be considered:

1. The patient's serum may have been taken too early in the primary immune response. Serial serum specimens (i.e., acute, convalescent) should be examined for significant changes.
2. A negative or low antibody titer in immunosuppressed patients cannot exclude the diagnosis of mycotic infection. In these cases antigen detection methods should be considered.

3. Assay antigens that are used may be different from those eliciting the immune response. The assay antigens used should include ones endemic to the regions involved.

Blastomycosis

Blastomycosis is caused by the spherical multinucleated yeast *Blastomyces dermatitidis* and should be considered a systemic mycosis. The mycelial form of *B. dermatitidis* is found in the soil of riverbanks around the Great Lakes and south-central United States.

CLINICAL MANIFESTATIONS

Inhalation of the fungal microconidia can cause primary pulmonary infection or hematogenously disseminated disease. The target organs are the skin (granulomas are produced), bones, testis, prostate, and epididymis. Immunocompromised patients such as AIDS patients have a greater frequency of CNS infection (about 40%).

LABORATORY DIAGNOSIS

CULTURE. Culture consists of identification of large budding yeasts on smears from culture. False negative results can occur, and culture can be very time consuming.

ANTIBODY. Detection of antibody directed against the A antigen by complement fixation (CF), immunodiffusion (ID), or EIA is fairly specific. However, EIA tests have demonstrated crossreactivity with histoplasmosis.

DELAYED HYPERSENSITIVITY SKIN TEST. Blastomycin skin test lacks sensitivity and specificity and is not extremely useful.

TREATMENT

Chronic forms of blastomycosis can be treated with itraconazole. Amphotericin B is the drug of choice for more acute infections or meningitis.

Coccidioidomycosis

Coccidioidomycosis is caused by the inhalation of *Coccidioides immitis*. The mycelial form is found in soil and semidesert areas of the United States and Mexico. Inhalation of the arthroconidia causes infection. Once inhaled, the large spherules rupture and release endospores that mature and produce more spherules.

CLINICAL MANIFESTATIONS

The endospores and spherules are the invasive forms of this fungus and produce primary pulmonary infection and hematogenously disseminated disease. There may be involvement with skin, bones, joints, and meninges. Common clinical manifestations of infection include skin lesions, ulcers, and verrucous granulomas. More acute clinical manifestations are seen in patients with AIDS.

LABORATORY DIAGNOSIS

CULTURE. Identification of endosporulating spherules on smears and histologic sections retrieved from culture is diagnostic.

SPECIFIC IMMUNOLOGIC INFECTIOUS DISEASE TESTS (FUNGAL)

ANTIBODY. Detection of antibody by ID or CF is useful in the diagnosis. Demonstration of an elevated or rising titer of greater than 1:16 with CF, along with a negative delayed hypersensitivity skin test, suggests hematogenous dissemination. Significant CF titers in CSF are considered diagnostic of coccidioidal meningitis.

DELAYED HYPERSENSITIVITY SKIN TESTS. Coccidioidin is used for the mycelial phase, and spherulin is used for the spherule phase.

TREATMENT

For immunocompromised patients with hematogenous dissemination, amphotericin B is the drug of choice. For nonmeningeal disease and maintenance therapy, the drugs of choice are ketoconazole, fluconazole, and itraconazole.

Histoplasmosis

Histoplasmosis is caused by *Histoplasma capsulatum,* an intracellular yeast found in soil in mycelial form. It is common to southeastern and central states of the United States and is also found throughout the world. Inhalation of microconidia in endemic areas causes infection.

CLINICAL MANIFESTATIONS

The predominant infections are seen in mucous membranes, adrenals, and the reticuloendothelial system. Clinical manifestations may include anemia, leukopenia, thrombocytopenia, oronasopharyngeal ulcerations, and the formation of fibrous mediastinitis. Hematogenous pneumonia and meningitis can be seen in acutely ill AIDS patients.

LABORATORY DIAGNOSIS

CULTURES. Detection of intracellular yeast on blood smears or histologic specimens, or from cultures of sputum, bone marrow, or blood, is diagnostic.

ANTIBODY. Detection of antibodies is with ID, CF, and latex particle agglutination (LPA). Titers of greater than or equal to 1:32 with LPA suggest active infection. A titer of greater than or equal to 1:32 or a fourfold titer rise with CF suggests active infection.

ANTIGEN. Radioimmunoassays (RIAs) for antigen detection in urine, serum, and CSF are experimental and not commercially available.

DELAYED HYPERSENSITIVITY SKIN TEST. Histoplasmin is used for the mycelial phase and Histolyn-CYL is used to detect the yeast phase of infection.

TREATMENT

Amphotericin B is the drug of choice, especially in acutely ill immunocompromised patients with hematogenous dissemination. Itraconazole is effective for less severe forms of disease.

Candidiasis

The *Candida* species that most often cause human infection are *Candida albicans* and *Candida tropicalis.* They generally colonize mucous membranes and not the skin. The source of infection is usually the normal flora. Disseminated infections occur in immunocompromised patients, categorizing the *Candida* species as one of the opportunistic pathogens.

CLINICAL MANIFESTATIONS

Clinical manifestations include mucosal candidiasis, characterized by laryngitis, esophagitis, vaginitis, cystitis, and thrush. Acute hematogenously disseminated candidiasis is characterized by involvement of the eyes, skin, and muscles. Chronic disseminated candidiasis is most common in patients with neutropenia.

LABORATORY DIAGNOSIS

CULTURE. Demonstration of fungi in culture is diagnostic of candidiasis.

ANTIBODY. Indirect hemagglutination and LPA tests are available, but they lack sensitivity and specificity. These are not useful with immunosuppressed patients.

ANTIGEN. LPA and EIA antigen tests are available. They are generally positive in low titer and may become positive too late in the illness for diagnostic benefits.

DELAYED HYPERSENSITIVITY SKIN TESTS. Tests may show positivity with healthy persons and are only an indication of exposure and therefore are rarely a good diagnostic indicator.

TREATMENT

Amphotericin B is the drug of choice for deep invasive infection or hematogenous dissemination. Topical imidizoles are used for thrush and vaginitis.

Aspergillosis

Species of *Aspergillus* that are most often pathogenic for humans are *Aspergillus fumigatus*, *Aspergillus flavus*, and *Aspergillus niger*. Infection is caused by inhalation of conidia. In response, a phagocytic defense is mounted that attacks the mycelia by extracellular apposition. Patients with neutropenia or neutrophil dysfunction are especially susceptible to hematogenous dissemination and respiratory tract involvement. Allergic bronchopulmonary aspergillosis (ABPA) can develop in response to inhalation of conidia or fungi.

CLINICAL MANIFESTATIONS

Clinical manifestations include invasive pulmonary infection in immunocompromised patients. Necrotizing pneumonia leading to thrombosis and infarction of the lung may also occur. Occasionally, widespread infection throughout the body may occur.

LABORATORY DIAGNOSIS

CULTURE. When blood cultures are performed they are usually negative. However, evidence of tissue invasion by histologic methods is considered diagnostic.

ANTIBODY. Precipitin tests for antibody (i.e., ID) lack sensitivity.

ANTIGEN. Galactomannan antigen detection by EIA has not proved to be of value.

DELAYED HYPERSENSITIVITY SKIN TESTS. Aspergillin antigen tests are positive in more than 90% of the patients with ABPA.

TREATMENT

Amphotericin B is the drug of choice but needs to be administered early in the disease.

Cryptococcoses

Cryptococcosis is caused by *Cryptocococcus neoformans*. The portal of entry is inhalation into the lungs. This encapsulated yeast has four serotypes (A, B, C, and D). Serotype A can be found anywhere in the world. Types B and C are most often found in subtropical areas. The cryptococcal infections most often associated with immunocompromised patients are of the serotypes A and D.

CLINICAL MANIFESTATIONS

Cryptococcal meningitis is common. The clinical manifestations include headache, optic neuritis, cranial nerve palsies, and seizures. Meningeal involvement with AIDS patients is sometimes subtle. These patients may exhibit skin lesions, usually as a direct result of hematogenous dissemination. Dissemination to the spinal column may occur, resulting in osteolytic lesions.

LABORATORY DIAGNOSIS

CULTURE. The detection on blood agar plates of mucoid appearing colonies of cryptococci is very useful for diagnosis. Rapid examination with India ink stains for capsules is also useful for presumptive identification.

ANTIBODY. IFA, EIA, and the tube agglutination assay (TA) generally lack specificity and sensitivity.

ANTIGEN. LPA and EIA for cryptococcal antigen are both sensitive and specific.

DELAYED HYPERSENSITIVITY SKIN TEST. Cryptococcal skin tests lack sensitivity and specificity.

TREATMENT

Amphotericin B is the drug of choice for therapy of cryptococcoses.

SPECIFIC IMMUNOLOGIC INFECTIOUS DISEASE TESTS *(RICKETTSIA)*

Ehrlichiosis

Ehrlichiosis is a relatively new tick borne disease caused by an obligate intracellular (leukocytic) gram negative–like bacterium of the family Rickettsiaceae. It ranges in size from 0.5 to 1.5 μm and is variable in shape but is described as a coccus. The first human case was reported in 1986; since then 360 cases have been documented by the CDC (1995), mostly in the south central and southeastern United States. There are two human forms:

1. Human monocytic ehrlichiosis (HME) caused by *Ehrlichia chaffeensis* or *Ehrlichia sennetsu*
2. A newly described human granulocytic ehrlichiosis (HGE) caused by *Ehrlichia equii* or a closely related genotype. HGE is expanding geographically because of its tick habitat and is causing concern to public health officials.

CLINICAL MANIFESTATIONS

Clinically the symptoms are similar to those of Rocky Mountain spotted fever (RMSF) but range from no symptoms to death. Ehrlichiosis has also been called Rocky Mountain *spotless* fever. Symptoms include fever, malaise, myalgia, headache, rigors, diaphoresis, nausea, vomiting, cough, arthralgias, rash, and confusion. Most studies on ehrlichiosis have been from hospitalized patients, so there tends to be a bias of clinical symptomatology toward being more severe. In fact, most cases are thought to be asymptomatic. Persistent infection after treatment is not common.

LABORATORY DIAGNOSIS

TECHNICAL NOTE   The laboratory diagnosis of *Ehrlichia* infection is somewhat problematic since most specific methods are either low yield, too late to help clinically, or high tech and not routinely available.

Normally nonspecific tests can be helpful when coupled to the clinical findings. For example, in a patient clinically suspected of having ehrlichiosis the following laboratory findings are common: leukopenia, thrombocytopenia, anemia, elevated serum aspartate aminotransferase levels, and elevated serum creatine levels (especially in HGE).

CULTURE. The gold standard is not useful in ehrlichiosis since only about three cases have ever been reported to be culture confirmed. However, direct demonstration of the organism in the blood as inclusions called *morulae* (which are vacuolar microcolonies) is a diagnostic option. This procedure is laborious and specialized. The detection of morulae is not extremely sensitive in HME (monocytic) and HGE (granulocytic) (see Chapter 27).

ANTIBODIES
EIA and IFA. Antibodies to *E. chaffeensis* and *E. equii* can be demonstrated by IFA and EIA techniques. However, there are only a few commercial sources of diagnostic kits for *Ehrlichia*. Additionally, the CDC recommends a fourfold rise in IFA for *E. chaffeensis* and *E. equii*, respectively, as an indication of seroconversion, which is too late to be of general clinical utility since treatment must start before seroconversion occurs.

Western Blot. The Western blot can be used as a confirmation of infection as individuals may respond with antibodies to a 22 to 30 kDa specific protein in HME and a 44 kDa specific protein in HGE. Again this is of limited clinical utility.

POLYMERASE CHAIN REACTION. PCR of peripheral blood leukocytes appears to be one of the best laboratory diagnostic methods for both HME and HGE. This procedure has been reported to have a sensitivity of 80% to 87% and a specificity of 100% in the acute phase. Unfortunately, only a few laboratories are able to perform *Ehrlichia* PCR.

TREATMENT

Tetracycline or doxycycline for 5 to 7 days is the treatment of choice. It should be noted that β-lactam antimicrobials and chloramphenicol are not effective. This has implications for other tick borne diseases since they are often treated with β-lactam antimicrobials.

Rocky Mountain Spotted Fever

RMSF is a disease caused by an obligate intracellular parasite called *Rickettsia rickettsii,* a gram negative bacterium of the family Rickettsiaceae. *R. rickettsii* is a human pathogen found in the United States and can be fatal if untreated, even in the immunocompetent person. The incidence of disease is dependent on the geographic location of the arthropod vectors or ticks and the amount of exposure (wooded areas, campgrounds) to these vectors. There is a high incidence in children during spring and summer. The perpetuation of the organism depends on passage between animal and insect vectors and is not dependent on human host infection, which is accidental.

CLINICAL MANIFESTATIONS

The disease typically begins with fever, severe headaches, vomiting, nausea, and myalgias. A rash develops 2 to 6 days later beginning as macules in the areas of the wrists and ankles and then appearing on the arms and legs and inward to the trunk. As the disease progresses, there is CNS and renal involvement, edema develops, and circulatory collapse can occur.

LABORATORY DIAGNOSIS

Rickettsial disease diagnosis is most often done without laboratory evidence, usually relying on the clinical and epidemiologic picture of the patient. Serologic tests are not sensitive enough and usually are unable to detect specific antibodies for rickettsiae during the acute phase of illness when medical attention is sought. Other laboratory alternatives such as DNA probes, PCR, and immunohistologic assays are not widely available.

ANTIGEN. Immunofluorescence staining of skin from patients with RMSF yields a specificity of 100% and a sensitivity of 70%. Test reagents are not yet commercially available for immunohistologic testing of rickettsioses.

ANTIBODY. The IFA is considered to be the gold standard serologic assay for rickettsioses. Except in endemic areas where higher serologic titers are required for diagnosis, IFA titers of 1:64 or greater are considered diagnostic. A fourfold increase in IFA antibody titer between acute and convalescent specimens is usually an indication of seroconversion (as in most infectious disease serologic tests). The specificity is reported to be 100%, and sensitivity ranges from 94% to 100%. A similar alternative test is the indirect immunoperoxidase antibody assay.

LATEX AGGLUTINATION AND SOLID PHASE ENZYME IMMUNOASSAY. These assays are also useful diagnostically and are inexpensive to perform.

TREATMENT

Tetracycline is the treatment of choice. Alternatives are chloramphenicol and doxycycline.

Chlamydia

Chlamydiae are obligate intracellular parasites of eukaryotic cells. The genus *Chlamydia* contains three species: *Chlamydia psittaci*, causing pneumonia infection; *Chlamydia trachomatis*, one of the most common causes of sexually transmitted disease; and *Chlamydia pneumoniae*, believed to be responsible for about 10% of community acquired pneumonias and originally thought to be a strain of *C. psittaci*.

LABORATORY DIAGNOSIS—*CHLAMYDIA TRACHOMATIS*

ANTIGEN DETECTION. Direct fluorescent antibody (DFA) assays along with EIAs exist for antigen detection of *C. trachomatis*. Their sensitivities vary from 70% to 100% depending on the test and manufacturer.

POLYMERASE CHAIN REACTION. PCR is useful for direct detection of *C. trachomatis*. Although the test is commercially available, the sensitivity range is large (64%–97%), depending on specimen type, and the test is expensive. The clinical utility of this assay needs to be determined.

DNA PROBE. This testing is available commercially for *C. trachomatis*. The sensitivity varies with the specimen samples. The specificity is typically 97% or greater.

ANTIBODY DETECTION. Antibody detection tests such as CF and microimmunofluorescence (MI) are of little use because antibody to *C. trachomatis* is present after the infection resolves, making the discrimination between recent or past infection difficult. In addition, the antibodies detected are not species specific. High titers (1:64) can be an indication of either lymphogranuloma venereum (LGV), an infection caused by *C. trachomatis*, or psittacosis.

TECHNICAL NOTE False positive tests in *C. trachomatis* infection can have adverse medical, social, or psychologic consequences. Therefore, the CDC recommends that DFA and EIA positive results be verified if a false positive result is likely to have negative consequences. Methods for verification include EIA blocking assays, probe competition assays, and culture.

LABORATORY DIAGNOSIS—*CHLAMYDIA PSITTACI*

ANTIBODY DETECTION. A fourfold or greater rise in CF titer between acute and convalescent specimens of symptomatic patients supports the diagnosis. If only a single specimen can be obtained from a symptomatic patient, a titer of 1:32 or higher would need to be obtained to demonstrate infection.

LABORATORY DIAGNOSIS—*CHLAMYDIA PNEUMONIAE*

ANTIBODY DETECTION. Serologic testing is done for diagnosing patients with *C. pneumoniae*. As with *C. psittaci*, a fourfold rise in IgG titer with acute and convalescent specimens is indicative of acute infection. IgG antibodies can be detected 6 to 8 weeks after the onset of illness, and a single IgG titer of 1:512 or greater is evidence of infection. IgM antibodies can be detected about 3 weeks after primary illness. IgM titers of 1:16 or greater by serologic MI tests are indicative of infection. IgM antibodies usually disappear after 3 to 6 months.

TREATMENT

For chlamydial infections, the treatment is usually tetracycline. For infections caused by *C. pneumoniae*, erythromycin can also be used. For those infections caused by *C. trachomatis*, tetracycline, erythromycin, ofloxacin, and sulfisoxazole are considered effective. Although effective for *C. trachomatis* infection, sulfonamides are not effective against *C. psittaci* and *C. pneumoniae*.

SPECIFIC IMMUNOLOGIC INFECTIOUS DISEASE TESTS (PARASITIC)

Introduction

Immunologic methods for the detection of parasitic disease have recently improved considerably. Assays are more sensitive and there are more characterized specific antigenic components, allowing test results to be more accurate. Although serologic methods have improved, they are limited in that they cannot distinguish between active and past infections. Therefore, serologic tests, as always, should be used in adjunct to the gold standard of demonstration of organisms in blood, tissue, stool, and body fluids. Those specific parasitic diseases that are discussed include amebiasis, babesiosis, and toxoplasmosis.

Amebiasis

The causative agent of amebiasis is the intestinal parasite *Entamoeba histolytica*. Infections caused by *E. histolytica* are often due to ingestion of food or water that is contaminated. The parasite is endemic in the United States and can also be acquired while traveling in foreign countries.

CLINICAL MANIFESTATIONS

Diseases caused by *E. histolytica* include amebic colitis, amebic dysentery, and liver abscesses. Amebic dysentery is an acute disease with symptoms of abdominal cramping and bloody diarrhea. The parasite can be invasive; in the intestinal mucosa it can cause ulcerations. Amebic liver abscess can also occur with symptoms of fever and abdominal pain. Abscesses of other organs are rare. More frequently seen in the United States is amebic colitis, with symptoms of nonbloody diarrhea and abdominal cramping.

LABORATORY DIAGNOSIS

DIRECT VISUALIZATION. The method of choice is direct visualization of trophozoites or cysts in stool.

ANTIBODY. Detection of antibody is performed by EIA and IFA.

ANTIGEN. Detection of antigen is available by EIA.

TREATMENT

Metronidazole plus iodoquinol is the treatment of choice.

Babesiosis

Babesiosis is a tick borne disease caused by the intraerythrocytic protozoan parasite of the genus *Babesia*. The first human case was described in 1957; however, there is speculation that it has been known since biblical times (possible reference in the book of Exodus). In the United States the geographic distribution is concentrated in the northeast and upper Midwest. There are over 100 species of *Babesia*, but most cases in the United States are due to *Babesia microti*. Since the tick vector *(Ixodes scapularis)* is common to *Ehrlichia* infection (HGE) and Lyme disease, coinfection with any combination of these diseases is theoretically possible.

CLINICAL MANIFESTATIONS

In most cases infection with *Babesia* is occult and self-limiting with few known sequelae. However, in compromised patients (advanced age, asplenic, or immunosuppressed) it can be a potentially life threatening hemolytic disease. Symptoms include low grade fever, malaise, fatigue, headache, rigor, nausea, vomiting, and musculoskeletal problems. Patients also exhibit jaundice, hepatomegaly, splenomegaly, hemolytic anemia, hemoglobinuria, thrombocytopenia, and increases in liver enzyme levels. Persistent infections have been reported.

LABORATORY DIAGNOSIS

The laboratory diagnosis of *Babesia* infection is certainly helped by the clinical findings and patient history. That is, it is extremely rare to find *Babesia* in patients outside the previously mentioned high risk group and without known travel to or residence in an endemic area.

CULTURE. Culture is seldom done for diagnostic purposes in *Babesia* infection since it is an intracellular parasite and inoculation of golden hamsters is used to culture it. However, the Wright-Giemsa stained peripheral blood smear and subsequent identification of the parasite is good and is the method of choice. The parasitemia ranges from 1% to 50%. A cruciate, Maltese cross tetrad form that lacks pigment is diagnostic of *B. microti*. Ring variants can be confused with *Plasmodium falciparum* (malaria); however, there is usually only one per cell. Even in difficult cases the smear is almost always positive after 2 to 4 weeks.

ANTIBODIES. Antibodies to *B. microti* can be demonstrated by IFA during or after the late acute phase. Crossreactivity is known to occur with other species and malaria. Antibody titers usually show a 10- to 20-fold rise between the acute and convalescent phases. EIA and Western blots are not commercially available. The serologic tests are of limited clinical utility since the smear is usually adequate.

SPECIFIC IMMUNOLOGIC INFECTIOUS DISEASE TESTS (PARASITIC)

POLYMERASE CHAIN REACTION. PCR of peripheral blood is more sensitive for acute disease than the smear and hamster culture, and it is equal in specificity. However, it has limited availability and is expensive.

TREATMENT

Clindamycin and quinine for 7 to 10 days is the treatment of choice. In unresponsive patients erythrocyte exchange may be required.

Toxoplasmosis

Toxoplasmosis is a disease caused by the protozoan parasite *Toxoplasma gondii*. Prevalence is worldwide in humans and domestic and wild animals. The disease causes serious complications in immunocompromised persons, such as those with AIDS. In utero toxoplasmosis may result in serious congenital infection or stillbirth. Infection in humans is by ingestion of *T. gondii* from partially cooked or uncooked meats that contain tissue cysts or by ingesting infective oocysts from material contaminated with cat feces, as from cat litter boxes. Transmission from blood transfusion is also possible.

CLINICAL MANIFESTATIONS

If fetal infection occurs early in pregnancy, death of the fetus, brain damage, hydrocephaly, fever, jaundice, splenomegaly, and convulsions at birth can occur. If fetal infection is later in pregnancy, a milder subclinical fetal disease can occur. Serologic testing is recommended for all pregnant women. With immunodeficient individuals, reactivated or primary infection may cause chorioretinitis, pneumonia, myocarditis, lymphadenopathy, cerebritis, and possibly death.

LABORATORY DIAGNOSIS

CULTURE. Routine cultures can be done but usually require long incubation. Identification in body fluid, tissues, and blood of tachyzoites or tissue cysts can be definitive. Fluorescent or immunoperoxidase stains are also quite useful.

ANTIBODY. IFA and the Sabin-Feldman dye test are the gold standards for diagnosis of toxoplasmosis, although the former is offered by only a few laboratories. EIAs are routinely used for laboratory diagnosis. IgM antibodies appear approximately 5 days after infection and can be indicative of congenital or acute infection, although caution must be used since IgM titers have been known to last for up to a year. IgM titers in the cord blood can also be useful in suspected neonates. The serologic positivity may suppressed if the patients are immunosuppressed (i.e., AIDS, transplant patients, and so forth). IgG appears 1 to 2 weeks after infection and may continue for months or years.

POLYMERASE CHAIN REACTION (PCR). Although offered by few laboratories, PCR shows high specificity and sensitivity for toxoplasmosis detection. False positives can occur if attention is not given to quality control.

TREATMENT

Pyrimethamine, along with sulfadiazine and folinic acid, are recommended treatments for toxoplasmosis.

SPECIFIC IMMUNOLOGIC INFECTIOUS DISEASE TESTS (VIRAL)

Infectious Mononucleosis

Infectious mononucleosis (IM) is a self-limiting systemic lymphoproliferative condition often occurring in early childhood and young adults and most often caused by Epstein Barr virus. EBV is a member of the herpesvirus family and often associated with Burkitt's lymphoma, nasopharyngeal carcinoma, and lymphocytic interstitial pneumonitis; infection is common in HIV infected patients. EBV is spread by contaminated saliva, with approximately 95% of the world's population being exposed. EBV infects B cells, initiating their proliferation and immortalizing them. In defense, natural killer cells and CD8 cytotoxic T lymphocytes aid in eradicating infected B cells. B cells, most likely, provide the reservoir for the virus, allowing EBV to remain latent.

CLINICAL MANIFESTATIONS

Children younger than 5 years usually demonstrate mild symptoms. Infectious mononucleosis has an incubation period of about 10 to 50 days, lasting about 1 to 4 weeks after it is fully developed. Pharyngitis, lymphadenopathy, extreme fatigue, and malaise are common in adolescents. Hepatitis is common, occasionally seen with jaundice, hepatomegaly, and splenomegaly.

LABORATORY DIAGNOSIS

Diagnosis of EBV in the laboratory is usually done by identification of atypical lymphocytes in the peripheral blood, along with a heterophile screening test. IgM and IgG anti–viral capsid antigen (VCA) titers are also occasionally useful. The serologic profile and culture technique are discussed later.

CULTURE. EBV can be cultured in lymphoblastoid cell lines. This testing is not timely and is impractical because it does not differentiate between primary and reactivated infections.

ANTIBODY DETECTION.
- *Heterophile antibodies* are highly specific but lack sensitivity: 85% to 90% detectable in adults and as low as 10% to 40% detectable in confirmed cases in children.
- *IFAs* are EBV specific assays using lymphoma cells expressing VCAs. Fluorescent antibody methods to detect antibodies to VCAs are commercially available when negative heterophile results are obtained in suspected cases of IM.
- *EIAs* are available for:
  Viral capsid antibody (IgG and IgM). VCA-IgM can be useful except that (1) false negatives are seen due to high titer IgG competitive binding, and (2) VCA-IgM is not always demonstrated in secondary reactivation. VCA-IgG titers rise early in infection and remain at high levels indefinitely, making it difficult to detect a fourfold rising titer.
  Early antigen (EA) antibodies. IgG to the EA is formed early in acute infection, demonstrating a fourfold rising titer.
  Epstein-Barr nuclear antigen (EBNA) antibodies. IgG does not appear until a patient enters the convalescent period. Note that immunocompromised patients

may not demonstrate EBNA antibodies, even when demonstrating VCA antibodies.

TREATMENT

Therapy is supportive and based on symptoms. Acyclovir offers no clinical benefits even though EBV is sensitive to acyclovir in vitro.

Cytomegalovirus

Cytomegalovirus (CMV) is a member of the herpesvirus family, including the human pathogens herpes simplex I and II, varicella-zoster virus, and EBV. One of the common characteristics CMV shares with these viruses is its ability to produce subclinical infections that are latent and then reactivated. The seroprevalence of CMV antibodies varies from 40% to 100% in healthy adults, depending on socioeconomic status.

CLINICAL MANIFESTATIONS

CONGENITAL INFECTION. In congenital CMV infection, 5% to 10% of infants infected during the perinatal period exhibit signs of severe infection with liver and CNS involvement. Convulsions, jaundice purpura, chorioretinitis, and intercerebral calcifications can occur in varied degrees. Death may occur in utero, and those who survive suffer mental retardation, motor disabilities, and chronic liver disease. Fetal infection can occur during primary or reactivated maternal infections, the former being at higher risk for greater severity of disease.

ADULT INFECTION. Those infections acquired later in life are usually subclinical and also include mononucleosis. In fact, CMV causes up to 10% of all cases of mononucleosis. Serious manifestations with immunoincompetent patients, such as AIDS patients are pneumonitis, chorioretinitis, gastrointestinal tract disorders, and hepatitis. Those immunosuppressed patients who are seronegative for CMV are at greater risk of developing CMV infection. CMV is a common post-transplantation infection. Seronegative patients who receive tissue from a seropositive donor are at greatest risk of mortality.

LABORATORY DIAGNOSIS

After initial infection, IgM antibodies are produced, last about 3 to 4 months, and generally do not appear with reactivation. IgG antibodies will also appear after initial infection and persist indefinitely.

CULTURE. Viral culture is the gold standard for confirming CMV infection. Isolation of CMV from amniotic fluid, cord blood, fetal tissues, and neonatal blood is diagnostic for congenital infection. Anti-CMV IgM antibodies detected in utero or at delivery are also indicative of congenital infection.

ANTIGEN DETECTION
- *Direct electron microscopy* for virus detection in urine is reliable when positive, but one cannot rule out CMV with negative results.
- *Direct fluorescent antibody* can detect early CMV in viral cultures and bronchoalveolar lavage specimens.

ANTIBODY DETECTION. EIA for detection of IgG (immune status and exposure) and IgM (acute infection) is the method of choice. LPA and indirect hemagglutination are often done for screening seronegative patients to be transplantation donors.

DNA PROBES. DNA probes for CMV detection are being developed.

IN SITU HYBRIDIZATION AND POLYMERASE CHAIN REACTION. These assays promise to be more sensitive than Northern blot assays and can be used for early CMV expression. When available, they will detect CMV DNA in peripheral blood.

Rubella

Rubella (German measles) is caused by an RNA virus of the togavirus family. This disease is highly contagious and is spread through respiratory secretions. Rubella infection is usually a self-limiting disease, with occasional complications in children and adults. Immunization against rubella virus has prevented the epidemics that once existed. Rubella can be devastating to fetuses, especially in the first trimester of the pregnancy. For this reason it is important to determine immune status and identify exposure to rubella virus in pregnant women.

CLINICAL MANIFESTATIONS

The incubation period for acquired rubella is generally 10 to 21 days. Adults experience low grade fever; malaise; headache; and involvement of the posterior, cervical, and occipital lymph nodes; with maculopapular rash in about 50% of the cases. Children exhibit a transient rash and mild fever. Exposure of the fetus during the first trimester can produce severe ocular and brain damage. Congenitally infected newborns may excrete virus for many months.

LABORATORY DIAGNOSIS

CULTURE. Tissue culture is very time consuming and not usually done by commercial laboratories.

ANTIBODY. EIAs for IgM antibodies as an indication of current infection, and IgG antibodies for immune status, are commonly done.

Viral Hepatitis

Viral hepatitis is the inflammation of the liver caused by the specific viruses hepatitis A (HAV), hepatitis B (HBV), hepatitis D (HDV), and hepatitis E (HEV). The hepatobiliary disease caused by these viruses can range from asymptomatic infections to fulminant life threatening infections. Diagnosis depends on the detection of antibodies and/or the presence of specific viral antigens.

CLINICAL MANIFESTATIONS

▌ *Hepatitis A* is caused by a small RNA picornavirus. The virus has a worldwide distribution and causes both epidemic and sporadic infection. HAV's incubation period is 7 to 42 days. The infection is usually acute and self-limiting. Symptoms may include nausea, vomiting, abdominal pain, dark urine, and fatigue. In severe disease massive liver damage can occur. Viral transmission is via the fecal-oral route, and it has no carrier state. No vaccine is presently available.

▮ *Hepatitis B* is caused by a double stranded DNA virus and is a member of the hepadena family. The virus consists of a central core (hepatitis B core antigen [HB Ag] and hepatitis B early antigen [HB Ag]), double stranded DNA, and DNA polymerase, the latter being responsible for viral replication. The core is surrounded by a protein capsid (hepatitis B surface antigen [HB Ag]). The virus also has a worldwide distribution, with hepatitis B infections being a leading cause of liver carcinoma worldwide. The incubation period is 30 to 180 days. The clinical outcome of hepatitis B is highly variable. As many as 50% of the patients are asymptomatic or exhibit a mild nonspecific viral-like illness. Viral transmission is percutaneous, transmucosal, and transplacental.

▮ *Hepatitis C* (also previously known as non-A, non-B) is a small lipid envelope enclosed single stranded RNA virus. It is related to the flaviviruses and has a worldwide distribution with an estimated 100,000,000 carriers. The majority of cases are asymptomatic; however, when symptoms occur chronic hepatitis is common. As with HBV there is considerable risk for progression to serious hepatobilary disease, including cirrhosis and liver carcinoma. Transmission is by exposure to blood or blood products, and the frequency of HCV in unscreened blood or blood products is 0.3% to 1.5%. Health care workers, intravenous drug abusers, and patients receiving blood products are at risk. Placental transmission is not known to occur.

▮ *Hepatitis D* virus contains circular RNA. It requires HB Ag in order to replicate and therefore requires coinfection with HBV. The mode of transmission is parenteral, and in endemic areas it is associated with high mortality epidemics. The clinical symptoms are similar to those of HBV.

▮ *Hepatitis E* (also previously known as non-A, non-B) is a 32 nm spherical nonenveloped RNA virus. This virus is restricted to developing countries and is not worldwide in distribution. The clinical manifestations include acute hepatitis that is generally self-limiting. However, fulminate cases can occur and have a 20% to 40% mortality rate in pregnant women.

LABORATORY DIAGNOSIS

The clinical manifestations of the different viral hepatitis infections are similar and are often indistinguishable from one another. Therefore, the diagnosis often depends on the detection of specific antibodies produced in response to exposure and infection by each particular virus and by detection of viral specific antigens. These serologic markers are not only useful in making a definitive diagnosis but also in helping to define the progression of the infection.

HEPATITIS A VIRUS. Detection of IgM antibodies to HAV indicates subclinical or acute disease. However, detection of IgG to HAV may indicate convalescent or immune status (see "Diagnostic Tests and Methodologies" on p 370).

HEPATITIS B VIRUS. The laboratory diagnosis of HBV is much more complex and consists of many antibody and antigen detection methods (see "Diagnostic Tests and Methodologies" on p 338. The time frame for the appearance of these antigens and the corresponding antibodies over the course of infection is best described in the form of a graph (see "Viral Markers in Hepatitis B Infection" on p 363).

HEPATITIS C VIRUS. Antibodies to HCV and elevated alanine aminotransferase (ALT) levels are the primary tests used to diagnose HCV. However, the time for seroconversion is generally 3 to 6 months in transfusion acquired infection and 6 to 9 months in non–transfusion related cases. The detection of HCV RNA by PCR has been used to monitor therapy. More recently, quantitative HCV RNA measurement by PCR (viral load studies) has been used in the management of these patients and may predict response to therapy (see "Diagnostic Tests and Methodologies" on p 370).

HEPATITIS D VIRUS. HDV only occurs with coinfection with HBV; therefore, it should only be considered in HBV cases. It can be demonstrated by the detection of the HDAg or by the detection of antibodies to this antigen (see "Diagnostic Tests and Methodologies" on p 370).

HEPATITIS E VIRUS. Antibodies to HEV are used to obtain laboratory evidence for HEV infection. PCR has also been used but is still considered a research tool (see "Diagnostic Tests and Methodologies" on p 370).

Viral Markers in Hepatitis B Infection

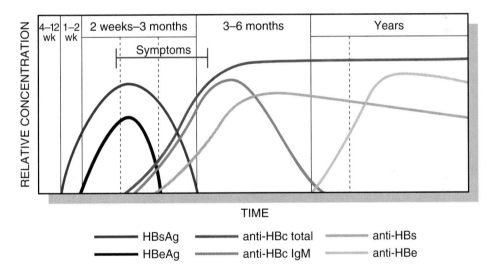

TREATMENT

In general, the treatment for hepatitis is supportive. However, in severe cases, treatment with interferon alpha has been used with some beneficial effect.

Human Immunodeficiency Virus

AIDS is the most common secondary immunodeficiency known. As of 1994 over 17 million individuals have been infected, with an estimated 6000 new cases occurring daily. AIDS is the leading cause of death in adolescents and in the 25 to 44 year old age group. Although the most severe manifestation of this disease is its profound effect on the immune system, this effect is secondary to infection with HIV. Therefore, it would be considered a secondary immunodeficiency.

CLINICAL MANIFESTATIONS

The clinical manifestations of HIV infection vary considerably depending on the stage of the disease (early versus late) and the genetic makeup of the individual infected. After the primary infection, there is a relatively asymptomatic period during which significant immune system damage occurs primarily in the lymph nodes. The patient then progresses to a more symptomatic stage that eventually leads to classic AIDS with its associated opportunistic infections and malignancies. There is evidence that asymptomatic carriers or resistant individuals exist, and this is one avenue that researchers are hoping will lead to knowledge of how to control the disease. The first clinical symptoms in HIV patients is usually fever, night sweats, lymphadenopathy, and fatigue. This is generally followed by extreme weight loss, diarrhea, opportunistic infections, and malignancies (Kaposi's sarcoma and lymphoma). The most common infection in HIV is *Pneumocystis carinii* pneumonia; however, toxoplasmosis, atypical and rare tuberculosis, cryptosporidiosis, and fungal, bacterial, and concomitant viral infections also occur. As in most immunodeficiencies, infections are the leading cause of death in AIDS. The pathogenesis is essentially related to the cytopathic effects of HIV on the various cells that it infects. The main target for HIV is the T helper cell. HIV undergoes rapid viral replication in these cells, which results in cell death shortly after infection. Under certain conditions a chronic viral infection may also be established, but the exact mechanism for this is not clear. It has been postulated that B cells and macrophages that also can become infected may play a role in chronic infection.

LABORATORY DIAGNOSIS

The actual laboratory diagnosis of HIV infection is usually not complicated and is straightforward. However, the testing is so highly regulated that it can become complex and laborious because of the shear regulatory requirements regarding testing procedures and confidentiality issues.

ANTIBODIES. The primary screening test for HIV is the determination of HIV directed antibodies, usually by EIA. A positive EIA must be confirmed by a Western blot to eliminate false positives and the associated sociologic ramifications. Serologic diagnosis of HIV infected infants presents a diagnostic problem not dissimilar to that other infectious diseases transmitted in utero. IgG assays on the newborn are inaccurate because of placental transfer of HIV specific maternal IgG, which may interfere for up to 18 months. IgA and IgM HIV assays have had problems with sensitivity. Many ancillary tests are performed in HIV positive individuals.

FLOW CYTOMETRY (T CELL SUBSETS CD4/8). Since the primary HIV target is the T helper cell (CD4), there is usually a marked reduction in the percentage and absolute numbers of T helper cells. This usually results in the classic inversion of the T helper to T cytotoxic (CD8) cell ratio and a decrease in the absolute lymphocyte count. In fact, this is so characteristic that CD4 T helper cell counts below $200/mm^3$ are considered a diagnostic test for HIV and subject to the same regulations as HIV antibody testing. Early in the disease the number and percentage of CD8 T cytotoxic cells may actually increase. All of the immune system functions and numbers (including the T cytotoxic cells) eventually deteriorate as the disease progresses. Although immunoglobulin levels are frequently elevated early on due to a polyclonal B cell activation, later in the disease these levels also deteriorate.

CELLULAR IMMUNE FUNCTION TESTS. The cellular immune function tests (antigen and mitogen proliferation studies) are decreased as the disease progresses.

ANTIGEN DETECTION. The newer technologies are proving themselves to be useful both in the diagnosis of difficult cases and for prognostic purposes. These include determinations of P24 antigenemia, PCR amplification of HIV DNA and/or mRNA, and viral culture studies.

PROGNOSTIC TESTS. For prognostic purposes only, a few adjuvant specific and nonspecific tests have been employed with the CD4 absolute counts. Until recently these were limited to p24 antigenemia, serum β_2-microglobulin determinations, or neopterin measurement. It has now been shown that the plasma viral load (viremia) by a quantitative branched DNA signal amplification assay is a better predictor for progression to AIDS and death than the absolute CD4 counts. This is not to say that CD4 counts are not still important as they still do provide important information to the clinician.

TREATMENT

Treatment for HIV and the induced immunodeficiency is still experimental with many clinical trials under way. Unfortunately, despite all the research and experimental protocols an effective treatment that significantly alters the long term disease progression has not been found. The sensitive quantitative viral load assays that can detect less than 500 molecules per milliliter should be a tremendous help in the evaluation of new therapies and vaccine development.

Human T Cell Leukemia Virus Types I and II

Human T cell leukemia virus types I and II (HTLV-I and HTLV-II) are type C retroviruses of the oncovirus subfamily. The distribution of HTLV-I infection is worldwide, with endemic areas including central Africa, southwestern Japan, the Caribbean basin, and southeastern United States. The HTLV-I virus is spread through infected blood, from mother to infant, through the mother's milk, and through sexual contact.

CLINICAL MANIFESTATIONS

These viruses target T lymphocytes, transforming and immortalizing them. Both HTLV-I and HTLV-II have been linked to T cell malignancies. HTLV-I has been linked to adult T cell leukemia and tropical spastic paraparesis. The HTLV-II retrovirus has been associated to unusual T cell malignancies in humans. Symptoms may be only flulike syndromes. With the more progressive leukemia there can be involvement of skin, lymph nodes, blood, and bone marrow. Life expectancy for the acute form is less than 1 year, and 1 to 2 years for the chronic form. HTLV-II is seen with intravenous drug users.

LABORATORY DIAGNOSIS

ANTIBODY. EIA, particle agglutination, and immunoblotting for the detection of antibodies to HTLV-I and HTLV-II are commercially available. Detection of antibodies is not diagnostic of leukemia or the neurologic disorder and does not mean the patient will develop these conditions.

PCR. PCR is not routinely available in general diagnostic laboratories.

TREATMENT

Treatment is experimental.

SPECIFIC IMMUNOLOGIC INFECTIOUS DISEASE TESTS (VIRAL)

SPECIMEN COLLECTION, STORAGE, AND REFERENCE RANGE

TEST	SPECIMEN REQUIREMENT	SPECIMEN STORAGE (°C)	REFERENCE RANGES
Infectious Disease (Fungal)			
Aspergillosis Antibodies Complement fixation (CF)	CSF Serum; minimum fast of 4 hr	4 4	None detected Titers <1:8
Immunodiffusion (ID)	Serum; minimum fast of 4 hr	4	Negative
Coccidioidomycosis CF	CSF Serum	4 4	None detected Titers <1:2
ID	Serum	4	Negative
Histoplasmosis CF yeast	Serum	4	Titers <1:8
CF histoplasmin	Serum	4	Titers <1:8
ID	Serum	4	Negative
Blastomycosis CF	Serum	4	Titers <1:8
ID	Serum	4	Negative
Cryptococcosis Latex agglutination (LA)	Serum	4	Negative
Infectious Disease (Parasitic)			
Amebiasis Indirect immunofluorescent antibody (IFA)	Serum	4	Titers <1:8
Toxoplasmosis SEROLOGIC TESTS: Enzyme immunoassay (EIA)	Serum	4	IgG = positive or negative, dependent on exposure IgM = no antibody detected
IFA	Serum	4	ADULT: IgG < 1:64 IgM <1:1024 NEONATE: IgM undetectable

Continued ▶

► Continued **SPECIMEN COLLECTION, STORAGE, AND REFERENCE RANGE**

TEST	SPECIMEN REQUIREMENT	SPECIMEN STORAGE (°C)	REFERENCE RANGES
Infectious Disease (Viral)			
Cytomegalovirus SEROLOGIC TESTS:			
IgG by EIA	Serum	4	IgG = positive or negative, dependent on exposure*
IgM by EIA	Serum	4	IgM = negative
IFA	Serum	4	IgG <1:16, for those exposed* IgM <1:8*
Rubella EIA:	Serum	4	
IgG antibody			IgG antibody = positive or negative, dependent on exposure
IgM antibody			IgM antibody = no antibody detected
Hepatitis A IgM: EIA and radioimmunoassay (RIA)	Serum	4	IgM = negative
IgG: EIA and RIA	Serum	4	IgG = positive, recent or prior exposure; negative if not exposed
Hepatitis B (HBV) Anticore antibody, total (anti-HB$_c$): EIA and RIA	Serum	4	Negative
Anticore antibody, IgM (anti-HBc): EIA and RIA	Serum	4	IgM = negative
Surface/Antigen (HB$_s$Ag): EIA and RIA			Negative
Antisurface (HB$_s$Ag) antibody: EIA and RIA			Negative
HB$_e$Ag: EIA and RIA			Negative
Anti-HBeAg: EIA and RIA	Serum	4	Negative
Hepatitis C (HCV) Anti-HCV: EIA and RIA	Serum	4	Negative
HCV RNA: PCR methodology			Negative
Hepatitis D (HDV) Anti-HDV: EIA and RIA	Serum	4	Negative
HDAg: EIA and RIA			Negative

Continued ►

SPECIMEN COLLECTION, STORAGE, AND REFERENCE RANGE

▶ Continued **SPECIMEN COLLECTION, STORAGE,
AND REFERENCE RANGE**

TEST	SPECIMEN REQUIREMENT	SPECIMEN STORAGE (°C)	REFERENCE RANGES
Infectious Disease (Viral)			
Hepatitis E (HEV) Viral RNA: PCR	Serum	4	Negative
Anti-HEV: EIA and RIA			Negative
Human Immunodeficiency Virus (HIV) EIA	Serum	4	Negative
Western blot			Negative
Quantitative branched DNA signal amplification by PCR			Negative
Human T-Cell Leukemia Virus (HTLV-I) EIA	Serum	4	Negative
Human T-Cell Leukemia Virus (HTLV-II) EIA	Serum	4	Negative
Infectious Disease (Bacterial)			
Syphilis VDRL (Venereal Disease Research Lab)	Serum CSF	4	Nonreactive Nonreactive
Rapid plasma reagin (RPR)	Serum		Nonreactive
Fluorescent treponemal antibody absorption (FTA)	Serum		Nonreactive
Lyme Borreliosis EIA	Serum CSF	4	Negative Negative
Western blot	Serum CSF		Negative Negative
Chlamydia CF	Serum; 4 hr fasting required	4	Titers <1:8
IFA	Serum		IgG: titers <1:16 IgA: titers <1:16 IgM: titers <1:10
Rickettsia (Rocky Mountain Spotted Fever) IFA	Serum	4	IgG: titer <1:64 IgM: titer <1:64

Continued ▶

▶ Continued **SPECIMEN COLLECTION, STORAGE, AND REFERENCE RANGE**

TEST	SPECIMEN REQUIREMENT	SPECIMEN STORAGE (°C)	REFERENCE RANGES
Infectious Disease (Bacterial)			
Erhlichiosis EIA, IFA, Western blot	Serum	4	IgG = negative or positive depending on exposure IgM = negative
Streptococcal Streptozyme slide agglutination	Serum	4	Negative
Anti-streptolysin O (ASO)			Titer <200 IU/mL
Anti–DNase			Pre–school age: titer <1:64 School age: titer <1:192 Adult: titer <1:96
Staphylococcal Teichoic acid antibody	Serum	4	Negative: titer <1:3

DIAGNOSTIC TESTS AND METHODOLOGIES

TEST	METHOD	INTERFERENCE	COMMENTS
		Infectious Disease (Fungal)	
Aspergillosis Serologic tests	Complement fixation (CF)	Nonfasting specimens may cause method interference. Falsely elevated titers may occur from recent skin testing with fungal antigens.	Titers of >1:8 suggest infection. CF has lower sensitivity than immunodiffusion. Fourfold rise or greater in titer between acute and convalescent specimens is indicative of infection. Culture for identification in addition to significantly elevated serologic titers may indicate infection. Negative test does not exclude aspergillosis.
	Immunodiffusion (ID)		One or more precipitin bands suggest infection. Negative test does not exclude aspergillosis.
Delayed Hypersensitivity Skin Test (DHST)	Intradermal injection with aspergillin antigen		>90% of patients with allergic bronchopulmonary aspergillosis are found to have positive tests. Induration of 5 mm or more in diameter is considered positive reaction. Test does not distinguish between past and present infection.
Coccidioidomycosis Serologic test	CF	Same as above	Titers of >1:16 suggest infection. Paired sera for detecting rising titers (2–3 wk apart), is recommended. Negative test does not exclude coccidioidomycosis.
	ID		Generally used as screening test. CF test used for confirmatory test. Negative test does not exclude coccidioidomycosis.
DHST	Intradermal injection with coccidioidin (mycelial phase) spherulin (spherulin phase)		Negative skin test (coccidioidin, spherulin) can suggest hematogenous dissemination if accompanied by high titer in complement fixation test.

Continued ▶

▶ Continued **DIAGNOSTIC TESTS AND METHODOLOGIES**

TEST	METHOD	INTERFERENCE	COMMENTS
		Infectious Disease (Fungal)	
Histoplasmosis Serologic tests	CF	Falsely elevated titers may occur from recent skin testing with fungal antigens.	CF antibody titers with fourfold titer or titers of ≥1:32 suggest active infection.
	ID		ID antibody "h" band suggests active infection.
	Latex particle agglutination (LPA)		LPA antibody titer ≥1:32 suggests active infection. Positive LA tests should be confirmed with CF or ID to rule out false positive results.
DHST	Intradermal injection with histoplasmin (mycelial phase) Hystolyn-CYL (yeast phase)		Positive histoplasmin skin tests can falsely elevate CF antibody titers.
Blastomycosis Serologic tests	CF	Falsely elevated titers may occur from recent skin testing with fungal antigens.	Titer of 1:8 to 1:16 suggests infection. Paired sera for detecting rising titers (2–3 wk apart), are recommended.
	ID		ID antibody to A antigen is highly specific.
Cryptococcosis Serologic tests	Indirect fluorescent antibody (IFA)	Presence of rheumatoid factor may cause false positive reaction.	Cryptococcal antibody tests lack sensitivity and specificity.
	Tube agglutination (TA)		
	LPA antigen		LPA and EIA tests or cryptococcal antigen is highly sensitive and specific. Patients with cryptococcal meningoencephalitis demonstrate capsular antigen in CSF, about 90%.
	Enzyme immunoassay (EIA) antigen		

Continued ▶

DIAGNOSTIC TESTS AND METHODOLOGIES

► Continued **DIAGNOSTIC TESTS AND METHODOLOGIES**

TEST	METHOD	INTERFERENCE	COMMENTS
Infectious Disease (Parasitic)			
Amebiasis Serologic tests	Indirect hemagglutination (IHA)		IHA test is used to support diagnosis of systemic amebiasis, caused by *Entamoeba histolytica*. ID and CF assays are also available. Titers of 1:256 to 1:512 indicate old or new infection. Titers may persist for up to 2 yr after curative treatment.
Toxoplasmosis Serologic tests	EIA		EIAs are routinely used for laboratory diagnosis. IgM antibodies appear approximately 5 days after infection and can be indicative of congenital or acute infection. Caution must be used because IgM titers have been known to last for up to 1 year. IgG titers may not be detectable very early in course of infection. IgM usually appears 1–2 wk after infection and may continue for months to years.
Infectious Disease (Viral)			
Cytomegalovirus Serologic tests	EIA and IFA		EIA and IFA are used to demonstrate IgG and IgM antibodies. Detection of CMV IgG antibodies indicates immune status and exposure. Detection of IgM antibodies indicates current infection.
Rubella	EIA		IgG antibody detection is generally used to determine immune status. IgM antibody detection is recommended for diagnosis of acute infection only.
Hepatitis A (HAV)	IgM: EIA and radioimmunoassay (RIA)		IgM assays detect acute and subclinical cases. It does not determine immune status to HAV.
	IgG: EIA and RIA		IgG assays are used to determine immune status.
Hepatitis B (HBV)	Anticore antibody, total (anti-HB$_c$): EIA and RIA		Anticore antibodies are not always associated with recovery or immunity. Lifelong persistence of antibody occurs.
	Anticore antibody, IgM (anti-HB$_c$): EIA and RIA		IgM antibodies are present during the acute phase and remain positive for 6 months.
	HDAg: EIA and RIA		Can detect HDAg antigens.

Continued ▶

▶ Continued **DIAGNOSTIC TESTS AND METHODOLOGIES**

TEST	METHOD	INTERFERENCE	COMMENTS
		Infectious Disease (Viral)	
Hepatitis E (HEV)	Viral RNA: PCR		Research use only. Can detect viral product in acute infection.
	Anti-HEV: EIA and RIA		Assay used to determine immune status. Useful in screening pregnant women in endemic regions.
Human Immunodeficiency Virus (HIV)	EIA		Primary screening test for HIV is determination of HIV directed antibodies usually performed by EIA.
	Quantitative branched DNA signal amplification		Plasma viral load (viremia) by quantitative branched DNA signal amplification is better predictor for progression to AIDS and death than absolute CD4 counts.
Human T cell Leukemia Virus (HTLV-I)	EIA	None found	Detection of antibodies is not diagnostic for leukemia or neurologic disorder.
	Surface antigen (HB$_s$Ag): EIA and RIA		HBV surface antigen is first marker detectable during incubation period and peaks during acute phase.
	Antisurface (HB$_s$Ag) antibody: EIA and RIA		Convalescent antibody indicates resolution and immunity.
	HB$_e$Ag: EIA and RIA		Short lived core protein whose detection indicates HBV DNA presence or replication and higher infectivity.
	Anti-HB$_e$Ag: EIA and RIA		Indicates infection resolution and precedes anti-HB$_s$.
Hepatitis C (HCV)	Anti-HCV: EIA and RIA		Useful in determining chronic infections. Assays are varible in antigens used; however, specific assays are available.
	HCV RNA: PCR methodology		Research use only. Can detect viral product in acute infection. May be useful in monitoring treatment.
Hepatitis D (HDV)	Anti-HDV: EIA and RIA		Used to detect antibodies in HDV and demonstrate infection.

Continued ▶

► Continued **DIAGNOSTIC TESTS AND METHODOLOGIES**

TEST	METHOD	INTERFERENCE	COMMENTS
		Infectious Disease (Bacterial)	
Syphilis Rapid Plasma Reagin (RPR) Screening test	Flocculation	Hemolyzed specimens should not be used. False positives can be caused by infectious and noninfectious diseases and conditions (e.g., measles, mononucleosis, leptospirosis, malaria, autoimmune disorders, pregnancy, and drug addiction).	Reactive tests results should be confirmed by FTA-ABS or MHA-TP test. Quantitative RPR test is primarily used in monitoring therapy of primary and secondary syphilis. Tertiary syphilis patients revert to being nonreactive, with or without treatment.
VDRL (Venereal Disease Research Lab) test	Flocculation	Biologic false positive results may occur as with the RPR. See RPR test, serum, above.	Positive test results should be confirmed by FTA-ABS or MHA-TP test. VDRL test is primarily used as screening test in suspected cases of primary or secondary syphilis. VDRL test is used for testing CSF specimens.
Fluorescent Treponemal Antibody Absorption (FTA-ABS)	Fluorescent antibody absorption test	Hemolyzed specimens should not be used.	FTA-ABS test is a treponemal test used to confirm reactive nontreponemal procedures. Positive FTA-ABS almost always remains positive, so not recommended for monitoring therapy. This test should be used if tertiary syphilis is suspected and nonreactive RPR is obtained.
Microhemagglutination *Treponema pallidium* (MHA-TP)	Hemagglutination test	False positive results may occur in patients with infectious mononucleosis, and connective tissue disease.	MHA-TP test is treponemal test used to confirm reactive nontreponemal procedures. This test should not be used as screening test.
Lyme Borreliosis	EIA, WB		
Chlamydia	CF, IFA	None found	
Rickettsia (Rocky Mountain Spotted Fever)	IFA	None found	

Continued ▶

▶ Continued **DIAGNOSTIC TESTS AND METHODOLOGIES**

TEST	METHOD	INTERFERENCE	COMMENTS
Infectious Disease (Bacterial)			
Erhlichiosis	EIA, IFA, WB	None found	FDA has not approved assay. Centers for Disease Control and Prevention recommends fourfold rise in IFA for *E. chaffeenis* and *E. equii*. Western blot can be used as confirmatory test.
Streptococcal Streptozyme	Slide agglutination		This test is not specific marker for group A streptococcal infection. Primarily used to exclude prior infection.
Anti-Streptolysin O (ASO)	Nephelometry		Carrier status is indicated in patients with positive streptococci group A culture having negative test result.
Anti-DNase (streptococcal)	Inhibition of DNA hydrolysis		Titers peak in 4–6 wk. Rising titers document exposure to group A streptococci, especially in pyoderma.
Staphylococcal Teichoic Acid	ID	None found	Titers of 1:3 are considered weak response. Titers ≥1:6 indicate staphylococcal infection.

Test method explanations: CF, assay for detection on antigen-antibody reaction using complement fixation; RIA, a category of immunologic techniques using radioactive isotopes for detection of antigens and antibodies; TA, tube agglutination test; IHA, indirect hemagglutination; PCR, polymerase chain reaction; LPA, latex agglutination reaction using latex particles; Nephelometry, Method of quantitating proteins by measuring turbidity or cloudiness in a suspension or a solution; IFA, fluorescent tagged antibody reacts with antigen. Antigen-antibody complex is visible as microscopic fluorescence by ultraviolet light; EIA, use of a conjugated enzyme to a known antigen or antibody for quantification of antigen or antibody; ID, detects reaction of antigen and antibody by precipitation reaction; Bioassay, a category of techniques involving in vivo cell lines; WB, Western blot technique detects specific proteins within a complex after separation by gel electrophoresis.

BIBLIOGRAPHY

Bakken JS, Krueth J, Wilson-Nordskog C, et al: Clinical and laboratory characteristics of human granulocytic ehrlichiosis. JAMA 275(3):199–205, 1996.

Bianco C: Hepatitis testing. Immunol Invest 24(1–2):155–61, 1995.

Clementi M, Menzo S, Manzin A, Bagnarelli P: Quantitative molecular methods in virology. Arch Virol 140(9):1523–1539, 1995.

Czaja AJ, Carpenter HA, Santrach PJ, Moore SB: Immunologic features and HLA associations in chronic viral hepatitis. Gastroenterology 108(1):157–164, 1995.

Golightly MG: Laboratory considerations in the diagnosis and management of Lyme borreliosis. Am J Clin Pathol 99(2):168–174, 1993.

Hopfer RL: Use of molecular biological techniques in the diagnostic laboratory for detecting and differentiating fungi. Arch Med Res 26(3):287–292, 1995.

Jensen HE, Schonheyder HC, Hotchi M, Kaufman L: Diagnosis of systemic mycoses by specific immunohistochemical tests. APMIS 104(4):241–258, 1996.

Kaell AT, Redecha PR, Elkon KB, et al: Occurrence of antibodies to *Borrelia burgdorferi* in patients with nonspirochetal subacute bacterial endocarditis. Ann Intern Med 119(11):1079–1083, 1993.

Katzenstein DA, Holodniy M: HIV viral load quantification, HIV resistance, and antiretroviral therapy. AIDS Clin Rev 277–303, 1995–1996.

Larsen SA, Steiner BM, Rudolph AH: Laboratory diagnosis and interpretation of tests for syphilis. Clin Microbiol Rev 8(1):1–21, 1995.

Magnarelli LA, Stafford KC 3rd, Mather TN, et al: Hemocytic rickettsia-like organisms in ticks: serologic reactivity with antisera to Ehrlichiae and detection of DNA of agent of human granulocytic ehrlichiosis by PCR. J Clin Microbiol 33(10):2710–2714, 1995.

Nandwani R, Evans DT: Are you sure it's syphilis? A review of false positive serology. Int J STD and AIDS 6(4):241–248, 1995.

Neuschwander-Tetri BA: Common blood tests for liver disease. Which ones are most useful? Postgrad Med 98(1):49–63, 1995.

Nuwayhid NF: Laboratory tests for detection of human immunodeficiency virus type 1 infection. Clin Diagnos Lab Immunol 2(6):637–645, 1995.

Tomee JF, van der Werf TS, Latge JP, et al: Serologic monitoring of disease and treatment in a patient with pulmonary aspergilloma. Am J Respir Crit Care Med 151(1):199–204, 1995.

Yang G, Vyas GN: Immunodiagnosis of viral hepatitides A to E and non-A to -E. Clin Diagn Lab Immunol 3(3):247–256, 1996.

Chapter **22**

TRANSPLANTATION IMMUNOLOGY

Candace Breen, BS, MLT (ASCP)
Marc Golightly, PhD

Q U I C K   C O N T E N T S

INTRODUCTION

The beginning of transplantation immunology started in 1911 when Lexner recognized that skin could not be successfully transplanted from one individual to another. By the early 1950s the knowledge of immunology had become sufficient that there was a theoretic basis for clinical transplantation. The first successful renal transplantation was performed in 1954. Since that time great advances have been made in surgical techniques, donor-recipient tissue typing, and circumventing and/or appropriately suppressing the immune system. Clinical transplantation in many cases is no longer experimental but a recognized effective treatment modality for organ failure and genetic diseases as well as cancer. Although kidney transplantation is the most established organ transplantation being performed, heart, liver, lung, pancreas, and bone marrow transplantation are now also common. A discussion of the specific diseases leading to organ transplantation is beyond the scope of this chapter. There are texts and journals devoted entirely to this subject, and the interested reader is referred to these references.

LABORATORY DIAGNOSIS

This chapter examines the testing and testing schemes that are done before and after the transplantation (see "Assessment of Histocompatibility Testing for Transplantation," p 378). It should be realized that most testing for transplantation immunology is controlled and dictated by the transplantation service. In most cases, there is a specific transplantation laboratory where the testing is performed and few tests (except for routine serologic tests) are performed by the general laboratory.

Assessment of Histocompatibility Testing for Transplantation

PATIENT PRELIMINARY TESTING INCLUDES

- Human leukocyte antigen (HLA) typing
- ABO/Rh typing
- HLA antibody screening
- Autoantibody screening
- Infectious disease panel to include human immunodeficiency virus (HIV) antibody, cytomegalovirus (CMV) antibody, hepatitis B surface antigen, hepatitis A antibody (total and IgM), hepatitis C antibody, human T cell leukemia virus (HTLV-I) antibody, syphilis antibody (rapid plasma reagin [RPR], Venereal Disease Research Laboratory [VDRL] tests), herpesvirus antibody.

SELECTED OR POTENTIAL DONOR TESTING INCLUDES

- HLA typing for matching recipient HLA antigens
- ABO/Rh typing for compatibility with patient
- Mixed lymphocyte culture (MLC) testing for determining amount of stimulation with patient cells
- Crossmatching for compatibility with patient
- Infectious disease panel (same as previous)

The following sections examine the specific testing that is performed before and after the transplantation. Kidney transplantation is used as an example with the knowledge that other organ transplantation testing is quite similar. The exception is bone marrow transplantation, which has the added complexity that it is the transplantation of immunocompetent cells. As a result, this type of transplantation has additional obstacles to overcome.

Pretransplantation Testing

The evaluation of the transplant recipient includes a complete medical evaluation to rule out contraindications to the transplantation, which vary with the type of transplantation being considered. The patient then undergoes an extensive immunologic evaluation. This includes ABO/Rh blood group typing, histocompatibility tissue typing, a determination of preformed antibodies to histocompatibility antigens and autoantibodies (crossmatching), and a large panel of viral serologic tests.

ABO/Rh BLOOD GROUP TESTING. The most important antigens to match between the donor and the recipient are the ABO/Rh blood group antigens. This is because the ABO/Rh blood group antigens are present not only on blood cells but also on the vascular endothelium. A mismatch here results in rapid organ rejection due to the preformed antibodies in the recipient, which immediately attack the vascular endothelium of the transplanted organ. The specifics of this testing are covered in Chapter 24 and the same blood banking transfusion rules apply.

HISTOCOMPATIBILITY TISSUE TYPING (see "Immunologic Methods Used for Histocompatibility Testing for Transplantation," p 380). Histocompatibility antigens, also referred to as *human leukocyte antigens* (HLAs) comprise six main recognized groups controlled by genetically coded polymorphic alleles. These groups are known as HLA-A, -B, -C, -DR, -DQ, and -DP antigens. The actual possible specificities within each group are numerous, which is the reason for the extreme polymorphism (variation) between individuals. It is the individual HLA antigens that are determined in histocompatibility tissue typing. HLA donor-recipient matching is important to the long term graft survival. The half-life of a renal graft is over 12 years when there are no HLA mismatches; however, with six mismatches it drops to under 8 years. With the advent of the third generation immunosuppressive therapies, short term (less than a year) renal graft survival appears to be independent of histocompatibility tissue matches. The traditional method for HLA tissue typing is by lymphocytotoxicity tests in microtiter plates. In this procedure, the purified lymphocytes of the patient or donor to be typed are exposed to a panel of different antisera with known HLA specificities. A source of complement is then added, followed by a vital dye. If the antibody recognizes an antigen on the cell surface, it binds and fixes complement, and the cell dies. The vital dye then stains the dead cells, and this is visualized microscopically and graded as to the positivity (1 to 8). Although this seems fairly straightforward, the interpretation and assignment of the full HLA type can be difficult as a very large number of typing sera (up to 200) with multiple specificities are used.

TECHNICAL NOTE HLA typing is generally performed by specialized tissue typing laboratories with highly trained personnel.

For HLA-DR and -DQ typing, the patients lymphocytes must be purified further to enrich for B cells, which are then used in the assay. Laboratories performing these tests are accredited and tightly regulated by the American Society for Histocompatibility and Immunogenetics. Other assays using the newer technologies of molecular biology, flow cytometry, and enzyme immunoassay have been developed but generally are not currently in wide use.

DETERMINATION OF PREFORMED ANTIBODIES (See "Immunologic Methods Used for Histocompatibility Testing for Transplantation," p 380). This is referred to as *crossmatching* and determines the presence of antibodies in the patient's serum that may be directed against antigens on the graft. These preformed antibodies indicate prior sensitization and may contribute to rejection and damage of the graft. Crossmatching is performed the same as the HLA tissue typing by lymphocytotoxicity except that the donor's lymphocytes are reacted with the recipient's serum instead of recipient lymphocytes with typing sera. If a weak cytotoxicity is observed (possibly due to antibodies to DR/DQ antigens on B cells), the crossmatching is performed on donor purified T and B cells to clarify the specificity of the reactivity. Crossmatching can also be performed by flow cytometry, which is more sensitive. In flow cytometry it is unnecessary to purify the T and B cells, since they can be identified by dual color analysis (see Chapter 20). False positives can occur because of antilymphocyte autoantibodies in the recipient's serum. These are controlled for by testing the recipient's cells with the recipient's serum. Autoantibodies may also interfere with the detection of donor specific antibodies.

CELLULAR ASSAYS IN HISTOCOMPATIBILITY TISSUE TYPING. Mixed lymphocyte culture reactions are important in determining discrepancies in the HLA class II (D locus), which the standard tissue typing may not detect. Clinically this is used in several

PRE-TRANSPLANTATION TESTING

situations. It has been used to confirm HLA identity, in both related and unrelated individuals. It has also been used to assess the best donor among several nonmatched family members. This assay is very labor intensive and costly. Basically, the recipient's lymphocytes are mixed with the potential donor's lymphocytes (which have been irradiated or otherwise treated so they cannot proliferate in response to the recipient) and cultured 4 to 5 days. Proliferation of the recipient's lymphocytes as measured by the uptake of a radioactive DNA precursor is a positive indication of the recipient's responsiveness to the donor. An alteration of this test is determination of the formation of cytotoxic T lymphocytes in response to the potential donor lymphocytes.

INFECTIOUS DISEASE SEROLOGIC TESTS. Both the recipient and the donor are evaluated for infectious diseases that may adversely effect the outcome of the graft. These include but may not be limited to CMV, hepatitis of various serologic types, HIV, and Epstein-Barr virus (EBV). See the section "Specific Immunologic Infectious Disease Tests (Viral)" in Chapter 21.

OTHER TESTS. The previously listed tests are the major immunologic tests that are performed in kidney transplantations. However, depending on the individual patient and the transplantation program, the list may be altered to include additional tests. This testing also varies with the type of transplantation.

IMMUNOLOGIC METHODS USED FOR HISTOCOMPATIBILITY TESTING FOR TRANSPLANTATION

TEST	METHODS	UTILITY
Tissue Typing Complement dependent lymphocyto-toxicity test	Serologic	Human leukocyte antigen (HLA) class I and II antigen identification
Mixed lymphocyte culture (MLC)	Cellular (tissue culture)	Determines HLA class II antigen
Crossmatching T and B cell crossmatching	Serologic	Detection of antidonor HLA class I antibodies (T) Detection of antidonor HLA class I and II antibodies (B)
Peripheral blood (PBL) crossmatching	Serologic	Detection of antibodies in patient's serum directed against donor antigens
Cell mediated lympholysis	Cellular	Detection of antidonor cytotoxic T lymphocytes
Flow cytometry crossmatching	Cellular (fluorescent antibody)	Sensitive assay for detection of HLA antibodies on lymphocytes
Screening HLA class I antibody screening	Serologic (T cell) DNA, polymerase chain reaction (PCR) is available	Detection of HLA class I antibodies for antibody specificity
HLA class II antibody screening	Serologic (B cell)	Detection of HLA class II antibodies for antibody specificity

POST-TRANSPLANTATION TESTING AND MONITORING

The immunologic tests performed after transplantation are the viral serologic tests, monitoring the appearance of HLA antibodies to the donor HLA antigens, and monitoring various peripheral blood T cells and natural killer cell populations by flow cytometry. Again, as with pretransplantation testing, the actual tests performed depend on the type of transplantation and the program in which the patient is enrolled.

BIBLIOGRAPHY

Antman K: When are bone marrow transplants considered? Sci Am 275:124–125, 1996.

Ball ST, Dallman MJ: Transplantation immunology. Curr Opin Nephrol Hypertens 4:465–471, 1995.

Brent L: Medawar Prize Lecture: tolerance and graft-vs-host disease: two sides of the same coin. Transplant Proc 27:12–14, 1995.

Burdick JF: What's new in transplantation. J Am Coll Surg 182:170–176, 1996.

Chaignaud BE, Vacanti JP: Opportunistic infections in immunocompromised patients. Semin Pediatr Surg 4:245–251, 1995.

Champlin R, Giralt S, Gajewski J: T cells, graft-versus-host disease and graft-versus-leukemia: innovative approaches for blood and marrow transplantation. Acta Haematol 95:157–163, 1996.

Dyer PA, Martin S, Sinnott P: Histocompatibility testing for kidney transplantation: an update. Nephrol Dial Transplant 10(suppl 1): 23–28, 1995.

Halloran PF, Batiuk TD, Goes NB, Campbell P: Strategies to improve the immunologic management of organ transplants. Clin Transplant 9(3 pt 2):227–236, 1995.

Haeney M: The immunological background to transplantation. J Antimicrob Chemother 36(suppl B):1–9, 1995.

Kontoyiannis DP, Rubin RH: Infection in the organ transplant recipient. An overview. Infect Dis Clin North Am 9:811–822, 1995.

Lee HM: Chronic rejection: pathogenesis and treatment. Transplant Proc 28:1146–1147, 1996.

Reisner Y, Martelli MF: Bone marrow transplantation across HLA barriers by increasing the number of transplanted cells. Immunol Today 16:437–440, 1995.

Remuzzi G, Perico N: Immunotolerance: from new knowledge of mechanisms of self-tolerance to future perspectives for induction of renal transplant tolerance. Exp Nephrol 3:319–330, 1995.

Schlitt HJ: Clinical and immunological aspects of liver allograft rejection. Transplant Proc 28:514–516, 1996.

Sullivan KM: Immunomodulation in allogeneic marrow transplantation: use of intravenous immune globulin to suppress acute graft-versus-host disease. Clin Exp Immunol 104(suppl 1):43–48, 1996.

Truong L, Shappell S, Solez K: Adhesion molecules as markers of acute cellular rejection of renal allografts. Transplant Proc 28:519–522, 1996.

Walter EA, Bowden RA: Infection in the bone marrow transplant recipient. Infect Dis Clin North Am 9:823–847, 1995.

METHODS USED FOR HISTOCOMPATIBILITY TESTING FOR TRANSPLANTATION

Section

III

IMMUNO-HEMATOLOGY

Elizabeth Cascone, MT(ASCP), SBB

Chapter *23*

BASIC CONCEPTS OF IMMUNOHEMATOLOGY

INTRODUCTION

Antibodies in the prenatal patient, pretransfusion recipient, and some patients with hematologic disorders are capable of destroying red blood cells that possess the corresponding antigen(s). The characteristics of antibodies produced in response to exposure to RBC antigens, as well as the biologic factors that influence the binding of antibody to antigen, are important considerations for all individuals employed in the transfusion service.

SOME IMPORTANT TERMS AND DEFINITIONS

TERM	DEFINITION
Agglutination	"Clumps" of red blood cells (RBCs). These "clumps" are a result of the formation of "bridges" between antibody molecules bound to antigens on the surface of different RBCs.
Antibody	A molecule produced in response to exposure to an antigen. These molecules bind specifically to the substance that generated their production.
Antigen	A substance capable of eliciting an immune response.
Immune Response	A reaction characterized by production of antibody (immunoglobulins) as a result of exposure to an antigen (immunogen).
Immunoglobulins (Igs)	Biologic molecules, consisting of five classes, that share a common basic structure and behave as antibodies.
In Vivo	Occurring in a living organism.
In Vitro	Occurring in a test tube or other laboratory vessel.
Isoagglutinin	An antibody produced in an individual that agglutinates RBCs that express the complementary antigen(s).
Isotonic Saline	A solution containing predominantly sodium chloride and water, in a concentration (0.85%) compatible with the normal function of living human cells.
Plasma	The liquid portion of blood.
Serum	The liquid portion of a blood sample that has been allowed to coagulate; plasma without fibrinogen.
Standard Operating Procedure (SOP)	A document that clearly defines a process, protocol, or procedure so that when the SOP is used, the outcome is a quality product. The SOP, when prepared and used in the appropriate manner, ensures standardization of the performance of the procedure that it addresses.
Zeta Potential	The difference in the density of electric charge between the inner and outer layer of ions that arrange themselves around an RBC in solution.

NOTE The terms *normal saline, physiologic saline,* and *isotonic saline* are used interchangeably in this text.

NOTE The terms *serum* and *plasma* may be used interchangeably throughout this section of the text.

One factor determining the in vivo survival of transfused RBCs is the presence or absence of recipient antibodies to antigens present on the transfused RBCs. Antigens are molecules that, by definition, elicit an immune response and are inherited traits.

Antibodies are immunoglobulins, molecules produced by the immune system in response to exposure to a specific antigen recognized by the antibody maker as nonself. These antibodies bind specifically to the antigen that elicited their production.

Immunoglobulins belong to one of five classes:

IgA
IgD
IgE
IgG
IgM

Each class has its own characteristics and properties. Antibodies produced in response to exposure to RBC antigens almost always belong to the IgG and/or IgM class.

CHARACTERISTICS OF IgG AND IgM MOLECULES

CHARACTERISTICS	IgG	IgM
Type of heavy chains	γ (gamma)	μ (mu)
Number of subunits	1	5
Normal adult serum concentration	16%	4%
Able to cross placenta (cause HDN)	Yes	No
Serologic designation	Incomplete antibody Nonagglutinating	Complete antibody Saline agglutinin
Serologic behavior	Agglutinates RBCs when intracellular distance is spanned	Agglutinates directly in an isotonic saline environment
Capable of fixing complement (cause intravascular hemolysis)	Variable (some specificities and/or subclasses)	Yes
Optimal temperature of reactivity	37°C	≤20°C
Usual mode of antigenic stimulation	Pregnancy or transfusion	Exposure to environmental substances
Degraded by sulfhydryl reagents (dithiothreitol, 2-mercaptoethanol)	No	Yes

From Vengelen-Tyler V, ed: Technical Manual, 12th ed. Bethesda, Md, American Association of Blood Banks, 1996.

CHARACTERISTICS OF IgG AND IgM MOLECULES

Schematic Illustration of Basic Four Chain Immunoglobulin Unit

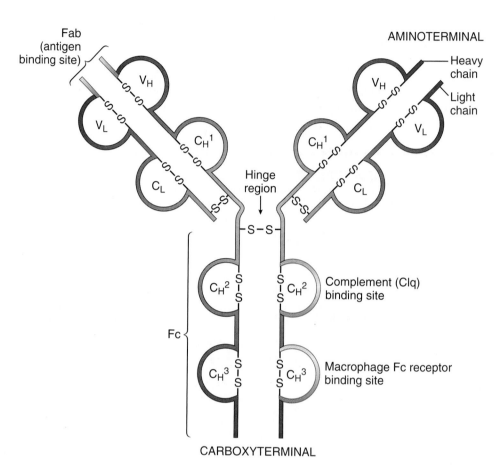

Schematic Illustration of Pentamer IgM Immunoglobulin Unit

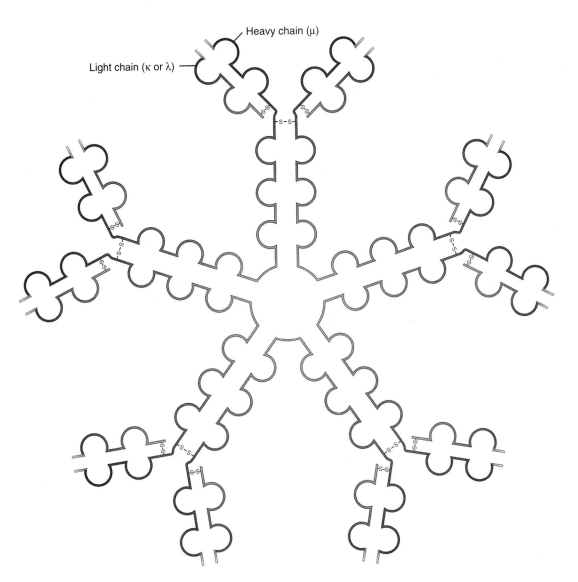

AGGLUTINATION REACTIONS

The agglutination reaction is the method most often used in the blood bank laboratory to visualize antigen-antibody reactions. This technique is used to detect and identify plasma antibodies in the recipient that could damage or destroy transfused RBCs.

Effects of Antigen-Antibody Reactions on Red Blood Cells

▌ Agglutination is the "clumping" of antigen bearing cells by their corresponding antibody. It occurs in two stages:
  1. Sensitization, the binding of antibody to RBCs
  2. Formation of bridges or lattices between antibody sensitized cells
▌ Lysis is the breakdown of RBCs (hemolysis).

Characteristics of the Antigen-Antibody Reaction

▌ RBCs carry a negative surface charge.
▌ RBCs in solution are surrounded by ions that arrange themselves in layers around the RBC.
▌ The resultant electrostatic potential (zeta potential) impedes spontaneous agglutination of adjacent RBCs.
▌ The electrostatic repulsive forces must be overcome for RBCs sensitized with antibody to approach each other and crosslink.
▌ When RBCs overcome the electrostatic repulsive forces, antibody molecules can bind to antigen sites on different RBCs, forming crosslinks (lattices, bridges) between RBCs. The environment of the reaction can be manipulated by physical and/or chemical processes to reduce the naturally occurring intercellular forces and promote the formation of visible agglutinates.

> **NOTE** In some cases, the antibody molecule (IgM) is large enough or antibody concentration is high enough to effect visible agglutination *without* manipulating the environment. These antibodies are called *"saline agglutinins"* or *"complete antibodies."*

Some intrinsic properties of antigens and/or antibodies contribute to their ability to combine and subsequently engage in lattice formation.

Biologic Factors Influencing Antigen-Antibody Reactions

FACTOR	EFFECT
Antibody size	IgM (pentamer) effectively spans distance between RBCs, causing direct agglutination. IgG (monomer) is too small to overcome electrostatic forces between RBCs.
Number of antigen sites	Increased number of antigen sites increases the possibility or likelihood of the antibody's encountering an available receptor with which to bind, e.g.: A antigen sites = >1.5 million/RBC K antigen sites = ~3500–6000/RBC
Availability of antigen binding sites	Some antigens are projected from RBC surface; others are more embedded in cellular membrane. Antigens on surface of RBC membrane are more available for antibody binding than those antigens closer to or partially contained in RBC membrane.
Arrangement of antigen on RBC surface (clustering)	This biologic property of an antigen is related to its mobility on or within RBC membrane. Antigen that is mobile within RBC membrane is more likely to overcome steric hindrances to antibody binding.

Methods and Techniques to Reduce the Zeta Potential

PROCEDURE	ACTION OR EFFECT
Enzyme Pretreatment of RBC	Removes negatively charged sialic acid residues from cell surface
Addition of Albumin or other Colloids	Increases electric conductivity (dielectric constant) of the environment
Centrifugation	Mechanical process that forces RBCs closer together

AGGLUTINATION REACTIONS

Schematic of the Zeta Potential Concept

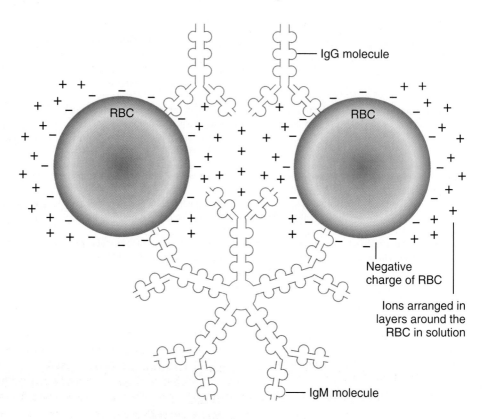

The zeta potential (electrostatic potential) impedes
the spontaneous agglutination of IgG sensitized RBCs.
Frequently, IgM molecules are large enough to span the distance
between adjacent RBCs and cause agglutination.

Methods and Techniques to Enhance and Visualize in Vitro Antigen-Antibody Reactions

Most antibodies directed at RBC antigens known to cause increased RBC damage or destruction, with the exception of ABO antibodies, belong to the IgG class of immunoglobulins. Antibodies of this class are called *sensitizing* antibodies; they bind at 37°C but they do not cause direct agglutination. Because of their clinical importance, every effort must be made in the blood bank laboratory to detect and identify antibodies of this type. A variety of methods and techniques are available to enhance and visualize the reaction between antigens on the RBC membrane and their corresponding antibodies in the serum:

VARIABLE	CHARACTERISTICS
pH	Binding of most blood group antibodies is optimal at pH of 6.5–7.5.
Temperature	*"Cold" agglutinins* (IgM antibodies) react optimally at ≤20°C. *Warm reactive* antibodies (IgG) react optimally at 37°C.
Time	Selecting optimal time of reaction promotes maximum antibody binding.
Antigen/Antibody Ratio	Increased serum to cell ratio allows more antibody molecules to bind to RBC antigens.
Ionic Strength	Lower ionic concentration in reaction environment disburses ionic cloud that surrounds RBCs, allowing more efficient antigen-antibody complexing.
Alteration or Modification of Ig Molecule	Chemical modification of IgG molecule to break the disulfide bonds responsible for its structure. This results in an IgG molecule with greater capacity to span the distance between RBCs. This process is used in manufacturing reagents for use in the blood bank laboratory.
Antigen Dosage	RBCs with two doses of antigen react more readily with its corresponding antibody than those RBCs that carry single dose of antigen.
Use of Colloids (Albumin, polyethylene glycol [PeG], polyvinylpyrrolidone [PVP], hexadimethrine bromide [Polybrene])	Reduces degree of repulsion between RBCs, allowing antibody molecules to approach and bind to their corresponding antigens.
Use of Proteolytic Enzymes (Ficin, Papain)	Reduces negative repulsive forces separating RBCs. Removes some structures from RBC surface, increasing accessability of other antigens.
Use of Antihuman Globulin	Forms crosslinks between antibody molecules that have sensitized (bound to the surface of) RBCs. This promotes formation of agglutinates and allows visualization of antigen-antibody reaction.

AGGLUTINATION REACTIONS

Reading Agglutination

▌ Grading the strength of agglutination reactions requires that the serologist assign a "standardized" number that relates to the size and amount of agglutinates that have formed.
▌ Although there is variability to be expected among individuals when grading serologic reactions, a descriptive guideline follows:

READING AGGLUTINATION

GRADE	DESCRIPTION		APPEARANCE	
	Cells	Supernate	Macroscopic*	Microscopict
0	No agglutinates	Dark, turbid, homogeneous		
w+	Many tiny agglutinates Many free cells May not be visible without microscope	Dark, turbid		
1+	Many small agglutinates Many free cells	Turbid		

Continued ▶

▶ Continued **READING AGGLUTINATION**

| GRADE | DESCRIPTION | | APPEARANCE | |
	Cells	**Supernate**	**Macroscopic***	**Microscopic†**
2+	Many medium sized agglutinates Moderate number of free cells	Clear		
3+	Several large agglutinates Few free cells	Clear		
4+	One large, solid agglutinate No free cells	Clear		

*For any one grade, readings can be on a scale from weak+ to strong+ (e.g., grade 2 can be scored as 2+w, 2+, or 2+s depending on the number and size of agglutinates).
†Microscopic readings are generally performed to differentiate pseudoagglutination (rouleaux) from true agglutination, to detect mixed field reactions, and to confirm a negative reaction.

AGGLUTINATION REACTIONS

> **REMEMBER** Both agglutination and hemolysis are indicators of antigen-antibody binding.

Additional considerations when reading agglutination reactions:

▌ *Hemolysis,* which is recognized as a pink to red supernate, can occur with any grade of agglutination.

▌ *Rouleaux,* recognized as small, isolated refractile aggregates that have a "rolled coin" appearance, and *mixed field,* which is recognized as small isolated agglutinates among many free cells, are commonly seen in w+ reactions but may also occur in 1+, 2+, and 3+ reactions.

Factors Leading to Invalid or Falsely Interpreted Agglutination Reactions[1]

SAMPLE PROBLEMS

▌ There are small fibrin strands in plasma samples or samples that have not completely coagulated.

▌ There are increased amounts of protein or the presence of an abnormal protein in the patient's serum or plasma.

▌ Patient's serum contains unexpected antibodies that react at room temperature.

▌ Patient's RBCs may be coated with antibody in vivo.

▌ Patient's sample may contain transfused or transplanted RBCs or plasma.

REAGENT PROBLEMS

▌ Potency of reagent has degraded due to improper storage.

▌ Reagents or saline have been contaminated during use.

▌ Reagent antisera contains antibodies to antigens other than those expected.

EQUIPMENT PROBLEMS

▌ Centrifuge is incorrectly calibrated.

▌ Pipette or glassware is dirty.

BIBLIOGRAPHY

Roitt IM: Essential Immunology, 8th ed. Oxford, Blackwell Scientific, 1994.

Rudmann SV: Textbook of Blood Banking and Transfusion Medicine. Philadelphia, WB Saunders, 1995.

Vengelen-Tyler B, ed: Technical Manual, 12th ed. Bethesda, Md, American Association of Blood Banks, 1996.

Widmann FK: An Introduction to Clinical Immunology. Philadelphia: FA Davis, 1989.

---

[1]The reader is referred to the American Association of Blood Banks Technical Manual, 12th edition, 1996, for a complete discussion of factors affecting agglutination.

24

COMPATIBILITY TESTING

Robert J. Borley, MS, MT (ASCP), SBB

Elizabeth Cascone, MT (ASCP), SBB

Q U I C K   C O N T E N T S

INTRODUCTION

Routine compatibility testing is the most important function provided by the hospital blood bank or transfusion medicine department. This importance is not because of the difficulty of the testing procedures but rather attests to the critical nature of all the steps in this process, the methodic approach that should be used, and the meticulous accuracy required in their performance.

FUNCTIONS INCLUDED IN COMPATIBILITY TESTING

The following functions and processes should be considered part of compatibility testing:

1. Patient specimen collection, submission requirements, and test requisition requirements (including patient transfusion related history review)
2. Donor unit testing, the extent of which depends on the nature of the transfusing facility (e.g., minimal testing requirements in the transfusion service include retyping blood center supplied donor units)
3. Patient testing, including antibody identification
4. Crossmatching
5. Donor unit selection, antigen typing, donor labeling, and issuing of blood and blood components.

In this chapter, the authors consider pretransfusion testing as a subset of the process of compatibility testing. This subset deals directly with the intended recipient, including functions 1 and 2 above, although many blood bankers freely interchange this terminology.

PATIENT SPECIMEN COLLECTION AND REQUISITION REQUIREMENTS

NOTE Most transfusion accidents occur due to:
- Errors in patient identification or labeling of the patient specimens
- Errors in identifying the intended recipient or the donor unit before transfusion.

In general, all patient specimens collected for submission to the blood bank must include a mechanism to positively identify the phlebotomist collecting that specimen. A requisition signed by the phlebotomist must be linked by a number or some other acceptable identification mechanism to the specimen that accompanies it. If this practice is not used, then both specimen and requisition must be signed by the phlebotomist to link this important identification information.

The blood specimen should be collected in an evacuated tube system or with syringe and needle and then transferred to an evacuated tube. Samples may be collected into tubes with or without anticoagulant.

Caution should be exercised to avoid damage to the red blood cells (RBCs) during collection; a hemolyzed sample is unacceptable for serologic testing in the blood bank laboratory. The specimen tube must be labeled *before leaving the bedside.*

Specimen Labeling Requirements

The following information must be clearly written or printed legibly on a label firmly affixed to each blood bank specimen:

- Patient's first and last name
- Patient's identification number
- Date (and time, if required) of collection
- Phlebotomist's signature or some other method to conclusively link the specimen to the phlebotomist

Other information may be required by state or local regulations or may be convenient to have available on the label, depending on individual laboratory or hospital requirements.

Blood Bank Test Requisitions

Test requisitions are submitted with samples as an additional means of identifying the patient; they also specify tests and/or blood products that are needed. Test requisitions also provide a formal record of the physician's order for the requested procedures and/or products. This satisfies federal law prohibiting the dispensing of blood or blood products without a prescription. Test requisitions may be recorded and transmitted on paper forms or on electronic media; any record must be traceable to a written physician order to satisfy federal dispensing laws.

INFORMATION ON REQUISITION FORMS

The following information must be included on the test requisition form:

- Patient identification matching the identification on the blood specimen label
- Date (and time if required) when the requisition was generated
- Ordering physician
- Blood bank tests and/or blood products requested
- Phlebotomist's identifier

Other information required by state and local codes should be included on the requisition, as well as information addressing internal needs as required by the individual laboratory or hospital.

After the specimen label and requisition are carefully examined for accuracy and completeness, the specimen itself must be examined and meet an additional set of criteria.

Blood Bank Specimen Requirements

The blood in the specimen tube should be:

- Free of excessive hemolysis caused by traumatic phlebotomy. Traumatic hemolysis could obscure hemolysis caused by antibody-antigen interaction in subsequent testing.
- Completely clotted when a sample tube without anticoagulant is used. Clotting of the sample during the test procedures may invalidate results or make them difficult to interpret.
- Free of visible contaminants such as gels or talc.
- Of normal consistency and free of obvious contamination with intravenous fluid. The serum should not appear watery or very light in color.

Either clotted or anticoagulated specimens may be submitted to the blood bank laboratory, depending on individual laboratory preference or reagent or instrument manufacturer's requirements. Clotted samples are required to detect complement dependent antibody reactions. The detection of such antibodies in this way is of limited use; powerful enhancement media and improved reagent red cells provide an increase in test sensitivity that permits detection and identification of these antibodies without relying on complement activation. In addition, the use of semiautomated or automated blood bank instruments may require the use of plasma samples in the not too distant future.

REQUIREMENTS FOR OUTDATING SAMPLES USED FOR CROSSMATCHING

Outdate or *expiration* of a patient sample refers to the date (and time) at which it is no longer acceptable for use in pretransfusion testing or crossmatching.

WAS PATIENT TRANSFUSED WITHIN PAST 3 MO? →	WAS PATIENT PREGNANT WITHIN PAST 3 MO? →	WAS AN ACCURATE PATIENT TRANSFUSION HISTORY OBTAINED? →	SET SAMPLE OUTDATE TO:
No	No	Yes	Determined by blood bank medical director
Yes	No	Yes	3 days* (from date of collection)
No	Yes	Yes	3 days* (from date of collection)
Yes	Yes	Yes	3 days* (from date of collection)
No	No	No†	3 days† (from date of collection)

*Three days is a somewhat arbitrary time limit allowed for detecting newly developing antibodies due to recent contact with foreign RBC antigens.
  †Uncertain history requires 3 day outdate.

All patient samples used for pretransfusion testing and crossmatching for patients who receive a transfusion must be stored for a minimum of 7 days after the date of transfusion. This requirement ensures that the sample will be available for testing in the event that the transfused patient's symptoms suggest a delayed hemolytic transfusion reaction.

PATIENT PRETRANSFUSION TESTING AS A PART OF COMPATIBILITY TESTING

Patient Tests Included in Pretransfusion Testing

Patient pretransfusion testing consists of a battery of test procedures. These procedures, each of which is fully described in a later section, include:

- ABO and $Rh_0(D)$ typing.
- Antibody screening to detect atypical clinically important serum antibodies in the patient's serum directed against an antigen that may be present on the RBCs of the donor unit selected for transfusion. Clinically important antibodies are those that are known to cause reduced survival or increased destruction of transfused donor RBCs. They are generally detected at 37°C or in the indirect antiglobulin test.
- Identification of clinically important antibodies detected in the antibody screen.
- Phenotyping of the patient's RBCs for antigens corresponding to identified antibodies.
- Crossmatching using one of several techniques selected by various parameters.

The method selected for crossmatching depends on the patient's serologic status; selection is determined by and must comply with prescribed regulatory requirements that define acceptable crossmatching procedures and when their use is appropriate.

> **NOTE** Current testing guidelines do not require a direct antiglobulin test in pretransfusion testing. This test is more appropriately considered a part of antiglobulin testing, performed only when indicated, or as part of antibody identification. The reader should refer to "Antiglobulin Test" on p 439 for more information regarding this test.

Donor Testing as a Part of Compatibility Testing

Blood donors, at minimum, must be tested for blood type (ABO group and $Rh_0(D)$ type), atypical serum antibodies, and transfusion transmitted disease markers. In addition, other pre- and postdonation screening, such as the test for sickle hemoglobin or antibodies to cytomegalovirus, may be indicated, depending on the intended recipient. In general, unless the hospital blood bank or transfusion service is also the collecting facility, it plays a minor role in this part of compatibility testing. The most common test procedure performed on donor RBCs in the transfusion service is retyping the donor RBCs received from a regional blood center for ABO group and $Rh_0(D)$ type (when necessary).

GENERAL COMPATIBILITY TESTING REQUIREMENTS FOR BLOOD DONORS

FUNCTION	REQUIRED OF COLLECTING FACILITY	REQUIRED OF TRANSFUSING FACILITY	REQUIRED BY
Donor History	Yes	No	FDA, American Association of Blood Banks (AABB)
Donor Physical	Yes	No	FDA, AABB
Donor Self-Deferral	Yes	No	FDA, AABB
ABO and Rh$_0$(D) Typing (Including Testing for Weak D)	Yes	Yes Retype ABO on all units Retype Rh$_0$(D) on Rh$_0$(D) negative only Weak D testing not required*	FDA,† AABB
Antibody Screen	Yes	No	FDA, AABB
Syphilis Serologic Tests	Yes	No	FDA
Transfusion Transmitted Viral Testing‡	Yes	No	FDA,§ AABB
Alanine Aminotransferase Surrogate Testing	Yes	No	Some states may require testing
Antigen Typing of Donor RBCs	No‖	Yes‖	AABB

*Weak D was formerly known as D^u.

†FDA does not require retesting by the transfusion facility.

‡Transfusion transmitted viral testing includes hepatitis B surface antigen, hepatitis B core antibody testing, hepatitis C antibody testing, HIV-1 and -2 antibody testing, HTLV-I and II antibody testing, HIV-1 (p-24) antigen testing.

§FDA does not require hepatitis B core antibody testing.

‖Responsibility lies with the transfusion service; however, the collecting facility may provide antigen screened units on the request of the transfusing facility. Usually the transfusion service retypes these units on receipt.

ABO BLOOD GROUP SYSTEM

Typing potential transfusion recipients for their ABO group and Rh$_0$(D) type is the most important and, by far, the most critical, testing performed in the blood bank laboratory.

WARNING The vast majority of transfusion accidents that cause serious patient injury are due to an error in identifying patient samples or donor units that results in the transfusion of an ABO incompatible blood product. A significant number of transfusion accidents occur, however, due to ABO typing errors in the transfusion service laboratory. *The ABO typing test is the most critical procedure encountered and performed in the blood bank laboratory!*

Basic Structures and Nature of ABO Blood Group System Antigens

The presence or absence of two antigens (A and B) defines the four blood types of the ABO blood group system. The ABO blood groups are determined genetically by the inheritance of a gene or genes that code for the production of transferase enzymes. These enzymes, known as *glycosyltransferases,* add specific hexoses (6 carbon sugars) to oligosaccharide chains present on the RBC membrane. In a series of enzymatic reactions, the ABH antigens are formed. The first of these enzyme reactions is the addition of fucose to oligosaccharide chains on the red cell membrane by the action of fucosyltransferase produced by the *H* gene. This creates the H antigen structure that is the substrate for further transferase activity associated with the A and B genes. Two other genetically controlled enzymes, group A transferase (*N*-acetylgalactosaminyltransferase) and group B transferase (D-galactosyltransferase), control the addition of the terminal sugars *N*-acetylgalactosamine and D-galactose, respectively, to the oligosaccharide chain that has acquired H antigen specificity.

GENETIC CONTROL OF THE ABO BLOOD GROUP ANTIGENS

GENES PRESENT	TRANSFERASE PRODUCED	TERMINAL SUGAR	RED BLOOD CELL PHENOTYPE
HH or *Hh*	Fucosyltransferase	Fucose	O
HH and *A,* or *Hh* and *A*	Fucosyltransferase and *N*-acetylgalac-tosaminyltransferase	Fucose and *N*-acetyl-galactosamine	A
HH and *B,* or *Hh* and *B*	Fucosyltransferase and D-galactosyl-transferase	Fucose and D-galactose	B
HH and *A* plus *B,* or *Hh* and *A* plus *B*	Fucosyltransferase and *N*-acetylgalac-tosaminyltransferase and D-galactosyl-transferase	Fucose and *N*-acetyl-galactosamine and D-galactose	AB
hh, or *hh* and any other gene (*A* and/or *B*)	None or *N*-acetylgalactosaminyltrans-ferase and/or D-galactosyltransferase	None	Bombay

TABLE OF ABO BLOOD GROUP FREQUENCIES (IN PERCENT) IN US POPULATION

BLOOD GROUP	WHITES	BLACKS	NATIVE AMERICANS	ASIANS
O	45	49	79	40
A	40	27	16	28
B	11	20	4	27
AB	4	4	<1	5

Modified from Vengelen-Tyler V (ed): Technical Manual, 12th ed. Baltimore, American Association of Blood Banks, 1996, p 230.

ABO BLOOD GROUP SYSTEM

Nature of ABO Blood Group System Antibodies

ABO blood group system antibodies are significantly different from those directed at other blood group system antigens because they are potent, naturally occurring antibodies found universally in immunocompetent persons. Current thinking indicates that the A and B antigen structure on RBC membranes is similar to bacterial antigen structures found in the environment; these bacterial antigens stimulate production of the "naturally occurring" antibodies of the ABO blood group system. In addition to natural environmental stimulation, "immune" antibodies of the ABO blood group system may be produced after exposure to foreign red blood cells.

Those individuals lacking A antigen produce anti-A and those lacking B antigen produce anti-B. Group O individuals lack both A and B antigen and thus produce anti-A and anti-B, whereas group AB persons have both A and B antigen and produce no ABO blood group antibodies.

BLOOD GROUP	ANTIBODY PRODUCED	PREDOMINANT IMMUNOGLOBULIN	SPECIAL CHARACTERISTICS
A	Anti-B	IgM*	Reacts better at room temperature or below "Natural" type antibody in ABO blood group system Rarely causes hemolytic disease of the newborn (HDN) or positive direct antiglobulin test (DAT) in newborns Is inactivated by 2-mercaptoethanol (2-ME) or dithiothreitol (DTT) treatment†
B	Anti-A	IgM*	Reacts better at room temperature or below "Natural" type antibody in ABO blood group system Rarely causes HDN or positive DAT in newborns Is inactivated by 2-ME or DTT treatment†
AB	None	NA	
O	Anti-A, anti-B and	IgM* and	Reacts better at room temperature or below "Natural" type antibody in ABO blood group system Rarely causes HDN or positive DAT in newborns Is inactivated by 2-ME and DTT treatment.†
	Anti-A,B (single antibody having both anti-A and anti-B specificity)	IgG*	Reacts better at physiologic temperatures (37°C) "Immune" antibody in ABO blood group system Is the predominant cause of ABO HDN Is not inactivated by 2-ME or DTT treatment.†

*In group A and B individuals, IgM class tends to predominate (unless immunization to ABO incompatible RBCs occurred due to exposure to fetal RBCs during a prior pregnancy or transfusion, in which case the immunoglobulin class is predominantly IgG). In group O individuals, IgG is generally the predominant immunoglobulin class.

†2-ME and DTT are thiol reagents capable of cleaving the disulfide bonds of IgM molecules.

ABO Donor—Recipient Compatibility Chart

DONOR *→	GROUP O	GROUP A	GROUP B	GROUP AB
RECIPIENT ↓	No A or B Antigen	A Antigen but no B Antigen	B Antigen but no A Antigen	Both A and B Antigens
Group O Both anti-A and anti-B in serum	Compatible	Incompatible	Incompatible	Incompatible
Group A Only anti-B in serum	Compatible	Compatible	Incompatible	Incompatible
Group B Only anti-A in serum	Compatible	Incompatible	Compatible	Incompatible
Group AB No anti-A or anti-B in serum	Compatible	Compatible	Compatible	Compatible

*Donor units supplied as RBCs.
Whole blood for transfusion should be type specific only.

ABO Typing

Although ABO typing is the most critical testing performed in the blood bank, the test has an inherent check system. The check system allows the blood bank technologist to compare the cell typing (front or forward type) with the serum typing (back or reverse type). The pattern of agglutination in the forward and reverse typing tests must match an established pattern (see "Expected Reactions with Commercial ABO Typing Reagents" on p 406), e.g., the RBCs from a patient who is group A will be agglutinated by anti-A but not anti-B; the serum of the same patient will agglutinate group B RBCs, but not RBCs that are group A.

If the expected reactions are not observed, this is called an *ABO typing discrepancy*; ABO typing discrepancies must be resolved before the patient can be transfused with type specific donor RBC units.

Expected reactions of patient red blood cells and patient serum with commercial ABO typing reagents can be found in the chart below.

EXPECTED REACTIONS WITH COMMERCIAL ABO TYPING REAGENTS

REAGENTS → PATIENTS ↓	ANTI-A WITH PATIENT'S CELLS	ANTI-B WITH PATIENT'S CELLS	ANTI-A,B* WITH PATIENT'S CELLS	A₁ CELLS WITH PATIENT'S SERUM	B CELLS WITH PATIENT'S SERUM
Group O Patient	Negative	Negative	Negative	Positive	Positive
Group A Patient	Positive	Negative	Positive	Negative	Positive
Group B Patient	Negative	Positive	Positive	Positive	Negative
Group AB Patient	Positive	Positive	Positive	Negative	Negative

*Routine testing with this reagent is not required.

☐ Cell Typing

☐ Serum Typing

Problems Encountered in ABO Typing

Problems encountered in ABO typing are frequently described as *ABO typing discrepancies.* The term *discrepancy* is used because problems are usually first seen when the cell type and the serum type do not match the previously described pattern. An example of such a case is a patient with a cell type of group A and a serum type of group O (patient's red blood cells are agglutinated by anti-A but not by anti-B; both A₁ and B reagent RBCs are agglutinated by the patient's serum). Beyond recognizing that cell and serum ABO blood typing does not match an expected pattern, the blood bank technologist must recognize any variations from expected strength or quality of reactivity normally seen in ABO testing and be aware that a problem exists.

Examples of these variations include:

▌ Abnormally weak agglutination. Generally ABO testing produces strong 3+ to 4+ agglutination (see "Estimated Number of ABO Antigen Sites on Different Blood Groups in Adults and Infants" on p 409).

▌ Mixed field agglutination. Some patients' RBCs are agglutinated by reagent antiserum whereas others are not.

Sometimes seen as a "halo" effect of unagglutinated RBCs adhering to the bottom of the test tube surrounding a "clump" of agglutinated cells.

When the tube is gently agitated to dislodge the cell button, the agglutinated portion in the center dislodges in a clump or several clumps from the central portion of the "halo."

Sometimes better visualized using the low power lens on the microscope.

▌ Rouleaux or RBC aggregation as opposed to true agglutination, characterized by stacked strings of RBCs or "stack of coins" appearance.

▌ "Clumping" due to blood clotting in the test procedure.

Characterized by odd formations of aggregated RBCs held together by fibrin strands; best visualized under the microscope

▌ RBCs trapped as "bystanders" to antibody-antigen complexes that do not involve RBC antigens have an appearance similar to that of mixed field agglutination.

▌ No agglutination (all cell and serum ABO typing tests are nonreactive).

▌ Agglutination in all cell and serum ABO typing tests.

COMMON CAUSES OF ABO BLOOD TYPING PROBLEMS

1. Incorrect use of reagents, contamination of reagents, or use of wrong or outdated reagents.
2. Failure to add reagents, patient's serum, or patient's cells.
3. Failure to follow manufacturer's instructions. The directions in the manufacturer's package insert must be followed for all testing procedures to avoid problems such as:

   Overcentrifugation or undercentrifugation causing false positive or false negative reactions, respectively.

   Incorrect incubation temperatures or time.

   Improper serum (commercial) to cell ratio in the test. Too many patient RBCs may cause a false negative result and too few cells make it difficult for the technologist to properly identify agglutination.

4. Typographic or transcription error in recording reactions or results.

NOTE   The results of *all* testing must be recorded immediately after reading *each* tube!

5. Incorrectly identified or switched specimens.
6. Dirty or contaminated glassware or supplies.
7. Incorrect or careless reading of weak agglutination. The anticipation of the normally strong ABO test agglutination can cause errors when weak agglutination is encountered.
8. Failure to identify hemolysis as a positive reaction.

CELL TYPING PROBLEMS: PATIENT'S RED CELLS WITH COMMERCIAL ANTISERUM

Type 1 Problem: Unexpected Agglutination in the Cell (Front or Forward) Typing

Agglutination of the patient's RBCs by commercial anti-A and/or anti-B does not correspond to agglutination of the reagent RBCs by the patient's serum, e.g., the patient's RBCs type as AB; the patient's serum types as B.

ABO BLOOD GROUP SYSTEM

	PATIENT'S CELLS WITH:		PATIENT'S SERUM WITH:	
Reagent	Anti-A	Anti-B	A₁ cells	B cells
Expected Reactions	+	0	0	+
Type 1 Problem Reactions	+	+	0	+

Causes

1. Antibody coated patient RBCs may cause spontaneous agglutination, e.g., cold reactive autoagglutinin. The patient may or may not have a positive direct antiglobulin test.
2. Recent blood transfusions or bone marrow transplant—transplant chimerism.
3. RBC polyagglutination, see "Identify and Characterize ABO Typing Problems Due to Polyagglutination" and discussion on causes and identification of polyagglutination on p 415.
4. Genetic or "acquired" anomalies affecting ABO type such as:

   Chimerism, caused most often by in utero transfer of blood group forming tissue from one twin to another creating a two cell population in the affected twin.

   Acquired B antigen, caused by deacetylase enzyme produced by bacteria. The enzymatic activity removes the acetyl group from the N-acetylgalactosamine of group A₁ RBCs. This results in a molecule that closely resembles galactosamine. This "galactosamine" can crossreact with antigalactose (anti-B), making it appear the B antigen is present.

5. Patient has antibody to a component in the reagent added during manufacturing, e.g., antiacriflavin (yellow dye used in some anti-B reagents). These antibodies can produce antibody-antigen complexes that are adsorbed onto the patient's RBCs, resulting in RBC agglutination (Rudmann, 1995).
6. Abnormally high levels of serum proteins or macromolecules may cause RBC aggregation mimicking true agglutination. Aggregation can also be caused by other contaminants like Wharton's jelly, a substance commonly found in cord blood.

Type 2 Problem: Lack of Expected Agglutination in the Cell (Forward or Front) Typing

The patient's RBCs are not agglutinated or are weakly agglutinated by commercial anti-A and/or anti-B, and the serum type does not correspond to the lack of agglutination in the cell type, e.g., the patient's cells type as group O and serum types as A.

	PATIENT'S CELLS WITH:		PATIENT'S SERUM WITH:	
Reagent	Anti-A	Anti-B	A₁ cells	B cells
Expected Reactions	+	0	0	+
Type 1 Problem Reactions	0/w+	0	0	+

Causes

1. Disease conditions, including leukemias and Hodgkin's disease, may result in weak expressions of A and B antigens (Beattie, 1972; Mollison et al, 1993).
2. RBCs of newborns, especially premature infants, may express A and B antigens weakly. This condition may persist until 6 months of age.
3. An ABO subgroup or some other genetic anomaly may cause weakened expression of A and B antigens. This may be due to:

   A reduced number of antigen sites on the RBCs of individuals of subgroups of A and B; refer to chart below.

   Qualitative differences in the ABO transferases produced

4. Recent blood transfusions, principally of group O red blood cells to patients of a different ABO type
5. Abnormally high concentrations of A and/or B substance in the patient's serum, which sometimes, although rarely, may neutralize the ABO typing reagent (Vengelen-Tyler, 1996).

*Estimated Number of ABO Antigen Sites on Different Blood Groups in Adults and Infants**

ANTIGENS	NUMBER OF SITES
A_1 (adults)	810,000–1,170,000 A
A_1 (newborns)	250,000–370,000 A
A_2 (adults)	240,000–290,000 A
A_2 (newborns)	140,000 A
A_3 (adults)	35,000 A
A_x (adults)	4,800 A
A_{end} (adults)	3,500 A
A_m (adults)	700 A
A_1B (adults)	460,000–850,000 A
A_1B (adults)	310,000–560,000 B
A_1B (newborns)	220,000 A
B (adults)	750,000 B
B (newborns)	200,000 B

(Bryant, 1982)

*This table demonstrates the differences in the number of antigen sites available for antibody binding and, therefore, a potential cause of variability in the strength of reactivity displayed in typing tests of various A and B blood groups.

SERUM TYPING PROBLEMS: PATIENT'S SERUM WITH COMMERCIAL RED BLOOD CELLS

Type 3 Problem: Unexpected Agglutination in the Serum (Reverse or Back) Typing

Patient's serum agglutinates commercial A_1 and/or B cells, and the patient's cell type does not correspond to the agglutination pattern in the serum type, e.g., the patient's serum types as group A and cells type as group O.

	PATIENT'S CELLS WITH:		PATIENT'S SERUM WITH:	
Reagent	Anti-A	Anti-B	A_1 cells	B cells
Expected Reactions	+	0	0	+
Type 1 Problem Reactions	+	0	+	+

Causes

1. Contaminants in the patient's serum, e.g.:

   Intravenous (IV) fluids used as plasma expanders, such as dextran or hetastarch (Hespan)

   Certain drugs that cause RBC aggregation or rouleaux

2. Abnormal serum protein levels or elevated fibrinogen levels found in some disease conditions, e.g., multiple myeloma or Waldenström's macroglobulinemia.

3. Unexpected alloantibody in the patient's serum, e.g.:

   An individual who belongs to a subgroup of A (e.g., A_2 or A_3) produces alloanti-A_1.

   Cold reactive alloantibody, other than anti-A or anti-B, reacts with reagent RBCs, e.g., anti-P_1, anti-Le^b, anti-M.

   Cold reactive autoantibody reacts with reagent RBCs.

NOTE Commercial reagent RBCs are *pooled cells,* a mixture of several donor RBCs; these RBC pools, unlike reagent RBCs used for antibody detection and antibody investigation testing, frequently express most of the antigens whose antibodies are commonly encountered.

4. Recent plasma transfusion. The patient's serum contains a passively acquired atypical cold reacting antibody, such as anti-M or anti-I, that was present in the transfused plasma.
5. Formation of fibrin strands that mimic agglutination when the test is centrifuged. This is usually due to incomplete clotting of the patient's "serum" before use in testing, especially when the patient is on heparin therapy.
6. Serum antibodies to chemicals used as a preservative in reagent RBCs. This can result in the formation of antibody-antigen complexes in the patient's serum that trap bystander RBCs, mimicking true agglutination (Vengelen-Tyler, 1996).

Type 4 Problem: Unexpected Lack of Agglutination in the Serum (Reverse or Back) Typing

The patient's serum does not agglutinate or weakly agglutinates commercial A_1 and/or B cells, and the patient's cell type does not correspond to the agglutination pattern in the serum type, e.g., the patient's serum types as group AB and cells type as group B.

	PATIENT'S CELLS WITH:		PATIENT'S SERUM WITH:	
Reagent	Anti-A	Anti-B	A$_1$ cells	B cells
Expected Reactions	0	+	+	0
Type 1 Problem Reactions	0	+	0/w+	0

Causes

1. Recent plasma transfusion with compatible but not group specific plasma, causing weakening of the patient's ABO test reactions, e.g., transfusion of large amounts of group AB plasma to a patient whose ABO group is not AB
2. Hypogammaglobulinemia (diminished production, inherited or acquired, of gamma globulins) This condition may be found in patients:

   Being treated with immunosuppressive drugs

   With congenital agammaglobulinemia

   With leukemias, i.e., chronic lymphocytic leukemia, and malignant lymphomas

   With immunodeficiency disease

3. Low isoagglutinin titers in newborns and elderly patients
4. Bone marrow or progenitor cell transplants
5. Unusual inheritance involving blood forming tissue, e.g., inherited chimerism—the result of in utero transfer and engraftment of blood forming tissue from one twin to another creating a two cell population

SUGGESTED APPROACHES TO SOLVING ABO TYPING PROBLEMS

PROBLEM	DISCREPANCY OBSERVED
Type 1	Unexpected agglutination of patient's RBCs with reagent antiserum
Type 2	Lack of expected reactions of patient's RBCs with reagent antiserum
Type 3	Unexpected agglutination of reagent RBCs with patient's serum
Type 4	Lack of expected agglutination of reagent RBCs with patient's serum

The determination or suspicion of a problem is usually based on one or more of several indicators, e.g.:

- A historical record of the patient's blood type that does not match current test results
- Weak agglutination in the cell and/or serum typing that does not match strong(er) agglutination patterns in the complementary reverse or cell typing
- Suspicious or abnormal looking agglutination (aggregation or rouleaux) in the discrepant (cell or serum) typing
- All positive or all negative reactions in both cell and serum tests

ABO BLOOD GROUP SYSTEM

ABO Typing Problem Solution Guide

PROBLEM	DESCRIPTION	GENERAL SOLUTION TECHNIQUE (REFER TO FOLLOWING SECTIONS)	SPECIFIC SOLUTION TECHNIQUE (REFER TO FOLLOWING SECTIONS)
Type 1	Unexpected agglutination in the cell (front) typing	1.1, 1.2, 1.5, 1.6, 1.7, 1.8	2.1, 2.2, 2.3
Type 2	Unexpected negative results (lack of agglutination) Expected agglutination significantly weaker than those in other typing reactions	1.1, 1.2, 1.3, 1.4, 1.5, 1.6, 1.7, 1.9	3.1, 3.2, 3.3, 3.4
Type 3	Unexpected agglutination in serum (back or reverse) typing	1.1, 1.2, 1.6, 1.9, 1.10	4.1, 4.2, 4.3, 4.4
Type 4	Unexpected negative results (lack of agglutination) Expected agglutination significantly weaker than those in other typing reactions	1.1, 1.2, 1.3, 1.4, 1.6	5.1, 5.2

NOTE Generally, the resolution method or technique with lower numbers within each category should be considered and, if necessary, investigated before continuing to the resolution method or technique with the next higher number.

1.0 General Solutions to ABO Blood Typing Problems

The following are some of the initial and basic steps that should be taken to resolve ABO typing discrepancies. It is prudent, in most cases, to consult this list and take the action described before undertaking the more demanding and labor intensive test procedures described in Sections 2.0, 3.0, 4.0, and 5.0.

1.1 Consult Reagent Manufacturer's Instructions Located in Reagent Package Insert and Repeat the Test Procedure

In addition to other interesting and useful information, the package insert defines specimen requirements, the concentration of the cell suspension to be used, centrifugation requirements, the incubation temperature and time, the detailed test procedure, controls to be used, interpretation of results, and limitations of the reagents and/or test procedure.

1.2 Obtain a New Patient Sample

Obtaining a new patient sample corrects for the cases in which the original specimen was collected incorrectly or was contaminated with IV fluid; cord blood can be contaminated with Wharton's jelly and/or mother's blood, causing incorrect or misleading results.

1.3 Inspect Sample Collection Date and Determine Its Age

Consult the reagent manufacturer's instructions for use to determine the sample storage recommendations for best testing results.

1.4 Determine or Confirm the Patient's Age

Infants and very young children may demonstrate weak expression of A and/or B antigens; in addition, their serum may contain insufficient titers of anti-A and/or anti-B to agglutinate reagent RBCs in routine serum typing (reverse or backtype) methods. It is also common for elderly patients to experience a significant reduction in antibody production resulting in weak or undetectable reactivity in serum typing tests.

1.5 Obtain Patient's Diagnosis

Patients with certain diseases, such as leukemia, may demonstrate weak expression of ABO antigens.

1.6 Obtain Patient's Transfusion History and Current Status

Patients who have been recently transfused with type compatible RBCs (not type specific) may demonstrate mixed field reactions in cell typing tests, e.g., a group A individual transfused with several units of group O RBCs. Patients who have undergone bone marrow transplantation may demonstrate a two cell population. This is known as *transplant chimerism.*

1.7 Wash Patient's Red Blood Cells with Normal Saline

Washing the patient's RBCs four times or more:

1. Removes some contaminants and abnormal serum proteins that could cause RBC aggregation. This allows recognition of true agglutination.
2. Removes plasma that may be contained in the RBC suspension. This resolves discrepancies (false negative results) due to an abnormally high concentration of A and/or B soluble blood group substance in the patient's serum that can neutralize the reagent antibodies.
3. Corrects discrepancies due to antibodies present in the patient's serum directed against dyes or other components in commercial reagents.

1.8 Determine if Polyagglutination is Present

Use commercially available plant lectins for those cases in which the patient's cells are agglutinated by all reagent and human sera. RBCs from these patients are agglutinated by those sera not expected to react with normal RBCs (e.g., AB plasma containing no detectable alloantibodies). See the section on polyagglutination and "Identify and Characterize ABO Typing Problems Due to Polyagglutination" on p 415.

1.9 Investigate the Sample for Possibility of A or B Subgroups

1. Consult "A and B Subgroup Typing Reactions with Common ABO Typing Reagents" on p 414 to determine if the reactions are in accordance with the patterns listed.
2. Test the patient's RBCs and serum with reagents other than those used for routine testing (e.g., anti-AB, anti-H, tests for transferases) if further information is necessary for characterization.

ABO BLOOD GROUP SYSTEM

A and B Subgroup Typing Reactions with Common ABO Typing Reagents

SUBGROUP	CELL TYPING				SERUM TYPING		COMMENTS
	Anti-A Human	Anti-A Monoclonal	Anti-B	Anti-A₁ Lectin	A₁ Cells	B Cells	
A₁	Strong	Strong	Negative	Strong	Negative	Positive	Reactions weak with anti-H
A₂	Strong	Strong	Negative	Negative	Negative (see comments)	Positive	1%–8% positive due to anti-A₁
A₃	Moderate mixed field	Strong	Negative	Negative	Negative	Positive	
Aint	Strong	Strong	Negative	Moderate	Negative	Positive	
Am	Weak	Data not available	Negative	Negative	Negative	Positive	
Ax	Weak to negative	Moderate	Negative	Negative	Positive (see comments)	Positive	Serum usually contains anti-A₁
Ael	Negative	Negative	Negative	Negative	Positive (see comments)	Positive	Serum usually contains anti-A₁
Aend	Weak	Data not available	Negative	Negative	Negative (see comments)	Positive	Serum does not contain anti-A₁
Abantu	Weak	Moderate	Negative	Negative	Positive (see comments)	Positive	Serum usually contains anti-A₁
Afinn	Weak	Data not available	Negative	Negative	Positive (see comments)	Positive	Serum usually contains anti-A₁
B₃	Negative	Negative	Mixed field	Negative	Positive	Negative	Secretes B and H substance
Bm	Negative	Negative	Negative	Negative	Positive	Negative	Secretes B and H substance
Bx	Negative	Negative	Weak	Negative	Positive	Positive	Secretes only H substance

1.10 Identify Interference Due to Cold Antibody

Perform an antibody screen, including the room temperature phase, to determine if an interfering cold reacting antibody is present in the patient's serum.

1.11 Identify and Characterize ABO Typing Problems Due to Polyagglutination

1. Polyagglutination occurs when RBC membranes are modified in vivo because of:

   A disease or some other process

   An inherited membrane abnormality

   With the exception of the Cad type, polyagglutination occurs because of exposure of antigen receptor sites on the RBC membrane that are normally hidden from the immune system. These exposed antigen sites cause agglutination by naturally occurring antibodies present in most adult human serum.
   There are four common types of polyagglutination: T, Tk, Tn, and Cad.

   T and Tk polyagglutination are caused by bacterial enzymatic activity, in vivo or in vitro. These types of polyagglutination are most often transient and are associated with patients infected with gram negative organisms. They can also occur in an old, bacterially contaminated blood sample.

   Cad polyagglutination is an inherited condition. Cad is believed to represent an enhanced form of Sd^a expression, in which Sd^a antigen sites are exposed and strongly agglutinated by most human sera. Anti-Sd^a is found in many adult human sera.

   Tn polyagglutination is due to a somatic mutation in a clone of hematopoietic cells. The line of cells derived from the mutation are Tn activated whereas other populations of cells are not. This gives rise to the classic mixed field appearance of the RBCs of Tn activated subjects when tested with ABO typing reagents. One population of cells is affected and has Tn activated characteristics (A-like), and the other population of cells is not affected.

   Characteristics of Tn polyagglutination:

   It is frequently associated with some hematologic disorder (Mollison et al, 1993).

   It has "A-like" characteristics: An *N*-acetylgalactosamine molecule is exposed, resulting in an A-like antigen. This causes Tn activated RBCs to react with anti-A, making group O cells appear as A cells and group B cells appear as AB (Harmening, 1994).

   It is a common cause of polyagglutination problems encountered in ABO blood typing.

   It is frequently persistent but has been known to disappear in some subjects.

2. Polyagglutination problems can be resolved. Increased use of monoclonal typing reagents has nearly eliminated polyagglutination as a cause for concern when performing routine blood typing tests. The antibodies found in normal adult human sera that are responsible for the detection of some forms of polyagglutination are no longer present in routinely used commercial monoclonal preparations.

ABO BLOOD GROUP SYSTEM

When detected, polyagglutination can be isolated as a cause of typing problems by the use of one of several methods:

Tn activation can be resolved by using enzyme premodified RBCs. Pretreating RBCs with proteolytic enzymes degrades the exposed antigens (cryptantigens) responsible for the interfering agglutination in the Tn activated RBCs. Enzyme pretreatment of the RBCs also enhances reactivity of true ABO agglutinins with their membrane determinants.

Polyagglutinable cells do not react with most cord sera.

Polyagglutinable cells can be identified and classified using commercially prepared lectin kits.

Characterizing Polyagglutination with Lectins

REACTIONS WITH:	NORMAL CELLS	TN+	CAD+	T+	TK+
Lectins					
Arachis hypogea	0	0	0	4+	2+
Salvia sclarea	0	4+	0	0	0
Salvia hominum	0	4+	4+	0	0
Glycine soja	0	4+	4+	4+	0

RESOLVING ABO BLOOD TYPING PROBLEMS

2.0 Procedures to Determine ABO Type in Samples Demonstrating Type 1 Discrepancies: Unexpected Agglutination of Patient's Red Blood Cells with Reagent Antiserum

2.1 Acquired "A-like" Antigen

Tn activation due to bacterial infection, among other factors, causes the appearance of an acquired "A-like" antigen (see the discussion of polyagglutination, Tn activation on p 415). Tn activation can be resolved by pretreatment of the patient's RBCs with proteolytic enzymes, principally papain. A-like antigen of Tn activated cells is destroyed by proteolytic enzymes, whereas true A antigen is enhanced.

2.2 Spontaneous Agglutination Due to Antibody Coated Red Blood Cells

Antibody coated RBCs can cause spontaneous agglutination in ABO testing, especially if the causative antibody is a strong IgM cold reacting autoantibody. Gentle elution with warm (37°–45°C) saline washes is the simplest method to remove these antibodies. This method sometimes requires repetition (two or more washes) but should be effective in removing sufficient antibody for accurate ABO typing. If elution methods fail, the RBCs can be treated with dithiothreitol (DTT). DTT destroys IgM antibody pentameric molecules by cleaving the disulfide bonds that connect its five subunits.

2.3 Acquired B Antigen

Acquired B antigen occurs only in group A_1 individuals. The serologic picture of acquired B antigen is that of a group AB patient in the cell typing (commonly weak reactions with anti-B) and a group A patient in the serum typing (agglutination of group B test RBCs).

The solution to the problem of obtaining an accurate ABO type of patients who have, or are suspected to have, an acquired B antigen involves both serologic testing and a thorough investigation of the patient's clinical history.

Many patients with acquired B antigen have an active infection, or a history of infection, with a gram negative organism; intestinal obstruction; or carcinoma of the rectum or colon. Bacterial enzymes (deacetylases) reach the circulation and act on RBCs to cleave the acetyl group from the group A blood group determinant (N-acetylgalactosamine). The resulting altered RBC antigen resembles the blood group B determinant (D-galactose), leading to agglutination of the patient's RBCs by commercial anti-B reagent or anti-B in the serum of other group B individuals. Characteristically, the anti-B detected in these patients is not an autoantibody and does not agglutinate their own RBCs that express the acquired B antigen.

Serologic testing helpful in resolving ABO discrepancies due to, or suspected to be due to, acquired B antigen includes:

1. Testing with a variety of commercially prepared monoclonal anti-B reagents, if available. Some of these reagents react with acquired B antigen, and some do not. The manufacturer's directions for reagent use includes information regarding the expected reactivity of that particular reagent with the acquired B antigen.
2. Testing the patient's RBCs with reagent or commercially prepared anti-B antiserum acidified to a pH of 6.0. Acidified anti-B will not agglutinate acquired B antigen; it will agglutinate RBCs that express true B antigen.
3. Testing the patient's saliva for the presence of soluble B blood group substance.
4. Treating the patient's RBCs with acetic anhydride. This reagent provides a source of the acetyl group that was removed from the RBC in vivo. If the patient is not genetically group B, the N-acetylgalactosaminyl transferase acts to attach the acetyl group provided by the acetic anhydride to the altered group A determinant. Acquired B antigen becomes nonreactive with reagent anti-B when reacetylation of the B-like antigen takes place, whereas true B RBCs, used as a control, continue to react with anti-B (Beattie, 1993).

3.0 Procedures to Determine ABO Type in Samples Demonstrating Type 2 Discrepancies: Lack of Expected Reactions of Patient's Red Blood Cells with Reagent Antiserum

3.1 Use of Extended Incubation Periods to Enhance Weak Cell Reactions

Incubate ABO typing test for an extended period (a half hour) at room temperature, or even at 4°C to enhance weak agglutination in cell testing.

ABO BLOOD GROUP SYSTEM

NOTE   Because of the prevalence of cold reactive autoantibodies, tests performed at 22° or 4°C must be accompanied by appropriate controls. Informative controls, such as group O reagent RBCs (antibody screening cells) and an autologous control, must be tested in parallel with the investigation of the patient's RBCs.

3.2 Use of Proteolytic Enzymes to Enhance Weak Agglutination

To enhance weak or absent reactions in ABO forward typing tests, the patient's RBCs can be treated with proteolytic enzymes before testing. RBCs treated with enzymes such as ficin, papain, or bromelain react more strongly with anti-A and anti-B reagents. Group O RBCs pretreated with the same proteolytic enzyme used for treatment of the patient's RBCs and tested in the same way as the patient's RBCs are an appropriate control for this procedure.

3.3 Adsorption and Elution of Anti-A and/or Anti-B from Patient's Red Blood Cells

Adsorption and subsequent elution of antibody contained in reagent antiserum is one definitive test to determine the ABO type of patient RBCs that fail to demonstrate agglutination with reagent anti-A and/or anti-B but are suspected to belong to a blood group other than group O.

1. Washed patient RBCs are incubated at room temperature with anti-A and anti-B and are then thoroughly washed after adsorption.
2. An eluate is prepared from the patient's adsorbed RBCs. Heat elution is the method of choice.
3. The eluate is tested against group A_1 and B reagent RBCs.
4. Agglutination in any test indicates that the patient's RBCs possessed the corresponding antigen, e.g.:

   Agglutination was noted in the tube containing A_1 but not B reagent RBCs.

   This agglutination indicates that the original sample of the patient's RBCs adsorbed anti-A but not anti-B.

   The patient appears to be group A.

NOTE   To validate the results obtained from this procedure, group O RBCs should be treated and tested in the same manner as the patient's RBCs

3.4 Determination of ABO Blood Group by Testing the Patient's Saliva

Seventy-eight percent of the population secrete ABH soluble blood group antigen in their body fluids. Testing the saliva of a secretor for the presence of soluble ABH antigens is another definitive test to resolve ABO discrepancies of this type. Briefly,

1. The saliva of a secretor contains A, B, or H (group O) antigen, depending on the genetic blood type.
2. The saliva is concentrated and enzymes are inactivated.
3. Soluble antigen in the concentrated saliva inhibits its complementary antibody contained in reagent anti-A, anti-B, and/or anti-H.

4. The reagent mixed with the patient's saliva will fail to agglutinate RBCs known to express the corresponding antigen, e.g.:

The saliva is concentrated and salivary enzymes are inactivated.

The treated saliva is added to separate test tubes containing diluted anti-A, anti-B, and anti-H and is incubated.

RBCs are added to the tube containing the complementary antisera (e.g. A_1 RBCs are added to the tube containing anti-A).

The test is centrifuged and read for agglutination. Results:

The tube with anti-A was agglutinated; the tubes with anti-B and anti-H were not. Interpretation:

The patient is blood group B and secretes B and H soluble blood group substances.

The B and H soluble blood group substances present in the patient's saliva inhibited the reactivity of the antibody in the diluted reagent anti-B and anti-H, rendering them nonreactive in the final test with B and O RBC samples.

Agglutination in the tube with the reagent anti-A and the group A test cell sample indicates there was no soluble blood group substance present in the patient's saliva that could bind to the anti-A antibody in the reagent.

5. The control system for this test, which must be run in parallel to validate the test results, is a set of tests that includes all the test components mentioned with the exception that saline is used instead of the patient's saliva. Appropriate agglutination in the control tubes indicates that the dilution of reagent antiserum did not abolish its ability to cause visual agglutination with the test RBC samples.

4.0 Procedures to Determine ABO Type in Samples Demonstrating Type 3 Discrepancies: Unexpected Agglutination of A_1 and B Reagent Red Cells by the Patient's Serum

4.1 Characterization of Serum Agglutination Reactions Due to Subgroups (A Subgroups Are Used in this Instance)

Unexpected agglutination with A_1 reagent RBCs is most often due to allo-anti-A_1 in the serum of a patient whose RBCs belong to a subgroup of A. After initial testing, the first step to resolve this problem should be to test:

▊ The patient's RBCs with anti-A_1 lectin
▊ The patient's serum with group A_2 and O reagent RBCs

Interpretation:

1. Lack of agglutination with anti-A_1 indicates that the RBCs do not express detectable A_1 antigen; the patient may be some other subgroup of A, group O, or group B.
2. Lack of agglutination with the A_2 cells indicates that the patient is not group B or O; serum from these individuals normally agglutinates A_2 RBCs.
3. Lack of agglutination with group O RBCs serves as a negative control and indicates that there are no detectable reactions attributable to other alloantibodies or to an autoantibody.

ABO BLOOD GROUP SYSTEM

The reaction pattern described is an indication that the antibody agglutinating the A_1 RBCs in the initial testing is most likely anti-A_1 found as an alloantibody in the serum of a patient who belongs to a subgroup of A.

If the reaction pattern in the testing described does *not* indicate the presence of anti-A_1, see later sections for additional suggestions.

NOTE It is important and informative to:
1. Test group O reagent RBCs (antibody screening cells) and an autologous control in parallel with the patient's serum grouping tests to control for and identify reactions due to the presence of autoantibodies and other, potentially misleading, cold reactive alloantibodies.
2. Test at least two additional group A_1 and two group A_2 reagent RBCs to comply with the requirement of the "rule of threes." See "Antibody Identification" in Chapter 26.

Refer to "A and B Subgroup Typing Reactions with Common ABO Typing Reagents" on p 414.

4.2 Characterization of Reactions Due to Cold Reactive Alloantibodies (Other Than Anti-A_1)

Cold reactive alloantibodies may, on occasion, react strongly with reagent RBCs used in ABO typing. Antibodies reacting in this way may appear to be anti-A or anti-B when, in fact, the observed reactions are due to an antibody directed at an antigen other than A or B. Antibodies with specificity for antigens such as I, P_1, or antigens in the MNS blood group system (especially M and N) are commonly the cause of this problem. This problem can be resolved by:

1. ABO typing tests performed at temperatures warmer than room temperature (e.g., 37°C) when cold agglutinins are present in the patient's serum is not recommended; ABO agglutination can be significantly diminished when testing is conducted at warmer temperatures. If ABO typing is attempted in this manner, it is essential to validate results with a positive control to avoid misinterpreting tests as negative. More suitable methods are described later.
2. Limiting the room temperature incubation of the serum (reverse or back) typing test to the minimal time required in the manufacturer's directions for reagent use. Appropriate controls to validate the test reactions should be tested in parallel with the serum typing test.

   If the interfering antibody continues to react strongly enough to obscure the interpretation of the patient's true ABO serum type:

   It must be identified.

   A_1 and/or B RBCs that lack the offending antigen must be selected for the serum (reverse) typing test.

NOTE RBCs from donor units or employees may be used for this purpose.

3. Using a commercial preparation of rabbit erythrocyte stroma (REST, Organon Teknika Corporation, Durham, N.C.). These stroma contain molecular structures that are similar to those of the human I and H antigen. This is useful

when anti-I in a patient's serum causes reactivity that makes identifying clinically significant IgG antibodies difficult. This preparation is not known to adsorb clinically important antibodies directed against antigens of the major blood group systems such as:

D, C, E, e, c, f, K, k, Kp^a, Kp^b, Js^a, Js^b, Fy^a, Fy^b, Jk^a, Jk^b, Le^a, Le^b, M, N, S, s

> **NOTE**   REST may adsorb anti-B from patient serum.

4.3 Characterization of Reactions Due to Cold Reacting Autoantibodies (Autoagglutinins)

Cold-reactive autoagglutinins may, on occasion, react strongly with reagent RBCs used in ABO typing. This problem can be resolved by:

1. Diluting the patient's serum and retesting. Normally, the patient's anti-A and/or anti-B is present in a significantly higher concentration than an autoagglutinin. The patient's serum may be diluted with normal saline to a point where the autoantibody is no longer reactive (usually 1:5 is sufficient), but reactivity of the patient's anti-A and anti-B is still detectable.
2. Autoadsorption of the patient's serum autoagglutinin with the patient's RBCs. A more technically demanding and longer but more reliable method to remove the autoantibody is adsorption of the autoantibody with the patient's RBCs. Group O donor RBCs may be substituted if there is an insufficient quantity of patient RBCs to perform this procedure.

> **NOTE**   Substituting group O donor RBCs for patient RBCs precludes testing the adsorbed serum for antibodies other than anti-A and anti-B.

This method reduces the amount of autoagglutinin in the patient's serum without appreciably reducing the reactivity of anti-A or anti-B.

> **NOTE**   1. The use of higher temperature reaction phases in ABO typing to reduce or abolish interfering reactions from a cold agglutinin may also reduce or abolish the reactivity of anti-A and/or anti-B.
>
> 2. Treatment of the patient's serum with DTT to destroy IgM cold agglutinins will destroy IgM anti-A and anti-B. This is a dangerous choice of a method to resolve this type of discrepancy as some patients have very little IgG anti-A or anti-B.

4.4 Removing Interference from Transfused Macromolecules (Intravenous Solutions), Abnormal Serum Proteins, or an Elevated Concentration of Serum Proteins

Tests using serum from patients who have abnormal or elevated levels of serum proteins or who have been treated with infusion of plasma expanders containing macromolecules may exhibit aggregation or rouleaux formation (a "stack" or chain formation of RBC aggregates) when tested with reagent, or even autologous, RBCs. This aggregation that in

ABO BLOOD GROUP SYSTEM

no way involves antigen-antibody binding can be mistaken for true agglutination in ABO serum typing tests. Aggregation can be differentiated from agglutination in the following manner:

1. "Saline displacement"

    Dilute the patient's serum to a point at which the aggregation no longer occurs (usually 1:2 or 1:4 is sufficient)

    Test the diluted serum against reagent A_1 and B RBCs

Commonly, the patient's anti-A and anti-B react at a significantly higher dilution than that required to disperse aggregation of this type.

2. "Saline replacement"

    Centrifuge the test serum–cell mixture a second time after observation of the suspected aggregation reaction

    Carefully remove the patient's supernatant serum with a Pasteur pipette

    Replace the patient's serum with an equal volume of normal saline

    Resuspend the test cell button in the saline

Aggregation will be dispersed by the addition of this small amount of saline; true agglutination will remain.

5.0 Procedures to Determine the ABO Type in Samples Demonstrating Type 4 Discrepancies: Lack of Expected Agglutination of Patient's Serum with Reagent A_1 and B Red Blood Cells

5.1 Obtain Precise and Accurate Patient Medical History and/or Clinical Information

Most problems of this type are more easily understood by collecting and assessing information about the patient's medical history. This problem most often occurs in the newborn (up to 6 months of age) and in the elderly patient. It may occur in immunocompromised patients or in patients with immunodeficiency diseases.

Low levels of anti-A and/or anti-B are often undetectable in routine ABO testing procedures. Reactivity can be enhanced by:

1. Using extended room temperature incubation periods (30 minutes°) of the serum-reagent red cell mixture
2. Incubating the test at 4°C°

5.2 Resolving Interference from an Abnormally High Concentration of Anti-A and/or Anti-B

Rarely, a patient's serum may contain abnormally high concentrations of anti-A and/or anti-B. In these cases all available antigen sites on the reagent RBCs are coated with antibody. As a result, no antigen sites are available to form lattices or antibody bridges that lead to visible agglutination. This phenomenon is called *prozone;* it can be resolved by

---

°Care must be taken to include controls (group O cells) that will detect auto and allo cold agglutinins (other than anti-A or anti-B) in the patient's serum.

diluting the patient's serum to a point at which the agglutination can be visualized. Testing doubling dilutions of the patient's serum in normal saline is useful in resolving this problem.

> **NOTE** Excellent methods for the procedures discussed in the section on resolving ABO typing problems are described in detail in the *Technical Manual* of the American Association of Blood Banks. Laboratory technologists wishing more information on these procedures should consult this publication.

$Rh_0(D)$ BLOOD GROUP SYSTEM

The $Rh_0(D)$ blood group system was named following the 1940 experiments of Karl Landsteiner and Alexander Wiener (Landsteiner and Wiener, 1940). In these experiments they immunized rabbits and guinea pigs by injecting them with rhesus monkey RBCs and discovered that the antibodies produced in experimental animals strongly agglutinated approximately 85% of human RBCs. Further investigation by Wiener (Wiener et al, 1940) and Philip Levine (Levine et al, 1940) determined that the "rhesus" antibody stimulated was indistinguishable from one that was produced in humans. This antibody causes severe hemolytic transfusion reactions and hemolytic disease of the newborn. The original antigen detected in the Rh blood group system was named $Rh_0(D)$ antigen (this antigen was later determined to be different from the $Rh_0(D)$ antigen and named LW, for Landsteiner and Wiener; see the section on the LW antigen on p 428).

The Rh blood group system is one of the most complex human blood group systems known. There are more than 40 antigens assigned to this system. In addition, it is a vitally significant blood group system, surpassed only in clinical importance by the ABO blood group system. Despite the complexity of this system, blood bank investigators are primarily concerned with its five major antigens, D, C, c, E, e. It is interesting that these were the first five antigens assigned to the Rh blood group system.

D, C, E, c, and e Antigens

COMPARISON OF ANTIBODY STIMULATING CHARACTERISTICS OF THE FIVE MAJOR Rh ANTIGENS

(Mollison et al, 1993)

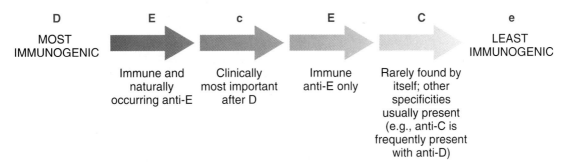

D	E	c	E	C	e
MOST IMMUNOGENIC	Immune and naturally occurring anti-E	Clinically most important after D	Immune anti-E only	Rarely found by itself; other specificities usually present (e.g., anti-C is frequently present with anti-D)	LEAST IMMUNOGENIC

$Rh_0(D)$ ANTIGEN

The significance of the $Rh_0(D)$ antigen involves its intense immunogenicity and the consequences of immunization to the $Rh_0(D)$ antigen. It has been reported that over 80% of

$Rh_0(D)$ negative individuals produce anti-D after receiving a single unit of $Rh_0(D)$ positive RBCs. $Rh_0(D)$ testing must be performed on the sample of every patient and donor for whom routine pretransfusion, presurgical, or prenatal testing is requested.

The immediate spin technique is sufficient to determine the $Rh_0(D)$ type of most prospective transfusion recipients. Agglutination of the test RBCs by reagent anti-D is interpreted as $Rh_0(D)$ positive; lack of agglutination is interpreted as $Rh_0(D)$ negative (see the section on ABO and $Rh_0(D)$ typing procedure on p 434).

RBCs from pregnant patients having prenatal or antepartum testing must be tested by the indirect antiglobulin test (IAT) when the immediate spin is nonreactive. This test identifies those individuals whose RBCs express "weak D" antigen.

WEAK D

The *weak D* terminology is currently used in place of the previous term, D^u. The designation *weak D* is applied when reagent anti-D fails to agglutinate test RBCs in the immediate spin test but they are subsequently agglutinated when the test is continued through the antiglobulin phase (indirect antiglobulin test [IAT]). Potent and specific monoclonal anti-D reagents now widely in use have the ability to detect $Rh_0(D)$ antigen in the immediate spin test on the RBCs of most individuals formerly classified as D^u.

The weak D phenotype occurs through one of several mechanisms:

1. The *C* gene is in the trans position (on the opposite chromosome) to the *D* gene. It is believed the *C* gene in trans position exerts a weakening influence on the *D* gene. Examples of genotypes giving rise to this type of weak D are *CDe/Ce* and *Dce/Ce*.

2. Weak D antigen is genetically transmitted. Inheritance of *D* genes that produce weakened forms of D antigen expression occurs most frequently in blacks of the $R^0(cDe)$ genotype; much less frequently, it occurs in whites with the $R^1(CDe)$ or $R^2(cDE)$genotypes.

3. The D antigen consists of multiple "pieces." Occasionally one or more of these pieces is missing. When this type of weak D is present, the RBCs are said to have *partial D.* $Rh_0(D)$ typing tests performed on the RBCs of these individuals may be positive, or the partial D antigen may result in initially negative typing tests with reagent anti-D, i.e., the individual who is a partial D can type either $Rh_0(D)$ positive or $Rh_0(D)$ negative. Individuals of the weak D phenotype can produce anti-D; in fact, partial D was recognized when potent anti-D was identified in the serum of apparently $Rh_0(D)$ positive individuals. In these cases, the anti-D is directed at the missing portion(s) of the $Rh_0(D)$ antigen; the antibody reacts with all common $Rh_0(D)$ positive RBCs. It is believed that some RBCs that express weak D antigen may elicit an immune response to the D antigen. It is important, therefore, to consider all factors in the criteria presented in the following section regarding indicated circumstances for weak D typing.

TESTING FOR $Rh_0(D)$ ANTIGEN IN THE HOSPITAL BLOOD BANK

1. The immediate spin technique is acceptable testing to determine the $Rh_0(D)$ type on prospective transfusion recipients.

2. In pregnant women whose samples are being investigated for prenatal or antenatal serologic problems, RBCs that test negative for $Rh_0(D)$ in the immediate spin test must be tested for weak D.

3. Obstetric patients who test negative for $Rh_0(D)$ and weak D are considered $Rh_0(D)$ negative and are candidates for Rh immune globulin (RhIg) prophylactic treatment.

4. There is controversy regarding RhIg candidacy of obstetric patients who belong to the weak D phenotype. It is unlikely that an individual of the weak D phenotype will produce anti-D. This issue should be clearly addressed by the laboratory standard operating procedure as determined by the blood bank medical director.

5. Newborns of $Rh_0(D)$ negative mothers should be tested for weak D. Mothers of infants negative for $Rh_0(D)$ and weak D are not candidates for RhIg prophylaxis. Mothers of infants positive for $Rh_0(D)$ or weak D are candidates for RhIg prophylaxis

6. Weak D testing is always performed on blood donors. A blood donor must be D and weak D negative to be considered $Rh_0(D)$ negative.

C, E, c, AND e ANTIGENS

1. There is no requirement to test for or match these antigens in transfusion therapy unless the patient develops the complementary antibody or the antibody is suspected to be present in the serum.

2. Potent commercial reagent antisera are readily available for typing patients and donors for these Rh antigens when necessary.

3. These antigens are immunogenic to varied degrees and often cause antibody production in antigen negative patients transfused with antigen positive RBCs.

4. These antigens, in conjunction with the $Rh_0(D)$ antigen, are the cause of production of many of the serum antibodies detected in routine blood bank testing.

CcEe ANTIGEN TESTING IN THE HOSPITAL OR CLINICAL BLOOD BANK

The commercially prepared reagent antisera used to test for these antigens are similar in nature to those available for $Rh_0(D)$ typing (see the section on ABO and $Rh_0(D)$ typing methods on p 432).

> **NOTE** The manufacturer's directions for the use of these reagents should be carefully followed. This is particularly true of high protein reagents since the recommended temperature and time of incubations can vary. Recommended controls vary with the composition of the reagent selected, and, in some cases, the use of the reagent in the IAT may or may not be indicated.

Other Rh Blood Group System Antigens

The routine hospital blood bank or transfusion service is rarely required to test patients or donors for Rh antigens other than D, C, c, E, or e. Antisera to identify other antigens in this blood group system are very rare. However, all technologists working in the blood bank must be aware of the polymorphism in the Rh blood group system and the fact that the uncommon antigens can stimulate an immune response in the antigen negative transfusion recipient. Many of the antibodies produced in response to exposure to antigens of the Rh blood group system are capable of causing accelerated in vivo RBC destruction and/or hemolytic disease of the newborn (HDN).

G ANTIGEN

The G antigen is found on most C positive and/or $Rh_0(D)$ positive RBCs. Originally anti-G was thought to be anti-D plus anti-C. The true specificity of the antigen was determined when $Rh_0(D)$ negative, C negative (rr) individuals transfused only with $Rh_0(D)$ positive, C negative donors developed apparent anti-D and anti-C.

Absorptions and elutions of this serum with r'r and Ro RBCs were inconsistent with the presence of only anti-D+anti-C. In addition, an r^Gr individual was found. The antibody was determined to be anti-G, an antibody directed against a single antigenic determinant. Anti-G can occur in conjunction with anti-D and/or anti-C. Transfusion of patients with these antibodies is not a problem since the patient can be transfused with rr (G negative) donor RBCs.

C^W ANTIGEN

The C^W antigen is associated in an undefined way with the C antigen. C^W is found in approximately 2% of whites and rarely in blacks. Anti-C^W can be produced after exposure to the antigen through transfusion or pregnancy. It has also been reported in individuals with no known exposure to foreign RBCs (Harmening, 1994). In the hospital blood bank or transfusion service, anti-C^W is not a transfusion problem since 98% of random donors are compatible.

COMPOUND OR *Cis* PRODUCT ANTIGENS

These antigens are more interesting than problematic in the hospital blood bank setting. They represent distinct specificities encoded by the same haplotype, hence the *cis* product designation. Their incidence may be higher than the relatively rare rate of encounter reported because they are commonly detected along with Rh antibodies. Their presence must be defined by testing serum after adsorption with RBCs of selected Rh phenotypes that possess only one of the compound antigenic determinants.

Nomenclature of More Common Compound or *Cis* Product Antigens

NUMERICAL DESIGNATION	CDE (FISHER-RACE)	RH-HR (WEINER)
Rh6	ce(f)	hr
Rh7	Ce	rh_i
Rh22	CE	rh_y
Rh27	cE	rh

Providing compatible donor blood to patients with antibodies to compound antigens is no more difficult than providing donor RBCs compatible with the serum of patients with distinct antibodies to the same antigens. The interesting aspect of these compound antigens lies in their complementary antibodies rather than the antigens themselves. These antibodies enable the blood bank technologists, especially those involved in parentage testing, to establish the specific genotype of an individual when ordinarily only the phenotype can be determined.

Anti-f(ce) serves as an example of this determination:

Anti-f + RBCs of phenotype CcDEe
$$= \text{agglutination with genotype CDE/ce}$$
$$= \text{no agglutination with genotype CDe/cDE}$$

GENE DELETIONS AND Rh NULL

Gene deletions are a rare genetic anomaly infrequently encountered in the hospital blood bank. These phenotypes occur because of the inheritance of genes at the Rh locus that fail to encode for detectable Rh antigens on the RBC membrane. This condition is detected in the blood bank laboratory when a complex allotypic antibody is detected, generally in routine antibody screening. These antibodies are extremely difficult to identify and/or specify in the routine testing laboratory. There may also be evidence of an apparently incomplete Rh phenotype in RBC testing, e.g., in the phenotype $-D-$ (D deleted) when the results of testing RBCs with anti-C, anti-c, anti-E, and anti-e all appear to be negative.

Rh$_{null}$

Rh$_{null}$ is an extremely rare genetic condition affecting the formation of all Rh antigens. This syndrome arises by one of two genetic pathways:

1. Absence of a modifier gene that does not directly code for Rh antigens but is required for their expression. This modifier gene, $X^l r$, is absent in Rh$_{null}$ individuals and is replaced by the rare $X^0 r$ gene ($X^0 r/X^0 r$). The lack of this modifier gene prevents the expression of all Rh antigens in an individual who usually possesses the commonly inherited Rh genes.
2. Inheritance, in the homozygous state, of an amorphic gene, $\overline{rr}$, at the Rh locus that prevents production of all Rh antigens.

Because the Rh protein appears to be an integral part of the RBC membrane, RBCs of individuals of the Rh$_{null}$ phenotype are structurally abnormal; stomatocytes are apparent on smears made from peripheral blood. Rh$_{null}$ individuals experience a persistent chronic hemolytic anemia, the severity of which varies. These individuals are generally recognized when unusual antibodies are detected in their serum during routine pretransfusion testing. Their antibodies, and subsequent characterization of the Rh$_{null}$ syndrome, are difficult to characterize in the routine hospital blood bank laboratory. The services of the regional reference laboratory are generally required in these cases. Transfusion of these individuals is difficult; they must receive RBCs from another individual of the Rh$_{null}$ phenotype. Regional or national suppliers of rare blood must be involved in this process.

For a more complete discussion on Rh$_{null}$ the reader is encouraged to review *Blood Transfusion in Clinical Medicine* by Mollison and colleagues.

Rh$_o$(D) BLOOD GROUP SYSTEM

Rh$_{mod}$

Rh$_{mod}$ individuals do not completely lack Rh antigen products, but the expression of the Rh antigens is so depressed that they are undetectable in routine Rh typing tests. More complex serologic techniques must be used to detect and characterize Rh antigens in these individuals.

LW BLOOD GROUP SYSTEM

The antibody identified as anti-Rh in the early research in which rabbits produced antibody after exposure to RBCs from rhesus monkeys (Landsteiner and Wiener) was later determined to be different from the antibody produced in humans.

It was observed that the antibody described by Landsteiner and Wiener reacted more strongly with true Rh$_0$(D) positive human RBCs; but this original antibody was also found to react, although very weakly, with many Rh$_0$(D) negative human RBCs. Levine later identified an antibody that failed to agglutinate approximately 16% of human RBCs. This new antibody was found to define the Rh[Rh$_0$(D)] human antigen and was named anti-D. The LW blood group was then named to honor its discoverers, Landsteiner and Wiener.

LW Genes and Inheritance

The LW blood group system contains two antithetical alleles, LW^a and LW^b. LW genes and their encoded antigens are inherited separately from the Rh system, and although not completely understood, it is apparent that the formation of LW antigen requires a form of regulator influence by Rh genes for their full expression. Rh$_{null}$ cells are also LW(a−b−), and anti-LW^a binds more readily and completely to Rh$_0$(D) positive LW(a+) RBCs than it does to Rh$_0$(D) negative LW(a+) RBCs. The inheritance and frequencies of the LW antigens are illustrated in the chart below.

Antibodies to LW Antigens

Antibodies to LW antigens generally do not cause difficulties in transfusion. Transient forms of anti-LW^a produced by LW(a+) individuals (autoanti-LW) present no transfusion problems. No significant adverse effects have been reported when these patients are transfused with LW(a+) blood; these antibodies have not been implicated in hemolytic transfusion reactions (HTRs) or in HDN. Anti-LW^a and anti-LW^{ab} produced respectively in LW(a−) and LW(a−b−) individuals must be considered potentially hemolytic. However, reports of HTR or HDN, even in these patients, is rare.

Identifying Anti-LW$^{a(ab)}$

- Anti-LW reacts more strongly with Rh$_0$(D) positive RBCs than with Rh$_0$(D) negative cells.
- Anti-LW reacts equally well with cord cells, regardless of Rh$_0$(D) type.
- LW antigen is not destroyed by enzyme treatment with ficin or papain.
- LW antigen is denatured by sulfhydryl reagents such as DTT.

All these characteristics help differentiate anti-LW from anti-D.

PHENOTYPES AND FREQUENCIES IN THE LW SYSTEM

REACTIONS WITH		GENOTYPE	PHENOTYPE	PHENOTYPE FREQUENCY (%)
Anti-LWª	**Anti-LWᵇ**			
+	0	*LWªLWª* or *LWªLW*	LW(a+b−)	Very rare
0	0	*LWLW*	LW(a−b−)	Very rare
+	+	*LWªLWᵇ*	LW(a+b+)	<1
0	+	*LWᵇLWᵇ* or *LWᵇLW*	LW(a−b+)	>99

Clinical Significance of the Rh System in Routine Transfusion Therapy

The Rh system is an extremely important consideration to the transfusion service for three main reasons:

1. The system has a high degree of polymorphism (many various combinations of Rh system antigenic determinants that are either present in a homozygous or heterozygous state or absent).
2. Unlike those in the ABO system, antibodies in the Rh blood group system are not naturally occurring. Antibody production is stimulated through contact with foreign RBCs in pregnancy or transfusion. Antibody production can occur after a single blood transfusion and is even more likely when a second contact occurs. This leads to transfusion complications and the need for frequent antibody screening on multiply transfused patients (see the section on antibody detection testing on p 456).
3. The $Rh_0(D)$ antigen is second only to the antigens in the ABO blood group system in its ability to stimulate an antibody response. Similarly, the C, E, c, and e antigens are known to be highly immunogenic (though not on a level with D antigen). In addition, these antigens frequently stimulate a combination of antibodies, e.g. anti-E and anti-c are frequently found together, as are anti-D and anti-C.

In routine clinical practice the Rh system is defined through the use of five readily available commercial typing sera. These reagents meet all the requirements of the routine transfusion service and hospital blood bank.

NOMENCLATURE OF THE MAJOR Rh SYSTEM ANTIGENS

FISHER-RACE CDE	WIENER RH-HR	ROSENFIELD NUMERICAL
D	Rh_0	Rh1
C	rh′	Rh2
E	rh″	Rh3
c	hr′	Rh4
e	hr″	Rh5

$Rh_0(D)$ BLOOD GROUP SYSTEM

Rh SYSTEM REACTION PATTERNS WITH ROUTINE ANTISERA AND GENOTYPE FREQUENCIES*

REACTIONS WITH ROUTINE TYPING SERA					MOST COMMON GENOTYPE			OTHER GENOTYPES	
Anti-D	Anti-C	Anti-E	Anti-c	Anti-e	Rh-hr	CDE	Frequency (%)	CDE	Combined Frequency
+	+	−	+	+	R^1r	CDe/ce	32.68	CDe/cDe cDe/Ce	2.21
+	+	−	−	+	R^1R^1	CDe/Ce	17.68	CDe/Ce	0.83
−	−	−	+	+	rr	ce/ce	15.10	None	NA
+	+	+	+	+	R^1R^2	CDe/cDE	11.86	CDe/cE Ce/cDE CDE/ce CDE/cDe CE/cDe	1.50
+	−	+	+	+	R^2r	cDE/ce	10.97	cDE/cDe cDe/cE	0.79
+	−	−	−	+	R^0r	cDe/ce	2.00	cDe/cDe	0.07
+	+	+	−	−	R^2R^2	cDE/cDE	1.99	cDE/cE	0.34
−	−	+	−	+	r″r	cE/ce	0.92	None	NA
−	+	−	−	+	r′r	Ce/ce	0.76	None	NA
+	+	+	−	+	R^ZR^1	CDE/CDe	0.20	CDE/Ce	<0.01
+	+	+	+	−	R^ZR^2	CDE/cDE	0.07	CDE/cE	<0.01

*Genotypes shown represent >99.9% of the population

NATURE OF ANTIBODIES TO ANTIGENS OF THE Rh BLOOD GROUP SYSTEM

1. Rh antibodies are usually produced as a result of exposure to foreign RBCs.
2. Antibodies are, with few exceptions, IgG and react optimally at 37°C with antiglobulin reagent.
3. Rh antibodies do not bind complement.
4. Most Rh antibodies persist for many years.
5. Rh antibodies cause HDN.
6. Rh antibody cell destruction is extravascular, frequently of the delayed hemolytic type. These reactions may proceed rapidly, once begun, and can be severe and life threatening.
7. Rh antibodies may be any one of the four IgG subclasses (IgG_1, IgG_2, IgG_3, IgG_4), with those in subclasses IgG_1 and IgG_3 being far more destructive.

Practical Aspects of Rh Blood Typing

The blood bank technologist should not expect to encounter the number of problems in Rh typing tests that might be encountered when determining an ABO type. Monoclonal Rh typing antisera have improved to such an extent that false positive or false negative reactions due to the reagent used are rarely encountered.

> **NOTE** It is important for the blood bank technologist to refer to the individual manufacturer's instructions for the use of each individual Rh typing reagent. This review should include careful consideration of the negative Rh control to be employed with each type of reagent.

PROBLEMS ENCOUNTERED IN Rh TYPING

False Positive Reactions

PROBLEM	NEGATIVE RH CONTROL	SOLUTION
1. Wrong reagent used (i.e., anti-A,B), or failure to follow reagent manufacturer's instructions for use.	0	Select correct reagent and repeat test. Read manufacturer's reagent package insert and follow instructions.
2. Positive direct antiglobulin test on cells to be Rh typed.	+	Use low protein or saline based reagent. In severe cases, heat elution or chloroquine treatment can be used to dissociate IgG antibody coating cells. *Weak D testing is invalid.*
3. Abnormally high protein level or macromolecules (dextran) in patient's serum causes aggregation or rouleaux.	+	Wash test cells in normal saline minimum of four times and repeat typing.
4. Cold autoagglutinin causes agglutination.	+	Wash test cells in warm (37°–45°C) normal saline at least four times and repeat typing.
5. Contaminated reagent vial containing foreign substances, bacteria, or crosscontamination with other reagents.	0	Inspect vial for foreign objects, tubidity, or discoloration. Look at reagent under high power microscope. Institute meticulous procedures to avoid crosscontamination of reagent vials. Keep reagents in refrigerator storage when not in use.
6. Patient may have polyagglutinable cells.	+	Try monoclonal reagent or reagent not based on human serum as diluent medium. See discussion on polyagglutination on p 415.
7. Reagent may have contaminating antibody of another specificity.	0	This rare occurrence usually involves antibody to very low frequency antigen that was not detected by manufacturer. Select different manufacturer's reagent or at minimum different lot number of same manufacturer. Report incident to manufacturer.

Rh₀(D) BLOOD GROUP SYSTEM

False Negative Reactions

PROBLEM	NEGATIVE RH CONTROL	SOLUTION
1. Failure to add antisera to test or adding wrong reagent	0	Select and add correct reagent and repeat typing.
2. Failure to follow manufacturer's directions, i.e., undercentrifugation or incorrect incubation time	0	Read manufacturer's package insert instruction for that particular reagent and repeat typing.
3. RBC suspension is too heavy	0	Read manufacturer's cell suspension requirements and adjust cell suspension and repeat typing.
4. Improper technique used, e.g., cell button suspended from bottom of tube too vigorously, agglutination broken up	0	Use proper technique to resuspend cell buttons.
5. Impotent, old, or outdated reagent used or reagent stored improperly	0	Use fresh reagent and test against known control cells; then repeat typing.

NOTE In the case of false negative Rh typings, the negative Rh control provides no help in problem recognition. In this case a known Rh positive control can be run along with the test procedure, or the technologist should refer to the daily reagent quality control performed on the reagent vial in use.

ROUTINE ABO AND RH₀(D) TYPING METHODS AND REAGENTS

ABO Typing Reagents

ABO blood group typing reagents are obtained from two sources, human and murine monoclonal. Monoclonal ABO antiserum reagents will soon completely replace human source reagents. Monoclonal reagents of this type have several advantages over human source reagents. These advantages include the following:

1. They are easier and cheaper to manufacture.
2. They are free from transmissible viral diseases.
3. They are more potent and specific.
4. They contain less potentially contaminating interfering antibodies.

Further discussion on ABO typing and typing procedures assumes the use of murine monoclonal ABO antisera.

Serum typing is performed with pools of A and B $Rh_0(D)$ negative human RBCs that are suspended in a diluent (Alsever's solution with other bactericidal chemicals and preservatives) in a concentration of approximately 3% to 5%.

Rh Typing Reagents

Two basic types of commercial Rh typing reagents are available, and are classified by their protein content as *high protein* or *low protein* reagents.

HIGH PROTEIN REAGENTS

High protein anti-D reagents are specifically used in slide or tube testing. These reagents typically contain about 20% to 30% protein or other high molecular weight additive. This concentration of protein varies somewhat between different manufacturers. The protein is added to reduce the zeta potential between RBC membranes and increase the strength of immediate spin agglutination. The disadvantage to a high protein reagent is that the increase in Rh antibody-antigen interaction can also cause spontaneous agglutination of RBCs. This is especially true of those cells coated with immunoglobulin (whether by antigen-antibody interaction, adsorption, or other means) that have a positive direct antiglobulin test. This introduces the potential for a false positive Rh typing and demonstrates the need (and requirement) to run an Rh control with each Rh typing test performed with this reagent. Because of this and the fact that high protein reagents are of human source, they are quickly fading from use.

LOW PROTEIN REAGENTS

Low protein reagents can be further broken down into three types, chemically modified reagents, saline reagents, and monoclonal or blended monoclonal-polyclonal reagents.

Chemically Modified Reagents

Chemically modified reagents contain IgG anti-Rh antibodies obtained from a human source that have been converted to direct agglutinating antibodies by sulfhydryl reduction of their interchain disulfide bonds. This allows the antibody to "span" a far greater distance between antigens located on different RBC membranes. Chemically modified reagents do not always fall strictly into the low protein category and might be better characterized as medium protein, depending on the manufacturer. Therefore, an Rh control is necessary if no negative test is encountered in the ABO and Rh typing procedure (i.e., AB, Rh positive typing), but for A, B, O, or Rh negative patients, no Rh control is required. Chemically modified reagents are rarely used and will probably soon be unavailable.

Saline Reagents

Saline reagents are obtained from relatively rare donors that produce IgM anti-Rh antibodies. The donor serum containing the antibody is prepared in a saline medium and is equivalent to an approximately 6% albumin solution that can be used (though not required) as a control. Saline reagents are very useful to solve an Rh typing problem when the Rh control is positive in an Rh typing test using a high protein reagent. Saline reagents cannot be used for the weak D (D^u) test.

Monoclonal, Monoclonal-Polyclonal Blend Reagents

Monoclonal anti-Rh reagents are prepared from an IgM antibody produced by a single human clone. These antibodies have a very narrow specificity and react strongly at room temperature with short incubation periods. Most manufacturers use a blended reagent for anti-D, which may contain a single monoclonal IgM anti-D or a blend of several monoclonal IgM anti-Ds as well as some form of IgG anti-D for use in the weak D (D^u) test. This IgG antibody may be obtained from human serum or it may also be a monoclonal antibody. The monoclonal source reagents are the most potent Rh typing reagents available and eventually will be manufactured entirely from sources that are virtually incapable of transmitting disease. It is now the most popular anti-D reagent and will, like ABO reagents, probably be the only continuous source of commercial anti-D reagent. Manufacturers generally do not require an Rh control for these reagents except when an AB Rh positive patient is encountered. In this case, a 6% to 8% albumin (in normal saline) control is recommended.

SUGGESTED ABO AND Rh TYPING PROCEDURE

NOTE This procedure has been adapted from a manufacturer's package insert directions. It should not be used universally without comparing it with the manufacturer's package insert directions for the specific set of reagents to be used. *Failure to follow the manufacturer's specific directions may lead to erroneous ABO and/or Rh typing results.*

Text continued on page 439

| Author: | | New | | Reviewed | | | | |
| Version: | | Revised | | Reviewed | | | | |

CMC TECHNICAL MANUAL

City Medical Center **Blood Bank** Riverside Lane New City, CA 99999	Subject: **Routine ABO and Rh$_o$(D) Typing**	
	Procedure # 999.999.99.99	Page 1 of 4
	Approved by: M.D.	Document #

PURPOSE:
To determine the ABO blood group and Rh$_o$(D) type of patients or whole blood donors.

PRINCIPLE:
Direct agglutination of red cells with a particular reagent antibody indicates the presence of the corresponding antigen. No agglutination generally indicates the absence of the corresponding antigen (see "Notes and Limitations"). Agglutination of reagent red cells of a known ABO type generally indicates the presence of an antibody against that ABO type of red blood cells. The ABO group can be determined by the combination of reagents used and their reactions based on an established pattern of the reagent antibodies and reagent red cells used to test the blood sample. The Rh type is determined by the presence (positive test) or the absence of the D antigen when reacted against reagent anti-D (see "Results and Interpretations").

STAFF RESPONSIBILITY:
All blood bank technologists are required to perform this testing.

MATERIALS:
1. Reagents:
   - Commercial anti-A, monoclonal
   - Commercial anti-B, monoclonal
   - Commercial anti-A,B, monoclonal, OPTIONAL for patient testing—REQUIRED for donor testing
   - Commercial A$_1$ human red blood cells
   - Commercial B human red blood cells
   - Commercial anti-D, monoclonal-polyclonal blend
2. 10 x 75 mm test tubes
3. Test tube rack
4. Plastic transfer pipets
5. Serologic centrifuge
6. Isotonic saline
7. Timer
8. Glassware marking pen
9. Saline filled wash bottle
10. Incubator, 37°C, optional for test for weak D
11. Anti-human globulin—anti-IgG, optional for test for weak D
12. Coombs control cells, optional for test for weak D

SPECIMEN:
Normal approved phlebotomy technique is sufficient for specimen collection. Specimens may be collected in any of the following media but should be tested in the appropriate time limit for the collection media.

City Medical Center **Blood Bank** Riverside Lane New City, CA 99999	Subject: **Routine ABO and Rh$_o$(D) Typing**
	Procedure # 999.999.99.99 Page 2 of 4

Approved Collection Media	Must Be Tested Within:
Clotted whole blood	14 days
Sodium citrate	14 days
Oxalate	14 days
ACD	28 days
CPD	28 days
CPDA-1	35 days

NOTE: Other collection media may be appropriate for the reagents used but are not approved by City Medical Center Blood Bank

METHOD:

ABO Red Cell Testing—Front (Forward) Type

1. Prepare a 3% to 5% cell suspension (in saline) of the red cells to be tested.
2. Label 2 or 3 clean test tubes as follows : tube #1: anti-A or (A), #2: anti-B or (B) and OPTIONALLY (required with donor testing) label tube #3: anti-A,B or (A,B).
3. Place 1 drop of commercial anti-A in tube #1 (A), 1 drop of commercial anti-B in tube #2 (B) and OPTIONALLY 1 drop of commercial anti-A,B in tube #3 (A,B)
4. Using a transfer pipet, add to each of the tubes 1 drop of the 3% to 5% cell suspension of the red cells to be tested.
5. Mix the contents of each tube thoroughly and centrifuge for 15 to 30 seconds at high speed. Use centrifuge calibrated for 900–1000 x g.
6. Gently agitate each tube to resuspend the red cell buttons.
7. Read macroscopically; interpret and record the results of each tube.

Rh$_o$ (D) Testing

8. Label 1 or 2 clean test tubes as follows : tube #4: Anti-D or (D), and OPTIONALLY label tube #5: Rh control or (CRL).
9. Place 1 drop of commercial anti-D in tube #4 (D).
10. Place 1 drop of a 6% to 8% albumin or isotonic saline solution in tube #5 (CRL) if optional Rh control is used.
11. Using a transfer pipet, add to each of the tubes 1 drop of the 3% to 5% cell suspension of the red cells to be tested.
12. Mix the contents of each tube thoroughly and centrifuge for 15 to 30 seconds at high speed. Use centrifuge calibrated for 900–1000 x g.
13. Gently agitate each tube to resuspend the red cell buttons.
14. Read macroscopically; interpret and record the results of each tube. If the test is negative, the weak D test must be completed on all donor samples and cord samples of Rho(D) negative mothers. Continue with step 23 for the weak D test.

ABO Serum Testing—Back (Reverse) Type

15. Label 2 clean test tubes as follows : tube #6: A$_1$ Cells or (A$_1$), and tube #7: B Cells or (B).
16. Using a transfer pipet, add to each of the tubes 2 or 3 drops of serum from the sample to be typed.
17. Add 1 drop of commercial A$_1$ cells to tube #6 (A$_1$).
18. Add 1 drop of commercial B cells to tube #7 (B).
19. Mix the contents of each tube thoroughly and centrifuge for 15 to 30 seconds at high speed. Use centrifuge calibrated for 900–1000 x g.
20. Examine tubes for any hemolysis in the supernatant prior to resuspending cell buttons.
21. Gently agitate each tube to resuspend the red cell buttons.
22. Read macroscopically, interpret and record the results of each tube.

Weak D Test—For additional information see section on antiglobulin testing beginning on p 439.

23. Incubate tube #4 (D) at 37°C for a minimum of 15 minutes and a maximum of 60 minutes.
24. After incubation, wash tube #4 (D) 4X in normal saline, decanting saline completely between washes and after the last wash.

City Medical Center **Blood Bank** Riverside Lane New City, CA 99999	Subject: **Routine ABO and Rh₀(D) Typing**	
	Procedure # 999.999.99.99	Page 3 of 4

25. Add 2 drops of anti-human globulin (anti-IgG).
26. Mix the contents of each tube thoroughly and centrifuge for 15 to 30 seconds at high speed. Use centrifuge calibrated for 900–1000 x g.
27. Gently agitate each tube to resuspend the red cell buttons.
28. Read macroscopically; interpret and record the results of each tube.

NOTE: All samples tested for weak D must have a negative direct antiglobulin test prior to reporting a positive weak D interpretation. A positive DAT makes the interpretation of a positive weak D test invalid.

Suggested Serologic Rack Arrangement—Shaded tubes are optional

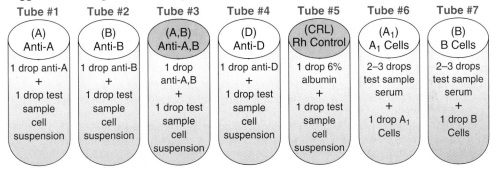

Tube #1	Tube #2	Tube #3	Tube #4	Tube #5	Tube #6	Tube #7
(A) Anti-A	(B) Anti-B	(A,B) Anti-A,B	(D) Anti-D	(CRL) Rh Control	(A₁) A₁ Cells	(B) B Cells
1 drop anti-A + 1 drop test sample cell suspension	1 drop anti-B + 1 drop test sample cell suspension	1 drop anti-A,B + 1 drop test sample cell suspension	1 drop anti-D + 1 drop test sample cell suspension	1 drop 6% albumin + 1 drop test sample cell suspension	2–3 drops test sample serum + 1 drop A₁ Cells	2–3 drops test sample serum + 1 drop B Cells

RESULTS AND INTERPRETATIONS:

ABO Typing

29. Agglutination and/or hemolysis constitutes a positive test result.
30. A red cell button that resuspends smoothly with no agglutination or hemolysis constitutes a negative test result.
31. Interpretation of cell and serum tests for ABO is given below.
32. Any discrepancies between the cell and serum types must be resolved before reporting results.

NOTE: In emergencies, group O red blood cells must be provided until ABO discrepancies are resolved.

Normal Reactions With Commercial ABO Typing Reagents

	Anti-A with patient's cells	Anti-B with patient's cells	Anti-A,B with patient's cells	A₁ cells with patient's serum	B cells with patient's serum	
Group O Patient	Negative	Negative	Negative	Positive	Positive	Cell Typing
Group A Patient	Positive	Negative	Positive	Negative	Positive	
Group B Patient	Negative	Positive	Positive	Positive	Negative	
Group AB Patient	Positive	Positive	Positive	Negative	Negative	Serum Typing

Rh₀(D) Typing

33. Agglutination of the test sample red cells is a positive test indicating the sample is Rh₀(D) positive.
34. No agglutination of the test sample red cells is a negative test indicating the sample is Rh₀(D) negative. Red cells appearing to be Rh₀(D) negative by this test method can be

<table>
<tr><td rowspan="2">City Medical Center
Blood Bank
Riverside Lane
New City, CA 99999</td><td colspan="2">Subject: Routine ABO and Rh_o(D) Typing</td></tr>
<tr><td>Procedure # 999.999.99.99</td><td>Page 4 of 4</td></tr>
</table>

Subject: **Routine ABO and Rh$_o$(D) Typing**

Procedure # 999.999.99.99 — Page 4 of 4

further tested for weak D. This testing is required in the case of blood donors and cord bloods of Rh$_o$(D) negative mothers.

35. Agglutination in the anti-human globulin phase of the weak D test is a positive test and the sample is considered weak D positive. Weak D positive donors are considered Rh$_o$(D) positive as are weak D positive babies of Rh$_o$(D) negative mothers for the purpose of Rh immune globulin administration.

36. No agglutination in the anti-human globulin phase of the weak D test indicates a true Rh$_o$(D) negative sample.

NOTES AND LIMITATIONS:

This section of the sample SOP should contain a description of the possible difficulties, errors, and pitfalls that could be encountered when performing this procedure or using these reagents. To avoid duplication, the reader is directed to the sections titled "Problems Encountered in ABO Typing" on p 406, and "Problems Encountered in Rh Typing" on p 431.

QUALITY CONTROL:

1. Each ABO reagent must be checked against a known positive and negative control on each day of use; i.e., anti-A must be tested with group A cells (+ control) and group B cells (– control).

2. Each anti-D reagent must be checked against a known Rh$_o$(D) positive and Rh$_o$(D) negative sample on each day of use. If weak D testing is required using the antiglobulin test, the Rh$_o$(D) negative control should be carried to the antiglobulin phase using the weak D procedure and a known weak D sample should also be tested using the weak D procedure. See section on antiglobulin testing on p 439.

3. An autocontrol should be run with ABO discrepancies where the cell type appears to be group AB and the serum type appears to be O, A, or B. The autocontrol can identify false positive agglutination/aggregation in the cell type.

4. An Rh control (6% albumin) should be run when an AB Rh$_o$(D) positive sample is typed. This control, similar to the autocontrol above, is used to rule out false positive agglutination/aggregation.

BIBLIOGRAPHY: Vengelen-Tyler V (ed): Technical Manual, 12th ed. American Association of Blood Banks, 1996. Rudmann SV: Textbook of Blood Banking and Transfusion Medicine. Philadelphia, WB Saunders, 1995. Harmening DM: Modern Blood Banking and Transfusion Practices, 3rd ed. Philadelphia, FA Davis, 1994.

SOP CROSS-REFERENCES: Routine Type and Screen, procedure number – 111.111.11.11
Cord Blood Testing, procedure number – 111.111.11.12
Typing Blood Donors, procedure number – 111.112.11.11

DISTRIBUTION:

1. Place a check mark (√) beside each area to which this document has been distributed.

2. The site number corresponds to the site number on the **"DOCUMENT CONTROL FORM"**

3. Enter the location if "OTHER" is selected

SITE NUMBER	LOCATION	√
01	Laboratory Office SOP Manual	
02	Laboratory SOP Manual	
03	Laboratory Office Training Manual	
04	Laboratory QC Manual	
05	Laboratory Staff Copy	
06	Donor Room Office SOP Manual	
07	Donor Room SOP Manual	
08	Donor Room Training Manual	
09	Donor Room QC Manual	
10	Donor Room Staff Copy	
11	"Capture R" Manual	
12	Other:	

ANTIGLOBULIN TEST

Introduction

Antihuman globulin (AHG) reagents (antiglobulin reagent, antihuman globulin, antihuman serum) are reagents that contain antibody directed at human protein molecules; specifically, immunoglobulins (Igs) and complement (C) components. These reagents detect Ig and/or C bound to the RBC membrane. AHG may be produced in animals or by monoclonal technology.

Principle of the Antiglobulin Test

1. Animals (usually rabbits) are injected with human serum that contains Ig and/or C. These components act as immunogens in the injected animal.
2. The animal produces antibodies directed at the substances that were injected. When purified, this is the reagent known as *antihuman globulin.*
3. In the antiglobulin test, the AHG that contains anti-IgG or anticomplement (anti-C3b, or anti–C3b-C3d) reacts with those specific proteins when bound to the RBC membrane or in solution in human plasma or serum.
4. RBCs coated with Ig and/or C are agglutinated by AHG.

Basic Antiglobulin Test Procedure

NOTE   The following steps should be specifically defined in the laboratory standard operating procedure manual. The laboratory standard operating procedures and manufacturer's directions for reagent use must always be followed when performing tests in the immunohematology laboratory.

1 Prepare the RBCs to be tested by washing in physiologic saline (0.9%) at least four times. Washing can be performed manually or in a mechanical cell washer. A dry cell button should remain after the wash procedure.

NOTE   Washing with physiologic (0.9%) saline removes human protein in the plasma in which the RBCs are suspended; RBCs remain intact. Residual protein in solution may combine with antibody in the reagent. When this occurs, antibody in the reagent may be "neutralized" by plasma proteins leaving insufficient reagent antibody to produce a positive test, *even when the RBCs are coated with IgG or complement.*

2 Add AHG.

3 Centrifuge the test.

4 Read carefully for agglutination and grade the observed reaction (see Chapter 23, "Basic Concepts of Immunohematology," on p 6).

5 Add IgG coated RBCs (O check cells) to all negative tests.

6 Centrifuge.

7 Read for agglutination.

> **NOTE**   In the *direct antiglobulin test* (DAT), the washing step is performed *as the first step,* i.e., an aliquot of the RBCs to be tested is removed from the sample tube and washed immediately. In the *indirect antiglobulin test* (IAT), the washing step is performed *after incubation of the serum and RBCs at 37°C,* before addition of AHG reagent.

> **NOTE**   O Check Cells (OCC or CC) are group O RBCs sensitized with IgG. *They must be added to negative antiglobulin tests, direct and indirect, to validate the negative reaction.*
> In a true negative test, IgG antibody bound to O check cells combines with anti-IgG in the AHG to form agglutinates.
> After the addition of O check cells and centrifugation of the mixture:
> Agglutination indicates that:
>
> 1. AHG was added.
> 2. AHG was not neutralized before or during testing.
>
> Lack of agglutination indicates:
>
> 1. Failure to add AHG
> 2. Inactivation of the AHG reagent
>
> *Lack of agglutination indicates an invalid test. All invalid antiglobulin tests must be repeated.*

Components of Antihuman Globulin Reagents

1. Anti-IgG: Antibody directed against the IgG molecule. Reagents that contain this antibody react only with IgG; they will *not* detect C components or other Igs (e.g., IgM or IgA) bound to the RBC membrane.
2. Anti-C3d, anti–C3b-C3d: Antibody directed against specific C components. C is activated and bound to the RBC membrane by the interaction of some blood group antigens and their antibodies. Reagents that contain these antibodies react with C components; they will *not* detect Ig bound to the RBC membrane.

Types of Antihuman Globulin Reagents

▌ Polyspecific (polyclonal, broad spectrum) AHG *must contain* anti-IgG and anti-C3d. Other C components or Igs may be present but are not required. This reagent detects either IgG or C bound to the RBC surface.

▌ Monospecific AHG contains *one* antibody, either anti-IgG, anti-C3d, or anti–C3b-C3d.

Anti-IgG: Detects only IgG bound to the RBC surface; no C detected.

Anti-C3d: Detects only C3d bound to the RBC surface; no Ig or other C components detected.

Anti–C3b-C3d: Detects only C3b and/or C3d bound to the RBC surface; no Ig or other C components detected.

All AHG reagents must be evaluated and approved for use by the Food and Drug Administration before being distributed for commercial use.

Types of Antiglobulin Tests

DIRECT ANTIGLOBULIN TEST

The DAT is used to detect IgG and/or C bound to the RBC membrane in vivo. It is principally used to diagnose:

- HDN
- Autoimmune hemolytic anemia (AIHA)
- Drug induced hemolytic anemia
- HTRs

INDIRECT ANTIGLOBULIN TEST

The IAT is used to detect IgG and/or C bound to the RBC membrane in vitro. RBCs are incubated with serum at 37°C to allow IgG antibodies to bind to their respective membrane-bound antigens or to activate C, which binds to RBCs. This test is used principally for:

- Antibody detection in the antibody screen
- Antibody investigation
- Phenotyping for some RBC antigens
- Antibody titration
- Compatibility testing (crossmatching)

One of the constituents used in this test is usually a "known" and one is an "unknown." The RBC antigen phenotype in the antibody detection and antibody identification procedures is *known;* the serum RBC antibody contents are *unknown.* Reagent antiserum in the RBC antigen phenotype test is *known;* the antigens present on the RBCs being tested are *unknown.*

 RBCs that demonstrate a positive DAT (i.e., coated in vivo with IgG or C) may not be accurately tested by the IAT e.g., *An individual's RBCs are positive in the DAT when using anti-IgG AHG.* The IAT using anti-IgG AHG reagent (antibody screen, antigen phenotyping, crossmatching) will be positive when testing with anti-IgG AHG; the patient or donor RBCs were coated with antibody *before beginning the IAT.* The agglutination that results when anti-IgG AHG is added after incubation at 37°C can lead to a false positive interpretation of the IAT.

See "Sources of Error in Antiglobulin Tests" in *Technical Manual* of the American Association of Blood Banks, 12th ed, pp. 218–221.

RELEVANCE OF THE DIRECT ANTIGLOBULIN TEST AS PART OF PRETRANSFUSION TESTING

1. Serologic tests *required* as part of pretransfusion testing:

   ABO and Rh typing

   Antibody detection

   Compatibility tests on blood components containing more than 5 mL of RBCs

ANTIGLOBULIN TEST

2. The DAT detects IgG or C components on the patient's or donor's RBCs; the autologous control or autocontrol is an IAT using a mixture of the patient's or donor's own RBCs and serum. Although they are somewhat different, these tests are generally used interchangeably. *Neither test is required as part of pretransfusion testing (Vengelen-Tyler, 1996).*

3. When the DAT is included as part of routine pretransfusion testing, its goal is to identify those patients who:

   Demonstrate a *clinically important* autoantibody

   Are experiencing an immune response, in an early stage, to recently transfused RBCs

CONSIDERATIONS REGARDING *ROUTINE* PERFORMANCE OF THE DIRECT ANTIGLOBULIN TEST

1. A positive DAT result in a patient or donor, an in vitro determination, is *not* always an indicator of the clinical importance of the in vivo process that is its cause.

2. Many individuals with a positive DAT experience no hemolysis or decreased RBC survival.

3. Clinical importance of an autoantibody is characterized by:

   Clinical signs and symptoms

   Results of other laboratory tests (hemoglobin concentration, hematocrit determination, haptoglobin level, lactate dehydrogenase (LDH) and bilirubin concentrations)

   The positive DAT provides *additional assurance* that an immune process is a likely cause of the hemolysis; it is not the sole determining factor of this diagnosis.

4. An alloantibody must be completely adsorbed from the serum by transfused RBCs for a transfusion reaction to be recognized by a positive DAT alone. Most patients who experience immune destruction of ABO compatible transfused RBCs have a positive antibody detection test as well as a positive DAT, that is, alloantibody is present and detectable on RBCs *and* in serum.

5. When clinical signs, results of laboratory tests, the appearance of the patient's serum, and/or routine pretransfusion testing identify a patient with possible immune-related RBC destruction, a DAT or autocontrol can be included as part of the serologic investigation in this targeted population.

6. Routine performance of the DAT or autocontrol to detect this patient population identifies so few individuals that the advisability of continuing the practice as a routine test should be evaluated carefully.

NOTE In the current health care climate of cost containment and cost effectiveness, the benefits and practicality of performing the DAT as part of pretransfusion testing, when its relevance in this patient population is questionable, is a matter to be evaluated and decided by the medical director of each individual institution.

APPLICATIONS OF THE DIRECT ANTIGLOBULIN TEST

1. To detect passively acquired maternal IgG on the RBCs of a neonate in suspected cases of HDN.
2. To detect IgG or C on the surface of transfused RBCs in suspected delayed or acute transfusion reaction (see Chapter 27, "Transfusion Reactions").
3. To detect IgG or C on the patient's RBCs in suspected cases of autoimmune hemolytic anemia.
4. To detect IgG or C on the patient's RBCs induced by therapy with some drugs or other preparations (intravenous immunoglobulin, intravenous Rh immune globulin, antilymphocyte globulin [ALG], antithymocyte globulin [ATG]).

NOTE The DAT "panel" should be performed when:

1. A DAT is specifically requested by a physician to investigate the cause of suspected RBC hemolysis.
2. The patient's transfusion history and/or the appearance and reactivity of the patient's serum sample indicate the need for performing the DAT.

This procedure includes testing the patient's RBCs with a variety of AHG reagents in order to characterize the nature of the protein present on the patient's RBCs.

Facts about Autoantibodies

1. Autoantibodies may be:

   Primary or idiopathic: arising spontaneously with no apparent precipitating event or underlying disease process

   Secondary to another disease: chronic lymphocytic leukemia (CLL), lymphoma, systemic lupus erythematosus (SLE), rheumatoid arthritis (RA), ulcerative colitis, some viral infections

   Secondary to drug therapy: methyldopa (Aldomet), levodopa, ibuprofen (Motrin), sulindac (Clinoril), procainamide (Pronestyl)

   Secondary to treatment with ALG or ATG

2. Autoantibodies in the serum of patients who have had no previous exposure to RBC antigens (have never been transfused or pregnant) are of little serologic interest or importance in the transfusion service.

   Involved serologic investigations on the serum and/or RBCs of these patients is generally inappropriate.

   There is no evidence that transfused RBCs survive longer than autologous RBCs while the autoantibody is circulating (Mollison et al, 1993).

3. The object of serologic studies on patients with a positive DAT and/or circulating autoantibodies to RBC antigens is *to detect alloantibodies* whose reactivity may be masked by the reactivity of the autoantibody.

ANTIGLOBULIN TEST

Points for Consideration When Dealing with Strongly Reactive Autoantibodies

1. Although transfusion therapy is occasionally required to relieve the cardiac and/or respiratory symptoms caused by the anemia resulting from the cellular destruction precipitated by some warm reactive (or cold reactive) autoantibodies, *in general, treatment is directed at suppressing antibody production.*
2. The goal of pretransfusion serologic investigation in patients who may have been sensitized from previous transfusion or pregnancy is to detect and identify alloantibodies whose reactivity may be masked by the reactivity of the autoantibody.
3. The complexity of the serologic investigation and amount of serologic manipulation that must be undertaken introduces an increased risk of failure to detect *alloantibodies.*
4. One or more techniques that could introduce a dilution factor are often required in the attempt to identify alloantibodies; the concentration of alloantibodies could be reduced to an undetectable level.
5. Information regarding the patient's diagnosis, and a history of drug or transfusion therapy, should be evaluated to interpret the relevance of the positive DAT and the appropriate serological investigation.

INTERPRETING THE RESULTS OF THE DIRECT ANTIGLOBULIN TEST

	REACTION WITH		PROTEIN(S) DETECTED	INTERPRETATION
	Anti-IgG	Anti-C		
1	Neg	Neg	None	1. No IgG or complement *detectable* on RBC membrane. 2. Some Ig other than IgG (e.g., IgA, IgM) or serum protein other than C3b or C3d may be present on the RBC membrane.
2	Pos	Neg	IgG	1. Possible transfusion reaction. (Agglutination should have mixed field appearance.) 2. Warm autoimmune hemolytic anemia (WAIHA). 3. Drug induced IgG adsorption, e.g., penicillin. 4. Drug induced hemolytic anemia, e.g., methyldopa (Aldomet).
3	Pos	Pos	1. IgG and C3d 2. IgG, C3b, and C3d 3. IgG, C3b, C3d, and other C components (The presence of anti-C in the AHG is not required. Detection depends on the type of reagent being used.)	1. Possible transfusion reaction. (Agglutination should have mixed field appearance.) 2. WAIHA (mixed type). 3. Membrane modification or other mechanism due to drug therapy, e.g., the cephalosporins. C components bind to the RBC membrane due to changes in the membrane caused by the drug.

Continued ▶

▶ Continued **INTERPRETING THE RESULTS OF THE DIRECT ANTIGLOBULIN TEST**

	REACTION WITH		PROTEIN(S) DETECTED	INTERPRETATION
	Anti-IgG	**Anti-C**		
4	Neg	Pos	1. C3d 2. C3b and C3d 3. C3b, C3d, and other C components (The presence of anti-C in the AHG is not required. Detection depends on the type of reagent being used.)	1. WAIHA. Only C is detected on the RBCs of a small percentage of patients with WAIHA. 2. Cold autoimmune hemolytic anemia (CAIHA, cold agglutinin syndrome, cold hemagglutinin disease, cold agglutinin disease). 3. Paroxysmal cold hemoglobinuria (PCH). 4. Formation of drug-antidrug complexes due to therapy with some drugs (e.g., the cephalosporins) may activate C, which binds to the RBC membrane. 5. C is present on the RBC membrane due to activation by some disease process. 6. C is present on the RBC membrane due to an undetermined process.

SUGGESTED APPROACH TO FOLLOW-UP TESTING WHEN THE DIRECT ANTIGLOBULIN TEST IS POSITIVE

NOTE This process should be defined by laboratory standard operating procedure. The laboratory standard operating procedure must *always* be followed.

Text continued on page 456

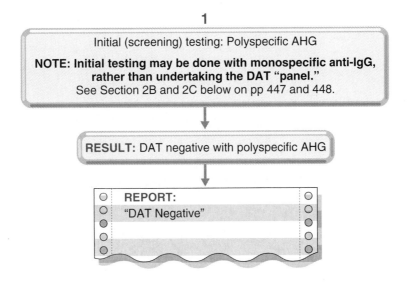

1

Initial (screening) testing: Polyspecific AHG

NOTE: Initial testing may be done with monospecific anti-IgG, rather than undertaking the DAT "panel."
See Section 2B and 2C below on pp 447 and 448.

RESULT: DAT negative with polyspecific AHG

REPORT:
"DAT Negative"

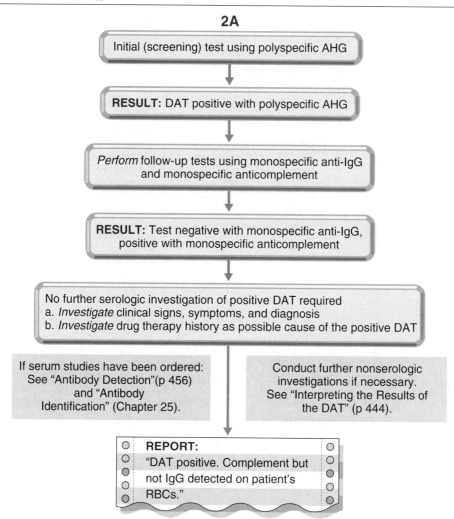

2A

Initial (screening) test using polyspecific AHG

↓

RESULT: DAT positive with polyspecific AHG

↓

Perform follow-up tests using monospecific anti-IgG and monospecific anticomplement

↓

RESULT: Test negative with monospecific anti-IgG, positive with monospecific anticomplement

↓

No further serologic investigation of positive DAT required
a. *Investigate* clinical signs, symptoms, and diagnosis
b. *Investigate* drug therapy history as possible cause of the positive DAT

If serum studies have been ordered: See "Antibody Detection"(p 456) and "Antibody Identification" (Chapter 25).

Conduct further nonserologic investigations if necessary. See "Interpreting the Results of the DAT" (p 444).

REPORT:
"DAT positive. Complement but not IgG detected on patient's RBCs."

ANTIGLOBULIN TEST

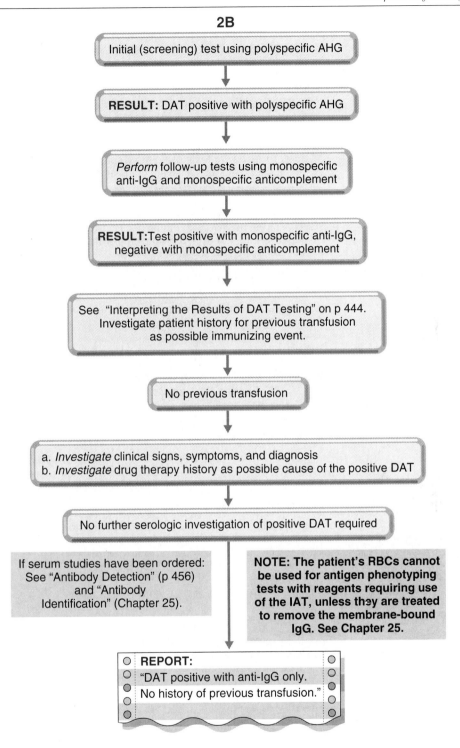

2B

Initial (screening) test using polyspecific AHG

RESULT: DAT positive with polyspecific AHG

Perform follow-up tests using monospecific anti-IgG and monospecific anticomplement

RESULT: Test positive with monospecific anti-IgG, negative with monospecific anticomplement

See "Interpreting the Results of DAT Testing" on p 444. Investigate patient history for previous transfusion as possible immunizing event.

No previous transfusion

a. *Investigate* clinical signs, symptoms, and diagnosis
b. *Investigate* drug therapy history as possible cause of the positive DAT

No further serologic investigation of positive DAT required

If serum studies have been ordered: See "Antibody Detection" (p 456) and "Antibody Identification" (Chapter 25).

NOTE: The patient's RBCs cannot be used for antigen phenotyping tests with reagents requiring use of the IAT, unless they are treated to remove the membrane-bound IgG. See Chapter 25.

REPORT:
"DAT positive with anti-IgG only. No history of previous transfusion."

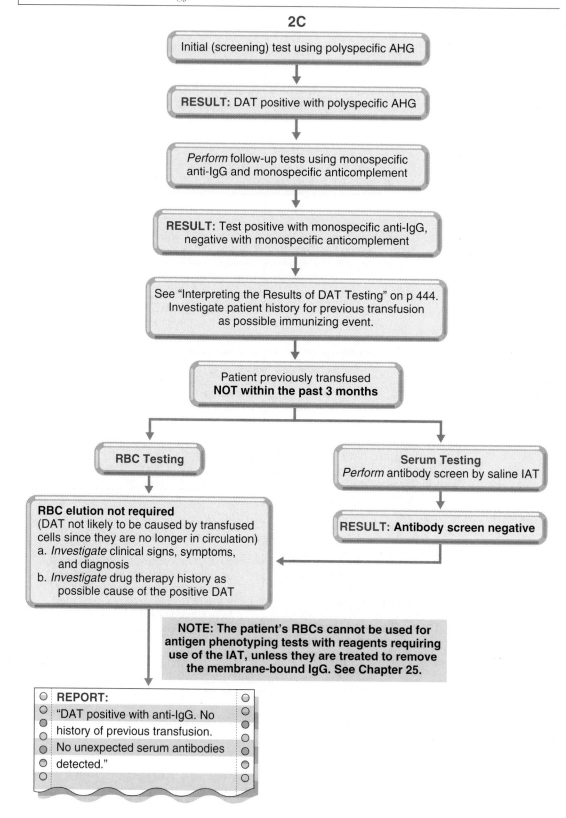

2C

Initial (screening) test using polyspecific AHG

RESULT: DAT positive with polyspecific AHG

Perform follow-up tests using monospecific anti-IgG and monospecific anticomplement

RESULT: Test positive with monospecific anti-IgG, negative with monospecific anticomplement

See "Interpreting the Results of DAT Testing" on p 444. Investigate patient history for previous transfusion as possible immunizing event.

Patient previously transfused **NOT within the past 3 months**

RBC Testing

Serum Testing *Perform* antibody screen by saline IAT

RBC elution not required (DAT not likely to be caused by transfused cells since they are no longer in circulation) a. *Investigate* clinical signs, symptoms, and diagnosis b. *Investigate* drug therapy history as possible cause of the positive DAT

RESULT: Antibody screen negative

NOTE: The patient's RBCs cannot be used for antigen phenotyping tests with reagents requiring use of the IAT, unless they are treated to remove the membrane-bound IgG. See Chapter 25.

REPORT: "DAT positive with anti-IgG. No history of previous transfusion. No unexpected serum antibodies detected."

ANTIGLOBULIN TEST

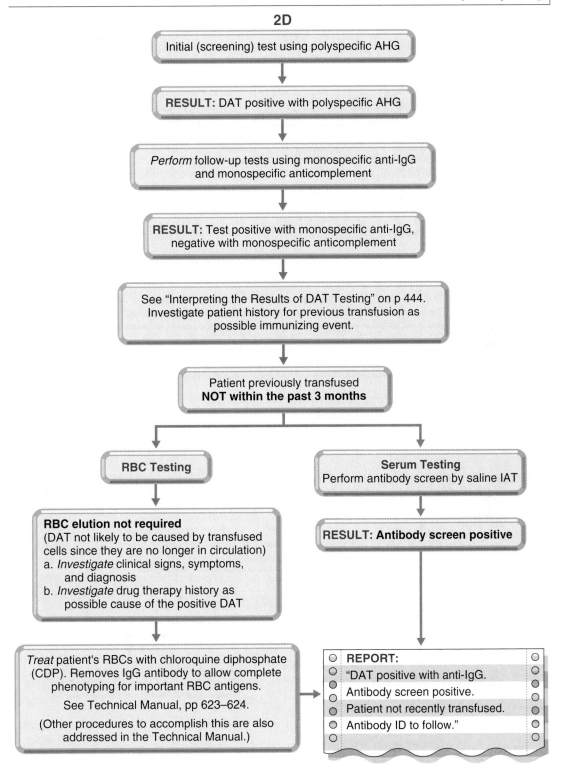

2D

Initial (screening) test using polyspecific AHG

RESULT: DAT positive with polyspecific AHG

Perform follow-up tests using monospecific anti-IgG and monospecific anticomplement

RESULT: Test positive with monospecific anti-IgG, negative with monospecific anticomplement

See "Interpreting the Results of DAT Testing" on p 444. Investigate patient history for previous transfusion as possible immunizing event.

Patient previously transfused **NOT within the past 3 months**

RBC Testing

Serum Testing Perform antibody screen by saline IAT

RBC elution not required (DAT not likely to be caused by transfused cells since they are no longer in circulation) a. *Investigate* clinical signs, symptoms, and diagnosis b. *Investigate* drug therapy history as possible cause of the positive DAT

RESULT: Antibody screen positive

Treat patient's RBCs with chloroquine diphosphate (CDP). Removes IgG antibody to allow complete phenotyping for important RBC antigens.

See Technical Manual, pp 623–624.

(Other procedures to accomplish this are also addressed in the Technical Manual.)

REPORT: "DAT positive with anti-IgG. Antibody screen positive. Patient not recently transfused. Antibody ID to follow."

FOLLOW-UP TESTING

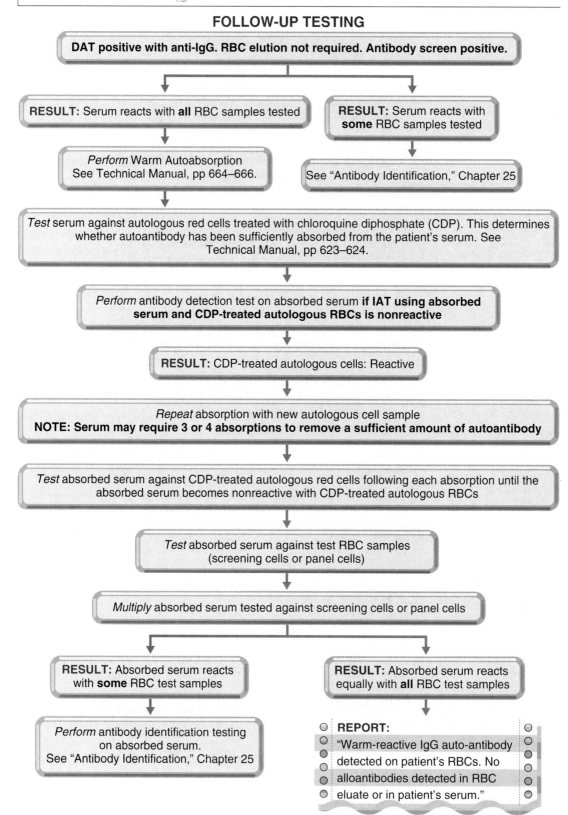

DAT positive with anti-IgG. RBC elution not required. Antibody screen positive.

RESULT: Serum reacts with **all** RBC samples tested

RESULT: Serum reacts with **some** RBC samples tested

Perform Warm Autoabsorption
See Technical Manual, pp 664–666.

See "Antibody Identification," Chapter 25

Test serum against autologous red cells treated with chloroquine diphosphate (CDP). This determines whether autoantibody has been sufficiently absorbed from the patient's serum. See Technical Manual, pp 623–624.

Perform antibody detection test on absorbed serum **if IAT using absorbed serum and CDP-treated autologous RBCs is nonreactive**

RESULT: CDP-treated autologous cells: Reactive

Repeat absorption with new autologous cell sample
NOTE: Serum may require 3 or 4 absorptions to remove a sufficient amount of autoantibody

Test absorbed serum against CDP-treated autologous red cells following each absorption until the absorbed serum becomes nonreactive with CDP-treated autologous RBCs

Test absorbed serum against test RBC samples (screening cells or panel cells)

Multiply absorbed serum tested against screening cells or panel cells

RESULT: Absorbed serum reacts with **some** RBC test samples

RESULT: Absorbed serum reacts equally with **all** RBC test samples

Perform antibody identification testing on absorbed serum.
See "Antibody Identification," Chapter 25

REPORT:
"Warm-reactive IgG auto-antibody detected on patient's RBCs. No alloantibodies detected in RBC eluate or in patient's serum."

2E

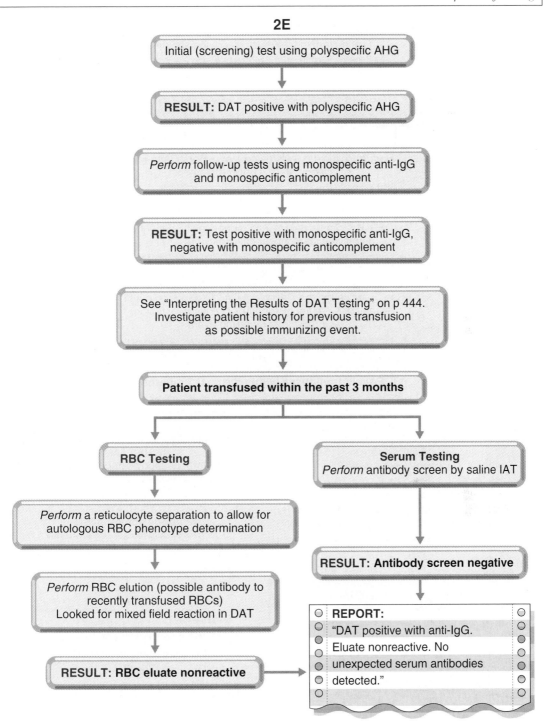

Initial (screening) test using polyspecific AHG

RESULT: DAT positive with polyspecific AHG

Perform follow-up tests using monospecific anti-IgG and monospecific anticomplement

RESULT: Test positive with monospecific anti-IgG, negative with monospecific anticomplement

See "Interpreting the Results of DAT Testing" on p 444. Investigate patient history for previous transfusion as possible immunizing event.

Patient transfused within the past 3 months

RBC Testing

Perform a reticulocyte separation to allow for autologous RBC phenotype determination

Perform RBC elution (possible antibody to recently transfused RBCs) Looked for mixed field reaction in DAT

RESULT: RBC eluate nonreactive

Serum Testing
Perform antibody screen by saline IAT

RESULT: Antibody screen negative

REPORT:
"DAT positive with anti-IgG. Eluate nonreactive. No unexpected serum antibodies detected."

ANTIGLOBULIN TEST

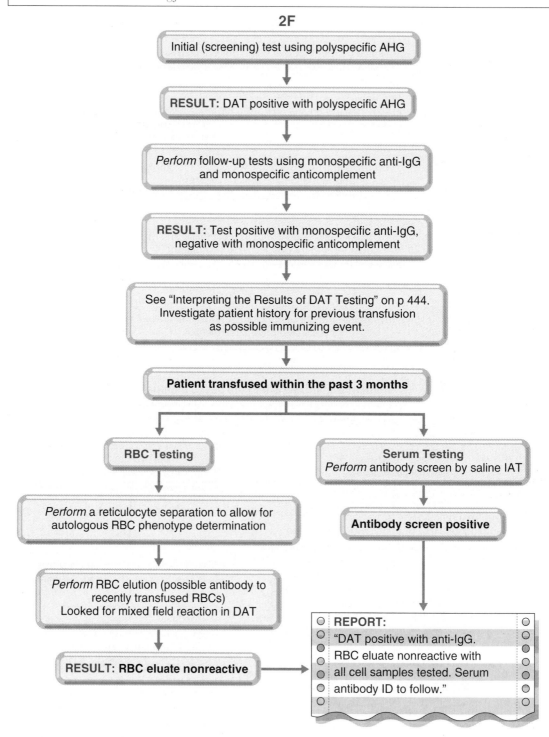

FOLLOW-UP TESTING

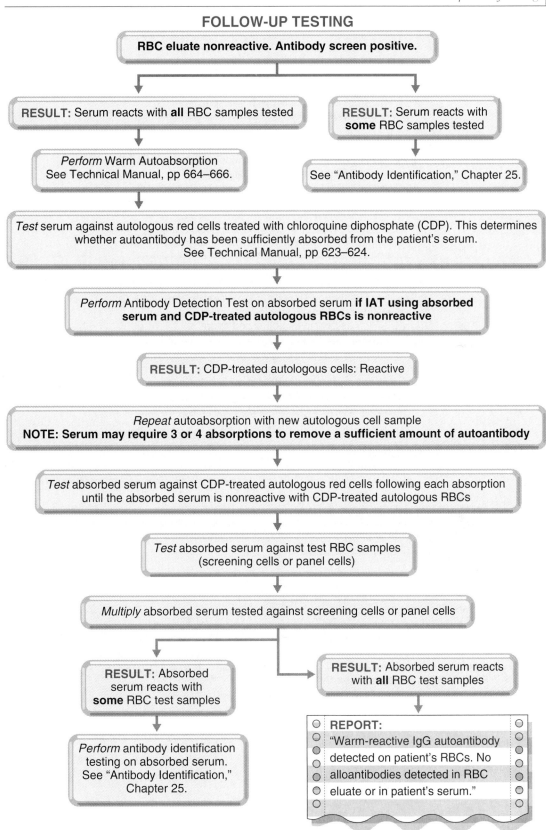

RBC eluate nonreactive. Antibody screen positive.

RESULT: Serum reacts with **all** RBC samples tested

RESULT: Serum reacts with **some** RBC samples tested

Perform Warm Autoabsorption
See Technical Manual, pp 664–666.

See "Antibody Identification," Chapter 25.

Test serum against autologous red cells treated with chloroquine diphosphate (CDP). This determines whether autoantibody has been sufficiently absorbed from the patient's serum.
See Technical Manual, pp 623–624.

Perform Antibody Detection Test on absorbed serum **if IAT using absorbed serum and CDP-treated autologous RBCs is nonreactive**

RESULT: CDP-treated autologous cells: Reactive

Repeat autoabsorption with new autologous cell sample
NOTE: Serum may require 3 or 4 absorptions to remove a sufficient amount of autoantibody

Test absorbed serum against CDP-treated autologous red cells following each absorption until the absorbed serum is nonreactive with CDP-treated autologous RBCs

Test absorbed serum against test RBC samples
(screening cells or panel cells)

Multiply absorbed serum tested against screening cells or panel cells

RESULT: Absorbed serum reacts with **some** RBC test samples

RESULT: Absorbed serum reacts with **all** RBC test samples

Perform antibody identification testing on absorbed serum.
See "Antibody Identification," Chapter 25.

REPORT:
"Warm-reactive IgG autoantibody detected on patient's RBCs. No alloantibodies detected in RBC eluate or in patient's serum."

ANTIGLOBULIN TEST

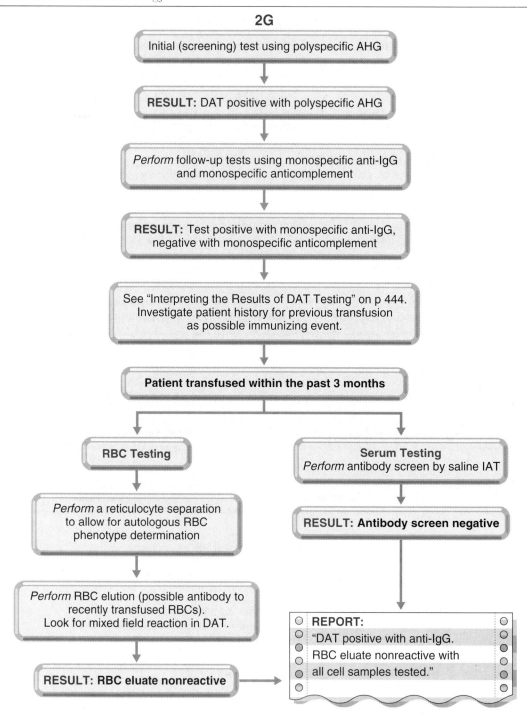

2G

Initial (screening) test using polyspecific AHG

↓

RESULT: DAT positive with polyspecific AHG

↓

Perform follow-up tests using monospecific anti-IgG and monospecific anticomplement

↓

RESULT: Test positive with monospecific anti-IgG, negative with monospecific anticomplement

↓

See "Interpreting the Results of DAT Testing" on p 444. Investigate patient history for previous transfusion as possible immunizing event.

↓

Patient transfused within the past 3 months

RBC Testing

Perform a reticulocyte separation to allow for autologous RBC phenotype determination

↓

Perform RBC elution (possible antibody to recently transfused RBCs). Look for mixed field reaction in DAT.

↓

RESULT: RBC eluate nonreactive

Serum Testing
Perform antibody screen by saline IAT

↓

RESULT: Antibody screen negative

↓

REPORT:
"DAT positive with anti-IgG.
RBC eluate nonreactive with
all cell samples tested."

FOLLOW-UP TESTING

RBC eluate reactive. Serum nonreactive.

If the DAT on the patient's RBCs is positive with anti-IgG AHG **AND** the patient has been very recently transfused (about 3–14 days), there is some chance that antibody produced in an anamnestic response may be present in a titer so low that it is only detectable on the surface of the transfused RBCs. **Under these circumstances**, it is appropriate to take the following measures.

Absorb the *eluate* with *selected allogeneic RBC samples*
See Technical Manual, pp 666–667

Perform **antibody detection test on absorbed eluate**
Test the absorbed serum against individual samples of each of the RBCs used for the absorption. This determines whether autoantibody has been sufficiently absorbed from the RBC eluate

RESULT: Eluate reacts with **all** test cell samples

RESULT: Eluate reacts with **some** test cell samples

RESULT: Eluate nonreactive with test cell samples

Repeat allogeneic absorption of the eluate with new aliquots of the absorbing cells.

NOTE: Several absorptions may be required to remove a sufficient amount of autoantibody

Perform antibody identification testing on absorbed eluate reactive with test cell samples.
See "Antibody Identification," Chapter 25.

REPORT:
"Warm-reactive IgG autoantibody detected on patient's RBCs. No alloantibodies detected in RBC eluate or in patient's serum."

Repeat tests of the multiply absorbed eluate against individual samples of the absorbing cells following each absorption until the absorbed serum becomes nonreactive with at least one test cell sample or ceases to react with all test cell samples
(no alloantibody detected**).

Perform antibody identification testing on absorbed serum if eluate reacts with one or more test cell samples.

**Antibodies directed against antigens of high incidence can be inadvertently absorbed in this process; this is unavoidable, but the appearance of absence of alloantibodies is misleading. This fact should be kept in mind if there is any evidence of new or continuing post-transfusion hemolysis.

ANTIGLOBULIN TEST

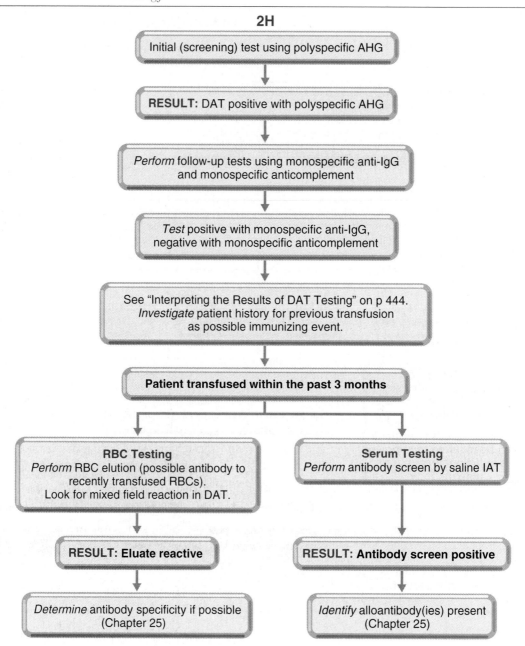

2H

Initial (screening) test using polyspecific AHG

↓

RESULT: DAT positive with polyspecific AHG

↓

Perform follow-up tests using monospecific anti-IgG
and monospecific anticomplement

↓

Test positive with monospecific anti-IgG,
negative with monospecific anticomplement

↓

See "Interpreting the Results of DAT Testing" on p 444.
Investigate patient history for previous transfusion
as possible immunizing event.

↓

Patient transfused within the past 3 months

RBC Testing
Perform RBC elution (possible antibody to
recently transfused RBCs).
Look for mixed field reaction in DAT.

↓

RESULT: Eluate reactive

↓

Determine antibody specificity if possible
(Chapter 25)

Serum Testing
Perform antibody screen by saline IAT

↓

RESULT: Antibody screen positive

↓

Identify alloantibody(ies) present
(Chapter 25)

ANTIBODY DETECTION TESTING

Antibody Detection in the Hospital Transfusion Service

The goal of individuals employed in the transfusion medicine service is to provide patients with blood products and components that are "safe, pure, and potent." Performing the "antibody screen" in the preliminary pretransfusion testing is one process that helps to achieve that goal.

Although most fatal transfusion reactions are caused by transfusion of *ABO* incompatible RBCs, circulating plasma antibodies in the recipient directed against RBC antigens of other blood groups are capable of causing significant RBC destruction or reduction in the survival of the transfused product. Antibodies that cause hemolysis or reduced survival of transfused RBCs are called *clinically significant* or *clinically important*. The antibody screen is designed to detect clinically important antibodies in the serum or plasma of the intended transfusion recipient.

Requirements of Antibody Detection Testing (Standards for Blood Banks and Transfusion Services)

- ▌ Reagent RBCs cannot be pooled when used for pretransfusion or prenatal testing. The sensitivity of individual donor test cells is required for this determination.
- ▌ Reagent RBCs used for donor antibody detection testing may be pooled RBCs.

> **NOTE** It is not a life threatening situation when an unexpected clinically important serum antibody to an RBC antigen in a unit of donor RBCs is not detected; the volume of serum in a unit of donor RBCs is small, and an RBC antibody in that serum is unlikely to cause significant destruction of the recipient's RBCs when transfused. However, plasma from a donor with a clinically important antibody directed at an RBC antigen should be discarded.

- ▌ Testing must be performed by a method known to detect clinically important antibodies and should include incubation at 37°C and an IAT.
- ▌ Testing must be sensitive enough to detect antibodies that are present in very low concentration.

> **NOTE** The medical director of the transfusion service must decide:
> What antibodies are considered clinically important
> What specific methods will be used in antibody screening tests

Reagents Used for Antibody Detection Testing

Reagent RBCs used for antibody detection testing are commercially prepared group O cells available in sets of two or three.

Characteristics of Reagent RBCs Used for Antibody Detection Testing

1. RBC antigens corresponding to clinically important antibodies must be present on the reagent test cells. In addition, antibody screening cells are positive for several antigens whose antibodies are frequently encountered but are not considered clinically important.
2. The reagent cells are suspended in saline in a concentration of about 2% to 5%. Antibiotics, nutrients, and/or other substances may be added to retard bacterial growth and hemolysis.
3. Some antigens on reagent RBCs stored for prolonged periods may deteriorate. It is difficult to predict the rate or extent of deterioration. All reagent RBCs should be stored at 1° to 6°C to delay the deterioration.
4. Reagents RBCs should not be used *for routine testing* past their expiration date. Some workers believe that expired reagent RBCs, when used for supplementary tests (e.g., selected cell panels), should be used with appropriate control antisera to ensure their reactivity.
5. All reagent RBCs used for testing should be inspected for hemolysis, discoloration, or turbidity before use. All of the above indicate that the reagents are unsuitable for use in testing.

ANTIGLOBULIN TEST

6. An *antigram* that defines the phenotype of reagent screening cells is included with every set. The antigram is used to interpret reactions.

NOTE *All reagents should be used according to the manufacturer's directions.*

Some Elements to Be Considered When Performing Antibody Detection Testing

1. The DAT or autocontrol is not required as part of routine pretransfusion or prenatal testing. The laboratory standard operating procedure must be followed with regard to this issue.
2. Procedures, reagents, and techniques used in the blood bank laboratory should be used in a uniform manner by all technical staff members. All personnel in the laboratory should perform tests and grade reactions according to well defined standard operating procedures. Standardization reduces additional variability in an inherently imprecise test and allows continuity of interpretation among investigators.
3. The patient's historical records must be consulted before beginning the current testing. A comparison of previous test results provides some assurance of correct patient identification, as well as information about serologic problems encountered in the previous testing. This can prevent problems that occur due to failure to detect low titer antibodies.

NOTE RBCs selected for transfusion to an individual whose serum contains a clinically important antibody must lack the offending antigen, regardless of whether the antibody is reactive or undetectable.

4. Techniques used to detect serum antibodies should be capable of identifying the greatest number of clinically significant RBC antibodies and the fewest clinically unimportant ones.

NOTE The room temperature (RT) and immediate spin (IS) test phases are not required in routine antibody detection testing. Performing these procedures may delay the process of providing blood for transfusion when antibodies reactive at low temperatures, generally of no clinical significance, are detected at crossmatch and require further testing for identification. When the IS crossmatch is used as the routine compatibility test, it may be beneficial to include this phase as part of antibody detection testing, when the antibody detection test is being performed as pretransfusion or presurgical testing.

5. Because most clinically significant antibodies, other than anti-A and anti-B, bind to their corresponding antigens at 37°C and require the addition of AHG to agglutinate, regulatory agencies require that antibody detection tests:

   Be performed at 37°C

   Include the IAT

6. The only component required to be included in the AHG reagent used in antibody detection procedures is anti-IgG. Polyspecific or broad spectrum AHG

reagent detects C on the surface of reagent RBCs bound during the incubation phase of the IAT. Although some clinically significant antibody specificities activate C at 37°C in vivo and in vitro, there is no requirement that anti-C be included in the AHG reagent used for antibody detection testing. In some rare cases, when the concentration of IgG antibody in a patient's serum is very low, anti-C in polyspecific AHG may be the only component that detects that antibody's reactivity (e.g., some examples of Kidd blood group system antibodies). In addition, anti-C activity may enhance detection of weak reactions of other antibody specificities. Frequently, anti-C in the AHG reagent enhances the detection of cold reactive serum antibodies (reacting optimally at 30°C or less). These antibodies, such as anti-I, and anti-P_1, are not important in transfusion therapy because they are not known, except in rare cases, to cause increased destruction of transfused RBCs. Agglutination that is the result of C components bound to RBC membranes in the antibody screening test may require an inappropriate amount of time and resources in identifying the cause of the serologic problem; when a serologic problem is detected, further investigation is required to determine that the reactivity observed is not the result of RBC antibody that may be clinically significant. The follow-up investigation often leads to delays in providing transfusion to trauma and surgical patients who may need treatment as quickly as possible. Currently available reagents, testing techniques, and enhancement media make the IAT test system using monospecific anti-IgG AHG more sensitive and are more likely to detect those low titered IgG complement-activating antibody specificities.

NOTE   Reagents, procedures, and techniques used for antibody detection and antibody investigation tests in each laboratory are selected by the blood bank director and should be clearly defined in the laboratory's standard operating procedures manual.

Commonly Used Techniques and Procedures for Antibody Detection Testing

Factors Affecting Detection of the Agglutination Reaction Are Described in Chapter 23 and Include:

1. The ionic concentration and pH of the test environment
2. The time and temperature of testing
3. The ratio of antibody to antigen in the reaction components
4. The dosage of the antigen on the test RBCs

Methods Frequently Used in the Blood Bank Laboratory to Enhance Detection of Agglutination of Serum Antibodies of Clinical Importance

1. Use of test reagents that express important antigens in double dose. Antigens *required by regulatory agencies* to be present on at least one of the reagent screening cells used include:

   Antigens corresponding to clinically important (37°C reactive) RBC antibodies: D, C, c, E, e, K, k, Jk^a, Jk^b, Fy^a, Fy^b, S, s

   Antigens corresponding to clinically unimportant but commonly encountered RBC antibodies include: P_1, Le^a, Le^b, M, N

ANTIGLOBULIN TEST

Other antigens often present on the screening cells and noted on the antigram include: C^W, V, Kp^a, Kp^b, Js^a, Js^b, Lu^a, Lu^b, Xg^a

Failure to detect clinically important serum antibodies present in low titer can sometimes be avoided by testing the serum with reagent RBCs that possess a double dose of the corresponding antigen. Commercially prepared three cell reagent sets are more likely to detect weakly reactive clinically important antibodies because the manufacturers usually include RBC samples that express important antigens in double dose, e.g., Jk(a+b−) and Jk(a−b+), Fy(a+b−) and Fy(a−b+) cell samples. The three cell reagent sets are more costly than two cell sets.

2. Use of low ionic strength solutions (LISS) or other macromolecular substances (e.g., polyethylene glycol) as additives to the test system. These reagents sometimes enhance reactivity of cold reactive antibodies and should only be used in conjunction with monospecific anti-IgG AHG.

NOTE These reagents are commercially available; they must be used in accordance with the manufacturer's instructions.

3. The serum to cell ratio can be adjusted in the saline IAT to increase the amount of antibody in the reaction, i.e., the number of drops of patient serum (antibody) may be increased to enhance antibody reactivity. This technique is not appropriate when using commercially prepared enhancement media that should be used in the manner precisely recommended by the manufacturer.

Other complex but more sensitive methods to enhance the reactivity of serum antibodies are available but may be more appropriately used for antibody identification (see Chapter 25).

Possible Explanations for Problems Encountered in Tests to Detect Unexpected Serum Antibodies (Direct Antiglobulin Test Included as Part of Routine Testing)

	REACTIVITY	IS	37°C/IgG AHG	POSSIBLE INTERPRETATION(S)
1	*Screening Cells*	Negative	Negative	No unexpected antibodies
	Autocontrol	Negative	Negative	
2	*Screening Cells*	Positive	Negative/w+	RT reactive alloantibody(ies) demonstrating "carryover" reactivity
	Autocontrol	Negative	Negative	
3	*Screening Cells*	Positive	Negative	RT reactive autoantibody
				or
	Autocontrol	Positive	Negative	RT reactive autoantibody + RT reactive alloantibody(ies)
4	*Screening Cells*	Negative	Positive	IgG autoantibody
				or
	Autocontrol	Negative	Positive	IgG autoantibody + IgG alloantibody(ies)
				or
				IgG alloantibody(ies) to recently transfused RBCs (autocontrol [AC] usually mixed-field appearance)

Continued ▶

► Continued **Possible Explanations for Problems Encountered in Tests to Detect Unexpected Serum Antibodies (Direct Antiglobulin Test Included as Part of Routine Testing)**

	REACTIVITY	IS	37°C/IgG AHG	POSSIBLE INTERPRETATION(S)
5	*Screening Cells*	Negative	Positive	RT reactive autoantibody + IgG autoantibody
	Autocontrol	Positive	Positive	*or* RT reactive autoantibody + IgG autoantibody + IgG alloantibody *or* RT reactive autoantibody (with carryover) + IgG alloantibody *or* IgG autoantibody (RBCs heavily coated with IgG) + IgG alloantibody *or* IgG alloantibody to recently transfused RBCs (AC usually mixed field appearance)
6	*Screening Cells*	Positive	Positive	RT reactive autoantibody + IgG alloantibody(ies)
	Autocontrol	Positive	Negative	*or* RT reactive autoantibody + RT reactive alloantibody(ies) + IgG alloantibody(ies)
7	*Screening Cells*	Positive	Positive	RT reactive alloantibody(ies) with carryover reactivity + IgG autoantibody
	Autocontrol	Negative	Positive	*or* RT reactive alloantibody(ies) + IgG autoantibody + IgG alloantibody(ies) *or* IgG alloantibody to recently transfused RBCs (AC usually mixed field appearance)
8	*Screening Cells*	Positive	Positive	RT alloantibody with carryover reactivity
	Autocontrol	Negative	Positive	*or* RT reactive alloantibody + IgG alloantibody
9	*Screening Cells*	Positive	Negative	RT reactive autoantibody + RT reactive alloantibody + IgG autoantibody
	Autocontrol	Positive	Positive	*or* RT reactive autoantibody + IgG alloantibody(ies) to recently transfused RBCs (AC usually mixed field appearance)
10	*Screening Cells*	Negative	Negative	IgG autoantibody (positive DAT)
	Autocontrol	Negative	Positive	*or* IgG antibody to transfused RBCs (AC usually mixed-field appearance)
11	*Screening Cells*	Negative	Positive	IgG alloantibody(ies)
	Autocontrol	Negative	Negative	

ANTIGLOBULIN TEST

Continued ►

► Continued **Possible Explanations for Problems Encountered in Tests to Detect Unexpected Serum Antibodies (Direct Antiglobulin Test Included as Part of Routine Testing)**

	REACTIVITY	IS	37°C/IgG AHG	POSSIBLE INTERPRETATIONS
12	*Screening Cells*	Positive	Positive	RT reactive autoantibody with carryover reactivity (e.g., cold agglutinin disease)
	Autocontrol	Positive	Positive	*or*
				RT reactive autoantibody with carryover reactivity + RT reactive alloantibody(ies)
				or
				RT reactive autoantibody + IgG autoantibody
				or
				RT reactive autoantibody + RT reactive alloantibody(ies) + IgG autoantibody + IgG alloantibody(ies)
				or
				RT reactive autoantibody with carryover reactivity + RT reactive alloantibody(ies) + IgG alloantibody(ies) to recently transfused RBCs (AC usually mixed field appearance)

Possible Explanations for Problems Encountered in Tests to Detect Unexpected Serum Antibodies (Direct Antiglobulin Test *Not* Included as Part of Routine Testing)

	REACTIVITY	IS	37°C/IgG AHG	POSSIBLE INTERPRETATIONS
1	*Screening Cells*	Negative	Negative	No unexpected antibodies
2	*Screening Cells*	Positive (not all cells reactive)	Negative/w+	RT reactive alloantibody
3	*Screening Cells*	Positive (all cells reactive)	Negative/w+	RT reactive alloantibody(ies)
				or
				RT reactive autoantibody (with carryover reactivity)
4	*Screening Cells*	Negative	Positive (not all cells reactive)	IgG autoantibody
				or
				IgG alloantibody(ies)
				or
				IgG autoantibody + IgG alloantibody(ies)
				or
				IgG alloantibody(ies) to recently transfused RBCs (AC usually mixed field appearance)
5	*Screening Cells*	Negative	Positive (all cells reactive)	IgG autoantibody
				or
				IgG autoantibody + IgG alloantibody

Continued ►

► Continued **Possible Explanations for Problems Encountered in Tests to Detect Unexpected Serum Antibodies (Direct Antiglobulin Test *Not* Included as Part of Routine Testing)**

	REACTIVITY	IS	37°C/IgG AHG	POSSIBLE INTERPRETATIONS
6	*Screening Cells*	Positive	Positive	RT reactive alloantibody with carryover reactivity *or* RT reactive autoantibody with carryover reactivity + RT reactive alloantibody with carryover reactivity *or* RT reactive autoantibody + IgG alloantibody *or* RT reactive alloantibody + IgG alloantibody RT reactive autoantibody + IgG autoantibody *or* RT reactive alloantibody + IgG autoantibody *or* RT reactive autoantibody + RT reactive alloantibody + IgG alloantibody *or* RT reactive autoantibody + RT reactive alloantibody + IgG autoantibody *or* RT reactive autoantibody + IgG autoantibody + IgG alloantibody and RT reactive alloantibody + IgG autoantibody + IgG alloantibody and RT reactive autoantibody + RT reactive alloantibody + IgG autoantibody + IgG alloantibody

CROSSMATCHING

General Guidelines for Compatibility Testing

Because blood components (especially group O and D negative RBCs) are often in short supply, units for transfusion should be selected with attention, care, and consideration paid to optimal inventory utilization:

1. RBCs ordered for "hold for possible transfusion" or "hold for surgery" *should not be selected* from units with a short outdate.
2. RBC units that are expected to be transfused to patients with very low hemoglobin concentrations or massive blood loss due to severe trauma or surgery should generally be selected from stock of units with shorter outdate.
3. Group specific RBCs may not be the best choice for transfusion if other group compatible units are in danger of expiring or if an inappropriate delay in providing transfusion therapy will be incurred, e.g.:

   An A negative patient requires transfusion; there are O negative units in stock that will expire at midnight on the day the unit is to be transfused. The O negative RBC units should be selected for transfusion to this patient.

A group B positive patient requires transfusion; several O positive RBCs will expire within the next 24 to 36 hours. The O positive units should be selected for transfusion to this patient.

A group B negative patient requires RBCs for emergency surgery; there are *no* B negative RBC units available in the hospital blood bank; group O negative RBCs should be selected for crossmatching for this patient.

The RBC sample used for compatibility testing should be obtained from a segment attached to the unit to be crossmatched.

It may be advisable to wash the suspension of donor RBCs to be used for the crossmatching procedure, especially if the IAT is used. Fibrin strands in the suspension prepared from the donor segment may:

1. Cause a fibrin clot to form during the 37°C incubation
2. Mimic microscopic agglutinins at the AHG phase
3. Neutralize the AHG reagent leading to invalid IAT (as evidenced by failure of O check cells to react)

Selection of Donor Red Blood Cell Components for Crossmatching

▮ Whole blood transfusions should be ABO specific to the patient's RBCs.
▮ Packed RBC transfusions must be ABO specific or ABO compatible with the patient's RBCs (see Chapter 26, "Component Therapy").
▮ The number of donor units that must be tested to obtain the quantity of units requested when those units must lack single or multiple antigens can be determined by considering the incidence of the antigen in the general population, e.g.:

Two units of K− RBCs are requested.

Approximately one in every 10 donors is expected to lack the K antigen.

Three units should be tested to fill this request.

Selection of Method for Crossmatching

The *minor crossmatch* (donor serum with patient RBCs) is not required for compatibility testing.

METHOD	PROCESS	REQUIREMENTS
AHG Crossmatch	Donor RBCs and recipient's serum are tested by IAT. *This test may be performed using an additive solution to increase test sensitivity and/or decrease time required for providing RBCs.*	This procedure is acceptable for all patients regardless of serologic status.
Abbreviated Crossmatch	Donor RBCs and patient's serum are tested only in IS phase. This is known as the *immediate Spin crossmatch.*	Patient's serum must be free of clinically important antibodies, with no historical record of clinically important serum antibodies
	Donor RBCs may be provided by selecting units through use of laboratory information system (computer). *No serologic testing is performed.* This is known as *computer* or *electronic crossmatch.*	1. Patient's serum must be free of clinically important antibodies, as determined by current serologic testing and historical records. 2. Blood group of donor unit must be confirmed by transfusing facility. 3. The above information must be recorded and stored by electronic information system in use. 4. The information system must be capable of preventing release for transfusion of *any* blood component when the above requirements are not met.

NOTE All of these issues should be specifically addressed by the blood bank medical director and clearly defined in laboratory standard operating procedures.

Interpretations of the Major Crossmatch (XM)

TYPE OF XM	REACTIONS			POSSIBLE INTERPRETATION
	Antibody Screen	Autocontrol	Crossmatch	
Immediate Spin	Negative	Negative	Negative	Serologic compatibility
	Negative	Negative	Positive	Alloantibody to room temperature reactive antibody Selection of donor unit of incorrect blood group Donor unit incorrectly typed Patient incorrectly typed

Continued ▶

ANTIGLOBULIN TEST

▶ Continued **Interpretations of the Major Crossmatch (XM)**

TYPE OF XM	REACTIONS			POSSIBLE INTERPRETATION
	Antibody Screen	**Autocontrol**	**Crossmatch**	
IAT	Negative	Negative	Negative	Serologic compatibility
	Negative	Negative	Positive	Alloantibody to RBC of low incidence Donor whose RBCs have positive DAT
	Positive	Negative	Positive	One or more antigens complementary to anti-body in patient's serum detected in antibody screening test are present on donor RBCs. One or more antibody(ies) in serum with multi-ple antibodies are not identified; comple-mentary antigen is present on donor RBCs.
	Positive	Positive	Positive	Autoantibody present in patient's serum and on patient's RBCs Autoantibody present on patient's RBCs; al-loantibody present in patient's serum Autoantibody present on patient's RBCs; au-toantibody and alloantibody present in pa-tient's serum Autoantibody and alloantibody present on pa-tient's RBCs (patient recently transfused); autoantibody and alloantibody present in patient's serum Contaminated patient sample

Labeling and Release of Blood and Components for Transfusion

Labeling

The final step in compatibility testing is the labeling and release of the blood compo-nent(s) selected for transfusion. All blood components drawn by the collecting facility are required to have the following information in legible form on a label that is firmly at-tached to the blood component:

▌ Numeric or alphanumeric identification that is unique for each individual unit of blood and its components

NOTE The transfusing facility may assign a local numeric or alphanumeric identifi-cation number to the unit of blood or component providing the facility as-signing the identification is clearly identified. No more than two numbers may be assigned to any given unit at any given time.

▌ Name of whole blood or component
▌ Name of the anticoagulant (not required for components in which the anticoag-ulant has been removed, e.g., deglycerolized RBCs)
▌ Approximate volume collected from the donor (approximate volume of the product must be recorded for platelets, low volume RBCs, fresh frozen plasma, pooled components, and components collected by apheresis.

▌ Sedimenting agent, if added
▌ Recommended temperature of storage
▌ Expiration date and, when applicable, the time of expiration
▌ ABO and Rh type and interpretation of antibody tests, when positive
▌ Instructions to the transfusionist that include: "See circular of information for the use of human blood and blood components," "Properly identify intended recipient," "This product may transmit infectious agents," and "Caution: federal law prohibits dispensing without a prescription"
▌ Statement identifying the blood donor as volunteer, paid, or autologous
▌ Identification of facility collecting, modifying, or preparing the final component
▌ Any additional identifying characteristics (e.g. cytomegalovirus negative, irradiation)

NOTE   Pooled components must be labeled with a unique identification number; the name and volume of the pooled component; the number of units in the pool; the ABO and Rh type (Rh type not required for pooled cryoprecipitated AHF [CRYO]); and the name of the facility preparing the pooled components. In addition, the preparing facility must keep records of the identification number of each unit contained in the pool and have a mechanism to identify the collecting facility for each unit in the pool.

Acceptable Modifications to the Label

Modifications to the label may include:

▌ Changes in the expiration date (to shorten the length of expiration)
▌ Changes in the expiration time
▌ Changes in the name of the blood or component

e.g., a unit of CPDA-1 whole blood is entered, using an open system, to prepare a unit of CPDA-1 RBCs. The expiration date, which was originally 35 days from the date of collection, is now changed to 24 hours from the time of preparation. The expiration time is indicated and a new label indicating the new name of the component, CPDA-1 RBCs, must be placed over the original name of the component. All changes made to the label must be legible and indelible.

Each unit of blood or component issued for transfusion by the transfusing facility must have the following information printed on a label or tag that is securely attached to the container:

▌ First and last name and identification number of the intended recipient
▌ Interpretation of compatibility tests (if performed)
▌ Donor unit number assigned by the collecting or transfusing facility
▌ Individual preparing the unit

The transfusion service must maintain a record for each unit of blood or component. This record must contain the following information:

▌ Intended recipient's first and last name, identification number, ABO type, and Rh type (if required)
▌ Results of compatibility testing (if performed)
▌ Donor ABO and Rh type
▌ Donor or pool identification number
▌ Identification of the tester

At the completion of the transfusion the transfusion record, or a copy, must be a permanent part of the patient's medical record.

Release of Blood and Components for Transfusion

The following steps must be followed by the transfusion service before the release of a unit of blood or component.

▌ The appearance of each unit of blood and component must be inspected and if found unacceptable (e.g., abnormal color, clots, hemolysis, evidence of bacterial growth, evidence of thawing in frozen components, platelet aggregates) must not be issued for transfusion.

▌ The expiration date and time (if applicable) must be inspected.

▌ The results of these inspections as well as the name of the person performing the inspection must be recorded.

In an emergency situation in which the clinical situation mandates the immediate release of RBC units, the patient's first and last name, identification number, and ABO and Rh type as well as the identification number of all donor components issued must be recorded. All units must be conspicuously labeled (e.g., a brightly colored tag attached to the unit). A complete description of what is to be included in the laboratory's standard operating procedure for emergency situations can be found in the section "Patients Requiring Immediate Transfusion" in Chapter 26.

BIBLIOGRAPHY

Beattie K (chair): Immunohematology Methods and Procedures, 1st ed. Rockville, Md, American Red Cross National Reference Laboratory, 1993.

Beattie KM: Discrepancies in ABO grouping. In A Seminar on Problems Encountered in Pretransfusion Tests. Washington, DC, American Association of Blood Banks, 1972, pp 129–165.

Bryant NJ: An Introduction to Immunohematology, 2nd ed. Philadelphia, WB Saunders, 1982.

Harmening DM: Modern Blood Banking and Transfusion Practices, 3rd ed. Philadelphia, FA Davis, 1994.

Issitt PD: Applied Blood Group Serology. Miami, Montgomery Scientific Publications, 1985.

Landsteiner K, Wiener A: An agglutinable factor in human blood recognizable by immune sera for rhesus blood. Proc Soc Exp Biol NY 43:223, 1940.

Levine P, Katsin EM: Isoimmunization in pregnancy and the variety of isoagglutinins observed. Proc Soc Exp Biol NY 43:343, 1940.

Mollison PL, Engelfriet CP, Contreras M: Blood Transfusion in Clinical Medicine, 9th ed. Oxford, Blackwell Scientific Publications, 1993.

Petz LD, Garratty G: Acquired Immune Hemolytic Anemias. New York, Churchill Livingstone, 1980.

Rossi EC, Simon TL, Moss GS, Gould SA: Principles of Transfusion Medicine, 2nd ed. Baltimore, Williams & Wilkins, 1996.

Rudmann SV: Textbook of Blood Banking and Transfusion Medicine, Philadelphia, WB Saunders, 1995.

Standards Committee of the American Association of Blood Banks: Standards for Blood Banks and Transfusion Services, 17 ed. Bethesda, Md, American Association of Blood Banks, 1996.

Vengelen-Tyler V (ed): Technical Manual, 12th ed. Bethesda, Md, American Association of Blood Banks, 1996.

Wiener AS, Peters HR: Hemolytic reactions following transfusions of blood of the homologous group, with three cases in which the same agglutinogen was responsible. Ann Intern Med 13:2306, 1940.

Chapter **25**

ANTIBODY IDENTIFICATION

Elizabeth Cascone, MT(ASCP), SBB

QUICK CONTENTS

INTRODUCTION

Approximately 0.3% to 2.8% of the population have produced antibodies known to cause decreased survival of transfused antigen-positive red blood cells (RBCs) and/or hemolytic disease of the newborn (Rudmann, 1995). Pregnancy and transfusion are the most common causes of immunization to RBC antigens. The purpose of performing antibody detection testing as part of the pretransfusion compatibility protocol is to identify those individuals who have produced clinically important antibodies to RBC antigens through some previous immunizing event.

COMMONLY ENCOUNTERED BLOOD GROUP SYSTEM ANTIBODIES (See previous chapters for ABO and Rh blood groups)

BLOOD GROUP	GENES	*MAJOR* ANTIGENS	PHENOTYPES	ANTIBODIES	COMMON SEROLOGIC CHARACTERISTICS
Lewis	*Le, le*	Le^a, Le^b *Plasma* antigens Adsorb to RBC surface Attachment reversible Poorly developed at birth	Le(a+b−) Le(a−b+) Le(a−b−)* Le(a+b+) (very rare)	Anti-Le^a Anti-Le^b Anti-Le^{a+b} Antibodies frequently found in pregnant women	ANTI-Le^a AND ANTI-Le^b: IgM saline agglutinins React better at <30°C Activate complement Do not cause hemolysis of transfused RBCs Do not cause HDN Reactivity enhanced by low ionic strength solution (LISS), enzymes (e.g., ficin, papain) May be neutralized by soluble blood group substance (human saliva) Provide crossmatch compatible RBCs
I/i	*I, i*	I, i Mostly i is present at birth. Antigen i converts to I. Conversion is complete at ~2 years of age. I antigen is usually undetectable on cord RBCs.	I, i	Anti-I Anti-i	IgM saline autoagglutinin. React best at <22°C. Reactivity is enhanced by LISS, enzymes. Do not cause hemolysis of transfused RBCs. Do not cause HDN. May interfere with identification of more important alloantibodies. Use prewarming techniques to avoid interference from these antibodies. ANTI-I: Cause of cold agglutinin disease (CAD) Also called: Cold autoimmune hemolytic anemia (CAIHA) Cold hemagglutinin disease (CHD) Cold agglutinin syndrome (CAS) Activates complement in vivo High titer, broad thermal range Neutralized by soluble blood group substance

Continued ▶

*Antibody maker: individuals who make Lewis antibodies usually lack both Le^a *and* Le^b.

▶ Continued **COMMONLY ENCOUNTERED BLOOD GROUP SYSTEM ANTIBODIES** (See previous chapters for ABO and Rh blood groups)

BLOOD GROUP	GENES	*MAJOR* ANTIGENS	PHENOTYPES	ANTIBODIES	COMMON SEROLOGIC CHARACTERISTICS
					ANTI-i: Weak autoantibody reactive at <30°C May be present in patients with infectious mononucleosis Reacts preferentially with cord RBCs
P	*P, P₁, Pᵏ* *p*	P₁, P, Pᵏ, p Poorly developed on cord RBCs.	P₁ (most common), P₂ p, P₁ᵏ, P₂ᵏ (rare)	Anti-P₁ (common) RARELY ENCOUN-TERED: Anti-P, Anti-P,P₁,Pᵏ (Anti-Tjᵃ)	ANTI-P₁: Found in P₂ individuals IgM agglutinin Reacts optimally at <30°C Rarely binds complement Rarely causes hemolysis of transfused RBCs Does not cause HDN Reactivity enhanced by LISS, enzymes Neutralized by soluble blood group substance Provide crossmatch compatible RBCs ANTI-Tjᵃ: Infrequently encountered antibody. *Potent, hemolytic IgM antibody.* Reacts with all RBCs except those of p pheno-type (lacks P₁, P, and Pᵏ antigens). Causes transfusion reactions and, occasionally, HDN. Transfuse RBCs of the p phenotype.

Continued ▲

► Continued **COMMONLY ENCOUNTERED BLOOD GROUP SYSTEM ANTIBODIES** (See previous chapters for ABO and Rh blood groups)

BLOOD GROUP	GENES	*MAJOR* ANTIGENS	PHENOTYPES	ANTIBODIES	COMMON SEROLOGIC CHARACTERISTICS
MNS (M, N)	MAJOR ALLELES: *M, N*	M, N Present during fetal life	M+N−, M−N+, M+N+ M−N− is rare. M−N− individuals are also Ena−.	anti-M, anti-N, anti-'N'	ANTI-M: IgM or IgG. Frequently encountered. Saline agglutinin. Demonstrates dosage. Not reactive with enzyme pretreated test RBCs. Reacts best at 22°C or 4°C. Reactivity is enhanced at lower pH (~6.5). Does not cause hemolysis of M+ transfused RBCs. Use prewarmed technique. Rare cases of HDN (IgG). Provide crossmatch compatible RBCs (in most cases). ANTI-N: Rarely encountered. IgM. Saline agglutinin. Demonstrates dosage. Not reactive with enzyme pretreated test RBCs. Typically weak cold-reactive antibody. Does not cause hemolysis of transfused N+ RBCs. Rare cases of HDN are reported. Provide crossmatch compatible RBCs. Potent examples are made by individuals of the M+N−S−s− phenotype (requires RBCs negative for N).

Continued ▲

▶ Continued **COMMONLY ENCOUNTERED BLOOD GROUP SYSTEM ANTIBODIES** (See previous chapters for ABO and Rh blood groups)

BLOOD GROUP	GENES	*MAJOR* ANTIGENS	PHENOTYPES	ANTIBODIES	COMMON SEROLOGIC CHARACTERISTICS
MNS	*S, s, U*	S, s, U Present during fetal life	S+s−, S+s+ S−s− is uncommon except in blacks; S−s− individuals are most often U−	anti-S, anti-s, anti-U	ANTI-'N': Produced by some patients undergoing hemodialysis Antibody causes hemolysis of N+ transfused RBCs ANTI-S: IgG, immune antibody. Reacts in IAT. May bind complement. May demonstrate dosage. Enhance reactivity by room temperature (RT) (22°C) incubation before IAT. Not reactive with enzyme pretreated test RBCs. May cause HDN. May cause hemolysis of S+ transfused RBCs. Provide S− RBCs for transfusion. ANTI-s: IgG, immune antibody Reacts in IAT May bind complement May demonstrate dosage Demonstrates variable reactivity with enzyme pretreated test RBCs May cause HDN May cause hemolysis of s+ transfused RBCs Provide s− RBCs for transfusion

Continued ▶

COMMONLY ENCOUNTERED BLOOD GROUP SYSTEM ANTIBODIES

▶ Continued **COMMONLY ENCOUNTERED BLOOD GROUP SYSTEM ANTIBODIES** (See previous chapters for ABO and Rh blood groups)

BLOOD GROUP	GENES	*MAJOR* ANTIGENS	PHENOTYPES	ANTIBODIES	COMMON SEROLOGIC CHARACTERISTICS
					ANTI-U: IgG, immune antibody. Causes HDN. Causes hemolysis of U+ transfused RBCs. May bind complement. May demonstrate dosage. Reacts with enzyme treated RBCs. Found only in blacks. May be identified as the cause of warm autoimmune hemolytic anemia. Provide U− crossmatch compatible RBCs for transfusion.
Kell	MAJOR ALLELES: *K, k, Kpª, Kpᵇ, Jsª, Jsᵇ*	K, k, Kpª, Kpᵇ, Jsª, Jsᵇ Appears early in gestation on fetal RBCs	K+k−, K+k+ K−k− (rare) Kp(a−b+), Kp(a+b+), Kp(a+b−) Kp(a−b−) rare Js(a−b+), Js(a+b+), Js(a+b−)	anti-K anti-k anti-Kpª anti-Kpᵇ anti-Jsª anti-Jsᵇ	IgG, immune antibodies; some IgM anti-K. React in IAT. Do not bind complement. Reactivity is not enhanced with enzyme pre-treated RBCs. Kell antigens are destroyed by sulfhydryl reagents (DTT, ZZAP, W.A.R.M.). Reactivity may be enhanced by increasing serum to cell ratio (4 or 5 drops serum to 1 drop of cells). Cause HDN. Cause hemolysis of antigen + transfused RBCs. Provide antigen negative RBCs for transfusion.

Continued ▶

▶ Continued **COMMONLY ENCOUNTERED BLOOD GROUP SYSTEM ANTIBODIES** (See previous chapters for ABO and Rh blood groups)

BLOOD GROUP	GENES	*MAJOR* ANTIGENS	PHENOTYPES	ANTIBODIES	COMMON SEROLOGIC CHARACTERISTICS
Kidd	*Jk^a, Jk^b, Jk*	Jk^a, Jk^b, Jk3 Well developed at birth	Jk(a+b−) Jk(a+b+) Jk(a−b+) Jk(a−b−) rare	anti-Jk^a anti-Jk^b anti-Jk3	IgG, immune antibodies. React in IAT. Titer frequently diminishes to undetectable level. Readily bind complement. May be more easily detected with polyspecific AHG reagents. Frequent cause of delayed hemolytic transfusion reactions. Reactivity enhanced with enzyme pretreated RBCs. Reactivity also increased with other enhancement media (PEG, LISS). Demonstrate dosage. Cause HDN. Cause hemolysis of antigen + transfused RBCs. Provide antigen-negative RBCs for transfusion.
Duffy	MAJOR ALLELES: *Fy^a, Fy^b, Fy^x, Fy*	Fy^a, Fy^b, Fy^x, Fy3, Fy4 Well developed at birth	Fy(a+b−) Fy(a+b+) Fy(a−b+) Fy(a−b−) is uncommon except in blacks.	anti-Fy^a anti-Fy^b	IgG, immune antibodies Detected by IAT May demonstrate dosage Rarely activates complement Not reactive with enzyme pretreated test RBCs Rare cause of HDN Only one reported case of HDN due to anti-Fy^b Cause hemolysis of antigen + transfused RBCs

Continued ▲

▶ Continued **COMMONLY ENCOUNTERED BLOOD GROUP SYSTEM ANTIBODIES** (See previous chapters for ABO and Rh blood groups)

BLOOD GROUP	GENES	*MAJOR* ANTIGENS	PHENOTYPES	ANTIBODIES	COMMON SEROLOGIC CHARACTERISTICS
Lutheran	MAJOR ALLELES: Lu^a, Lu^b, Lu	Lu^a, Lu^b Poorly developed at birth	Lu(a+b−) Lu(a+b+) Lu(a−b+) Lu(a−b−) rare	anti-Lu^a anti-Lu^b anti-Lu^{ab} (Lu3)	ANTI-Lu^a AND ANTI-Lu^b: Infrequently encountered IgG or IgM May be immune or nonimmune May directly agglutinate RBCs at RT or 37°C Nonreactive with DTT-treated test RBCs Do not cause HDN ANTI-Lu^a: Demonstrates mixed field agglutination pattern Does not cause hemolysis of Lu(a+) transfused RBCs Provide crossmatch compatible RBCs ANTI-Lu^b: May cause hemolysis of Lu(b+) transfused RBCs. Provide Lu(b−) RBCs for transfusion.

See references for additional information about the blood groups mentioned and additional blood groups whose antibodies are less frequently encountered.

GUIDELINES FOR PERFORMING AN ANTIBODY IDENTIFICATION INVESTIGATION

Some points for consideration when undertaking antibody identification investigations:

1. Remember that the goal of the investigation is to

   Identify antibody or antibodies detected in preliminary serum or plasma serologic studies

   Determine the clinical importance of these antibodies

   Ensure availability of compatible units of RBCs for pretransfusion or presurgical patients (the requirements regarding this issue are generally defined by laboratory standard operating procedure)

2. Evaluate results of antibody detection testing:

   Ascertain temperature and phase of reactivity.

   NOTE   Hemolysis is a positive reaction.

   Assess variability (or lack of variability) of reactions.

   If autocontrol was tested, compare its reactivity with that of test cells.

   (See the section "Suggested Approach to Follow-Up Testing When the DAT is Positive" in Chapter 24.)

3. Select the method that is most likely to produce detectable reactions, e.g., If reactions were observed at the immediate spin phase of the antibody detection procedure, continue testing at room temperature to identify antibody(ies) detected. If reactions were observed in the IAT using LISS, continue testing by that technique to identify antibody(ies) detected.

   In some cases, testing enzyme premodified test cells provides a great deal of information. If commercially prepared ficin-treated panel cells and sufficient serum or plasma are available, it may be beneficial to select some of these cells to be tested as part of the preliminary antibody investigation.

4. Always include an autocontrol with the panel studies for comparison with reactions of test RBCs.

5. Consider the amount of serum or plasma available before beginning preliminary investigation. It may be advisable to judiciously select a small number of test RBCs to begin the investigation, especially if the amount of serum or plasma is limited. Further testing can then be targeted at identifying particular antibody specificity(ies).

   NOTE   Waiting for an additional sample may cause a delay that could compromise patient safety.

6. Phenotype the patient's RBCs for common antigens to assist in ruling out antibody specificities.

NOTE Red cell phenotype results are unreliable when
  a. Testing samples from a patient who has been recently transfused. Transfused red cells may react with reagent antiserum causing incorrect interpretation of these tests
  b. The Direct Antiglobulin Test (DAT) is positive
  All cells positive in the DAT will be positive in the IAT.

7. Evaluate reactions observed in the serologic investigation (antibody screen and RBC panel).

Evaluating Results of Red Cell Panels

When a problem is encountered in antibody detection testing, i.e., the patient's serum or plasma reacts with reagent screening cells, in general, the problem may be attributed to

- Autoantibody: antibody directed at some component of all RBCs, including the individual's own (autologous) RBCs
- Alloantibody: antibody directed at a RBC antigen(s) missing from the RBCs of the antibody maker
- Combination of autoantibody and alloantibody

The following steps are a guideline to be used when evaluating the results of an RBC panel.

1. Nonreactivity with any test cell indicates that the serum antibody is not likely to be directed against an antigen present on that nonreactive test cell.
    Sources of error in interpretation:

    Some antibodies demonstrate dosage (Rh, Kidd, Duffy, MNS); i.e., reactivity is stronger with RBCs that have a double dose of the corresponding antigen than with those with a single dose. Consider using an enhancement technique to amplify reactions with single dose test cells.

    Some antigens are variably expressed on RBCs (P_1, Sd^a, Lewis).

    Some antigens deteriorate on storage (Duffy, P_1, M, Lewis).

2. Locate the line at the top of the antigram that defines each antigen in each blood group system. Move across the row of antigen headings and cross out any antigen present on a panel cell that fails to react with the serum being tested.
3. Reactions at different phases of testing may indicate the presence of more than one antibody specificity, each with different reaction characteristics.
4. Reactions that vary in strength may indicate that the antibody is reacting with more than one antigen present on the test cell, e.g.:

TEST CELL		REACTION
R_1R_1	DDCCee	3+
R_0r	Dccee	$1+^s$
Serum may contain anti-D + C. R_1R_1: cell has both D *and* C antigens. R_0r: cell has only D antigen.		

NOTE An antibody may be present in the serum and directed against any antigen that has *not* been eliminated in the "crossout" procedure!

5. Determine the antibody specificities that may be present, based on the crossed out antigens in step 2. Significant antibodies may be present in a serum along with antibodies *not* considered clinically important such as

Antibodies reactive only at room temperature (22°C) or lower

Autoantibodies—cold or warm

In these cases, only the clinically important antibody(ies) must be identified and honored when transfusion therapy is required. Differentiating the important antibodies from the unimportant antibodies is generally accomplished by removing or bypassing the reactivity of the interfering antibody. (See the section "Commonly Used Special Serologic Techniques" on p 488.)

6. Select panel cells positive for *each antigen that has not been eliminated*, e.g., anti-D is suspected, but all K positive (K+) and E positive (E+) RBCs are also D positive (D+). Select D negative (D−) cells from another panel:

At least one red cell sample that is   D−, E−,   and   K+
At least one red cell sample that is   D−, K−,   and   E+

NOTE If select cells are unavailable, consider
Techniques to remove antigens from the RBC membrane. For example, ficin removes, M, N, S, Duffy, Xgᵃ. W.A.R.M. (Organon Teknika Corporation, Durham, N.C.) removes Kell blood group system antigens as well as Ytᵃ, M, N, S, Duffy, Xgᵃ.
Inhibition with soluble blood group substances (P₁, Lewis, Chido, Rogers). (See "Commonly Used Special Serologic Techniques" on p 488.)

7. The RBC phenotype of the individual who has produced the antibody may be very useful in the "rule out" process. Antigens that cannot be ruled out with negative panel reactions can be eliminated if the antibody maker's RBCs possess those antigens.

NOTE Remember that the RBC phenotype of patients who have been recently transfused (within 3 months) cannot be reliably determined without some advanced serologic techniques.

8. To establish the validity of the identification of any antibody specificity, the *rule of threes* should be applied:

Three positive reactions should be obtained with RBCs possessing the antigen against which the antibody is directed, e.g., if anti-D is suspected, at least three test RBC samples that are D+ should be reactive when tested with the patient's serum.

and

Three negative reactions should be obtained with RBCs lacking the antigen against which the antibody is directed, e.g., if anti-D is suspected, at least three test RBC samples that are D− should be nonreactive when tested with the patient's serum.

If more than one specificity is suspected, select RBC samples that are *positive for only one of the antigens* under investigation. Each suspected specificity must be investigated separately in this way, e.g., Anti-D, −C and −K are suspected

NO. OF CELLS TO BE RUN	ANTIGEN ON CELL	ANTIGENS ABSENT FROM CELL
3	D	C, K
3	C	D, K
3	K	D, C
3	XXX	D, C, K

NOTE The goal of serologic investigations in the transfusion service laboratory is to identify alloantibody(ies), *known to cause RBC destruction or shortened RBC survival* in the serum or plasma of prospective transfusion recipients.

Sample Problem (refer to chart on facing page)

1. Cells 1, 4, and 7 are negative when reacted with the patient's serum and demonstrate that the serum antibody is not likely to be directed against antigens on these cells. These cells are known as "rule-out" cells.

2. The line at the top of the antigram is used to cross off any antigens that are present on cells 1, 4, and 7 since they were nonreactive with the patient's serum, e.g., using cell 1 as an example, the antigens D, C, e, K, k, Kp^a, Kp^b, Js^b, Fy^a, Jk^b, Le^b, P_1, N, s, Lu^b, and Xg^a can be crossed off on the top line as illustrated:

CELL	SPECIAL TYPE	DONOR	RH-HR								KELL						DUFFY		KIDD	
			D̸	C̸	c	E	e̸	f	V	Cw	K̸	k̸	Kp̸a	Kp̸b	Jsa	Js̸b	Fy̸a	Fyb	Jka	Jk̸b

LEWIS		P	M		N		LUTHERAN		Xg		PATIENT'S TEST RESULTS				
Lea	L̸eb	P̸1	M	M̸	S	s̸	Lua	L̸ub	X̸ga	Cell	IS	37	AHG	CC

This same cross-out procedure is repeated for the antigens present on cells 4 and 7.

3. The difference in the strength and phase of reactions observed in cells 2, 5, 8, 9, and 10 at the IS, 37, and antihuman globulin (AHG) phase may indicate the presence of more than one antibody specificity.

4. The antibody specificities that may be present, based on the crossed out antigens, include anti-E, anti-C^w, anti-Le^a, and anti-Lu^a.

5. Anti-Lu^a can be eliminated because the Lu^a antigen is absent from all panel cells and therefore cannot be responsible for the reactions.

Anti-C^w is an antibody to a low incidence antigen, and although it cannot be eliminated, select cells to confirm the presence or absence of this antibody are not routinely tested unless there is some serologic evidence to suggest the antibody is present. This antibody, if present, will be detected in the cross-

CELL	SPECIAL TYPE	DONOR	D	C	c	E	e	f	V	Cw	K	k	Kpa	Kpb	Jsa	Jsb	Fya	Fyb	Jka	Jkb	Lea	Leb	P1	M	N	S	s	Lua	Lub	Xga	Cell	IS	37	AHG	CC
1	Ch−	R₁R₁	+	+	0	0	+	0	0	0	+	+	+	+	0	+	+	0	0	+	0	+	+	0	+	0	+	0	+	+	1	0	0	0	2+
2	Co(b+)	R₁ʷR₁	+	+	0	0	+	0	0	+	0	+	0	+	0	+	+	0	0	+	+	0	+	+	0	+	+	0	+	+	2	2+	1+	0	2+
3		R₂R₂	+	0	+	+	+	0	0	0	0	+	0	+	0	+	0	+	0	+	0	+	+	+	0	+	+	0	+	+	3	0	0	3+	
4		R₀r	+	0	+	0	+	+	+	0	0	+	0	+	+	+	0	0	+	0	0	0	+	+	0	+	0	0	+	0	4	0	0	0	2+
5	Co(b+)	r′r	0	+	+	+	+	+	0	0	0	+	0	+	0	+	+	+	0	+	+	0	0	+	+	+	+	0	+	+	5	2+	1+	0	2+
6		r″r	0	0	+	0	0	+	0	0	0	+	0	+	0	+	+	0	0	+	0	0	0	+	0	+	+	0	+	+	6	0	0	3+	
7		rrK	0	0	+	0	+	+	0	0	+	+	0	+	0	+	0	0	+	0	0	+	w+	+	+	0	+	0	+	+	7	0	0	0	2+
8	Co(b+)	rrFyᵃ	0	0	+	0	+	+	0	0	0	+	0	+	0	+	+	0	+	0	+	0	+	+	+	0	+	0	+	+	8	2+	1+	0	2+
9	Bg(a+)	rr	0	0	+	0	+	+	0	0	0	+	0	+	0	+	+	+	+	0	+	0	0	+	0	0	0	0	+	+	9	2+	1+	0	2+
10	Yt(b+)	R₁R₂	+	+	+	+	+	0	0	0	+	0	0	+	0	+	+	+	+	0	+	0	+	+	0	0	+	0	+	+	10	2+	1+	3+	
11		Patient's cells																													11	0	0	0	2+

match if patient serum, tested against donor cells known to express the offending antigen, is reactive.

6. The antibody specificities remaining are anti-E and anti-Le^a. Anti-Le^a is responsible for the reactions seen with cells 2, 5, 8, 9, and 10 at IS and 37. Anti-E is reacting 3+ in the AHG phase with cells 3, 6, and 10.

7. It is now necessary to determine if these antibodies fulfill the probability requirements as defined by the *rule of threes*.

PANEL CELLS	ANTIGEN PRESENT ON CELL	ANTIGEN ABSENT FROM CELL	REACTION WITH PATIENT SERUM	TOTAL NUMBER OF CELLS TESTED
2, 5, 8, 9	Le^a	E	+	4
3, 6	E	Le^a	+	2
1, 4, 7	—	E, Le^a	0	3

One additional cell that is E+Le^a must be tested with the patient's serum to comply with the *rule of threes*.

NOTE Cell 10 *cannot* be used because it is positive for *both* the E and Le^a antigens.

8. The patient's RBCs must now be phenotyped (assuming there have been no transfusions in the past 3 months) with anti-E, anti-Le^a, and anti-Le^b. It is expected that the patient's cells will lack these antigens.

SUGGESTED PROTOCOLS TO FOLLOW FOR ANTIBODY IDENTIFICATION

PROTOCOL	ANTIBODY SCREEN	PATTERN OF REACTIONS	SPECIFICITY APPARENT	SECTION	PAGE
1	Positive	Reacts with some, but not all, test cells	Yes	1	
2	Positive	One test cell nonreactive; reactions *not* variable	No	2A	
3	Positive	Reacts with all test cells; reactions variable	Either	2B	
4	Positive	Reacts with one test cell	No	2C	

NOTE The DAT in each of the following examples is negative; see the section "The Antiglobulin Test" in Chapter 24 for handling samples with a positive DAT.

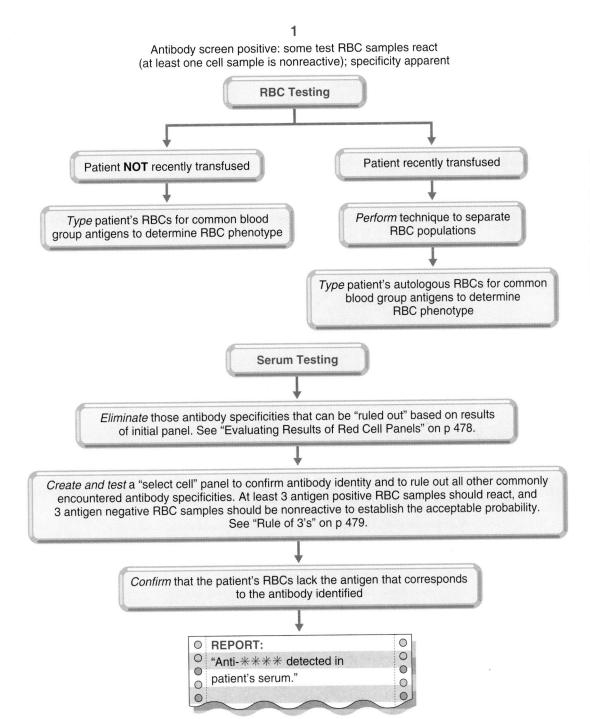

1

Antibody screen positive: some test RBC samples react
(at least one cell sample is nonreactive); specificity apparent

RBC Testing

Patient **NOT** recently transfused

Patient recently transfused

Type patient's RBCs for common blood group antigens to determine RBC phenotype

Perform technique to separate RBC populations

Type patient's autologous RBCs for common blood group antigens to determine RBC phenotype

Serum Testing

Eliminate those antibody specificities that can be "ruled out" based on results of initial panel. See "Evaluating Results of Red Cell Panels" on p 478.

Create and test a "select cell" panel to confirm antibody identity and to rule out all other commonly encountered antibody specificities. At least 3 antigen positive RBC samples should react, and 3 antigen negative RBC samples should be nonreactive to establish the acceptable probability. See "Rule of 3's" on p 479.

Confirm that the patient's RBCs lack the antigen that corresponds to the antibody identified

REPORT:
"Anti-✳✳✳✳ detected in patient's serum."

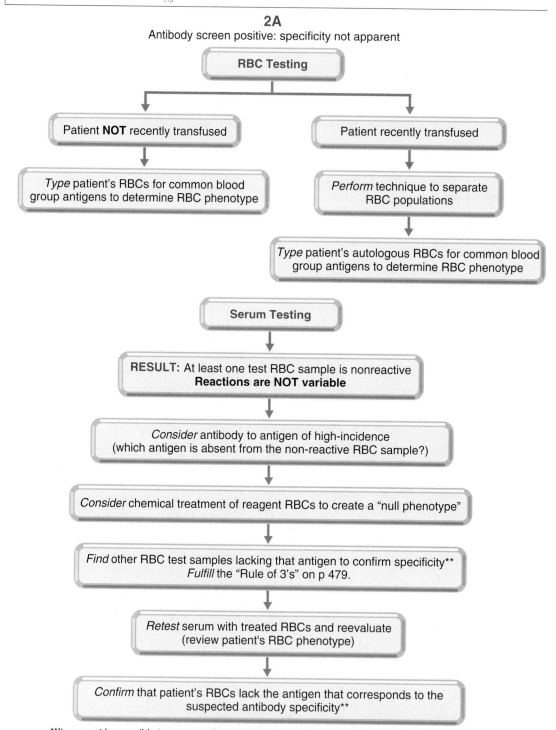

2A
Antibody screen positive: specificity not apparent

RBC Testing

Patient **NOT** recently transfused

Patient recently transfused

Type patient's RBCs for common blood group antigens to determine RBC phenotype

Perform technique to separate RBC populations

Type patient's autologous RBCs for common blood group antigens to determine RBC phenotype

Serum Testing

RESULT: At least one test RBC sample is nonreactive
Reactions are NOT variable

Consider antibody to antigen of high-incidence
(which antigen is absent from the non-reactive RBC sample?)

Consider chemical treatment of reagent RBCs to create a "null phenotype"

Find other RBC test samples lacking that antigen to confirm specificity**
Fulfill the "Rule of 3's" on p 479.

Retest serum with treated RBCs and reevaluate
(review patient's RBC phenotype)

Confirm that patient's RBCs lack the antigen that corresponds to the suspected antibody specificity**

**It may not be possible to carry out these processes in the routine hospital blood bank laboratory.
Refer sample to a Reference Laboratory for resolution/confirmation.
Generally, suitable RBCs for transfusion to a patient with this problem will be available only from a supplier of rare blood.

CONSULT LABORATORY SOPs FOR PROTOCOL THAT IS TO BE FOLLOWED IN THESE CASES

2B
Antibody screen positive: specificity not apparent

RBC Testing

Patient **NOT** recently transfused

Type patient's RBCs for commonly encountered blood group antigens to determine RBC phenotype

Patient recently transfused

Perform technique to separate RBC populations

Type patient's autologous RBCs for common blood group antigens to determine RBC phenotype

Serum Testing

RESULT: All RBCs react
Reactions demonstrate variability

Consider antibody to antigen of high incidence or multiple antibodies

1. *Test* sample in different environment, e.g., change temperature, add LISS or PEG

2. *Use* special serologic technique(s) known to abolish or enhance antibody reactivity e.g., antibody neutralization, test cell treatment with enzyme or sulfhydryl reagent (See "Commonly Used Special Serologic Techniques" on p 488.)

RESULT: Specificity apparent

See Case 1 on p 483.

○ **REPORT:**
○ "Anti-✳✳✳✳ detected
○ in patient's serum."
○

RESULT: Specificity NOT apparent

Refer sample to Reference Laboratory

CONSULT LABORATORY SOPs FOR PROTOCOL THAT IS TO BE FOLLOWED IN THESE CASES

SUGGESTED PROTOCOLS TO FOLLOW FOR ANTIBODY IDENTIFICATION

2C
Antibody screen positive: **one** test RBC sample reactive

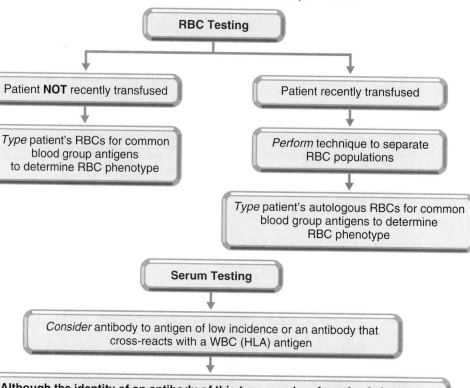

RBC Testing

Patient **NOT** recently transfused

Type patient's RBCs for common blood group antigens to determine RBC phenotype

Patient recently transfused

Perform technique to separate RBC populations

Type patient's autologous RBCs for common blood group antigens to determine RBC phenotype

Serum Testing

Consider antibody to antigen of low incidence or an antibody that cross-reacts with a WBC (HLA) antigen

1. **Although the identity of an antibody of this type may be of academic interest, pursuit of its identity is not required to provide safe transfusion if all clinically important antibody specificities are ruled out.**

2. Any unit of RBCs randomly selected is expected to be crossmatch compatible since, by definition, the antigen is present on a very small percentage (usually <1%) of the population.

3. The sample can be sent to a Reference Laboratory if identification is of interest.

4. Antibodies in this category can also be detected:
   a. in a crossmatch procedure when only one donor unit is incompatible.
   b. in babies born with a positive DAT with no apparent serologic cause.
      e.g., no ABO incompatibility with the mother
         no maternal serum antibody detected by prenatal antibody detection testing

SELECTION OF RED BLOOD CELL COMPONENTS FOR PATIENTS WITH SERUM ANTIBODIES

ANTIBODY REACTIVE ONLY AT IS OR RT PHASE	ANTIBODY REACTIVE (AGGLUTINATION OR HEMOLYSIS) AT 37°C AND/OR AHG PHASE
1. These antibodies are generally not important with regard to transfusion therapy; selection of crossmatch compatible RBCs is appropriate. 2. Prewarmed IAT crossmatch may be indicated when antibody reacts at IS phase or if carry-over reactions are observed.	1. Units of RBCs that lack the offending antigen should be selected for transfusion. 2. IAT crossmatching must be performed.

Selection of Appropriate Number of Donor Units to Screen

The number of donor units that must be tested to obtain the quantity of units requested when those units must lack single or multiple antigens can be determined by considering the number of donors in the general population that lack the relevant antigen(s).

The following formula may be used for this purpose:

$$\text{Number of units to test} = \frac{\text{number of units requested}}{\% \text{ donors with RBCs negative for the relevant antigen(s)}}$$

For example, 2 units of K negative RBCs are requested. Approximately 9% of random donor units selected are expected to lack the K antigen.

$$\text{Number of units to test} = \frac{2}{0.90} = 2.22$$

Screen 3 units to obtain 2 suitable units.

When filling requests for donor units whose RBCs lack more than one antigen, the incidence of units lacking each relevant antigen must be multiplied; the formula shown may then be applied, e.g., 2 units of $(E-Jk^a-)$ donor units are requested.

Approximately 70% of random donor units selected are expected to be $E-$.
Approximately 23% of random donor units selected are expected to lack Jk^a antigen.

$$\text{Number of units to test} = \frac{2}{0.70 \times 0.23} = 12.5$$

Screen 13 units to obtain 2 suitable units.

COMMONLY USED SPECIAL SEROLOGIC TECHNIQUES

Treatment of Red Blood Cells

PROCEDURE	PRINCIPLE
Chloroquine Diphosphate (CDP) Treatment It is not possible to obtain the RBC antigen phenotype of a patient whose RBCs have been coated in vivo with IgG antibody. The IgG present on the RBC membrane leads to a false positive result when these RBCs are tested with antisera that require testing by IAT.	IgG must be removed from surface of RBC before testing for RBC antigens by IAT. RBC must remain intact after treatment. CDP destroys only HLA antigens; other more important RBC antigens remain unaltered.
Separation of Red Cell Populations in a Patient Sample Autologous RBCs from patients who have been transfused within about 3 months cannot be reliably tested for RBC antigens because autologous RBCs are mixed with transfused RBCs in circulation.	
Separation by Hypotonic* Saline Wash	Normal RBCs are lysed when exposed to hypotonic saline. RBCs that contain hemoglobin S are resistant to hemolysis by hypotonic saline. RBC sample from a patient with sickle cell anemia who has been recently transfused can be washed with 0.3% saline solution: transfused RBCs will be hemolyzed and patient's autologous RBCs will remain intact after wash. Remaining autologous RBCs may be harvested and tested to determine RBC antigen phenotype.
Microhematocrit Centrifugation	Transfused RBCs are older than patient's own newly formed RBCs. Older RBCs are denser than neocytes. When centrifuged in microhematocrit tube, transfused RBCs occupy space at bottom of column of RBCs; least dense RBCs, patient's own neocytes, are contained in upper layer. Upper layer is harvested and phenotyped for RBC antigens.
Pretreatment of Test RBCs with Proteolytic Enzymes	Sometimes antibodies are present in a mixture of specificities, making identification of each individual specificity difficult. Treating test RBC samples with proteolytic enzyme (most commonly ficin or papain) alters some RBC antigens, especially M, N, Fy^a, Fy^b, S, and some examples of s, in a way that abolishes reactivity with their corresponding antibodies.

*Hypotonic saline: saline solution that has a lower ionic concentration than physiologic saline.

Continued ▶

► Continued **Treatment of Red Blood Cells**

PROCEDURE	PRINCIPLE
Elution of Antibody from RBCs (e.g., heat, CDP, commercial preparations) *Note:* Many chemicals that can be used effectively to produce RBC eluates are toxic and, therefore, unsuitable for routine use in the immunohematology laboratory.	Under certain circumstances (after recent transfusion or when HDN is suspected) it is important to determine specificity of antibody(ies) detected on RBC membrane in DAT. IgG antibody molecule can be dissociated from antigen that binds it to RBC membrane by physical or chemical means. Some procedures destroy RBC membrane; some leave membrane intact. Supernatant fluid (eluate) remaining after elution procedure can be tested to determine antibody specificity.
Treatment of RBCs with ZZAP ZZAP contains proteolytic enzyme (papain) and sulfhydryl reagent (dithiothreitol [DTT]) Commercial preparations of ZZAP are available	When used as preparation of autologous RBCs for serum absorption, ZZAP effectively removes autoantibody coating surface of autologous RBC, allowing more complete absorption of autoantibody from patient's serum.

Preparation of RBCs for autologous or allogeneic adsorption (see below)	Allogeneic RBCs can be prepared with ZZAP
	    To remove autoantibody from a mixture of antibodies in patient's serum, allowing detection of alloantibodies that may also be present in that serum
	    To selectively remove certain alloantibody specificities from a mixture of alloantibodies when select RBC test samples are unavailable
	    When sufficient amount of autologous RBCs is not available
	
	ZZAP *does not alter* expression of Rh and Kidd blood group antigens.
	
	When phenotype (Rh and Kidd) of adsorbing cell sample is known, serum can be investigated for presence of specific clinically significant alloantibodies after adsorption with ZZAP treated RBCs.

Serum Treatments and Antibody Enhancement Techniques

PROCEDURE	PRINCIPLE
Saline Replacement of Serum Causing Rouleaux *Note:* Rouleaux are not seen in the AHG phase of the IAT; all serum proteins should be removed by the washing process before addition of the AHG.	Abnormal proteins or synthetic plasma expanders may cause RBCs in suspension to aggregate, even when no antigen-antibody reaction has occurred; this aggregation may be mistaken for agglutination when samples being tested by the IAT are centrifuged and read for agglutination after 37°C incubation phase and before saline washing. Rouleaux can be differentiated from agglutination by replacing serum with normal saline. Rouleaux are dispersed when abnormal protein in test system is removed. True agglutination (due to antigen-antibody binding and lattice formation) remains after serum replacement.

Continued ►

▶ Continued **Serum Treatments and Antibody Enhancement Techniques**

PROCEDURE	PRINCIPLE
Prewarmed Technique for Performing IAT	Occasionally interference from cold reactive clinically unimportant antibodies is observed in the IAT. These antibodies may react in early phases of the IAT, forming agglutinates that subsequently fail to dissociate. This is known as "carry-over" reactivity. Environment (temperature) of the IAT can be controlled to remain at 37°C throughout testing; "carry-over" reactivity is prevented, whereas clinically significant IgG antibody specificities remain.
Saline IAT with Additive Solutions These additives are available as commercially prepared reagents.	Some antibodies to RBC antigens are present at very low concentration, making identification by routine IAT difficult. Use of certain additives in the IAT may enhance reactions between antigens and their corresponding antibodies and/or shorten the time required for antigens and antibodies to bind.
Low ionic strength solution (LISS) contains ionic salts, buffers, and sometimes other macromolecules	LISS reduces concentration of ions in reaction environment and reduces time required for testing.
Polyethylene glycol (PEG)	PEG enhances antigen-antibody reactivity by increasing the amount of antibody bound to RBC surface antigens.
Bovine serum albumin (22% or 30%)	Bovine serum albumin enhances agglutination seen after the 37°C phase of the IAT, but does not generally increase the amount of antibody bound to antigens on RBC membrane.
Inhibition of Antibody Reactions	Genes that code for production of some blood group antigens code for production of soluble blood group substance as well. Soluble forms of these blood group antigens can be found in certain body fluids: plasma, urine, breast milk, saliva. In addition, soluble blood group substances exist in other sources in nature; these solutions can be harvested and purified for use in the immunohematology laboratory.

Neutralizable Antibody Specificities	*Primary Source of Substance*	
ABO antibodies	Human saliva	When serum antibodies exist in a mixture, soluble blood group substances can be used to remove the reactivity seen with RBC panel samples that possess the corresponding antigen. This is especially useful when select test cell samples lacking the antigen in question are not available, e.g., E−, c−, K−, Jk(b−), P1− RBC samples are required for antibody investigation. E−, c−, K−, Jk(b−), P1+ cell samples can be chosen if testing is performed with patient's serum mixed with P$_1$ substance.
Anti-Le^a and/or anti-Le^b†	Human saliva	
Anti-P$_1$†	Hydatid cyst fluid Pigeon eggs	
Anti-Sd^a	Human urine	
Anti-Ch (Chido)	Human plasma	
anti-Rg (Rogers)	Human plasma	Soluble blood group substances can also be used to establish the identity of a particular neutralizable antibody, when reactions observed on the panel mimic reactions of a more clinically significant antibody specificity. It is imperative that serum mixed with normal saline instead of soluble blood group substance be tested in parallel with neutralized serum as a control of the dilution process. Positive reactions observed when antigen positive cell samples are tested with control serum validate negative reactions with those RBCs when tested with neutralized serum.

†Substance commercially available

Continued ▶

PROCEDURE	PRINCIPLE
Serum Antibody Adsorption	One basic principle of immunology is that serum or plasma antibodies recognize and bind to their corresponding antigens. Sometimes, serum for investigation contains antibody directed against the patient's own RBC antigens. Reactivity due to cold or warm reactive autoantibodies can be abolished by absorbing autoantibody from serum or plasma with autologous or allogeneic RBC samples, chemically treated to maximize the amount of antibody adsorbed.
Cold Autoantibody Adsorption	This procedure is appropriate when the prewarmed IAT technique combined with use of monospecific anti-IgG AHG fails to abolish reactivity caused by cold reactive autoantibody.
Warm Autoantibody Adsorption	This procedure is appropriate when warm reactive autoantibody present in patient's serum reacts with all RBC samples tested; reactions of a concomitant alloantibody in the serum of a patient previously transfused or pregnant could be undetectable under these circumstances.
Warm Allogeneic Adsorption	This procedure is appropriate when: ▮ Warm reactive autoantibody present *in a recently transfused patient's serum* reacts with all RBC samples tested; reactions of a concomitant alloantibody in the serum of this patient could be undetectable under these circumstances. Autologous RBCs are unsuitable for use in adsorption because the sample is a mixture of autologous and transfused RBCs. Transfused RBCs may possess antigen(s) that correspond to alloantibodies in the patient's serum. In these cases, alloantibody may not be identified because it could be adsorbed by transfused RBCs. ▮ Mixture of alloantibodies is present in patient's serum, making selection of antigen negative test samples difficult or impossible. Allogeneic RBC samples can be selected, by phenotype, to differentially adsorb suspected alloantibody specificities leaving others in plasma to be investigated and identified.

Note: Other methods of treating test samples, both RBCs and serum, are described in Section 6 of the AABB Technical Manual. The methods listed and described above are those that are most easily performed in the routine immunohematology laboratory, and/or the most commonly used procedures.

COMMONLY USED SPECIAL SEROLOGIC TECHNIQUES

BIBLIOGRAPHY

Anstall HB, Blaylock RC: The P blood group system: biochemistry, genetics and clinical significance. In Moulds JM, Woods LL, eds: Blood Groups P, I, Sd^a and Pr. Arlington, Va: American Association of Blood Banks, 1991, pp 1–22.

Beattie KM: The Duffy blood group system: distribution, serology and genetics. In Pierce P, Macpherson CR, eds: Blood Group Systems: Duffy, Kidd and Lutheran. Arlington, Va; American Association of Blood Banks, 1988, pp 1–20.

Crawford MN: The Lutheran blood group system: serology and genetics. In Pierce P, Macpherson CR, eds: Blood Group Systems: Duffy, Kidd and Lutheran. Arlington, Va, American Association of Blood Banks, 1988, pp 93–117.

Daniels G: The Kell blood group system: genetics. In Laird FB, Daniels G, Levitt J, eds: Blood Group Systems: Kell. Arlington, Va, American Association of Blood Banks, 1990, pp 1–36.

Graham HA, Williams AN: A genetic model for the inheritance of the P, P_1 and P^k antigens (abstract). Transfusion 18:638, 1978.

Holliman SM: The MN blood group system: distribution, serology and genetics. In Moulds JM, Woods LL, eds: Blood Group Systems: MN and Gerbich. Arlington, Va; American Association of Blood Banks, 1989, pp 1–29.

Judd WJ: Methods in Immunohematology. Durham, NC, Montgomery Scientific Publications, 1994.

Mallory D, ed: Immunohematology Methods. Rockville, MD, The American National Red Cross, 1993.

Marsh WL, Reid ME, Kuriyan M, Marsh NJ, eds: A Handbook of Clinical and Laboratory Practices in the Transfusion of Red Blood Cells. Moneta, Va, Moneta Medical Press, 1993.

Mougey R: The Kidd blood group system: serology and genetics. In Pierce P, Macpherson CR, eds: Blood Group Systems: Duffy, Kidd and Lutheran. Arlington, Va, American Association of Blood Banks, 1988, pp 53–71.

Nance ST: Serology of the ABH and Lewis blood group systems. In Wallace ME, Gibbs F, eds: Blood Group Systems: ABH and Lewis. Arlington, Va, American Association of Blood Banks, 1986, pp 57–77.

Rudmann SV: Textbook of Blood Banking and Transfusion Medicine. Philadelphia, WB Saunders, 1995.

Schultz MH: Serology and clinical significance of Kell blood group system antibodies. In Laird FB, Daniels G, Levitt J, eds: Blood Group Systems: Kell. Arlington, Va, American Association of Blood Banks, 1990, pp 37–64.

Vengelen-Tyler V, ed: Technical Manual, 12th ed. Bethesda, Md, American Association of Blood Banks, 1996.

Wallace ME, Green TS, eds: Selection of Procedures for Problem Solving. Arlington, Va, American Association of Blood Banks, 1983.

Chapter *26*

COMPONENT THERAPY

Elizabeth Cascone, MT(ASCP), SBB

Deborah Firestone, MA, MT(ASCP), SBB

Q U I C K   C O N T E N T S

INTRODUCTION

More than 22 million blood components are transfused in the United States each year. Blood components and derivatives are prepared from blood collected by whole blood or apheresis donation. Blood products can be divided into three groups: those that are prepared from whole blood donation and contain red blood cells (RBCs), those that are prepared from whole blood donation and do not contain RBCs, and blood derivatives that are commercially prepared. Commercially prepared blood derivatives are manufactured from large pools of human plasma and either do not transmit viral infections or have been processed in a manner known to significantly decrease the risk of spreading transfusion transmitted infections.

COMMON BLOOD PRODUCTS AVAILABLE FOR TRANSFUSION

COMPONENTS THAT CONTAIN RED BLOOD CELLS	COMPONENTS THAT DO NOT CONTAIN RED BLOOD CELLS	COMMERCIALLY PREPARED BLOOD DERIVATIVES
Whole blood (WB) or modified whole blood	Fresh frozen plasma (FFP)	Factor VIII concentrate (available as recombinant factor VIII and plasma derived factor VIII)
Red blood cells (RBCs)	Cryoprecipitated Antihemophilic Factor (AHF) (cryo)	Factor IX concentrate (available as high purity plasma derived factor IX concentrate and pro-thrombin complex concentrate)
Red blood cells, adenine saline added	Platelet concentrate (PC)	
Leukocyte reduced red blood cells (LR-RBC)	Platelets, Pheresis (SD-PC)*	Albumin solutions
Washed red blood cells (W-RBCs)	Granulocytes, pheresis (GC)*	Plasma protein fraction
Deglycerolized red blood cells (D-RBCs)		Immune serum globulin
		Antithrombin III concentrate
		Rh immune globulin
*Depending on the method of preparation, these products may contain >5mL of RBCs.		

The goal of component therapy is to provide the patient with the safest possible blood product that will achieve the desired clinical outcome. Each component has its own specific clinical indication(s) for use based on the composition of the product. Guidelines have been established (by state, federal, and professional organizations) that define the serologic testing that must be performed on blood products and components before transfusion (see Chapter 24). The benefits of transfusion (e.g., improved tissue oxygenation, control of bleeding) must be carefully weighed against the potential adverse effects (e.g., acute or delayed hemolytic transfusion reactions, transmission of infectious diseases, alloimmunization, immunosuppression). A number of organizations such as the National Institutes of Health, American Association of Blood Banks, and College of American Pathologists have issued clinical practice guidelines for blood component therapy. These guidelines are designed to improve transfusion practices, minimize the risks associated with transfusions, and decrease costs. Once a decision has been made to transfuse a particular blood component or derivative, the efficacy of each transfusion must be assessed. This can be accomplished by comparing the relevant pre- and post-transfusion laboratory data. All apparently unwarranted transfusions should be retrospectively reviewed by the hospital transfusion committee.

PREPARATION OF BLOOD AND COMPONENTS

Components That Contain Red Blood Cells

RBCs are prepared from a whole blood donation by sedimentation during refrigerated storage or centrifugation. Approximately 225 to 250 mL of plasma is removed before the expiration date of the blood.

RBCs adenine saline added are prepared from whole blood collected into an anticoagulant solution such as CPD or CP2D. After sedimentation or centrifugation and removal of plasma (see preparation of RBCs described previously), the additive contained in an attached satellite bag is added to the packed RBCs.

Leukocyte reduced RBCs are most commonly prepared by filtration of RBCs before or after storage using leukocyte depletion filters. This method removes 99% to 99.9% of the original number of white blood cells in the RBC unit. Other methods used in the preparation of leukocyte reduced RBCs include centrifugation of whole blood followed by removal of the buffy coat and saline washing of packed RBCs. These methods, however, are less effective in removing white blood cells than using a leukocyte depletion filter.

Washed RBCs are prepared by automated or manual techniques that add an RBC compatible solution, such as normal saline, to RBCs followed by mixing, centrifugation, and removal of the supernatant saline and plasma solution. The process is repeated until most leukocytes, platelets, and plasma are removed.

Frozen RBCs are most commonly prepared by adding a "high" concentration of glycerol to RBCs within 6 days of collection. The RBC glycerol solution is agitated, allowed to equilibrate for 5 to 30 minutes, and frozen at $-65°$ C or lower. The RBCs are *deglycerolized* by thawing the frozen unit at $37°$ C and washing the unit initially with 12% NaCl followed by subsequent washing with decreasing concentrations of saline. At the completion of the wash process, the deglycerolized RBCs are suspended in normal saline with 0.2% dextrose. The unit is then available for transfusion for up to 24 hours. Other less commonly used methods to prepare frozen RBCs include the addition of a "low" concentration of glycerol and agglomeration.

Components That Do Not Contain Red Blood Cells

Fresh frozen plasma (FFP) is prepared by centrifuging a unit of whole blood at $4°$ C using a "heavy" spin. The plasma is separated from the RBCs of an individual donor unit and placed at $-18°$ C or lower within 8 hours of the collection.

Cryoprecipitated antihemophilic factor (AHF) is prepared by thawing a unit of FFP between $1°$ and $6°$ C to a consistency of slush. The unit of thawed FFP is then centrifuged at $1°$ to $6°$ C, using a "heavy" spin; the FFP bag is then hung in an inverted position or placed in a plasma expressor so that approximately 90%

of the cryo poor plasma can be removed. The 10 to 15mL of supernatant plasma remaining in the original bag contains the cold insoluble material known as *cryoprecipitate*. The cryoprecipitated AHF is refrozen at −18° C or lower. The supernatant plasma in the transfer bag is labeled "cryo-depleted plasma" and refrozen at −18° C or lower.

Platelet concentrates are separated within 8 hours of collection from a unit of whole blood that has been kept at room temperature before the separation process. The unit of whole blood is centrifuged, using a "light" spin and the platelet rich plasma is separated into a transfer bag. The remaining RBCs are refrigerated at 1° to 6° C. The platelet rich plasma is centrifuged at 20° C using a "heavy" spin, and the majority of the supernatant platelet depleted plasma is expressed into a transfer bag, labeled "fresh frozen plasma" and frozen at −18° C or lower. The remaining platelets are then stored at 20 to 24° C with gentle agitation until use or expiration. The shelf life is determined by the composition of the plastic bag used for collection and storage. Six to 10 units of platelet concentrates are usually pooled for transfusion to an adult.

Platelets, pheresis and *granulocytes, pheresis* are prepared by cytapheresis. This process involves the use of an instrument that removes whole blood from a donor, mechanically separates the whole blood into components, retains the desired component (platelets or granulocytes), and returns the remaining fractions to the donor. One unit of single donor platelets is equivalent to 6 to 8 units of platelet concentrates.

PREPARATION OF COMMERCIALLY DERIVED BLOOD PRODUCTS

Commercially available blood derivatives are prepared by a process known as *plasma fractionation*. Methods of plasma fractionation include cold ethanol fractionation and affinity and ion exchange chromatography. The major adverse effect of transfusion of plasma derivatives is the transmission of viral diseases. Methods currently in place to decrease the risk of viral transmission due to the transfusion of plasma derivatives include:

▌ Predonation physical examination and health history
▌ Self-exclusion of blood donors (opportunity provided for donors to self-defer)
▌ Serologic testing of donor blood for viral markers
▌ Manufacturing processes used specifically to reduce transmissibility (e.g., heat treatment, ultraviolet light, chemical inactivation)

The preparation of plasma derivatives by recombinant DNA technology produces a product that carries minimal risk of disease transmission. This technology is currently being used to manufacture factor VIII concentrate.

COMPOSITION AND STORAGE OF COMPONENTS

Each blood component and derivative has its own unique composition and storage requirements.

Components That Contain Red Blood Cells

NAME OF COMPONENT	COMPOSITION	APPROXIMATE VOLUME (ML)	STORAGE TEMPERATURE (°C)	EXPIRATION DATE
Whole Blood (WB) or Whole Blood Modified	RBCs; few white blood cells (WBCs) and platelets	500	1–6	21 days after collection for *CPD* and *CP2D;* 35 days after collection for *CPDA-1*
Red Blood Cells (RBCs)	RBCs; reduced plasma; few WBCs and platelets	250	1–6	Same expiration date as WB from which it was prepared if separated in *closed system;* 24 hours if separated in *open system*
RBCs Adenine Saline Added	RBCs; reduced plasma; few WBCs and platelets; 100 mL additive solution	330	1–6	42 days
Leukocyte Reduced RBCs (LR-RBCs)	≥80% of original RBCs; few platelets; minimal plasma; product must contain $<5 \times 10^8$ WBCs if intended to prevent febrile transfusion reactions and $<5 \times 10^6$ WBCs if intended to decrease alloimmunization to HLA antigens and cytomegalovirus transmission	200	1–6	Same expiration date as RBCs if prepared in *closed system;* 24 hours if prepared in *open system*
Washed RBCs (W-RBCs)	RBCs; no plasma; $<5 \times 10^8$ WBCs	180	1–6	24 hours after entering unit
Deglycerolized RBCs (D-RBCs)	RBCs; $<5 \times 10^8$ WBCs; no platelets; no plasma	180	*Frozen:* ≤ -65 *Thawed:* 1–6	*Frozen:* up to 10 yr *Thawed:* transfuse within 24 hr of thawing

Components That Do Not Contain Red Blood Cells

NAME OF COMPONENT	COMPOSITION	APPROXIMATE VOLUME (ML)	STORAGE TEMPERATURE (°C)	EXPIRATION DATE
Fresh Frozen Plasma (FFP)	Plasma; all coagulation factors; complement	220	*Frozen:* ≤ -18 *Thawed:* thaw rapidly at 30–37; store at 1–6	*Frozen:* up to 1 yr *Thawed:* 24 hr after thawing

COMPOSITION AND STORAGE OF COMPONENTS

Continued ▶

▶ Continued **Components That Do Not Contain Red Blood Cells**

NAME OF COMPONENT	COMPOSITION	APPROXIMATE VOLUME (ML)	STORAGE TEMPERATURE (°C)	EXPIRATION DATE
Cryoprecipi-tated AHF (Cryo)	Fibrinogen; factor VIII, factor XIII, von Willebrand factor (vWF), fibronectin	15	*Frozen:* ≤ − 18	*Frozen:* up to 1 yr
			Thaw at 30–37; store at 20–24	*Thawed:* transfuse within 6 hr of thawing
			Pooled: 20–24	*Pooled:* transfuse within 4 hr of pooling
Platelet Concentrate (PC)	>5.5 × 10^{10} platelets/unit; trace RBCs; WBCs; plasma	50	20–24 with continuous gentle agitation	Up to 5 days (depending on collection method or storage bag)
			Pooled: 20–24 with continuous gentle agitation	*Pooled:* 4 hr after pooling
Platelets, Pheresis (SD-PC)	>3 × 10^{11} platelets/unit; plasma; amount of RBCs and leukocytes depends on method of collection	300	20–24 with continuous gentle agitation	24 hr if prepared in *open* system; 5 days if prepared in *closed* system
Granulocytes, Pheresis (GC)	>1 × 10^{10} granulocytes/unit; plasma; variable amounts of lymphocytes, RBCs (may be >5mL), and platelets	300	20–24	24 hr; however, should be administered as soon as possible after collection

Commercially Prepared Blood Derivatives

NAME OF DERIVATIVE	COMPOSITION
Factor VIII Concentrate	Lyophilized concentrate of FVIII; activity units on label
Factor IX Concentrate	Lyophilized concentrate of FIX; may be some FII, FVII, FX, protein C, and ABO antibodies depending on method of preparation
Albumin	5% or 25% protein solution containing 96% albumin and 4% globulins as well as other proteins
Plasma Protein Fraction	5% protein solution containing 83% albumin and 17% alpha and beta globulins
Immune Serum Globulin	Protein solution containing 95% IgG; trace amounts of other serum proteins; available for intramuscular or intravenous administration
Antithrombin III	Antithrombin III; trace amounts of other plasma proteins
Rh Immune Globulin	Concentrate containing primarily IgG anti-D; a full dose (300 μg) of Rh immune globulin protects against 15 mL of D positive cells, a microdose (50 μg) of Rh immune globulin protects against up to 2.5 mL of D positive cells; available as preparation for intramuscular or intravenous administration

The concentration of each individual blood derivative varies depending on the volume of the product. Storage temperatures and expiration dates are detailed in the package insert.

DONOR BLOOD GROUP COMPATIBILITY

ABO Compatibility

Whole blood for transfusion should be ABO group specific with the recipient; transfusions of packed cells should be ABO group compatible with the recipient. Since platelets carry ABH antigens, it is recommended that platelets be ABO compatible with the recipient's serum. In a clinical situation when there is a need for platelets, transfusion should not be delayed in order to obtain ABO compatible platelets. When transfusing infants and young children with pooled platelets or single donor platelets that contain ABO antibodies incompatible with the recipient's RBCs, it may be desirable to remove the majority of the plasma. Transfusions of FFP should be ABO compatible with the recipient's RBCs. ABO compatible cryoprecipitate should be transfused when large volumes of plasma are being transfused relative to the recipient's RBC mass. Granulocyte concentrates and platelet concentrates contain RBCs and therefore must be ABO compatible with the recipient. Blood derivatives are transfused without regard to ABO compatibility.

ABO Compatibility of Cellular and Plasma Containing Products

PATIENT ABO TYPE	CELLULAR PRODUCTS ABO TYPE				PLASMA PRODUCTS ABO TYPE			
	O	A	B	AB	O	A	B	AB
O	Y	N	N	N	Y	Y	Y	Y
A	Y	Y	N	N	N	Y	N	Y
B	Y	N	Y	N	N	N	Y	Y
AB	Y	Y	Y	Y	N	N	N	Y

Y, ABO type of cellular or plasma product is compatible; N, ABO type of cellular or plasma product is not compatible.

Rh Compatibility

Recipients who are D positive may receive D positive or D negative whole blood or RBC components. Recipients who are D negative must receive D negative whole blood or RBC components. FFP and cryoprecipitate do not contain RBCs and may be transfused without regard to $Rh_0(D)$ antigen type. Each unit of platelet concentrate may contain up to 0.5 mL of RBCs. It may be necessary therefore to consider $Rh_0(D)$ antigen incompatibility when selecting platelet products for transfusion to certain patient populations (e.g., D negative female of childbearing age). If D positive platelets are transfused to a D negative individual, administration of Rh immune globulin may be considered to prevent Rh immunization. A full dose of Rh immune globulin will protect against the RBC contamination in 30 units of D positive platelet concentrates or 3 units of D positive platelets, pheresis. Blood derivatives are transfused without regard to the patient's $Rh_0(D)$ antigen type.

SEROLOGIC TESTING OF BLOOD COMPONENTS BEFORE TRANSFUSION

The crossmatch test (donor RBCs with patient serum) is required before transfusion of whole blood and RBC containing components; this includes platelet and granulocyte products that contain more than the acceptable volume of RBCs. If the recipient has no clinically important antibodies and no history of such antibodies, a test to detect ABO incompatibility is required. If the recipient has a clinically important RBC antibody or a history of a previously detected clinically important antibody, the indirect antiglobulin test (IAT) must be used for crossmatching. The crossmatch is not required for non-RBC containing products such as platelets and plasma components; however, most facilities require that the ABO and $Rh_0(D)$ type of the recipient be known and/or confirmed before components are selected for transfusion. Refer to the section on crossmatching in Chapter 24 for additional discussion of required pretransfusion crossmatch tests.

INDICATIONS AND CONTRAINDICATIONS FOR TRANSFUSION OF COMPONENTS

The decision to transfuse a patient with a specific component is generally made after a review of the relevant laboratory data and a complete assessment of the patient's clinical needs and symptoms.

Components That Contain Red Blood Cells

NAME OF COMPONENT	INDICATIONS FOR TRANSFUSION	DO NOT TRANSFUSE:
Whole Blood or Whole Blood Modified	1. To provide blood volume expansion and RBC mass in acute (loss of >25% of blood volume) blood loss 2. For neonatal exchange transfusion	1. For volume replacement 2. When a specific component is suitable and available
RBCs or RBCs Adenine Saline Added	1. To increase RBC mass of symptomatic, normo-volemic patients	1. For anemia that can be treated pharma-cologically or nutritionally 2. To patients who are well compensated for their anemia

Continued ▶

▶ Continued **Components That Contain Red Blood Cells**

NAME OF COMPONENT	INDICATIONS FOR TRANSFUSION	DO NOT TRANSFUSE:
Leukocyte Reduced RBCs	1. To increase RBC mass in patients with severe and/or recurrent nonhemolytic febrile transfusion reactions due to leukocyte antibodies 2. To increase RBC mass in patients at risk for alloimmunization to leukocyte or HLA antigens or susceptible to cytomegalovirus infection	Same as RBCs
Washed RBCs	1. To increase RBC mass of symptomatic anemic patients with history of febrile, urticarial, and possibly anaphylactic transfusion reactions 2. To increase RBC mass of patients with paroxysmal nocturnal hemoglobinuria and IgA deficiency 3. For intrauterine transfusion	Same as RBCs
Deglycerolized RBCs	1. To increase RBC mass in patients with rare blood types, paroxysmal nocturnal hemoglobinuria, and certain allergic or febrile transfusion reactions 2. To prolong storage of rare or autologous units 3. For intrauterine transfusion	1. When cost precludes routine use in transfusion therapy

Components That Do Not Contain Red Blood Cells

NAME OF COMPONENT	INDICATIONS FOR TRANSFUSION	DO NOT TRANSFUSE:
Fresh Frozen Plasma	1. To reverse effects of Warfarin (Coumadin) or anticoagulant drugs 2. To replace antithrombin III 3. To correct multiple coagulation factor deficiencies (e.g., liver disease, disseminated intravascular coagulation) 4. To replace isolated factor deficiencies when specific component is not available 5. As replacement fluid in plasma exchange for TTP (thrombotic thrombocytopenic purpura) and HUS (hemolytic uremic syndrome)	1. For volume expansion 2. As nutritional supplement 3. As source of immunoglobulins 4. To enhance wound healing
Cryoprecipitated AHF	1. For treatment of hemophilia A, factor XIII deficiency, congenital or acquired fibrinogen deficiency, and von Willebrand's disease unresponsive to DDAVP 2. As source of fibrin glue	1. When safer, more concentrated factor concentrate is available
Platelet Concentrate	1. For bleeding due to thrombocytopenia or thrombocytopathy 2. For low platelet count	1. For treatment of idiopathic autoimmune thrombocytopenic purpura 2. For drug induced thrombocytopenia 3. For untreated DIC 4. For TTP

INDICATIONS AND CONTRAINDICATIONS FOR TRANSFUSION OF COMPONENTS

Continued ▶

▶ Continued **Components That Do Not Contain Red Blood Cells**

NAME OF COMPONENT	INDICATIONS FOR TRANSFUSION	DO NOT TRANSFUSE:
Platelets, Pheresis	1. For thrombocytopenic patients alloimmunized to HLA or platelet antigens; the donor should be HLA matched. 2. To limit donor exposure in thrombocytopenic patients who require long term platelet transfusions	1. Same as platelets
Granulocytes, Pheresis	1. Patients with documented granulocyte dysfunction or myeloid hypoplasia who are unresponsive to antibiotics and *have a good prognosis for recovering from the neutropenia*	1. To patients with poor chance of bone marrow recovery 2. To patients with infections that are responsive to antibiotic therapy

Commercially Prepared Blood Derivatives

NAME OF COMPONENT	INDICATIONS FOR TRANSFUSION	DO NOT TRANSFUSE:
Factor VIII Concentrate	1. To prevent or control bleeding in hemophilia A patients with moderate to severe deficiency of factor VIII 2. For patients with low titers of FVIII inhibitors	1. To treat von Willebrand's disease 2. When bleeding is not associated with deficiency of FVIII
Factor IX Concentrate	1. To prevent or control bleeding in patients with hemophilia B or with specific factor deficiencies 2. For selected patients with FVIII or FIX inhibitors	1. When bleeding is not associated with deficiency of FIX 2. To patients at risk of thrombosis or those with liver disease
Albumin; Plasma Protein Fraction	1. To replace loss of colloids in hypovolemic shock, severe burns, or for pressure support during hypotensive episodes 2. As replacement fluid in plasmapheresis	1. For nutritional support 2. When crystalloid replacement would be more appropriate 3. When patient's clinical condition dictates otherwise
Immune Serum Globulin	1. To patients with congenital hypogammaglobulinemia 2. As prophylaxis in certain diseases (e.g., hepatitis A, measles)	
Antithrombin III	1. To treat congenital deficiencies associated with thrombotic disease	
Rh Immune Globulin	1. To prevent immunization to $Rh_0(D)$ antigen of D negative females who are pregnant or have recently delivered 2. To treat patients with some hematologic disorders (e.g., idiopathic thrombocytopenic purpura, autoimmune hemolytic anemia) 3. To prevent immunization to D antigen when D negative patient has been intentionally or unintentionally transfused with limited amount of D positive blood products	1. To D negative female who has given birth to D negative baby 2. To D negative female immunized to the $Rh_0(D)$ antigen

BLOOD TRANSFUSION ALTERNATIVES

DDAVP (1-deamino-8-D-arginine vasopressin) is a synthetic analog of vasopressin. DDAVP promotes release of factor VIII (FVIII) and von Willebrand factor (vWF) from endothelial storage sites into the circulation. It is the drug of choice in the treatment of patients with mild cases of hemophilia A and type 1 or type 2 (with the exception of type 2B) von Willebrand's disease who have previously shown an adequate response to DDAVP. After infusion of DDAVP, levels of clotting factor peak at 30 to 60 minutes and have a half-life similar to that of endogenous clotting factors. DDAVP has also been shown to be useful in treating a variety of platelet function disorders.

Erythropoietin is a glycoprotein secreted by the kidney that stimulates RBC production by acting on erythroid committed stem cells (erythroid colony forming units, or CFU-E). Erythropoietin has been produced using recombinant DNA technology and is known as *recombinant human erythropoietin* (rHuEPO). rHuEPO has been effective in treating anemia associated with end stage renal disease and human immunodeficiency virus (HIV) infected patients receiving zidovudine (AZT). Other uses for rHuEPO therapy such as reducing the need for allogeneic blood transfusion in autologous blood donors undergoing elective surgery, anemia in the presurgical patient, and anemia subsequent to chemotherapy are under investigation.

GENERAL CONSIDERATIONS IN THE ADMINISTRATION OF BLOOD AND COMPONENTS

All blood and blood components *must* be transfused through a standard 170 to 260 micron filter. It is recommended that the filter be changed every 4 hours or after 2 to 4 units have been transfused. The manufacturer's instructions should be consulted for the appropriate use of filters in the administration of commercially prepared blood derivatives. The following chart identifies general considerations in the administration of blood and components.

ISSUE	CONSIDERATIONS
Compatible Fluids	No medications are to be added to blood or components. Normal saline is acceptable to add to blood or component container; fluids intended for IV use may be added to blood or components or come in contact with blood in administration set only if approved by FDA.
Leukocyte Reducing Filter	Administration of RBCs through leukocyte reducing filter eliminates need for standard blood filter.
Time Limits	Duration of rate of infusion varies with patient's clinical condition. 4 hr is commonly used as maximal time permitted for infusion to reduce risk of bacterial contamination.

Continued ▶

► Continued

ISSUE	CONSIDERATIONS
Reissue of Components	May only be reissued if the following conditions are met: 1. Container seal has not been penetrated. 2. Component has been maintained at temperature <10° C. 3. Not more than 30 min has elapsed from time of issue (unless stored in monitored refrigerator). 4. Records must indicate blood has been reissued and inspected before reissue.
Blood Warmers	May be indicated for: 1. Adult patients receiving rapid (>50 mL/kg/hr), multiple transfusions 2. Exchange or large volume transfusions in infants 3. Children being infused at rates >15 mL/kg/hr 4. Patients with cold agglutinins active in vitro at 37° C 5. Rapid infusion of blood through central venous catheter
Gamma Irradiation	To prevent graft versus host disease Required for cellular components (RBCs, platelets, granulocytes) when donor is blood relative of intended recipient or if recipient is immunocompromised (e.g. Hodgkin's disease, bone marrow transplantation, intrauterine transfusion, congenital immunodeficiency)

ASSESSING THE EFFICACY OF TRANSFUSION

COMPONENT	ASSESSMENT OF RESULTS OF TRANSFUSION	EXPECTED RESULTS WERE NOT SEEN
Red Blood Cells or Whole Blood	Perform hemoglobin and hematocrit within 24 hr after completion of transfusion. Expect increase of 1–1.5 g/dL hemoglobin and 3–5% hematocrit for each unit transfused in hematologically stable adult.	Consider: patient's clinical condition (e.g., bleeding)
Platelets	Observe for cessation of bleeding. Perform platelet count 10 min to 1 hr after completion of transfusion. Expect increase in platelets of $5–10 \times 10^9$/L per *platelet concentrate* in 70 kg adult. Expect increase of $30–60 \times 10^9$ platelets/L per unit of platelets, pheresis in a 70 kg adult. Perform corrected count increment (CCI*) to determine posttransfusion increment in platelets. CCI >4000–5000/μL is indicative of adequate response to platelets. Two consecutive CCI values <4000–5000/μL suggest platelet refractoriness. $$*CCI = \frac{[\text{platelet count after transfusion} - \text{platelet count before transfusion } (10^9/L)] \times \text{body surface area } (m^2)}{\text{number of units transfused}}$$	Consider: HLA antibodies, platelet antibodies, splenomegaly, DIC, infection, bone marrow transplantation, massive transfusion, active bleeding, drugs *Additional components to consider transfusing:* HLA matched platelets for patients with HLA antibodies, Crossmatch platelets for patients with platelet antibodies

Continued ►

▶ Continued **ASSESSING THE EFFICACY OF TRANSFUSION**

COMPONENT	ASSESSMENT OF RESULTS OF TRANSFUSION	EXPECTED RESULTS WERE NOT SEEN
Factor VIII	Expect posttransfusion activity levels of FVIII of 30%–100% depending on patient's clinical condition. Amount of FVIII to be transfused can be calculated using following formula: 1. Weight (kg) $\times$ 70 mL/kg = blood volume (mL) 2. Blood volume (mL) $\times$ (1.0 − hematocrit) = plasma volume 3. Units of FVIII required = (desired FVIII level in units/mL − initial FVIII level in units/mL) $\times$ plasma volume (mL) *Note:* Value obtained for amount of FVIII units is divided by 80 to calculate number of bags of cryoprecipitate required.	Consider: FVIII antibodies *Additional treatment strategies to consider:* 1. Induce immune tolerance using large infusions of FVIII. 2. Porcine FVIII. 3. Concentrates of activated FIX complex.

PATIENTS WITH SPECIAL TRANSFUSION NEEDS

Patients Requiring Immediate Emergency Transfusion

The process to provide care for patients who have an urgent need for transfusion should be clearly defined by a laboratory standard operating procedure (SOP). This SOP should address:

1. Conditions and situations that constitute emergency situations qualifying for immediate release of blood components
2. Official forms or requests that must be submitted
3. Information required to be present on the forms submitted
4. Patient sample requirements
5. Patient sample labeling requirements
6. Information required on the tag attached to the blood component, e.g.:

   Patient's name

   Patient's unique identifier

   "Uncrossmatched unit"

   "Partially crossmatched unit"

7. The amount, type, and sequence of components to be issued under emergency circumstances, including detailed guidelines addressing conditions under which D positive RBCs may be transfused to a D negative patient.

   Since emergency situations may arise at any time, it is critical that all transfusion service personnel be thoroughly familiar with the laboratory SOP for emergency release of blood components as described.

   Health care providers (nurses, physicians, residents, physician's assistants, and so forth) staffing areas such as the emergency service, surgical suite, and intensive care units may have a limited knowledge or understanding of the process required to obtain blood components quickly. In these circumstances, any delay can represent a life threatening event. Transfusion service staff thoroughly familiar with the protocol to provide blood components in an emergency can guide clinicians through the process of obtaining blood components in an orderly and timely way.

Patients Suffering Acute, Rapid Blood Loss (Hemorrhage)

Massive transfusion is the replacement of one or more blood volumes within a 24 hour period. Blood volume depends on body surface area and can be calculated as a function of height and weight. In general, a single volume replacement in the average adult is about 10 units of RBCs. The source of bleeding may not always be evident, e.g., gastric or intestinal bleeding, internal fractures, internal organ injury.

MANIFESTATIONS OF HEMORRHAGE:

- Rapid, thready pulse
- Low blood pressure
- Increased respirations
- Pallor
- Cold and clammy skin
- Decreased hemoglobin, hematocrit, and RBC count

TREATMENT OF HEMORRHAGE INCLUDES:

- Prevention of vascular collapse by administration of colloids or other solutions containing electrolytes.

 Transfusion of FFP is *not* recommended for the purpose of fluid replacement since it constitutes possible exposure to a blood borne transmissible disease.

- Restoration of oxygen carrying capacity by administration of RBCs.

COMPATIBILITY TESTING IN MASSIVE TRANSFUSION

When 10 or more units have been transfused, the patient's sample submitted before transfusion is not representative of the patient's post-transfusion status; most of the blood circulating is really the blood and fluids that have been transfused. A delay in issuing additional RBCs in order to complete serologic crossmatches using the patient's serum is generally not warranted.

POTENTIAL APPROACH TO COMPATIBILITY TESTING FOR PATIENTS WHO HAVE RECEIVED MASSIVE TRANSFUSION

PATIENT'S PRETRANSFUSION STATUS	COMPATIBILITY TEST OPTIONS
1. No detectable clinically important antibodies to RBC antigens	▎ "Immediate spin" crossmatch ▎ "Electronic (computer)" crossmatch ▎ Uncrossmatched ABO and Rh compatible RBCs
This approach precludes transfusion of donor RBCs that are ABO and/or Rh incompatible with isoagglutinins in the patient's plasma (determined by pretransfusion ABO and Rh testing).	
2. Clinically important antibodies to RBC antigens detected and identified Clinical situation allows time required for serologic testing	▎ Use commercial antiserum that detects offending antigen. ▎ Perform immediate spin serologic crossmatch confirmed with antigen negative donor RBCs (this step identifies only ABO incompatibilities).
Commercial antiserum generally has antibody titer equal to or greater than that of patient; detection of an antigen incompatible with patient's serum antibody is more likely using commercial antiserum than using patient's serum diluted with transfused components and other IV fluids.	

3. Clinically important antibodies to RBC antigens detected and identified
 	
Clinical situation *does not* allow time required for serologic testing
	1a. Select ABO/Rh_0(D) compatible donor units identified as negative for offending antigen in previous antigen screening efforts.
	  b. Perform immediate spin serologic crossmatching with antigen negative donor units. (This step identifies only ABO incompatibilities)
	2a. Select ABO/Rh_0(D) compatible donor units identified as negative for offending antigen in previous antigen screening efforts.
	  b. Issue antigen negative donor units without serologic crossmatching.
	3. Issue ABO/Rh_0(D) compatible donor units untested for offending antigen.

These are life-threatening situations, in which delay caused by serologic testing of any kind could cause or contribute to the death of a patient. The consequences of transfusing ABO compatible blood, even if there is Rh_0(D) or other antigen incompatibility, can be addressed at a later time, *providing the patient survives the massive hemorrhage!*	

PATIENTS WITH SPECIAL TRANSFUSION NEEDS

NOTE Prescribed procedures for providing RBCs in these situations depends on each blood bank director's discretion and preferences; *procedures MUST be clearly defined in laboratory SOP manual.* Laboratory SOP for emergency and/or massive transfusion must be followed!

ADVERSE EFFECTS OF MASSIVE TRANSFUSION

SIGN OR SYMPTOM	CAUSE	EFFECT	TREATMENT OR PREVENTION
Hypothermia	Rapid infusion of refrigerated RBCs	Decreased temperature at sinoatrial node of heart; cardiac arrhythmia	Use of blood warmer
Hypocalcemia	Citrate in donor unit complexing with circulating ionized calcium in recipient	Tetany in patient with severe liver disease, kidney disease, or other conditions that impair normal metabolism	Administration of IV calcium solution
Acid-Base Disturbances	Rapid transfusion of anticoagulated RBCs stored in citrate	Respiratory disturbances Inability to oxygenate tissues Cardiac disturbances	Restoration of acid-base balance
Depletion of 2,3-diphosphoglycerate	Transfusion of large amount of stored RBCs ($\geq$2 wks old) in short period of time	Decrease in oxygen carrying capacity of RBCs	Selection and issue of units that are a mixture of fresher and older RBCs
Dilutional Thrombocytopenia or Dilutional Coagulopathy	Transfusion of large amounts of stored blood	Inability to arrest bleeding	Effective fluid replacement and tissue perfusion Administration of platelet products Administration of fresh frozen plasma and/or cryoprecipitated AHF
Immune Suppression	Unknown	Decreased resistance to infection	Drug therapy

Neonatal Transfusion

Special problems of low birth weight (<1500 g) and seriously ill neonates include:

▌ Body size with concomitant small blood volume
▌ Unresponsive immune system
▌ Passive acquisition of maternal antibodies through placental transport
▌ Anemia induced by frequent testing of blood samples
▌ Increased affinity of fetal hemoglobin for oxygen

INDICATIONS FOR NEONATAL TRANSFUSION

1. Determination of anemia is based on:

   The age, weight, and physical condition of the infant

   Hemoglobin values that define anemia

> **NOTE** Hemoglobin values are normally much higher in infants than in adults or older children

2. Anemia in infants with HDN whose bilirubin concentrations are too low to necessitate an exchange transfusion

SPECIAL REQUIREMENTS FOR RBCS TO BE TRANSFUSED TO SICK NEONATES

> **NOTE** This protocol should be defined in a laboratory SOP.

RBC REQUIREMENTS	EFFECTS
Serologically compatible with mother and infant	Prevents destruction or reduced survival of RBCs due to passively acquired maternal antibodies
As fresh as possible	Contains reduced concentration of metabolic byproducts that increase with time of storage
Unlikely to transmit cytomegalovirus (CMV) (either seronegative or prefiltered to adequately reduce leukocytes)	Reduces chance of infection with CMV, which can cause life threatening pneumonia in immunocompromised recipient

In some cases in which the infant is physiologically compromised it may also be advisable to transfuse:

- RBCs negative for hemoglobin S (HbS) because reduced oxygen tension in the neonate may cause HbS RBCs to sickle
- Irradiated RBCs because some infants are susceptible to graft versus host disease (GVHD)
- RBC units free of adenine preservative solution (AS) to prevent the transfusion of increased amounts of some components of the preservative that may be detrimental to severely compromised infants

DOSAGE AND ADMINISTRATION OF RBCS FOR TRANSFUSION:

- Must be carefully calculated as a function of the infant's total blood volume
- About 3 mL of packed RBCs/kg of body weight should increase the infant's hemoglobin by about 1 g/dL
- RBCs should not be administered through a needle with a bore smaller than that of a 25 gauge needle to prevent mechanical hemolysis

POSSIBLE APPROACHES OF THE TRANSFUSION SERVICE TO NEONATAL TRANSFUSION:

1. One (D negative) or two (one D negative and one D positive) units of group O RBCs may be used for all neonatal transfusions until the unit(s) is (are) finished.

Features of This Practice:

▮ A sterile connecting device (SCD) can be used, if available, to connect additional satellite bags so that the unit may be used for multiple small volume transfusion

▮ Attached satellite bags can be used to preserve the unit for more than 24 hours, (shelf life of a unit of RBCs with a broken seal)

▮ This practice results in maximum utilization of a commodity (fresh, cytomegalovirus [CMV] negative pediatric unit) that may be chronically in short supply

▮ Virtually all transfusions are performed with fresh RBCs

2. One unit may be selected and reserved for each individual neonate requiring transfusion.

Features of This Practice:

▮ Small aliquots may be transferred to integral satellite bags and issued for transfusion.

▮ The expiration date of the remainder of the unit is unchanged, and the unit may be used until it is no longer suitable for a neonate (defined by SOP).

▮ Limits exposure of the infant to blood borne transmissible diseases.

PRETRANSFUSION TESTING FOR NEONATAL PATIENTS

Neonates require transfusion, in many cases, because of blood loss attributed to frequent phlebotomy or heel sticks for laboratory testing. Neonates do not generally produce antibodies of their own before about 6 months of age. In an effort to reduce the chances of inducing this type of anemia (iatrogenic anemia), regulatory agencies require a minimum of compatibility testing for those neonates who are to be treated with transfusion therapy.

1. Serologic testing required for neonates *once per admission* (provided only group O RBCs are transfused):

   ABO grouping (forward typing only)

   $Rh_0(D)$ typing

   Antibody detection testing

NOTE   Antibody detection testing may be performed on a serum sample from the mother *or* the infant.

2. Serologic testing that should be repeated at prescribed intervals:

▮ Indirect antiglobulin test to detect anti-A or anti-B in the infant's plasma if:

Group specific (other than group O) RBCs are transfused

Serologic studies (positive direct antiglobulin test [DAT] or incompatible cross-match with RBCs other than group O) indicate ABO incompatibility due to passively acquired maternal isoagglutinins

▮ Indirect antiglobulin test (IAT) to detect incompatibility due to a serum antibody directed against an antigen other than ABO if:

Clinically important antibodies are demonstrated in antibody detection testing of the mother's or infant's serum

3. Special considerations regarding serologic testing of samples from neonates:

Infants whose serum is incompatible with group specific RBCs because of anti-A, anti-B, and/or anti-A,B must be transfused with group O RBCs. It is unnecessary to perform serologic crossmatching of the group O RBCs with the patient's serum in these cases.

If the mother has a clinically important serum antibody to an RBC antigen other than A or B, the unit to be transfused must lack the offending antigen. To provide antigen negative RBCs for transfusion:

Antigen type RBCs from the donor unit for the offending antigen.

Or perform serologic crossmatching using the indirect antiglobulin test.

Testing should be performed and continued at intervals, defined by the laboratory SOPs, for as long as antibody is detectable in the infant's serum.

Neonates and Fetuses with Hemolytic Disease of the Newborn

DEFINITION

Hemolytic disease of the newborn (HDN) is a clinical condition caused by the immune destruction of fetal or neonatal RBCs due to the attachment of maternal antibody to an antigen present on the membrane of the fetal or neonatal RBCs.

ETIOLOGY AND CHARACTERISTICS OF HEMOLYTIC DISEASE OF THE NEWBORN AND FETUS

▮ The fetus inherits a gene from the father that codes for an RBC antigen that the mother's RBCs lack.

▮ The mother's immune system is exposed to the foreign antigen on the baby's RBCs (most frequently during birth but sometimes during gestation).

▮ The woman produces IgG antibody to the "foreign" RBC antigen.

▮ In subsequent pregnancies with fetuses whose RBCs carry the offending antigen, the maternal IgG antibody that crosses the placenta binds to the antigen on the surface of the fetal RBC and causes immune destruction.

▮ The disease becomes progressively more severe with subsequent pregnancies when fetal RBCs carry the offending antigen.

▮ HDN varies in severity based on antibody specificity, antibody class and subclass, serum antibody concentration, and the number of pregnancies with fetuses whose RBCs carry the offending antigen.

▮ HDN begins during gestation and continues even after birth, until the maternal antibody dissipates or is removed.

▌ The disease follows a course that leads to different features in the fetus and the newborn:

	PATHOLOGIC FEATURE	CHARACTERISTICS
In Utero	"Hydrops fetalis"	Anemia Cardiac insufficiency Accumulation of fluid in the tissues of the fetus (edema)
Neonatal Period	Permanent, irreversible brain damage	Antibody mediated RBC destruction (hemolysis) Accumulation of plasma bilirubin Absorption of bilirubin by body tissue containing lipids, including the brain

▌ When serum antibodies known to cause HDN are identified in antenatal testing, and/or the woman has a history of babies born with HDN, the woman is monitored closely during pregnancy to detect signs of fetal RBC destruction in utero.

INVESTIGATIONS AND PROCEDURES PERFORMED DURING PREGNANCY AS INDICATORS OF FETAL RBC DESTRUCTION INCLUDE:

▌ Periodic determination of maternal antibody titer
▌ Ultrasound imaging
▌ Amniocentesis (removal with a needle of a sample of the amniotic fluid for analysis)
▌ Percutaneous umbilical blood sampling (PUBS) (removal with a needle of a sample of fetal blood for analysis)

DIAGNOSIS OF HEMOLYTIC DISEASE OF THE NEWBORN

▌ A clinically important antibody to an RBC antigen(s) is detected in the mother's serum, usually in prenatal serologic studies.
▌ The presence of the antigen on the RBCs of the fetus.
▌ Previous baby (ies) diagnosed with HDN.

NOTE   Antibody produced in a previous immune response remains a potential problem for the antibody maker throughout life; the immune system retains its ability to destroy the target antigen once the individual is sensitized.

INDICATORS TO PREDICT THE SEVERITY OF THE EFFECTS OF CIRCULATING ANTIBODY ON THE FETUS

▮ Rising titer of serum antibody during gestation.

▮ Amniocentesis.

Elevated bilirubin level indicates RBC destruction. Critical values are determined from a graph (Liley graph) that relates the bilirubin concentration to gestational age.

L/S ratio (lecithin to sphingomyelin):

Indicator of fetal lung maturity

Predicts likelihood of pulmonary complications in a fetus if delivered before completion of gestation by cesarean section

L/S ratio less than 2.0: cesarean section contraindicated

▮ Cordocentesis (obtaining RBCs from the fetus in utero from a blood vessel in the umbilical cord). This procedure generally provides a very limited amount of sample, so testing must be selected to provide the greatest amount of information.

Serologic testing that can be performed on a sample obtained by cordocentesis to determine the likelihood of antigen-antibody reaction:

ABO group

$Rh_0(D)$ type

DAT

RBC typing for the offending antigen

Determination of hemoglobin concentration and hematocrit to detect anemia

NOTE The course of the pregnancy may or may not be interrupted by cesarean section, depending on the indications of the clinical and serologic evaluation and the likelihood of harming the fetus by premature delivery. A severely anemic fetus whose lungs are still immature must be allowed to remain in utero until the danger of respiratory problems becomes less likely. In these cases, the fetus must undergo treatment in utero.

TREATMENT OF HEMOLYTIC DISEASE OF THE NEWBORN

	INTRAUTERINE TRANSFUSION	EXCHANGE TRANSFUSION
Definition	Transfusion of packed RBCs to the fetus	Removal of infant RBCs coated with maternal antibody and replacement with antigen negative RBCs in 1 unit of whole blood
When performed	In utero	Neonatal period
Indications	Fetus <32 wk gestation Immaturity of fetal lungs	Hyperbilirubinemia Anemia

PATIENTS WITH SPECIAL TRANSFUSION NEEDS

Continued ▶

► Continued **TREATMENT OF HEMOLYTIC DISEASE OF THE NEWBORN**

	INTRAUTERINE TRANSFUSION	**EXCHANGE TRANSFUSION**
Goals	Correction of anemia	Removal of bilirubin Removal of antibody Removal of antibody coated RBCs Provision of antigen negative RBCs
Sample for crossmatching	Mother's serum	Mother's serum (preferred) *or* Infant's serum *or* Eluate made from cord RBCs
Selection of RBCs	As fresh as possible (preferably <5 days old) Group O, negative for offending antigen Irradiated CMV negative Negative for hemoglobin S Hematocrit 75% to 85%	As fresh as possible (preferably <5 days old) Group O or group specific* Negative for offending antigen Irradiated CMV negative Negative for hemoglobin S Hematocrit ~50%
Volume to be transfused	About 50 mL Calculated by physician as function of fetal age and/or size	"Double volume" exchange (usually 1 unit of RBCs reconstituted to whole blood (~500 mL) is provided.)

*Depends on sample used for compatibility testing.

PREVENTION OF HEMOLYTIC DISEASE OF THE NEWBORN

▮ No prevention exists for HDN except for those cases that are caused by maternal immunization to $Rh_0(D)$ antigen.

▮ Prevention of HDN due to anti-D (the most destructive RBC antibody) through the administration of Rh immune globulin (RhIg) is accomplished prophylactically.

Rh IMMUNE GLOBULIN

Composition	Anti-D made from pooled human plasma Not known to be source of viral transmission
Dosage	300 μg Covers fetal bleed of 30 mL of whole blood (15 mL RBCs) 50 μg Suitable for administration during first trimester
Mechanism of protection	Unknown

Administration	*Antepartum* at about 28 wk of gestation
	Postpartum within 72 hr of delivery
	After any event during pregnancy that could result in exposure of the mother's immune system to fetal RBCs (as little as 0.1 mL of fetal blood could immunize a woman to the $Rh_0(D)$ antigen).
	These events include:
	    Spontaneous or induced abortion
	    Trauma to the abdomen
	    Ectopic pregnancy
	    Chorionic villus sampling
	    Amniocentesis
	    Cordocentesis
	    Fetal hemorrhage

Determination of candidacy for RhIg	Woman must be $Rh_0(D)$ negative and must not be immunized to the $Rh_0(D)$ antigen,* and infant must be D positive†

Determination of volume of fetal bleed	Screening test
	    Rosette test (qualitative only)
	Quantitative test‡
	    Kleihauer-Betke acid elution test
	    Enzyme linked antiglobulin test (ELAT)
	    Flow cytometry

*Antepartum dose of RhIg may be detected in postpartum sample; this does not disqualify the woman as a candidate for RhIg therapy.

Note: RhIg should never be withheld when there is doubt about the source of the D antibody detected in the mother's serum or if more than 72 hr has elapsed since delivery.

†When the $Rh_0(D)$ type of fetus cannot be determined, the fetus is assumed to be $Rh_0(D)$ positive.

‡The dose of RhIg must be increased when the fetal bleed is determined to be >30 mL of whole blood. (Calculation for the administration of >1 vial of RhIG is found on p 475 of the *AABB Technical Manual.*)

Patients with Immune Hemolytic Anemia

PROBLEM	MOST LIKELY CAUSATIVE AGENT	FEATURES	TREATMENT
Warm Autoimmune Hemolytic Anemia	IgG antibody Reacts optimally at 37° C Specificity usually not apparent May demonstrate relative specificity for some antigen in Rh blood group system (e.g., e, E, or c)	1. Antibody usually causes extravascular hemolysis by cells of the reticuloendothelial system 2. Laboratory features: Positive DAT Some have IgG on RBCs Some have IgG + C3 Occasionally only C3 detectable Positive IAT Elevated reticulocyte count Decreased hemoglobin and hematocrit Decreased haptoglobin Increased serum bilirubin (indirect) Increased urine urobilinogen 3. Clinical signs of hemolysis (variable) Fatigue Pallor Shortness of breath Palpitations Tachycardia (rapid heart beat) Mild jaundice Enlarged spleen	1. Glucocorticosteroids 2. Splenectomy 3. Cytotoxins 4. Transfusion Not treatment of first choice. Often, donor RBCs cannot be found to be "compatible" with autoantibody. Transfused RBCs are usually destroyed at same rate as autologous RBCs. Serum alloantibody(ies) may be masked by reactivity of autoantibody. *Note:* See "Suggested Approaches to Follow-up Testing for the DAT" in Chapter 24 for approach to solving serologic problems seen in these patients. Although the warm reactive autoantibody occasionally demonstrates a relative specificity (often anti-e), it is generally not advisable to transfuse antigen negative donor RBCs. *Note:* Some patients with apparent autoantibody that appears to have specificity in the Kell blood group system should be given RBCs that lack the specific antigen.

REASONS FOR TRANSFUSING DONOR RED BLOOD CELLS THAT DO NOT LACK THE ANTIGEN COMPLEMENTARY TO THE SPECIFICITY OF THE WARM AUTOANTIBODY

1. The specificity demonstrated when investigating autoantibodies is frequently a "relative" in vitro specificity; the autoantibody is usually directed against some "core antigen" present on the membrane of *all* RBCs.
2. Most often, antigen negative donor RBCs survive no better than autologous or antigen positive allogeneic RBCs.
3. The patient's RBCs may lack the antithetical antigen; transfusion of donor RBCs negative for the apparently offending antigen could cause immunization to the antithetical antigen, (e.g., transfusing e−E+ donor RBCs could immunize an E− patient).

4. Selecting antigen negative donor RBCs for transfusion to a patient with an autoantibody demonstrating an apparent RBC antigen specificity removes that unit(s) for use by a patient who has produced an *alloantibody* to that antigen.

PROBLEM	MOST LIKELY CAUSATIVE AGENT	FEATURES	TREATMENT
Cold Agglutinin Syndrome Cold Hemagglutinin Disease Cold Agglutinin Disease	IgM antibody: Reacts optimally at 0°–4° C Is occasionally reactive up to 30° C Has a specificity usually for I/i antigens, but other blood group system autoantibodies have been reported Must be distinguished from benign form of anti-I present in most healthy individuals who suffer no adverse effects from antibody Pathologic form usually has titer >1000	1. Antibody usually binds to RBCs in microvasculature of skin and extremities; subsequently IgM dissociates but causes hemolysis by activating complement as RBCs reach 37° C. Hemolysis may be intravascular *and* extravascular. 2. Laboratory features: Positive DAT (only C3 detectable on RBCs) Negative IAT *Note:* Occasionally, in severe cases, RBCs may agglutinate immediately and irreversibly, appearing positive in the IAT. Reticulocytosis Increased serum bilirubin (indirect) Hemoglobinuria during hemolytic episodes Hemosiderosis Difficulty in obtaining accurate RBC indices because of spontaneous RBC agglutination Rouleaux formation on blood smear	Disease is usually self-limiting and generally does not require intervention. Treatment, when required, may include: 1. Fluid support to avoid renal failure secondary to hemolysis 2. Limitation of patient's exposure to cold environment 3. Plasmapheresis in extreme cases 4. Transfusion for patients whose cardiovascular or cerebrovascular system is compromised Use of blood warmer is appropriate. Washing RBCs will avoid transfusing additional complement.
Paroxysmal Cold Hemoglobinuria (PCH)	IgG antibody "Biphasic hemolysin" with behavior of CAD antibody (see above) Anti-P specificity	1. Onset following upper respiratory infection 2. Laboratory features Positive DAT (only C3 present on RBCs) *Note:* IgG is not usually detectable unless RBCs are washed in cold (4° C) normal saline; this is temperature of reactivity of IgG antibody associated with PCH). Hemoglobinemia Hemoglobinuria Reticulocytosis Leukocytosis Increased serum bilirubin (indirect) Rouleaux formation on blood smear 3. Clinical features: Shaking chills Back and leg pain Abdominal cramps Fever Hemoglobinuria 4. Positive Donath-Landsteiner test*	Disease is usually self-limiting and does not require intervention. 1. Avoid exposure to cold. 2. Administer only warm RBCs if transfusion is required.

PATIENTS WITH SPECIAL TRANSFUSION NEEDS

Continued ►

► Continued

PROBLEM	MOST LIKELY CAUSATIVE AGENT	FEATURES	TREATMENT
Drug Induced Hemolytic Anemia	1. May be due to binding of IgG antibody or activation of complement. 2. Method of RBC destruction is dependent on process initiated by formation of drug-antidrug complex or drug–RBC interaction	1. Laboratory features: Vary with mechanism involved† 2. Clinical features: May cause anemia with related symptoms	Generally self-limiting problem that ceases when drug is discontinued: 1. Discontinue drug 2. Glucocorticosteroids (occasionally necessary)

*The principle of the Donath-Landsteiner test is found on p 668 in the *AABB Technical Manual.*
†Methods to detect drug induced antibodies can be found on pp 669 to 672 in the *AABB Technical Manual.*

Oncology Patients

Treatment of the primary disease using radiation therapy and chemotherapy induces secondary conditions (e.g., anemia, thrombocytopenia, and leukopenia) requiring transfusion therapy.

POSSIBLE ADVERSE EFFECT OF TRANSFUSION	COMPONENT REQUIRED
Transfusion associated graft vs host disease	Irradiated cellular components: RBCs Platelet products Granulocyte products
CMV infection (especially pneumonia)	1. RBCs and platelet products from donors seronegative for the antibody to CMV 2. Leukocyte reduced RBCs and platelet products
Platelet refractoriness due to alloimmunization to HLA and/or platelet antigens	1. Leukocyte reduced RBCs and platelet products (prophylaxis) 2. HLA-matched single donor platelets 3. Crossmatch compatible platelets

Patients Requiring Plasma Exchange

Plasma exchange is the removal of a patient's plasma and replacement of the volume removed with normal donor plasma or human serum albumin. This process removes some pathologic substances in the patient's plasma and supplies a volume of compatible fluid in an attempt to correct the abnormality.

Plasma exchange is used to correct abnormal conditions due to pathologic substances such as:

> ▌ Abnormal serum proteins
> ▌ Circulating immune complexes
> ▌ Circulating plasma antibodies

Some diseases for which plasma exchange has been successfully used as treatment include:

> ▌ Thrombotic thrombocytopenic purpura (TTP)
> ▌ Waldenström's macroglobulinemia
> ▌ Multiple myeloma
> ▌ Systemic lupus erythematosus (SLE)
> ▌ Guillain-Barré syndrome
> ▌ Multiple sclerosis
> ▌ Myasthenia gravis

Plasma is used for TTP, liver disease, and coagulopathies

Normal human plasma is the product of choice for plasma exchange.

> ▌ The volume required for the procedure is calculated for each patient as a function of his or her body weight.
> ▌ One volume exchange is usually sufficient, although sometimes more than one volume is replaced.
> ▌ Frequently the treatment must be performed several times based on:
>
> The results of the monitors used to measure the indicator parameter
>
> A predetermined protocol for the course of treatment

Problems associated with providing blood products for patients undergoing plasma exchange:

> ▌ A significant amount of time is required to defrost the necessary volumes of FFP required for this procedure.
> ▌ A sufficient supply of blood product (FFP) must be available; this may be more units than the blood bank normally keeps in inventory.
> ▌ The procedure is generally performed several times; this requires that the blood bank keep a sufficient inventory of FFP to provide product for multiple procedures. This can present supply or storage problems.
> ▌ Advance notice of the intention to perform one or more procedures facilitates provision of the required components.

NOTE These patients generally do not require the coagulation factors present in FFP. The policy must be clearly defined in the laboratory SOP manual allowing that plasma intended for use in a plasma exchange procedure and thawed more than 24 hours before the procedure is suitable for use.

Patients with Sickle Cell Anemia

Sickle cell anemia is a condition caused by inheritance of a gene that codes for an abnormal hemoglobin (HbS). RBCs that contain HbS hemolyze, assume a sickled or crescent shape, and/or aggregate on sickling. Sickling of the patient's RBCs is the result of changes in the hemoglobin molecule that occur when the oxygen tension is low; the sickling is irreversible.

Characteristic changes in the HbS RBCs are brought about by any condition that results in reduced oxygen supply (hypoxia). These conditions include:

- Fever
- Stress
- Infection
- Respiratory disease
- Exposure to extremes of environmental temperature

Sickle cell crisis is a condition caused by an acute episode of sickling of RBCs containing HbS. Signs and symptoms of sickle cell crisis include:

- Severe pain in the extremities and abdomen (due to occlusion of small blood vessels by microaggregates of the sickled RBCs)
- Fever
- Fatigue
- Shortness of breath
- Pallor
- Rapid heartbeat
- Hematuria
- Priapism (prolonged, painful erection)

Possible serious complications of sickle cell crisis are:

- Stroke
- Acute chest syndrome

Treatment:

- Symptomatic treatments (e.g., oxygenation, hydration, management of pain) are used to manage this disease in its acute phase
- In the RBC exchange procedure:

  A volume of the patient's impaired RBCs that contain HbS is removed and replaced with donor RBCs that contain HbA (normal hemoglobin).

  The procedure is commonly performed with automated instruments (cytapheresis).

  The volume to be exchanged is calculated by the physician, based on the patient's blood volume and the amount of RBCs to be replaced.

Problems associated with transfusing patients with sickle cell anemia:

- Many of these patients are immunologic responders and frequently have produced alloantibodies to RBC antigens known to cause destruction of transfused antigen positive RBCs
- These patients are generally of African or Mediterranean origin and possess an ethnically characteristic RBC phenotype; some of the antigens against which these patients form alloantibodies are present in high incidence in ethnically dissimilar populations (e.g., Js^b,U).
- When these individuals produce multiple clinically significant alloantibodies, donor RBCs suitable for transfusion are most easily obtained from ethnically similar donors. These donor units may be in short supply.
- These patients often produce autoantibodies, warm and/or cold reactive, that are present in the serum along with alloantibodies.

  Identifying multiple antibodies in these patients may present a challenge for the routine hospital transfusion service due to reduced staff, unavailability of resources, and/or shortage of time required to complete the serologic investigation required in these cases.

Increased time may be required before compatible blood can be provided if the sample must be sent to a reference laboratory for serologic investigation.

▌ When these patients have produced one or more clinically significant RBC antibodies:

Obtaining a sufficient number of donor units negative for one or more RBC antigens may present a problem.

Advanced notification of the intention to perform an RBC exchange procedure on this type of patient allows time for a donor unit screening effort or to order RBCs from the blood bank's supplier of rare blood.

▌ When the patient has no detectable clinically significant RBC antibodies:

Some blood bank medical directors may prefer, when possible, to provide donor units that match, to some degree, the RBC phenotype of the intended recipient, to minimize the risk of alloimmunizing these patients. This decision must be carefully considered, since this practice may lead to what some suppliers call "unjustified use of a limited resource," by removing units from the available supply that may be needed for patients who have already produced alloantibodies. Patients who have produced multiple clinically significant alloantibodies often require transfusion with the same antigen negative donor units.

HOSPITAL TRANSFUSION COMMITTEE

The Joint Commission for Accreditation of Hospital Organizations requires that all blood transfusions be reviewed to ensure that they were used appropriately. The hospital transfusion committee may serve as the peer review group for blood transfusions in the hospital. The committee is most effective when composed of those individuals who are involved in the selection and administration of blood. The committee is charged with (1) ensuring that the appropriate indications for the transfusion of blood, blood components, and derivatives were met and (2) reviewing transfusion reactions and complications.

BIBLIOGRAPHY

American Society of Anesthesiologists Task Force on Blood Component Therapy: Practice guidelines for blood component therapy. Anesthesiology 84:732–747, 1996.

Association of Hemophilia Clinic Directors of Canada: Hemophilia and von Willebrands disease: 2. Management. Can Med Assoc J 153(2):147–157, 1995.

Butch SH, Tiehen A (eds): Blood Irradiation: A User's Guide. Bethesda, MD, American Association of Blood Bank Press, 1996.

Contreras M, Ala FA, Greaves M, et al: Guidelines for the use of fresh frozen plasma. British Committee for Standards in Haematology, Working Party of the Blood Transfusion Task Force: Transfus Med 2(1):57–63, 1992.

Development Task Force of the College of American Pathologists: Practice parameter for the use of fresh-frozen plasma, cryoprecipitate and platelets. JAMA 271:777–781, 1994.

Gill JC: Therapy of factor VIII deficiency. Semin Thromb Hemost 19(1):1–12, 1993.

Harmening DM: Modern Blood Banking and Transfusion Practices. Philadelphia, FA Davis, 1994.

Hutchinson RJ: Blood products. Semin Pediatr Surg 1(3):231–241, 1992.

PATIENTS WITH SPECIAL TRANSFUSION NEEDS

Klapper EB, Goldfinger D: Leukocyte-reduced blood components in transfusion medicine. Current indications and prospects for the future. Clin Lab Med 12(4):711–721, 1992.

Lane TA, Anderson KC, Goodnough LT, et al: Leukocyte reduction in blood component therapy. Ann Intern Med 117(2):151–162, 1992.

Miller JP, Mintz PD: The use of leukocyte-reduced blood components. Hematol Oncol Clin North Am 9(1):69–90, 1995.

Mollison PL: Blood Transfusion in Clinical Medicine. Oxford, Blackwell Scientific, 1993.

Muirhead N, Bargman J, Burgess E, et al: Evidence-based recommendations for the clinical use of recombinant human erythropoietin. Am J Kidney Dis 26(2 suppl 1):1–24, 1995.

Murphy MF, Brozovic B, Murphy W, et al: Guidelines for platelet transfusions. British Committee for Standards in Haematology, Working Party of the Blood Transfusion Task Force. Transfus Med 2(4):311–318, 1992.

Nacht A: The use of blood products in shock. Crit Care Clin 8(2):255–291, 1992.

Petz LD, Swisher SN, Kleinman S, et al: Clinical Practice of Transfusion Medicine. New York, Churchill Livingstone, 1996.

Rodeghiero F, Castaman G, Meyer D, Mannucci PM: Replacement therapy with virus-inactivated plasma concentrates in von Willebrand disease. Vox Sang 62(4):193–199, 1992.

Rosen NR, Bates LH, Herod G: Transfusion therapy: improved patient care and resource utilization. Transfusion 33(4):341–347, 1993.

Rossi EC, Simon TL, Moss GS, Gould SA: Principles of transfusion medicine, 2nd ed. Baltimore, Williams & Wilkins, 1996.

Rudman SV: Textbook of Blood Banking and Transfusion Medicine. Philadelphia, WB Saunders, 1995.

Shanberge JN, Quattrociocchi-Longe T: Analysis of fresh frozen plasma administration with suggestions for ways to reduce usage. Transfus Med 2(3):189–194, 1992.

Silver H, Tahhan HR, Anderson J, Lachman M: A non–computer-dependent prospective review of blood and blood component utilization. Transfusion 32(3):260–265, 1992.

Standards Committee of the American Association of Blood Banks: Standards of Blood Banks and Transfusion Services, 17th ed. Bethesda, Md, American Association of Blood Banks, 1996.

Pisciotto PT (ed): Blood Transfusion Therapy—A Physician's Handbook. Bethesda, Md, American Association of Blood Banks, 1993.

Tobias JD, Schleien C: Granulocyte transfusions—a review for the intensive care physician. Anaesth Intensive Care 19(4):512–520, 1991.

Vengelen-Tyler V (ed): Technical Manual 12th ed. Bethesda, Md, American Association of Blood Banks, 1996.

Williford PD, Bensky KP: Blood component therapy and changing transfusion triggers. Crna. 5(4):139–150, 1994.

Chapter **27**

TRANSFUSION REACTIONS

Deborah Firestone, MA, MT(ASCP), SBB

Q U I C K   C O N T E N T S

INTRODUCTION

A *transfusion reaction* is defined as any adverse effect that occurs as the result of the administration of blood or a blood component; transfusion reactions may occur in up to 10% of transfusion recipients. Patients must be advised by their physician of the risks and benefits of transfusion therapy and whether alternatives to transfusion exist. The chance of experiencing any adverse effect of transfusion can be minimized by reducing exposure to allogeneic blood components through judicious use of component therapy. Transfusion reactions can be initially classified as *immediate* or *delayed* and further classified as *immunologic* or *nonimmunologic*.

CLASSIFICATION OF TRANSFUSION REACTIONS

IMMEDIATE		DELAYED	
Immunologic	**Nonimmunologic**	**Immunologic**	**Nonimmunologic**

Hemolytic
Febrile nonhemolytic
Allergic
Transfusion related acute
   lung injury (TRALI)
	Bacterial contamination
	Circulatory overload
	Physical or chemical he-
	   molysis
		Hemolytic
		Transfusion associated
		   graft versus host
		   disease
		Post-transfusion purpura
			Transfusion induced
			   hemosiderosis
			Disease transmission

Immediate Transfusion Reactions

In immediate transfusion reactions, clinical signs and symptoms occur during the transfusion or shortly after (within 24 hours) its completion. Immediate transfusion reactions can be immunologic (mediated by antibody) or nonimmunologic.

IMMUNOLOGIC TRANSFUSION REACTIONS

Hemolytic

In an immediate hemolytic transfusion reaction, transfused donor RBCs are destroyed by preformed recipient antibody. The destruction of donor RBCs can be either intravascular, extravascular, or both.

Intravascular

Intravascular destruction of RBCs occurs within the blood vessels as the classic complement cascade is activated, the RBC membrane is lysed, and free hemoglobin is released into the plasma. The severity of these reactions is generally proportional to the amount of blood transfused and the rate of administration. The majority of immediate hemolytic intravascular transfusion reactions are due to antibodies in the ABO blood group system (anti-A, anti-B, anti-A,B) and are a direct result of human error in patient or specimen identification. An example is the transfusion of ABO incompatible blood (e.g., group A, B, or AB) to a group O individual. Most of these errors are due to a violation of existing operating protocols, such as, e.g., (1) failure to identify the patient correctly, before blood is drawn and (2) improper identification of intended transfusion recipient and/or donor unit at the bedside.

Extravascular

Donor RBCs destroyed extravascularly are removed from the circulation primarily in the liver and spleen with subsequent release of bilirubin into the plasma. Antibodies that destroy RBCs through this mechanism either fail to activate the classic complement cascade or activate only to the C3 stage. RBCs coated with complement components and/or IgG are then removed from the circulation by macrophages. Antibodies commonly associated with the immediate extravascular destruction of RBCs are in the Kell, Kidd, and Duffy blood group systems.

Febrile Nonhemolytic

A febrile nonhemolytic transfusion reaction is defined by the American Association of Blood Banks (AABB) *Technical Manual* as an increase in temperature of 1°C or more that is associated with a transfusion and cannot be explained by any other medical condition. These reactions are caused by recipient alloantibodies directed against antigens present on lymphocytes, granulocytes, or platelets transfused in leukocyte containing blood products (e.g., RBCs, platelets). This type of transfusion reaction occurs most often in transfusion recipients with a history of previous transfusions or multiple pregnancies.

Allergic

The etiology of allergic, or urticarial, transfusion reactions is not well understood but is believed to be a reaction between recipient antibody and transfused donor plasma proteins. Histamine release from the recipient's mast cells is the primary mediator of the allergic response.

Anaphylactic

Anaphylactic transfusion reactions can occur after the infusion of only a few millimeters of blood and can be life threatening. They are due to the reaction between potent class specific anti-IgA antibodies and IgA in transfused products. These antibodies, found in the plasma of some IgA deficient recipients, are produced after exposure to IgA through previous pregnancy or transfusion.

Transfusion Related Acute Lung Injury

Transfusion related acute lung injury (TRALI) is a potentially life threatening complication attributed to the transfusion of donor plasma containing high concentrations of leukoagglutinins directed against recipient leukocytes. These antibodies usually have specificity within the HLA system. Donor units involved in this type of transfusion reaction are typically from multiparous women. Proposed mechanisms to explain the lung injury seen in TRALI include the antigen-antibody reaction of leukocytes with their respective antibodies and the subsequent trapping of these white blood cell aggregates in the pulmonary microcirculation. This leads to pulmonary edema, activation of the complement cascade, and subsequent sequestration and degranulation of neutrophils in the lung. Pulmonary vascular damage results from these events (Anstall, 1993). These reactions are frequently not recognized as related to transfusion; however, when a donor unit is implicated, identification of leukocyte antibodies in the donor plasma reactive against recipient leukocytes may be helpful. It may be prudent to discard plasma components from donors from whom components from previous donations have been identified as the cause of this type of reaction.

NONIMMUNOLOGIC

Bacterial Contamination

The frequency of sepsis due to contamination of transfused RBCs has decreased over the past 30 years, whereas the number of cases of platelet contamination has increased. This is primarily due to increased usage of platelet components and increased room temperature storage time in containers with enhanced gas permeability. Principal causes of bacterial contamination of RBCs are transient bacteremia in asymptomatic donors and contamination of collection equipment during the manufacturing process. *Yersinia enterocolitica*, an intestinal parasite, is the organism most commonly implicated in units from asymptomatic donors. Contamination of platelet products occurs during phlebotomy as a result of insufficient skin decontamination. Components stored longer than 3 days at room temperature are more susceptible to bacterial growth. *Staphylococcus epidermidis* and *Bacillus aureus* are the organisms primarily associated with platelet contamination. It has been suggested that platelet concentrates stored for 3 days or more be tested before transfusion to detect bacterial contamination. The clinical signs and symptoms manifested by the patient after the transfusion of contaminated platelets are more varied than those displayed after the transfusion of contaminated RBCs and may therefore often be overlooked (Hogman, 1996). Fresh frozen plasma and cryoprecipitate are susceptible to bacterial contamination when thawed in a 37°C water bath. It is important to prevent water from contacting the entry port of the bag during thawing. This can be accomplished by placing the product in a plastic overwrap and thawing in an upright position in the waterbath.

Circulatory Overload

Circulatory overload is usually associated with the rapid infusion of large volumes of blood products. Populations at risk include the very young, the elderly, patients with cardiac disease, and patients with chronic anemia. These individuals are unable to tolerate rapid expansion in blood volume. In individuals with pre-existing cardiopulmonary disease, even transfusion of relatively small volumes of blood, especially when infused rapidly, can lead to congestive heart failure and pulmonary edema.

Physical or Chemical Hemolysis

In physically or chemically induced transfusion reactions, hemolysis of RBCs can be caused by mechanical damage (infusion of blood through a small bore needle, open heart surgery bypass machines), osmotic or chemical damage (addition of hypotonic or hypertonic solutions or drugs), or thermal trauma (freezing blood without a cryoprotective agent or warming blood above 45°C). If RBCs are subjected to any of the above, they may be hemolyzed before administration to the patient.

Delayed Transfusion Reactions

Clinical signs and symptoms of a delayed transfusion reaction may not be evident for days, weeks, months, or even years after the transfusion.

IMMUNOLOGIC

Delayed Hemolytic Transfusion Reaction

In a delayed hemolytic transfusion reaction the destruction of RBCs, which may be intravascular or extravascular, is primarily due to an anamnestic immune response in the recipient with subsequent destruction of donor cells. The recipient has previously been exposed to the implicated antigen through pregnancy or transfusion, but the antibody formed in the primary immune response is no longer at a level detectable in standard compatibility testing techniques. Subsequent transfusion of RBCs bearing the same antigen initiates an anamnestic response, resulting in the rapid production of IgG antibody specific for the antigen in question. These types of transfusion reactions are generally mild due to the gradual destruction of antibody coated donor RBCs, primarily by macrophages in the reticuloendothelial system, within approximately 14 days after transfusion. The majority of these reactions are, in fact, asymptomatic and might be more appropriately termed *delayed serologic transfusion reactions*. Antibodies most commonly implicated in this type of reaction include those to antigens in the Rh, Kidd, Duffy, and Kell blood group systems. Fatalities are rare. The diagnosis of delayed hemolytic transfusion reactions is most commonly made by detection of a positive direct antiglobulin test (usually mixed field), the appearance of a previously undetected RBC alloantibody in the recipient's serum, and/or RBC eluate and decreased survival of transfused donor cells as evidenced by lack of expected hemoglobin increase.

Transfusion Associated Graft Versus Host Disease

Transfusion associated graft versus host disease (TA-GVHD) occurs when certain susceptible recipients, with compromised immune systems, are transfused with blood or blood components containing immunocompetent lymphocytes. These lymphocytes engraft in the recipient's tissues and multiply. The engrafted donor cells react against the foreign tissues of the host-recipient, who is unable to recognize or destroy the donor lymphocytes.

Individuals most at risk for TA-GVHD include (Anstall, 1993; Standards, 1996):

▌ Recipients of bone marrow or peripheral stem cell transplants
▌ Transfusion recipients with inherited immunodeficiency syndromes
▌ Fetuses receiving intrauterine transfusions
▌ Recipients of donor units from a blood relative
▌ Newborns receiving exchange transfusions
▌ Patients with certain hematologic and oncologic disorders

TA-GVHD can be acute or chronic. Symptoms of acute TA-GVHD are generally manifested 2 to 30 days after transfusion, whereas symptoms of chronic TA-GVHD are generally not apparent until 100 days after transfusion. A diagnosis of TA-GVHD is generally made postmortem, and HLA typing can be performed to confirm the presence of donor lymphocytes.

Post-Transfusion Purpura

Most cases of post-transfusion purpura occur in middle-aged and elderly women after the transfusion of platelet concentrates. Individuals primarily at risk have been previously immunized to platelet antigens (most commonly HPA-1a) through pregnancy and/or previous transfusion. This antibody, once stimulated, causes destruction of the patient's own HPA-1a negative platelets either through crossreactivity of antibody with the patient's platelets or through nonspecific destruction. Transfusions of HPA-1a negative platelets are generally not beneficial and are usually reserved for severe cases. Patient's serum may be tested for platelet specific antibodies to confirm this diagnosis.

NONIMMUNOLOGIC

Hemosiderosis

A long term complication of RBC transfusion is iron overload, also known as *hemosiderosis*. Populations at risk of transfusion induced hemosiderosis are those that are chronically transfused (e.g., with thalassemia major, sickle cell anemia, other hemoglobinopathies) without a concomitant loss of blood. Each unit of RBCs contains approximately 200 mg of iron as part of the hemoglobin molecule. The daily excretion of iron in a patient who is not bleeding is approximately 1 mg. Since there is no way for the body to eliminate iron except through blood loss, excess iron accumulates in the mitochondria of cells in critical organs such as the liver, heart, and endocrine glands. This leads to organ failure. Symptoms of hemosiderosis are usually seen when a patient has received more than 100 units of blood. Iron storage levels (ferritin) and other iron analyses can be performed to establish this diagnosis.

Disease Transmission

The majority of deaths caused by blood transfusion are due to the transmission of viruses, bacteria, or protozoa. The transmission of disease by blood transfusion is largely prevented by the use of a totally volunteer donor supply. In addition, a comprehensive medical history, physical examination, and serologic testing for markers for the implicated diseases is required for all prospective allogeneic blood donors. It is still possible, however, for an asymptomatic blood donor to make it through the screening process and transmit pathogenic organisms to transfusion recipients.

Examples of diseases that can be transmitted through the blood supply include infection with:

- Hepatitis B, C, and D virus
- Cytomegalovirus
- Epstein-Barr virus
- Human T cell leukemia virus types I and II (HTLV I and II)
- Human immunodeficiency virus (HIV) 1
- *Treponema pallidum* parasite (syphilis)
- Malarial parasite
- *Babesia microti* parasite
- *Trypanosoma cruzi* parasite (Chagas' disease)
- *Toxoplasma gondii* parasite

A great deal of research is currently directed at developing effective methods to inactivate viruses and other organisms in blood and blood components implicated in disease transmission.

ESTIMATED RISK (PER UNIT TRANSFUSED)

Immediate Transfusion Reactions

CLASSIFICATION	REACTION	RISK
Immunologic	Acute hemolytic transfusion reaction	1:6,000–1:33,000
	Febrile	1:200
	Allergic	
	Mild	1:333
	Anaphylactic	1:20,000–50,000
	Transfusion related noncardiogenic pulmonary edema	1:5,000
Nonimmunologic	Bacterial contamination	RBCs 1:4,000,000
		Platelets 1:4,000–12,000
	Circulatory overload	Common, under-reported
	Physical or chemical hemolysis	NA; infrequent
NA, Numbers not available.		

From DeChristopher PJ, Anderson RR: Risks of transfusion and organ and tissue transplantation: Practical concerns that drive practical policies. Pathology Patterns, Am J Clin Pathol 1997, 107:S2–S11. Copyright © 1997, by the American Society of Clinical Pathologists. Reprinted with permission.

Delayed Transfusion Reactions

CLASSIFICATION	REACTION	RISK
Immunologic	Hemolytic transfusion reaction	1:4,000
	Transfusion-associated graft versus host disease	Rare
	Post-transfusion purpura	Rare
Nonimmunologic	Transfusion induced hemosiderosis	NA; uncommon*
	Infectious disease	
	HIV	1:450,000–660,000
	Hepatitis B	1:63,000
	Hepatitis C	1:103,000
	HTLV-I and -II	1:641,000
	Malaria, *Babesia microti*, *Trypanosoma cruzi*	<1:1,000,000
NA, Numbers not available.		

From DeChristopher PJ, Anderson RR: Risks of transfusion and organ and tissue transplantation: Practical concerns that drive practical policies. Pathology Patterns, Am J Clin Pathol 1997, 107:S2–S11. Copyright © 1997, by the American Society of Clinical Pathologists. Reprinted with permission.
*Lifelong risks high in chronically transfused patients such as those with thalassemias and sickle cell disease.

SIGNS AND SYMPTOMS, MANAGEMENT, AND PREVENTION OF IMMEDIATE TRANSFUSION REACTIONS

TYPE OF TRANSFUSION REACTION	SIGNS AND SYMPTOMS	MANAGEMENT	PREVENTION
Hemolytic	Fever, chills, flushing, nausea, dyspnea, chest pain, flank pain, hypotension, shock, hemoglobinemia, hemoglobinuria, disseminated intravascular coagulation, renal failure; in anesthetized or unconscious patient, may see hypotension, hemoglobinuria, anuria, bleeding	Adequate renal perfusion; induce diuresis, treat shock and manage DIC.	Avoid human error (e.g., computerized confirmation of recipient and donor). Use well written procedure manuals. Use highly trained clinical and laboratory staff. Use quality assurance and/or quality improvement program.
Febrile Nonhemolytic (FNHTR)	Chills, fever	Administer antipyretics.	Premedicate with antipyretics. Transfuse leukocyte reduced products to patients who have experienced two or more FNHTRs.
Urticarial	Hives	Administer antihistamine while blood flow is slowed or stopped.	In patients who have suffered multiple urticarial reactions, pretreat with antihistamines.
Anaphylactic	Flushing of skin, abrupt hypertension followed by hypotension, substernal pain, dyspnea, nausea, abdominal cramps, emesis, diarrhea	Give immediate treatment with epinephrine; IV corticosteroids and O_2 therapy may be indicated.	Transfuse washed RBCs or platelets or frozen RBCs and plasma from IgA deficient donors (e.g., autologous plasma).
Transfusion Related Acute Lung Injury (TRALI)	Chills, fever, nonproductive cough, dyspnea, cyanosis, bilateral pulmonary edema, severe hypoxemia, fever, hypotension	Give respiratory support, steroids, diuretics.	Use proper donor selection (recommended that RBCs from donors previously implicated in TRALI reaction who have circulating granulocyte or lymphocyte antibodies be administered as deglycerolized or washed RBCs).
Bacterial Contamination	Fever, chills, hypotension, tachycardia, shock (warm type), hemoglobinemia, hemoglobinuria, renal failure, DIC	Give IV antibiotics, fluids, and vasopressors to maintain blood pressure, appropriate therapy for DIC (if present).	Carefully monitor each step of blood collection, storage, and transfusion to prevent introduction of bacteria into unit. Carefully inspect blood products before distribution for transfusion.

Continued ▶

▶ Continued **SIGNS AND SYMPTOMS, MANAGEMENT, AND PREVENTION OF IMMEDIATE TRANSFUSION REACTIONS**

TYPE OF TRANSFUSION REACTION	SIGNS AND SYMPTOMS	MANAGEMENT	PREVENTION
Circulatory Overload	Anxiety, restlessness, coughing, tachycardia, dyspnea, cyanosis, severe headache, signs of congestive heart failure	Administer diuretics, place patient in upright position (O_2 by mask, IV morphine, phlebotomy of 200–400 mL of blood if necessary).	Identify susceptible individuals and transfuse blood and blood components slowly (1 mL/kg body weight/hr) and in most concentrated form available (when necessary, aliquot donor unit and refrigerate unused portion(s) at 1–6°C).
Physical or Chemical Hemolysis	Asymptomatic hemoglobinuria, (hemoglobinemia, DIC, and renal failure are rare)	Generally none needed; serious sequelae need to be treated immediately.	Adhere to established protocols outlined in laboratory policy and procedure manual for proper preparation, storage, and transfusion of blood components.

From Lane TA, ed: Blood Transfusion Therapy—A Physician's Handbook, 5th ed. Bethesda, Md, American Association of Blood Banks, 1996, pp 103–115; and Vengelen-Tyler V, ed: Technical Manual, 12th ed. Bethesda, Md, American Association of Blood Banks, 1996.

SIGNS/MANAGEMENT/PREVENTION: IMMEDIATE TRANSFUSION REACTIONS

SIGNS AND SYMPTOMS, MANAGEMENT, AND PREVENTION OF DELAYED TRANSFUSION REACTIONS

TYPE OF TRANSFUSION REACTION	SIGNS AND SYMPTOMS	MANAGEMENT	PREVENTION
Hemolytic	Fever, decreased hemoglobin, mild jaundice	Treatment is rarely necessary; give antigen negative blood for subsequent transfusions.	Check patient's previous records. Make notation of patient's antibody status in permanent laboratory record. Administer antigen negative blood for all subsequent transfusions (even if antibody screen is negative).
Transfusion Associated Graft Versus Host Disease	*Acute:* fever, diffuse skin rash, diarrhea, infection, abnormal liver function, pancytopenia, usually fatal *Chronic:* fever, scleroderma-like disease, sicca syndrome, interstitial pneumonitis, malabsorption	*Acute:* no adequate therapy. *Chronic:* no adequate therapy.	Irradiate all blood components containing lymphocytes with a dose of 25 Gy (1 gray = 100 rads) before transfusion to susceptible individuals.
Post-transfusion Purpura	Profound self-limiting thrombocytopenia, generalized purpura	Use corticosteroids, therapeutic plasma exchange, high dose intravenous immunoglobulins.	Difficult to prevent. Clinician should have thorough patient history and history of any adverse reactions to previous transfusions.
Transfusion Induced Hemosiderosis	Muscle weakness, weight loss, mild jaundice, fatigue, cardiac arrythmias, mild diabetes, growth retardation in children	Administer desferrioxamine (iron chelating agent).	Super- or hypertransfusions of neocytes.
Disease Transmission	Fever, fatigue, lymphadenopathy, adenopathy, malaise, arthralgias, icterus, hemolysis (malaria)	Notify facility responsible for drawing blood, quarantine all components in storage prepared from same unit.	Use volunteer blood supply. Do serologic testing of all donor units. Require medical and physical history of all potential donors. Give hepatitis B vaccine to all health care workers. Administer hepatitis prophylaxis after exposure to Hb_sAg positive blood.

From Lane TA, ed: Blood Transfusion Therapy—A Physician's Handbook, 5th ed. Bethesda, Md, American Association of Blood Banks, 1996, 103–115; Vengelen-Tyler V, ed: Technical Manual, 12th ed. Bethesda, Md, American Association of Blood Banks, 1996.

SYMPTOMS OR FINDINGS SUGGESTIVE OF AN ACUTE TRANSFUSION REACTION

The American Association of Blood Banks (AABB) *Standards of Blood Banks and Transfusion Services* requires that patients receiving transfusions be observed during and for an appropriate period of time after transfusion for suspected adverse reactions. A patient is suspected of experiencing an acute transfusion reaction when a qualified health care provider (physician, nurse, transfusionist) notices any unexpected sign(s) or symptom(s) that occurs during, or shortly after, the transfusion of blood or any one of its components. As seen in "Signs and Symptoms, Management, and Prevention of Immediate Transfusion Reactions" on p 530 and "Signs and Symptoms, Management, and Prevention of Delayed Transfusion Reactions on p 532, these signs and symptoms can range from mild to severe, and the initial presenting symptoms (e.g., fever, chills) can be the same for both a life threatening (hemolytic) and less serious (febrile) transfusion reaction. In all cases of suspected hemolytic transfusion reactions, the presenting signs and symptoms must be assumed to have been caused by the blood and/or component until proved otherwise and must be investigated as a potentially life threatening transfusion reaction. According to the AABB *Standards,* all adverse reactions must be investigated promptly. Both federal regulatory and voluntary accreditation agencies (e.g., AABB, College of American Pathologists) require written protocols and policies defining all steps to be taken in the detection, evaluation, and reporting of transfusion reactions. All transfusion reaction work-ups must be reviewed by the blood bank or transfusion service medical director. A recommended protocol for the investigation of a suspected hemolytic transfusion reaction is presented.

Preliminary Work-up on the Floor

1. Discontinue the transfusion.
2. Notify the patient's physician.
3. Maintain intravascular access with normal saline.
4. Perform a clerical check at the bedside (e.g., patient's armband, donor unit) to determine whether an error was made identifying the patient or donor unit.
5. Immediately report a suspected reaction to blood bank personnel.
6. Obtain a new, properly labeled nonhemolyzed EDTA and clotted sample from the patient; send promptly to the blood bank along with the discontinued blood container, administration set (without the needle), attached IV solutions, and all related forms and labels. The transfusion reaction form should contain the following information: pre- and post-transfusion vital signs, type and time of reaction, amount of product transfused, and any other relevant information.
7. Send other samples (e.g., clotted blood sample drawn 5 to 7 hours post-transfusion, first voided post-transfusion urine sample) to the blood bank for the evaluation of acute hemolysis as requested by the blood bank medical director or patient's physician.
8. Transfusion services and blood banks must have procedures readily available to all personnel detailing steps to be followed when investigating a transfusion reaction.

> NOTE Transfusion need not be discontinued if urticaria is the only finding. Stop the transfusion, administer antihistamines, and restart the transfusion when symptoms have subsided.

Preliminary Work-up in the Blood Bank

The following three steps should be performed as part of a preliminary transfusion reaction work-up in the blood bank:

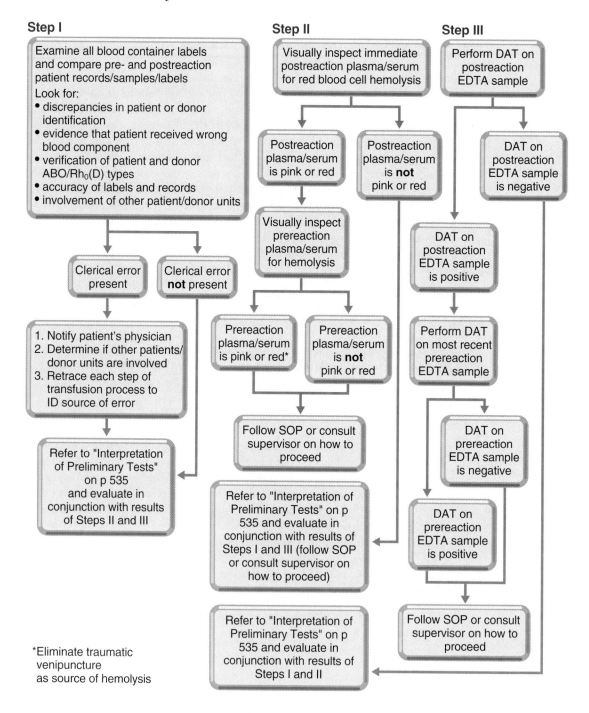

Step I

Examine all blood container labels and compare pre- and postreaction patient records/samples/labels
Look for:
- discrepancies in patient or donor identification
- evidence that patient received wrong blood component
- verification of patient and donor ABO/Rh$_0$(D) types
- accuracy of labels and records
- involvement of other patient/donor units

Clerical error present

Clerical error **not** present

1. Notify patient's physician
2. Determine if other patients/donor units are involved
3. Retrace each step of transfusion process to ID source of error

Refer to "Interpretation of Preliminary Tests" on p 535 and evaluate in conjunction with results of Steps II and III

*Eliminate traumatic venipuncture as source of hemolysis

Step II

Visually inspect immediate postreaction plasma/serum for red blood cell hemolysis

Postreaction plasma/serum is pink or red

Postreaction plasma/serum is **not** pink or red

Visually inspect prereaction plasma/serum for hemolysis

Prereaction plasma/serum is pink or red*

Prereaction plasma/serum is **not** pink or red

Follow SOP or consult supervisor on how to proceed

Refer to "Interpretation of Preliminary Tests" on p 535 and evaluate in conjunction with results of Steps I and III (follow SOP or consult supervisor on how to proceed)

Refer to "Interpretation of Preliminary Tests" on p 535 and evaluate in conjunction with results of Steps I and II

Step III

Perform DAT on postreaction EDTA sample

DAT on postreaction EDTA sample is negative

DAT on postreaction EDTA sample is positive

Perform DAT on most recent prereaction EDTA sample

DAT on prereaction EDTA sample is negative

DAT on prereaction EDTA sample is positive

Follow SOP or consult supervisor on how to proceed

INTERPRETATION OF PRELIMINARY TESTS

CLERICAL ERROR	VISIBLE HEMOLYSIS		POSITIVE DAT		INTERPRETATION
	Pre	Post	Pre	Post	
Yes	No	Yes	No	Yes or No*	Hemolysis has probably occurred.
No	No	Yes	No	Yes or No*	Hemolysis has probably occurred.
No	No	No	No	No	Hemolysis has probably not occurred.

*Post-transfusion direct antiglobulin test (DAT) may be negative if incompatible transfused cells were immediately destroyed.

Recommended Additional Laboratory Work-up When Hemolysis Is Suspected

If the results of preliminary laboratory tests indicate that hemolysis has probably occurred, if the results of any laboratory tests are doubtful, or if the patient's clinical condition suggests that a hemolytic transfusion reaction may have occurred, some or all of the following tests should be performed and the results and interpretations recorded. The following five steps are recommended when the preliminary work-up suggests that hemolysis has probably occurred:

Step 1: Examine blood in the administration tube and supernatant plasma from the donor bag for hemolysis.

Step 2: Repeat ABO/Rh$_0$(D) typing on the patient's pre- and post-transfusion sample.

Step 3: Repeat ABO/Rh$_0$(D) typing on the donor's blood and compare with the ABO/Rh$_0$(D) type on the label.

Step 4: Repeat crossmatching (including antihuman globulin [AHG] phase) using a pre- and post-transfusion sample tested against cells used in the original crossmatching.

Step 5: Repeat antibody tests on pre- and post-transfusion samples and donor unit(s).

A *flow chart* is included for each step on the following pages.

SYMPTOMS OR FINDINGS SUGGESTIVE OF AN ACUTE TRANSFUSION REACTION

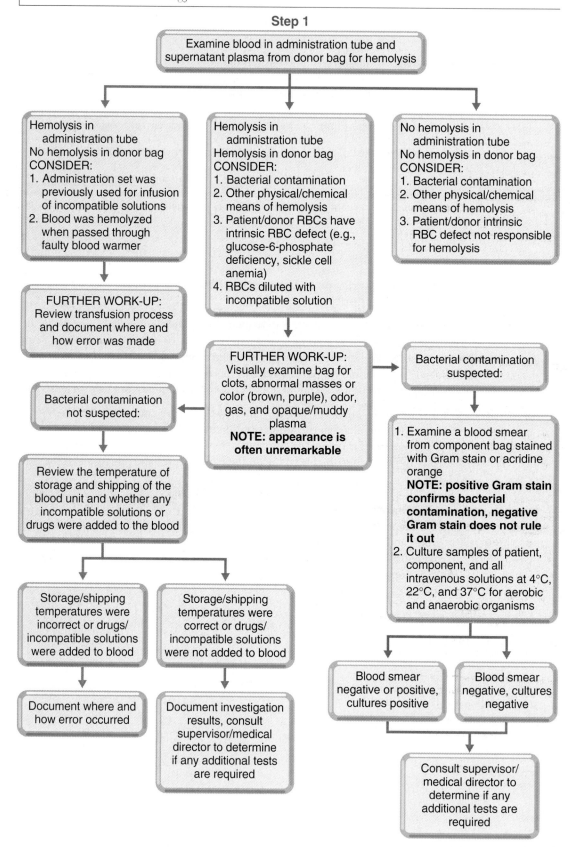

Step 1

Examine blood in administration tube and supernatant plasma from donor bag for hemolysis

Hemolysis in administration tube
No hemolysis in donor bag
CONSIDER:
1. Administration set was previously used for infusion of incompatible solutions
2. Blood was hemolyzed when passed through faulty blood warmer

Hemolysis in administration tube
Hemolysis in donor bag
CONSIDER:
1. Bacterial contamination
2. Other physical/chemical means of hemolysis
3. Patient/donor RBCs have intrinsic RBC defect (e.g., glucose-6-phosphate deficiency, sickle cell anemia)
4. RBCs diluted with incompatible solution

No hemolysis in administration tube
No hemolysis in donor bag
CONSIDER:
1. Bacterial contamination
2. Other physical/chemical means of hemolysis
3. Patient/donor intrinsic RBC defect not responsible for hemolysis

FURTHER WORK-UP:
Review transfusion process and document where and how error was made

FURTHER WORK-UP:
Visually examine bag for clots, abnormal masses or color (brown, purple), odor, gas, and opaque/muddy plasma
NOTE: appearance is often unremarkable

Bacterial contamination suspected:

Bacterial contamination not suspected:

Review the temperature of storage and shipping of the blood unit and whether any incompatible solutions or drugs were added to the blood

1. Examine a blood smear from component bag stained with Gram stain or acridine orange
   NOTE: positive Gram stain confirms bacterial contamination, negative Gram stain does not rule it out
2. Culture samples of patient, component, and all intravenous solutions at 4°C, 22°C, and 37°C for aerobic and anaerobic organisms

Storage/shipping temperatures were incorrect or drugs/ incompatible solutions were added to blood

Storage/shipping temperatures were correct or drugs/ incompatible solutions were not added to blood

Document where and how error occurred

Document investigation results, consult supervisor/medical director to determine if any additional tests are required

Blood smear negative or positive, cultures positive

Blood smear negative, cultures negative

Consult supervisor/ medical director to determine if any additional tests are required

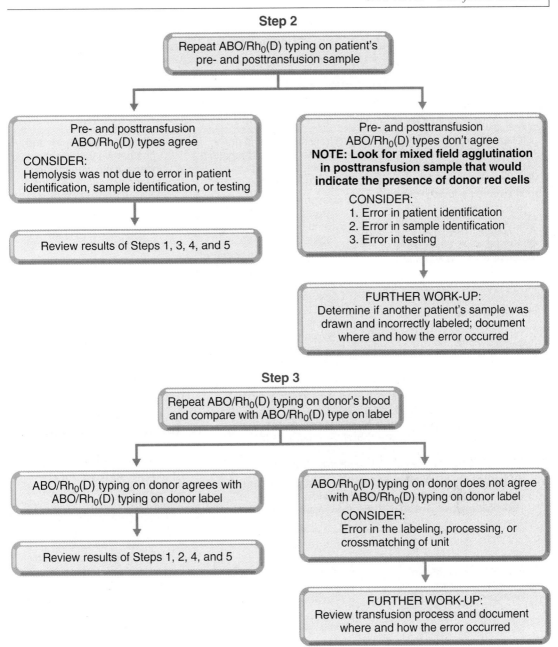

Step 2

Repeat ABO/Rh$_0$(D) typing on patient's
pre- and posttransfusion sample

Pre- and posttransfusion
ABO/Rh$_0$(D) types agree

CONSIDER:
Hemolysis was not due to error in patient
identification, sample identification, or testing

Review results of Steps 1, 3, 4, and 5

Pre- and posttransfusion
ABO/Rh$_0$(D) types don't agree
**NOTE: Look for mixed field agglutination
in posttransfusion sample that would
indicate the presence of donor red cells**

CONSIDER:
1. Error in patient identification
2. Error in sample identification
3. Error in testing

FURTHER WORK-UP:
Determine if another patient's sample was
drawn and incorrectly labeled; document
where and how the error occurred

Step 3

Repeat ABO/Rh$_0$(D) typing on donor's blood
and compare with ABO/Rh$_0$(D) type on label

ABO/Rh$_0$(D) typing on donor agrees with
ABO/Rh$_0$(D) typing on donor label

Review results of Steps 1, 2, 4, and 5

ABO/Rh$_0$(D) typing on donor does not agree
with ABO/Rh$_0$(D) typing on donor label

CONSIDER:
Error in the labeling, processing, or
crossmatching of unit

FURTHER WORK-UP:
Review transfusion process and document
where and how the error occurred

SYMPTOMS OR FINDINGS SUGGESTIVE OF AN ACUTE TRANSFUSION REACTION

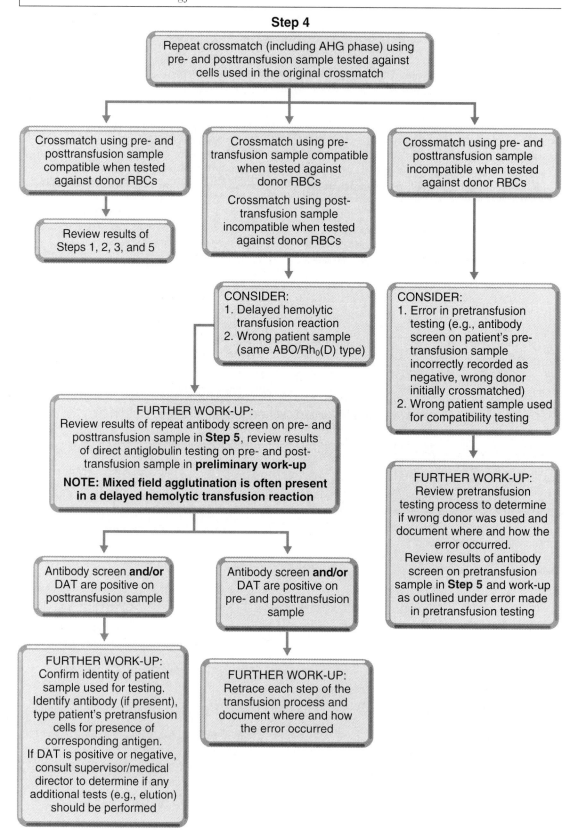

Step 4

Repeat crossmatch (including AHG phase) using pre- and posttransfusion sample tested against cells used in the original crossmatch

Crossmatch using pre- and posttransfusion sample compatible when tested against donor RBCs

Review results of Steps 1, 2, 3, and 5

Crossmatch using pretransfusion sample compatible when tested against donor RBCs

Crossmatch using posttransfusion sample incompatible when tested against donor RBCs

Crossmatch using pre- and posttransfusion sample incompatible when tested against donor RBCs

CONSIDER:
1. Delayed hemolytic transfusion reaction
2. Wrong patient sample (same ABO/Rh_0(D) type)

CONSIDER:
1. Error in pretransfusion testing (e.g., antibody screen on patient's pretransfusion sample incorrectly recorded as negative, wrong donor initially crossmatched)
2. Wrong patient sample used for compatibility testing

FURTHER WORK-UP:
Review results of repeat antibody screen on pre- and posttransfusion sample in **Step 5**, review results of direct antiglobulin testing on pre- and post-transfusion sample in **preliminary work-up**

NOTE: Mixed field agglutination is often present in a delayed hemolytic transfusion reaction

FURTHER WORK-UP:
Review pretransfusion testing process to determine if wrong donor was used and document where and how the error occurred.
Review results of antibody screen on pretransfusion sample in **Step 5** and work-up as outlined under error made in pretransfusion testing

Antibody screen **and/or** DAT are positive on posttransfusion sample

Antibody screen **and/or** DAT are positive on pre- and posttransfusion sample

FURTHER WORK-UP:
Confirm identity of patient sample used for testing. Identify antibody (if present), type patient's pretransfusion cells for presence of corresponding antigen.
If DAT is positive or negative, consult supervisor/medical director to determine if any additional tests (e.g., elution) should be performed

FURTHER WORK-UP:
Retrace each step of the transfusion process and document where and how the error occurred

Step 5

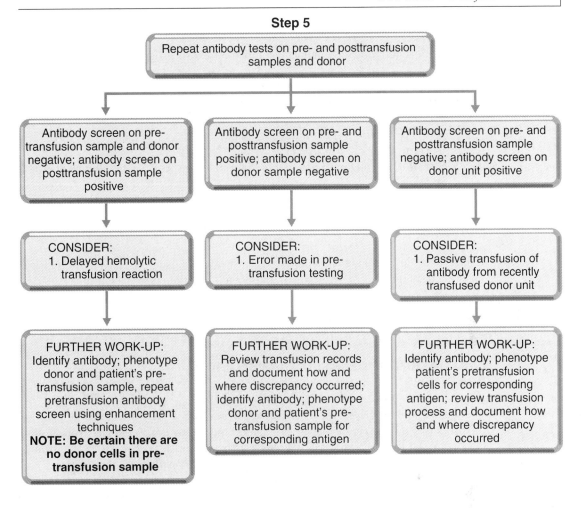

Repeat antibody tests on pre- and posttransfusion samples and donor

---

Antibody screen on pre-transfusion sample and donor negative; antibody screen on posttransfusion sample positive

Antibody screen on pre- and posttransfusion sample positive; antibody screen on donor sample negative

Antibody screen on pre- and posttransfusion sample negative; antibody screen on donor unit positive

---

CONSIDER:
1. Delayed hemolytic transfusion reaction

CONSIDER:
1. Error made in pre-transfusion testing

CONSIDER:
1. Passive transfusion of antibody from recently transfused donor unit

---

FURTHER WORK-UP:
Identify antibody; phenotype donor and patient's pre-transfusion sample, repeat pretransfusion antibody screen using enhancement techniques
NOTE: Be certain there are no donor cells in pre-transfusion sample

FURTHER WORK-UP:
Review transfusion records and document how and where discrepancy occurred; identify antibody; phenotype donor and patient's pre-transfusion sample for corresponding antigen

FURTHER WORK-UP:
Identify antibody; phenotype patient's pretransfusion cells for corresponding antigen; review transfusion process and document how and where discrepancy occurred

SYMPTOMS OR FINDINGS SUGGESTIVE OF AN ACUTE TRANSFUSION REACTION

Additional Tests That May Be Performed When Hemolysis Is Suspected

1. Perform urine tests on a first voided post-transfusion sample.

   Examine the supernate of a centrifuged sample for free hemoglobin.

   Examine urine for intact RBCs; if present, they represent bleeding, not hemolysis.

   Test for hemosiderin if the sample was collected more than 24 hours after the transfusion.

2. Perform bilirubin analyses on pre- and post-transfusion samples.

   NOTE Record the time on the sample, as bilirubin can be detected as early as 1 hour after transfusion; levels peak approximately 3 to 6 hours after a hemolytic transfusion reaction and can return to normal within 24 hours if liver function is normal.

3. Perform hemoglobin (Hb) and hematocrit (Hct) determinations at regular intervals. Note whether the transfusion produced the expected therapeutic bene-

fit and whether there was a decrease in Hb and Hct after the expected increase.

4. Repeat antibody screening and compatibility tests using more sensitive techniques.
5. Perform DAT and antibody detection tests at frequent intervals.
6. Compare the phenotype of the patient's pretransfusion sample to the phenotype of the donor RBCs. Note which antigen(s) is (are) absent from the patient's cells and present on the donor cells.
7. Perform RBC survival studies.
8. Perform pre- and posthaptoglobin determinations to evaluate minimal degrees of hemolysis.

NOTE The normal range for haptoglobin is 100 to 150 mg/dL.

If it has been determined that hemolysis has probably not occurred, consult the supervisor or medical director to determine if additional immunohematologic testing is necessary.

EVALUATION OF DELAYED TRANSFUSION REACTIONS

The diagnosis of a delayed transfusion reaction is often made retrospectively because the patient's signs and symptoms are not manifested until 1 to 2 weeks after transfusion. Generally, the clinical signs and symptoms associated with post-transfusion purpura, iron overload, and disease transmission are noticed by the patient and/or clinician.

The diagnosis of delayed hemolytic (serologic) transfusion reactions is more obscure because oftentimes the patient has been discharged from the hospital with no follow-up studies. In an asymptomatic patient, the blood bank may detect serologic findings indicative of a delayed transfusion reaction when subsequent requests for transfusions reveal the presence of a newly detected positive direct antiglobulin test (DAT), alloantibody(ies), or both, yet fail to associate these findings with a delayed hemolytic transfusion reaction. With this in mind, the following steps should be adhered to when testing all samples:

1. Perform pretransfusion studies on patient samples that are 72 hours old or less at the time of transfusion if the patient has previously been transfused or pregnant within the past 3 months or the history is unknown. This allows the detection of rapidly developing antibodies that may be missed if the sample wasn't representative of the patient's current immunologic status.
2. Compare the results of all ABO/Rh$_0$(D) typing, antibody screens, and compatibility tests with previous patient records. The detection of an alloantibody in a post-transfusion sample that is absent from the pretransfusion sample or a crossmatch that is incompatible with a post-transfusion sample that was compatible with a pretransfusion sample is strongly suggestive of a delayed transfusion reaction. The antibody must be identified and patient pretransfusion and donor cells phenotyped for the corresponding antigen.
3. If a DAT is performed, compare results with previous patient records. The presence of a positive DAT in the post-transfusion sample compared with a

negative DAT in a pretransfusion sample is, once again, strongly indicative of a delayed transfusion reaction. An elution should be performed and the antibody identified if IgG is coating the RBCs and the post-transfusion antibody screen is negative.

> **NOTE** If positive, the DAT may be mixed field because the antibody is reacting with donor, not patient cells. The DAT may be negative if cells are being rapidly destroyed. Early in the immune response, the DAT may be positive and the antibody screen negative because all available antibody is adsorbed onto donor cells. As the titer of the antibody increases and all antigen sites on donor cells are saturated, the antibody screen will then become positive.

REPORTING TRANSFUSION REACTIONS

An interpretation of the transfusion reaction work-up must be recorded in the patient's medical chart. If the results of the work-up suggest a hemolytic reaction or bacterial contamination, the patient's physician and blood bank or transfusion service medical director must be notified immediately. Blood banks and transfusion services must keep records of all transfusion complications. The AABB *Standards* requires that transfusion records be maintained for a minimum of 5 years. All confirmed cases of transfusion associated infections such as transfusion associated hepatitis, acquired immunodeficiency syndrome (AIDS), and other viral diseases (as well as those cases that cannot be ruled out) must be reported to the facility that drew the blood. Fatalities that occur as a direct result of blood transfusion must be reported within 24 hours to the Director, Center for Biologics Evaluation and Research. A written report must be received within 7 days. The facility responsible for collecting the unit must also be notified.

BIBLIOGRAPHY

Anderson KC, Ness PM, eds: Scientific Basis of Transfusion Medicine: Implications for Clinical Practice. Philadelphia, WB Saunders, 1994.

Anstall HB, Blaylock RC, Craven CM: Managing Hazards in the Transfusion Service. Chicago, American Society of Clinical Pathologists, 1993.

Barrett BB, Andersen JW, Anderson KC: Strategies for the avoidance of bacterial contamination of blood components. Transfusion 33(3):228–233, 1993.

Beauregard P, Blajchman MA: Hemolytic and pseudo-hemolytic transfusion reactions: an overview of the hemolytic transfusion reactions and the clinical conditions that mimic them. Transfus Med Rev 8(3):184–199, 1994.

DeChristopher PJ, Sosler SD: Discoveries and developments transforming blood banking and transfusion medicine—part 2. Lab Med 25:315–320, 1995.

DeChristopher PJ: Adverse effects of blood transfusion. In Summers SH, Smith DM, Agranenko VA, eds: Transfusion Therapy: Guidelines for Practice. Arlington, Va, American Association of Blood Banks, 1990.

Fakhry SM, Sheldon GF: Blood administration, risks, and substitutes. Adv Surg 28:71–92, 1995.

Harmening DM, ed: Modern Blood Banking and Transfusion Practices. Philadelphia, FA Davis, 1994.

Hogman CF: Adverse effects: bacterial contamination (including shelf life). A brief review of bacterial contamination of blood components. Vox Sang 70(suppl 3):78–82, 1996.

Jeter EK, Spivey MA: Noninfectious complications of blood transfusion. Hematol/Oncol Clin North Am 9:187–200, 1995.

Krishnan LA, Brecher ME: Transfusion-transmitted bacterial infection. Hematol/Oncol Clin North Am 9:167–184, 1995.

Linden JV, Kaplan HS: Transfusion errors: causes and effects. Transfus Med Rev 8(3):169–183, 1994.

Marcus RE, Huehns ER: Transfusional iron overload. Clin Lab Haematol 7:195–212, 1985.

Mollison PL, Engelfriet CP, Contreras M: Blood transfusion in clinical medicine. London, Blackwell Scientific, 1993.

Petz LD, Kleinman S, Swisher SN, Spence RK, eds: Clinical Practice of Transfusion Medicine, 3rd ed. New York, Churchill Livingstone, 1996.

Pisciotto PT, ed: Blood Transfusion Therapy—A Physician's Handbook. Bethesda, American Association of Blood Banks, 1993.

Popovsky MA, ed: Transfusion Reactions. Bethesda, American Association of Blood Banks, 1996.

Rossi EC, Simon TL, Moss GS, Gould SA, eds: Principles of Transfusion Medicine. Baltimore, Williams & Wilkins, 1996.

Rudmann SV, ed: Textbook of Blood Banking and Transfusion Medicine. Philadelphia, WB Saunders, 1995.

Standards Committee of the American Association of Blood Banks: Standards of Blood Banks and Transfusion Services, 17th ed. Bethesda, American Association of Blood Banks, 1996.

Steane EA: Bacterial contamination of cellular blood components. Vox Sanguinis 67(suppl 3): 33–35, 1994.

Vengelen-Tyler V, ed: Technical Manual, 12th ed. Bethesda, American Association of Blood Banks, 1996.

Wendel S: Current concepts on transmission of bacteria and parasites by blood components. Vox Sanguinis 67(suppl 3):161–174, 1994.

Chapter **28**

QUALITY ASSURANCE

Elizabeth Cascone, MT(ASCP), SBB

Q U I C K   C O N T E N T S

INTRODUCTION

Quality is the responsibility of every staff member in the blood bank or transfusion service. The quality of the product of the institution is only as good as the commitment to excellence of each individual employee. The quality assurance program is put in place to monitor and improve the quality of the services provided by the blood bank and improve them when necessary.

REGULATORY AGENCIES

A program of quality assurance (QA) is mandated by regulatory agencies that oversee laboratory operations. These regulatory agencies include:

1. Joint Commission on Accreditation of Healthcare Organizations (JCAHO)
2. Food and Drug Administration (FDA)
3. Health Care Financing Administration (HCFA)
4. College of American Pathologists (CAP)
5. American Association of Blood Banks (AABB)
6. Some state agencies

QUALITY ASSURANCE CONCEPTS

Quality Assurance (QA). Those activities incorporated into the standard operating procedures (SOPs) of the blood bank or transfusion service that ensure the quality of the final product.

Quality Control (QC). The process of monitoring and evaluating the performance of reagents, supplies, or equipment by measuring that performance against established standards.

Continuous Quality Improvement (CQI). Activities designed to review, evaluate, and *correct* laboratory processes to achieve maximal efficiency, suitability, and quality.

Quality Assurance Unit. The individual or group of individuals charged with the design, development, execution, and oversight of QA activities. This group should, ideally, be separated from the operational unit of the blood bank or transfusion service.

AREAS TO CONSIDER AS PART OF THE QUALITY ASSURANCE PROGRAM

AREA	ELEMENT*

System Processes	Procedure manual (SOPs)
	    Techniques
	    Protocols
	    Procedures
	Blood utilization
	Record keeping
	Error management
	Information management systems

Products, Equipment, Reagents, Technical Procedures	Blood components (QA may be performed pre- or post-transfusion) Scales Hemoglobinometer Refrigerators and freezers Thermometers Timers Incubators Heat blocks Centrifuges Serofuges Cell washers Reagent antiserum Reagent red cells Antiglobulin testing Elutions Chemical treatment of RBCs

Continued ▶

► Continued **AREAS TO CONSIDER AS PART OF THE QUALITY ASSURANCE PROGRAM**

AREA	ELEMENT*

Personnel	Job description and hiring practices
	Performance standards
	Employee performance assessment
	Training
	Competency assessment
	   Continuing education
	   Proficiency testing
	   Direct observation
	   Knowledge of laboratory SOPs

*These items represent a partial list of the elements monitored and measured by a QC program.

ACTIVITIES INVOLVING ALL STAFF MEMBERS ENGAGED IN PATIENT CARE

Process Quality Assurance

SYSTEM MONITORS (AUDITS). These are specific procedures designed to review critical points in the laboratory processes to identify points in the system that demonstrate a need for process improvement.

RECORD KEEPING:
- Handwritten
- Electronic (computer)

Product, Equipment, and Reagent Quality Assurance

QC activities are defined and governed by regulatory requirements and should be described in detail in the laboratory SOPs.

- Blood products
- Reagents
- Equipment
- Technical procedures

Personnel Quality Assurance

- Hiring guidelines, job descriptions, and performance programs.
- Training.

Staff members trained in laboratory procedures and techniques may be required to assist in training newer staff members.

Training documents and/or checklists should be defined and available to ensure complete and effective training of new employees and retraining of other employees whenever necessary.

▌ Competency assessment. The scope and details of these activities is defined in the laboratory SOPs. All employees must be called on, at least annually, to:

Demonstrate their ability to accurately and precisely perform, under observation, the technical procedures for which they are responsible (as described by performance standards)

Demonstrate their technical expertise by accurately analyzing unknown survey samples

Demonstrate their knowledge of the laboratory's SOPs (this may involve written test exercises)

Demonstrate development and advancement of professional knowledge and skills by participation in continuing education events

Demonstrate their ability to effectively solve problems related to technical procedures or patient care

SPECIFIC ACTIVITIES AND PROTOCOLS DEFINING A QUALITY ASSURANCE PROGRAM

Process and System Quality Assurance

SYSTEM MONITORS (AUDITS)

System monitors may be constructed by:

▌ Reviewing error logs or incidence reports to identify areas in which improvement is critical or desirable

▌ Identifying those steps in laboratory practices, protocols, or procedures that place the patient in a dangerous situation if an error is made (critical control points), even when errors have not been a problem in that particular area

System monitors should be designed to be:

▌ Uncomplicated
▌ Manageable
▌ Meaningful
▌ Flexible

System monitors should be clearly defined in a laboratory SOP, describing:

▌ The activity to be measured
▌ The tools and/or mechanisms (forms, reports) to be used in performing the activities of the monitor
▌ The exact measurement of failure of each individual element being measured
▌ The definition of "failure" in the process that is being measured
▌ Measures that must be undertaken to improve or correct the failed process
▌ The steps to be taken to reassess the corrected process for improvement

RECORD KEEPING

1. All requirements for record keeping activities are defined by federal, national, state, and/or local regulatory agencies.

2. Most regulatory requirements are in agreement with those that are described in the *Standards for Blood Banks and Transfusion Services* published by the AABB.

3. All activities performed by the blood bank and transfusion service must be documented in a way that ensures "traceability and trackability." According to the FDA, an agency of the federal government: *Traceability* provides the ability to follow an entire manufacturing process from its inception to its conclusion. *Trackability* provides the ability to follow a process or product, including the individuals involved in manufacturing, testing, and dispensing of product from start to finish. Complete, legible, and accurate records must be made and kept of significant blood bank activities (Quinley, 1994).

   These record keeping activities are defined and governed by regulatory requirements and defined in laboratory SOPs.

   Records may be recorded and stored as either handwritten documents or on electronic media.

   All personnel employed in the blood bank or transfusion service should be familiar with record keeping requirements defined by these agencies.

Product, Equipment, Reagent, and Testing Quality Assurance

QUALITY CONTROL

QC activities are constructed to provide the means for blood bank laboratory staff and management to measure, record, and amend processes or procedures that require improvement. These activities are defined and governed by regulatory requirements and should be defined by laboratory SOPs.

Blood Products

The reader is referred to the AABB *Standards* for a thorough discussion on QC and blood products.

Equipment

1. Specifications, calibration, performance, function, and repair of all equipment must be thoroughly documented.
2. Manufacturer's instructions should be followed with regard to frequency and scope of preventive maintenance on each piece of equipment or instrument.
3. Instrument function and/or performance should be monitored at intervals prescribed by regulatory agencies.
4. Exact parameters defining acceptable function of each instrument or piece of equipment must be defined in the laboratory SOP manual.
5. Clear and precise instructions for corrective action to be taken when an instrument or piece of equipment does not meet criteria for use must be defined in the laboratory SOP manual.
6. Clear and precise instructions for removal from service of malfunctioning instruments or equipment must be defined in the laboratory SOP manual.
7. Most equipment and instruments must be recalibrated when returned to service after repair.

SPECIFIC ACTIVITIES AND PROTOCOLS DEFINING A QUALITY ASSURANCE PROGRAM

8. The following table describes the intervals, as defined by the AABB, for monitoring the function of some commonly used blood bank and transfusion service equipment:

INSTRUMENT OR EQUIPMENT	PRESCRIBED MONITORING INTERVALS
Transfusion Service	
Mercury thermometers	Annually
Heating blocks	Daily when in use
Water baths	Daily when in use
Refrigerators and freezers (continuous monitors)	Daily
Alarm activation (refrigerators and freezers)	Monthly
Platelet incubators (ambient temperature storage)	Every 4 hr
Platelet incubators (enclosed, monitored chambers)	Daily

Centrifuges
  Speed, timer
  Temperature (refrigerated instruments)
	
	Quarterly
	Monthly

Cell washers (speed, timer)	Quarterly
Blood warmers	Quarterly

Irradiators
  Decay
  Leakage
	
	Defined by source of irradiation
	Biannually

Donor Facility	
Donor unit agitators (vacuum and nonvacuum type)	Daily when in use
Scales	Daily when in use
Balances	Daily when in use
Hemoglobinometers	Daily when in use
Microhematocrit centrifuges	Daily when in use

NOTE Each laboratory must conform to the strictest requirements defined by the agencies by which it is regulated!

Reagents

1. Most blood banks and transfusion services purchase commercially prepared reagents for use in serologic testing.
2. When a blood bank or transfusion service chooses to manufacture reagents for its own use, that laboratory is held to the federal requirements that apply to all

manufacturers of blood bank reagents. These are rigorous and detailed; the cost-effectiveness of this process, especially the time and technical resources spent in its execution, compared with purchasing approved commercial reagents should be carefully evaluated.

3. The following important information relating to commercially prepared reagents should be recorded on receipt:

   Manufacturer

   Date of receipt

   Date of expiration

   Lot number

   Visible damage, degradation, contamination (hemolysis, flocculation, cloudiness)

4. Although all commercially prepared reagents used in the blood bank for serologic testing must meet the standards of the Bureau of Biologics and be approved for use by the FDA, validation studies should be performed whenever a different manufacturer's reagents are chosen for use. The parameters, describing the validation of the study, must be clearly described, including the expected performance characteristics and measures to be taken when the reagent does not meet expectations.

5. All commercially prepared reagents must be stored at the temperature prescribed by the manufacturer.

6. The system for receipt and storage of reagents should provide for optimal use of the laboratory's reagent inventory.

7. *All reagents must be used strictly according to the manufacturer's instructions!*

8. The reagent inserts that contain the manufacturer's instructions for use must be available at all times for use by the laboratory staff.

9. Reagent inserts that are enclosed with each shipment of commercially prepared reagents must be carefully evaluated for changes from the instructions received with the previous shipment.

10. The table on p 550 describes a QC program, as defined by the AABB, for monitoring the function of some commonly used blood bank and transfusion service reagents.

REAGENTS	PRESCRIBED MONITORING INTERVALS
Red Blood Cells (for detecting presence of antibody in patient or reagent antiserum)	Daily, when in use.
Antisera (for detecting presence of antigen on patient or reagent RBCs)*	Daily, when in use.
Antihuman globulin	Daily, when in use. Every negative antiglobulin test must be validated with O check cells. See section on antiglobulin test in Chapter 24, p 439.

*The reagent RBC that should be selected as the positive control when assessing the performance of a reagent antiserum is one that expresses a single dose of the antigen complementary to the antibody contained in the antiserum. It is important to establish that the antiserum being controlled reacts with the weakest expression of an antigen on an RBC of unknown phenotype, e.g., when controlling anti-Fy^a, select an Fy(a+b+) RBC sample as the positive control. When controlling anti-K, select a K+k+ RBC sample as a positive control. This may not be possible in a situation when the reagent antiserum being controlled is one whose allelic antigen is a low incidence antigen, e.g., when controlling anti-$\bar{k}$, a K+$\bar{k}$+) RBC sample may not be available; a K−$\bar{k}$+) RBC sample must be used in this case.

Technical Procedures

Because of the critical nature of the testing performed in the immunohematology laboratory, it is important that adequate, accurate and informative controls be constructed and run with each test. Sometimes, the investigator is in the position to choose the controls appropriate to a particular testing situation.

To accomplish this, one must understand the concept of *test controls:*

1. The validity of the reactions observed with most blood bank reagents must be established.
2. The outcome of each procedure designed to manipulate a test system for the purpose of identifying alloantibodies must be confirmed.

NOTE
1. Most controls are appropriately tested in parallel with the test being controlled.
2. Inappropriate or unexpected results in any control indicates that the test being controlled must be repeated.

EXAMPLES OF TESTS AND PROCEDURES THAT REQUIRE CONTROLS

TEST OR PROCEDURE	CONTROL(S)	EXPLANATION
Forward Group (RBC Type) Testing	Reverse group determination. See section on "routine ABO and Rh typing methods and reagents" in Chapter 24, p 432.	Plasma of individuals who are genetically incapable of producing an RBC antigen of the ABO blood group system normally contains an antibody (isoagglutinin) directed at the antigen that their RBCs lack. The patient's plasma contains the antibody complementary to the RBC antigen(s) on that patient's RBCs, e.g., group A individuals produce anti-B. See section on ABO typing in Chapter 24, p 402.
$Rh_0(D)$ Antigen Typing	Reagent that contains all components in the diluent in which anti-D is prepared *except* anti-D, e.g.: 1. Rh control for anti-D used for slide and rapid tube testing contains bovine albumin in concentration of 22% or 30%, in addition to formula of preservatives and other additives usually patented by manufacturer. 2. Rh control reagent for saline, monoclonal, or chemically modified anti-D contains albumin in approximately 6% (normal serum albumin concentration), in addition to formula of preservatives and other additives usually patented by manufacturer.	Because of the negative consequences to the patient of identifying a D negative recipient as D positive, the $Rh_0(D)$ control must be performed with each patient antigen typing test when high protein reagents are used. This generally includes the reagents labeled "For Slide and Rapid Tube Tests," *but it should always be remembered that manufacturer's recommendations for reagent use must be followed whenever commercially prepared reagents are used.* A negative $Rh_0(D)$ control result validates the $Rh_0(D)$ antigen test result. A positive $Rh_0(D)$ control result, seen at any phase of testing, invalidates the $Rh_0(D)$ antigen test result. See section on problems encountered in Rh typing in Chapter 24, p 423.
Antihuman Globulin (AHG) Reagent	O check cells. See section on antiglobulin test in Chapter 24, p 439.	Because of the potentially harmful adverse consequences to the patient of a false negative antiglobulin test, each apparently negative test must be validated by using O check cells. These cells agglutinate when the AHG reagent contained in a completed test is reactive. See section on antiglobulin test in Chapter 24, p 439.

Crossmatch	Visual inspection of selected donor unit(s) as well as attached segments.	Donor unit must be inspected for:
		  Leaks and/or breaks in integrity of collection bag
		  Presence of clots
		  Abnormal color
		  Hemolysis
		  Any abnormality of color or appearance of donor red blood cells or plasma
		Any unit suspected of failing this QC process should not be used for transfusion. The supplier should be notified of the problem, and it may be prudent or required to return the unit to the supplier for follow-up investigation.

Continued ▶

► Continued **EXAMPLES OF TESTS AND PROCEDURES
THAT REQUIRE CONTROLS**

TEST OR PROCEDURE	CONTROL(S)	EXPLANATION
Antibody Identification	Autocontrol tested by same method used for investigation, e.g.: *Method:* Polyethylene glycol (PEG) indirect antiglobulin test (IAT) *Control:* Patient's serum + patient's RBCs + PEG *Method:* IAT with enzyme pretreated test RBCs *Control:* Patient's serum + patient's RBCs pretreated with enzyme used *Method:* 4°C incubation *Control:* Patient's serum + patient's RBCs incubated at 4°C	Negative autocontrol indicates that reactivity of the patient serum with test RBCs is most likely due to an alloantibody. Positive autocontrol indicates that an autoantibody is present and must be considered when attempting to identify alloantibodies that may be present in the patient's serum.
Cold RBC Adsorptions	Patient's RBCs + absorbed serum incubated at temperature of reactivity and read for agglutination. *NOTE:* If patient's RBCs spontaneously agglutinate when suspended in normal saline, they must be treated to remove antibody from RBC surface. See section on commonly used special serologic techniques in Chapter 25, p 488.	Negative result indicates that the autoantibody was successfully removed from the patient's serum. Positive result indicates incomplete adsorption of the autoantibody and the adsorption should be repeated.
Warm RBC Adsorptions	Patient's RBCs + absorbed serum tested by IAT. *NOTE:* Patient's RBCs that demonstrate positive direct antiglobulin test (DAT) must be treated to remove autoantibody. See section on commonly used special serologic techniques in Chapter 25, p 488.	Negative result indicates that the autoantibody was successfully removed from the patient's serum. Positive result indicates incomplete adsorption of the autoantibody, and the adsorption should be repeated.
Rosette Test for Fetal RBCs in a Mother's Sample	*Negative Control:* Saline suspension of RBCs known to be D negative. *Positive Control:* Saline suspension of mixture of negative and D positive RBCs. Concentration of D positive RBCs should be about 0.5%.	Appropriate reactions in the negative and positive controls indicate that the test reagents are performing as expected.

Continued ►

► Continued **EXAMPLES OF TESTS AND PROCEDURES
THAT REQUIRE CONTROLS**

TEST OR PROCEDURE	CONTROL(S)	EXPLANATION
RBC Elutions	Supernatant wash solution from last wash of RBCs to be used in elution procedure should be tested with representative test RBC samples by IAT in parallel with test on elution	Negative result indicates that any reactivity of the test RBC samples with the eluate is due to antibody that was bound to the RBC membrane. Positive result indicates that: 1. The cells used for the elution were not washed sufficiently (serum antibody still remained and was present in the last wash) *or* 2. Membrane bound antibody was shed from the RBC surface during the wash process. Either of these outcomes invalidates the elution test results; the reactivity seen in the IAT when testing the eluate may be attributed to the antibody detected in the test with the last wash or may be due to a mixture of antibody from the last wash and antibody removed from the RBC.
Proteolytic Enzyme Treatment of RBCs	Test RBC sample should be selected that expresses double dose of antigen known to be abolished or significantly reduced by pretreatment with proteolytic enzyme. *Untreated Control:* Selected RBC sample of *untreated* RBCs. *Treated Control:* Selected RBC sample pretreated with proteolytic enzyme. Test control samples with reagent antiserum containing relevant antibody.	*Untreated Control:* RBC sample should react when tested with antiserum containing the designated antibody. *Treated Control:* RBC sample should be nonreactive when tested with antiserum containing the designated antibody. If the treated RBC sample is reactive, the enzyme pretreatment was ineffective. The treatment should be repeated with a new vial or preparation of proteolytic enzyme. The patient investigation should also be repeated. *Note:* Enzymes characteristically degrade on storage.
Chemical Pretreatment of RBCs (ZZAP, dithiothreitol [DTT])	Treat aliquot or sample of RBCs known to express antigen whose reactivity is abolished by chemical being used: DTT Select RBC sample that expresses Kell blood group system antigen. ZZAP Select RBC sample that expresses Kell, Duffy, or MNS blood group system antigen. Test treated control sample with reagent antiserum containing relevant antibody.	Chemically treated control RBCs should be nonreactive when tested with the antiserum containing the complementary antibody. Reactivity with this RBC sample indicates ineffective treatment. The procedure should be repeated for a longer time (Always consult manufacturer's recommendations for use) or with new reagent.

EXAMPLES OF TESTS AND PROCEDURES THAT REQUIRE CONTROLS

> **NOTE** Construction of an appropriate control system may not be defined but left to the discretion of the investigator. The investigator should thoughtfully consider the expected or desired activity of the reagent or procedure undertaken and select controls accordingly.

PERSONNEL QUALITY ASSURANCE

1. Clearly defined and precise job descriptions in which the qualifications of the individual performing the tasks outlined are in compliance with the guidelines of all regulatory agencies governing the operation of the blood bank laboratory.
2. Hiring practices that conform to the job descriptions as described in step 1.
3. Training that is adequate and comprehensive enough to prepare the individual to perform the tasks outlined in his or her job description.
4. Monitoring each individual's competency to perform the tasks for which they were hired. This can be accomplished by:

   Proficiency testing—distribution of unknown and/or blind samples for investigation and interpretation

   Tests designed to assess the individual's knowledge of SOPs and ability to problem-solve

   Observation of the individual performing tasks as outlined in his job description

   This assessment is required to be performed and documented annually for each employee.

BIBLIOGRAPHY

Butch SH: Quality control, quality assurance, total quality improvement, and utilization review. In Rudmann SV, ed: Textbook of Blood Banking and Transfusion Medicine. Philadelphia, WB Saunders, 1995.

Quinley ED, Caglioti TA: GMP Fundamentals. Raritan, NJ, Ortho Diagnostic Systems, 1994.

Rock G, Seghatchian J, eds: Quality Assurance in Transfusion Medicine, Vols I and II. Boca Raton, Fla, CRC Press, 1992.

Sazama K, ed: Accreditation Requirements Manual, 6th ed. Bethesda, American Association of Blood Banks, 1995.

Standards Committee of the American Association of Blood Banks: Standards of Blood Banks and Transfusion Services, 17th ed. Bethesda, American Association of Blood Banks, 1996.

Snyder JR, Senhauser DA, eds: Administration and Supervision in Laboratory Medicine. Philadelphia, JB Lippincott, 1989.

Transfusion Service Quality Assurance Committee: Standard Operating Procedures, Training Guides and Competence Assessment Tools. Bethesda, American Association of Blood Banks, 1996.

Vengelen-Tyler B, ed: Technical Manual. American Association of Blood Banks, 12th ed. Bethesda, American Association of Blood Banks, 1996.

Section IV

MICROBIOLOGY

Chapter **29**

QUALITY CONTROL IN THE CLINICAL MICROBIOLOGY LABORATORY

Maria Reitano, PhD
Ronald Malowitz, PhD, MT(ASCP)

QUICK CONTENTS

INTRODUCTION

Quality control, a major part of quality assurance (a system of procedures used to ensure the quality of patient care), encompasses those procedures designed to ensure reliable laboratory testing. It involves monitoring the performance of media, reagents, stains, antimicrobial susceptibility testing, thermometers, automated and manual commercial systems, equipment, and personnel.

The purpose of this chapter is to give the reader, in flow chart form, the general guidelines for instituting quality control.

QUALITY CONTROL OF LABORATORY EQUIPMENT

Incubator

Temperature[1]

CO_2 Incubator

Temperature[1]
CO_2 content[2]

Refrigerator/ Freezer

Temperature[1]

Water Bath/ Heating Block

Temperature[1]

Biologic Safety Cabinet

Air Flow[3]
UV Light[4]

Anaerobic Glove Box

Temperature[1]
Anaerobiasis[5]
Humidity[6]

Anaerobic Jar/Gas Pak

Anaerobiasis[5]

Autoclave

Temperature[7]
Pressure[8]
Sterility[9]

pH Meter

pH Accuracy[10]

Balances

Weight Accuracy[11]

[1] Standardized thermometer in glycerol or water
[2] Fyrite (CO_2 measuring device)
[3] Air flow meter
[4] UV monitor
[5] Methylene blue indicator
[6] Drierite with indicator
[7] Temperature recording chart
[8] Pressure gauge
[9] Spore preparation (3M "Attest" ampules)
[10] Standardized acidic, neutral, and alkaline buffers
[11] Standardized weights

QUALITY CONTROL OF STAINS
AND REAGENTS

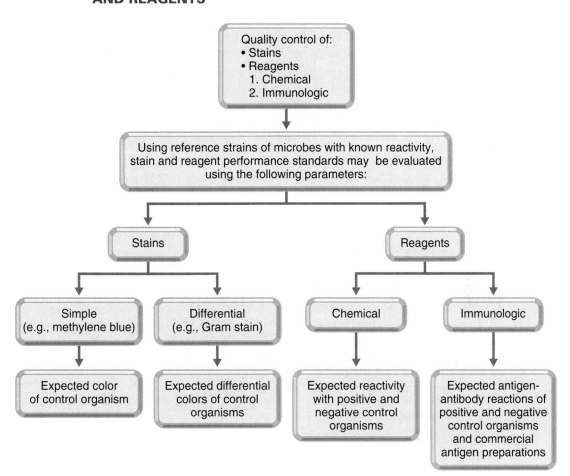

QUALITY CONTROL OF MEDIA

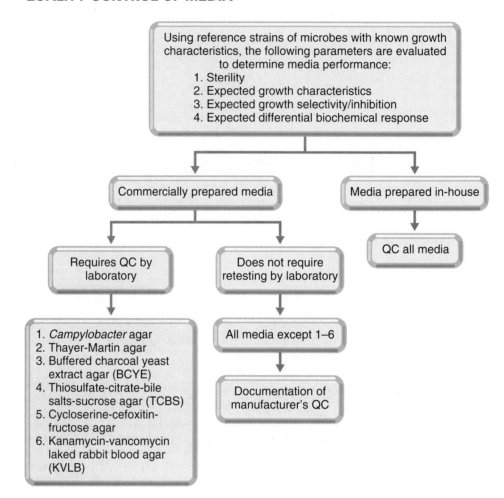

QUALITY CONTROL OF ANTIMICROBIAL SUSCEPTIBILITY TESTING

(For rapidly growing aerobic and facultative anaerobic bacteria and selected fastidious organisms based on National Committee for Clinical Laboratory Standards (NCCLS) guidelines.)

Disk Method*

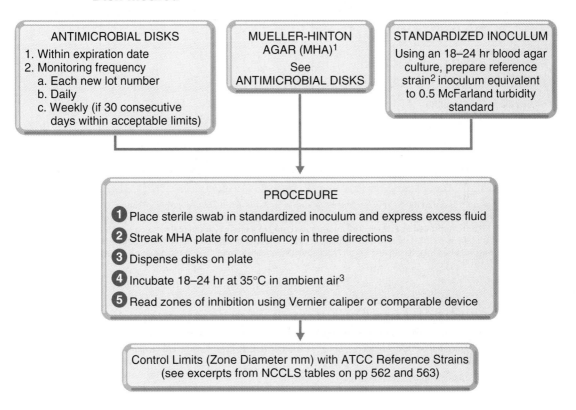

ANTIMICROBIAL DISKS
1. Within expiration date
2. Monitoring frequency
   a. Each new lot number
   b. Daily
   c. Weekly (if 30 consecutive days within acceptable limits)

MUELLER-HINTON AGAR (MHA)[1]
See
ANTIMICROBIAL DISKS

STANDARDIZED INOCULUM
Using an 18–24 hr blood agar culture, prepare reference strain[2] inoculum equivalent to 0.5 McFarland turbidity standard

PROCEDURE

1 Place sterile swab in standardized inoculum and express excess fluid

2 Streak MHA plate for confluency in three directions

3 Dispense disks on plate

4 Incubate 18–24 hr at 35°C in ambient air[3]

5 Read zones of inhibition using Vernier caliper or comparable device

Control Limits (Zone Diameter mm) with ATCC Reference Strains
(see excerpts from NCCLS tables on pp 562 and 563)

QUALITY CONTROL OF ANTIMICROBIAL SUSCEPTIBILITY TESTING

---

*NCCLS M2-A6.

CONTROL LIMITS FOR MONITORING ANTIMICROBIAL DISK SUSCEPTIBILITY TESTS; ZONE DIAMETER (mm) LIMITS FOR INDIVIDUAL TESTS ON MUELLER-HINTON MEDIUM WITHOUT BLOOD OR OTHER SUPPLEMENTS

ANTIMICROBIAL AGENT	DISK CONTENT (μg)	*ESCHERICHIA COLI* ATCC 25922	*STAPHYLOCOCCUS AUREUS* ATCC 25923	*PSEUDOMONAS AERUGINOSA* ATCC 27853	*ESCHERICHIA COLI* ATCC 35218
Amikacin	30	19–26	20–26	18–26	—
Amoxicillin/ clavulanic acid	20/10	19–25	28–36	—	18–22
Ampicillin	10	16–22	27–35	—	—
Ampicillin/ sulbactam	10/10	20–24	29–37	—	13–19
Azithromycin	15	—	21–26	—	—
Azlocillin	75	—	—	24–30	—

Permission to use portions of M100-S7 (*Performance Standards for Antimicrobial Susceptibility Testing;* Seventh Informational Supplement) has been granted by NCCLS. M100-S7 updates M2-A6 (Performance Standards for Antimicrobial Disk Susceptibility Tests - Sixth Edition; Approved Standard). The interpretive data are valid only if the methodology in M2-A6 is followed. NCCLS frequently updates the M2 tables to new editions of the standard and supplements. Users should refer to the most recent edition. The current standard may be obtained from NCCLS, 940 West Valley Road, Suite 1400, Wayne, PA 19087, United States.

ACCEPTABLE ZONE DIAMETER (mm) QUALITY CONTROL LIMITS FOR *HAEMOPHILUS INFLUENZAE*

ANTIMICROBIAL AGENT	DISK CONTENT (μg)	ATCC 49247	ATCC 49766
Amoxicillin/clavulanic acid	20/10	15–23	—
Ampicillin	10	13–21	—
Ampicillin/sulbactam	10/10	14–22	—
Azithromycin	15	13–21	—
Aztreonam	30	30–38	—
Cefaclor	30	—	25–31
Cefdinir	5	—	24–31

Permission to use portions of M100-S7 (*Performance Standards for Antimicrobial Susceptibility Testing;* Seventh Informational Supplement) has been granted by NCCLS. M100-S7 updates M2-A6 (Performance Standards for Antimicrobial Disk Susceptibility Tests - Sixth Edition; Approved Standard). The interpretive data are valid only if the methodology in M2-A6 is followed. NCCLS frequently updates the M2 tables to new editions of the standard and supplements. Users should refer to the most recent edition. The current standard may be obtained from NCCLS, 940 West Valley Road, Suite 1400, Wayne, PA 19087, United States.

ACCEPTABLE ZONE DIAMETER (mm) QUALITY CONTROL LIMITS FOR *NEISSERIA GONORRHOEAE*

ANTIMICROBIAL AGENT	DISK CONTENT (μg)	*NEISSERIA GONORRHOEAE* ATCC 49226
Cefdinir	5	40–49
Cefepime	30	37–46
Cefetamet	10	35–43
Cefixime	5	37–45
Cefmetazole	30	31–36

Permission to use portions of M100-S7 for use with M2-A6 (*Performance Standards for Antimicrobial Disc Susceptibility Tests,* 6th ed. Approved standard M2-A6) has been granted by the National Committee for Clinical Laboratory Standards. NCCLS is not responsible for errors or inaccuracies. The interpretive data are valid only if the methodology in M2-A6 is followed. These documents may be requested from The National Committee for Clinical Laboratory Standards, 940 West Valley Road, Suite 1400, Wayne, PA 19087-1898.

ACCEPTABLE ZONE DIAMETER (mm) QUALITY CONTROL LIMITS FOR DISK TESTS WITH *STREPTOCOCCUS* SPP

ANTIMICROBIAL AGENT	DISK CONTENT (μg)	*STREPTOCOCCUS PNEUMONIAE* (ATCC 49619)
Ampicillin	10	30–36
Azithromycin	15	19–25
Cefaclor	30	24–32
Cefdinir	5	26–31
Cefixime	5	16–23
Cefotaxime	30	30–35

Permission to use portions of M100-S7 for use with M2-A6 (*Performance Standards for Antimicrobial Disc Susceptibility Tests,* 6th ed. Approved standard M2-A6) has been granted by the National Committee for Clinical Laboratory Standards. NCCLS is not responsible for errors or inaccuracies. The interpretive data are valid only if the methodology in M2-A6 is followed. These documents may be requested from The National Committee for Clinical Laboratory Standards, 940 West Valley Road, Suite 1400, Wayne, PA 19087-1898.

1. For *N. gonorrhoeae,* GC (gonococcus) II agar with Isovitalex
   For *H. influenzae, Haemophilus* test agar
   For *S. pneumoniae,* Mueller-Hinton sheep blood agar plate
2. *E. coli,* ATCC 25922, ATCC 35218
   S. aureus, ATCC 25923
   P. aeruginosa, ATCC 27853
   N. gonorrhoeae, ATCC 49226
   H. influenzae, ATCC 49247, ATCC 49766
   S. pneumoniae, ATCC 49619
3. *H. influenzae,* 3%–7% CO_2
   N. gonorrhoeae, 3%–7% CO_2

QUALITY CONTROL OF ANTIMICROBIAL SUSCEPTIBILITY TESTING

QUALITY CONTROL OF PERSONNEL

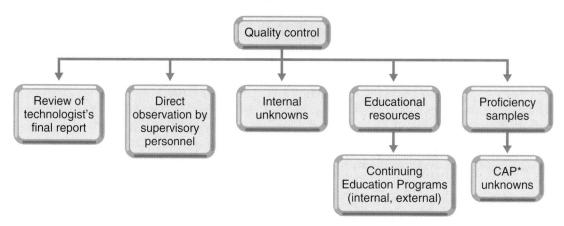

*CAP, College of American Pathologists

BIBLIOGRAPHY

August MJ, Hindler A, Huber TW, Sewell DL: In Weissfeld AS, ed: Cumitech 3A, Quality Control and Quality Assurance Practices in Clinical Microbiology. Washington, DC, American Society for Microbiology, 1990.

Bartlett RC, Mazens-Sullivan M, Tetreault S, et al: Evolving approaches to management of quality in clinical microbiology. Clin Microbiol Rev 7:55–88, 1994.

Bartlett RC et al: Clinical microbiology. In Inhorn SL, ed: Quality Assurance Practices for Health Laboratories. Washington, DC, American Public Health Association, 1978, pp 871–1005.

Eisenberg HD, ed: Clinical Microbiology Procedures Handbook. Washington, DC, American Society for Microbiology, 1992, secs 12–13.

Miller JM: Quality control of media, reagents, and stains. In Balows A, Hausler WJ Jr, Hermann KL, et al, eds: Manual of Clinical Microbiology, 5th ed. Washington, DC, American Society for Microbiology, 1991, pp 1203–1225.

Miller MJ, Wentworth BB, eds: Methods for Quality Control in Diagnostic Microbiology. Washington, DC, American Public Health Association, 1985.

National Committee for Clinical Laboratory Standards: Quality Assurance for Commercially Prepared Microbiological Culture Media, 2nd ed. Approved Standard M22-A2. Wayne, Pa, National Committee for Clinical Laboratory Standards, 1996.

National Committee for Clinical Laboratory Standards: Performance Standards for Antimicrobial Disc Susceptibility Tests, 6th ed. Approved Standard M2-A6. Wayne, Pa, National Committee for Clinical Laboratory Standards, 1997.

Sewell DL, Schifman RB: Quality assurance: quality improvement, quality control, and test validation. In Murray PR, Baron EJ, Pfaller MA, et al, eds: Manual of Clinical Microbiology, 6th ed. Washington, DC, American Society for Microbiology, 1995.

Chapter **30**

HANDLING AND PROCESSING SPECIMENS FOR BACTERIOLOGY, MYCOLOGY, AND PARASITOLOGY

Maria Reitano, PhD
Ronald Malowitz, PhD, MT(ASCP)

Q U I C K   C O N T E N T S

INTRODUCTION

The clinical microbiology laboratory plays a critical role in the diagnosis and treatment of the etiologic agents of infectious diseases. The principal functions of the laboratory include the microscopic examination and culture of specimens, accurate species identification of isolates, and antimicrobial susceptibility testing of those isolates. However, the effectiveness of the laboratory in most of these capacities is largely determined by proper specimen collection and the expeditious transport of the specimen to the laboratory. Proper techniques for specimen collection and specimen transport are critical for the recovery and accurate identification of microbial agents of infectious disease. Therefore, it is important for the clinical microbiology laboratory to provide guidelines for specimen collection and transport in order to ensure optimal recovery and identification.

Abbreviations

The following abbreviations are used throughout this chapter:
        AF = acid fast
        Bac = bacterial
        BAP = sheep blood agar
        BAP SXT = sheep blood agar with trimethoprim/sulfamethoxazole
        BBE = *Bacteroides* bile esculin agar
        BCYEa = buffered charcoal yeast extract agar with alpha ketoglutaric acid
        BHI = brain heart infusion agar
        CHOC = chocolate agar
        CIN = cefsulodin-irgasan-novobiocin agar
        CNA = colistin-nalidixic acid agar
        DFA = direct fluorescent microscopy
        EMB = eosin-methylene blue agar
        Fun = fungal
        7H11 = Middlebrook 7H11 medium
        HE = Hektoen enteric agar
        IMA = inhibitory mold agar
        KVA = kanamycin vancomycin agar
        LJ = Lowenstein-Jensen egg medium
        MAC = MacConkey agar
        MSDA = modified Sabouraud's dextrose agar
        NA = not applicable
        Para = parasitologic
        PAS = period acid-Schiff stain
        PEA = phenylethyl alcohol agar
        PVA = polyvinyl alcohol
        RT = room temperature
        SAB = Sabouraud's dextrose agar
        SS = *Salmonella-Shigella* agar
        TM = Thayer-Martin agar
        TSB = tryptic soy broth
        w/wo = with or without
        XLD = xylose-lysine-deoxycholate agar

RESPIRATORY TRACT

One of the most common sites of infection in the human body is the respiratory tract. This distinction can be attributed to its continuous exposure to the environment and thus its constant contact with a diverse variety of microorganisms. In addition, the human respiratory tract provides a warm environment for the multiplication of organisms. These factors contribute to make disease of the respiratory tract one of the greatest burdens on the American health care system.

The human respiratory tract is divided into two basic regions: the upper respiratory tract (URT) and the lower respiratory tract (LRT). The URT consists of a passageway that extends from the nose and lips to the trachea and bronchi. Secondary to this pathway are smaller side passages that lead to other air filled cavities such as the middle ear, paranasal sinuses, oropharynx, and nasopharynx. The LRT includes the bronchial tree, the pulmonary parenchyma, and the pleura.

Clinical manifestations of respiratory tract infection depend on the causative agent, localization of infection, and the condition of the host defense mechanisms. The primary causative agents of respiratory disease include the viruses, bacteria, and fungi. Protozoa and helminthic infections are rare.

Specimen Handling

SPECIMEN TYPE	COLLECTION	TRANSPORT/STORAGE	COMMENT
Throat Culture	Bac/Fun: Swab in transport medium Para: NA	Within 24 hr RT	*N. gonorrhoeae:* do not refrigerate
Ear	Bac/Fun: Fluid in sterile container or swab in transport medium Para: NA	See "Throat Culture" above	
Sputum	Bac–Fun/Para: 1–10 mL in sterile container	Within 2 hr–RT/24 hr–refrigerate	
Nasopharynx	Bac: Swab in transport medium	2 hr RT/24 hr: refrigerate	
Bronchoscopy (Bronchial Washings)	See "Sputum" above	Within 2 hr	
Aspirate: Nasotracheal/ Endotracheal/ Transtracheal/ Transthoracic	Bac/Fun/Para: Sterile container	Within 2 hr	Process ASAP
Pleural Fluid	Sterile container	Within 2 hr	Process ASAP
Lung Biopsy	Sterile container	Within 2 hr	Tissue in small amount of sterile *N*-saline. Store residual tissue at 5°C for 1–2 wk.

RESPIRATORY TRACT

Specimen Processing

	PROCESSING	DIRECT EXAM	CULTURE MEDIUM	COMMENTS
Throat				
Bacterial	Streak for isolation	None	BAP, BAP SXT	*C. diphtheriae:* BAP, Tellurite, aerobic, 35°C *N. gonorrhoeae:* T.M. agar, CO_2, 35°C
Fungal	Streak for isolation	None	IMA, or MSDA and Mycosel	
Parasitic	NA	None		
Ear				
Bacterial	Streak for isolation	Gram stain	BAP, CHOC, MAC, CNA or PEA, TSB with isovitalex 35°C, CO_2	
Fungal	Streak for isolation	KOH prep w/wo Calcofluor	IMA or MSDA, Mycosel, 30°C, aerobic	
Parasitic	NA			
Sputum/Bronchoscopy/Bronchoscopic washings, brushings				
Bacterial	Routine: streak for isolation	Routine: Gram stain	Routine: BAP, MAC, CHOC	
	Legionella sp.:	*Legionella* sp.: DFA	*Legionella* sp.: BCYE alpha	
	Mycobacteria sp.: decontaminate and concentrate	*Mycobacteria* sp.: AF stain	*Mycobacteria* sp.: LJ+7H11	
	Nocardia sp.: streak for isolation	*Nocardia* sp.: modified AF stain	*Nocardia* sp.: routine non-selective media, 7H11, MSDA	
Fungal	Streak for isolation	10% KOH prep w/wo Calcofluor	IMA or MSDA, Mycosel	Giemsa stain for *Pneumocystis* sp.
Parasitic		Direct preparation	NA	Acid fast stain for *Cryptosporidium* sp.

Continued ▶

▶ Continued **Specimen Processing**

	PROCESSING	DIRECT EXAM	CULTURE MEDIUM	COMMENTS
Aspirate				
Bacterial	Centrifuge, streak for isolation	Gram stain	BAP, CHOC, PEA or CNA, MAC, enriched broth media, anaerobic BAP, BBE, KVA, anaerobic PEA, supplemented thioglycolate	
Fungal	Centrifuge, streak for isolation	10% KOH prep w/wo Calcofluor	IMA or MSDA, and Mycosel	
Parasitic	Centrifuge specimen	Wet mount, w/wo iodine	NA	
Pleural Fluids				
Bacterial	Centrifuge	Gram stain	See "Aspirate" above	
Fungal	Centrifuge	India ink prep	IMA or MSDA, BHI with blood, Mycosel	
Parasitic	NA	NA		
Lung biopsy				
Bacterial	Touch prep, grind tissue	Gram stain	See "Aspirate" above	DFA for *Legionella* spp.
Fungal	See "Bacterial" above	Giemsa stain for *Pneumocystis* sp., PAS or methenamine silver	IMA or MSDA, Mycosel, BHI with blood	

RESPIRATORY TRACT

HAIR

A diverse, transient microbial population exists on hair. Infections at this site are superficial because they do not invade living tissue. The causative agents of hair infections are usually superficial mycotic agents and the dermatophytes.

Specimen Handling

SPECIMEN TYPE	COLLECTION	TRANSPORT/STORAGE	COMMENT
Hair	Bac: NA Fun: Epilate infected hairs and place in screw cap container. Para: Remove ectoparasite and infected hairs and place in screw cap container.	Fun: Within 24 hr at RT Para: Within 24 hr at RT	Para: Screen for parasitic lice.

Specimen Processing

	PROCESSING	DIRECT EXAM	CULTURE MEDIUM	COMMENTS
Bacterial	NA			
Fungal	Place several hairs on agar and press down gently.	Prepare wet prep using lactophenol cotton blue stain.	SAB, Mycosel	
Parasitic	Place hair and/or ectoparasite on slide.	Study under low power objective.	NA	Parasitic eggs are usually cemented to the hairs.

SKIN

The skin is the first line of defense against infection, for it provides a physical barrier against microbial penetration. The flora indigenous to the skin supports this antimicrobial barrier by contributing to the low pH of the skin and by the production of organic acids. The low pH of the skin inhibits the growth of most pathogenic bacteria and the organic acids produced by the indigenous microflora have a bactericidal effect on those organisms. The indigenous flora of the skin includes *Propionibacterium acnes* and the staphylococci. On occasion, these commensals are responsible for infection.

The microbial pathogens most commonly associated with skin infection are distributed according to the anatomic structure of the skin. Pathogenic bacteria occur primarily on the dead cells of the superficial squamous epithelium. These organisms include the staphylococci, hemolytic streptococci, and *Corynebacterium diphtheriae*. However, lipophilic anaerobes such as *P. acnes* are present in the deep sebaceous glands of the skin. Viruses, which require living cells for survival, infect those skin cells found in the basal germinal layers of the epithelium. Fungi, on the other hand, vary in their distribution. *Microsporum, Trichophyton,* and *Epidermophyton* are dermatophytic fungi that occur on the surface of the skin and cause scaling lesions known as tinea or ringworm. Those fungi that occur in moist areas between the fingers and toes include *Candida* sp. *Blastomyces dermatitidis* and *Pseudallescheria boydii* are responsible for systemic fungal infections with cutaneous manifestations.

Specimen Handling

SPECIMEN TYPE	COLLECTION	TRANSPORT/STORAGE	COMMENT
Vesicular Lesion	Bac/Fun: Sterile syringe	Bac: ASAP	Add small amount of sterile *N*-saline if no fluid is present and aspirate.
	Para: NA	Fun: Within 2 hr at RT	
Rash	Bac: Pus or fluid in sterile syringe	Bac: Within 2 hr at RT	
	Fun: Scrape active growing border into sterile container (for ringworm).	Fun: Within 24 hr at RT	
	Para: Remove ectoparasite and place into screw cap container.	Para: Within 24 hr at RT	Para: Principally for parasitic lice and ticks.

Specimen Processing

	PROCESSING	DIRECT EXAM	CULTURE MEDIUM	COMMENTS
Vesicular Lesion				
Bacterial	Streak for isolation	Gram stain	BAP, MAC, CHOC, enriched broth	For syphilis: darkfield microscopy of vesicular fluid
Fungal	Streak for isolation	10% KOH wet prep w/wo Calcofluor	IMA or MSDA, Mycosel, BHI with blood	
Parasitic	NA			
Rash				
Bacterial	See "Vesicular Lesion" above	See "Vesicular Lesion" above	See "Vesicular Lesion" above	
Fungal	Place skin scrapings on top of media.	10% KOH prep w/wo Calcofluor	SDA, Mycosel	Heat slide gently and let stand 10–15 min prior to microscopic study.
Parasitic	Place specimen on slide.	Study under low power objectives.	NA	

SKIN

NAILS

The nail is a thin horny plate on the end of a finger or toe, and as such is in frequent contact with the external environment and its diverse microflora.

Microbial infection of the nail is caused by both dermatophytic and nondermatophytic fungi (onychomycosis). The principal dermatophytic agents include *Trichophyton rubrum, T. mentagrophytes, T. tonsurans, T. violaceum, T. megninii, T. schoenleinii, T. concentricum,* and *Epidermophyton floccosum.* Prevalent among the nondermatophytic fungi causing onychomycosis are *C. albicans, Geotrichum candidum, Scopulariopsis brevicaulis, Aspergillus* sp., *Scytalidium* sp., and *Fusarium* sp.

Specimen Handling

SPECIMEN TYPE	COLLECTION	TRANSPORT/STORAGE	COMMENT
Nail	Bac: NA Fun: Scrape infected underside of nail. Scrape infected dorsal nail plate to clean outer surface and discard. Continue scraping for several minutes and collect scrapings in screw cap container. Para: NA	Fun: Within 24 hr at RT	

Specimen Processing

	PROCESSING	DIRECT EXAM	CULTURE MEDIUM	COMMENTS
Bacterial	NA			
Fungal	Place nail scrapings on top of media and press down gently.	10% KOH prep w/wo Calcofluor	SDA, Mycosel	Heat slide gently and let stand 10–15 min prior to microscopic study.
Parasitic	NA			

EYE

A variety of microbial agents are responsible for eye infections, including bacteria, fungi, viruses, and parasites. These infectious agents may be introduced by trauma, such as surgery, or by hematogenous spread from a focal site of infection. The most common eye infection is conjunctivitis. More serious infections include keratitis and endophthalmitis. Specimen collection can be a delicate procedure that often requires a specialized hospital setting. This factor, along with limitations on specimen volume, needs special consideration. In addition, knowledge of the indigenous flora of the conjunctiva is useful. These microorganisms include diphtheroids, coagulase negative staphylococci, viridans streptococci, *P. acnes, Staphylococcus aureus, Moraxella (Branhamella) catarrhalis,* and gram negative bacilli.

Specimen Handling

SPECIMEN TYPE	COLLECTION	TRANSPORT/STORAGE	COMMENT
Eye	Bac/Fun: Sterile, moistened swab of lesion or conjunctival and/or corneal scrapings. Swab is placed in sterile tube with small amount of nutrient broth. Scrapings are placed in sterile screw cap container.	Bac/Fun: Within 2 hr at RT	Corneal scrapings recommended for *Chlamydia* sp.
	Para: Corneal scrapings	Para: Immediately	Do not freeze

Specimen Processing

	PROCESSING	DIRECT EXAM	CULTURE MEDIUM	COMMENTS
Bacterial	Routine: streak for isolation.	Gram stain	BAP, CHOC, MAC, enriched broth	DNA probe preferred for *Chlamydia* sp.
	Chlamydia sp.: see "Vaginal/Cervix" on p 581.	*Chlamydia* sp.: DFA	*Chlamydia* sp.: see "Vaginal/Cervix" on p 581	
Fungal	Streak for isolation	10% KOH prep w/wo Calcofluor	IMA, BHI with blood	
Parasitic	Fix smear of corneal scrapings with methanol for staining. Culture corneal material	Stain with Hemacolor	Non-nutritive medium seed with *Enterobacter aerogenes* or *Escherichia coli*	For free-living amebae

EYE

EAR

Otitis media, one of the most common diseases of childhood, is an inflammatory infection of the mucosal lining of the middle ear. The warm, moist environment of the ear canal supports the multiplication of microorganisms. The principal etiologic agents responsible for acute otitis media include *Streptococcus pneumoniae, Haemophilus influenzae,* and *S. pyogenes.* In newborns, staphylococci and coliforms are often the causative agents of this disease. The major microorganisms responsible for chronic otitis media include *Proteus, Klebsiella, Enterobacter,* and *Pseudomonas* spp. Effusions of the middle ear should be cultured for bacteria and should include media that will support aerobic, anaerobic, and fastidious microbes such as *H. influenzae.* However, because specimen collection is an invasive procedure involving needle aspiration through the eardrum, laboratory culture is not common.

Otitis externa is an infection of the external auditory canal. Organisms responsible for this syndrome include the bacterial flora normally present on the skin, i.e., *S. aureus, S. epidermidis, Corynebacterium* sp., and to a lesser extent *P. acnes* and *Pseudomonas* sp. In the presence of an inflammatory condition, material from this site should be collected using a sterile swab and cultured for both bacteria and fungi.

Specimen Handling

SPECIMEN TYPE	COLLECTION	TRANSPORT/STORAGE	COMMENT
Ear	Bac/Fun: Sterile swab in transport medium Para: NA	Within 24 hr at RT	

Specimen Processing

	PROCESSING	DIRECT EXAM	CULTURE MEDIUM	COMMENTS
Bacterial	Streak for isolation	Gram stain	BAP, CHOC, MAC, enriched broth	
Fungal	See "Bacterial"	10% KOH prep w/wo Calcofluor	IMA or MSDA, Mycosel	
Parasitic	NA			

CEREBROSPINAL FLUID (CSF)

Infections of the central nervous system (CNS) are serious and life threatening. Factors such as age, time of year, and geographic location influence the etiologic agents of CNS infections. The standard diagnostic procedures for the determination of these infections include microscopic examination of spinal fluid for the presence of microorganisms and leukocytes, bacterial and cryptococcal antigen detection, and culture.

The principal bacterial pathogens involved in meningitis are *Neisseria meningitidis, S. pneumoniae, H. influenzae, Listeria monocytogenes,* and *Streptococcus agalactiae.* Other pathogens include viruses, *Mycobacterium tuberculosis, E. coli, C. neoformans, Naegleria* sp., and *Acanthamoeba* sp.

Specimen Handling

SPECIMEN TYPE	COLLECTION	TRANSPORT/STORAGE	COMMENT
CSF	Bac/Fun/Para: Collect several milliliters in sterile, screw cap tube.	Immediately	Do not refrigerate

Specimen Processing

	PROCESSING	DIRECT EXAM	CULTURE MEDIUM	COMMENTS
Bacterial	Centrifuge, streak sediment for isolation	Gram stain of sediment	BAP, CHOC, enriched broth	Filde's enriched broth recommended
Fungal	See "Bacterial"	India ink prep	IMA or MSDA, and BHI with blood	India ink prep: 50% sensitive; cryptococcal antigen method of choice
Parasitic	See "Bacterial"	Wet mount prep	Non-nutritive medium seeded with *E. aerogenes* or *E. coli*	For free-living amebae

BODY FLUIDS

Body fluids may collect at various sites, including synovial, pleural, pericardial, and peritoneal spaces. These fluids are aseptically collected by needle aspiration and processed immediately. Bile, another body fluid, is produced by the liver, and injury or obstruction to this system can result in infection, primarily bacterial. The most common pathogens recovered from these sites include the following:

BODY FLUID	PATHOGEN(S)
Synovial Fluid	*S. aureus, H. influenzae, N. gonorrhoeae*
Pleural Fluid	*S. pneumoniae, S. aureus, H. influenzae,* mixed anaerobic flora
Pericardial Fluid	Viruses, especially Coxsackie A and B
Peritoneal Fluid	*S. pneumoniae, S. pyogenes,* Enterobacteriaceae
Bile Fluid	*Bacteroides* sp., *Clostridium* sp., members of the Enterobacteriaceae, *Enterococcus* sp.

Specimen Handling

SPECIMEN TYPE	COLLECTION	TRANSPORT/STORAGE	COMMENT
Body fluids other than blood, urine, CSF	Aseptically collect several milliliters preferably by syringe aspiration.	Within 2 hr at RT	

CEREBROSPINAL FLUID

Specimen Processing

	PROCESSING	DIRECT EXAM	CULTURE MEDIUM	COMMENTS
Bacterial	Centrifuge, streak sediment for isolation	Gram stain of sediment	BAP, CHOC, PEA or CNA, MAC, enriched broth, anaerobic BAP, BBE, KVA, anaerobic PEA, supplemented thioglycolate	
Fungal	See "Bacterial"	10% KOH prep w/wo Calcofluor	IMA or MSDA, and Mycosel, BHI with blood	
Parasitic	NA			

URINARY TRACT

Urinary tract infections (UTIs) may occur in both males and females, but incidence is far greater in the female population.

The urinary tract is divided into two parts: the upper, which includes the kidneys and ureters, and the lower, which includes the urethra and urinary bladder. Under normal conditions, the urinary tract is free of microorganisms. Symptoms indicative of upper UTI include fever, chills, and flank pain. Dysuria and frequent urination are more characteristic of lower UTI. The microbial pathogens most often involved in these infections are the enteric gram negative bacilli. Of these, *E. coli* is the most common organism associated with urinary tract infection.

Specimen Handling

SPECIMEN TYPE	COLLECTION	TRANSPORT/STORAGE	COMMENT
Clean catch midstream urine	Bac/Fun: Clean genital area thoroughly. Collect at least 1 ml of midstream urine in a sterile screw cap container. Para: Collect in screw cap container.	Bac/Fun: Within 2 hr of collection or refrigerate Para: Refrigerate up to 24 hr	For *Schistosoma haematobium*
Catheter/Bladder/ Suprapubic Aspirate	Bac/Fun: Collect at least 1 ml of urine aseptically Para: NA	Within 2 hr	

Specimen Processing

	PROCESSING	DIRECT EXAM	CULTURE MEDIUM	COMMENTS
Clean catch midstream specimen				
Bacterial	Mix urine and inoculate using 1 µl calibrated loop	Gram stain	BAP, MAC	
Fungal	See "Bacterial" above	Not routinely done	IMA or MSDA, and Mycosel	
Parasitic	Centrifuge	Wet prep for *Trichomonas vaginalis* and *S. haematobium*	NA	*Onchocerca volvulus* microfilariae may be found in urine.
Catheter/Bladder/Suprapubic Aspirate				
Bacterial	Mix urine and inoculate 0.1 mL onto media.	Gram stain	BAP, MAC	
Fungal	See "Bacterial" above	NA	IMA or MSDA, and Mycosel	
Parasitic	NA			

URINARY TRACT

BLOOD

Microbial infection of the blood is referred to as bacteremia. The sources of these infectious agents include focal sites of infection most often associated with the respiratory tract, the genitourinary tract, and the abdomen as well as the skin and soft tissues. The pathogens involved often reflect the indigenous microflora present at these focal sites. *E. coli* and other enteric gram negative rods are the most common cause of bacteremia. These organisms represent the microbial flora indigenous to the gastrointestinal (GI) and genitourinary tracts. *S. pneumoniae* and *H. influenzae* are the most common etiologic agents of bacteremia in the pediatric population. *S. aureus* and the streptococci are usually the cause of bacteremia in association with indwelling catheters and implants.

Owing to their intermittent nature, most bacteremias are detected using three sets of blood culture bottles taken during a given episode of elevated temperature. A blood volume of 10 to 20 mL per culture is necessary for adequate recovery and detection of the pathogen. The significant consequences of bacteremia make detection a matter of critical concern to the microbiology laboratory.

Specimen Handling

SPECIMEN TYPE	COLLECTION	TRANSPORT/STORAGE	COMMENT
Peripheral	Bac: 10 mL for adults and older children; 1–5 mL for infants and young children. For routine culture: 3 samples per 24 hr. Inoculate directly into aerobic and anaerobic culture bottle or into isolator system.	Bac: Keep at RT or preferably at 35°C and transport ASAP.	Skin must be decontaminated with 70% alcohol and povidone-iodine solution prior to blood withdrawal. Do not refrigerate blood cultures. Automated blood culture systems available
	Fun: See "Bac"	Fun: See "Bac"	Isolator system recommended for fungi
	Para: Thick and thin blood smears from fingerstick and/or 5 mL of blood into EDTA collection tube.	Para: Transport within 24 hr.	

Specimen Processing

	PROCESSING	DIRECT EXAM	CULTURE MEDIUM	COMMENTS
Bacterial	Automated: If positive for growth, subculture. Nonautomated: Blind subculture at 24, 48, and 120 hr.	Automated: If positive for growth, Gram stain. Nonautomated: Gram stain done simultaneously with subculture	Aerobic bottle: Subculture to CHOC, BAP, and as Gram stain indicates. Anaerobic bottle: Subculture to CHOC, BAP, anaerobic BAP, and as Gram stain indicates.	Inspect blood culture bottles daily for evidence of growth. If growth is observed, Gram stain and subculture.
Fungal	See "Bacterial" above	NA	IMA or MSDA, and BHI with blood	
Parasitic	Air dry thin and thick smears. Fix thin smear in absolute methanol. Stain both thin and thick smear with Giemsa stain	NA	NA	

TISSUE

In the microbiology laboratory, the most common surgical specimens include intra-abdominal, thoracic, obstetric, gynecologic, CNS, and pleuropulmonary specimens. Operative tissue specimens are difficult to obtain and are unlikely to be repeatable specimens. Therefore, once collected in a sterile container, these specimens should be immediately transported to the laboratory and processed upon arrival. Special consideration should be given to techniques for the collection, transport, and recovery of anaerobic bacteria, since they have a high likelihood of being the infecting organism at these sites.

Specimen Handling

SPECIMEN TYPE	COLLECTION	TRANSPORT/STORAGE	COMMENT
Tissue	Bac/Fun: Sterile gassed out vial containing small amount of sterile *N*-saline	Bac/Fun/Para: Transport immediately at RT	Store residual tissue for up to 2 wk at 5°C.
	Para: Sterile container		For *Toxoplasma* sp.

Specimen Processing

	PROCESSING	DIRECT EXAM	CULTURE MEDIUM	COMMENTS
Bacterial	Grind tissue with sterile tissue grinder.	Gram stain; acid fast stain for *Mycobacterium* sp., DFA for *Legionella* sp.	See "Body Fluids" on p 576	Touch prep for *Legionella* sp. and *Mycobacterium* sp.
Fungal	Mince tissue with sterile scalpel.	10% KOH wet prep w/wo Calcofluor; Giemsa stain for *Pneumocystis* sp.	See "Body Fluids" on p 576	Touch prep for *Pneumocystis* sp.
Parasitic	Touch prep	Giemsa stain	NA	For *Toxoplasma* sp.

TISSUE

GENITAL

The potential microbial pathogens of the female and male genital tracts are greatly influenced by anatomic and physiologic differences. The female genital tract has two subdivisions, the upper and lower tract. The upper female genital tract includes the uterus, fallopian tubes, and ovaries. Infections are named according to the nature of the infection and the anatomic site. The lower female genital tract includes the vulva, vagina, and cervix. These sites have a diverse indigenous microbial population that includes *Lactobacillus* sp., *Corynebacterium* sp., coagulase-negative staphylococci, *Streptococcus* sp., *E. coli*, *Bacteroides* sp., *Fusobacterium* sp., and (less commonly) *Clostridium* sp. These organisms, as well as various fungi, protozoa, and viruses, are potential agents of genital tract disease. Predisposing conditions that may be responsible for infection with these organisms include malignancy, malnutrition, surgery, pregnancy, and intrauterine devices. The principal pathogens of the genital tract that are associated with sexually transmitted disease are *Treponema pallidum, Neisseria gonorrhoeae, Haemophilus ducreyi, Chlamydia trachomatis, Ureaplasma urealyticum,* human immunodeficiency virus, and genital herpes.

The anatomy and microbial dynamics of the male genital tract differ significantly from those of the female genital tract. The microorganisms most often involved in male genital tract infections are facultative gram negative rods and those agents of sexually transmitted disease listed on p 579. The specimens most often submitted for culture include the urethral exudate, prostatic secretions, and testicular aspirates.

Specimen Handling

FEMALE GENITAL TRACT

SPECIMEN TYPE	COLLECTION	TRANSPORT/STORAGE	COMMENT
Vaginal/Cervix	Bac:	Bac:	Culture of external vaginal orifice not useful. Specimen must not dry out. Endocervical cells must be collected for NGU.
	T. pallidum: Scrape and collect exudate from hard chancre; place on slide, add small amount of sterile *N*-saline, coverslip.	*T. pallidum:* immediate transport to lab for darkfield microscopy	
	H. ducreyi: Swab moistened with sterile *N*-saline.	*H. ducreyi:* Sterile, screw cap container within 2 hr at RT	
	N. gonorrhoeae: Endocervical exudate plated directly on JemBec or Transgrow	*N. gonorrhoeae:* Within 2 hr at 35°C or RT	
	Nongonococcal urethritis (NGU): Culture CTM-2-SP media Probepace specimen collection kit.*		
	Fun: *C. albicans:* swab of vaginal secretions	Fun: within 2 hr at RT	
	Para: *T. vaginalis:* Sterile tube of vaginal secretions; swab of vaginal material in sterile *N*-saline.	Immediate transport at RT	
Urethra	Bac: See "Vaginal/Cervix" above for *N. gonorrhoeae*		
*Gen-Probe Inc, San Diego, CA.			

▶ Continued **Specimen Handling**

MALE GENITAL TRACT

SPECIMEN TYPE	COLLECTION	TRANSPORT/STORAGE	COMMENT
Urethra	Bac: *N. gonorrhoeae:* urethral exudate plated directly on JemBec or Transgrow. NGU: Same as female Fun/Para: NA	Bac: same as female	
Penile Lesion	Bac: *T. pallidum:* See "Vaginal/Cervix" above *H. ducreyi:* Same as female for "Vaginal/Cervix" Fun/Para: NA	Bac: *T. pallidum:* same as female for "Vaginal/Cervix" *H. ducreyi:* same as female for "Vaginal/Cervix"	Specimen must not dry out.

Specimen Processing

FEMALE GENITAL TRACT

	PROCESSING	DIRECT EXAM	CULTURE MEDIUM	COMMENTS
	Vaginal/Cervix			
Bacterial	*T. pallidum:* Make wet prep of exudate. *H. ducreyi:* Inoculate media. *N. gonorrhoeae:* Transgrow—loosen cap and place in CO_2 incubator. Jembec: remove plastic bag and place in CO_2 incubator. *Chlamydia* sp.: Culture: inoculate cells.	*T. pallidum:* darkfield exam *H. ducreyi:* Gram stain *N. gonorrhoeae:* Gram stain	*T. pallidum:* NA *H. ducreyi:* Supplemented CHOC (1% Isovitalex + 3 μg vancomycin/mL) *N. gonorrhoeae:* TM or Martin Lewis agar *Chlamydia* sp.: McCoy cells	 DNA probe preferred for *Chlamydia* sp.

Continued ▶

GENITAL

► Continued **Specimen Processing**

FEMALE GENITAL TRACT

	PROCESSING	DIRECT EXAM	CULTURE MEDIUM	COMMENTS
Vaginal/Cervix				
Fungal	Inoculate media	10% KOH prep w/wo Calcofluor	IMA, Mycosel	Examine immediately
Parasitic	NA	Wet mount prep		
Urethra				
Bacterial	*N. gonorrhoeae, Chlamydia* sp. (NGU): see "Vaginal/Cervix"	Gram stain for *N. gonorrhoeae*	*N. gonorrhoeae:* TM or Martin Lewis agar *Chlamydia* sp.: McCoy cells	DNA probe preferred for Chlamydia sp.
Fungal	NA			
Parasitic	NA			

Specimen Processing

MALE GENITAL TRACT

	PROCESSING	DIRECT EXAM	CULTURE MEDIUM	COMMENTS
Urethra				
Bacterial	Same as female	Same as female	Same as female	
Fungal	Same as female	Same as female	Same as female	
Parasitic	Same as female	Same as female	Same as female	
Penile Lesion				
Bacterial	*T. pallidum:* Scrape chancre and make wet prep of exudate. *H. ducreyi:* See "Vaginal/Cervix"	*T. pallidum:* darkfield microscopy *H. ducreyi:* See "Vaginal/Cervix"	*T. pallidum:* NA *H. ducreyi:* See "Vaginal/Cervix"	
Fungal	NA			
Parasitic	NA			

WOUNDS

A significant number of specimens received in the microbiology laboratory are wound cultures. A diverse spectrum of microorganisms are responsible for these infections, including bacteria, fungi, viruses, and parasites. Among the bacteria, both fastidious aerobes, facultative anaerobes, and anaerobes may be involved.

Deep wounds and abscesses may be obtained surgically or by needle aspiration after skin decontamination. Adequate specimen volume is essential for optimal recovery of pathogens. Since there is a high likelihood of anaerobic bacteria being present, special techniques regarding specimen collection and transport must be considered. Gram stain of specimens prior to media inoculation is recommended.

Superficial wound infections are usually collected by swab after skin decontamination. The microorganisms involved include aerobic, facultative anaerobic, and anaerobic bacteria and usually reflect the indigenous flora present.

Specimen Handling

SPECIMEN TYPE	COLLECTION	TRANSPORT/STORAGE	COMMENT
Deep Wounds	Bac/Fun: Needle aspirate	Bac/Fun: within 2 hr at RT	Do not refrigerate
	Para: NA		
Superficial Wounds			
Pus	Bac/Fun: Sterile swab in transport media	Bac/Fun: within 24 hr at RT	
	Para: NA		
Biopsy	Bac/Fun: Sterile container	Bac/Fun: within 2 hr at RT	
	Para: NA		

Specimen Processing

	PROCESSING	DIRECT EXAM	CULTURE MEDIUM	COMMENTS
Deep Wounds				
Bacterial	Streak for isolation	Gram stain	See "Body Fluids" on p 576	If *Mycobacterium* sp. suspected, perform acid fast stain.
Fungal	See "Bacterial" above	10% KOH prep w/wo Calcofluor	See "Body Fluids" on p 576	
Parasitic	NA			

Continued ▶

WOUNDS

► Continued **Specimen Processing**

	PROCESSING	DIRECT EXAM	CULTURE MEDIUM	COMMENTS
Superficial wounds: Pus				
Bacterial	Streak for isolation	Gram stain	BAP, CHOC, MAC, enriched broth	If *Mycobacterium* sp. suspected, perform acid fast stain.
Fungal	See "Bacterial" above	10% KOH prep w/wo Calcofluor	IMA or MSDA, Mycosel, BHI with blood	
Parasitic	NA			
Superficial wounds: Biopsy				
Bacterial	Grind tissue with sterile tissue grinder. Streak for isolation.	Gram stain	See "Body Fluids" on p 576	If *Mycobacterium* sp. suspected, perform acid fast stain.
Fungal	Mince tissue with scalpel. Streak for isolation.	10% KOH prep w/wo Calcofluor	See "Body Fluids" on p 576	
Parasitic	NA			

GASTROINTESTINAL TRACT

The GI tract is one of the most prevalent sites of microbial encounter in the human body. The oral cavity is the portal that allows entry of these microorganisms via food, fluid, or hand to mouth contamination. This results in a transient microbial population that varies in number and composition depending on diet, geographical location, sanitary habits, and host health status.

There exists a disparity in the distribution of microorganisms in the GI tract. The upper GI tract, which includes the esophagus and stomach, has few microorganisms relative to the lower GI tract. This is due primarily to the low pH of the stomach, which destroys nearly all the bacteria that enter the alimentary tract. This low concentration of bacteria continues in the duodenum as long as the health of the host is not compromised. The lower GI tract, beginning with the distal ileum, reflects a dense microbial population consisting of bacteria, fungi, protozoa, and viruses. Of these, bacteria are the most abundant in the colon and represent approximately one third of the dry weight of fecal matter.

Microorganisms indigenous to the GI tract form a symbiotic relationship with the host, where they contribute to digestive processes and defense mechanisms. However, microbial disease of the GI tract is a significant concern in industrialized nations and a major cause of morbidity and mortality worldwide. These infections can be categorized into three distinct groups: (1) those caused by ingestion of classic pathogens, (2) those caused by ingestion of preformed microbial toxins, and (3) those caused by dissemination of indigenous flora to extraintestinal sites. There is also evidence to support intestinal pathogens in ulcerative disease and neoplasia.

In most areas of the United States, the bacterial pathogens responsible for infectious diarrhea are *Salmonella, Shigella, Campylobacter, Yersinia,* and enteropathogenic and enterotoxigenic *E. coli,* while the parasitic agents are *Entamoeba histolytica* and *Giardia duodenalis.* The viruses causing infectious diarrhea are generally the parvovirus-like agents and, in the very young, rotavirus.

Specimen Handling

SPECIMEN TYPE	COLLECTION	TRANSPORT/STORAGE	COMMENT
Stool	Bac: Cary Blair Transport Media	Bac: RT within 24 hr, room temp	
	Fun: NA	Para: fresh specimen within 2 hr at RT. PVA, formalin, 48 hr at RT.	
	Para—Sterile screw cap container		
Rectal Swab	Bac: See "Stool" above		
	Fun/Para: NA		
Scotch Tape	Bac/Fun: NA		
	Para: Press tape against perianal area and transfer tape sticky side down on clear glass slide.	Para: Place slide in envelope and transport within 24 hr.	Use clear Scotch tape only.
Duodenal Material			
Aspirate	Bac: NA		
	Fun: NA		
	Para: Sterile screw cap container	RT, within 2 hr	Process immediately.
String Test	Place string in sterile screw cap container.	RT, within 2 hr	Process immediately.

Specimen Processing

	PROCESSING	DIRECT EXAM	CULTURE MEDIUM	COMMENTS
Stool				
Bacterial	Inoculate media with specimen using sterile swab.	Gram stain for leuko-cytes	BAP, MAC, HE, SS, CIN, Campy BAP, Sorbitol MAC, Selenite broth, Campy thio	Alternative media, EMB, XLD, bismuth sulfite
Fungal	NA			
Parasitic	Formalin ethyl acetate concentration; trichrome stain	0.85% saline or io-dine prep	NA	Trichrome stain for loose stool only. Acid fast stain for *Cryptosporidium* and *Cyclospora* spp.
Rectal Swab				
Bacterial	See "Stool" above	NA	See "Stool" above	Roll swab over medium.
Fungal	NA			
Parasitic	NA			
Scotch Tape Prep				
Bacterial	NA			
Fungal	NA			
Parasitic	NA	Examine entire slide under 400× mag-nification.		
Duodenal Material: Aspirate				
Bacterial	NA			
Fungal	NA			
Parasitic	Centrifuge nonvis-cous material.	Prepare wet mount using 0.85% saline. For trichrome prep, 1 drop sample in 3 drops PVA. Mix. Make thin smear. Air dry, stain.	NA	Iodine prep may be used to detect *Strongyloides* sp.

Continued ▶

▶ Continued **Specimen Processing**

	PROCESSING	DIRECT EXAM	CULTURE MEDIUM	COMMENTS
Duodenal Material: String Test				
Bacterial	NA			
Fungal	NA	See "Aspirate" on p 586		
Parasitic	Remove material from string.			

BIBLIOGRAPHY

Bannatyne RM, Clausen C, McCarthy LR: Cumitech 10, Laboratory Diagnosis of Upper Respiratory Tract Infections. Coordinating ed, Duncan IBR. American Society for Microbiology, Washington, DC, 1979.

Bartlett JG, Ryan KJ, Smith TF, Wilson WR: Cumitech 7A, Laboratory Diagnosis of Lower Respiratory Tract Infections. Coordinating ed, Washington JA II. American Society for Microbiology, Washington, DC, 1987.

Braude AI, Davis CE, Fierer J, eds: Infectious Diseases and Medical Microbiology, 2nd ed. Philadelphia, WB Saunders, 1986.

Clarridge JE, Pezzlo MT, Vosti KL: Cumitech 2A, Laboratory Diagnosis of Urinary Tract Infections. Coordinating ed, Weissfeld AS. American Society for Microbiology, Washington, DC, 1987.

Clyde WA, Kenny GC, Schachter J: Cumitech 19, Laboratory Diagnosis of Chlamydial and Mycoplasma Infections. Coordinating ed, Drew WL. American Society for Microbiology, Washington, DC, 1984.

Drasar BS, Hill MJ: Human Intestinal Flora. London, Academic Press, 1974.

Eisenberg HD, Schoenknecht FD, von Graevenitz A: Cumitech 9, Collection and Processing of Bacteriological Specimens. Coordinating ed, Baron SJ. American Society for Microbiology, Washington, DC, 1979.

Eschenbach D, Pollack HM, Schachter J: Cumitech 17, Laboratory Diagnosis of Female Genital Tract Infections. Coordinating ed, Baron SJ. American Society for Microbiology, Washington, DC, 1983.

Haley LD, Callaway CS: Laboratory Methods in Medical Mycology, 4th ed. U.S. Department of Health, Education and Welfare, Public Health Service, Centers for Disease Control, Bureau of Laboratories, Atlanta, GA, 1978.

Haley LD, Trandel J, Coyle MB: Cumitech 11, Practical Methods for Culture and Identification of Fungi in the Clinical Microbiology Laboratory. Coordinating ed, Sherris JC. American Society for Microbiology, Washington, DC, 1980.

Holden J: Collection and transport of clinical specimens for anaerobic culture. In Isenberg HD, ed: Clinical Microbiology Handbook, vol 1. American Society for Microbiology, Washington, DC, 1992.

Jones DB, Liesegang TJ, Robinson NM: Cumitech 13, Laboratory Diagnosis of Ocular Infections. Coordinating ed, Washington JA II. American Society for Microbiology, Washington, DC, 1981.

Markell EK, Voge M, John DT: Medical Parasitology, 7th ed. Philadelphia, WB Saunders, 1986.

Murray PR, Baron EJ, Pfaller MA, et al, eds: Manual of Clinical Microbiology, 6th ed. American Society for Microbiology, Washington, DC, 1995, Chapters 3, 21, 60, and 101.

Ray CG, Wasilauskas BL, Zabransky R: Cumitech 14, Laboratory Diagnosis of Central Nervous System Infections. Coordinating ed, McCarthy LR. American Society for Microbiology, Washington, DC, 1982.

GASTROINTESTINAL TRACT

Reller LB, Murray PR, MacLowry JD: Cumitech 1A, Blood Cultures 11. Coordinating ed, Washington JA II. American Society for Microbiology, Washington, DC, 1982.

Sack RB, Tilton RC, Weissfeld AS: Cumitech 12, Laboratory Diagnosis of Bacterial Diarrhea. Coordinating ed, Rubin SJ. American Society for Microbiology, Washington, DC, 1980.

Simor AE, Roberts FJ, Smith JA: Cumitech 23, Infections of the Skin and Subcutaneous Tissues. Coordinating ed, Smith JA. American Society for Microbiology, Washington, DC, 1988.

Sommers HM, McClatchy JK: Cumitech 16, Laboratory Diagnosis of Mycobacteriosis. Coordinating ed, Morello JA. American Society for Microbiology, Washington, DC, 1983.

Tilton RC, Balows A, Hohnadel DC, Reiss RF, ed: Clinical Laboratory Medicine, Part 7, Microbiological Analysis of Clinical Specimens. St. Louis, Mosby–Year Book, 1992.

Chapter *31*

CLINICAL BACTERIOLOGY

Maria Reitano, PhD

QUICK CONTENTS

AEROBIC AND FACULTATIVE ANAEROBIC GRAM POSITIVE COCCI

Introduction

Clinically relevant aerobic and facultative anaerobic gram positive cocci encompass several genera including *Staphylococcus, Micrococcus, Streptococcus,* and *Enterococcus.* These organisms are widespread in nature and can be found on the skin and mucosal surfaces of both humans and animals.

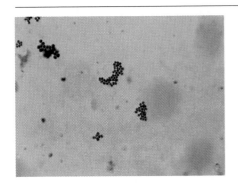

Characteristics of *Staphylococcus* Species and *Micrococcus* Species

Staphylococcus is a relatively large, gram positive coccal bacterium that occurs in groups of varied numbers, some resembling grapelike clusters (see left).

They are nonmotile, catalase positive, facultative anaerobes that belong to the family Micrococcaceae. The genus *Micrococcus* is also a member of the Micrococcaceae family. Members of this genus are small coccal bacteria that, unlike *Staphylococcus*, are obligate aerobes. They can be further differentiated from clinically relevant species of *Staphylococcus* on the basis of several characteristics (see figure on next page). Both genera grow well on 5% sheep blood agar and thioglycollate broth, but an incubation period of 48 hours may be required for *Micrococcus* species. Yellow pigmented and rose pigmented colonies of *M. luteus* and *M. roseus*, respectively, may be used as a tool in preliminary differentiation.

AEROBIC AND FACULTATIVE ANAEROBIC GRAM POSITIVE COCCI

DIFFERENTIATION OF SELECTED MEMBERS OF MICROCOCCACEAE CLINICALLY RELEVANT IN HUMANS

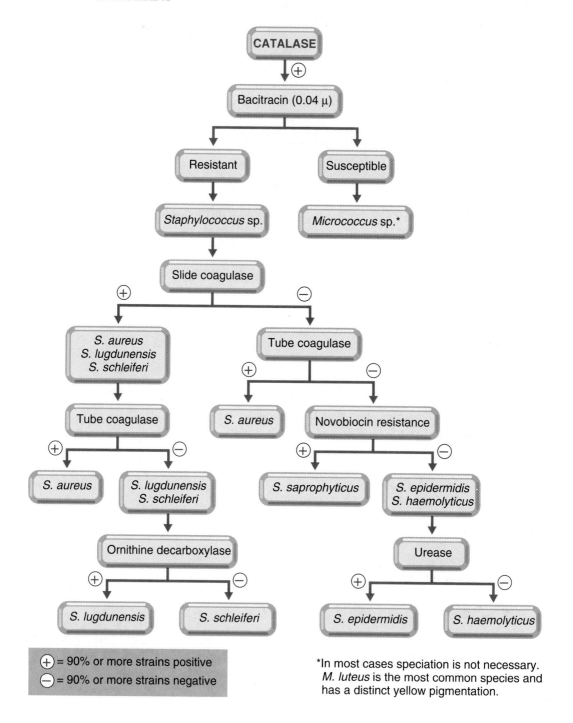

⊕ = 90% or more strains positive
⊖ = 90% or more strains negative

*In most cases speciation is not necessary. *M. luteus* is the most common species and has a distinct yellow pigmentation.

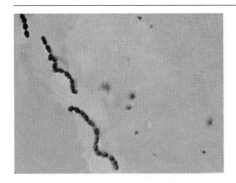

From Mahon CR, Manuselis G: Textbook of Diagnostic Microbiology. Philadelphia, WB Saunders, 1995, p 340.

Characteristics of *Streptococcus* Species and *Enterococcus* Species

Streptococci and enterococci are a diverse group of small, gram positive cocci that occur singly or in pairs, or in long chains when viewed microscopically (see left).

These organisms are nonmotile, catalase negative, facultative anaerobes that belong to the family Streptococcaceae. Preliminary classification of *Streptococcus* and *Enterococcus* is based on hemolysis on 5% sheep blood agar. Biochemical characteristics and differentiation of clinically relevant species are presented on the next page.

AEROBIC AND FACULTATIVE ANAEROBIC GRAM POSITIVE COCCI

DIFFERENTIATION OF SELECTED MEMBERS OF STREPTO-COCCACEAE CLINICALLY RELEVANT IN HUMANS

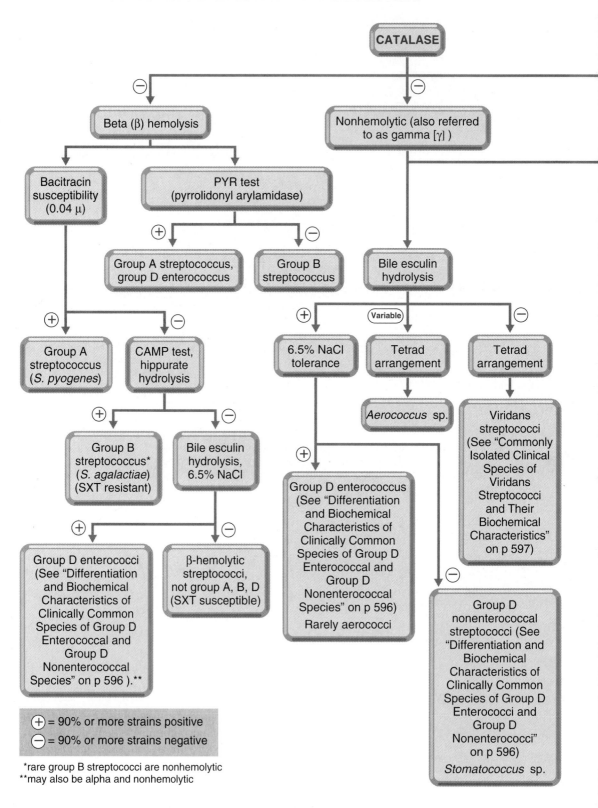

⊕ = 90% or more strains positive
⊖ = 90% or more strains negative

*rare group B streptococci are nonhemolytic
**may also be alpha and nonhemolytic

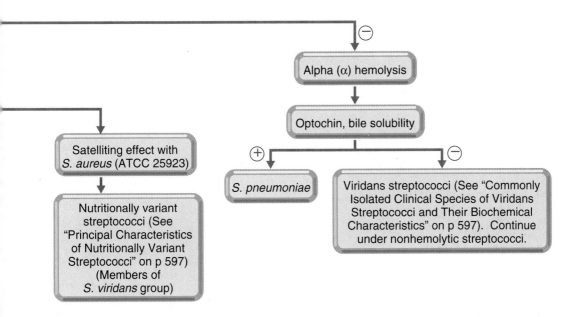

LANCEFIELD CLASSIFICATION

In addition to genus and species, classification of the streptococci may also be based on an antigenic C carbohydrate present on the streptococcal cell wall. Serologic differences in this carbohydrate, which was first detected by Rebecca Lancefield, resulted in distinct serologic groups classified as A to H and K to T. Thus, *S. pyogenes*, for example, is also referred to as *group A streptococcus*.

GROUP D STREPTOCOCCI

Group D streptococci are divided into two groups, namely, the *Enterococcus* species and the nonenterococci, which can be differentiated on the basis of certain biochemical properties (see p 596).

AEROBIC AND FACULTIVE ANAEROBIC GRAM POSITIVE COCCI

Differentiation and Biochemical Characteristics of Clinically Common Species of Group D Enterococci and Group D Nonenterococci

CHARACTERISTIC	GROUP D ENTEROCOCCI				GROUP D NONENTEROCOCCI
	E. faecalis	*E. faecium*	*E. durans*	*E. avium*	*Streptococcus bovis*
Hemolysis on 5% Sheep Blood Agar	α, β, none	α, none	α, β, none	α, none	α,* none
Bile Esculin	+	+	+	+	+
6.5% NaCl	+	+	+	+	−
PYR	+	+	+		−
LAP	+	+	+	+	+
Growth at: 10°C	+	+	+	−	−
45°C	+	+	+	+	+
Vancomycin	Susc	Susc	Susc	Susc	Susc
Penicillin	Resis	Resis	Resis	Resis	Susc
Lactose	+	+	+	+	+
Arabinose	−	+	−	+	−
Arginine	+	+	+	−	−
Sorbitol	+	−	−	+	−

PYR, production of pyrrolidonyl arylamidase; LAP, production of leucine aminopeptidase; Susc, susceptible; Resis, resistant; +, >90% positive; −, <10% positive.
   *Uncommon.

The viridans streptococci are nonhemolytic, and their biochemical properties are listed in the chart on the facing page.

One group of viridans streptococci are the nutritionally variant streptococci that require thiol derivative supplements for growth. The following chart lists the principal characteristics of these organisms.

Commonly Isolated Clinical Species of Viridans Streptococci and Their Biochemical Characteristics*

SPECIES	BIOCHEMICAL CHARACTERISTICS					
	Voges-Proskauer	**Mannitol**	**Sorbitol**	**Arginine**	**Esculin**	**Urease**
S. milleri Group (*S. anginosus, S. constellatus, S. intermedius*)	+	±†	−	+	±	−
S. mitis Group (*S. mitior, S. oralis, S. sanguis* II)	−	−	−	−	−	−
S. mutans Group (*S. cricetus, S. mutans, S. rattus, S. sobrinus*)	+	+	+	−‡	+	−
S. salivarius (*S. vestibularis*)	+§	−	−	−	+	±
S. sanguis Group (*S. crista, S. gordonii, S. parasanguis, S. sanguis*)	−	−	−	+‖	+¶	−

*Adapted from Facklan RR, Washington AA: In Balows A, et al, eds: Manual of Clinical Microbiology, 5th ed. Washington, DC: American Society for Microbiology, 1991, p 250.

　†+, >90% positive; −, <10% positive; ±, variable.

‡*S. rattus* is arginine positive.

§*S. vestibularis* is VP variable.

‖*S. crista* is arginine variable.

¶*S. crista* is esculin negative; *S. parasanguis* is esculin variable.

Principal Characteristics of Nutritionally Variant Streptococci ("Satelliting Streptococci," "Thiol-Dependent Streptococci")*

1. Fermentation of glucose and sucrose
2. Growth in thioglycollate medium
3. Failure to grow in: 6.5% NaCl, 10%–40% bile esculin
4. Inability to hydrolyze hippurate

Rapid Test Methods for Identification

In addition to conventional biochemical assays, numerous commercial kits, automated systems, and genetic probes are available for the identification of Micrococcaceae and the Streptococcaceae (see p. 598). Quality control with appropriate reference strains is an important criterion in the interpretation of any of these assays.

*Adapted from Brown S, Fuchs PC: ASCP Microbiology Check Sample exercise MB 80-4. Thiol-Dependent Streptococci (Nutritionally Variant Streptococci). Check sample MB 180-107. Copyright 1980, American Society of Clinical Pathologists, Chicago, Illinois. Reproduced with permission.

AEROBIC AND FACULTATIVE ANAEROBIC GRAM POSITIVE COCCI

SELECTED COMMERCIAL KITS, PROBES, AND AUTOMATED METHODS FOR THE IDENTIFICATION OF THE MICROCOCCACEAE AND STREPTOCOCCACEAE*

IDENTIFICATION SYSTEM	MANUFACTURER	ORGANISMS IDENTIFIED
Chromogenic Enzyme Substrate Tests		
api STAPH-IDENT	bioMérieux Vitek, Hazelwood, MO	*Staphylococcus* species
api STAPH	bioMérieux Vitek, Hazelwood, MO	*Staphylococcus* species *Micrococcus* species
Vitek Gram-Positive Identification Card (GPI): Used with AutoMicrobic System (AMS)	bioMérieux Vitek, Hazelwood, MO	*Micrococcus* species *Staphylococcus* species *Streptococcus* species *Enterococcus* species
MicroScan Pos ID Panel	Dade International, Chicago, IL	See above
Minitek Gram-Positive System	Becton Dickinson Microbiology Systems, Sparks, MD	See above
api 20 strep	bioMérieux Vitek, Hazelwood, MO	*Streptococcus* species *Enterococcus* species
Rapid ID STREP System	Innovative Diagnostic Systems, Atlanta, GA	*Streptococcus* species *Enterococcus* species
Coagglutination Test		
Phadebact System	Pharmacia Diagnostic, Piscataway, NJ	Groups A, B, C, D, and G streptococci
Agglutination Tests		
Streptex	Wellcome Laboratories, Research Triangle Park, NC	Group A, B, C, D, F, or G streptococci
Molecular Assays		
AccuProbe Culture ID Test	Gen-Probe, San Diego, CA	*S. aureus*
Nucleic Acid Probe	See above	Group A streptococcus

*Refer to manufacturer's guidelines regarding procedure, interpretation, and specificity and sensitivity of each assay.

Pathogenicity

The disease syndromes for the micrococci, staphylococci, streptococci, and enterococci are presented in the chart below. *Micrococcus* species are seldom associated with disease but may cause opportunistic infection in immunocompromised patients. Staphylococci, on the other hand, are significant agents of human disease. *S. aureus* is the most pathogenic species and a major agent of nosocomial infection. *S. epidermidis* is a pathogenic, coagulase negative species known to cause infections associated with implanted devices such as shunts, intravenous catheters, heart valves, and prostheses. *S. saprophyticus* is the causative agent of urinary tract infections in young sexually active women. Of clinical and epidemiologic significance are strains of methicillin resistant *S. aureus* and *S. epidermidis* (MRSA and MRSE, respectively). These strains are most common in hospitals and large institutions and are an important health care concern. Streptococci and enterococci are a diverse, well recognized group of pathogens responsible for a wide range of diseases. *Leuconostoc* species, *Pediococcus* species, and *Stomatococcus* species are aerobic gram positive cocci that are not considered in this chapter. These organisms rarely cause disease, and only in an opportunistic setting.

DISEASE SPECTRA OF SELECTED MEMBERS OF THE MICROCOCCACEAE AND STREPTOCOCCACEAE

ORGANISM	DISEASE(S)
Micrococcaceae	
***Micrococcus* species**	Opportunistic pathogens: pneumonia, meningitis, bacteremia, abscesses
Staphylococcus aureus	Cutaneous infections: carbuncles, impetigo, cellulitis, scalded skin syndrome Other infections: abscesses, enterocolitis, food poisoning, pneumonia, meningitis, bacteremia, osteomyelitis, toxic shock syndrome
Staphylococcus epidermidis	Endocarditis, peritonitis, bacteremia from indwelling catheters, infections associated with shunts, valves, and orthopedic devices
Staphylococcus saprophyticus	Urinary tract infections and cystitis in young sexually active women
Streptococcaceae	
S. pyogenes (group A streptococcus)	Suppurative infections (pus producing): pharyngitis, otitis media, pneumonia, meningitis, and puerperal fever Nonsuppurative infections: rheumatic fever, acute glomerulonephritis, and scarlet fever Cutaneous infections: impetigo, erysipelas, and cellulitis
S. agalactiae (group B streptococcus)	Neonatal sepsis, neonatal pneumonia, neonatal meningitis, cellulitis, pneumonia, meningitis, endocarditis
Groups C and G Streptococcus (large colony)	Rare cause of human disease: pharyngitis, pneumonia, meningitis, bacteremia, cellulitis, acute glomerulonephritis
***Enterococcus* species**	Urinary tract infections, endocarditis, neonatal meningitis, hospital associated infections
Nonenterococcal Group D Streptococcus	*S. bovis*—bacteremia

AEROBIC AND FACULTATIVE ANAEROBIC GRAM POSITIVE COCCI

Continued ▶

► Continued **DISEASE SPECTRA OF SELECTED MEMBERS OF THE MICROCOCCACEAE AND STREPTOCOCCACEAE**

ORGANISM	DISEASE(S)
Micrococcaceae	
Viridans Streptococci	Opportunistic pathogens: subacute bacterial endocarditis, dental caries
Nutritionally Variant Streptococci	Endocarditis in association with prosthetic valves
Streptococcus pneumoniae	Pneumonia, otitis media, and bacteremia in infants and children, meningitis in adults and children

GRAM POSITIVE BACILLI

Introduction and Distribution

Aerobic and facultatively anaerobic gram positive bacilli represent a diverse group of common laboratory isolates that are ubiquitous in both aquatic and terrestrial environments. The majority of these laboratory isolates represent contaminants. The most common genera included in this category are *Bacillus, Listeria, Corynebacterium,* and *Lactobacillus.*

Morphology and Biochemical Characteristics of Endospore Forming Bacilli

The endospore forming gram positive bacilli belong to the genus *Bacillus.* These organisms exhibit notably large, dull, spreading colonies that are beta hemolytic (except *B. anthracis*). They are Gram stain variable with subterminal, unstained endospores. Significant *Bacillus* species can be differentiated on the basis of several biochemical properties as well as other characteristics (see figure on facing page).

BIOCHEMICAL DIFFERENTIATION OF SEVERAL CLINICALLY SIGNIFICANT SPECIES OF BACILLUS

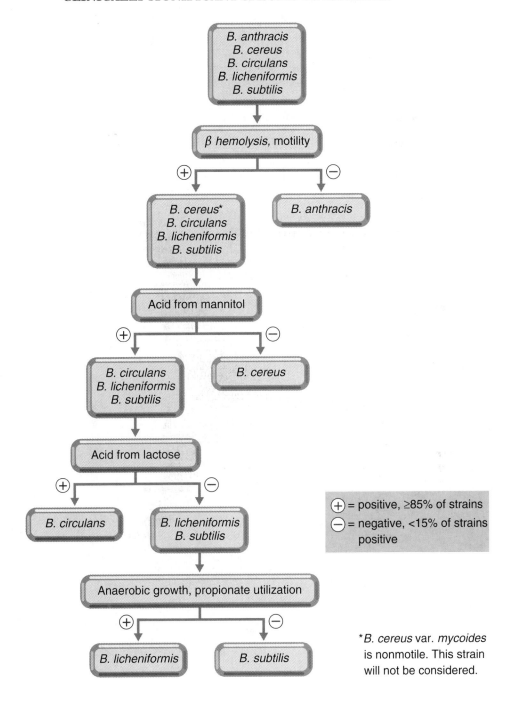

B. anthracis
B. cereus
B. circulans
B. licheniformis
B. subtilis

β *hemolysis*, motility

(+) *B. cereus**
B. circulans
B. licheniformis
B. subtilis

(−) *B. anthracis*

Acid from mannitol

(+) *B. circulans*
B. licheniformis
B. subtilis

(−) *B. cereus*

Acid from lactose

(+) *B. circulans*

(−) *B. licheniformis*
B. subtilis

Anaerobic growth, propionate utilization

(+) *B. licheniformis*

(−) *B. subtilis*

(+) = positive, ≥85% of strains
(−) = negative, <15% of strains positive

**B. cereus* var. *mycoides* is nonmotile. This strain will not be considered.

GRAM POSITIVE BACILLI

Morphology and Differentiation of Non–Spore Forming Bacilli

The more clinically common, non–spore forming, morphologically regular gram positive bacilli belong to the genera *Listeria, Lactobacillus, Erysipelothrix,* and *Kurthia.* On Gram stain, these organisms appear as straight or slightly curved rods, with uniform, parallel sides. Variability in morphology does occur, and coccobacillary forms may be evident. Generally, these organisms are shorter and thinner than *Bacillus* species. Various biochemical characteristics can be used for the differentiation of these genera (see p 603).

PRESUMPTIVE DIFFERENTIATION OF SELECTED AEROBIC AND FACULTATIVE ANAEROBIC GRAM POSITIVE BACILLI

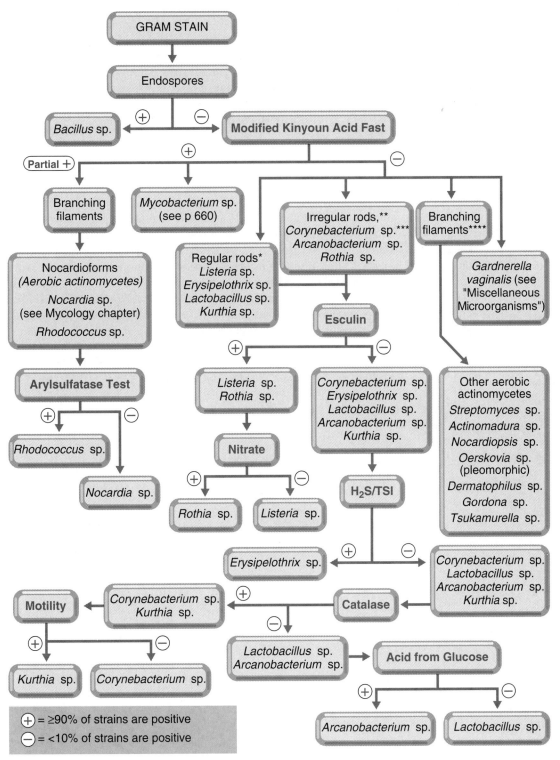

*Regular rods: usually straight or slightly curved rods with somewhat uniform, parallel sides.

**Irregular rods: morphology more variable; usually club-shaped rods with rounded ends and uneven sides.

***Also referred to as coryneform or diphtheroid bacilli.

****Morphologic and biochemical overlap and variability between regular rods and branching filaments known to occur.

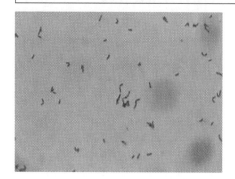

Irregular Bacilli or "Coryneforms"

The irregular, non–endospore forming gram positive bacilli are referred to as *diphtheroids* of *"coryneforms."* These organisms are pleomorphic, ranging from coccal to bacillary forms of various sizes. They exhibit variability and "Chinese letter" morphology on Gram stain. A beaded appearance due to dark staining metachromatic granules is characteristic of diphtheria bacilli (see left).

Pathogenicity

The clinical manifestations of the aerobic and facultative anaerobic gram positive bacilli are diverse (see chart below). Pathogenicity can range from normal commensals of the skin and mucous membranes to significant agents of disease, especially in the immunocompromised host. The clinical setting, as well as recovery from normally sterile body sites (blood, cerebrospinal fluid, and so forth), determines the clinical significance of these organisms. The most notable presentation within the *Bacillus* genus is anthrax, whereas other more common syndromes include food poisoning, bacteremia, and wound infections. Meningitis and abortion due to *Listeria monocytogenes*, and diphtheria caused by *Corynebacterium diphtheriae* are also notable.

KEY CHARACTERISTICS AND CLINICAL SIGNIFICANCE OF SELECTED AEROBIC AND FACULTATIVE ANAEROBIC GRAM POSITIVE BACILLI

GENUS	MORE COMMON SPECIES	NOTABLE CHARACTERISTICS	RAPID IDENTIFICATION SYSTEMS	CLINICAL SIGNIFICANCE
Bacillus	*anthracis*			Inhalation anthrax, or woolsorters' disease: hemorrhaging and edema of respiratory tract. Complications include septicemia and meningitis. Cutaneous anthrax: necrotic skin lesions with consequent bacteremia. Gastrointestinal anthrax: necrotic lesions in intestinal tract.
	cereus	Ubiquitous in nature; common laboratory contaminant. Rare cause of human disease; opportunistic pathogen associated with gastrointestinal food poisoning. Invasive disease in immunocompromised host.		TOXIN MEDIATED FOOD POISONING: Vomiting syndrome—associated with ingestion of contaminated fried rice Diarrheal syndrome—associated with ingestion of cooked meats, soups, mashed potatoes OTHER: Wound infections, bacteremia, septicemia, respiratory infection, osteomyelitis, myonecrosis
	circulans			Wound infections, bacteremia, septicemia
	licheniformis			Bacteremia, septicemia
	subtilis	*B. thuringenensis* used as environmental pesticide		Bacteremia, septicemia, endocarditis
Arcanobacterium	*haemolyticum*			Found in oral cavity; causative agent of pharyngitis
Corynebacterium	*diphtheriae*	Highly pleomorphic; "Chinese letter" morphology on Gram stain. Selective media include Loeffler's serum medium, potassium tellurite medium; gray-black colonies evident.	Rapid CORYNE (bioMérieux, Hazelwood, MO) not recommended	May be carried on skin, mucous membranes, and gastrointestinal tract of humans. Toxin producing strains are causative agents of diphtheria, communicable airway obstruction, and congestive heart failure.

Continued ▶

GRAM POSITIVE BACILLI

▶ Continued **KEY CHARACTERISTICS AND CLINICAL SIGNIFICANCE OF SELECTED AEROBIC AND FACULTATIVE ANAEROBIC GRAM POSITIVE BACILLI**

GENUS	MORE COMMON SPECIES	NOTABLE CHARACTERISTICS	RAPID IDENTIFICATION SYSTEMS	CLINICAL SIGNIFICANCE
Erysipelothrix	*group JK*	Resistant to many antibiotics		Causative agent of bacterial endocarditis
	rhusiopathiae (uncommon)			Causative agent of erysipeloid, a cutaneous inflammatory disease of hands and fingers associated with animal and fish contact
Kurthia	*bessonii*			Rare pathogen; prosthetic heart valve infection
Lactobacillus	*casei*	*Lactobacillus* selective medium (BBL Microbiology Systems, Cockeysville, MD)		Indigenous flora of oral cavity, mucosal membranes, gastrointestinal tract, and vagina. Rare pathogen; endocarditis, meningitis
Listeria	*monocytogenes*	Tumbling motility in wet preparations Growth at 4°C	api-Listeria (bio-Mérieux Vitek, Hazelwood, MO) Listeria-Tek (Organon Technika Corp,, Durham, NC) PCR Gene-Trak *Listeria* assay (Gene-Trak Systems, Framingham, MA)	Food borne gastroenteritis; placental infections resulting in abortion, bacterial meningitis, listeriosis; complications include lymphadenitis, conjunctivitis, endocarditis, cutaneous infections, encephalitis, septicemia
Rhodococcus	*equi*	Orange, pinkish, reddish colonies Related genera include *Gordona* and *Tsukamurella*		Opportunistic pathogen in immunocompromised population, especially AIDS patients. Causative agent of pulmonary disease, especially pneumonia, and bacteremia
Rothia	*dentocariosa*			Present in oral cavity May cause prosthetic valve endocarditis

NEISSERIA, MORAXELLA (BRANHAMELLA)

Introduction

Neisseria and the genus *Branhamella*, which contains the single species *catarrhalis*, are aerobic, oxidase positive, gram negative cocci or diplococci (*N. elongata* is a coccobacillus). Both genera belong to the family Neisseriaceae, and there are several key characteristics that can be used for their differentiation (see figure and charts on following pages). Other genera that belong to the Neisseriaceae family include *Moraxella*, *Kingella*, and *Acinetobacter.*

DIFFERENTIAL CHARACTERISTICS OF NEISSERIA SPECIES AND *MORAXELLA (BRANHAMELLA) CATARRHALIS* INVOLVED IN HUMAN INFECTION

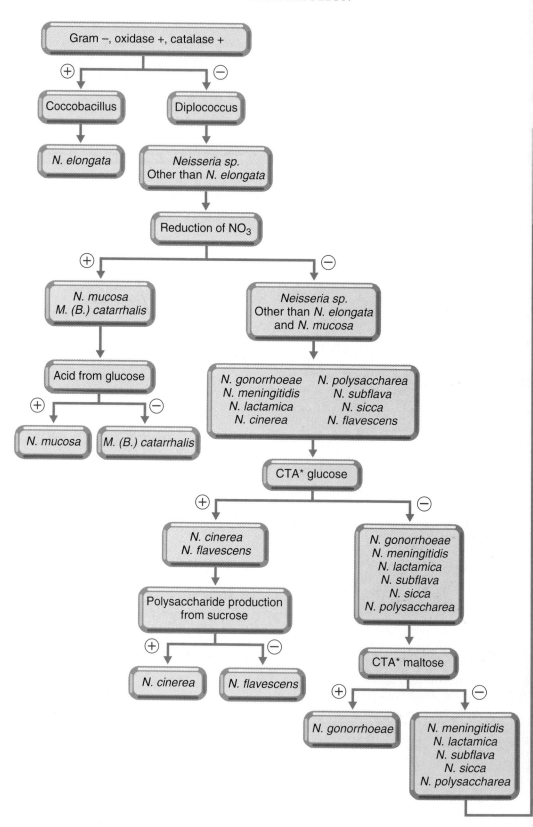

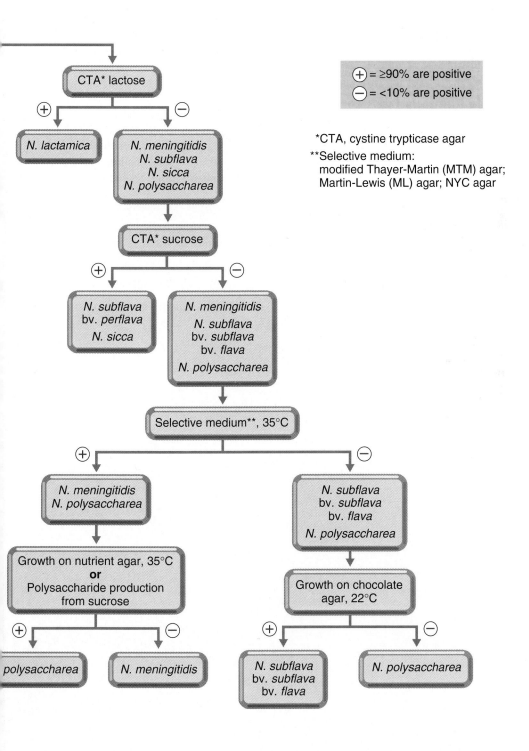

+ = ≥90% are positive
− = <10% are positive

*CTA, cystine trypticase agar

**Selective medium:
  modified Thayer-Martin (MTM) agar;
  Martin-Lewis (ML) agar; NYC agar

CTA* lactose

+ → N. lactamica

− → N. meningitidis
N. subflava
N. sicca
N. polysaccharea

CTA* sucrose

+ → N. subflava
bv. perflava
N. sicca

− → N. meningitidis
N. subflava
bv. subflava
bv. flava
N. polysaccharea

Selective medium**, 35°C

+ → N. meningitidis
N. polysaccharea

− → N. subflava
bv. subflava
bv. flava
N. polysaccharea

Growth on nutrient agar, 35°C
or
Polysaccharide production
from sucrose

+ → polysaccharea

− → N. meningitidis

Growth on chocolate
agar, 22°C

+ → N. subflava
bv. subflava
bv. flava

− → N. polysaccharea

NEISSERIA, MORAXELLA (BRANHAMELLA)

Taxonomy

Recent molecular studies have resulted in extensive reclassification of the microorganisms belonging to this family. Based on genetic relatedness, the families Moraxellaceae and Branhamellaceae have been proposed, and *B. catarrhalis* has been reclassified in the *Moraxella* genus. The nomenclature employed in this text is based on common usage in the clinical laboratory as well as common biochemical characteristics. Therefore, *B. catarrhalis* is used because it is more universally accepted in the clinical laboratory setting. In addition, the genera *Moraxella* and *Acinetobacter* are considered under the discussion of nonfermentative gram negative bacteria and the genus *Kingella* is included with miscellaneous bacteria.

Rapid Methods for Identification

There are several rapid methods that are used for the presumptive identification of *Neisseria* species and *M.(B.) catarrhalis* (see chart on facing page). These methods include enzyme and serologic tests, carbohydrate utilization tests, and molecular and fluorescent assays. The accurate interpretation of these assays requires routine testing of *Neisseria* reference strains and experienced laboratory personnel.

RAPID TEST METHODS FOR THE IDENTIFICATION OF *NEISSERIA MENINGITIDIS, NEISSERIA GONORRHOEAE,* AND *BRANHAMELLA CATARRHALIS*

TEST	COMMENTS
Carbohydrate Utilization Tests Minitek System (Becton Dickinson, Sparks, MD) RIM-N (Rapid Identification Method–*Neisseria*) (Austin Biologicals, Austin TX) QuadFERM+ system (bioMérieux Vitek, Hazelwood, MO)	Determine carbohydrate utilization patterns for *N. meningitidis, N. gonorrhoeae,* and *M.(B.) catarrhalis,* within approximately 4 hr
Latex Agglutination Tests Wellcome Diagnostics (Research Triangle Park, NC) Becton Dickinson, Sparks, MD	Detect *N. meningitidis* in body fluids; permits rapid *presumptive* diagnosis
Coagglutination Tests Phadebact GC test (Pharmacia, Piscataway, NJ) GonoGen test (New Horizons Diagnostics, Columbia, MD)	Presumptive identification of *N. meningitidis* and *N. gonorrhoeae*
Fluorescent Antibody Test Behring Diagnostics, San Jose, CA	Utilizes a fluorescein isothiocyanate conjugated monoclonal antibody reagent for culture confirmation of *N. gonorrhoeae*
Enzyme Immunoassay Gonozyme test (Abbott Labs, Abbott Park, IL)	Detects *N. gonorrhoeae* antigens in swab specimens from endocervical and urethral sites. For presumptive identification only.
Chromogenic Enzyme Substrate Tests Gonochek II (du Pont de Nemours, Wilmington, DE)	Identification of *N. meningitidis* and *N. gonorrhoeae.* Only presumptive diagnosis of *M.(B.) catarrhalis.*
Other Tests NHI card (bioMérieux Vitek, Hazelwood, MO) HNID panel (Dade International, Chicago, IL) RapID NH panel (Innovative Diagnostic Systems, Atlanta, GA)	Reliable identification of *Neisseria* species, *Haemophilus* species, and some fastidious gram negative bacteria in approximately 4 hr
Nucleic Acid Probe Test (PACE, Gen-Probe, San Diego, CA): Probe assay chemiluminescence	*N. gonorrhoeae* screening; presumptive identification only
DNA Probe test (AccuProbe, Gen-Probe, San Diego, CA)	Culture confirmation test for *N. gonorrhoeae*
PCR: polymerase chain reaction	Detection of *N. meningitidis;* not commercially available

NEISSERIA, MORAXELLA (BRANHAMELLA)

Pathogenicity

The genus *Neisseria* contains two species pathogenic to humans, namely, *N. meningitidis* and *N. gonorrhoeae.* In addition to being the causative agents of meningitis and gonorrhea, respectively, these species are responsible for a wide range of diseases (see chart on p 612). Both species are highly fastidious with special growth requirements. Knowledge of these requirements is critical for the recovery and subsequent identification of these organisms from clinical specimens (see "Important Considerations for the Recovery of *N. gonorrhoeae, N. meningitidis,* and *M.(B.) catarrhalis* from Clinical Specimens" on p 613). The remaining *Neisseria* species are normal inhabitants of mucosal surfaces of the respiratory tract. These commensals occasionally cause disease. *M.(B.) catarrhalis,* which is part of the normal flora of the nasopharynx and the upper respiratory tract, has also been associated with a wide range of diseases including otitis media and sinusitis.

HUMAN DISEASE SYNDROMES ASSOCIATED WITH SELECTED *NEISSERIA* SPECIES AND *MORAXELLA (BRANHAMELLA) CATARRHALIS*

SPECIES	DISEASE SYNDROME(S)
N. gonorrhoeae	Gonorrhea—infectious, sexually transmitted disease usually involving mucosal surface of genitourinary tract. May result in urethritis, pharyngitis, and proctitis in males; complications include epididymitis and periurethral abscess. May result in cervicitis, proctitis, and pharyngitis in females; complications include peritonitis and bartholinitis. Pelvic inflammatory disease (PID)—fallopian tube infection (salpingitis), endometritis. Disseminated gonococcal infection (DGI)—arthritis, dermatitis, endocarditis, tenosynovitis. Ophthalmia—conjunctivitis, "conjunctivitis neonatorum," conjunctivitis in newborns.
N. meningitidis	Meningitis—symptoms include headache, stiff neck, sometimes petechial rash. Shock, DIC (disseminated intravascular coagulation) possible. Meningococcemia—usually in individuals with underlying health problems. Disseminated disease—arthritis, osteomyelitis, pericarditis, pneumonia, cervicitis.
N. cinerea *N. elongota* *N. flavescens* *N. lactamica* *N. mucosa* *N. polysaccharea* *N. sicca* *N. subflava*	Nonpathogenic species. Normal inhabitants of upper respiratory tract. *Rare* disease syndromes including meningitis, proctitis, bacteremia, pericarditis, pneumonia, and endocarditis. Differentiation of pathogenic species from nonpathogenic species is critical.
M.(B.) catarrhalis	Otitis media and sinusitis in children. *M.(B.) catarrhalis* is resistant to amoxicillin and ampicillin, which are usually used in treatment of otitis media and sinusitis. Opportunistic pathogen in individuals with underlying disease or advanced age. In this clinical setting, disease syndromes may include meningitis, endocarditis, and chronic bronchitis.

IMPORTANT CONSIDERATIONS FOR THE RECOVERY OF *NEISSERIA GONORRHOEAE, NEISSERIA MENINGITIDIS,* AND *MORAXELLA (BRANHAMELLA) CATARRHALIS* FROM CLINICAL SPECIMENS

ORGANISM	TRANSPORT	MICROSCOPIC MORPHOLOGY	SPECIMEN TYPES	MEDIA	INOCULATION INCUBATION
*N. gonorrhoeae**	1. Use nontoxic swabs, i.e., Dacron, rayon, or calcium alginate. 2. Immediate inoculation of specimen onto prewarmed media plate optimal. For blood, use sterile syringe. 3. If transport necessary, recommended transport systems: JEMBEC (Ames Co., Elkhart, IN) and Gono-Pak (Becton Dickinson, Sparks, MD) 4. Avoid extremes of temperature and drying of specimen (do not refrigerate).	Kidney or bean shaped diplococcus. Organisms may appear within polymorphonuclear neutrophils (PMNs) in smears prepared from clinical specimens.	Endocervix Anterior urethra, 1 hr after urination Oropharynx Rectum Blood for disseminated gonococcal infection (DGI) Conjunctiva Joint fluid Skin lesion	Selective† Selective Selective Selective Aerobic blood culture bottle; use without SPS (sodium polyanetholsulfonate) or with 1% gelatin (Carr Scarborough, Microbiologic, GA) Nonselective‡ Nonselective Selective	Make Z pattern with swabs onto media, cross-streak with inoculating loop, place in high humidity, 3%–5% CO_2, 35°C–37°C.
N. meningitidis		See *N. gonorrhoeae*	CSF Skin lesion Blood Nasopharynx	Nonselective Nonselective Aerobic blood culture (see *N. gonorrhoeae*) Selective, nonselective	
M.(B.) catarrhalis		See *N. gonorrhoeae*	Sputum, transtracheal aspirates	Nonselective	

N. gonorrhoeae auxotypes are strains that have specific nutritional growth requirements. One example is the AHU (arginine, hypoxanthine, and uracil) requiring strains. These strains cause DGI and are penicillin susceptible. PPNG (penicillinase producing *N. gonorrhoeae*) strains are detected using Cefinase disks (Becton Dickinson, Sparks, MD).

†Selective media (usually used for contaminated specimens): modified Thayer-Martin agar, Martin-Lewis agar, NYC agar.

‡Nonselective media: chocolate agar, blood agar.

NEISSERIA, MORAXELLA (BRANHAMELLA)

ENTEROBACTERIACEAE

Introduction

The Enterobacteriaceae family includes a diverse membership of organisms that range from enteric pathogens to extraintestinal opportunistic pathogens. In addition to the human intestinal tract, these organisms are ubiquitous in nature and can be found in soil, water, plants, and animals. Members of this family are also the most frequently recovered organisms from clinical specimens. They account for nearly half of all clinically significant laboratory isolates.

Taxonomy

Classification of the members of this family is a continually evolving process due to expansive technologic progress, especially in the area of deoxyribonucleic acid (DNA) hybridization techniques. This has resulted in some confusion as new genera and species of bacteria belonging to the Enterobacteriaceae are increased and existing members are renamed and sometimes reclassified.

Principal Characteristics

The Enterobacteriaceae represent a heterogeneous group that have the following properties in common. They

1. Are gram negative rods
2. Ferment glucose, usually with gas production
3. Grow well on MacConkey agar
4. Are catalase positive
5. Are oxidase negative
6. Reduce nitrate to nitrite

Identification and Biochemical Differentiation of Common Laboratory Isolates

Identification and differentiation of the Enterobacteriaceae can be tedious and labor intensive. In order to simplify this task several flow charts for the differentiation of major laboratory isolates are presented on the following pages. However, owing to strain variability, interpretation of many of the biochemical reactions is not straightforward; that is, there is no clear-cut positive or negative reaction. Commercial identification systems, such as the api 20E (bioMérieux Vitek, Hazelwood, MO) and automated instrumentation, such as the AutoMicrobic System (AMS) (bioMérieux Vitek, Hazelwood, MO), provide computer assisted interpretation of the biochemical reactions and, in most cases, accurate identification of the Enterobacteriaceae.

ENTEROBACTERIACEAE

IDENTIFICATION AND BIOCHEMICAL DIFFERENTIATION OF COMMON LABORATORY ISOLATES

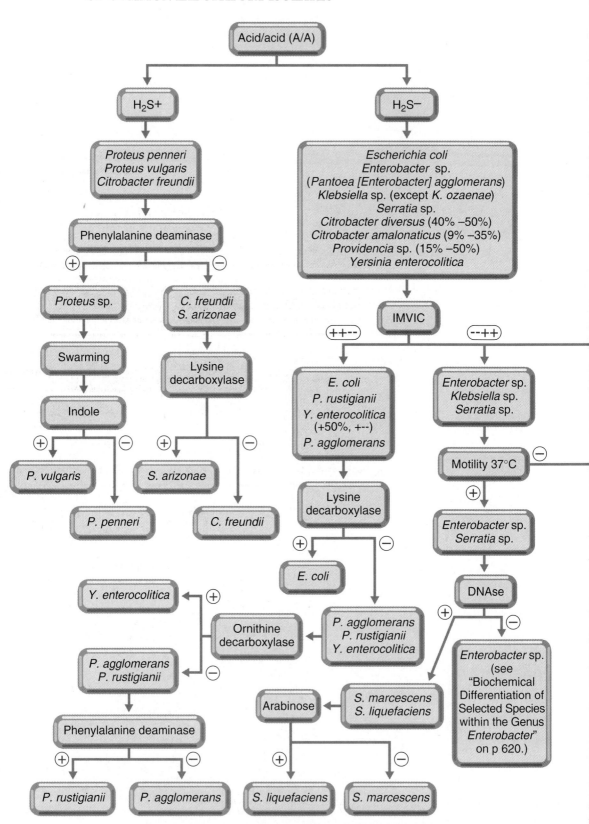

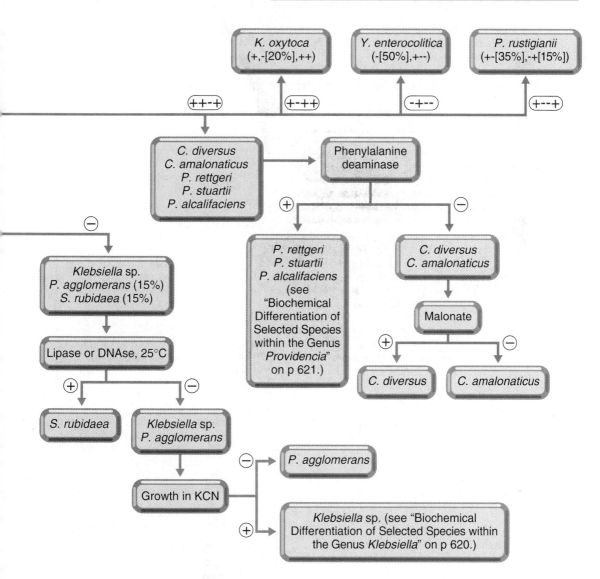

+ = ≥90% of strains are positive

− = <10% of strains are positive

IMVIC = Indole, Methyl Red, Voges Proskauer, Citrate

K. oxytoca
(+,-[20%],++)

Y. enterocolitica
(-[50%],+--)

P. rustigianii
(+-[35%],-+[15%])

++-+

+-++

-+--

+--+

C. diversus
C. amalonaticus
P. rettgeri
P. stuartii
P. alcalifaciens

Phenylalanine
deaminase

+

−

P. rettgeri
P. stuartii
P. alcalifaciens
(see
"Biochemical
Differentiation of
Selected Species
within the Genus
Providencia"
on p 621.)

C. diversus
C. amalonaticus

Malonate

+

−

C. diversus

C. amalonaticus

−

Klebsiella sp.
P. agglomerans (15%)
S. rubidaea (15%)

Lipase or DNAse, 25°C

+

−

S. rubidaea

Klebsiella sp.
P. agglomerans

−

P. agglomerans

Growth in KCN

+

Klebsiella sp. (see "Biochemical
Differentiation of Selected Species within
the Genus *Klebsiella*" on p 620.)

ENTEROBACTERIACEAE

IDENTIFICATION AND BIOCHEMICAL DIFFERENTIATION OF COMMON LABORATORY ISOLATES

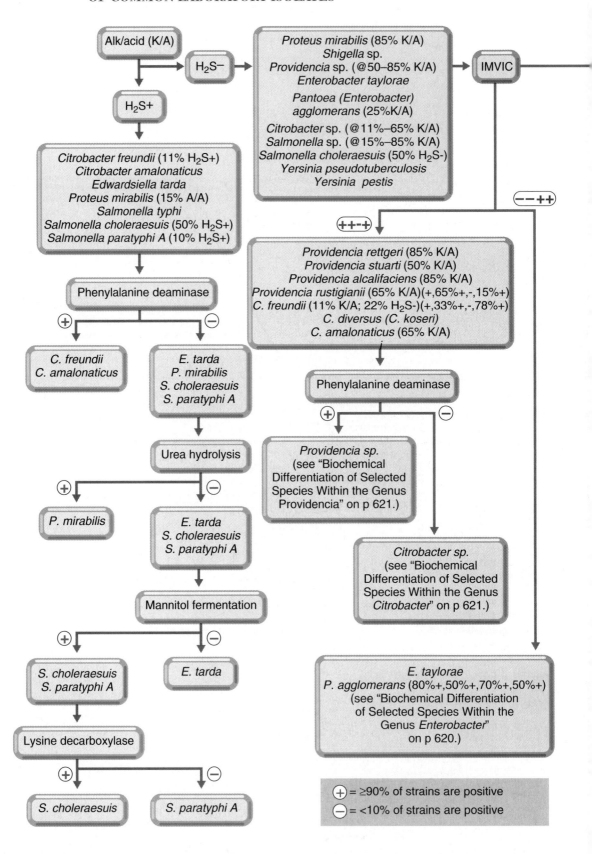

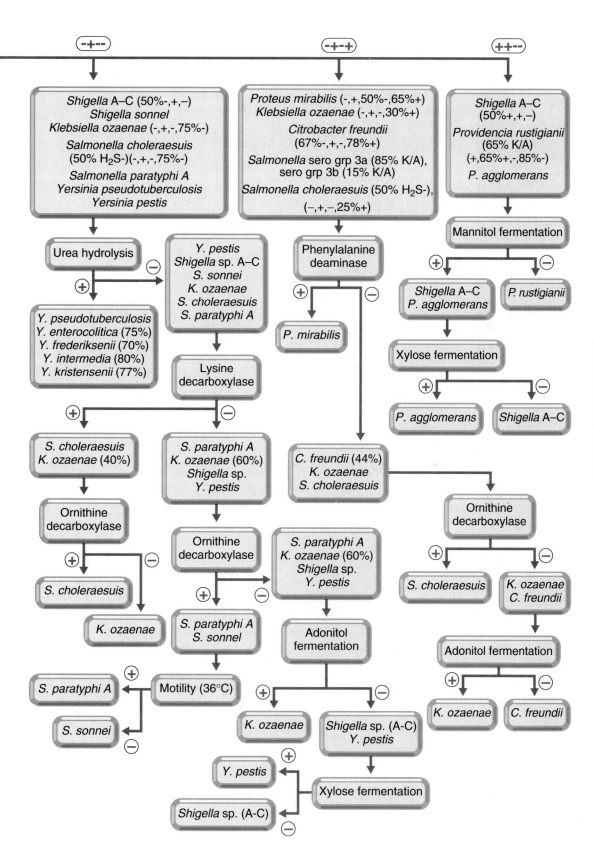

BIOCHEMICAL DIFFERENTIATION OF SELECTED SPECIES WITHIN THE GENUS *ENTEROBACTER*

BIOCHEMICAL ASSAY	SPECIES						
	aerogenes	*cloacae*	*Pantoea (E.) agglomerans*	*amnigenus*	*gergoviae*	*sakazakii*	*taylorae*
Lysine Decarboxylase	+	−	−	−	+	−	−
Arginine Dihydrolase	−	+	−	−	−	+	+
Ornithine Decarboxylase	+	+	−	55%	+	+	+
Urea Hydrolysis	−	65%	20%	−	+	+	
Growth in KCN	+	+	35%	+	−	+	+
Fermentation of:							
Adonitol	+	25%	−	−	−	−	−
Inositol	+	15%	15	−	−	75	−
Sorbitol	+	+	30	−	−	−	−
Raffinose	+	+	30	+	+	+	−
Arabitol	+	15	50	−	+	−	−

+, 90% or more strains are positive; −, 90% or more strains are negative.

BIOCHEMICAL DIFFERENTIATION OF SELECTED SPECIES WITHIN THE GENUS *KLEBSIELLA*

BIOCHEMICAL ASSAY	SPECIES			
	pneumoniae	*oxytoca*	*ozaenae*	*rhinoscleromatis*
Indole	−	+	−	−
Voges-Proskauer	+	−	−	−
Malonate	+	+	−	+
Glucose fermentation at 10°C	−	+	−	−

+, 90% or more strains positive; −, 90% or more strains negative.

BIOCHEMICAL DIFFERENTIATION OF SELECTED SPECIES WITHIN THE GENUS *PROVIDENCIA*

BIOCHEMICAL ASSAY	SPECIES			
	retteri	*stuartii*	*alcalifaciens*	*rustiganii*
Citrate	+	+	+	− (85%)
Urea Hydrolysis	+	− (70%)	−	−
Fermentation of:				
Mannitol	+	−	−	−
Adonitol	+	−	+	−
Inositol	+	+	−	−
Trehalose	−	+	−	−
Arabitol	+	−	−	−
+, 90% or more strains positive; −, 90% or more strains negative.				

BIOCHEMICAL DIFFERENTIATION OF SELECTED SPECIES WITHIN THE GENUS *CITROBACTER*

BIOCHEMICAL ASSAY	SPECIES		
	freundii	*diversus*	*amalonaticus*
Ornithine Decarboxylase	−	+	+
Growth in KCN	+	−	+
Malonate Utilization	11%	+	−
Adonitol Fermentation	−	+	−
Melibiose Fermentation	+	−	−
+, 90% or more strains positive; −, 90% or more strains negative.			

ENTEROBACTERIACEAE

Pathogenicity

Clinically relevant members of the Enterobacteriaceae are listed in the chart below. They are responsible for a wide range of human infections, especially intestinal and extraintestinal disease. The most clinically significant genera are *Escherichia, Salmonella, Shigella,* and *Yersinia.* These organisms are notorious pathogens responsible for serious and life threatening gastrointestinal and systemic disease. Of most recent notoriety, in association with the ingestion of undercooked ground beef, is enterohemorrhagic *E. coli,* serotype 0157:H7. This pathogen can cause hemolytic uremic syndrome and hemorrhagic colitis.

SELECTED GENERA OF ENTEROBACTERIACEAE AND CLINICALLY SIGNIFICANT LABORATORY ISOLATES°

GENUS	SPECIES	COMMENTS
Citrobacter	*freundii* * *diversus* *amalonaticus*	Clinical manifestations include sepsis, meningitis, and gastrointestinal disease.
Edwardsiella	*tarda* * *ictaluri* *hoshinae*	*E. tarda* most common species associated with human infection. Other species are pathogenic in aquatic setting.
Enterobacter	*aerogenes* * *agglomerans* *† *cloacae* * *gergoviae* * *sakazakii* *asburiae*	Broad range of infections, especially nosocomial.
Escherichia	*coli* * *fergusonii* *hermannii* *vulneris*	Most commonly recovered genus in clinical laboratory. *E. coli* is significant pathogen responsible for broad range of clinical manifestations, especially urinary tract infection and gastrointestinal illness.
Hafnia	*alvei*	Opportunistic pathogen.
Klebsiella	*oxytoca* * *pneumoniae* * *ozaenae* * *rhinoscleromatis* * *planticola* *terrigena* *group 47*	Important cause of pulmonary and extrapulmonary infections.
Morganella	*morganii*	Associated with urinary tract and wound infections as well as diarrheal disease.
Proteus	*vulgaris* * *mirabilis* * *penneri*	Clinically relevant as cause of urinary tract and wound infections.
Providencia	*alcalifaciens* * *stuartii* * *rustigianii* *rettgeri*	Not frequently isolated. Associated with urinary tract and, less often, diarrheal disease.
Salmonella	*enteritidis* * *cholerasuis* * *typhi* * *paratyphi* *	Clinically relevant as causative agent of gastroenteritis, enteric fever, and bacteremia.
Serratia	*marcescens* *liquifaciens* *rubidaea*	Nosocomial, opportunistic pathogen.
Shigella	*dysenteriae* *flexneri* *boydii* *sonnei*	Most commonly associated with dysentery. Extraintestinal disease rare.

Continued ►

▶ Continued **SELECTED GENERA OF ENTEROBACTERIACEAE AND CLINICALLY SIGNIFICANT LABORATORY ISOLATES°**

GENUS	SPECIES	COMMENTS
Yersinia	*enterocolitica* *pseudotuberculosis* *pestis*	Causative agent of enterocolitis, ileitis, and septicemia. Causative agent of mesenteric lymphadenitis usually in 5–15 yr olds. Causative agent of plague.

*More common isolates.
†Pantoea (E.) agglomerans.

NONFERMENTATIVE GRAM NEGATIVE BACILLI

Introduction

The gram negative bacilli that do not ferment glucose are referred to as *nonfermenters*. The nonfermenters degrade glucose oxidatively or not at all. They constitute a large and diverse group of organisms. These organisms are found widespread in nature including soil and aquatic environments. They also occur on the mucosal membranes of humans and animals.

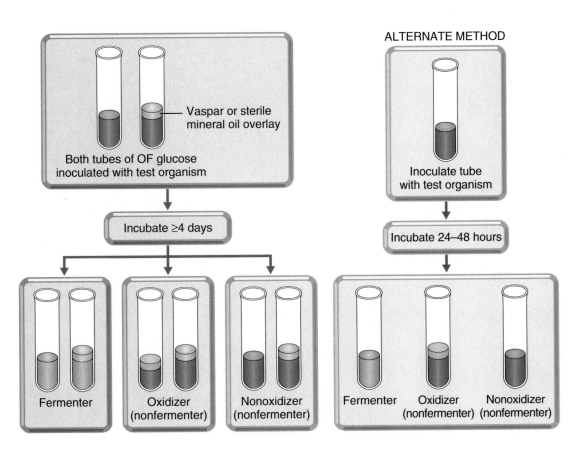

ALTERNATE METHOD

Vaspar or sterile mineral oil overlay

Both tubes of OF glucose inoculated with test organism

Incubate ≥4 days

Fermenter   Oxidizer (nonfermenter)   Nonoxidizer (nonfermenter)

Inoculate tube with test organism

Incubate 24–48 hours

Fermenter   Oxidizer (nonfermenter)   Nonoxidizer (nonfermenter)

NONFERMENTATIVE GRAM NEGATIVE BACILLI

Taxonomy

Advances in applied molecular biology have resulted in the extensive reclassification of many microorganisms, but most especially the nonfermenters. Nomenclature of this particular group of microorganisms is consistently changing, resulting in some confusion, and readers are referred to reference texts for definitive classification.

Identification and Biochemical Properties

In most clinical laboratories, microorganisms are categorized according to morphologic, microscopic, and traditional biochemical properties. The nonfermenters are aerobic, non–spore forming gram negative bacilli that do not utilize carbohydrates fermentatively. The classic characteristics used in the identification of these organism include the failure to acidify the butt of oxidative-fermentative media (OF media), Kligler iron (KIA), or triple sugar iron (TSI) agar. This characteristic is perhaps the most important criterion for classification. Another definitive characteristic is the positive oxidase test (except *Acinetobacter* species). These characteristics differentiate the nonfermenters from the Enterobacteriaceae (see p 614), which do ferment glucose and therefore acidify TSI, KIA, or OF medium and are oxidase negative. Additional biochemical characteristics and the differentiation of selected genera of nonfermenters are presented in the two charts on pp 626 and 627. *Neisseria, Vibrio,* and *Campylobacter* have the general characteristics of nonfermenters but have special growth requirements. They are discussed elsewhere in this text.

Rapid Test Methods for Identification

Several commercial test systems are available for the identification of gram negative, nonfermentative rods, namely:

1. The AutoMicrobic System Gram-Negative Identification card and Rapid NFT (bioMérieux Vitek, Hazelwood, MO).
2. The RapID NF Plus (Innovative Diagnostic Systems, Atlanta, GA).
3. The N/F System (Remel Labs, Lenexa, KA).
4. The autoSCAN W/A Rapid Neg Combo (RNC) (DADE International, Chicago, IL).

Of these, the Rapid NFT system is the only system capable of rapidly identifying *Pseudomonas aeruginosa, P. fluorescens, P. putida,* and *B. pseudomallei.* DNA probes and direct fluorescent antibody assays are not yet commercially available for *Pseudomonas* species and *Burkholderia* species.

Pathogenicity

Generally, the nonfermentative gram negative bacilli are causative agents of disease in a postsurgical setting, in the immunocompromised population, or after a traumatic event. The most clinically significant and the most frequently isolated nonfermenter is *Pseudomonas aeruginosa.* It is second only to *E. coli* as a common cause of nosocomial infection, and it is the leading cause of nosocomial disease of the respiratory tract. Other frequently isolated nonfermenters include *Acinetobacter calcoaceticus, Burkholderia (Pseudomonas) cepacia,* and *Stenotrophomonas (Xanthomonas) maltophilia.* The clinical manifestations of these and other clinically relevant nonfermentative gram negative bacilli are presented in the charts on pp 628 to 630.

NONFERMENTATIVE GRAM NEGATIVE BACILLI

DIFFERENTIATION OF SELECTED NONFERMENTATIVE GRAM NEGATIVE BACILLI

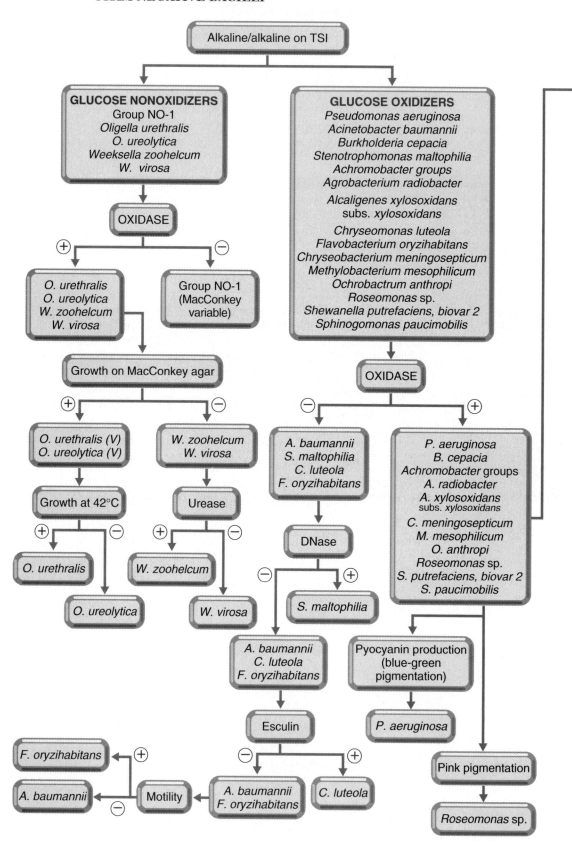

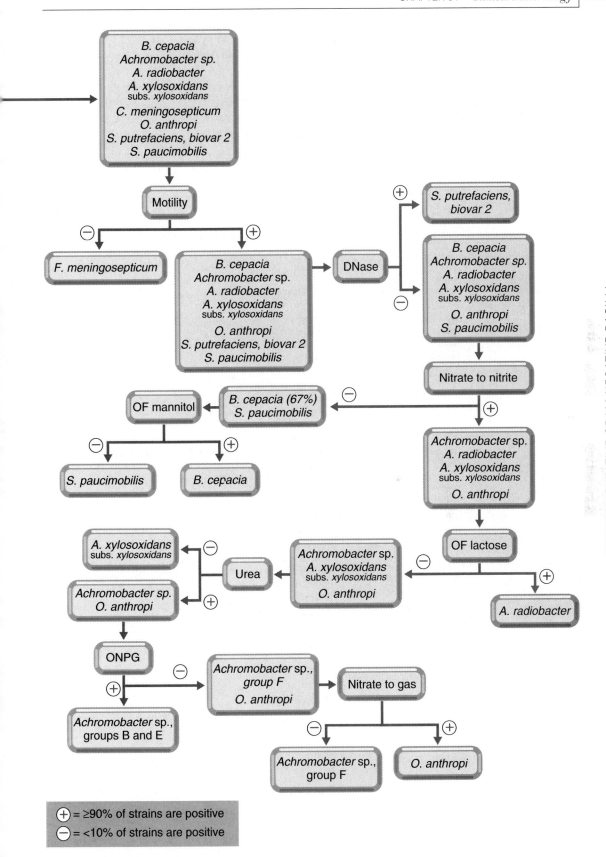

NONFERMENTATIVE GRAM NEGATIVE BACILLI

⊕ = ≥90% of strains are positive
⊖ = <10% of strains are positive

KEY CHARACTERISTICS AND CLINICAL MANIFESTATIONS OF THE NONFERMENTATIVE GRAM NEGATIVE BACILLI FREQUENTLY ISOLATED IN THE CLINICAL LABORATORY

ORGANISM	KEY CHARACTERISTICS	CLINICAL MANIFESTATIONS	COMMENTS
Pseudomonas aeruginosa	Oxidase positive Motile (polar flagella) Strict aerobe Blue-green pigmentation (most isolates) Grapelike odor	Nosocomial infections; indwelling catheters Burn wound infections Water borne infections, swimmer's ear, folliculitis (from hot tubs) Eye infections, often from contact lenses Urinary tract infections Lower respiratory infections, especially individuals with cystic fibrosis	INFREQUENTLY ISOLATED PATHOGENS: *P. fluorescens* *P. stutzeri* LESS FREQUENTLY ISOLATED PATHOGENS: *P. alcaligenes* *P. putida* RARELY ISOLATED PATHOGEN: *P. vesicularis*
Acinetobacter calcoaceticus	Coccobacillus, often diplococcus (similar to *Neisseria*) Oxidase negative Nonmotile Penicillin resistant	Widespread in nature Usually a hospital acquired infection in the setting of surgery and/or instrumentation Pneumonia, usually in association with tracheotomies Cellulitis Urinary tract infections Multiply resistant strains: *A. haemolyticus, A. calcoaceticus, A. baumannii*	LESS FREQUENTLY ISOLATED PATHOGENS: *A. baumannii* *A. iwoffi* *A. haemolyticus* *A. johnsonii* *A. genospecies* 3 & 6
Burkholderia (Pseudomonas) cepacia	Oxidase negative Motile	Pneumonia in patients with cystic fibrosis Wound infections associated with water, e.g., drug use, irrigation fluids, nebulizers	*B. pseudomallei,* cause of melioidosis
Stenotrophomonas (Xanthomonas) maltophilia	Oxidase negative Motile Ammonia-like smell	Widespread in nature Usually a hospital acquired infection in the setting of surgery and/or instrumentation Urinary tract infections Oral cavity colonizer when there is therapy with antimicrobial agents	

KEY CHARACTERISTICS AND CLINICAL MANIFESTATIONS OF THE NONFERMENTATIVE GRAM NEGATIVE BACILLI LESS FREQUENTLY ISOLATED IN THE CLINICAL LABORATORY

ORGANISM	KEY CHARACTERISTICS	CLINICAL MANIFESTATIONS	COMMENTS
***Achromobacter* species groups A through F**	Biochemically similar to *Ochrobactrum anthropi* Utilize glucose oxidatively Oxidase positive	Septicemia	Taxonomy uncertain with regard to *Alcaligenes* species
***Agrobacterium* (radiobacter) tumefaciens**	Utilize glucose oxidatively Oxidase positive Indole positive Motile	Infection usually associated with peritoneal and intravenous catheters Pathogenicity uncertain	
Alcaligenes xylosoxidans* subspecies *xylosoxidans	Nonoxidizer Oxidase positive Indole negative Motile	Not uncommon; opportunistic pathogen Associated with nosocomial infection, especially septicemia	RARE HUMAN PATHOGENS: *A. faecalis* *A. piechaudii* *A. xylosoxidans* subspecies *dentrificans*
Chryseobacterium meningosepticum	Indole positive Oxidase positive Oxidizer Nonmotile	Associated with neonatal meningitis and sepsis	
***Chryseomonas* (Pseudomonas) luteola**	Oxidase negative Oxidizer Motile	Found in both environment and hospital settings Associated with catheter infections, peritonitis, and septicemia	
***Comamonas* (Pseudomonas) species**	Oxidase positive Nonoxidizer Motile	Rare opportunistic pathogen	*C. acidovorans* *C. testosteroni* *C. terrigena*
***Flavimonas* (Pseudomonas) oryzihabitans**	See *Chryseomonas* species	Found in both environment and hospital settings Associated with catheter infections, peritonitis, and septicemia	RARE HUMAN PATHOGENS: *F. breve* *F. indologenes* *F. odoratum*
Group NO-1	Nonoxidizer Oxidase negative Nonmotile	Infection associated with dog and cat bites	
***Methylobacterium* (Pseudomonas) mesophilicum**	Weak oxidizer Oxidase positive Indole negative Motile	Opportunistic pathogen Peritonitis associated with continuous ambulatory peritoneal dialysis (CAPD)	
Ochrobactrum anthropi	Oxidizer Oxidase positive Indole negative Motile	Associated with bacteremia in catheterized patients	

NONFERMENTATIVE GRAM NEGATIVE BACILLI

Continued ▶

▶ Continued **KEY CHARACTERISTICS AND CLINICAL MANIFESTATIONS OF THE NONFERMENTATIVE GRAM NEGATIVE BACILLI LESS FREQUENTLY ISOLATED IN THE CLINICAL LABORATORY**

ORGANISM	KEY CHARACTERISTICS	CLINICAL MANIFESTATIONS	COMMENTS
Oligella urethralis	Nonoxidizer Oxidase positive Indole negative Nonmotile		
Oligella ureolytica	Nonoxidizer Oxidase positive Indole negative Motile Phenylalanine positive Urease positive	Genitourinary tract inhabitants Pathogenicity uncertain	
Roseomonas species	Oxidizer Oxidase positive Indole negative	Opportunistic pathogen Associated with bacteremia	
Shewanella (Pseudomonas) putrefaciens (Biovar 2)	Oxidizer Oxidase positive Indole negative Motile	Septicemia, cellulitis, otitis media	Rare in humans Biovar 1
Sphingomonas (Pseudomonas) paucimobilis	Oxidizer Oxidase positive Indole negative Motile	Wound infection, sepsis, pneumonia, endocarditis	LESS COMMON PATHOGENS: *S. multivorum* *S. spiritovorum*
Weeksella zoohelcum	Nonoxidizer Oxidase positive Indole negative Nonmotile Unable to grow on MacConkey agar	Wound infections as consequence of animal scratches and/or bites	
Weeksella virosa	Nonoxidizer Oxidase positive Indole negative Nonmotile Unable to grow on MacConkey agar	Vaginal and urine isolates	

VIBRIO, AEROMONAS, PLESIOMONAS

Taxonomy and General Characteristics

The family Vibrionaceae has included three clinically relevant genera in humans, namely, *Vibrio*, *Aeromonas*, and *Plesiomonas*. Members of these genera are distributed in both fresh and marine bodies of water. Based on molecular studies, a separate Aeromonadaceae family as well as possible reclassification of *Plesiomonas* as a member of the Enterobacteriaceae has been proposed. Historical classification of the three clinically relevant genera as one family has been based on the following common characteristics. They

Are gram negative rods
Are oxidase positive (except *V. metschnikovii*)
Are facultative anaerobes
Ferment glucose
Are motile by polar flagella

Biochemical Properties

Vibrio species, *Aeromonas* species, and *Plesiomonas* species can be differentiated from the Enterobacteriaceae, which are oxidase negative, and from *Pseudomonas* species, which do not ferment glucose. Differentiating characteristics are presented on the next page.

BIOCHEMICAL DIFFERENTIATION OF *VIBRIO* SPECIES, *AEROMONAS* SPECIES, AND *PLESIOMONAS* SPECIES

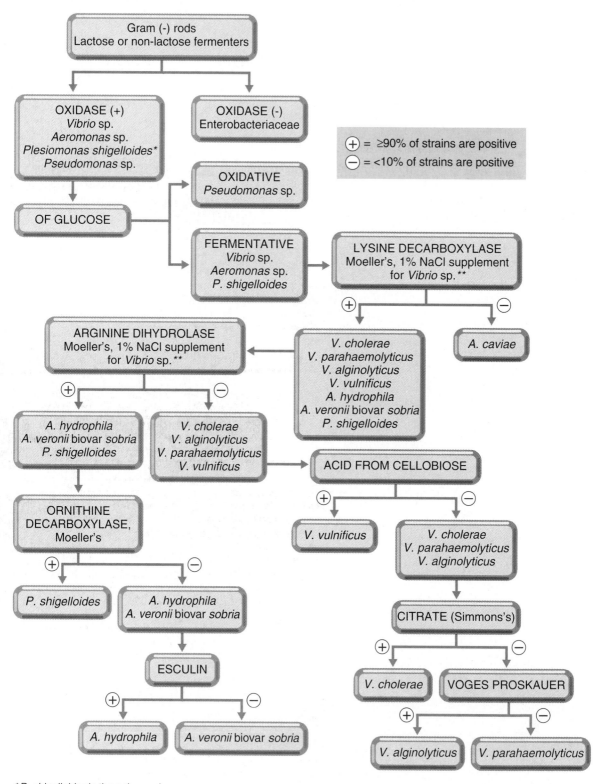

* *P. shigelloides* is the only species.

**Most *Vibrio* spp. are halophiles. NaCl supplement to basic media enhances their biochemical reactions.

Rapid Test Methods for Identification

Two methods are available for the direct detection of *V. cholerae* 01 in stool specimens, namely, the antigen capture test (New Horizons Diagnostics Corp., Columbia, MD), and a latex agglutination test (Denka Seiken Co., Tokyo, Japan). Neither assay is extensively used in the clinical laboratory. Polymerase chain reaction (PCR) for *V. cholerae* is not yet commercially available. Serologic and molecular assays for *Aeromonas* species and *Plesiomonas* species have not been standardized and are not routinely used.

Pathogenicity

Disease syndromes of the three genera include gastroenteritis, wound, and systematic infections (see chart below). These organisms are natural inhabitants of aquatic environments, and their disease syndromes are usually a result of contact or ingestion of contaminated water or seafood, including shellfish. Of notable significance is cholera, an acute, infectious diarrheal disease caused by *V. cholerae*. This disease is responsible for worldwide epidemics that have been documented since 1817 and still remain a major public health concern. *Aeromonas* infections in humans include bacteremia, gastroenteritis, and wound infections. *Plesiomonas* disease syndromes include diarrheal syndromes, septicemia, and meningitis.

HUMAN DISEASE SYNDROME(S) OF SELECTED *VIBRIO* SPECIES

DISEASE SYNDROME(S)			
Gastroenteritis and Related Symptoms	**Syndrome Other Than Gastroenteritis**	**Medical History**	**Likely Species**
Cholera: severe watery diarrhea, "rice water" stool—watery stool with mucus. Vomiting, dehydration		Travel to endemic areas: Bengal region of Bangladesh; India; Asia; Latin America; US Gulf Coast states. Ingestion of contaminated shellfish or seafood	*V. cholerae* 01
Diarrhea: not as severe as with 01 strain	Septicemia, wound infection, ear infection	Extraintestinal: infections usually occur in immunocompromised patients.	*V. cholerae* non01
Cholera: severe watery diarrhea, vomiting, dehydration		Travel to endemic areas: Bengal, Bangladesh; India. Occurs mostly in adults	*V. cholerae* 0139
	Septicemia, wound infections	Contact with contaminated water. Ingestion of contaminated, raw seafood and shellfish. Liver disease is risk factor.	*V. vulnificus*
Acute, sometimes bloody diarrhea; usually short lived	Septicemia (wound and ear infections less common)	Travel to endemic area: Japan. Sporadic cases in United States	*V. parahaemolyticus*
	Wound and ear infection, septicemia, conjunctivitis less common	Exposure to seawater	*V. alginolyticus*

VIBRIO, AEROMONAS, PLESIOMONAS

MISCELLANEOUS BACTERIAL SPECIES ASSOCIATED WITH HUMAN DISEASE

The organisms discussed in this section are taxonomically unrelated bacteria that are infrequent agents of human disease. This list of pathogens is not complete, nor is it exclusive, since the organisms discussed in other chapters may be comparable in their general characteristics. Basically, they represent random agents of disease that are not especially familiar or notorious but emerge periodically as a health care challenge. Often the most important factor in the identification of these organisms is clinical history and symptomatology effectively communicated by the physician to laboratory personnel.

ORGANISM	NOTABLE CHARACTERISTICS	CLINICAL MANIFESTATIONS
Gram Negative		
Agrobacterium species	Gram negative rod resistant to multiple antibiotics	Nosocomial infections, especially bacteremia in patients with indwelling plastic catheters
Bordetella pertussis	Gram negative, oxidase positive, urease negative, nonmotile, nonoxidizer Grows well on Bordet-Gengou agar	Whooping cough: highly contagious respiratory infection characterized by flu-like symptoms. Complications include severe coughing possibly leading to pneumonia and central nervous system involvement.
B. bronchiseptica	Gram negative, oxidase positive, urease positive, motile, nonoxidizer Grows well on MacConkey agar	Rare cause of respiratory infection, endocarditis, septicemia, and wound infection
Brucella species	Gram negative, oxidase positive, urease variable, nonmotile, oxidizer Grows well on selective buffered charcoal yeast extract (BCYE) and Thayer-Martin medium	Brucellosis: febrile illness associated with animal or animal product (milk) contact. Septicemia and wound infections. Complications include osteomyelitis.
Capnocytophaga ochracea	Gram negative, gliding motility; indigenous flora of human oral cavity	Bacteremia in immunocompromised patients. Juvenile periodontosis.
Cardiobacterium hominis	Gram negative, pleomorphic, nonmotile, indigenous flora of human respiratory and intestinal tracts	Endocarditis
Chromobacterium violaceum	Gram negative, slightly curved, motile rod, oxidase positive, catalase negative, found in environment (soil, water). Produces purple pigment in culture Optimal temperature for growth is 25°C.	Bacteremia, septicemia, abscess formation, especially in granulomatous disease. Infections are often fatal.
Eikenella corrodens	Oxidase positive, nonmotile, nonoxidizer	Normal flora of oral cavity and gastrointestinal tract. Associated with intra-abdominal abscesses, peritonitis, endocarditis, meningitis, and wound infections resulting from human bites.

Continued ▶

▶ Continued

ORGANISM	NOTABLE CHARACTERISTICS	CLINICAL MANIFESTATIONS
Gram Negative		
Francisella tularensis	Gram negative, small, nonmotile, pleomorphic or coccobacillary, oxidase negative Diagnosis through febrile agglutinins or ELISA	Tularemia: generally a flulike illness characterized by fever, headache, and lymphadenopathy. Ulcerative lesion at focal site of penetration (usually). There are many different kinds with various clinical presentations. Infection is through animal or animal product contact (especially rabbits), tick and deerfly bites, and aerosols. Known as *hunters' disease.*
Pasteurella multocida	Small, nonmotile, gram negative rod; oxidase, catalase, and indole positive, penicillin susceptible Normal respiratory and gastrointestinal flora of animals and birds	Majority of human infections is through animal bites.
Stomatococcus mucilaginosus	Gram positive coccus, catalase negative, esculin and PYR positive Doesn't grow in 5% NaCl Normal oral flora	Bacteremia, endocarditis in intravenous drug abusers, dialysis associated peritonitis
Gram Positive		
Dermatophilus congolensis	Gram positive, but optimal stain is Giemsa or methenamine silver. Hyphal-like, septate forms with coccoid spores.	Dermatophilosis: scabbing dermatitis
Kingella	Gram positive, nonmotile rods, oxidase positive, nitrate positive, catalase negative Grow on Thayer-Martin media	*K. indologenes:* associated with eye infections *K. kingae:* septic arthritis, skin lesions, bacteremia
Streptobacillus moniliformis	Pleomorphic rod; catalase, oxidase, indole, and nitrate negative. Normal flora of rat nasopharynx and throat Ascitic fluid supplementation facilitates growth.	Rat bite fever characterized by fever, headache, arthritis, and rash on extremities, palms, and soles
Gram Variable		
Gardnerella vaginalis	Gram variable, coccobacilli and short rods; oxidase and catalase negative	Bacterial vaginosis: sexually transmitted disease characterized by malodorous discharge. Postpartum sepsis. UTI in males.

BYCE, buffered charcoal yeast extract; VCNT, vancomycin, nystatin, colistin, trimethoprim; UTI, urinary tract infection; ELISA, enzyme linked immunosorbent assay; PYR, pyrrolidonyl arylamidase.

MISCELLANEOUS BACTERIAL SPECIES ASSOCIATED WITH HUMAN DISEASE

CAMPYLOBACTER, ARCOBACTER, HELICOBACTER, SPIRILLUM

Taxonomy

Curved rod and spiral shaped gram negative bacteria that are motile via polar flagella are included in the genera *Campylobacter, Arcobacter, Helicobacter,* and *Spirillum.* These organisms are morphologically similar to the spirochetes, namely, *Treponema* species, *Borrelia* species, and *Leptospira* species that are motile via axial filaments (see p 653). As with many other groups of bacteria, there has been extensive reclassification within the family Campylobacteraceae. Several species of *Campylobacter* have been reclassified to the genus *Arcobacter,* namely *A. butzleri, A. nitrotigilis,* and *A. cryaerophilus. Helicobacter* is a relatively new genus and species important in human disease including *H. pylori, H. fennelliae,* and *H. cinaedi* (formerly known as *C. pylori, C. fennelliae,* and *C. cinaedi,* respectively). Furthermore, two species of *Wolinella* have been reclassified as *Campylobacter,* namely *W. curva* and *W. recta.*

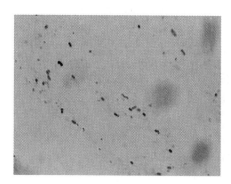

Morphology

The characteristic curved or spiral morphology of the *Campylobacter* species, *Arcobacter* species, *Helicobacter* species, and *Spirillum* species is best visualized using carbol fuchsin or basic fuchsin as the counterstain in the gram stain procedure rather than safranin (see left). It is important to note that *Campylobacter* species, *Arcobacter* species, and *Helicobacter* species deviate from the expected curved rod or spiral shaped morphology in older cultures and cultures exposed to air. Under these conditions they may appear as coccal forms. Furthermore, *Spirillum* species, which cannot be cultured in vitro are seen only in biopsy samples stained with Giemsa or Wright's stain. In unstained preparations, darting motility is characteristic of *Campylobacter* species.

Characteristics and Biochemical Properties

Campylobacter species, *Arcobacter* species, and *Helicobacter* species are non–spore forming, microaerophilic organisms that vary in their atmospheric requirements as well as their optimal temperatures for growth. Differential characteristics and biochemical properties of the three genera are presented in the figure on p 637. Generally, *Campylobacter* species and *Arcobacter* species may be recovered from stool specimens and blood cultures, whereas gastrointestinal biopsies are the specimen of choice for *Helicobacter* species recovery. Selective agar used for recovery include Campy-BAP, Skirrow agar, and Butzler medium.

DIFFERENTIAL CHARACTERISTICS AND BIOCHEMICAL PROPERTIES OF SELECTED *CAMPYLOBACTER* SPECIES, *ARCOBACTER* SPECIES, AND *HELICOBACTER* SPECIES

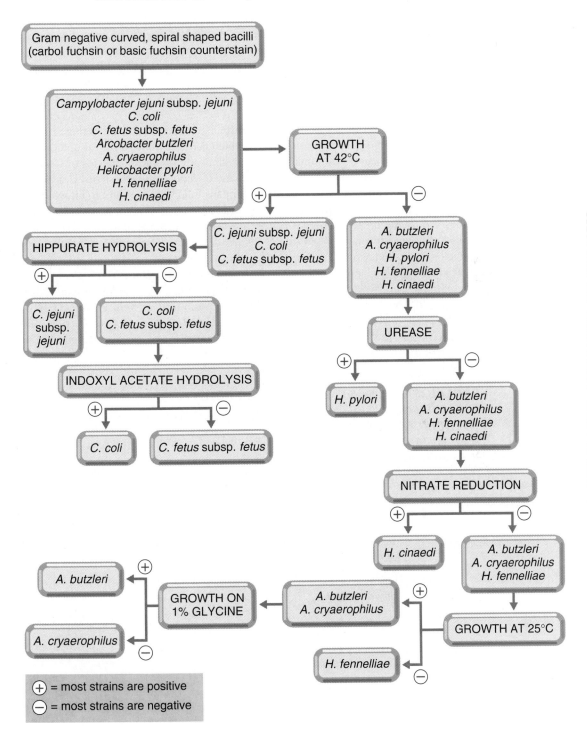

CAMPYLOBACTER, ARCOBACTER, HELICOBACTER

Rapid Test Methods for Identification

Latex agglutination assays for the detection of *C. jejuni* and *C. coli* are the Meritec Campy (jcl) test (Meridian Diagnostics, Cincinnati, OH) and the Campy slide (Becton Dickinson, Sparks, MD) for the detection of *C. jejuni*, *C. coli*, and *C. fetus*. DNA probes (Gen-Probe, San Diego, CA) are available for *C. jejuni* and *C. coli* but are not routinely used. Serologic tests for *Helicobacter* species include enzyme immunoassay and latex agglutination. Polymerase chain reaction (PCR) is available for *H. pylori* identification.

Pathogenicity

Intestinal and extraintestinal illnesses are the primary disease syndromes of these organisms with the exception of *Spirillum* species, which causes rat bite fever (also known as sodoku) (see chart below). In humans the most clinically significant species of *Campylobacter* are *C. jejuni* subspecies *jejuni*, *C. coli*, and *C. fetus* subspecies *fetus*. *C. jejuni* is the most common cause of gastroenteritis in humans following exposure to infected animals, contaminated meat, especially poultry, and contaminated water as well. Some infections are asymptomatic, whereas others are severe, accompanied by diarrhea, abdominal pain, and fever. *C. jejuni* and *C. fetus* are a cause of proctitis in homosexual men, and *C. jejuni* may play a role in Guillain-Barré syndrome (a neuromuscular condition accompanied by paralysis). *C. coli* is clinically similar to *C. jejuni*. *A. butzleri* and *A. cryaerophilus* are associated with diarrhea and bacteremia, and the latter species has been isolated from patients with endocarditis and peritonitis as well. Significant *Helicobacter* species associated with human disease include *H. pylori*, *H. fennelliae*, and *H. cinaedi*. *H. pylori* is the causative agent of chronic gastritis and has been implicated in peptic ulcer disease as well.

SPIRILLUM MINUS AND THE MAJOR SPECIES OF *CAMPYLOBACTER*, *ARCOBACTER*, AND *HELICOBACTER* ASSOCIATED WITH HUMAN DISEASE

ORGANISM	DISEASE AND SYMPTOMATOLOGY	MECHANISM OF TRANSMISSION
Spirillum minus	Rat bite fever (sodoku): ulceration and swelling of wound bite; maculopapular rash, fever	Infected rat or infected cat bite
C. jejuni subspecies *jejuni*	Gastroenteritis: diarrhea containing blood or mucus accompanied by abdominal pain and fever Proctitis in homosexual men Guillain-Barré syndrome: neuromuscular condition with paralysis	Food borne: contaminated meat (especially poultry), milk, and water Perinatal
C. coli	See *C. jejuni*	See *C. jejuni*
C. fetus subspecies *fetus*	Septicemia in immunocompromised population; proctitis and proctocolitis in homosexual men	Food borne
A. butzleri	Diarrhea, bacteremia	Food borne
A. cryaerophilus	Diarrhea, bacteremia (endocarditis and peritonitis not common)	Food borne

Continued ▶

▶ Continued ***SPIRILLUM MINUS* AND THE MAJOR SPECIES OF *CAMPYLOBACTER*, *ARCOBACTER*, AND *HELICOBACTER* ASSOCIATED WITH HUMAN DISEASE**

ORGANISM	DISEASE AND SYMPTOMATOLOGY	MECHANISM OF TRANSMISSION
H. pylori	Chronic gastritis Possibly peptic ulcer disease	Possibly fecal-oral or oral-oral
H. fennelliae	Proctitis, proctocolitis, and enteritis in AIDS population	Uncertain
H. cinaedi	Gastroenteritis Bacteremia, proctitis, proctocolitis, and enteritis in AIDS population	Uncertain

HAEMOPHILUS

Introduction and Taxonomy

The genus *Haemophilus* belongs to the family Pasteurellaceae, which also includes the genera *Pasteurella* and *Actinobacillus*. However, owing to incomplete DNA homology studies, investigators are not in agreement regarding the classifications of these organisms. Therefore *Pasteurella* and *Actinobacillus* species are discussed in the sections "Miscellaneous Bacterial Species Associated with Human Disease" and "Nonfermentative Gram Negative Bacilli," respectively.

Biochemical Properties

Haemophilus species are facultatively anaerobic, gram negative coccobacilli that are normal inhabitants of the human upper respiratory tract. Biochemical differentiation of *Haemophilus* species recovered in human specimens is presented in the figure on p 640. Generally, these organisms are oxidase positive, catalase positive, ferment carbohydrates, and reduce nitrates to nitrites. All species need 5% to 10% CO_2 for growth. They are nutritionally fastidious and require X factor (hemin) and/or V factor (nicotinamide adenine dinucleotide [NAD]), (with the exception of *H. aphrophilus*). The X and V factors can be provided in several ways, namely, through the use of

1. chocolate agar.
2. 5% sheep blood cross-streaked with V factor–producing *S. aureus* (ATCC 25923). The staphylococci produce V factor, and X factor is provided by the lysed erythrocytes. *Haemophilus* species appear as pinpoint "satellite" colonies within the hemolytic zone of staphylococcal growth.
3. X or V discs (Difco Labs). Additional tests may be employed for species differentiation such as β-hemolysis on horse or rabbit blood agar.

HAEMOPHILUS

DIFFERENTIATION OF SELECTED *HAEMOPHILUS* SPECIES ISOLATED FROM HUMANS

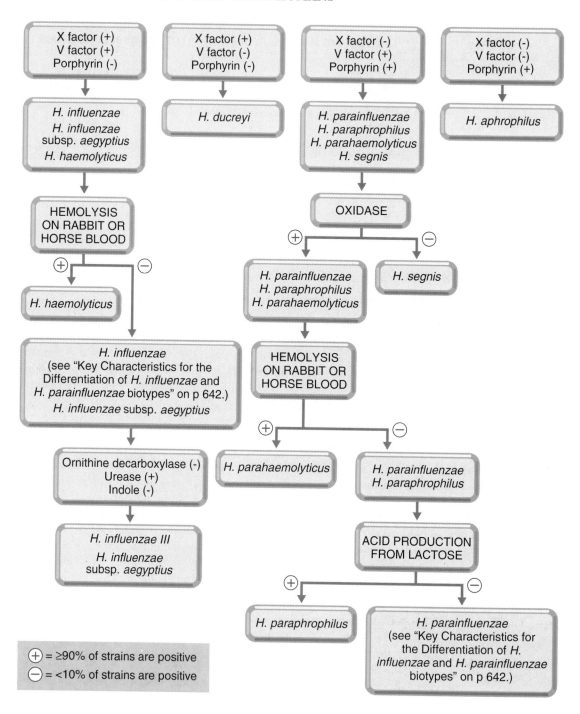

+ = ≥90% of strains are positive
− = <10% of strains are positive

Rapid Test Methods for Identification

Several rapid methods for the identification and/or biotyping of *Haemophilus* species are shown in the charts on pp 641 and 642. These methods include chromogenic enzyme substrate tests, agglutination tests, serotyping kits, immunoassays, and molecular assays. Appropriate controls, with known reference strains, should be used with each diagnostic assay.

RAPID TEST METHODS FOR THE IDENTIFICATION
OF *HAEMOPHILUS* SPECIES

TEST	COMMENTS
Chromogenic Enzyme Substrate Tests RapID NH panel (Innovative Diagnostic Systems, Atlanta, GA)	Identification and biotyping of pure isolates of *Haemophilus* species and *Neisseria* species within approximately 4 hr
NHI Card (bioMérieux Vitek, Hazelwood, MO)	
HNID panel (American MicroScan, West Sacramento, CA)	
Latex Agglutination Tests	
Wellcogen Bacterial Antigen Kit (Murex, Norcross, GA)	Detection of *H. influenzae,* type b antigen in body fluids, sensitivity 97%.
Coagglutination Test Phadebact Haemophilus Test (Pharmacia, Piscataway, NJ)	Culture confirmation of *Haemophilus* species and serotyping of *H. influenzae,* type b strains
Serotyping Kits Wellcome Diagnostics	Polyvalent and group specific *H. influenzae* antisera used for serotyping
Difco Laboratories (Detroit, MI)	Same as above
Other Methods Counterimmunoelectrophoresis (CIE)	Available, but limited clinical application for *H. influenzae,* type b antigen detection
Indirect immunofluorescence	Sensitivity and specificity ranging from 50% to 100% for *H. ducreyi*
Enzyme immunoassay (EIA)	Sensitivity and specificity of 100% for *H. ducreyi* (30 reported patients)
Molecular Assays PCR DNA probe	High sensitivity (98%), but low specificity (51%) for *H. ducreyi*

HAEMOPHILUS

KEY CHARACTERISTICS FOR THE DIFFERENTIATION
OF *H. INFLUENZAE* AND *H. PARAINFLUENZAE* BIOTYPES

ORGANISM	CHARACTERISTICS			COMMENTS
	Urease	Indole	Ornithine Decarboxylase	
H. influenzae				RAPID KITS AVAILABLE FOR BIOTYPING:
Biotype: I	+	+	+	HNID (Dade International, Chicago, IL)
II	+	+	−	api 10E, api NH (bioMérieux, LaBalme-las-Grottes,
III	+	−	−	France)
IV	+	−	+	
V	−	+	+	
VI	−	−	+	
VII	−	+	−	
VIII	−	−	−	
H. parainfluenzae				
Biotype: I	−	−	+	
II	+	−	+	
III	+	−	−	
IV	+	+	+	
V	−	+	+	
VI	+	+	−	
VII	−	+	−	

+, ≥90% of strains are positive; −, <10% of strains are positive.

Table adapted from Kilian M: *Haemophilus.* In Balows A, Hausler WJ Jr, Herrmann HD, Shadomy HJ, eds: Manual of Clinical Microbiology, 5th ed. Washington, DC, American Society for Microbiology, 1991.

Pathogenicity

Clinically relevant species include, *H. influenzae, H. parainfluenzae, H. aphrophilus, H. paraphrophilus, H. ducreyi, H. parahaemolyticus,* and *H. segnis. H. influenzae* has six serotypes, with serotypes b most often associated with infection. The presence of a polysaccharide capsule is a major factor associated with virulence. *H. haemolyticus, H. parahaemolyticus, H. paraphrophilus,* and *H. segnis* seldom cause disease, whereas *H. influenzae, H. ducreyi,* and *H. aphrophilus* are more common agents of infection. The disease spectra associated with these species range from relatively innocuous infection to serious, potentially fatal disease such as acute meningitis in young children (see chart on facing page).

Disease Spectra of Selected *Haemophilus* Species Associated with Human Infection

SPECIES	DISEASE SYNDROME(S)
H. influenzae, type b	Meningitis (usually in children up to 2 yr of age), pharyngitis, laryngotracheobronchitis, epiglottitis, pneumonia (in elderly), endocarditis (rare)
H. influenzae, capsular types other than b	Meningitis (rare), epiglottitis (rare)
H. influenzae, nontypable strains	Bronchitis, pneumonia
H. influenzae, biogroup aegyptius	Conjunctivitis and otitis media (in children)
H. influenzae, nonencapsulated strains	Pneumonia and chronic bronchitis in adults
H. parainfluenzae	Endocarditis, urethritis (in adults), bacteremia
H. aphrophilus	Brain abscess, endocarditis
H. ducreyi	Chanchroid

LEGIONELLA

Introduction

After the 1976 outbreak of Legionnaire's disease at an American Legion convention in Philadelphia, there was a rebirth of a bacterial pathogen, and a new genus, *Legionella,* was established. *Legionella* species are widespread in nature, especially in aquatic environments. Reservoirs for these organisms include air conditioners, water cooling towers, and other water devices, fresh water lakes, hot springs, tap water plumbing, and whirlpools. The notoriety of their outbreaks and their ubiquity in the environment has made this genus the target of intense investigation.

Taxonomy

Based on serologic techniques and DNA relatedness studies, innumerable species and subspecies have been identified, and two additional genera within the family Legionellaceae have been proposed. Until these taxonomic issues are resolved, only the *Legionella* genus will be recognized, and only two species with major involvement in human disease, namely *L. pneumophila* and *L. micdadei,* are considered in this chapter.

Characteristics

Legionella species are aerobic, non–spore forming, motile and slender, gram negative rods that, for the most part, are biochemically inactive. Some of the characteristic features of this genus and assays that are used for identification are presented in the chart on the next page.

LEGIONELLA

Rapid Test Methods for Identification

Culture is the most definitive form of identification of *Legionella* species. There are several diagnostic assays available for identification (see chart below), but some exhibit low sensitivity and/or specificity. Detection of *Legionella* antigen by radioimmunoassay has a sensitivity of ≥80% and a high specificity.

CHARACTERISTIC FEATURES AND ASSAYS USED IN THE IDENTIFICATION OF *LEGIONELLA* SPECIES

FEATURE	DESCRIPTION
Gram Stain Morphology	Faint staining, slender gram negative rods
Biochemical Properties	Oxidase positive Catalase positive Relatively inactive
Other Properties	Motile Non–spore forming Aerobic Widespread in nature—reservoirs include bodies of water and potable water sources
Growth on Selective Agar	Require L-cysteine for growth. Iron salts enhance growth. 5% CO_2 enhances growth. *Buffered charcoal yeast extract agar or broth—culture is most definitive form of identification.*
Disease Spectra	Subacute illness—recognized on basis of antibody titers. Pontiac fever—epidemic illness characterized by fever, cough, and flu-like symptoms devoid of pulmonary involvement. Pneumonia—characterized by nonproductive cough, high fever, headache, pulmonary infiltrates; sporadic or epidemic occurrence. Community acquired or nosocomial infection. Extrapulmonary illness—bacteremia, pericarditis, cellulitis, gastrointestinal and hepatic abscess.

DIAGNOSTIC ASSAYS	COMMENT
Antigen Detection	
Direct Immunofluorescence	Commercially available, but not recommended due to sensitivity and specificity problems
Radioimmunoassay	Commercially available for *L. pneumophila*—relatively high sensitivity and specificity
Enzyme Immunoassay	Not commercially available—high sensitivity and specificity
Latex Agglutination	Commercially available, but not recommended due to low sensitivity
DNA Probe	Commercially available, sensitivity of 70%
Antibody Detection	
Indirect Fluorescent Antibody	Sensitivity 75%–80%, specificity 96%

Pathogenicity

Legionellosis is an inclusive term that refers to any infection caused by *Legionella* species. Disease syndromes include subclinical illness, Pontiac fever, pneumonia, and extrapulmonary illness (see chart above). Infections may be sporadic, epidemic, or nosocomially acquired. Human to human transmission has not been documented.

ANAEROBIC BACTERIA

Introduction and Occurrence

Anaerobic bacteria are widespread in the environment, including soil, bodies of water (both fresh and salt water), sewage, plants, and animals. In humans, anaerobes are part of the normal flora of the skin, oral cavity (especially gingival crevices surrounding the teeth), gastrointestinal tract (especially the colon), and genitourinary tract. Infections caused by this indigenous microflora are referred to as *endogenous infections*. Factors that may be responsible for endogenous infections include trauma, surgery, immunosuppressive agents (chemotherapy and radiation), immunosuppressive diseases (AIDS), and debilitating diseases such as diabetes and renal failure. The less common exogenous infections, which are caused by anaerobes, originate from sources outside the body and include food borne botulism, tetanus, and gas gangrene. Owing to the potential fatality associated with these infections, laboratory identification of these organisms to the genus level is essential in order that appropriate antimicrobial therapy be determined.

ENDOGENOUS AND EXOGENOUS ANAEROBIC INFECTIONS

ENDOGENOUS ANAEROBIC INFECTIONS	EXOGENOUS ANAEROBIC INFECTIONS
Abscess, especially brain	BOTULISM:
Actinomycosis (see Chapter 42)	Food borne
Appendicitis and cholecystitis complications	Infant
Cellulitis, crepitant and noncrepitant	Wound
Colitis and diarrhea associated with antibiotic usage	Crepitant cellulitis
Dental and periodontal infection	Gastroenteritis, caused by *C. perfringens*
Endocarditis	Gas gangrene
Gas gangrene (myonecrosis)	Infections following human or animal bites
Meningitis (usually associated with brain abscess)	Septic abortion
Pneumonia, aspiration and necrotizing	Tetanus
Osteomyelitis	
Otitis media	
Septic arthritis	
Sinusitis	

Adapted from Koneman EW, Allen SD, Dodwell VR Jr, et al: Color Atlas and Textbook of Diagnostic Microbiology, 3rd ed. New York, JB Lippincott, pp 396–397, 1988.

Classification of More Common Clinically Relevant Species

Anaerobic bacteria exhibit varied degrees of tolerance to the presence of oxygen and on this basis can be classified into several categories, namely, strict obligate anaerobes,

ANAEROBIC BACTERIA

moderate obligate anaerobes, and aerotolerant anaerobes. Facultative anaerobes such as *S. aureus* and *E. coli*, and microaerophiles such as *C. jejuni* are discussed elsewhere. Most clinical anaerobic isolates are moderate obligate anaerobes, which include *Bacteroides fragilis, Fusobacterium nucleatum,* and *Clostridium perfringens.* The anaerobes most commonly recovered in a routine laboratory, and two of notorious reputation (*C. botulinum* and *C. tetanus*), are classified on the basis of gram stain morphology and spore formation. It is important to note that gram stain and morphology may exhibit variability in older cultures.

ANAEROBIC BACTERIA THAT ARE MORE COMMONLY ENCOUNTERED IN THE ROUTINE CLINICAL LABORATORY

GRAM POSITIVE SPORE FORMING BACILLI	GRAM POSITIVE NON–SPORE FORMING BACILLI	GRAM POSITIVE NON–SPORE FORMING COCCI	GRAM NEGATIVE NON–SPORE FORMING BACILLI	GRAM NEGATIVE NON–SPORE FORMING COCCI
*Clostridium perfringens** *C. botulinum†* *C. tetani†* *C. difficile* *C. ramosum* *C. innocuum*	*Actinomyces* species *Bifidobacterium* species *Eubacterium lentum* *Lactobacillus* species (80% facultative, 20% obligate anaerobe) *Mobiluncus* species *Propionibacterium acnes, P. propionicum* *Rothia* species (see p 606)	*Peptococcus niger* *Peptostreptococcus magnus* *P. tetradius* *P. asaccharolyticus* *P. anaerobius* *P. prevotii*	*Bacteroides fragilis* *B. melaninogenicus* *Fusobacterium nucleatum* *Prevotella* species *Porphyromonas* species	*Veillonella* species

*Most commonly isolated anaerobe.
†Not commonly isolated, but renowned pathogens.

Identification

Identification of anaerobes is neither simple nor straightforward. Their involvement in infectious processes is usually concomitant with that of other pathogens. In addition, they are part of the normal microbial flora of the skin and mucous membranes, which makes interpretation of cultures difficult.

Before culture, proper collection, transport, and processing of clinical specimens with minimal exposure to atmospheric oxygen is critical. Inoculation of fresh or prereduced anaerobic media is important. The most widely recommended anaerobic medium is CDC anaerobic blood agar as well as enriched thioglycollate medium. In most routine laboratories anaerobic conditions are achieved using a GasPak anaerobic jar together with an active catalyst as an optimal means of anaerobic recovery.

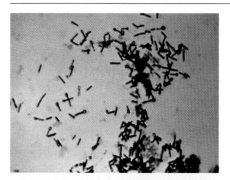

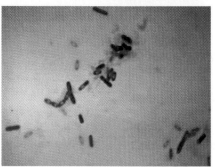

Microscopic Morphology

One of the first indications of an anaerobic isolate is growth on anaerobic medium incubated anaerobically, together with a lack of microbial growth on media inoculated aerobically. A pungent odor and the presence of gas in an inoculated specimen are valuable clues. On microscopic evaluation the presence and position of spores, sulfur granules, and filamentous and branching forms should be noted. The photograph on the left indicates the terminal and subterminal spores of *C. tetani* and *C. sordellii*, respectively.

Courtesy of Suzette L. Bartley, James D. Howard, and Ray Simon, Centers for Disease Control and Prevention, Atlanta, GA.

Rapid Test Methods for Identification

The extent of identification of a pure, anaerobic, clinical isolate beyond colonial and microscopic morphology is dependent on the capabilities of the laboratory. Where there are limited resources, reference laboratories are used for identification. Commercially available kits are listed below.

Commercial kits for anaerobic identification:

api-20A (bioMérieux Vitek, Hazelwood, MO)
Minitek Anaerobe (Becton Dickinson Sparks, MD)
api-ZYM (bioMérieux Vitek, Hazelwood, MO)
api AnIdent system (bioMérieux Vitek, Hazelwood, MO)
RapID ANA (Innovative Diagnostic Systems, Atlanta, GA)

The api-20A and Minitek systems both identify approximately 50% of the anaerobes present in clinical specimens, with deficiencies most pronounced in the identification of gram positive non–spore forming bacilli and anaerobic cocci. The api-ZYM AnIdent system and RapID ANA are 4 hour identification systems based on enzymatic profiles of the anaerobes. There is no database for the api-ZYM. The AnIdent system has an overall accuracy of 71% in the identification of anaerobes to the species level, whereas accuracy reports for the RapID ANA system are in the range of 63%–92%. Ideally, supplemental tests, especially gas liquid chromatography (GLC), would greatly enhance the accuracy. GLC is an invaluable tool in the identification of anaerobes and the only definitive means of *Bacteroides* and *Fusobacterium* speciation. Schematic diagrams for the presumptive identification of the more common clinically significant anaerobes follow.

ANAEROBIC BACTERIA

DIFFERENTIATION OF THE MORE COMMON CLINICALLY SIGNIFICANT GRAM POSITIVE, SPORE FORMING, ANAEROBIC BACILLI

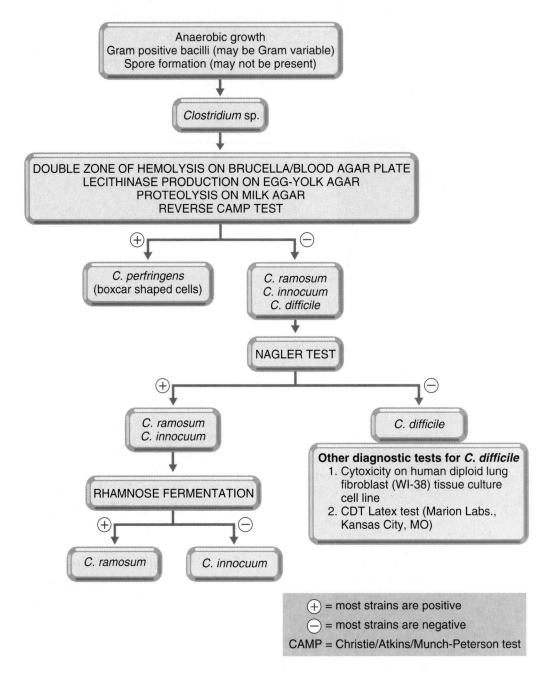

DIFFERENTIATION OF THE MORE COMMON CLINICALLY SIGNIFICANT GRAM POSITIVE, NON–SPORE FORMING BACILLI

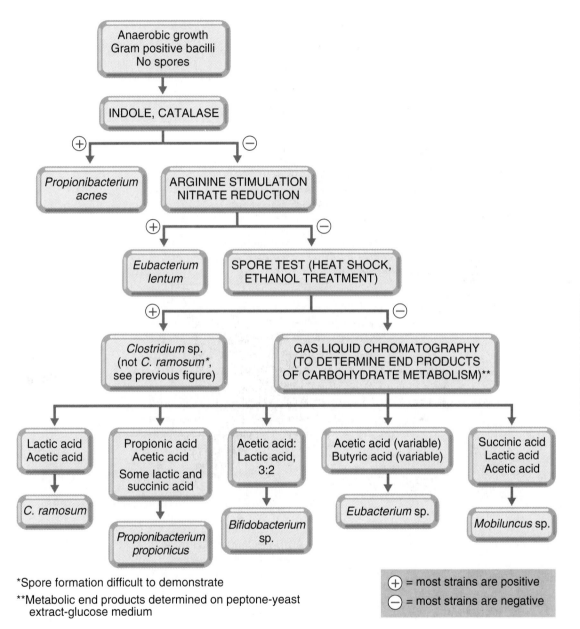

*Spore formation difficult to demonstrate

**Metabolic end products determined on peptone-yeast extract-glucose medium

⊕ = most strains are positive

⊖ = most strains are negative

ANAEROBIC BACTERIA

DIFFERENTIATION OF THE MORE COMMON
CLINICALLY SIGNIFICANT GRAM POSITIVE COCCI

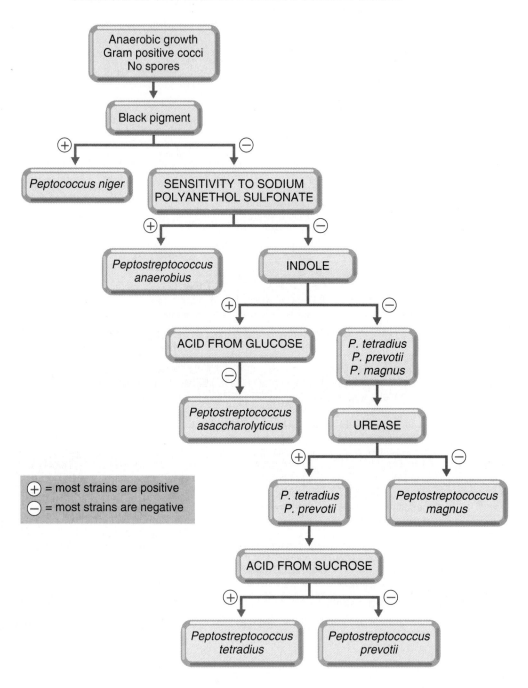

DIFFERENTIATION OF THE MORE COMMON CLINICALLY SIGNIFICANT GRAM NEGATIVE NON–SPORE FORMING BACILLI

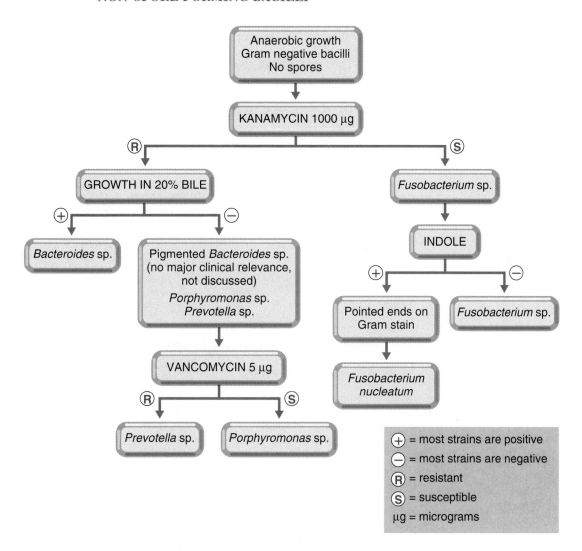

IDENTIFICATION OF GRAM NEGATIVE NON–SPORE FORMING COCCI

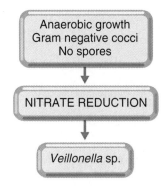

ANAEROBIC BACTERIA

Pathogenicity

The clinical manifestations of the more common anaerobic pathogens are presented in the chart below. Most infections are polymicrobic, and others are difficult to interpret due to the presence of normal, indigenous flora. Communication of the physician with laboratory personnel regarding the specimen and symptomatology is recommended.

CLINICAL MANIFESTATIONS OF PRINCIPAL ANAEROBIC PATHOGENS

ORGANISM	CLINICAL MANIFESTATION
Gram Positive Spore Forming Bacilli	
Clostridium	
perfringens	ENDOGENOUS INFECTIONS ESPECIALLY ASSOCIATED WITH COLON: Intra-abdominal abscess, peritonitis, gangrenous cholecystitis, myonecrosis (gas gangrene) EXOGENOUS INFECTIONS: Wound infections, crepitant cellulitis, food poisoning, bacteremia, and necrotizing bowel disease
botulinum	BOTULISM—NEUROPARALYTIC DISEASE: Food borne—ingestion of preformed toxin Infant—results from in vivo multiplication of *C. botulinum* in infant gut Wound—from in vivo toxin production
tetani	Tetanus—infectious disease characterized by muscle spasm, lockjaw, and back spasms
difficile	Pseudomembranous colitis, antibiotic associated diarrhea, colitis
ramosum	Intra-abdominal infections, bacteremia
innocuum	Gastrointestinal infections, empyema
Gram Positive Non–Spore Forming Bacilli	
Actinomyces israelii	Actinomycosis—chronic granulomatous disease due to infection of the gingivodental crevices and tonsillar crypts; facial, thoracic, abdominal, and genital involvement most common
Bifidobacterium	
dentium *eriksonii*	Rare pathogens, isolated from lower respiratory tract, dental caries, and vaginal and fecal clinical specimens
Eubacterium lentum	Most common species, rare pathogen; abscess and wound infection
Lactobacillus species	Rare pathogens; neonatal meningitis, endocarditis, chorioamnionitis, bacteremia
Mobiluncus species	Role in bacterial vaginosis unclear
Propionibacterium acnes	Associated with polymicrobic skin infections, acne, surgical infections, bacteremia, endocarditis
propionicum	Actinomycosis, lacrimal canaliculitis
Rothia species	See "Gram Positive Bacilli" on p 600.

Continued ▶

► Continued   **CLINICAL MANIFESTATIONS OF PRINCIPAL
ANAEROBIC PATHOGENS**

ORGANISM	CLINICAL MANIFESTATION
Gram Positive Non–Spore Forming Cocci	
Peptococcus niger	Rare cause of postpartum endometritis
Peptostreptococcus	
magnus *tetradius* *asaccharolyticus* *anaerobius* *prevotii*	Usually polymicrobic infections: postpartum endometritis, septic abortions, amnionitis, brain abscesses, sinusitis, otitis media, pneumonitis, bacteremia, intra-abdominal abscesses *P. magnus* especially associated with bone and joint infection
Gram Negative Non–Spore Forming Bacilli	
Bacteroides	
fragilis	Intra-abdominal and other infections
thetaiotaomicron	Intra-abdominal and other infections
ureolyticus	Head and neck infections; pulmonary, urogenital, and intra-abdominal infections
gracilis	Head and neck infections
Fusobacterium	
nucleatum	Oral cavity abscesses, polymicrobic infections
necrophorum	Peritonsillar abscesses
mortiferum	Intra-abdominal abscesses
varium	Intra-abdominal abscesses
Prevotella species	Infections associated with bites; oral, dental, and lower respiratory tract infections
Porphyromonas species	Animal bite infections
Gram Negative Non–Spore Forming Cocci	
Veillonella species	Oral abscesses, head, neck, and pulmonary infections

ANAEROBIC BACTERIA

SPIROCHETES

Introduction

The spirochetes are long, slender, helically curved bacteria that are motile via axial filaments or fibrils that are attached at each end of the organism. These filaments (fibrils) allow their rotational and corkscrew motility. Both their morphology and method of movement differentiate the spirochetes from other bacteria.

Taxonomy

The taxonomic classification of spirochetes includes the families Spirochaetaceae and Leptospiraceae. In the Spirochaetaceae family there are five genera, namely *Borrelia, Treponema, Spirochaeta, Serpulina,* and *Cristispira.* Included in the Leptospiraceae family are the genera *Leptospira* and *Leptonema. Borrelia, Treponema,* and *Leptospira* are the genera pathogenic to humans.

Morphology

The three pathogenic genera are all gram negative, but *Treponema* species and *Leptospira* species do not stain readily with routine laboratory stains and can best be differentiated on the basis of helical morphology and movement using darkfield microscopy. The treponemes are slender and have regularly spaced spirals and tapered ends; characteristic flexing may be evident. The spirals of *Leptospira* species are tightly coiled and have hooked ends, and *Borrelia* species are broader, less tightly coiled and more irregular (see figure below).

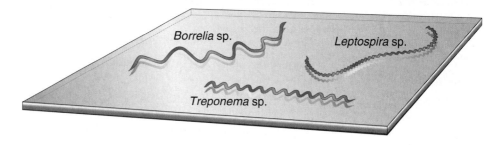

Pathogenic Spirochetes

The disease spectra of the pathogenic spirochetes are presented in the chart on p 656. Diseases caused by *Borrelia* species are transmitted to humans via arthropod vectors. These diseases include human relapsing fever and Lyme disease.

HUMAN RELAPSING FEVER

The vectors responsible for the transmission of human relapsing fever are the body louse *Pediculus humanus humanus* and the tick *Ornithodoros* species. As the table below indicates, human relapsing fever is caused by several species of *Borrelia.* The illness is characterized by chills and fever lasting several days to a week with possible organ involvement (liver, spleen) and rash development. There is then an asymptomatic period followed by several more febrile relapses that are less severe and of shorter duration.

LYME DISEASE

The spirochete that causes Lyme disease is *Borrelia burgdorferi,* which is transmitted to humans through the bite of an infected *Ixodes* tick. Rodents and deer serve as the natural reservoirs for these ticks. Lyme disease is a chronic inflammatory disorder that may first present as a distinctive red skin lesion (erythema migrans) with a central clearing at the site of the bite. Characteristic symptoms include fever, stiff neck, headache, fatigue, and muscle and joint pain. The second stage of the disease may be marked by arthritis and neurologic disorders such as meningitis.

VENEREAL SYPHILIS

The causative agent of venereal syphilis is *T. pallidum.* Syphilis is a histologically significant disease that can be transmitted by several means: sexual contact, congenitally, or through direct contact with infected lesions. There are three distinct stages, each with a unique clinical presentation.

Primary Stage

Primary syphilis presents with a firm, usually painless lesion that develops into an ulcerated sore called a *chancre.* This lesion usually appears on the penis or cervix but may also occur on any mucous membrane or cutaneous surface. Enlarged lymph nodes may also occur near the chancre and act as a portal of infection to other sites in the body.

Secondary Stage

Secondary syphilis is characterized by the appearance of lesions on mucous membranes and cutaneous surfaces. A macular papular skin rash on the trunk, limbs, palms, and soles of feet is common. Condylomata, or large mucous membrane lesions, may also be evident. Latent syphilis is characterized by a lack of symptoms but high serologic titers.

Tertiary Stage

Tertiary or late syphilis is a noninfectious stage. Characteristic granulomatous skin lesions called *gummas* may occur on mucous membranes, subcutaneous tissues, bone, and viscera. Visceral involvement, with lesions of the central nervous or cardiovascular system, has a high morbidity.

CONGENITAL SYPHILIS

Congenital syphilis occurs when treponemes from an infected mother pass to the fetus via the placenta. The disease is extensive with the potential of mucocutaneous, bone, nerve, and central nervous system involvement.

PINTA, YAWS, AND ENDEMIC SYPHILIS

Other pathogenic treponemes include *T. pallidum* subspecies *carateum,* the causative agent of pinta, *T. pallidum* subspecies *pertenue,* the causative agent of yaws, and *T. pallidum* subspecies *endemicum,* which causes endemic syphilis (bejel). Pinta, yaws, and endemic or bejel syphilis are somewhat similar in clinical presentation to venereal syphilis, but transmission is oral in endemic regions with poor hygiene. Pinta is a chronic skin disease that presents in Central and South America. Yaws is a tropical disease, and endemic syphilis is restricted to North Africa and the Middle East.

LEPTOSPIROSIS

Leptospirosis is a zoonotic illness transmitted to humans directly or indirectly by contaminated rodents and domestic animals. Direct contamination occurs as a consequence

SPIROCHETES

of animal contact. Therefore, veterinarians, herders, and meat, poultry, and fish processors are especially at risk. Indirect contamination occurs through exposure to water or soil contaminated with leptospires as a consequence of animal urination. The incidence of this disease is especially high in the summer months in association with swimming.

Leptospires enter the body through mucosal surfaces or skin abrasions, multiply in the blood, and then travel to other body sites such as kidneys, liver, and meninges, where they cause infection. Leptospirosis is a biphasic illness; the initial phase is similar to a flu-like syndrome with fever, muscle aches, headache, and chills. The second phase is often characterized by renal and hepatic involvement, meningitis, and skin rash. This phase has a relatively high mortality.

DISEASE SYNDROMES AND KEY CHARACTERISTICS OF SELECTED SPIROCHETAL PATHOGENS

SPIROCHETE	DISEASE	MODE OR VECTOR OF TRANSMISSION	KEY CHARACTERISTICS
Borrelia recurrentis	Human relapsing fever	*Pediculus humanus humanus* (body louse)	Febrile relapses, possible organ involvement
B. hermsii *B. parkeri* *B. turicatae* *B. mazzotti*	American relapsing fever	*Ornithodoros* species (tick)	Febrile relapses, possible organ involvement
B. burgdorferi *B. afzelii* *B. garinii*	Lyme disease	*Ixodes* species (tick)	Erythema migrans
Treponema pallidum subspecies *pallidum*	Syphilis	Sexual	Primary, secondary, latent, tertiary phases; congenital
T. pallidum subspecies *pertenue*	Yaws	Skin contact	Children, tropical areas
T. carateum	Pinta	Skin contact	Central and South America
T. pallidum subspecies *endemicum*	Endemic syphilis, bejel	Mucous membrane	Africa, Middle East
Leptospira interrogans	Leptospirosis	Skin, mucosal surfaces	Biphasic illness

Diagnostic Procedures

Procedure for the diagnosis of the spirochetal disease are listed in the chart below. Treponemal spirochetes cannot be cultured in vitro as readily as *Borrelia* species and *Leptospira* species. Direct examination of potentially infected material using darkfield microscopy or direct fluorescent antibody methods is an important diagnostic criterion. Molecular assays as well as commercially available serologic tests vary in uniformity and standardization from one laboratory to the next and must be evaluated on an individual basis.

PROCEDURES FOR THE DIAGNOSIS OF SELECTED SPIROCHETAL SYNDROMES

DISEASE	SPECIMEN	DIRECT EXAMINATION	STAINS	IN VITRO CULTURE	IN VIVO CULTURE	MOLECULAR ASSAYS	SEROLOGIC TESTS
Human Relapsing Fever	Blood; infecting tick—less optimal	Light or darkfield microscopy, direct fluorescent antibody (DFA)	Aniline dyes, Leishman's, Geimsa's, Wright's stains; Warthin-Starry silver stain; fluorescein conjugated polyclonal antibody stain	Barbour-Stoenner-Kellyll BSK-II medium, BSK-H medium (Sigma, St Louis, MO); 30°–37°C, 4–6 wk	Rodents, arthropod vectors, embryonated chicken eggs	DNA probes, PCR	Indirect immunofluorescence assays (IFAs)
Lyme	Skin biopsies of area surrounding erythema migrans; tissues, blood—less optimal	Light microscopy; darkfield microscopy—both less optimal than serologic testing	Aniline dyes, Leishman's, Geimsa's, Wright's stains; Warthin-Starry silver stain; fluorescein conjugated polyclonal antibody stain				Serologic testing is method of choice for Lyme disease IFA, ELISA, recombinant antigenic techniques, Western immunoblot technique
Syphilis: Primary	Lesion exudate, lymph node aspirate, tissue; blood, CSF—less optimal	Darkfield microscopy, DFA	Silver	None	Animal inoculation (rabbit)	PCR	NONTREPONEMAL: Venereal Disease Research Laboratory (VDRL) Rapid plasma reagin (RPR) Unheated serum reagin (USR) Toluidine red unheated serum test (TRUST) TREPONEMAL: Fluorescent treponemal antibody absorption (FTA-ABS) Microhemagglutination test (MHA-TP)

Continued ▶

SPIROCHETES

▶ Continued **PROCEDURES FOR THE DIAGNOSIS OF SELECTED SPIROCHETAL SYNDROMES**

DISEASE	SPECIMEN	DIRECT EXAMINATION	STAINS	IN VITRO CULTURE	IN VIVO CULTURE	MOLECULAR ASSAYS	SEROLOGIC TESTS
Syphilis: Secondary	Same as primary	Same as primary	Same as primary	Same as primary			Nontreponemal assays: see p. 657
Syphilis: Latent Early	None	None	None	None			Nontreponemal and treponemal assays: see p. 657
Syphilis: Latent Late	Tissue, CSF	DFAT-TP (direct fluorescent antibody test for *T. pallidum*					VDRL on CSF, treponemal assays
Syphilis: Congenital	Placenta, umbilical cord, lesion exudate, nasal discharge	Darkfield microscopy					
Yaws Pinta Endemic Syphilis (Bejel)	Diagnosis is based on geographic region and clinical presentation, transmission mode, and patient age.						
Leptospirosis	Blood, CSF, urine; tissue (kidney, liver, brain)—fatal cases only	Darkfield microscopy, DFA	Silver—tissue only	Ellinghausen's, Fletcher's, Polysorbate 80 medium, 5°–20°C, up to 4 mo		DNA PCR	Microscopic agglutination test (MAT)

MYCOPLASMA AND UREAPLASMA

Distribution and Unique Characteristics

Mycoplasma and *Ureaplasma* are clinically significant genera within the class Mollicutes and collectively are referred to as *mycoplasmas*. These organisms are the smallest free living bacteria and are found widespread in nature, including both the animal and the plant kingdoms. Due to the absence of a cell wall they are pleomorphic in shape, not visible on Gram stain, and resistant to β-lactamase antibiotics. Filamentous and coccal forms may be evident using phase contrast and darkfield microscopy.

Culture and Growth Requirements

Mollicutes are aerobes or facultative anaerobes and have fastidious growth requirements. Media for their isolation require supplementation with nucleic acid and/or lipid precursors or fatty acids. Antibiotics such as penicillin may be added to inhibit bacterial contaminants. Commercially available media include SP4, PPLO broth, and Shepard's A7-B agar.

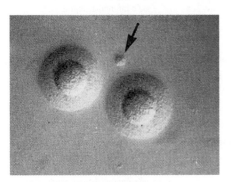

From Mahon CR, Manuselis G: Textbook of Diagnostic Microbiology. Philadelphia, WB Saunders, 1995, p 631.

Colonial Morphology

Mycoplasma species exhibit a typical "fried egg" appearance on selective agar (see left). *Ureaplasma* species appear as smaller, granular spheres.

Identification

M. pneumoniae and *M. genitalium* take as long as several weeks to several months, respectively, to grow, and therefore culture of these species may not be optimal for diagnostic purposes. *M. hominis* grows in less than 7 days and *Ureaplasma* species in 24 to 48 hours. Thus, culture is the method of choice for the identification of these latter organisms. Other methods, both serologic and nonserologic, are available (see chart on p 660).

MYCOPLASMA, UREAPLASMA, ACHOLEPLASMA

KEY FEATURES AND IDENTIFICATION METHODS FOR SELECTED *MYCOPLASMA* SPECIES AND *UREAPLASMA UREALYTICUM*

ORGANISM	NOTABLE BIOCHEMICAL CHARACTERISTICS	CLINICAL LABORATORY METHODS FOR IDENTIFICATION	CLINICAL MANIFESTATIONS
M. pneumoniae	Fermentation of glucose H_2O_2 production Hemadsorption	Culture: difficult LOW SENSITIVITY: Latex agglutination Complement fixation Cold agglutination antibody titer Enzyme immunoassay Direct immunofluorescence DNA probe test (PACE, Gen-Probe) PCR: good sensitivity	Atypical pneumonia Walking pneumonia Acute upper and lower respiratory tract infection
M. hominis	Arginine hydrolysis	Culture on colistin nalidixic agar (CNA) Indirect hemagglutination: low sensitivity ELISA	UROGENITAL: Pyelonephritis Pelvic inflammatory disease Postpartum fever
M. genitalium	Fermentation of glucose H_2O_2 production Hemadsorption	Culture Micro IF (immunofluorescence) Nucleic acid dot-blot hybridization (research only) PCR: good sensitivity	Genitourinary tract disease Nongonococcal urethritis (NGU)
U. urealyticum	Urea hydrolysis	Culture on ureaplasma agar: not difficult ELISA PCR: good sensitivity	NGU in men Chorioamnionitis in women Pneumonia, septicemia, and meningitis in newborns

Pathogenicity

The most notable disease associated with this category of organisms is walking pneumonia or atypical pneumonia. *M. pneumoniae,* the causative agent of this disease, is responsible for acute upper and lower respiratory tract infection. *M. hominis* and *U. urealyticum* are commensals of the urogenital tract of both men and women. *M. hominis* has been implicated as a rare cause of pyelonephritis and postpartum fever. *M. genitalium* may be associated with genitourinary disease, particularly nongonococcal urethritis (NGU). Evidence indicates *U. urealyticum* is a cause of NGU in men, chorioamnionitis in women, and pneumonia, septicemia, and meningitis in premature infants (see chart above).

MYCOBACTERIA

Introduction and Morphology

Mycobacteria are well known agents of disease that remain a major health concern in the United States, but more especially in developing nations. They are nonmotile, slender, rod shaped organisms. Although they stain Gram positive, this is not a valid technique due to their resistance to acid alcohol decolorization. They are also strict aerobes and non–spore formers.

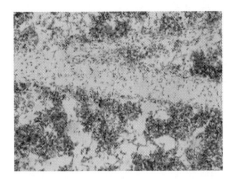

Unique Characteristics

Several unique characteristics distinguish *Mycobacterium* species from other bacteria, namely:

1. Acid fastness (exception: *Nocardia* species are also acid fast): these organisms resist acid alcohol decolorization and must be stained with acid fast stains such as Kinyoun's and Ziehl-Nielsen acid fast stain. The organisms stain red and appear as slender rods (see left).
2. High cell wall lipid content: the majority of these lipids are mycolic acid.
3. Cording factor: the ability of some species (e.g., *M. tuberculosis*) to form rough, serpentine colonies on certain media.
4. Very slow growth rate resulting in visible colonial growth within several days or up to 8 weeks, depending on the species.
5. Pigment production, in certain species, which may or may not be light dependent. Scotochromogens are those species that produce pigment independent of environmental condition. Photochromogens are those species in which pigment production is light dependent.

Identification

Identification of *Mycobacteria* species is based on:

1. The identification of acid fast bacilli in stained smears of clinical specimens.
2. Growth of the microorganism on suitable media; Löwenstein-Jensen or Middlebrook 7H10 or 7H11 media (Becton Dickinson, Sparks, MD).
3. Biochemical tests, such as niacin and catalase (see p 662), DNA probes, high performance liquid chromotography (HPLC), or automated systems such as the BACTEC AFB system (Becton Dickinson Diagnostic Instruments, Sparks, MD).

MYCOBACTERIA

KEY BIOCHEMICAL TESTS FOR THE DIFFERENTIATION OF SELECTED MYCOBACTERIUM SPECIES THAT ARE CLINICALLY RELEVANT

	NIACIN	NITRATE REDUCTION	CATALASE 68°C	CATALASE SEMIQUANTITATIVE	TELLURITE REDUCTION	TWEEN 80	UREASE	NaCl	AR	Fe	M
M. tuberculosis	+	+	–	89%	36%	68%	64%	–	–	–	–
M. bovis	–	–	–	69%	–	21%	50%	–	–	–	–
M. avium complex (MAC)	–	–	60%	+	81%	–	–	–	–	–	±
M. genavense	–	–	+	–	–	+	+	–	–	–	–
M. haemophilum	–	–	–	–	–	–	–	–	–	–	–
M. xenopi	–	–	31%	85%	65%	–	–	–	36%	–	–
M. kansasii	–	+	+	+	31%	+	49%	–	–	–	–
M. marinum	21%	–	30%	98%	39%	+	83%	–	41%	–	–
M. scrofulaceum	–	–	+	84%	64%	–	31%	–	–	–	–

+, ≥90% of strains are positive; –, <10% of all strains are positive; NaCl, sodium chloride; AR, arylsulfatase; Fe, iron; M, growth on MacConkey agar

Adapted from Roberts GD, Koneman EW, Kim YK: *Mycobacterium*. In Balows A, Hausler WJ Jr, Hermann KL, et al, eds: Manual of Clinical Microbiology, 5th ed. Washington, DC, American Society for Microbiology, 1991, pp 304–339.

Pathogenicity

At least 14 species have been commonly encountered in human infection. The most recognized of these species are *M. tuberculosis* and *M. leprae*, the causative agents of tuberculosis and leprosy, respectively. In recent years, several factors including the AIDS epidemic, drug resistance, immigration, and nosocomial transmission have contributed to the increased incidence of tuberculosis and disseminated disease due to *M. avium-intracellulare* complex (MAC). Other species, pathogenic to humans, are presented in the chart below.

CLINICAL MANIFESTATIONS OF *MYCOBACTERIUM* SPECIES MOST OFTEN ASSOCIATED WITH DISEASE

GROUP	SPECIES	CLINICAL MANIFESTATION
M. tuberculosis complex	*tuberculosis*	Pulmonary tuberculosis: highly communicable disease of respiratory tract Extrapulmonary tuberculosis (most often in children and AIDS patients), cutaneous tuberculosis, synovitis, lymphadenitis
	bovis	Pulmonary tuberculosis Attenuated strain, bacille Calmette-Guérin (BCG), used for vaccine
Nonphotochromogen (Other than *M. tuberculosis* complex)	*M. avium complex (MAC)*	Pulmonary disease similar to tuberculosis. Most likely to occur in immunocompromised population, in which infection of any organ is possible.
	genavense	Disseminated disease in AIDS population, similar in presentation to MAC
	haemophilum	Cutaneous disease and disseminated disease most commonly in immunocompromised population
	xenopi	Pulmonary disease; rare extrapulmonary infection, with lymph node and bone involvement, usually in immunocompromised individuals
Photochromogen	*kansasii*	Pulmonary disease similar to tuberculosis. Extrapulmonary infection includes cutaneous and musculoskeletal disease, and lymphadenitis in children. These manifestations are not common.
	marinum	Cutaneous and, rarely, disseminated disease as a consequence of exposure to contaminated fish or saltwater
Scotochromogen	*scrofulaceum*	Cervical lymphadenitis in children; less often pulmonary and disseminated disease
Rapid Growers (Growth within 7 days)	*M. fortuitum complex* (*M. fortuitum, M. chelonae, M. abscessus*)	Wound infections, pulmonary and cutaneous disease
Nongrower in vitro	*M. leprae*	Leprosy, or Hansen's disease: cutaneous lesions, infection of peripheral nerves and mucous membranes

MYCOBACTERIA

CHLAMYDIAE, RICKETTSIAE, AND RELATED ORGANISMS

General Characteristics

Chlamydia species, *Rickettsia* species, *Coxiella* species, and *Ehrlichia* species are obligate intracellular parasites, a feature that distinguishes them from other bacteria. All four genera grow well in the yolk sac of embryonated hen eggs. *Chlamydia* are gram negative, nonmotile organisms that form intracellular inclusion bodies on replication within the host cell cytoplasm. These characteristic inclusion bodies are visible using Giemsa, iodine, and fluorescent antibody staining of appropriate specimens.

Clinically significant members of the order Rickettsiales include *Rickettsia* species, *Coxiella* species, and *Ehrlichia* species. *Rickettsia* species and *Coxiella* species are short gram negative rods or coccobacilli. These organisms are only transmitted through arthropod vectors, except for *C. burnetii*, which may also be transmitted via infected milk or by aerosol. Vascular endothelial cells are targets of infection. *Ehrlichia* species are pleomorphic organisms with no well defined life cycle.

Identification

Identification of *Chlamydia* species is through either serologic or nonserologic methods, including culture, which is the optimal method. The most common cultural technique involves inoculation of McCoy cells with the clinical specimen, incubation for 48 to 72 hours, followed by staining with fluorescein conjugated monoclonal antibodies. Commercial cell culture systems are also available, but culture techniques are generally very time consuming and not available in routine laboratories. Nonserologic diagnostic assays include direct fluorescent antibodies (DFAs) (Syva Microtak DFA, Palo Alto, CA), enzyme immunoassays (Abbott Chlamydiazyme EIA), and nucleic acid probes (PCR and ligase chain reaction [LCR]). These diagnostic tools are applicable for *C. trachomatis*, but not *C. pneumoniae* or *C. psittaci* identification. Serologic tests include complement fixation and microimmunofluorescence (micro-IF). For rickettsial infection, isolation is not recommended owing to their high level of infectivity. Serologic techniques such as complement fixation (CF) and microagglutination, and nonserologic assays including ELISA and radioimmunoassay (RIA), are limited in terms of sensitivity, specificity, and availability. Indirect immunofluorescence assay (IFA) is the most widely used serodiagnostic tool (see chart on p 665).

LABORATORY DIAGNOSIS OF THE *CHLAMYDIA* SPECIES AND *RICKETTSIA* SPECIES

TECHNIQUE	*CHLAMYDIA* SPECIES	*RICKETTSIA* SPECIES
Direct Examination	DETECTION OF INCLUSION BODIES: Cytologic examination of conjunctiva of newborns useful with Giemsa staining—not sensitive in adults DETECTION OF *CHLAMYDIA* ELEMENTARY BODIES: DFA of smears using monoclonal antibodies (Syva Microtrak DFA), highly specific Fluorescein conjugated monoclonal antibodies or iodine stain for *C. trachomatis* inclusion bodies in cell culture Monoclonal antibodies or Giemsa's stain for *C. pneumoniae* in cell culture Enzyme immunoassays (Abbott Chlamydia EIA) for *C. trachomatis*—less sensitive and specific than DFA and micro-IF	Immunofluorescence of cutaneous lesions and biopsy specimens—lacks sensitivity Immunofluorescence of circulating endothelial cells using monoclonal antibodies—approximately 50% accurate, not currently available Immunofluorescence of postmortem tissue, especially spleen, kidney, and lung—approximately 66% accurate
Culture	Cycloheximide treated McCoy cells most frequently used for *C. trachomatis* and *C. psittaci* HL and Hep-2 cells used for *C. pneumoniae*	Not recommended
Serologic Assays		
Complement Fixation	Most frequently used serologic test—useful for diagnosis of psittacosis; less useful for diagnosis of trachoma or inclusion bodies	Specific, but not sensitive
ELISA		Highly sensitive in IgM capture assays, but antigens not commercially available
Indirect Immunofluorescence (IFA)		Most widely used test due to sensitivity and cost
Indirect Hemagglutination (IHA)		As sensitive as IFA; however, rickettsial erythrocyte sensitive antigen not commercially available
Immunoperoxidase		Used for scrub typhus in situations outside laboratory
Latex Agglutination		Low sensitivity for convalescent sera More optimal than Weil-Felix test
Microagglutination		Lacks sensitivity
Microimmunofluorescence	Useful for psittacosis, but less useful for lymphogranuloma venereum (LGV), trachoma, genital tract infections, inclusion conjunctivitis; very useful in neonatal infections	
Radioimmunoassay		May be useful for disease of early onset

CHLAMYDIAE, RICKETTSIAE, AND RELATED ORGANISMS

Continued ▶

► Continued **LABORATORY DIAGNOSIS OF THE *CHLAMYDIA* SPECIES AND *RICKETTSIA* SPECIES**

TECHNIQUE	*CHLAMYDIA* SPECIES	*RICKETTSIA* SPECIES
Serologic Assays		
Weil-Felix		Low sensitivity and specificity, but simple to use in routine laboratory
Molecular Assays		
PCR	Available only for *C. trachomatis*—most sensitive method for diagnosis of male urethritis	High specificity, low sensitivity in patients seriously ill with Rocky Mountain spotted fever
LCR	Less sensitive than PCR	
DNA-RNA Hybridization	Commercially available (Gen-Probe), as sensitive as antigen detection techniques, relatively good specificity	

Pathogenicity

CHLAMYDIA SPECIES

Within the *Chlamydia* genus four species are recognized, but only three are associated with human disease, namely, *C. trachomatis*, *C. psittaci*, and *C. pneumoniae*. *C. trachomatis* is the leading bacterial pathogen responsible for sexually transmitted disease, including NGU in males and pelvic inflammatory disease (PID) in females. Other bacterial agents that cause PID are *N. gonorrhoeae*, *M. hominis*, and *U. urealyticum*. A frequent complication associated with *C. trachomatis* infections is infertility and ectopic pregnancy. Other *C. trachomatis* disease syndromes include trachoma, inclusion conjunctivitis, and lymphogranuloma venereum (LGV). *C. psittaci* is responsible for psittacosis, a disease transmitted by birds that may lead to atypical pneumonia. *C. pneumoniae* (formerly known as *Chlamydia* species strain TWAR) causes pneumonia and bronchitis.

RICKETTSIA SPECIES

Rickettsial disease syndromes most often involve the skin and the brain and are characterized by headache, fever, and a rash that usually spreads in the direction of the extremities to the trunk (ehrlichiosis and Q fever are usually rashless). Of exceptional notoriety are typhus, Rocky Mountain spotted fever (RMSF), and Q fever.

Typhus

There are several types of typhus, a disease that is transmitted through arthropod vector. Epidemic typhus is caused by *R. prowazekii* and is transmitted by the body louse *Pediculus humanus*. It occurs most frequently in areas of Africa and South America where there are overcrowding, poverty, and poor sanitary conditions. Symptoms includes high fever (102°–104°F), headache, and a rash that spreads over the entire body except rarely the face, palms, and soles. Endemic or murine typhus is caused by *R. typhi* and is transmitted to humans via a rat flea. The symptoms are similar but milder than those of epidemic typhus. Brill-Zinsser disease is a relapse of epidemic typhus without the characteristic rash. Scrub typhus is caused by *R. tsutsugamushi* and is transmitted to humans by rodent mites. Symptoms include body rash and spleen enlargement in 50% of the cases. Death may result from neurologic and cardiovascular complications.

Rocky Mountain Spotted Fever

RMSF is caused by *R. rickettsii*, which is transmitted primarily to children and young adults by various ticks. Symptoms include headache, fever, and a rash that usually begins at the wrists and spreads to the trunk, extremities, and face. Death occurs within 2 weeks of onset of symptoms when not treated. Other types of spotted fever are presented in the chart.

Q Fever

Coxiella burnetii is the causative agent of Q fever, which is transmitted to humans via infected animals, usually through inhalation of aerosols or dust generated from infected animal byproducts.

Ehrlichiosis

Ehrlichia chaffeensis is the causative agent of human ehrlichiosis, the symptoms of which are similar to those of RMSF, but it is usually rashless. Sennetsu ehrlichiosis occurs primarily in Japan and is a self-limiting disease characterized by fever, headache, chills, and lymphadenopathy. The causative agent is *E. sennetsu*.

CHLAMYDIAL AND RICKETTSIAL INFECTIONS

ORGANISM	DISEASE	SYMPTOMS
C. trachomatis	**OCULAR DISEASE**	
	Trachoma	Chronic disease of conjunctiva and cornea; may cause blindness
	Inclusion conjunctivitis	May occur in infants during passage through infected birth canal. May lead to neonatal pneumonia. In adults, infection is through genital contamination and is usually self-limited.
	SEXUALLY TRANSMITTED DISEASE	
	Lymphogranuloma venereum	Lesions of femoral or inguinal lymph nodes occur. May lead to fistulas and perianal abscesses.
	Nongonococcal urethritis (NGU)	Self-limiting, sexually transmitted disease characterized by white discharge. May develop into epididymitis.
	Pelvic inflammatory disease (PID)	Sexually transmitted disease of women that usually involves the cervix. May result in infertility.

Continued ▶

▶ Continued **CHLAMYDIAL AND RICKETTSIAL INFECTIONS**

ORGANISM	DISEASE	SYMPTOMS
C. psittaci	Psittacosis	Asymptomatic infection that may lead to atypical pneumonia characterized by headache, fever, and cough. Associated with bird (especially poultry) contact.
C. pneumoniae	Pneumonia, bronchitis	Cough, fever, sore throat
R. prowazekii	Typhus	
	Epidemic typhus	High fever, headache, and rash over entire body except face, palms, and soles
	Brill-Zinsser	Relapse of epidemic typhus without rash
R. typhi	Endemic or murine typhus	Similar to epidemic typhus, but milder
R. tsutsugamushi	Scrub Typhus	Body rash and spleen enlargement
R. rickettsii	Spotted Fever	
	Rocky Mountain Spotted fever (RMSF)	Fever, headache, rash that covers the trunk, extremities, and face. Occurs primarily in children and young adults.
R. conorii	Boutonneuse fever	Similar to RMSF except with eschar at site of tick bite and milder symptoms. Occurs primarily near Mediterranean.
R. akari	Rickettsial pox	Mild rickettsial disease
R. australis	Queensland tick typhus	Mild rickettsial disease. Occurs primarily in Australia.
R. sibirica	Siberian tick typhus	Mild rickettsial disease. Occurs primarily in Asia, Siberia.
C. burnetii	Q fever	Fever, headache, malaise. Acquired through inhalation of animal contaminated aerosols or dust.
E. chaffeensis	Human ehrlichiosis	Symptoms similar to those of RMSF, with infrequent rash
E. sennetsu	Sennetsu ehrlichiosis	Fever, headache, chills, and lymphadenopathy. Most frequently occurs in Japan.

ANTIMICROBIAL SUSCEPTIBILITY TESTING

Introduction

Antimicrobial susceptibility testing of microbial isolates is an essential function of the clinical microbiology laboratory. This information provides the clinician with a therapeutic guideline with which to treat the infectious process. Chemotherapeutic agents must be used knowledgeably in order to control disease. In addition, due to the problematic emergence of resistant bacterial strains and their constantly changing susceptibility patterns, testing of individual bacteria against specific antimicrobial agents is critical.

Antimicrobial Assays Used in the Clinical Laboratory

The major antimicrobial assays used in the clinical laboratory are presented in the following table:

SELECTED ANTIMICROBIAL ASSAYS FOR FAST GROWING AEROBIC AND FACULTATIVE ANAEROBIC BACTERIA

PROCEDURE	PURPOSE	NECESSARY SPECIMEN
Minimum Inhibitory Concentration (MIC)	To determine lowest concentration of antibiotic needed to inhibit visible growth	
Broth Dilution	To determine MIC of an isolate	Bacterial isolate
Agar Dilution	To determine MIC for large number of isolates	Bacterial isolate
Minimum Bactericidal Concentration	To determine lowest antibiotic concentration that results in 99.9% kill of bacterial isolate	Bacterial isolate
Disk Diffusion Susceptibility Test	More rapid, cost effective procedure for susceptibility determination. Based on growth inhibition surrounding antibiotic impregnated disks.	Bacterial isolate
E Test	To determine MIC of single antimicrobial agent	Bacterial isolate
Serum Bactericidal Test (Schlichter test)	To determine highest serum dilution needed to kill 99.9% of isolated bacterial pathogen. Important in cases of endocarditis, osteomyelitis, and gram negative bacteremia.	Peak serum Trough serum Bacterial isolate
Serum Antimicrobial Levels	To determine antibiotic concentration in patient's serum. Necessary assay when there is narrow range between therapeutic and toxic antibiotic concentration; especially with aminoglycoside, chloramphenicol, and vancomycin	Peak serum Trough serum

Quantitative Assays

BROTH DILUTION SUSCEPTIBILITY TEST

This test, based on NCCLS M7-T2 guidelines, is an assay used to determine both minimal inhibitory concentration (MIC) and the minimal bactericidal concentration (MBC). For MIC determination, serial dilutions of the antibiotic, in decreasing concentrations, are made in sterile broth. The last tube, which serves as a growth control, is free of antibiotic. A standardized inoculum of the test organism is added to each tube, and the tubes are then incubated at 35°C for 18 to 24 hours. The MIC is the lowest concentration of antibiotic that inhibits bacterial growth in the tube. Microdilution trays and dispensing tools have helped expedite the application of this assay by cutting labor time and cost and by increasing the number of organisms tested. Commercially available systems include MIC-2000 (Dynatech Labs, Alexandria, VA) and Pasco system (Difco Labs, Detroit, MI).

The MBC is the lowest antibiotic concentration that results in the death of the test isolate. This assay is performed by plating broth from the tubes showing no visible growth and incubating the plates overnight at 35°C. The lowest concentration of antibiotic that results in 99.9% killing of the isolate is the MBC.

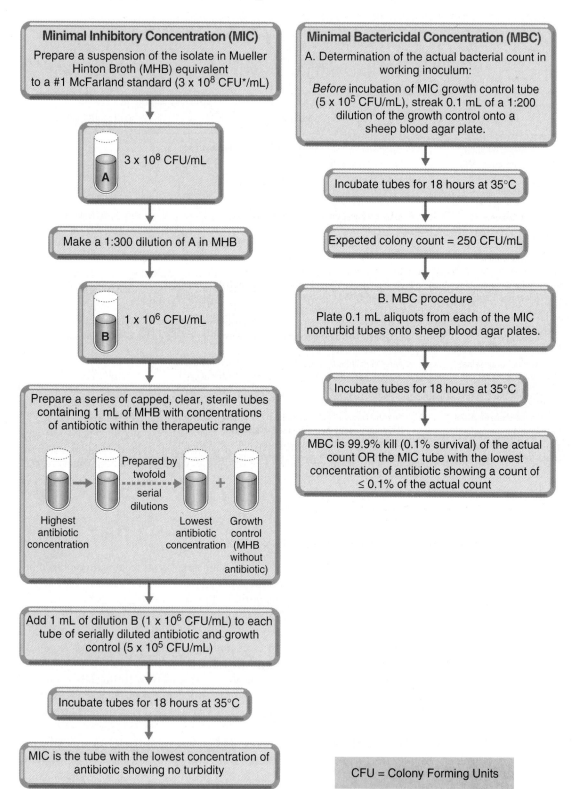

Minimal Inhibitory Concentration (MIC)

Prepare a suspension of the isolate in Mueller Hinton Broth (MHB) equivalent to a #1 McFarland standard (3 x 10^8 CFU*/mL)

3×10^8 CFU/mL
A

Make a 1:300 dilution of A in MHB

1×10^6 CFU/mL
B

Prepare a series of capped, clear, sterile tubes containing 1 mL of MHB with concentrations of antibiotic within the therapeutic range

Prepared by twofold serial dilutions

Highest antibiotic concentration
Lowest antibiotic concentration
Growth control (MHB without antibiotic)

Add 1 mL of dilution B (1 x 10^6 CFU/mL) to each tube of serially diluted antibiotic and growth control (5 x 10^5 CFU/mL)

Incubate tubes for 18 hours at 35°C

MIC is the tube with the lowest concentration of antibiotic showing no turbidity

Minimal Bactericidal Concentration (MBC)

A. Determination of the actual bacterial count in working inoculum:

Before incubation of MIC growth control tube (5 x 10^5 CFU/mL), streak 0.1 mL of a 1:200 dilution of the growth control onto a sheep blood agar plate.

Incubate tubes for 18 hours at 35°C

Expected colony count = 250 CFU/mL

B. MBC procedure

Plate 0.1 mL aliquots from each of the MIC nonturbid tubes onto sheep blood agar plates.

Incubate tubes for 18 hours at 35°C

MBC is 99.9% kill (0.1% survival) of the actual count OR the MIC tube with the lowest concentration of antibiotic showing a count of ≤ 0.1% of the actual count

CFU = Colony Forming Units

AGAR DILUTION SUSCEPTIBILITY TEST

This assay determines the MIC of an antimicrobial agent for a large number of bacterial isolates. A series of antibiotic concentrations, within a therapeutic range, are prepared. Each concentration is then mixed with individual tubes of molten agar, poured into Petri dishes, and allowed to harden. A 36-well seed tray, with as many as 33 standardized bacterial suspensions, is then prepared. Three wells in the seed plate are used for positive controls: *Staphylococcus aureus*, ATCC 25923; *Escherichia coli*, ATCC 25922; and *Pseudomonas aeruginosa*, ATCC 27853. The negative control is an agar plate without antibiotic. Using a 36 prong Steer replicator, standardized aliquots of the test organism are transferred to each of the agar plates. The inoculated plates are incubated at 35°C for 18 hours. The MIC is the lowest antibiotic concentration that inhibits bacterial growth.

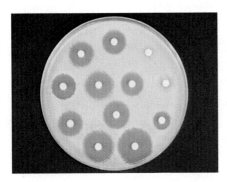

From Mahon CR, Manuselis G: Textbook of Diagnostic Microbiology. Philadelphia, WB Saunders, 1995, p 68.

Qualitative Assays

DISK DIFFUSION SUSCEPTIBILITY TEST

This test is a widely used, cost effective procedure for determining the susceptibility of bacterial pathogens to antimicrobial agents. The Kirby-Bauer method is a standardized disk diffusion susceptibility test for fast growing aerobic and facultative anaerobic organisms. One prepares Mueller-Hinton agar plates (MHAPs) that have been standardized for several factors, namely, depth, pH, and cation content. These plates are seeded with a standardized bacterial test inoculum. Inoculation of the plates is achieved by using a sterile swab that is dipped into standardized bacterial suspension, rimmed against the tube, and streaked for confluency in three directions across the plate. Then disks impregnated with an antimicrobial of known amount (usually 30 μg) are placed on the seeded MHAPs. The plates are inverted and incubated for 18 hours at 35°C (see left). Interpretation of the zones of growth inhibition are based on standards of the National Committee for Clinical Laboratory Standards (NCCLS). These standards are derived from regression curve analysis of the MIC, obtainable blood levels of antibiotic, and zone size.

E TEST

The E test is an effective, widely used assay that determines the MIC of a single antimicrobial agent. This assay is based on the diffusion of an antibiotic gradient from a plastic strip into agar inoculated with the isolated pathogen.

Less Common Antimicrobial Susceptibility Tests

SERUM BACTERICIDAL ASSAY

The serum bactericidal test (SBT), also known as the Schlichter test, determines the highest dilution of patient's serum needed to kill the isolated bacterial pathogen. This information is useful in monitoring therapy in serious infections such as bacterial endocarditis, osteomyelitis, and gram negative bacteremia and when host defense mechanisms are compromised. Based on NCCLS M21-P guidelines, serial twofold dilutions of

ANTIMICROBIAL SUSCEPTIBILITY TESTING

the patient's sera, both trough and peak, are made. A standardized inoculum of the patient's isolated bacterial pathogen is prepared, and an aliquot is added to each dilution. The tubes are then incubated overnight. All tubes that show no visible bacterial growth are subcultured to agar plates. The highest dilution of serum that shows no growth is the serum bactericidal level. A trough titer of 1:32 or greater and a peak titer of 1:64 or greater are optimal. Microdilution methods with microtiter plates may also be used.

SERUM ANTIMICROBIAL LEVELS

This assay determines the concentration of antibiotic present in a patient's serum. Testing is indicated when antibiotics, such as aminoglycosides, chloramphenicol, and vancomycin, have a narrow range between therapeutic and toxic levels. Enzyme immunoassays (EIAs), radioimmunoassays (RIAs), and fluorescent immunoassays are commonly used to determine antimicrobial levels in serum and other body fluids.

Automated Methods for Antimicrobial Susceptibility Testing

VITEK SYSTEM (bioMérieux Vitek, Hazelwood, MO)

This system is capable of determining susceptible, intermediate, or resistant strains as well as MICs for isolated bacterial pathogens that are rapidly growing gram positive and gram negative aerobes or facultative anaerobes. It provides rapid (4 to 10 hours), accurate results for as many as 240 isolates and is a widely used system in most clinical laboratories.

BAXTER MICROSCAN AUTO SCAN WALKAWAY (Baxter Healthcare Corp., West Sacramento, CA)

In addition to determining MICs this system can identify the isolate. This information can be available within 3.5 to 7 hours for gram negative bacteria.

Antimicrobial Susceptibility Testing of Selected Fastidious Microorganisms

MYCOBACTERIA

In determining the susceptibility of *Mycobacterium* species to various antimicrobial agents, an awareness of in vivo or in vitro correlatives as well as drug resistant mutants is necessary. The assay itself is performed by incorporating various concentrations of antimicrobial agents into Middlebrook 7H11 agar and pouring the agar into Petri dishes divided into quadrants. A second method utilizes antimicrobial impregnated filter paper disks within poured agar plates. With this elution technique the antimicrobial agent diffuses from the disk into the agar. Plates are incubated for approximately 3 weeks, and the number of colony forming units (CFUs) is determined.

ANAEROBES

Disk elution techniques, similar to those used for mycobacteria, involve the flow of antimicrobial agents from impregnated filter disks into agar. This methodology is the basis of techniques such as the microbial procedure for anaerobic antimicrobial susceptibility testing as well as automated susceptibility testing systems for anaerobes. The latter include the Autobac (Organon-Technika, Durham, NC). Control strains include *B. fragilis*

ATCC 25285 and *C. prefringens* ATCC 13124. This procedure for the broth-disk elution method for anaerobes is described in the NCCLS publications on anaerobic susceptibility testing.

STREPTOCOCCUS PNEUMONIAE, NEISSERIA GONORRHOEAE, AND HAEMOPHILUS INFLUENZAE

These fastidious bacteria are tested for antimicrobial susceptibility by NCCLS modification of disk diffusion and microdilution methods. The following table provides highlights of this information.

Disk Diffusion Antimicrobial Susceptibility Testing of *Haemophilus influenzae, Streptococcus pneumoniae,* and *Neisseria gonorrhoeae*

ORGANISM	TEST MEDIUM	DISK(S)	ZONE INTERPRETATION (MM)	
			Susceptible	Resistant
S. pneumoniae	Mueller-Hinton agar supplemented with 5% sheep blood	Oxacillin (1 μg)	≥20	≤19
N. gonorrhoeae	GC agar (Difco Labs) supplemented with isovitalex or supplement VX	Penicillin (10 μg)	≥20	≤19
H. influenzae	Haemophilus test medium	Amoxicillin (20 μg)—clavulanic acid (10 μg)	≥20	≤19
		Ampicillin (10 μg)	≥25	
		Cefotaxime (30 μg)	≥26	
		Cefuroxime (30 μg)	≥24	≤20
		Chloramphenicol (30 μg)	≥29	≤25
		Ciprofloxacin (5 μg)	≥21	
		Trimethoprim (1.25μg)-sulfamethoxazole (23.75 μg)	≥16	≤10

Special Considerations in Antimicrobial Susceptibility

β-LACTAMASE PRODUCTION

β-Lactamases are enzymes produced by various gram positive and gram negative bacteria. These enzymes have the ability to inactivate penicillin and cephalosporin antibiotics by cleaving the β-lactam rings. Organisms such as *Staphylococcus* species, *Neisseria gonorrhoeae, Haemophilus* species, *Moraxella* species, *Enterococcus* species, and some *Bacteroides* species are significant β-lactamase producers. Testing these isolates for β-lactamase production is critical. The most commonly used test to detect for β-lactamase production is a chromogenic cephalosporin test using nitrocefin (Cefinase) (Becton Dickinson Microbiology Systems, Sparks, MD). Other tests include iodometric and acidometric methods.

METHICILLIN RESISTANT *STAPHYLOCOCCUS*

Chromosomally mediated heteroresistance of *S. aureus* and *S. epidermidis* to methicillin, oxacillin, and other penicillinase resistant penicillins is difficult to detect using the standard procedures previously described. The following modifications are necessary to enhance detection:

1. Oxacillin is the drug of choice used for testing.
2. Inoculum should be prepared by a direct method using colonies from a fresh overnight plate.
3. Supplementation of Mueller-Hinton broth with 2% sodium chloride and Mueller-Hinton agar with 4% sodium chloride should be done.
4. Plates should be incubated at 35°C, no higher, to enhance growth of resistant strains.
5. Plates are incubated for a full 24 hours.
6. For disk diffusion assays, the periphery of the zone of inhibition should be closely examined using transmitted light.

BIBLIOGRAPHY

General

Baron EJ, Finegold S: Bailey and Scott's Diagnostic Microbiology, 8th ed. Philadelphia, CV Mosby, 1990.

Boyd RF: Medical Microbiology, 5th ed. Boston, Little, Brown, 1995.

Koneman EW, Allen SD, Dowell VR, et al: Color Atlas and Textbook of Diagnostic Microbiology, 3rd ed. Philadelphia, JB Lippincott, 1988.

Koneman EW, et al: Color Atlas and Textbook of Diagnostic Microbiology, 4th ed. Philadelphia, JB Lippincott, 1992.

Koneman EW, Allen SD, Janda WM, et al: Color Atlas and Textbook of Diagnostic Microbiology, 5th ed. Philadelphia, JB Lippincott, 1997.

Mahon CR, Manuselis G: Textbook of Diagnostic Microbiology. Philadelphia, WB Saunders, 1995.

Murray PR, Baron EJ, Pfaller MA, et al, eds: Manual of Clinical Microbiology, 6th ed. Washington, DC, American Society for Microbiology, 1995.

Schaechter M, Medoff G, Eisenstein BI: Mechanisms of Microbial Disease. Philadelphia, Williams & Wilkins, 1993.

Aerobic and Facultative Anaerobic Gram Positive Cocci

Archer GL, Pennell E: Detection of methicillin resistance in staphylococci by using a DNA probe. Antimicrob Agents Chemother 34:1720–1724, 1990.

Baker JS: Comparison of various methods for differentiation of staphylococci and micrococci. J Clin Microbiol 19:875–879, 1984.

Brown S, Fuchs PC: Thiol-dependent streptococci (nutritionally variant streptococci). Chicago, American Society of Clinical Pathologists, 1980.

Chambers HF: Methicillin resistant staphylococci. Clin Microbiol Rev 1:173–186, 1988.

Coykendall AL: Classification and identification of the viridans streptococci. Clin Microbiol Rev 2:315–328, 1989.

Crouch SF, Pearson TA, Parham DM: Comparison of modified Minitek system with Staph-Ident system for species identification of coagulase negative staphylococci. J Clin Microbiol 25:1626–1628, 1987.

Davis TE, Fuller DD: Direct identification of bacterial isolates in blood cultures by using a DNA probe. J Clin Microbiol 29:2192–2196, 1991.

Devriese LA: A review. Identification of pathogenic staphylococci from animals and foods derived from animals. J Appl Bacteriol 49:1–11, 1980.

Enns RK: DNA probes: an overview and comparison with current methods. Lab Med 19:295–300, 1988.

Evans JB: Genus *Aerococcus*. Williams, Hirch, and Cohen 1953, 475[AL]. In Sneath PHA, Mair NS, Sharpe ME, Hott JG, eds: Bergey's Manual of Clinical Microbiology, 5th ed. Washington, DC, American Society for Microbiology, 1986, p 1080.

Facklam RR, Washington AA: In Balows AA, Hausler WJ, Hermann KL, et al, eds: Manual of Clinical Microbiology, 5th ed. Washington, DC: American Society for Microbiology, 1991, p. 250.

Fleurette J, Bes M, Brun Y, et al: Clinical isolates of *Staphylococcus lugdunensis* and *S. schleiferi*: bacteriological characteristics and susceptibility to antimicrobial agents. Res Microbiol 140:107–118, 1989.

Herbert GA, Crowder CG, Hancock GA, et al: Characteristics of coagulase-negative staphylococci that help differentiate these species and other members of the family Micrococcaceae. J Clin Microbiol 26:1939–1949, 1988.

Hinnebusch CJ, Nikolai DM, Bruckner DA: Comparison of API Rapid STREP, Baxter Microscan Rapid Pos ID Panel, BBL Minitek Differential Identification System, IDS RapID STR System, and Vitek GPI to conventional biochemical tests for identification of viridans streptococci. Am J Clin Pathol 96:459–463, 1991.

Kalina AP: The taxonomy and nomenclature of enterococci. Int J Syst Bacteriol 20:185–189, 1970.

Kloos WE, Schleifer KH: *Staphylococcus*. In Sneath PHA, Mair NS, Sharpe ME, et al, eds: Bergey's Manual of Systemic Bacteriology, Vol 2. Washington, DC, American Society for Microbiology, 1986, pp 1013–1015.

Kloos WE: Natural populations of the genus *Staphylococcus*. Annu Rev Microbiol 34:559–592, 1980.

Kloos WE, Schleifer KH: Simplified scheme for routine identification of human *Staphylococcus* species. J Clin Microbiol 1:82–88, 1975.

Lowy FD, Hammer SM: *Staphylococcus epidermidis* infections. Ann Intern Med 99:834–839, 1983.

Mahon CR, Manuselis G: Textbook of Diagnostic Microbiology. Philadelphia, WB Saunders, 1995.

Moellering RC Jr: Emergence of *Enterococcus* as a significant pathogen. Clin Infect Dis 14:1173–1178, 1992.

Parker MT, Ball LC: Streptococci and aerococci associated with systemic infection in man. J Med Microbiol 9:275–302, 1976.

Pfaller MA, Herwaldt LA: Laboratory, clinical, and epidemiological aspects of coagulase-negative staphylococci. Clin Microbiol Rev 1:281–299, 1988.

Ruoff KL: Nutritionally variant streptococci. Clin Microbiol Rev 4:184–190, 1991.

Ruoff KL: Dealing with viridans streptococci in the clinical laboratory: the continuing challenge. Clin Microbiol Newsl 15:73–76, 1993.

Ruoff KL, De La Maza L, Murtaugh MJ, et al: Species identities of enterococci isolated from clinical specimens. J Clin Microbiol 28:435–437, 1990.

Ruoff KL: *Streptococcus*. In Murray PR, Baron EJ, Pfaller MA, et al, eds: Manual of Clinical Microbiology, 6th ed. Washington, DC, American Society for Microbiology, 1995, pp 299–307.

Schaechter M, Medoff G, Eisenstein BI: Mechanisms of Microbial Disease. Baltimore, Williams & Wilkins, 1993, p 188.

Schleifer KH: Family I. Micrococcaceae Prevot 1961, 31[AL]. In Sneath PHA, Mair NS, Sharpe ME, Hott JG, eds: Bergey's Manual of Systemic Bacteriology, Vol 2. Baltimore, Williams & Wilkins, 1986, pp 1003–1035.

Schleifer KH, Kloos WE, Kocur MP: The genus *Micrococcus*. In Starr MP, Stolp H, Truper HG, et al, eds: The Procaryotes: A Handbook of Habitats, Isolation, and Identification of Bacteria. New York, Springer-Verlag, 1981.

Gram Positive Bacilli

Barksdale L: *Corynebacterium diphtheriae* and its relatives. Bacteriol Rev 34:378–422, 1970.

Clarridge JE: When, why, and how far should coryneforms be identified? Clin Microbiol Newsl 8:32–34, 1986.

Coyle MB, Lipsky BA: Coryneform bacteria in infectious disease: clinical and laboratory aspects. Clin Microbiol Rev 3:227–246, 1990.

BIBLIOGRAPHY

Dan J: *Corynebacterium* group JK septicemia: community-acquired infection in an apparently immunocompromised patient. Isr J Med Sci 20:1107–1108, 1984.

Doyle MP, Schoeni JL: Selective enrichment procedure for isolation of *Listeria monocytogenes* from fecal and biological specimens. Appl Environ Microbiol 51:1127–1129, 1986.

Drobniewski FA: *Bacillus cereus* and related species. Clin Microbiol Rev 6:324–338, 1993.

Gavin SE, Leonard RB, Briselden AM, Coyle MB: Evaluation of the rapid CORYNE identification system for *Corynebacterium* species and other coryneforms. J Clin Microbiol 30:1692–1695, 1992.

Gillies RR, Dodds TC: Bacteriology illustrated. In Boyd RF, ed: Medical Microbiology, 5th ed. Boston, Little, Brown, 1976, p 285.

Hayes PS, Feeley JC, Graves LM, et al: Isolation of *Listeria monocytogenes* from raw milk. Appl Environ Microbiol 51:438–440, 1986.

Hayes PS, Graves LM, Swaminathan B, et al: Comparison of three selective enrichment methods for the isolation of *Listeria monocytogenes* from naturally contaminated foods. J Food Prot 55:952–959, 1992.

Holbrook R, Anderson JM: An improved selective and diagnostic medium for the isolation and enumeration of *Bacillus cereus* in foods. Can J Microbiol 263:753–759, 1980.

Lipsky BA, Goldberger AC, Tompkins LS, et al: Infections caused by non-diphtheria *Corynebacteria*. Rev Infect Dis 4:1220–1235, 1982.

Marshall RJ, Johnson E: Corynebacteria: incidence among samples submitted to a clinical laboratory for culture. Med Lab Sci 47:36–41, 1990.

Niaman RE, Lorber B: Listeriosis in adults, a changing pattern: report of eight cases and a review of the literature, 1968–1978. Rev Infect Dis 2:207–227, 1980.

Priest FG: Isolation and identification of aerobic endospore-forming bacteria. In Harwood CR, ed: Bacillus. Biotechnology Handbooks No. 2. New York, Plenum Press, 1989, pp 27–56.

Reboli AC, Farrar WE: *Erysipelothrix rhusiopathiae:* an occupational pathogen. Clin Microbiol Rev 2:354–359, 1989.

Rodriguez LD, Fernandez GS, Garayzabal JF, et al: New methodology for the isolation of *Listeria* microorganisms from heavily contaminated environments. Appl Environ Microbiol 47:1188–1190, 1984.

Schlech WF: Listeriosis: new pieces to an old puzzle. Arch Intern Med 146:459–460, 1986.

Schuchat A, Swaminathan B, Broome CV: Epidemiology of human listeriosis. Clin Microbiol Rev 4:169–183, 1991.

Slifkin M, Gil G, Endwall C: Rapid identification of group JK and other corynebacteria with the Minitek system. J Clin Microbiol 24:177–180, 1986.

Neisseria, Moraxella (Branhamella)

Catlin BW: Branhamaceae fam nov, a proposed family to accommodate the genera *Branhamella* and *Moraxella.* Int J Syst Bacteriol 41:320–323, 1991.

Dalabetta G, Hook EW III: Gonococcal infections. Infect Dis Clin North Am 1:25–54, 1987.

Dillon JR, Pauze M, Yeung KH: Evaluation of eight methods for identification of pathogenic *Neisseria* species: *Neisseria* Kwik, RIM-N, Gonobio-Test, Minitek, Gonochek II, GonoGen, Phadebact Monoclonal GC OMNI test, and Syva MicroTrak test. J Clin Microbiol 26:493–497, 1988.

D'Amato RF, Eriquez LA, Thomfohrde KM, Singerman E: Rapid identification of *Neisseria gonorrhoeae* and *Neisseria meningitidis* by using enzyme profiles. J Clin Microbiol 7:77–81, 1978.

Granato PA, Franz MR: Use of the Gen-Probe PACE system for the detection of *Neisseria gonorrhoeae* in urogenital samples. Diagn Microbiol Infect Dis 13:217–221, 1990.

Herbert DA, Ruskin J: Are the "nonpathogenic" Neisseriae pathogenic? Am J Clin Pathol 75:739–742, 1981.

Janda WM, Bradna JJ, Ruther P: Identification of *Neisseria* spp, *Haemophilus* spp, and other fastidious gram-negative bacteria with the MicroScan *Haemophilus-Neisseria* identification panel. J Clin Microbiol 27:869–873, 1989.

Janda WM, Malloy PJ, Schreckenberger PC: Clinical evaluation of the Vitek *Neisseria-Haemophilus* identification card. J Clin Microbiol 25:37–41, 1987.

Koneman EW, Allen SD, Janda WM, et al: Color Atlas and Textbook of Diagnostic Microbiology, 5th ed. Philadelphia, JB Lippincott, 1997.

Lewis JS, Fakile O, Foss E, et al: Direct DNA probe assay for *Neisseria gonorrhoeae* in pharyngeal and rectal specimens. J Clin Microbiol 28:2783–2785, 1993.

Mahon CR, Manuselis G: Textbook of Diagnostic Microbiology. Philadelphia, WB Saunders, 1995, p 400.

Martin JE Jr, Jackson RL: A biological environmental chamber for the culture of *Neisseria gonorrhoeae.* J Am Vener Dis Assoc 2:28–30, 1985.

Panke ES, Yang LI, Leist PA, et al: Comparison of Gen-Probe DNA probe test and culture for the detection of *Neisseria gonorrhoeae* in endocervical specimens. J Clin Microbiol 29:883–888, 1991.

Rossau RG, van Landschoot A, Gillis M, de Ley J: Taxonomy of Moraxellaceae fam nov, a new bacterial family to accommodate the genera *Moraxella, Acinetobacter,* and *Psychobacter* and related organisms. Int J Syst Bacteriol 41:310–319, 1991.

Enterobacteriaceae

Balows AH, Truper HG, Dworkin M, et al, eds: The Prokaryotes, 2nd ed, Vol 3. Berlin, Springer-Verlag, 1992, pp 2673–2737.

Castillo CB, Bruckner DA: Comparative evaluation of the Eiken and API 20E systems and conventional methods for the identification of members of the family Enterobacteriaceae. J Clin Microbiol 20:754–757, 1984.

DeGiorlami PC, Eichelberger KA, Salfity LC, et al: Evaluation of the AutoScan-3 device for reading microdilution trays. J Clin Microbiol 18:1292–1295, 1983.

DuPont HL, Formal SB, Hornick RB, et al: Pathogenesis of *Escherichia coli* diarrhea. N Engl J Med 285:1–9, 1971.

Edwards PR, Ewing WH: Identification of Enterobacteriaceae, 3rd ed. Minneapolis, Burgess, 1972.

Ewing WH: Edwards and Ewing Identification of Enterobacteriaceae, 4th ed. New York, Elsevier Science, 1986.

Farmer JJ III, Davis RB, Hickman-Brenner FW, et al: Biochemical identification of new species and biogroups of Enterobacteriaceae isolated from clinical specimens. J Clin Microbiol 21:46–76, 1974.

Greene LC, Applebaum PC, Kellogg JA: Evaluation of a two-hour method for screening pathogens from stool specimens. J Clin Microbiol 20:285–287, 1984.

Hickman FW, Farmer JJ III: *Salmonella typhi:* identification, antibiograms, serology, and bacteriophage typing. Am J Med Technol 44:1149–1159, 1978.

Kauffmann F: The Bacteriology of Enterobacteriaceae. Baltimore, Williams & Wilkins, 1966.

Kay BA, Griffin PM, Strockbine NA, Wells JG: Too fast food: bloody diarrhea and death from *Escherichia coli* 0157:H7. Clin Microbiol Newsl 16:17–19, 1994.

Kelly MT, Matsen JM, Morello JA, et al: Collaborative clinical evaluation of the Autobac IDX system for identification of gram-negative bacilli. J Clin Microbiol 19:529–533, 1984.

Murray PR, Gauthier A, Niles A: Evaluation of Quantum II and Rapid E identification systems. J Clin Microbiol 20:509–514, 1984.

Nadler HL, Dolan C, Mele L, et al: Accuracy and reproducibility of the AutoMicrobic system gram-negative general susceptibility-plus card for testing selected challenge organisms. J Clin Microbiol 22:336–338, 1985.

Overman TL, Pumley D, Overman SB, et al: Comparison of the API Rapid E four-hour system with API 20E overnight system for the identification of routine isolates of the family Enterobacteriaceae. J Clin Microbiol 21:542–545, 1985.

Rhoden DL, Smith PB, Baker CN, et al: AutoScan-4 system for the identification of gram-negative bacilli. J Clin Microbiol 22:915–918, 1985.

Sack RB: Human diarrheal disease caused by enterotoxigenic *Escherechia coli.* Annu Rev Microbiol 29:333–353, 1975.

Schaberg DR: Major trends in microbial etiology of nosocomial infections. Ann Intern Med 91(suppl 3B):72S–75S, 1991.

Woolfrey BF, Lally RT, Ederer MN, et al: Evaluation of the AutoMicrobic system for identification and susceptibility testing of gram-negative bacilli. J Clin Microbiol 20:1053–1059, 1984.

Nonfermentative Gram Negative Bacilli

Baron EJ, Finegold S: Bailey and Scott's Diagnostic Microbiology, 8th ed. Philadelphia, CV Mosby, 1990, p 389.

Burdash NM, Bannister ER, Manos JP, West ME: A comparison of four commercial systems for the identification of non-fermentative gram-negative bacilli. Am J Clin Pathol 73:564–569, 1980.

Clark WA, Hollis DG, Weaver RE, Riley P: Identification of Unusual Pathogenic Gram-Negative Aerobic and Facultatively Anaerobic Bacteria. Atlanta, Centers for Disease Control, 1984.

Freney J, Hansen W, Ploton C, et al: Septicemia caused by *Sphingobacterium multivorum.* J Clin Microbiol 25:1126, 1987.

Gerner-Smidt P, Tjernberg I, Ursing J: Reliability of phenotypic tests for identification of *Acinetobacter* species. J Clin Microbiol 29:277–282, 1991.

Gilardi GL, ed: Nonfermentative Gram-negative Rods: Laboratory Identification and Clinical Aspects. New York, Marcel Dekker, 1985.

Gilardi GL: *Flavobacterium.* Clin Microbiol Newsl 8:143, 1986.

Gilardi GL: Identification of glucose non-fermenting gram-negative rods. New York, Department of Laboratories, North General Hospital, 1989.

Gilligan PH, Gage PA, Bradshaw LM, et al: Isolation medium for the recovery of *Pseudomonas cepacia* from respiratory secretions of patients with cystic fibrosis. J Clin Microbiol 22:5–8, 1985.

Holmes BC, Pinning A, Dawson CA: A probability matrix for the identification of gram-negative, aerobic, non-fermentative bacteria that grow on nutrient agar. J Gen Microbiol 132:1827–1842, 1986.

Kim JH, Cooper RA, Welty-Wolf KE, et al: *Pseudomonas putrefaciens* bacteremia. Rev Infect Dis 11:97–104, 1989.

Kitch TT, Jacobs MR, Applebaum PC: Evaluation of the 4-hour RapID NF Plus method for identification of 345 gram-negative nonfermentative rods. J Clin Microbiol 30:1267–1270, 1992.

Krieg NR, Holt JG, eds: Bergey's Manual of Systematic Bacteriology, Vol 1, Sec 4. Baltimore, Williams & Wilkins, p 140.

Martin R, Siavoshi F, McDougal DL: Comparison of rapid NFT system and conventional methods for identification of nonsaccharolytic gram-negative bacteria. J Clin Microbiol 24:1089–1092, 1986.

Morrison AJ Jr, Wenzel RP: Epidemiology of infections due to *Pseudomonas aeruginosa.* Rev Infect Dis 6(suppl 3):S627–S642, 1984.

Osterhout GJ, Shull VH, Dick JD: Identification of clinical isolates of gram-negative nonfermentative bacteria by an automated cellular fatty acid identification system. J Clin Microbiol 29:1822–1830, 1991.

Pfaller MA, Sahm D, O'Hara C, et al: Comparison of the autoSCAN-W/A rapid bacterial identification system and the Vitek AutoMicrobic system for identification of gram-negative bacilli. J Clin Microbiol 29:2322–2325, 1991.

Pickett MJ: Methods for identification of flavobacteria. J Clin Microbiol 27:2309–2315, 1989.

Plorde JJ, Gates JA, Carlson LG, Tenover FC: Critical evaluation of the AutoMicrobic system gram-negative identification card for the identification of glucose-non-fermenting gram-negative rods. J Clin Microbiol 23:251–257, 1986.

Schaberg GL, Culver DH, Gaynes RP: Major trends in the microbial etiology of nosocomial infection. Am J Med 91(suppl 3B):72S–75S, 1991.

Tablan OC, Carlson LA, Cusick LB, et al: Laboratory proficiency test results on use of selective media for isolating *Pseudomonas cepacia* from simulated sputum specimens of patients with cystic fibrosis. J Clin Microbiol 25:485–487, 1987.

Tenover FC, Mizuki TS, Carlson LG: Evaluation of autoSCAN-W/A automated microbiology system for the identification of non-glucose-fermenting gram-negative bacilli. J Clin Microbiol 28:1628–1634, 1990.

Vibrio, Aeromonas, Plesiomonas

Abbott SL, Cheung WKW, Kroske-Bystrom S, et al: Identification of *Aeromonas* strains to the genospecies level in the clinical laboratory. J Clin Microbiol 30:1261–1266, 1992.

Almeida RJ, Hickman-Brenner FW, Sowers ED, et al: Comparison of a latex agglutination assay and an enzyme-linked immunosorbent assay for detecting cholera toxin. J Clin Microbiol 28:128–130, 1990.

Altwegg M, Steigerwalt AG, Altwegg-Bissis R, et al: Biochemical identification of *Aeromonas* genospecies isolated from humans. J Clin Microbiol 28:258–264, 1991.

de la Morena ML, Van R, Singh K, et al: Diarrhea associated with *Aeromonas* species in children in day care centers. J Infect Dis 168:215–218, 1993.

Janda JM, Powers C, Bryant RG, Abbott SL: Current perspectives on the epidemiology and pathogenesis of clinically significant *Vibrio* spp. Clin Microbiol Rev 1:245–267, 1988.

Janda JM: Recent advances in the study of taxonomy, pathogenicity, and infectious syndromes associated with the genus *Aeromonas*. Clin Microbiol Rev 4:397–410, 1991.

Johnston JM, Becker SF, McFarland LM: Gastroenteritis in patients with stool isolates of *Vibrio vulnificus*. Am J Med 80:336–338, 1986.

Manafi M, Rotter ML: Enzymatic profile of *Plesiomonas shigelloides*. J Microbiol Methods 16:175–180, 1992.

Martinez-Murcia AJ, Benlloch S, Collins MD: Phylogenetic interrelationships of members of the genera *Aeromonas* and *Plesiomonas* as determined by 16S ribosomal DNA sequencing: lack of congruence with results of DNA-DNA hybridizations. Int J Syst Bacteriol 42:412–421, 1992.

Ramamurthy T, Pal A, Bag PK, et al: Detection of cholera toxin gene in stool specimens by polymerase chain reaction: comparison with bead enzyme-linked immunosorbent assay and culture method for laboratory diagnosis of cholera. J Clin Microbiol 31:3068–3070, 1993.

Safrin S, Morris JG Jr, Adams M, et al: Non-0:1 *Vibrio cholera* bacteremia: case report and review. Rev Infect Dis 10:1012–1017, 1988.

Tison DL, Kelly MT: *Vibrio* species of medical importance. Diagn Microbiol Infect Dis 2:263–276, 1984.

Wright AC, Guo Y, Johnson JP, et al: Development and testing of a nonradioactive DNA oligonucleotide probe that is specific for *Vibrio cholerae* cholera toxin. J Clin Microbiol 30:2302–2306, 1992.

Miscellaneous Bacterial Species Associated with Human Disease

Banai M, Mayer I, Cohen A: Isolation, identification and characterization in Israel of *Brucella melitensis* biovar 1 atypical strains susceptible to dyes and penicillin, indicating the evolution of a new variant. J Clin Microbiol 28:1057–1059, 1990.

Campbell PB, Masters PL, Rohwedder E: Whooping cough diagnosis: a clinical evaluation of complementing and immunofluorescence with enzyme-linked immunosorbent assay of pertussis immunoglobin A in nasopharyngeal secretions. J Med Microbiol 27:247–254, 1988.

Catlin W: *Gardnerella vaginalis*: characteristics, clinical considerations, and controversies. Clin Microbiol Rev 5:213–237, 1992.

Chen CK, Wilson ME: *Eikenella corrodens* in human oral and non-oral infections: a review. J Periodontol 63:941–953, 1992.

Chooromoney KN, Hampson DJ, Eamens GJ, Turner MJ: Analysis of *Erysipelothrix rhusiopathiae* and *Erysipelothrix tonsillorum* by multilocus enzyme electrophoresis. J Clin Microbiol 32:371–376, 1994.

Clark WA, Hollis DG, Weaver RE, Riley P: Identification of Unusual Pathogenic Gram-Negative Aerobic and Facultatively Anaerobic Bacteria. Atlanta, Centers for Disease Control, 1984.

Dewhirst FE, Paster BJ, Olsen I, Fraser GJ: Phylogeny of 54 representative strains of species in the family Pasteurellaceae as determined by comparison of 16S rRNA sequences. J Bacteriol 21:39–42, 1992.

Edwards R, Finch RG: Characterization and antibiotic susceptibilities of *Streptobacillus moniliformis*. J Clin Microbiol 27:2606–2608, 1986.

Etemadi H, Raissadat A, Pickett MJ, et al: Isolation of *Brucella* spp from clinical specimens. J Clin Microbiol 20:586, 1984.

Evans ME, Gregory DW, Schaffner W, McGee ZA: Tularemia: a 30 year experience with 88 cases. Medicine 64:251–269, 1985.

Ewanowich CA, Chui LWL, Paranchych MG, et al: Major outbreak of pertussis in northern Alberta, Canada: an analysis of discrepant direct fluorescent-antibody and culture results by using polymerase chain reaction methodology. J Clin Microbiol 31:1715–1725, 1993.

Farizo KM, Cochi SL, Zell ER, et al: Epidemiological features of pertussis in the United States, 1980–1989. Clin Infect Dis 14:708–719, 1992.

Gotuzzo E, Carrillo C, Guerra J, Llosa L: An evaluation of diagnostic methods for brucellosis—the value of bone marrow culture. J Infect Dis 153:122–125, 1986.

Halperin SA, Bortolussi R, Wort AJ: Evaluation of culture, immunofluorescence and serology for the diagnosis of pertussis. J Clin Microbiol 27:752–757, 1989.

Herman L, DeRidder H: Identification of *Brucella* spp by using the polymerase chain reaction. Appl Environ Microbiol 58:2099–2101, 1992.

Holt SC, Kinder SA: Genus II. *Capnocytophaga* Leadbetter, Holt and Socransky 1982. In Staley JT, Bryant MP, Pfennig N, Holt JG, eds: Bergey's Manual of Systematic Bacteriology, Vol 3. Baltimore, Williams & Wilkins, 1989, pp 2052–2058.

BIBLIOGRAPHY

Khwaja KJ, Parish P, Aldred MJ, Wade WG: Protein profiles of *Capnocytophagia* species. J Appl Bacteriol 68:385–390, 1990.

Lambe DW Jr, McPhedran AW, Mertz JA, Stewart P: *Streptobacillus moniliformis* isolated from a case of Haverhill fever: biochemical characterization and inhibitory effect of sodium polyanethol sulfonate. Am J Clin Pathol 60:854–860, 1973.

Morrison VA, Wagner KF: Clinical manifestations of *Kingella kingae* infections: case report and review. Rev Infect Dis 11:776–782, 1989.

Moyer NP, Evans GM, Pigott NE, et al: Comparison of serologic screening tests for brucellosis. J Clin Microbiol 25:1969–1972, 1987.

Peiris V, Fraser S, Fairhurst M, et al: Laboratory diagnosis of *Brucella* infection: some pitfalls. Lancet 339:1415, 1992.

Sato T, Fujita H, Ohara Y, Homma M: Microagglutination test for early and specific serodiagnosis of tularemia. J Clin Microbiol 28:2372–2374, 1990.

Ti TY, Tan WC, Chong APY, Lee EH: Nonfatal and fatal infections caused by *Chromobacterium violaceum*. Clin Infect Dis 17:505–507, 1993.

Westerman EL, McDonald J: Tularemia pneumonia mimicking Legionnaires' disease: isolation of organism on CYE agar and successful treatment with erythromycin. South Med J 76:1169–1170, 1986.

Young EJ: Serologic diagnosis of human brucellosis: analysis of 214 cases by agglutination tests and review of the literature. Rev Infect Dis 13:359–372, 1991.

Campylobacter, Arcobacter, Helicobacter, and Spirillum

Baker CN: The E-test and *Campylobacter jejuni*. Diagn Microbiol Infect Dis 15:469–472, 1992.

Barrett TJ, Patton CM, Morris GK: Differentiation of *Campylobacter* species using phenotypic characterization. Lab Med 19:96–102, 1988.

Bell GD: Clinical aspects of infection with *Helicobacter pylori*. Commun Dis Rep 3:R59–R62, 1993.

Blaser MJ: *Helicobacter pylori:* its role in disease. Clin Infect Dis 15:386–393, 1992.

Endtz HP, Ruijs CJ, Zwinderman AH, et al: Comparison of six media, including a semisolid agar, for the isolation of various *Campylobacter* species from stool specimens. J Clin Microbiol 29:1007–1010, 1991.

Goodwin CS, Worsley BW: The *Helicobacter* genus: the history of *H. pylori* and taxonomy of current species. In Goodwin CS, Worsley BW, eds: *Helicobacter pylori:* Biology and Clinical Practice. Boca Raton, FL, CRC Press, 1993.

Goodwin CS, Worsley BW: Microbiology of *Helicobacter pylori*. Gastroenterol Clin North Am 22:5–19, 1993.

Gun-Monro J, Rennie RP, Thornley JH, et al: Laboratory and clinical evaluation of isolation media for *Campylobacter jejuni*. J Clin Microbiol 25:2274–2277, 1987.

Hodinka RL, Gilligan PH: Evaluation of the Campyslide agglutination test for confirmatory identification of selected *Campylobacter* species. J Clin Microbiol 26:47–49, 1988.

Hutchinson DN, Bolton FJ: Improved blood free selective medium for the isolation of *Campylobacter jejuni* from faecal specimens. J Clin Pathol 37:956–957, 1984.

Johnson CC, Finegold SM: Uncommonly encountered motile, anaerobic gram-negative bacilli associated with infection. Rev Infect Dis 9:1150–1162, 1987.

Koneman EW, Elmer SD, Allen VR, et al: Color Atlas and Textbook of Diagnostic Microbiology, 3rd ed. Philadelphia, JB Lippincott, 1988, p 230.

Nachamkin I, Barbagallo S: Culture confirmation of *Campylobacter* spp by latex agglutination. J Clin Microbiol 28:817–818, 1990.

Owens RJ: Microbiological aspects of *Helicobacter pylori* infection. Commun Dis Rep 3:R51–R56, 1993.

Parsonnet J: *Helicobacter pylori* and gastric cancer. Gastroenterol Clin North Am 22:89–104, 1993.

Schembri MA, Lin SK, Lambert JR: Comparison of commercial diagnostic tests for *Helicobacter pylori* antibodies. J Clin Microbiol 31:2621–2624, 1993.

Haemophilus

Albritton WL: Infections due to *Haemophilus* species other than *H. influenzae*. Annu Rev Microbiol 36:199–216, 1982.

Barbe G, Babolat M, Monget D, Freney J: Evaluation of API NH, a new 2-hour system for identification of *Neisseria* and *Haemophilus* species and *Moraxella catarrhalis* in a routine clinical laboratory. J Clin Microbiol 32:187–189, 1994.

Bieger RC, Brewer NS, Washington JA: *Haemophilus aphrophilus:* a microbiologic and clinical review and report of 42 cases. Medicine 57:345–355, 1978.

Chui L, Albritton W, Paster B, et al: Development of the polymerase chain reaction for diagnosis of chancroid. J Clin Microbiol 31:659–664, 1993.

Collins JK, Kelly MT: Comparison of Phadebact coagglutination, Bactigen latex agglutination, and counterimmunoelectrophoresis for detection of *Haemophilus influenzae* type b antigens in spinal fluid. J Clin Microbiol 17:1005–1008, 1983.

Daly JA, Clifton NL, Seskin KC, Gooch WM III: Use of rapid, nonradioactive DNA probes in culture confirmation tests to detect *Streptococcus agalactiae, Haemophilus influenzae,* and *Enterococcus* spp from pediatric patients with significant infections. J Clin Microbiol 29:80–82, 1991.

Doern GV, Chapin KC: Laboratory identification of *Haemophilus influenzae:* effects of basal media on the results of satellitism test and evaluation of the RapID NH system. J Clin Microbiol 20:599–601, 1984.

Durfee KK, Alexander H, Smith JP, et al: Comparison of methods for the identification of *Haemophilus influenzae.* Lab Med 17:275–277, 1986.

Edberg SE, Melton E, Singer JM: Rapid biochemical characterization of *Haemophilus* species by using the Micro-ID. J Clin Microbiol 11:22–26, 1980.

Hannah P, Greenwood JR: Isolation and rapid identification of *Haemophilus ducreyi.* J Clin Microbiol 16:861–864, 1982.

Ingram DL, Pearson AW, Occhiuti AR: Detection of bacterial antigens in body fluids with the Wellcogen *Haemophilus influenzae* b, *Streptococcus pneumoniae,* and *Neisseria meningitidis* (ACYW135) latex agglutination tests. J Clin Microbiol 18:1119–1121, 1983.

Kilian M: *Haemophilus.* In Balows A, Hausler WJ Jr, Herrmann KL, et al, eds: Manual of Clinical Microbiology, 5th ed. Washington, DC, American Society for Microbiology, 1991, pp 463–470.

Kilian M, Sorenson I, Frederiksen W: Biochemical characterization of 130 recent isolates from *Haemophilus influenzae* meningitis. J Clin Microbiol 9:409–412, 1979.

Macone AB, Arakere G, Letourneau JM, et al: Comparison of a new, rapid enzyme-linked immunosorbent assay with latex particle agglutination for the detection of *Haemophilus influenzae* type b infections. J Clin Microbiol 21:711–714, 1985.

Marcon MJ, Hamoudi AC, Cannon HJ: Comparative laboratory evaluation of three antigen detection methods for diagnosis of *Haemophilus influenzae* type b disease. J Clin Microbiol 19:333–337, 1984.

Möller LVM, Ruijs GJ, Heijerman HGM, et al: *Haemophilus influenzae* is frequently detected with monoclonal antibody 8BD9 in sputum samples from patients with cystic fibrosis. J Clin Microbiol 30:1952–1954, 1992.

Morse TF, Apicella MAA: Nontypable *Haemophilus influenzae:* a review of clinical aspects, surface antigens, and the human immune response to infection. Rev Infect Dis 9:1–15, 1987.

Oberhofer TR, Back AE: Isolation and cultivation of *Haemophilus ducreyi.* J Clin Microbiol 15:625–629, 1982.

Palladino S, Leahy BJ, Newall TL: Comparison of the RIM-H rapid identification kit for the identification of *Haemophilus* spp. J Clin Microbiol 28:1862–1863, 1990.

Rennie R, Gordon T, Yaschuk Y, et al: Laboratory and clinical evaluations of media for the primary isolation of *Haemophilus* species. J Clin Microbiol 30:1917–1921, 1992.

Riera L: Detection of *Haemophilus influenzae* type b antigenuria by Bactigen and Phadebact kits. J Clin Microbiol 21:638–640, 1985.

Turk DC: The pathogenicity of *Haemophilus influenzae.* J Med Microbiol 18:1–16, 1984.

Legionella

Dowling JN, Saha AK, Glew RH: Virulence factors of the family Legionellaceae. Microbiol Rev 56:32–60, 1992.

Edelstein PH, Meyer RD, Finegold SM: Laboratory diagnosis of Legionnaire's disease. Am Rev Respir Dis 121:317–327, 1980.

Edelstein PH, Edelstein MAC: Evaluation of the Merifluor-*Legionella* immunofluorescent reagent for identifying and detecting 21 *Legionella* species. J Clin Microbiol 27:2455–2458, 1989.

Edelstein PH, Edelstein MAC: Comparison of three buffers used in the formulation of buffered charcoal yeast extract medium. J Clin Microbiol 31:3329–3330, 1993.

Fraser DW, Tsai TR, Orenstein W, et al: Legionnaire's disease: description of an epidemic of pneumonia. N Engl J Med 297:1189–1197, 1977.

Garrity GM, Brown A, Vickers RM: *Tatlockia* and *Fluoribacter:* two new genera of organisms resembling *Legionella pneumophila.* Int J System Bacteriol 30:609–614, 1980.

Kaufmann AF, McDade JE, Patton CM, et al: Pontiac fever: isolation of the etiologic agent *(Legionella pneumophila)* and demonstration of its mode of transmission. Am J Epidemiol 114:337–347, 1981.

Keathey JD, Winn WC Jr: Comparison of media for recovery of clinical isolates of *Legionella pneumophila.* Am J Clin Pathol 83:498–499, 1985.

Kirby BD, Snyder KM, Meyer RD, Finegold SM: Legionnaire's disease: report of sixty-five nosocomially acquired cases and review of the literature. Medicine (Baltimore) 59:188–205, 1980.

Lee TC, Vickers KM, Yu VL, Wagener MM: Growth of 28 *Legionella* species on selective culture media: a comparative study. J Clin Microbiol 31:2764–2768, 1993.

Pasculle AW, Veto GE, Krystofiak S, et al: Laboratory and clinical evaluation of a commercial DNA probe for the detection of *Legionella* spp *Legionella pneumophila.* J Clin Microbiol 27:2350–2358, 1989.

Sathapatayavongs B, Kohler RB, Wheat LJ, et al: Rapid diagnosis of Legionnaire's disease by latex agglutination. Am Rev Respir Dis 127:559–562, 1983.

Tenover FC, Carlson L, Goldstein L, et al: Confirmation of *Legionella pneumophila* cultures with a fluorescein-labeled monoclonal antibody. J Clin Microbiol 21:983–984, 1985.

Wilkinson HW, Sampson JS, Plikaytis BB: Evaluation of a commercial gene probe for identification of *Legionella* cultures. J Clin Microbiol 23:217–220, 1986.

Anaerobic Bacteria

Brook I: Recovery of anaerobic bacteria from clinical specimens in 12 years at two military hospitals. J Clin Microbiol 26:1181–1188, 1988.

Brook I, Frazier EH: Significant recovery of nonsporulating anaerobic rods from clinical specimens. Clin Infect Dis 16:476–480, 1993.

Brook I: Comparison of two transport systems for recovery of aerobic and anaerobic bacteria from abscesses. J Clin Microbiol 24:2020–2022, 1987.

Burlage RS, Ellner PD: Comparison of PRAS II, AN-Ident, and RapID-ANA systems for identification of anaerobic bacteria. J Clin Microbiol 22:32–35, 1985.

Celig DM, Schreckenberger PC: Clinical evaluation of the RapID-ANA II panel for identification of anaerobic bacteria. J Clin Microbiol 29:457–462, 1991.

Engelkirk PG, Duben-Engelkirk J, Dowell VR Jr: Principles and Practice of Clinical Anaerobic Bacteriology. Belmont, CA, Star Publishing, 1992.

Finegold SM: Anaerobic Bacteria in Human Disease. New York, Academic Press, 1977.

Finegold SM, Baron EJ, Wexler HM: A Clinical Guide to Anaerobic Infections. Belmont, CA, Star Publishing, 1991.

Finegold SM, George WL, eds: Anaerobic Infections in Humans. San Diego, CA, Academic Press, 1989.

Holdeman LV, Cato EP, Moore WEC, eds: Anaerobic Laboratory Manual, 4th ed. Blacksburg, VA, Virginia Polytechnic Institute and State University, 1977.

Kitch TT, Applebaum PC: Accuracy and reproducibility of the 4-hour ATB 32A method for anaerobe identification. J Clin Microbiol 27:2509–2513, 1989.

Koneman EW, Elmer SD, Allen VR, et al: Color Atlas and Textbook of Diagnostic Microbiology, 3rd ed. Philadelphia, JB Lippincott, 1988, pp 396–397.

Li N, Hashimoto Y, Adnan S, et al: Three new species of the genus *Peptostreptococcus* isolated from humans: *Peptostreptococcus vaginalis* sp nov, *Peptostreptococcus lacrimalis* sp nov, and *Peptostreptococcus lactolyticus* sp nov. Int J Syst Bacteriol 42:602–605, 1992.

Mahon CR, Manuselis G: Textbook of Diagnostic Microbiology. Philadelphia, WB Saunders, 1995.

Murray PR, Weber CJ, Niles AC: Comparative evaluation of three identification systems for anaerobes. J Clin Microbiol 22:52–55, 1985.

Ng J, Ng LK, Chow AW, Dillon JR: Identification of five *Peptostreptococcus* species isolated predominantly from the female genital tract by using the rapid ID32A system. J Clin Microbiol 32:1302–1307, 1994.

Quentin C, Desailey-Chanson MA, Bebear C: Evaluation of AN-Ident. J Clin Microbiol 29:231–235, 1991.

Schreckenberger PC, Celig DM, Janda WM: Clinical evaluation of the Vitek ANI card for identification of anaerobic bacteria. J Clin Microbiol 26:225–230, 1988.
Shah HN, Gharbia SE: Biochemical and chemical studies on strains designated *Prevotella intermedia* and proposal of a new pigmented species, *Prevotella nigrescens* sp nov. Int J Syst Bacteriol 42:542–546, 1992.
Summanen P, Jousimies-Somer H: Comparative evaluation of RapID ANA and API 20A for identification of anaerobic bacteria. Eur J Clin Microbiol Infect Dis 7:771–775, 1988.

Spirochetes

Barbour AG: Laboratory aspects of Lyme borreliosis. Clin Microbiol Rev 1:399–414, 1988.
Barbour AG: The diagnosis of Lyme disease: rewards and perils. Ann Intern Med 110:501–502, 1989.
Barbour AG, Hayes SF: Biology of *Borrelia* species. Microbiol Rev 50:381–400, 1986.
Duffy J, Mertz LE, Wobig GH, Katzmann JA: Diagnosing Lyme disease: the contribution of serologic testing. Mayo Clin Proc 63:1116–1121, 1988.
Felsenfeld O: *Borrelia.* Strains, Vectors, Human and Animal Borreliosis. St. Louis, Warren H Green, 1971, p 180.
Hanff PA, Fernandez C, Folds JD: Percoll-purified *T. pallidum*, an improved fluorescent treponemal antibody–absorbed antigen. J Clin Microbiol 23:980–982, 1986.
Hook EW III, Roddy RE, Lukehart SA, et al: Detection of *Treponema pallidum* in lesion exudate with a pathogen-specific monoclonal antibody. J Clin Microbiol 22:241–244, 1985.
Hyde FW, Johnson RC: Genetic relationship of Lyme disease spirochetes to *Borrelia, Treponema,* and *Leptospira* species. J Clin Microbiol 20:151–154, 1984.
Johnson RC: The spirochetes. Annu Rev Microbiol 31:89–106, 1977.
Larsen SA, Hambie EA, Pettit DE, et al: Specificity, sensitivity and reproducibility among the fluorescent treponemal antibody–absorption test, the microhemagglutination assay for *Treponema pallidum* antibodies, and the hemagglutination treponemal test for syphilis. J Clin Microbiol 14:441–445, 1981.
Malloy DC, Nauman RK, Paxton H: Detection of *Borrelia burgdorferi* using the polymerase chain reaction. J Clin Microbiol 28:1089–1093.
Manca N, Columrita VD, Ravizzola G, et al: Radiometric method for rapid detection of *Leptospira* organisms. J Clin Microbiol 23:401–403, 1986.
Merien F, Amouriax P, Perolat P, et al: Polymerase chain reaction detection of *Leptospira* spp in clinical samples. J Clin Microbiol 30:2219–2224, 1992.
Miller BC, Chappel RJ, Adler B: Detection of leptospires in biological fluids using DNA hybridization. Vet Microbiol 15:71–78, 1987.
Millner AR, Jackson KB, Woodruff K, et al: Enzyme linked immunosorbent assay for determining specific immunoglobulin in infections caused by *Leptospira interrogans* serovar *hardjo.* J Clin Microbiol 22:539–542, 1985.
Norgard MV, Fortgang JC, White KE, et al: Sensitivity and specificity of monoclonal antibodies directed against antigenic determinants of *Treponema pallidum* Nichols in the diagnosis of syphilis. J Clin Microbiol 20:711–717, 1984.
Schmid GP, Steigerwalt AG, Johnson SE, et al: DNA characterization of the spirochete that caused Lyme disease. J Clin Microbiol 20:155–158, 1984.
Schwan TG, Simpson WJ, Schrumpf ME, Karstens RH: Identification of *Borrelia burgdorferi* and *B. hermsii* using DNA hybridization probes. J Clin Microbiol 27:1734–1738, 1989.
Skilbeck NW, Chappel RJ: Immunogold silver staining for visualization of leptospires in histologic sections. J Clin Microbiol 25:85–86, 1987.
Soneshine DE: Biology of Ticks. New York, Oxford University Press, 1991.
Wilkinson HW: Immunodiagnostic tests for Lyme disease. Yale J Biol Med 57:567–572, 1984.

Mycoplasma, Ureaplasma

Barker CE, Sillis M, Wreghitt TG: Evaluation of Serodia Myco II particle agglutination test for detection of *Mycoplasma pneumoniae* antibody: comparison with μ-capture ELISA and indirect immunofluorescence. J Clin Pathol 43:163–165, 1990.
Bernet C, Garret M, de Barbeyrac B, et al: Detection of *Mycoplasm pneumoniae* by using the polymerase chain reaction. J Clin Microbiol 27:2492–2496, 1989.

Blanchard A, Hentschel J, Duffy J, et al: Detection of *Ureaplasma urealyticum* by polymerase chain reaction in the urogenital tract of adults, in amniotic fluid, and in the respiratory tract of newborns. Clin Infect Dis 17(suppl 1):148–153, 1993.

Clyde WA: Clinical overview of typical *Mycoplasma pneumoniae* infections. Clin Infect Dis 17(suppl 1):32–36, 1993.

de Barbeyrac B, Bernet-Poggi C, Febrer F, et al: Detection of *Mycoplasma genitalium* in clinical samples by polymerase chain reaction. Clin Infect Dis 17(suppl 1):83–39, 1993.

Eschenbach DA: *Ureaplasma urealyticum* and premature birth. Clin Infect Dis 17(suppl 1):100–106, 1993.

Foy HM: Infections caused by *Mycoplasma pneumoniae* and possible carrier states in different populations of patients. Clin Infect Dis 17(suppl 1):37–46, 1993.

Freundt EA: Culture media for classic mycoplasmas. In Razin S, Tully JG, eds: Methods in Mycoplasmology, Vol 1. New York, Academic Press, 1983, pp 127–135.

Harris R, Marmion BP, Varkanis G, et al: Laboratory diagnosis of *M. pneumoniae* infection. II. Comparison of methods for direct detection of specific antigens or nucleic acid sequences in respiratory exudates. Epidemiol Infect 101:685–694, 1988.

Jacobs E: Serologic diagnosis of *Mycoplasma pneumoniae* infections: a critical review of current procedures. Clin Infect Dis 17(suppl 1):79–82, 1993.

Kenny GE: Serodiagnosis. In Maniloff J, McElhaney RN, Finch LR, Baseman JB, eds: Mycoplasmas: Molecular Biology and Pathogenesis. Washington, DC, American Society for Microbiology, 1992, pp 505–512.

Kok TW, Varkanis G, Marmion BP, Martin J, et al: Laboratory diagnosis of *Mycoplasma pneumoniae* infection. I. Direct detection of antigen in respiratory exudates by enzyme immunoassay. Epidemiol Infect 101:669–684, 1988.

Mahon CR, Manuselis G Jr: Textbook of Diagnostic Microbiology. Philadelphia, WB Saunders, 1995, p 631.

Marmion BP, Williamson J, Worswick DA, et al: Experience with newer techniques for the laboratory detection of *Mycoplasma pneumoniae* infection: Adelaide, 1978–1992. Clin Infect Dis 17(suppl 1):90–99, 1993.

Razin S, Barile MF, eds: The Mycoplasmas, Vol 4. New York, Academic Press, 1985.

Taylor-Robinsons D: Serologic identification of ureaplasmas from humans. In Tully JG, Razin S, eds: Methods in Mycoplasmology, Vol 2. New York, Academic Press, 1983, pp 57–63.

Tully J: Current status of the mollicute flora of humans. Clin Infect Dis 17(suppl 1):2–9, 1993.

Tully J, Whitcomb RF, eds: The Mycoplasmas, Vol 2. New York, Academic Press, 1979.

Whitcomb RF, Tully JG, eds: The Mycoplasmas, Vol 5. New York, Academic Press, 1989.

Mycobacteria

Agy MB, Wassis CK, Plorde JJ, et al: Evaluation of four mycobacterial blood culture media: BACTEC 13A, Isolator/BACTEC 12 B, Isolator/Middlebrook Agar and a biphasic medium. Diagn Microbiol Infect Dis 12:303–308, 1989.

Altamirano M, Kelly MT, Wong A, et al: Characterization of a DNA probe for detection of *Mycobacterium tuberculosis* complex in clinical samples by polymerase chain reactions. J Clin Microbiol 30:2173–2176, 1992.

Barksdale L, Kim KS: *Mycobacterium.* Bacteriol Rev 21:217, 1977.

Butler WR, Jost KC, Kilburn JO: Identification of mycobacteria by high performance liquid chromotography. J Clin Microbiol 29:2468–2472, 1991.

Centers for Disease Control: Diagnosis of tuberculosis by nucleic acid amplification methods applied to clinical specimens. MMRW Morb Mortal Wkly Rep 42:686, 1993.

Clarridge J, Shawar R, Shinnick T, Plikaytis B: Large scale use of polymerase chain reaction for detection of *Mycobacterium tuberculosis* in a routine mycobacteriology laboratory. J Clin Microbiol 31:2049–2056, 1993.

D'Amato JJ, Collins MT, Rothlauf MV, et al: Detection of mycobacteria by radiometric and standard plate procedures. J Clin Microbiol 17:1066–1073, 1983.

Daniel T: Rapid diagnosis of tuberculosis: laboratory techniques applicable in developing countries. Rev Infect Dis 11:S471–S478, 1989.

Forbes B, Hicks K: Direct detection of *Mycobacterium tuberculosis* in respiratory specimens in a clinical laboratory by polymerase chain reaction. J Clin Microbiol 31:1688–1694, 1993.

Gross WM, Hawkins JE: Radiometric selective inhibition tests for differentiating *Mycobacterium tuberculosis, Mycobacterium bovis* and other mycobacteria. J Clin Microbiol 21:565–568, 1985.

Havlik J, Horsburch C, Metchock B, et al: Disseminated *Mycobacterium avium* complex infection: clinical identification and epidemiologic trends. J Infect Dis 165:577–580, 1992.

Huebner RE, Good RC, Tokar JI: Current practices in mycobacteriology: results of a survey of state public health laboratories. J Clin Microbiol 31:771–775, 1993.

Inderlied C, Kempler C, Bermudez L: The *Mycobacterium avium* complex. Clin Microbiol 38:151–156, 1993.

Kirihara JM, Hillier SL, Coyle MG, et al: Improved detection times for *Mycobacterium avium* complex and *Mycobacterium tuberculosis* with BACTEC radiometric system. J Clin Microbiol 22:841–845, 1985.

Koneman EW, Elmer SD, Allen VR, et al: Color Atlas and Textbook of Diagnostic Microbiology, 3rd ed. Philadelphia, JB Lippincott, 1988, color plates 13–35.

Lipsky BA, Gates JA, Tenover FC, et al: Factors affecting the clinical value of microscopy for acid-fast bacilli. Rev Infect Dis 6:214–222, 1984.

Morgan MA, Horstmeir CD, DeYoung DR: Comparison of a radiometric method (BACTEC) and conventional culture media for recovery of mycobacteria from smear negative specimens. J Clin Microbiol 18:384–388, 1983.

Noordhoek GT, Holk AHJ, Bjune G, et al: Sensitivity and specificity of PCR for detection of *Mycobacterium tuberculosis:* a blind comparison study among seven laboratories. J Clin Microbiol 32:277–284, 1994.

Roberts GD, Koneman EW, Kim YK: *Mycobacterium.* In Balows A, Hausler WJ Jr, Hermann KL, et al, eds: Manual of Clinical Microbiology, 5th ed. Washington, DC, American Society for Microbiology, 1991, pp 304–339.

Sewell D, Rashad A, Rourke W, et al: Comparison of the Septi-Chek AFB and BACTEC systems and conventional culture for recovery of mycobacteria. J Clin Microbiol 31:2689–2691, 1993.

Teirstein A, Damsker B, Kischner P, et al: Pulmonary infection with MAI: diagnosis, clinical patterns, treatment. Mt Sinai J Med 57:209–215, 1990.

Tenover F, Crawford J, Huebner R, et al: The resurgence of tuberculosis: is your lab ready? J Clin Microbiol 32:767–770, 1993.

Wayne L: The "atypical" mycobacteria: recognition and disease association. Crit Rev Microbiol 12:185–222, 1985.

Wolinsky E: Mycobacterial diseases other than tuberculosis. Clin Infect Dis 15:1–12, 1992.

Chlamydiae, Rickettsiae, and Related Organisms

Baron EJ, Finegold S: Bailey and Scott's Diagnostic Microbiology, 8th ed. Philadelphia, CV Mosby, 1990, p 563.

Bauwens JE, Clare AM, Loeffelholz MJ, et al: Diagnosis of *Chlamydia trachomatis* urethritis in men by polymerase chain reaction assay of first catch urine. J Clin Microbiol 31:3013–3016, 1993.

Bell TA, Kuo CC, Stamm WE, et al: Direct fluorescent monoclonal antibody stain for rapid detection of infant *Chlamydia trachomatis* infections. Pediatrics 74:224–228, 1984.

Chernesky MA, Mahony JB, Castriciano S, et al: Detection of *Chlamydia trachomatis* antigens by enzyme immunoassay and immunoflourescence in genital specimens from symptomatic and asymptomatic men and women. J Infect Dis 154:141–148, 1986.

Clarke LM, Sierra MF, Daidone BJ, et al: Comparison of the Syva MicroTrak enzyme immunoassay and Gen-Probe PACE 2 with culture for diagnosis of cervical *Chlamydia trachomatis* infection in a high-prevalence population. J Clin Microbiol 31:968–971, 1993.

Clyde WA Jr, Kenny GE, Schachter J: CUMITECH 19: Laboratory Diagnosis of Chlamydial and Mycoplasmal Infections. Washington, DC, American Society for Microbiology, 1984.

Coudron PE, Fedorko DP, Dawson DS, et al: Detection of *Chlamydia trachomatis* in genital specimens by Microtrak direct specimen test. Am J Clin Pathol 85:89–92, 1986.

Fishbein DB, Kaplan JE, Bernard KW, Winkler WG: Surveillance of Rocky Mountain spotted fever in the United States, 1981–1983. J Infect Dis 150:609–611, 1984.

Godfrey E, Winn W Jr, Keathley JD: Performance of Microtrak direct test for *Chlamydia trachomatis* in a prevalence study. Diagn Microbiol Infect Dis 5:313–316, 1986.

Grayston JT: Infections caused by *Chlamydia pneumoniae* strain TWAR. Clin Infect Dis 15:757–763, 1992.

Horn JE, Hammer ML, Falkow S, et al: Detection of *Chlamydia trachomatis* in tissue culture and cervical scrapings by in situ DNA hybridization. J Infect Dis 153:1155–1159, 1986.

Jones MF, Smith TF, Houglum AJ, et al: Detection of *Chlamydia trachomatis* in genital specimens by Chlamydiazyme test. J Clin Microbiol 20:465–467, 1984.

Kaplan JE, Schonberger LB: The sensitivity of various serologic tests in the diagnosis of Rocky Mountain spotted fever. Am J Trop Med Hyg 35:840–844, 1986.

McCutchan JA: Epidemiology of venereal urethritis: comparison of gonorrhea and nongonococcal urethritis. Rev Infect Dis 6:669–688, 1984.

Rikihisa Y: The tribe Ehrlichieae and ehrlichial disease. Clin Microbiol Rev 4:286–308, 1991.

Schachter J: Chlamydial infections. N Engl J Med 298:428–435, 490–495, 540–549, 1978.

Tzianabos T, Anderson BE, McDade JE: Detection of *Rickettsia rickettsii* DNA in clinical specimens by using polymerase chain reaction technology. J Clin Microbiol 27:2866–2868, 1989.

Antimicrobial Susceptibility Testing

Baron EJ, Finegold S: Bailey and Scott's Diagnostic Microbiology, 8th ed. Philadelphia, CV Mosby, 1990.

Boyce JM: Increasing prevalence of methicillin-resistant *Staphylococcus aureus* in the United States. Infect Control Hosp Epidemiol 11:639–642, 1990.

Brown BA, Swenson JM, Wallace RJ Jr: Agar disk elution test for rapidly growing mycobacteria. In Isenberg HD, ed: Clinical Microbiology Procedures Handbook. Washington, DC, American Society for Microbiology, 1992, pp 5.11.1–5.11.10.

Brown BA, Swenson JM, Wallace RJ Jr: Agar disk elution test for rapidly growing mycobacteria. In Isenberg HD, ed: Clinical Microbiology Procedures Handbook. Washington, DC, American Society for Microbiology, 1992, pp 5.10.1–5.10.11.

Chambers HF: Methicillin-resistant staphylococci. Clin Microbiol Rev 1:173–186, 1988.

Hindler J: Strategies for antimicrobial susceptibility testing of fastidious aerobic bacteria. Am J Med Tech 49:761, 1983.

Mahon CR, Manuselis G: Textbook of Diagnostic Microbiology. Philadelphia, WB Saunders, 1995, p 68.

National Committee for Clinical Laboratories: Methods for Dilution Antimicrobial Susceptibility Tests for Bacteria That Grow Aerobically. M7-A. Villanova, PA, NCCLS, 1985.

National Committee for Clinical Laboratories: Performance Standards for Antimicrobial Disk Susceptibility Tests, 3rd ed. M2-A3. Villanova, PA, NCCLS, 1984.

National Committee for Clinical Laboratories: Methodology for the Serum Bactericidal Test; Proposed Guideline. M21-P. Villanova, PA, NCCLS, 1987.

National Committee for Clinical Laboratories: Methods for Dilution Antimicrobial Susceptibility Tests for Bacteria That Grow Aerobically, 2nd ed. Tentative Standard M7-T2. Villanova, PA, NCCLS, 1988.

National Committee for Clinical Laboratories: Methods for Antimicrobial Susceptibility Testing of Anaerobic Bacteria, 2nd ed. Tentative Standard M11-T2. Villanova, PA, NCCLS, 1989.

National Committee for Clinical Laboratories: Reference Agar Dilution Procedure for Antimicrobial Susceptibility Testing of Anaerobic Bacteria. Approved Standard M11-A. Villanova, PA, NCCLS, 1985.

National Committee for Clinical Laboratories: Performance Standards for Antimicrobial Disk Susceptibility Tests, 4th ed. M2-A4. Villanova, PA, NCCLS, 1990.

Chapter 32

CLINICAL PARASITOLOGY

Ronald Malowitz, PhD, MT(ASCP)

Q U I C K   C O N T E N T S

INTRODUCTION

Parasitic disease occurs worldwide and is responsible for significant morbidity and mortality. For example, each year intestinal parasites infect 1800 million humans and the malarial parasite attacks 20 million humans. Two relatively recent factors have significantly affected clinical parasitology. The rapid movement of people from widely distant geographic areas into different areas has brought people with parasitic disease that is endemic to their area of origin but relatively unknown in their area of destination. Newly emerging diseases such as acquired immunodeficiency syndrome (AIDS); the use of drugs such as broad spectrum antibiotics and corticosteroids; patients receiving transplants; and patients requiring oncology services have all led to increased susceptibility to parasitic infection and an increased morbidity and mortality from these infections.

The parasite is in a symbiotic relationship in which the parasite benefits while its host is in some manner harmed. The parasite may be a very simple one celled protozoon or a complex organism such as a helminth or ectoparasite. These organisms may have a very simple life cycle in which an intimate relationship is formed with only one host, whereas others may have complicated life cycles in which free living forms and/or one to several intermediate hosts are involved.

In this chapter the major internal parasites are discussed with regard to the disease they cause, the clinical laboratory diagnosis, diagnostic morphology, life cycle, epidemiology, and control. The "Clinical Laboratory Diagnosis" segment identifies the procedures that are usually performed in a clinical microbiologic setting and afford good to excellent results. Other procedures are available, and some of those that are more frequently used are listed in the section "Selected Diagnostic Procedures." The "Diagnostic Morphology" segment identifies those characteristics that are most useful in the clinical microbiology setting for the identification of a particular parasite.

The section on ectoparasites is in the same format as that of the endoparasites and has been limited to those parasites that are occasionally seen in the clinical microbiology laboratory. Discussions on other ectoparasites are available in the parasitology textbooks listed in the bibliography.

INTESTINAL PROTOZOA

AMEBA

Entamoeba histolytica

DISEASE. Intestinal amebiasis (amebic dysentry) and extraintestinal amebiasis (invasion of the liver and rarely other organs)

CLINICAL LABORATORY DIAGNOSIS
▮ Wet mount of a formalin–ethyl acetate concentrate of fecal sample stained with D'Antoni's iodine
▮ Smear of a polyvinyl alcohol (PVA) preserved fecal sample stained with Gomori's trichrome stain

DIAGNOSTIC MORPHOLOGY. See "Differential Characteristics of *Entamoeba histolytica* and the Nonpathogenic Amebae (Trophozoite Form)" on p **691** and "Differential Characteristics of *Entamoeba histolytica* and the Nonpathogenic Amebae (Cyst Form)" on p **693.**

LIFE CYCLE
1. The mature resistant infective cysts, which are formed in the lumen of the large intestine, are passed into the external environment.
2. The mature cyst is ingested by the host (humans) and passes into the lower part of the small intestine. Under the influence of digestive juices and the activity of the ameba, the cyst wall disintegrates, allowing the quadrinucleated ameba to escape through the wall, ultimately forming eight trophozoites.
3. The young trophozoites move to the large intestine, and due to intestinal stasis establish a site of infection in the colon (especially the cecal area).
4. Trophozoites may penetrate the intestinal mucosa and may also multiply by binary fission in the submucosa and form flasklike ulcers.
5. From these ulcers, the trophozoites may enter the circulation and form extraintestinal abscesses.
6. Trophozoites are stimulated to encyst due to a decrease in water availability in the lower colon and are passed out in the stool into the environment.

EPIDEMIOLOGY
▮ Cosmopolitan
▮ Higher incidence in tropical and subtropical regions, especially with contaminated water and poor sanitation

AMEBA

CONTROL

- Avoidance of fecal contamination of food and water
- Purification of water by boiling or treatment with iodine
- Washing fruits and vegetables with noncontaminated water
- Not using night soil (human feces) as a fertilizer
- Protection of food from flies and cockroaches
- Screening of food handlers for asymptomatic carriage of *E. histolytica*
- Sanitary methods of sewage disposal
- Safe sexual practices
- Public education on the transmission and methods of avoidance of *E. histolytica*

Differential Characteristics of *Entamoeba histolytica* and the Nonpathogenic Amebae

TROPHOZOITE FORM (STAINED)

ORGANISM	SIZE (μm)	NO. OF NUCLEI	KARYOSOME	PERIPHERAL CHROMATIN	CYTOPLASMIC INCLUSIONS	MICROSCOPIC VIEW
Entamoeba hartmanni	5–12	1	Small, usually eccentric	Similar to that of *E. histolytica*	Bacteria	*
Entamoeba coli	15–25	1	Large, usually eccentric	Coarsely granular, unevenly distributed	Bacteria and other microorganisms	*
Endolimax nana	6–12	1	Very large, round, irregular, or blotlike	None	Bacteria	*

Continued ▶

AMEBA

▲ Continued **TROPHOZOITE FORM (STAINED)**

ORGANISM	SIZE (μm)	NO. OF NUCLEI	KARYOSOME	PERIPHERAL CHROMATIN	CYTOPLASMIC INCLUSIONS	MICROSCOPIC VIEW
Iodamoeba butschlii	12–15	1	Very large, round, and surrounded by indistinct refractile granules	None	Bacteria and other microorganisms	*
Dientamoeba fragilis†	5–12	2 Sometimes 1	Large, fragmented into cluster of 4–8 granules	Finely granular, inapparent	Bacteria	*
Entamoeba histolytica	15–20	1	Small, usually central	Finely granular, evenly distributed	Occasionally RBCs; may have bacteria	*

†This organism is now considered to be a flagellate; may possess some pathogenicity.

* Photomicrographs from Markell EK, Voge M: Medical Parasitology (a slide presentation). Philadelphia, WB Saunders, 1976.

CYST FORM (STAINED)

ORGANISM	SIZE (μm)	SHAPE	NUMBER OF NUCLEI	KARYOSOME	PERIPHERAL CHROMATIN	CHROMATOID BODIES	GLYCOGEN	MICROSCOPIC VIEW
Entamoeba hartmanni	6–8	Spherical	1–4; 4 in mature cyst	Similar to that of *E. histolytica*	Similar to that of *E. histolytica*	Similar to that of *E. histolytica*	Similar to that of *E. histolytica*	*
Entamoeba coli	15–25	Spherical, sometimes oval	2–8; 8 in mature cyst	Large, usually eccentric	Coarsely granular, unevenly distributed	Seldom seen; splinter-like with pointed ends	Usually diffuse	*
Endolimax nana	6–8	Ellipsoid, spherical, or ovoid	4 in mature cyst	Large, usually central	None	None	Usually diffuse	*

Continued ▶

AMEBA

► Continued **CYST FORM (STAINED)**

ORGANISM	SIZE (μm)	SHAPE	NUMBER OF NUCLEI	KARYOSOME	PERIPHERAL CHROMATIN	CHROMATOID BODIES	GLYCOGEN	MICROSCOPIC VIEW
Iodamoeba butschlii	10–12	Irregular	1 in mature cyst	Large, usually eccentric	None	None	Large, spherical, compact mass	*
Dientamoeba fragilis	No cyst stage	—	—	—	—	—	—	
Entamoeba histolytica	12–15	Spherical	1–2; 4 in mature cyst	Small, usually central	Finely granular, evenly distributed	Rodlike structures with blunt or rounded ends	Usually diffuse	*

* Photomicrographs from Markell EK, Voge M: Medical Parasitology (a slide presentation). Philadelphia, WB Saunders, 1976.

FLAGELLATES

Giardia duodenalis (lamblia)

DISEASE. Giardiasis, lambliasis

CLINICAL LABORATORY DIAGNOSIS

▋ Direct saline wet mount of loose stool, duodenal contents, or material from the "string test" (Enterotest, International Health Services, Mountainview, CA)

▋ Wet mount of a formalin–ethyl acetate concentrate of a formed fecal sample stained with D'Antoni's iodine

DIAGNOSTIC MORPHOLOGY. See "Differential Characteristics of the Common Intestinal Flagellates" on p **696.**

LIFE CYCLE

1. By hand to mouth or through contaminated food or water, mature cysts are ingested and pass through the stomach into the small intestine.
2. In the duodenum excystation occurs.
3. The released trophozoites can migrate and inhabit most of the small intestine.
4. By adhering to the intestinal epithelial cell with its ventral sucking disc, the trophozoite resists peristalsis and remains in the upper intestinal tract. Here it feeds and may reproduce by longitudinal binary fission.
5. As feces with entrapped trophozoites enter the colon, encystment with concurrent mitotic division occurs.
6. The cysts enter the external environment, and the cycle is repeated.

EPIDEMIOLOGY

▋ Cosmopolitan.

▋ Infection more common in children, particularly the 6 to 10 year old age group.

▋ *Giardia* is highly infectious and is principally transmitted by the ingestion of food or water contaminated by the cyst.

▋ Beavers, muskrats, and other water rodents are believed to be sources of *Giardia* contamination of streams and other bodies of fresh water.

▋ *Giardia* may be sexually transmitted.

CONTROL

▋ Avoidance of fecal contaminated water and food

▋ Use of a portable water purification unit for hikers or campers

▋ Safe sexual practices

▋ Public education on transmission and methods of avoidance of *Giardia*

FLAGELLATES

Differential Characteristics of the Common Intestinal Flagellates†

TROPHOZOITE FORM (STAINED)

ORGANISM	SIZE (μm)	SHAPE	NUCLEI	OTHER FEATURES	MICROSCOPIC VIEW
Giardia duodenalis	12–15	Pyriform	2	Large, ovoid, ventral sucking disc; 4 pairs of flagella; 2 curved median bodies	*
Chilomastix mesnili	10–15	Pyriform	1	Prominent cytostome; ventral spiral groove; 4 flagella	*

* Photomicrographs from Markell EK, Voge M: Medical Parasitology (a slide presentation). Philadelphia, WB Saunders, 1976.

CYST FORM (STAINED)

ORGANISM	SIZE (μm)	SHAPE	NUCLEI	OTHER FEATURES	MICROSCOPIC VIEW
Giardia duodenalis	11–12	Ellipsoid	Usually 4, sometimes 2	Lengthwise running central fibrils; short fibers laterally or obliquely across fibrils in lower half of cyst	*
Chilomastix mesnili	6–10	Lemon shaped with anterior "nipple"	1	Sausage shaped cytostome located toward one side of cyst	*

* Photomicrographs from Markell EK, Voge M: Medical Parasitology (a slide presentation). Philadelphia, WB Saunders, 1976.

†The intestinal flagellates **Enteromonas hominis** and **Retortamonas intestinalis** are rarely seen and nonpathogenic and are not described.

CILIATES

Balantidium coli

DISEASE. Balantidiasis, balantidiosis, balantidial dysentery

CLINICAL LABORATORY DIAGNOSIS. See *"Entamoeba histolytica."*

DIAGNOSTIC MORPHOLOGY

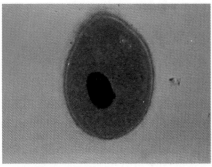

From Markell EK, Voge M: Medical Parasitology (a slide presentation). Philadelphia, WB Saunders, 1976.

Trophozoite Stage

- Size: 50 to 70 µm long by 40 to 50 µm wide.
- Shape: bag- or saclike.
- Rows of cilia surround the entire organism.
- At the anterior end, a ciliated lined triangular opening, known as a *peristome,* leads into a ciliated funnel shaped cytostome.
- In the cytoplasm are the large kidney shaped macronucleus, a small spherical micronucleus that lies very close to the macronucleus, and two contractile vacuoles.

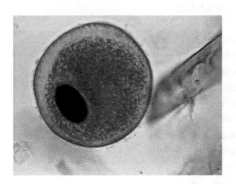

From Markell EK, Voge M: Medical Parasitology (a slide presentation). Philadelphia, WB Saunders, 1976.

Cyst Stage

- Size: 45 to 65 µm in diameter.
- Shape: spherical to oval.
- Cilia are present in the young cyst but are absent in older forms.
- In the cytoplasm are the large kidney shaped macronucleus and contractile vacuoles.

LIFE CYCLE

1. The infective cysts are ingested by the host (humans) and excyst in the small intestine.
2. The released trophozoites migrate to the large intestine, where they invade and multiply by transverse fission in the intestinal wall. Sexual reproduction by conjugation may also occur.
3. Encystment occurs as the trophozoites are passed with the feces into the external environment. No reproduction occurs in the cyst stage.

EPIDEMIOLOGY

- Cosmopolitan. Endemic in New Guinea.
- Principal host is the hog, but other mammals may be infected.
- Incidence of human infection is low.
- Human infection is acquired by ingestion of cysts in contaminated food and water. Hand to mouth transmission is also believed to occur.
- *B. coli* infection has occurred in epidemic form in U.S. mental hospitals.

CILIATES

CONTROL. Similar to the control measures listed for *E. histolytica*

INTESTINAL COCCIDIA, MICROSPORIDIA, AND *BLASTOCYSTIS HOMINIS*

Isospora belli

DISEASE. Isosporiasis, intestinal coccidiosis

CLINICAL LABORATORY DIAGNOSIS
- Wet mount of a formalin–ethyl acetate concentrate of fecal sample stained with D'Antoni's iodine
- Modified acid fast stain of a smear from a fecal formalin–ethyl acetate concentrate

DIAGNOSTIC MORPHOLOGY. See "Differential Characteristics of the Intestinal Coccidia, Microsporidia, and *Blastocystis hominis*" on p **701.**

LIFE CYCLE
1. Mature oocysts or sporocysts are ingested.
2. Sporozoites are released from the sporocyst in the intestine.
3. In the intestinal epithelial cells, repeated asexual (schizogony) reproduction occurs, resulting in the spread of the infection.
4. Along with the asexual phase occurring in the intestinal epithelium, sexual reproduction (sporogony) also takes place, resulting in the formation of the oocyst.
5. The oocyst is passed out in the feces and the cycle is repeated.

EPIDEMIOLOGY
- Cosmopolitan.
- Transmission is by hand to mouth or through contaminated food or water.
- Infection rate is low except in the immunocompromised.

CONTROL. Similar to that of *E. histolytica*

Sarcocystis **Species**

DISEASE. Sarcosporidiasis

CLINICAL LABORATORY DIAGNOSIS. Wet mount of a formalin–ethyl acetate concentrate of fecal sample stained with D'Antoni's iodine

DIAGNOSTIC MORPHOLOGY. See "Differential Characteristics of the Intestinal Coccidia, Microsporidia, and *Blastocystis hominis*" on p **701.**

LIFE CYCLE
1. The sporocyst is ingested by the intermediate vertebrate host (i.e., a variety of mammals and birds)
2. Initially, asexual reproduction (schizogony) occurs in the endothelial cells of the liver and brain.
3. This is followed by invasion of the muscle cells and the development of cysts containing trophozoites.

4. The cyst is transmitted to the definitive host (i.e., humans) by eating the muscle infected with the cysts.
5. Within the definitive host, sexual reproduction occurs (sporogony), resulting in the formation of oocysts.
6. Mature oocysts, or more likely sporocysts, are excreted with the feces and the cycle is repeated.

NOTE   Humans may also serve as an intermediate host.

EPIDEMIOLOGY
▐ Cosmopolitan
▐ Transmission by eating raw or undercooked meat (definitive host) or by hand to mouth or through contaminated water or food (intermediate host)

CONTROL
▐ Similar to that of *E. histolytica*
▐ Eating fully cooked meat

Cyclospora cayetanensis

DISEASE. Cyclosporiasis

CLINICAL LABORATORY DIAGNOSIS
▐ Wet mount of a formalin–ethyl acetate concentrate of a fecal sample viewed under light microscopy or with an epifluorescent microscope
▐ Modified acid fast stain of a smear from a fecal formalin–ethyl acetate concentrate

DIAGNOSTIC MORPHOLOGY. See "Differential Characteristics of the Intestinal Coccidia, Microsporidia, and *Blastocystis hominis*" on p **701.**

LIFE CYCLE. The life cycle has not been detailed.

EPIDEMIOLOGY
▐ Reported as a cause of traveler's diarrhea in areas of Asia and South America.
▐ Evidence points to transmission through contaminated water.

CONTROL. Probably similar to that of *E. histolytica*

Cryptosporidium parvum

DISEASE. Cryptosporidiosis

CLINICAL LABORATORY DIAGNOSIS. Modified acid fast stain of a fecal smear made from a formalin–ethyl acetate concentrate of the stool

DIAGNOSTIC MORPHOLOGY. See "Differential Characteristics of the Intestinal Coccidia, Microsporidia and *Blastocystis hominis*" on p **701.**

LIFE CYCLE
1. Oocysts are ingested.
2. Excystation occurs in the upper intestinal tract, releasing sporozoites.

COCCIDIA, MICROSPORIDIA, AND BLASTOCYSTIS HOMINIS

3. The sporozoites infect the brush border of the intestinal columnar epithelial cells, where both asexual and sexual reproduction occurs.
4. The asexual phase produces merozoites, which both spread the infection to neighboring cells and also produce the male and female gamonts (sexual phase), which fuse, ultimately forming the oocyst.
5. Both thin and thick walled oocysts are produced. The thin walled oocysts are believed to release their sporozoites before leaving the host and therefore cause autoinfection. The thick walled oocysts are passed out with the stool and reinitiate the cycle.

EPIDEMIOLOGY

- Cosmopolitan.
- A zoonosis, infecting a wide variety of animals.
- Children are more commonly infected.
- Outbreaks reported in day care centers.
- A common cause of traveler's diarrhea.
- Transmission is primarily through contaminated food or water or by person to person contact.

CONTROL. Similar to that of *Giardia duodenalis*

Microsporidia

Genera found in humans: *Enterocytozoon, Encephalitozoon, Pleistophora, Nosema,* and *Microsporidium*

DISEASE. Microsporidiosis

CLINICAL LABORATORY DIAGNOSIS. Unconcentrated, formalin fixed, thin fecal smear stained with the modified trichrome stain

DIAGNOSTIC MORPHOLOGY. See "Differential Characteristics of the Intestinal Coccidia, Microsporidia, and *Blastocystis hominis*" on p **701.**

LIFE CYCLE

1. After the spore is ingested, a polar filament is extruded.
2. The tubular filament penetrates the host cell, and its infectious material is injected.
3. Within the infected cell, asexual and sexual reproduction occur with the production of new spores.
4. The spores are passed out in the feces or urine or are liberated after the death of the host.

EPIDEMIOLOGY

- Principally affects immunologically compromised hosts, but may cause disease in normal hosts.
- Except for *Enterocytozoon bieneusi,* which has been found only in humans and is the most frequent cause of microsporidian enteritis in AIDS patients, other microsporidia parasitize other mammals and insects.

CONTROL. Precautions should be taken on disposal of excreta and fomites from patients diagnosed with microsporidiosis.

Differential Characteristics of the Intestinal Coccidia, Microsporidia, and *Blastocystis hominis*

ORGANISM	SIZE (μm)	SHAPE	OTHER FEATURES	MICROSCOPIC VIEW
Isospora belli	Average: 29 by 14	Elongated or ovoid	Three oocyst forms may be found in feces: 1. Unicellular form with single large oval mass of protoplasm 2. Oocyst containing two oval sporoblasts 3. Mature oocyst with two oval spores, each containing four sausage shaped sporozoites Oocysts are acid fast with modified stain.	
Sarcocystis	Average: 15 by 9 (sporocyst)	Ovoid	Released sporocysts, either singly or in pairs, each containing four sporozoites, are found in feces.	*
Cryptosporidium	4–5	Round	Four sausage shaped sporozoites within oocyst may be visible. Oocysts are acid fast with modified stain.	

Continued ▶

▶ Continued **Differential Characteristics of the Intestinal Coccidia, Microsporidia, and *Blastocystis hominis***

ORGANISM	SIZE (μm)	SHAPE	OTHER FEATURES	MICROSCOPIC VIEW
Cyclospora	8–10	Round	Immature oocyst found in feces. Acid fast variable with modified stain. May appear similar to *Cryptosporidium*, but twice the size.	
Microsporidia	2–4	Ovoid or rodlike	Stained by modified trichrome stain, spore wall is pink-red. Interior of cell is transparent, or with pink-red line across cell.	
Blastocystis hominis†	6–40	Round	Organism has large, central, vacuole-like body. Around periphery of cell are many small nuclei.	*

†Currently classified as an ameba; may be pathogenic.

* Photomicrographs from Markell EK, Voge M: Medical parasitology (a slide presentation). Philadelphia, WB Saunders, 1976.

OTHER PROTOZOA

BLOOD AND TISSUE PROTOZOA

Plasmodium

vivax, malariae, falciparum, and *ovale*
DISEASE. Malaria

> *P. vivax:* Benign tertian malaria
> *P. malariae:* Quartan malaria
> *P. falciparum:* Malignant tertian malaria
> *P. ovale:* Ovale tertian malaria

CLINICAL LABORATORY DIAGNOSIS. Giemsa stained thick and thin blood smears

DIAGNOSTIC MORPHOLOGY. See "Differential Characteristics of *Plasmodium* Species" on p **706.**

LIFE CYCLE
Mosquito (Sexual Cycle, Sporogony)
1. The female anopheline mosquito (definitive host) bites an infected person and withdraws into her stomach blood containing macro- and microgametocytes.
2. In the midgut of the mosquito, the microgametocyte matures and by the process known as *exflagellation* produces microgametes (structures with flagella).
3. The microgametes detach from the parent cell and swim actively in search of the macrogamete.
4. The macrogametocyte, during the maturation of the microgametocyte, becomes spherical and matures, finally extruding a macrogamete.
5. The motile microgamete fuses with the macrogamete and forms a zygote.
6. The zygote elongates and becomes a motile ookinete.
7. The ookinete penetrates the mosquito's stomach wall, rounds up, and becomes the oocyst.
8. The oocyst produces many filamentous sporozoites, which finally rupture the oocyst.
9. The released sporozoites wander throughout the body of the mosquito, finally locating in the salivary glands, and are injected into a host at the next feeding.

Humans (Asexual Cycle, Schizogony)
1. While feeding on the human host, the infected female anopheline mosquito injects motile sporozoites into the host's bloodstream.
2. Within 1 hour the sporozoites leave the blood vascular system and enter the parenchymal cells of the liver, where they begin the initial phase of asexual reproduction, exoerythrocytic schizogony.
3. The infected liver cell yields upon rupture from 2000 to 40,000 merozoites, depending on the malarial species.
4. The released merozoites enter the circulation and begin the asexual cycle in the erythrocyte.

> In *P. vivax* and *P. ovale* infections, a portion of the infecting sporozoites enters a resting stage, the hypnozoite, within the liver parenchymal cells. After a period of weeks, months, or years, this latent form begins the process of asexual multiplication, ultimately releasing thousands of merozoites into the general

circulation. This process is responsible for the relapses seen in vivax and ovale malarias.

Although true relapses do not occur in falciparum or malarial malaria, periodic recrudescences may occur with falciparum malaria in the first year and for as long as 40 years with malarial malaria. This recurrence of symptoms is believed to happen as a result of a small number of erythrocytic parasites that have survived the immune response of the host.

5. Within the erythrocyte the malarial parasite matures and then enters the schizont stage, where the single nucleus of the trophozoite divides repeatedly, forming merozoites, the number of which is species dependent.

After several hours into the asexual cycle, granules of brownish pigment, known as hemazoin, accumulate within the infected erythrocyte.

a) *P. vivax* and *P. ovale* prefer to invade reticulocytes.

b) *P. malariae* prefers to invade senescent erythrocytes.

c) *P. falciparum* invades erythrocytes of all ages.

P. falciparum infected erythrocytes develop knobs on their surface inducing adherence of these infected cells to the endothelium of capillaries in the internal organs. Thus, in the peripheral blood only the young trophozoite and on occasion the gametocyte are seen. In the moribund patient, however, the more mature forms may appear in the peripheral blood.

6. Once the full complement of merozoites is formed within the schizont, the erythrocytes rupture, releasing the merozoites into the circulation to infect new erythrocytes.

7. The cyclic process of merozoite invasion of the erythrocyte through the parasites' maturation and asexual reproduction with final release of daughter merozoites results in a cyclic paroxysm of fever. Malarial schizogony in the red blood cell with the resulting fever pattern occurs during specific intervals of time and is species dependent.

ORGANISM	CYCLIC PAROXYSM
P. falciparum	Every 36–48 hr
P. vivax and *P. ovale*	Every 48 hr
P. malariae	Every 72 hr

8. After several erythrocytic cycles, in response to an unknown stimulus, merozoites mature into micro- and macrogametocytes.

EPIDEMIOLOGY

▌ *P. vivax* is present in the tropics, subtropics, and temperate regions. This species is the most prevalent and has the widest geographic distribution.

▌ *P. ovale* is present primarily in tropical Africa. It may be found in Asia and South America.

▌ *P. malariae* is found in subtropical and temperate regions.

▌ *P. falciparum* is found in tropical and subtropical regions.

▌ Areas of significant incidence of malaria:

Africa: present in countries north of the Sahara and in the sub-Saharan countries. The highest levels of endemic malaria in the world are found in the sub-Saharan countries.

South-central Asia: Afghanistan.

Southeast Asia: Bangladesh, India, Nepal, and Sri Lanka.

Eastern Asia and Oceania: China, Indonesia, Philippines, Solomon Islands, Thailand, Myanmar, Vietnam, and Laos.

Europe: southeastern Turkey and Republics of Azerbaijan and Tadjik.

The Americas: French Guiana, Guyana, Nicaragua, Honduras, Brazil, Colombia, and Mexico.

CONTROL
Mosquito Control
▌ Residual insecticides:

Example: DDT

Factors influencing use:

Vector must be susceptible.

Vector must feed and rest indoors.

Abode must be of a construction suitable for residual insecticide use (houses should have walls, limited windows, limited open areas).
▌ Elimination of breeding places:

Land reclamation

Filling vacant land and pumping out water

Intermittent irrigation of rice fields

Removal of junk and water-retaining debris
▌ Destruction of larvae:

Adding larva-eating fish

Cleaning drains

Removing vegetation (algae) from ponds

Mechanical Barriers to Human-Vector Contact
▌ Insecticide impregnated (see "Mosquito Repellents" below) or unimpregnated mosquito bed nets and wall mats
▌ Screening of dwellings
▌ Clothing to prevent mosquito bites

Mosquito Repellents
▌ N,N-diethylmetatoluamide (DEET)
▌ Pyrethroid repellents (permethrin)

Assessment
▌ Assessment of epidemiologic risk factors to select appropriate control measures for a *particular* locality

Experts Both Public and Private, to:
▌ Train personnel in malaria surveillance (i.e., emergence of parasite resistance to antimalarial drugs)
▌ Train in malaria detection, clinical treatment, and follow-up

BLOOD AND TISSUE PROTOZOA

Differential Characteristics of *Plasmodium* Species

	P. VIVAX	P. MALARIAE	P. FALCIPARUM	P. OVALE
Early Trophozoite (Ring Form)	Thick ring, one sometimes two chromatin dots	Thick ring, one chromatin dot	Thin, delicate ring, accolé forms, multiple infections	Thick ring, one chromatin dot
Mature Trophozoite	Irregular, ameboid shape	Compact, band forms	Compact, not usually in peripheral blood	Compact
Immature Schizont	Chromatin divided into numerous irregular masses	Chromatin divided into few irregular masses	Chromatin divided into numerous irregular masses, rarely in peripheral blood	Chromatin divided into few irregular masses

Continued ▶

► Continued **Differential Characteristics of *Plasmodium* Species**

	P. VIVAX	P. MALARIAE	P. FALCIPARUM	P. OVALE
Mature Schizont	12–18 merozoites	6–12 merozoites, usually in rosette	8–32 merozoites, rarely in peripheral blood	6–12 merozoites
Gametocyte	Round, oval, or compact, diffuse (male) or compact (female) chromatin	Round compact, diffuse (male) or compact (female) chromatin	Crescentic, diffuse (male) or compact (female) chromatin	Round compact diffuse (male) or compact (female) chromatin
Size of RBC	Enlarged	Normal or smaller	Normal	Enlarged
Pigment	Schüffner's dots	Rarely Ziemann's dots	Sometimes Maurer's dots	Schüffner's dots

Photomicrographs from Markell EK, Voge M: Medical Parasitology (a slide presentation). Philadelphia, WB Saunders, 1976.

Babesia

DISEASE. Babesiosis

CLINICAL LABORATORY DIAGNOSIS. Giemsa stained thick and thin blood smears

DIAGNOSTIC MORPHOLOGY. This organism resembles *Plasmodium falciparum*.
See "Differential Characteristics of *Babesia* and *Plasmodium falciparum* in Peripheral Blood" on p 709.

LIFE CYCLE

1. The *Ixodes* tick feeds on the reservoir vertebrate host that harbors the parasite (i.e., deer and mice).
2. After entering the tick, the parasite begins a complex asexual and sexual cycle. Finally the parasite enters the channels of the salivary glands for transmission to a vertebrate host. In addition, the parasite is transmitted transovarially in the tick, thereby increasing the effectiveness of its transfer to the vertebrate host.
3. While feeding, the tick injects the parasite into the vertebrate host (i.e., a human, an accidental host).
4. The parasite enters the erythrocyte and undergoes asexual reproduction, producing merozoites, which infect new cells.

EPIDEMIOLOGY

▮ The majority of cases of babesiosis have been reported from North America and Europe.
▮ In Europe, *B. divergens (bovis)* parasitizes cattle, and of the several human cases reported, most have had fatal outcomes.
▮ In North America, particularly in the northeastern United States, *B. microti* parasitizes mice and deer and causes a nonfatal disease in the immunocompetent human host, but it may be fatal in the splenectomized or otherwise immunocompromised patient.

CONTROL

▮ Avoid wooded endemic areas during tick season.
▮ Wear protective clothing and tick repellent in areas of tick infestation.
▮ Examine for ticks all household pets that are allowed outdoors.

Differential Characteristics of *Babesia* and *Plasmodium falciparum* in Peripheral Blood

ORGANISM	FORMS PRESENT	TROPHOZOITE (RING FORM) CHARACTERISTICS	HEMAZOIN	MULTIPLE INFECTIONS	EXTRACELLULAR FORMS (OUTSIDE ERYTHROCYTE)	MICROSCOPIC VIEW
Babesia	Trophozoite (ring form)	Pleomorphic; one to three chromatin dots; tetrad (four organisms linked by cytoplasm); usually smaller than *P. falciparum*	No	Yes, usually two to five or more	Yes	* *
Plasmodium falciparum	Trophozoite (ring form) and gametocyte	One to three chromatin dots, no tetrad forms	Yes	Yes, usually two to three, occasionally more	No	*

* Photomicrographs from Markell EK, Voge M: Medical Parasitology (a slide presentation). Philadelphia, WB Saunders, 1976.

BLOOD AND TISSUE PROTOZOA

Trypanosoma brucei

T. b. gambiense and *rhodesiense*

DISEASE. African trypanosomiasis

T. b. gambiense: Gambian trypanosomiasis, West and Mid-African sleeping sickness

T. b. rhodesiense: Rhodesian trypanosomiasis, East African sleeping sickness

CLINICAL LABORATORY DIAGNOSIS

▮ Early stage disease: Giemsa stained thick and thin blood smears; Giemsa stained smears of lymph exudate

▮ Late stage disease: Giemsa stained smears of cerebrospinal fluid (CSF)

DIAGNOSTIC MORPHOLOGY

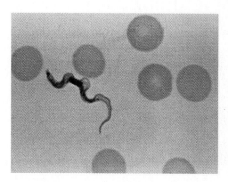

From Markell EK, Voge M: Medical Parasitology (a slide presentation). Philadelphia, WB Saunders, 1976.

Trypomastigote Stage

▮ Size: average 25 μm in length.

▮ Shape: slender to fat and stumpy forms; in Giemsa stained films: **C** or **U** shaped forms are *not* seen (see *"Trypanosoma cruzi"* on p **711.**)

▮ Nucleus: oval and central.

▮ Kinetoplast: small, oval, and located posterior to the nucleus; subterminal.

▮ Flagellum: anterior, long free flagellum.

▮ Undulating membrane: delicate (visualized by scanning electron microscope [EM]).

LIFE CYCLE. The life cycles of the African trypanosomes are very similar and are discussed as one.

1. The stumpy trypomastigotes are ingested by the tsetse fly (*Glossina* species) from the blood of the infected mammalian host (i.e., humans).
2. The parasites migrate to the gut of the fly, where they transform into the epimastigote form and multiply.
3. After migrating to the salivary glands, the epismastigotes transform into the infective, metacyclic trypomastigotes.
4. On feeding on a mammalian host, the metacyclic forms are injected into the host with the fly's saliva.
5. At first, the parasite remains at the site of injection in the subcutaneous tissue fluid. Here it becomes long and slender and divides by binary fission.

6. Over time the parasite enters the blood and lymphatic systems.
7. Some of the slender trypomastigotes transform into the nondividing (in the mammalian host) stumpy form.
8. Eventually the parasite enters the central nervous system (CNS).

EPIDEMIOLOGY

▌ *T. b. gambiense* is found in West and Central Africa, and *T. b. rhodesiense* is endemic in East Africa.
▌ *T. b. gambiense* infection is prevalent in river areas where the insect vector resides. Humans are the primary reservoir host, and transmission is principally human to fly to human.
▌ *T. b. rhodesiense* infection occurs in the woodland areas where the insect vector and its reservoir hosts (wild animals) are found.

CONTROL

▌ Avoid contact with the vector by wearing protective clothing and through the use of repellents.
▌ Exterminate or control the vector by the use of insecticides and the destruction of the vector's habitat.

Trypanosoma cruzi

DISEASE. American trypanosomiasis, Chagas' disease

CLINICAL LABORATORY DIAGNOSIS

▌ Giemsa stained thick and thin blood smears for the trypomastigote
▌ Histopathologic examination for the amastigote

DIAGNOSTIC MORPHOLOGY

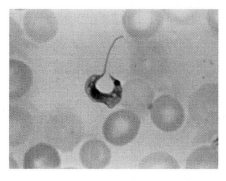

From Markell EK, Voge M: Medical Parasitology (a slide presentation). Philadelphia, WB Saunders, 1976.

Trypomastigote Stage
▌ Size: average 20 μm in length
▌ Shape: short and stubby to long and slender; in Giemsa stained blood films: **C** or **U** shaped
▌ Nucleus: oval and central
▌ Kinetoplast: large, oval and located posterior to the nucleus; subterminal
▌ Flagellum: anterior long free flagellum
▌ Undulating membrane: delicate (visualized by scanning EM)

BLOOD AND TISSUE PROTOZOA

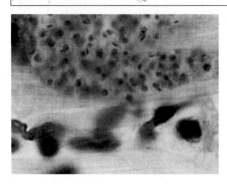

From Markell EK, Voge M: Medical Parasitology (a slide presentation). Philadelphia, WB Saunders, 1976.

Amastigote Stage
- Size: 3 to 5 μm
- Shape: ovoid
- Nucleus: large and eccentric
- Kinetoplast: small rodlike structure positioned opposite the nucleus
- Axoneme: rodlike structure perpendicular to the kinetoplast

LIFE CYCLE

1. The nocturnally active infected insect vector, the blood sucking reduviid bug (genera: *Triatoma, Panstrongylus,* and *Rhodnius*) bites the host, usually near the eye, or about the nose or lips (thus the name *kissing bug*).
2. During the blood meal, the vector usually defecates, and the fecal material containing the infective metacyclic trypomastigotes enters the host through the bite or may be rubbed into skin abrasions or intact mucous membranes.
3. At the site of inoculation, an edematous swelling occurs, the *chagoma*, which represents the area where the parasites (as amastigotes) are colonizing the tissue cells.
4. The amastigotes multiply by binary fission within the cells until the cells are almost completely filled with the amastigotes, forming a pseudocyst, which eventually ruptures, releasing the parasites.
5. After rupture, transformation of the amastigote to both the transitional form (the epimastigote) and the trypomastigote form occurs.
6. The nonmultiplying trypomastigotes enter the bloodstream and lymphatics and are disseminated throughout the body. The parasite preferentially invades the fixed phagocytic cells of the reticuloendothelium system (RES), cardiac muscle, and neuroglial cells of the CNS.
7. In addition to disseminating the infection in the host, the circulating trypomastigotes are infective for susceptible insect vectors. On feeding upon an infected host, the vector ingests the trypomastigote, which in the midgut transforms into the epimastigote, which then multiplies by asexual division. The epimastigote then transforms into the infective metacyclic trypomastigote and migrates to the hindgut of the insect, and the cycle repeats itself.

EPIDEMIOLOGY

- Significant human infections with *T. cruzi* are found in Central and South America.
- Reservoirs of *T. cruzi* are opossums, raccoons, woodrats, armadillos, dogs, and cats.
- The infected vector, the reduviid bug, is found, not only in South and Central America but in the United States as well. The feeding habits of the vector (to be an effective transmitter of the parasite the vector must defecate while feeding), the domiciliation of the vector (favored by poorly constructed homes that provide crevices for the vector), strain differences in the virulence of the parasite, and poor sanitation practices favor the transmission of the parasite in the rural and poor areas of Central and South America.

- The disease is more common in children.
- Congenital transmission has been reported.

CONTROL

- Use of insecticides to control the vector (DTT, lindane, dieldrin)
- Avoidance of contact with animal reservoirs
- Construction of better housing that prevents the nesting of the vector in the home
- Education of the populace about the preventive measures to control the disease.

Toxoplasma gondii

DISEASE. Toxoplasmosis

CLINICAL LABORATORY DIAGNOSIS. It is difficult to identify the parasite in tissue, and therefore serologic tests are often relied upon for diagnosis.

- The two serologic tests most often used for the measurement of antibodies to *T. gondii* are the indirect fluorescent antibody test and the enzyme linked immunosorbent assay (ELISA). To diagnose congenital toxoplasmosis, the measurement of IgM with the double sandwich ELISA test is recommended.
- Giemsa stained smears of exudates, aspirates, or tissues are used.

DIAGNOSTIC MORPHOLOGY

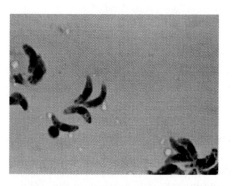

From Markell EK, Voge M: Medical Parasitology (a slide presentation). Philadelphia, WB Saunders, 1976.

Tachyzoite Form
- Size: 3×6 μm
- Shape: crescentic to pyriform
- Nucleus: large and centrally located

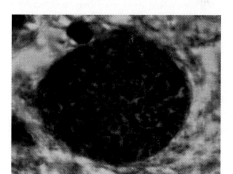

From Markell EK, Voge M: Medical Parasitology (a slide presentation). Philadelphia, WB Saunders, 1976.

Cyst (Bradyzoite) Form
- Shape: oval
- Size: up to 200 μm
- Contents: many spherical bradyzoites

BLOOD AND TISSUE PROTOZOA

LIFE CYCLE

1. Domestic cats and several other members of the family Felidae (definitive host) become infected by eating infected rodents (intermediate host) harboring the cyst form of *T. gondii.*
2. The cyst wall is digested and liberates bradyzoites that enter the epithelial cells of the small intestine.
3. Intracelluar multiplication occurs, terminating with the production of micro- and macrogametes.
4. Fusion of the gametes occurs, resulting in the formation of the oocyst.
5. The immature oocyst is released from the intestinal epithelial cells and is excreted with the feces into the external environment.
6. After several days the oocyst matures.
7. The mature oocyst (oval, 10×13 µm), containing four sporozoites, may be ingested by a variety of animals (intermediate hosts), including humans (accidental intermediate host).
8. The sporozoites are released in the small intestine and enter the host cells.
9. Asexual reproduction occurs, forming tachyzoites, which fill and finally rupture the cell, liberating the progeny, which in turn infect new cells.
10. As the disease proceeds to the chronic stage, the infection may spread to multiple organ systems such as skeletal muscle, brain, and heart, where the rapidly dividing tachyzoites become less active and are termed *bradyzoites.*
11. These bradyzoites gather in large numbers and form cysts.

> **NOTE** The cat may also ingest the oocyst and have a cycle similar to that of other animals (intermediate hosts), except that a sexual cycle also occurs with the formation of the oocyst.
>
> Humans and other carnivores may also become infected by eating *T. gondii* infected meat.
>
> *T. gondii* may be congenitally acquired by transplacental passage of the parasite.

EPIDEMIOLOGY

- Cosmopolitan.
- A wide variety of mammals and birds are susceptible to *T. gondii* infection.
- Infection may be acquired by (1) ingestion of oocyst contaminated water, (2) aerosolization of oocyst contaminated dust or litter, (3) consumption of raw or undercooked cyst infected meat, or (4) transplacental passage of the tachyzoite.

CONTROL

- Cats' litter boxes should be cleaned and disinfected daily.
- Children's sandboxes should be covered when not in use to prevent cats from defecating in them.
- After handling meat, hands should be washed thoroughly.
- All meat should be thoroughly cooked before consumption.
- Pregnant women should avoid contact with cats, litter boxes, or sandboxes.

Leishmania

tropica complex, *mexicana* complex, *braziliensis* complex, *donovani*

DISEASES

L. tropica complex causes Old World cutaneous leishmaniasis (Oriental sore, Aleppo boil, Delhi ulcer, Baghdad boil).

L. mexicana causes New World cutaneous leishmaniasis (chiclero ulcer, bay sore).

L. braziliensis causes mucocutaneous leishmaniasis (espundia, uta).

L. donovani causes visceral leishmaniasis (kala-azar or black disease, Dumdum fever).

CLINICAL LABORATORY DIAGNOSIS. Giemsa stained tissue sections or impression smears

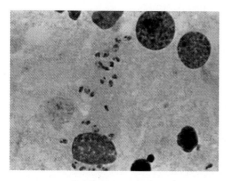

From Markell EK, Voge M: Medical Parasitology (a slide presentation). Philadelphia, WB Saunders, 1976.

DIAGNOSTIC MORPHOLOGY
Amastigote Stage

▌ Size: 2–4 μm in diameter
▌ Shape: ovoid
▌ Nucleus: large and eccentric
▌ Kinetoplast: small rodlike structure positioned opposite the nucleus
▌ Axoneme: rodlike structure perpendicular to the kinetoplast

LIFE CYCLE

1. The infected female sandfly of the genus *Phlebotomus* in the Old World and the genus *Lutzomyia* in the New World bites a susceptible host (humans, reservoir vertebrates: dogs, foxes, marsupials, and a number of small forest animals), and during the blood meal leishmanial promastigotes are dislodged from the insect's foregut and proboscis and are swept into the puncture wound.

2. The promastigotes are ingested by mononuclear phagocytic cells and transform into amastigotes and divide. When the cell is full of amastigotes, it ruptures and the released parasites infect nearby macrophages. In this manner, depending on the species of *Leishmania,* the infection may be spread to extensive areas of the skin and mucous membranes or may be transmitted throughout the body and infect cells in many of the internal organs of the reticuloendothelial system.

3. The cycle is completed when a female sandfly takes a blood meal (a requirement for egg maturation) from an infected host and ingests macrophages containing amastigotes.

4. After the amastigotes are released from the host cell in the midgut of the fly, they transform into promastigotes and actively divide by binary fission.

5. The promastigotes migrate to the pharynx and buccal cavity of the fly, where they can be transmitted during the next bite. The cycle within the sandfly takes approximately 10 days.

BLOOD AND TISSUE PROTOZOA

EPIDEMIOLOGY

▌ *L. donovani* is endemic in India, the Mediterranean countries, China, Middle Asia, East Africa, Central and South America.

In India, the human is the only apparent host.

In other countries dogs, wild canids, and rodents may serve as reservoir hosts.

Around the Mediterranean area, children are the more commonly infected age group. This is probably because dogs are the primary reservoir host.

▌ *L. tropica* is endemic in Asia, India, the Mediterranean basin, and the north and west coasts of Africa.

Gerbils (rural leishmaniasis) and dogs (urban leishmaniasis) are the primary reservoir hosts.

▌ *L. brasiliensis* is endemic in South and Central America.

Rodents are the reservoir hosts.

▌ *L. mexicana* is endemic in rural areas of South and Central America. It also has occurred in south-central Texas.

Wild rodents are the reservoir hosts.

CONTROL

▌ Protection from sandfly bites. The use of repellents such as diethyltoluamide (Off) has proved effective.
▌ Spraying of houses with insecticides such as DDT.
▌ Destruction, where possible, of infected reservoir hosts (i.e., infected dogs).
▌ Treatment of infected people.
▌ Protection of leishmanial lesions from sandflies.

PROTOZOA FROM OTHER BODY SITES

Free Living Amebae

NAEGLERIA

DISEASE. Primary amebic meningoencephalitis (PAM)

ACANTHAMOEBA

DISEASE. Chronic granulomatous amebic encephalitis (GAE) and keratitis

DIFFERENTIAL CHARACTERISTICS OF THE FREE LIVING AMEBAE

ORGANISM	TROPHOZOITE FORM			CYST FORM		FLAGELLATE STAGE	MICROSCOPIC VIEW
	Size (μm)	Pseudopodia	Motility	Size (μm)	Features	Presence	
Naegleria	10–35	Broad	Active	7–15	Smooth walled	Yes	*
Acanthamoeba	15–45	Filamentous	Sluggish	10–25	Double walled	No	*

* Photomicrographs courtesy of David T. John, PhD, Oklahoma State University, College of Osteopathic Medicine, Tulsa, OK.

PROTOZOA FROM OTHER BODY SITES

CLINICAL LABORATORY DIAGNOSIS

❚ Direct microscopic examination of sample as a wet mount in suspected cases of PAM or GAE.

❚ Permanent stained smears using Wheatley's trichrome stain.

❚ Culture of organism by inoculation of sample (spinal fluid, corneal scrapings) onto nonnutritive agar seeded with *E. coli* or *E. aerogenes*.

See "Differential Characteristics of the Free Living Amebae" on p 717.

LIFE CYCLE
Naegleria

1. In its natural habitat, this organism alternates between the ameboid and cyst phases and the ameboid and biflagellate phases.
2. Infection occurs when the ameba enters the nose, penetrates the cribiform plate, and multiplies in the brain.

Acanthamoeba

1. In its natural habitat, this organism alternates between the ameboid phase and the cyst phase.
2. Infection occurs when the organism enters the body via the respiratory tract or through ulcers in the skin or mucosa, often followed by hematogenous spread to the CNS. Direct invasion of the eye may also occur, resulting in *Acanthamoeba* keratitis.
3. Within the human host, both ameboid and cyst stages occur.

EPIDEMIOLOGY
Naegleria

❚ Worldwide distribution.

❚ Parasite may be present in warm lakes, streams, ponds, backwater bays, and heated, inadequately chlorinated indoor swimming pools.

❚ Infections have occurred mainly in children and young adults.

Acanthamoeba

❚ Epidemiology has not been adequately described.

❚ GAE has not been linked to swimming; it occurs in the immunocompromised or debilitated host.

❚ *Acanthamoeba* keratitis is associated with trauma to the eye with contaminated materials and with contact lenses that were immersed in improperly sterilized normal saline solutions.

CONTROL
Naegleria

❚ Avoid swimming in warm, muddy, or stagnant bodies of water.

❚ Use adequate levels of chlorination in swimming pools.

Acanthamoeba

❚ Disinfect contact lenses as directed by the manufacturer; use only certified sterile normal saline solutions for contact lens immersion.

Trichomonas vaginalis

DISEASE. Trichomonad vaginitis

CLINICAL LABORATORY DIAGNOSIS. Wet mount of vaginal exudate, prostatic fluid, fresh urine sample

DIAGNOSTIC MORPHOLOGY. Microscopic examination of the wet mount: large, 15 to 18 by 5 to 15 μm, pyriform, flagellate exhibiting rapid and jerky motility. The wavelike motion of the undulating membrane is often apparent.

LIFE CYCLE

1. The trophozoite of *T. vaginalis* (there is no cyst stage) is transmitted from the infected to the noninfected host. In females the usual habitat is the vagina and urethra, and in the male it is the urethra and the prostate.
2. Asexual reproduction occurs by binary longitudinal fission within the infected host.

EPIDEMIOLOGY

▌ Cosmopolitan.
▌ The human is the sole source of infection.
▌ Incidence of infection in females approaches 25%.
▌ Transmission occurs principally through sexual intercourse; also may be transmitted to newborns from infected mothers during delivery and by fomites.

CONTROL

▌ Attention to personal hygiene.
▌ Use of condoms during sexual intercourse.

HELMINTHS

INTESTINAL NEMATODES

Enterobius vermicularis

DISEASE. Enterobiasis, oxyuriasis, pinworm infection, seatworm infection

CLINICAL LABORATORY DIAGNOSIS. Microscopic examination of a cellophane tape preparation of the perianal area

DIAGNOSTIC MORPHOLOGY. See "Differential Morphology of the Intestinal Nematode Ova" on p **725.**

LIFE CYCLE

1. Infective ova containing the rhabditiform larva (first stage larva) are ingested by the human host.
2. The larvae are released in the duodenum and molt twice during their migration to the lower intestine.
3. The worms attach to the intestinal mucosa and feed on epithelial cells and bacteria.
4. The mature adults copulate in the cecum, where soon afterward the male worm dies.
5. The gravid females migrate to the perianal regions, deposit their ova, and die.
6. Within a few hours the ova mature and become infective.

EPIDEMIOLOGY

▌ Cosmopolitan, with greater prevalence in temperate regions.
▌ Greatest incidence in schoolchildren.
▌ Sources of infection: oral-fecal route, through contaminated food or fomites, inhalation followed by ingestion of airborne ova, and retroinfection, whereby some larvae hatch and migrate back into the intestine.

CONTROL

❚ Attention should be paid to personal hygiene.
❚ Children with pinworm infection should wear tight fitting pajama pants to prevent, by hindering hand contact with the anal area, both reinfection and the dissemination of infective ova.
❚ All bedding should be washed in hot water, and the entire household should be cleaned thoroughly to reduce the prevalence of infective ova in the household.

Ascaris lumbricoides

DISEASE. Ascariasis, roundworm infection

CLINICAL LABORATORY DIAGNOSIS. Wet mount of a formalin–ethyl acetate concentrate of a fecal sample stained with D'Antoni's iodine

DIAGNOSTIC MORPHOLOGY. See "Differential Morphology of the Intestinal Nematode Ova" on p **725.**

LIFE CYCLE

1. Unsegmented ova are passed admixed with fecal material by the infected host (human) into the external environment.
2. Under favorable conditions (i.e., moisture and a temperature of 21° to 30°C) in the soil, the first stage larva is formed. Formation of the infective second stage larva occurs after its first molt. The process from unsegmented ova to infective larvae takes about 2 to 3 weeks.
3. After the ingestion of ova containing infective larvae, they hatch in the upper small intestine, and the freed larvae penetrate the intestinal wall and enter the portal circulation via the blood and/or lymphatic vessels.
4. From the liver the larvae are carried to the heart and via the pulmonary artery to the lungs, where they undergo their second and third molts.
5. Since the larvae are larger in diameter than the diameter of the pulmonary capillaries, the larvae break out into the alveoli.
6. The larvae then migrate or are carried to the bronchi, then to trachea, and then to the glottis and finally pass down the esophagus to the intestine, where they undergo a fourth molt.
7. Maturation to adult males and females occurs in the lower small intestine.
8. Mating occurs, and about 2.5 months after infection, ovipositing females develop.
9. The life span of the adult worms is about 12 to 18 months.

EPIDEMIOLOGY

❚ Ascariasis is present in both temperate and tropical zones, but more common in warm countries, especially where sanitation is poor.
❚ Infection occurs at all ages, but it is usually more common in preschool and early school aged children.
❚ The prevalence of ascariasis is dependent on socioeconomic, educational, and sanitary factors. Ascaris infection is prominent in poor and rural communities, where there is heavy soil pollution and poor hygiene.

CONTROL

❚ Family hygiene: Sanitary disposal of feces
❚ Avoidance of using night soil (human feces) as fertilizer unless treated to destroy parasites (compost manuring, chemicals).

- Eating of cooked food and avoidance or thorough washing of green vegetables or salads where night soil is used as a fertilizer.
- Educational programs
- Regular chemotherapy to reduce the intensity and prevalence of infection

Necator americanus

DISEASE. New World hookworm disease

CLINICAL LABORATORY DIAGNOSIS. Wet mount of a formalin–ethyl acetate concentrate of a fecal sample stained with D'Antoni's iodine

DIAGNOSTIC MORPHOLOGY. See "Differential Morphology of the Intestinal Nematode Ova" on p **725** and "Differential Morphology of the Rhabditiform Larvae of the Intestinal Nematodes" on p **727.**

LIFE CYCLE

1. *Necator* ova are passed in the feces into the environment.
2. Under favorable conditions (loose soil, high humidity, warm and shady), embryonation continues, followed by the hatching of the ova and the release of the first stage larva, the rhabditiform larva.
3. The first stage larva actively feeds on organic debris and bacteria in the soil.
4. After 2 to 3 days there is a molt into a second rhabditiform larva, which continues feeding.
5. After 2 to 5 days, another molt occurs to produce the third stage infective, nonfeeding larva, the filariform larva.
6. The filariform larvae climb up on moist soil particles, moist vegetative debris, and so forth, and extend themselves in the air awaiting a host to penetrate (i.e., foot, ankle, and so forth).
7. The filariform larvae, on contact with human skin, penetrate the skin and burrow until they enter a lymph or blood vessel.
8. The larvae are carried to the right side of the heart and enter the alveoli.
9. The ciliary movement of the bronchial and tracheal epithelium carries the larvae to the throat.
10. The larvae are swallowed and pass down the esophagus to the stomach and finally to the intestines.
11. The larvae bury themselves between the intestinal (jejunum) villi, where they molt.
12. The larvae grow rapidly and molt once more and acquire adult characteristics. They attach to the intestinal mucosa by their buccal capsule and suck blood and mucosal substances.
13. About 5 weeks after infection, fertilization occurs and the female worms begin to release ova.

EPIDEMIOLOGY

- Endemic to South America, Africa (south of the Sahara), parts of India, North America (especially southeast sections)
- Also found with *Ancylostoma duodenale* in China, Southeast Asia, islands of the South and Southwest Pacific, and parts of Australia

CONTROL

- Personal protection: wearing of shoes and other protective clothing to prevent contact with soil laden with hookworm

INTESTINAL NEMATODES

▌ Chemical disinfection of feces in areas where hookworm is endemic and where human feces are deposited directly into the soil

▌ Public education about the transmission of the disease and its prevention

▌ In areas of high incidence of infection (>50%), mass institution of chemotherapeutic measures accompanied by improvements in sanitation

Ancylostoma duodenale

DISEASE. Old World hookworm disease

CLINICAL LABORATORY DIAGNOSIS. Wet mount of a formalin–ethyl acetate concentrate of a fecal sample stained with D'Antoni's iodine

DIAGNOSTIC MORPHOLOGY. See *"Necator americanus"* on pp **725** and **727**.

LIFE CYCLE. See *"Necator americanus"* on p **721**.

EPIDEMIOLOGY. Endemic to India, northern Africa, Southeast Asia, southern Europe, China, and scattered areas within the Caribbean islands and North and South America.

CONTROL. See *"Necator americanus"* on p **721**.

Trichostrongylus **Species**

DISEASE. Trichostrongyliasis

CLINICAL LABORATORY DIAGNOSIS. Wet mount of a formalin–ethyl acetate concentrate of fecal sample stained with D'Antoni's iodine

DIAGNOSTIC MORPHOLOGY. See "Differential Morphology of the Intestinal Nematode Ova" on p **726**.

LIFE CYCLE

1. Ova, admixed with feces, are passed into the external environment.
2. Larvae hatch out of the ova, undergo two molts, and become infective larvae.
3. Infection is acquired by the ingestion of the infective larvae in fecal contaminated foodstuffs.
4. The larvae pass directly to the upper intestine, where they attach and feed.
5. After two molts the adult worms detach, pass into the lumen, and produce ova.

EPIDEMIOLOGY

▌ Common in many parts of the world, especially the Far East.

▌ A common parasite of many mammals, including farm animals, rodents, and birds.

▌ In endemic areas, humans are frequently an accidental host.

CONTROL

▌ Avoidance of the use of human fecal fertilizer.

▌ Soil fumigation

▌ Avoidance of the consumption of raw vegetable material from contaminated areas.

Trichuris trichiura

DISEASE. Trichuriasis, trichocephaliasis, whipworm infection

CLINICAL LABORATORY DIAGNOSIS. Wet mount of a formalin–ethyl acetate concentrate of a fecal sample stained with D'Antoni's iodine

DIAGNOSTIC MORPHOLOGY. See "Differential Morphology of the Intestinal Nematode Ova" on p **726.**

LIFE CYCLE
1. Single stage ova are passed, admixed with feces, by the infected host (i.e., a human) into the external environment.
2. Under favorable conditions (i.e., warmth, moist soil, dense shade, high humidity), the ova undergo embryonic development and contain, after several weeks to several months, first stage infective larvae.
3. After ingestion, the activated larvae escape from their weakened eggshell in the upper small intestine, penetrate intestinal villi, and develop there for about 10 days.
4. On reaching adolescence, the parasites migrate to the cecum. Here they embed a spearlike projection, which is located at their anterior end, into the intestinal mucosa.
5. After mating, the females produce ova in 2 to 3 months.

EPIDEMIOLOGY
▌ Cosmopolitan parasite
▌ Most common in warm, moist climates, especially where sanitation is poor

CONTROL
▌ Sanitary disposal of human feces
▌ Washing of hands before meals
▌ Thorough washing and scalding of raw vegetables
▌ Treatment of infected individuals

Strongyloides stercoralis

DISEASE. Strongyloidiasis, Cochin-China diarrhea

CLINICAL LABORATORY DIAGNOSIS
▌ Wet mount of a formalin–ethyl acetate concentrate of a fecal sample stained with D'Antoni's iodine
▌ Direct saline or iodine stained wet mount of duodenal contents, or material from the "string test."*
▌ Direct saline or iodine stained wet mount of sputum in disseminated strongyloidiasis

DIAGNOSTIC MORPHOLOGY. See "Differential Morphology of the Intestinal Nematode Ova" on p **725** and "Differential Morphology of the Rhabditiform Larvae of Intestinal Nematodes" on p **727.**

---

*Enterotest, International Health Services, Mountainview, CA.

INTESTINAL NEMATODES

LIFE CYCLE. *Strongyloides* larvae (free living rhabditiform larvae) are passed with the feces into the external environment.

> **NOTE** Two different cycles may occur, direct or indirect. Which cycle takes place is believed to be dependent on the existing environmental conditions. The indirect cycle is favored by warm, moist tropical climates, whereas the direct cycle is favored by suboptimal conditions such as those found in more temperate climates.

Indirect (Free Living) Cycle

1. The rhabditiform larvae molt and differentiate into free living, sexually mature males and females.
2. After fertilization, the female deposits her ova.
3. The ova hatch into rhabditiform larvae and thence into either free living males and females or into the infective filariform larvae.
4. The filariform larvae penetrate the human skin, enter the venous circulation, migrate to the lungs, and pass into the alveoli. During the course of this migration the larvae molt twice and become adolescent worms.
5. The parasites then ascend to the glottis, are swallowed, and on reaching the upper intestine burrow into its mucosa.
6. Parthenogenetic females deposit their ova in the mucosa.
7. The ova hatch into rhabditiform larvae and eventually are passed out with the feces.
8. Within the intestinal mucosa, the rhabditiform larvae may quickly develop into the filariform stage, penetrate the intestinal mucosa or the perianal skin, and repeat steps 4 through 8. This process is termed *autoinfection* and is responsible for hyperinfection and the persistence of infection in nonendemic areas.

Direct Cycle

1. The rhabditiform larvae molt into the infective filariform larvae.
2. See steps 4 through 8 under "Indirect (Free Living) Cycle" above.

EPIDEMIOLOGY

- Cosmopolitan with a distribution similar to that of hookworm
- Found in long term care facilities and in institutions where hygienic measures are not maintained

CONTROL

- Proper sanitary techniques in the disposal of fecal debris
- Wearing of shoes in endemic areas

Differential Morphology of the Intestinal Nematode Ova

ORGANISM	AVERAGE SIZE (μm)	SHAPE	IMPORTANT FEATURES AND COMMENTS	MICROSCOPIC VIEW
Enterobius vermicularis	55 × 26	Oval, asymmetric with one side noticeably flattened	Smooth, thin shelled; may contain embryo	*
Ascaris lumbricoides	Fertile ovum: 60 × 45 Infertile ovum: 90 × 40	Fertile ovum: broadly oval; thick shell Infertile ovum: elongated with thin shell	Fertile ovum: thick shell, often surrounded by bumpy outer layer (mammillated, albuminous covering); albuminous layer may be absent (decorticated) Infertile ovum: surrounded by irregular albuminous layer	*
Hookworm *Necator americanus* *Ancylostoma duodenale*	60–65 × 40	Oval or ellipsoid; thin shell	Usually embryo at four cell stage. Ovum of *Strongyloides stercoralis* is morphologically identical to hookworm ova but is rarely found in stool.	*

Continued ▶

INTESTINAL NEMATODES

▲ Continued **Differential Morphology of the Intestinal Nematode Ova**

ORGANISM	AVERAGE SIZE (μm)	SHAPE	IMPORTANT FEATURES AND COMMENTS	MICROSCOPIC VIEW
Trichostrongylus **Species**	89 × 48	Oval with thin shell; one end more pointed	Similar to hookworm ova except for size and asymmetry at poles	*
Trichuris trichiura	52 × 23	Barrel shaped with distinctive plugs at both ends	Intestinal nematode ova of *Capillaria hepatica* and *Capillaria philippinensis* are similar to *T. trichiura* ova but are rarely encountered and are not discussed further.	*

* Photomicrographs from Markell EK, Voge M: Medical Parasitology (a slide presentation). Philadelphia, WB Saunders, 1976.

Differential Morphology of the Rhabditiform Larvae of the Intestinal Nematodes

ORGANISM	USUAL SIZE (μm)	SHAPE	BUCCAL CAVITY	GENITAL PRIMORDIUM	COMMENTS	MICROSCOPIC VIEW
Strongyloides stercoralis	225 × 16	Cylindric	Short (10 μm), 1/3 to 1/2 as long as width of anterior end of body	Prominent, approximately 35 μm	This form is usually passed in stool.	
Hookworm *Necator americanus* *Ancylostoma duodenale*	250 × 17	Cylindric	Long (20 μm), about as long as width of body	Small and inconspicuous, approximately 20 μm	This form is rarely passed in stool.	

INTESTINAL CESTODES

Taenia saginata

DISEASE. Taeniasis, beef tapeworm infection

CLINICAL LABORATORY DIAGNOSIS

▮ Perianal swabbing for the gravid prolottid. Clear the proglottid in warm normal saline followed by carbol-xylene; press between two glass sides and study microscopically.

▮ Wet mount of a formalin–ethyl acetate concentrate of a fecal sample stained with D'Antoni's iodine. Study microscopically for *Taenia* ova (less sensitive than swabbing technique).

DIAGNOSTIC MORPHOLOGY. See "Differential Morphology of the Intestinal Cestode Ova" on p **733** and "Differential Morphology of Cestode Gravid Proglottids" on p **735.**

LIFE CYCLE

1. The definitive host, a human, ingests raw or undercooked beef containing the cysticercus, which is also known as a *bladder worm.*
2. In the small intestine, the invaginated scolex and neck within the cysticercus evaginate and the bladder is digested or absorbed by the scolex.
3. The scolex of the adult tapeworm attaches to the wall of the small intestine by means of its four suckers.
4. It develops into an adult worm in several weeks and begins shedding gravid proglottids.
5. The gravid proglottids actively crawl out of the anus or may be passed out with the stool.
6. The proglottids begin to dry in the external environment, rupture, and release several hundred infective ova.
7. The ova are ingested by grazing cattle (intermediate host).
8. The ova hatch in response to gastric secretions and pass into the intestine.
9. The hexacanth embryo leaves the ova, enters the intestinal wall, and reaches the muscles by means of the circulatory system.
10. Within the muscle, the embryo develops into a mature cysticercus (cysticercus bovis).

EPIDEMIOLOGY

▮ Cosmopolitan in beef eating countries.

▮ Humans acquire the infection by eating raw or undercooked beef containing cysticerci.

▮ Cattle acquire the infection from grazing on land contaminated with ova from sewage or from human feces used as fertilizer (night soil).

CONTROL

▮ Prevent contamination of grazing land by treating infected humans and by the disuse of night soil.

▮ Inspect beef for cysticerci.

▮ Thoroughly cook all beef before consumption.

Taenia solium

DISEASE. Taeniasis, pork tapeworm infection

CLINICAL LABORATORY DIAGNOSIS

▌ Search fecal material for the gravid proglottid and procede as explained under *"Taenia saginata"* on p **728.**

▌ Wet mount of a formalin–ethyl acetate concentrate of a fecal sample stained with D'Antoni's iodine. Study microscopically for *Taenia* ova.

DIAGNOSTIC MORPHOLOGY. See "Differential Morphology of the Intestinal Cestode Ova" on p **733** and "Differential Morphology of Cestode Gravid Proglottids" on p **735.**

LIFE CYCLE

1. The definitive host, a human, eats raw or undercooked pork infected with the larval stage (cysticercus) of *T. solium.*
2. The scolex evaginates in the small intestine and becomes attached to the intestinal mucosa via its four suckers and two rows of hooks.
3. After several weeks, it develops into an adult worm and begins shedding gravid proglottids.
4. The gravid proglottids and their liberated ova are released with the stool into the external environment.
5. The intermediate host, a pig, ingests the ova. Humans may also ingest the ova and act like an intermediate host. See "Cysticercosis in Humans" below.
6. The hexacanth embryo escapes from the ova in the small intestine.
7. The embryo penetrates the intestinal wall and is transported via the circulation to the voluntary muscles, where the mature cysticercus (bladder worm) forms.

Cysticercosis in Humans

1. A human may ingest *T. solium* ova from the following sources:

   Fecally contaminated food or water

   Ova on the hands of individuals infected with the adult worm

   Regurgitation of proglottids from the intestine into the stomach, followed by the release of ova (autoinfection)

2. The hexacanth embryos escape from the ova in the small intestine, penetrate the intestinal wall, and are transported via the circulation to various parts of the body to form mature cysticerci.

EPIDEMIOLOGY

▌ Worldwide distribution where pigs have access to human feces and where cured or undercooked pork is eaten.

▌ Endemic in Latin America, China, India, and Africa.

▌ Principal intermediate hosts are the pig and boar.

CONTROL

▌ Thorough cooking of pork and pork products
▌ Inspection of pork for cysticerci
▌ Treatment of infected people
▌ Sanitary disposal of human fecal waste

Hymenolepis nana

DISEASE. Hymenolepiasis, dwarf tapeworm infection

INTESTINAL CESTODES

CLINICAL LABORATORY DIAGNOSIS. Wet mount of a formalin–ethyl acetate concentrate of a fecal sample stained with D'Anotoni's iodine

DIAGNOSTIC MORPHOLOGY. See "Differential Morphology of the Intestinal Cestode Ova" on p **733** and "Differential Morphology of Cestode Gravid Proglottids" on p **735.**

LIFE CYCLE

1. Ova are ingested by the definitive host (humans, mice, and rats).
2. The ova hatch in the upper small intestine, releasing the hexacanth embryo.
3. The embryo penetrates a villus and develops into a cysticercoid larva.
4. After several days, the larva leaves the villus and enters the lumen of the small intestine, where it attaches and matures into an adult.
5. After several weeks, gravid proglottids are liberated.
6. On reaching the large intestine, the proglottids disintegrate and release their ova.
7. The ova are passed with the stool and are immediately infective.

> **NOTE**   *H. nana* does not require an intermediate host. However, insect intermediate hosts, such as the grain beetle, do exist, and infection may be acquired when these insects are ingested.

EPIDEMIOLOGY

- Cosmopolitan.
- More prevalent in young children.
- Principal routes of infection are hand to mouth and contaminated food and water.

CONTROL

- Instruction in good personal hygiene, especially to young children
- Treatment of infected children to prevent autoinfection as well as the spread of infection to others
- Protection of food from rodents and insects

Hymenolepis diminuta

DISEASE. Hymenolepiasis, rat tapeworm infection

CLINICAL LABORATORY DIAGNOSIS. Wet mount of a formalin–ethyl acetate concentrate of a fecal sample stained with D'Antoni's iodine

DIAGNOSTIC MORPHOLOGY. See "Differential Morphology of the Intestinal Cestode Ova" on p **734** and "Differential Morphology of Cestode Gravid Proglottids" on p **736.**

LIFE CYCLE

1. Ova are passed in the fecal material of the definitive host (rat, mouse, and human) into the external environment.
2. The ova are ingested by a variety of insects (the intermediate host), principally the rat and mouse flea, the flour moth and flour beetle.
3. Within the insect, the ovum hatches into a hexacanth embryo.
4. The embryo penetrates the insect's body cavity, where it develops into a cysticercoid.

5. On ingestion of the infected insect by the definitive host, the cysticercoid is liberated and attaches to the small intestine, where it develops into an adult worm.
6. The gravid proglottids detach from the worm, disintegrate, and release the infective ova.

EPIDEMIOLOGY

▮ Cosmopolitan
▮ More prevalent in young children
▮ Principal sources of infection are infected insect contaminated grains and rice; also transfer of infected insects by unclean hands to the mouth (primarily in children).

CONTROL

▮ Protect grains and rice from insects, rats, and mice.
▮ Control insects by the use of pesticides and rodents by the use of traps or poison.

Diphyllobothrium latum

DISEASE. Diphyllobothriasis, fish tapeworm infection, broad tapeworm infection

CLINICAL LABORATORY DIAGNOSIS. Wet mount of a formalin–ethyl acetate concentrate of a fecal sample stained with D'Antoni's iodine

DIAGNOSTIC MORPHOLOGY. See "Differential Morphology of the Intestinal Cestode Ova" on p **734** and "Differential Morphology of Cestode Gravid Proglottids" on p **736.**

LIFE CYCLE

1. Immature ova are passed with the feces by the definitive host (human, dog, cat, and many other mammals) into fresh water.
2. After nine days to several weeks, a ciliated embryo, the coracidium, escapes the ovum through its operculum.
3. The randomly swimming coracidium is ingested by a crustacean belonging to the genera *Cyclops* or *Diaptomus* (first intermediate host).
4. The coracidium penetrates the body cavity of the crustacean and transforms into a procercoid larva.
5. When the infected crustacean is eaten by a suitable fresh water fish (second intermediate host), it is digested and the released procercoid larva penetrates the intestinal wall and enters the viscera, connective tissue, and muscles.
6. After one to several weeks, the procercoid larva transforms into a plerocercoid larva.
7. The infected fish may be eaten by a definitive host or it may be devoured by a larger carnivorous fish such as the pike, salmon, trout, or whitefish. Within the larger fish the released plerocercoid larva does not develop further and is infectious for the definitive host.
8. On consumption and digestion of raw or undercooked plerocercoid infected fish by the definitive host, the larva is released and attaches to the small intestine. Maturity is reached in several weeks.
9. The ova are discharged from the gravid proglottids of the adult worm through their uterine pore and are evacuated with the stool.

EPIDEMIOLOGY

▌ Primarily found in the northern temperate and subarctic regions.

▌ Source of infection is the consumption of raw or partially cooked contaminated fish.

▌ More prevalent in young children.

▌ Discharge of untreated sewage into lakes or rivers may result in infection of large numbers of susceptible fish.

CONTROL

▌ Thorough cooking of all fish

▌ Adequate treatment of sewage

Dipylidium caninum

DISEASE. Dipylidiasis, dog tapeworm infection

CLINICAL LABORATORY DIAGNOSIS

▌ Search fecal material for the gravid proglottid and procede as explained under *"Taenia saginata"* on p **728.**

▌ Wet mount of a formalin–ethyl acetate concentrate of a fecal sample stained with D'Antoni's iodine. Study microscopically for the packets of ova.

DIAGNOSTIC MORPHOLOGY. See "Differential Morphology of the Intestinal Cestode Ova" on p **734** and "Differential Morphology of Cestode Gravid Proglottids" on p **736.**

LIFE CYCLE

1. Gravid proglottids detach from the adult worm and actively creep out of the anal orifice of the definitive host (dog and cat; the human is an occasional host).
2. The ova are either released by the contractions of the proglottid or by the proglottid's disintegration.
3. The larval flea, the usual intermediate host, ingests the ova.
4. The hexacanth embryo leaves the ova and penetrates the intestine, where it develops into a cysticercoid.
5. The definitive host ingests the infected flea.
6. The cysticercoid is freed and attaches to the upper intestinal wall, where it develops into an adult worm.

EPIDEMIOLOGY

▌ Worldwide; very common in dogs.

▌ Humans acquire the infection by the ingestion of infected dog or cat fleas.

▌ Most prevalent in young children.

CONTROL

▌ Do not allow children to play with pets infested with fleas.

▌ Treat flea infested pets and surroundings with insecticide.

▌ Treat infected pets with anthelmintic drugs.

Differential Morphology of the Intestinal Cestode Ova

ORGANISM	AVERAGE SIZE (μm)	SHAPE	IMPORTANT FEATURES	MICROSCOPIC VIEW
Taenia saginata	35 × 25	Spherical	Thick, radially striated shell containing six hooked embryo (hexacanth embryo)	*
Taenia solium	See *T. saginata*	See *T. saginata*	Indistinguishable from *T. saginata*	
Hymenolepis nana	47 × 37	Oval	Shell is composed of two membranes enclosing hexacanth embryo. Outer shell membrane is separated by clear space from inner membrane. Inner membrane has two polar thickenings with several filaments emanating from them.	*

Continued ▶

INTESTINAL CESTODES

▶ Continued **Differential Morphology of the Intestinal Cestode Ova**

ORGANISM	AVERAGE SIZE (μm)	SHAPE	IMPORTANT FEATURES	MICROSCOPIC VIEW
Hymenolepis diminuta	72 × 65	Oval	Thick, striated outer membrane is separated by granular space from thick inner membrane. Enclosed is hexacanth embryo. Lack of polar filaments and its size distinguish it from *H. nana*.	*
Diphyllobothrium latum	70 × 45	Oval to elliptic	At one pole there is indistinct operculum. At opposite pole there is knoblike thickening.	*
Dipylidium caninum	40 × 36	Spherical	Ovum contains hexacanth embryo. 8–15 ova are usually enclosed within saclike membrane.	*

* Photomicrographs from Markell EK, Voge M: Medical Parasitology (a slide presentation). Philadelphia, WB Saunders, 1976.

Differential Morphology of Cestode Gravid Proglottids

ORGANISM	AVERAGE SIZE (mm)	APPEARANCE OF UTERUS	IMPORTANT FEATURES	MICROSCOPIC VIEW
Taenia saginata	18 long × 6 wide	15–30 main uterine branches on each side of central stem	Proglottids are much longer than wide. They are distinguished from those of *T. solium* by larger number of uterine branches.	
Taenia solium	11 long × 6 wide	7–13 main uterine branches on each side of central stem	Proglottids are longer than wide. They are distinguished from those of *T. saginata* by smaller number of uterine branches.	
Hymenolepis nana	0.3 long × 0.85 wide	Sacculate uterus; single lateral gonopore	Proglottids are broader than long and are filled with 80–180 ova.	

Continued ▲

INTESTINAL CESTODES

▲ Continued **Differential Morphology of Cestode Gravid Proglottids**

ORGANISM	AVERAGE SIZE (mm)	APPEARANCE OF UTERUS	IMPORTANT FEATURES	MICROSCOPIC VIEW
Hymenolepis diminuta	0.75 long × 2.5 wide	Sacculate uterus; single lateral gonopore	Proglottids are broader than long.	✚
Diphyllobothrium latum	3 long × 11 wide	Rosette shaped and coiled; absence of lateral gonopore	Proglottids are broader than long.	✚
Dipylidium caninum	11 long × 2.8 wide	Barrel shaped; two gonopores on each proglottid; packed with sacs of ova	Proglottids are much longer than broad.	◆

✳ Photomicrograph from Markell EK, Voge M: Medical Parasitology (a slide presentation). Philadelphia, WB Saunders, 1976.
◆ Photomicrographs courtesy of Edward K. Markell, PhD, MD, Berkeley, CA.
✚ Photomicrographs by Eugene Wienke, MD, Pathology Laboratory, Deaconess Hospital Systems–Central Campus, St Louis, MO.

INTESTINAL TREMATODES

Clonorchis sinensis

Chinese or oriental liver fluke

DISEASE. Clonorchiasis

CLINICAL LABORATORY DIAGNOSIS
- Wet mount of a formalin–ethyl acetate concentrate of a fecal sample stained with D'Antoni's iodine
- Duodenal aspirate or material from the "string test"°

DIAGNOSTIC MORPHOLOGY. See "Differential Morphology of the Trematode Ova" on p **744.**

LIFE CYCLE
1. Ova with fully developed miracidia are passed with the stool into the external environment by the definitive host (human, dog, cat, and several other mammals).
2. After the ova are ingested by the first intermediate host, a fresh water snail (*Bulinus, Parafossarulus*), the miracidia escape the ova.
3. Within the snail's tissues, each miracidium forms a sporocyst, then rediae, and finally cercariae, which escape into the water.
4. On encountering the second intermediate host, a fresh water fish of the family *Cyprinidae,* the free swimming cercariae penetrate its skin and encyst as metacercariae, primarily in its muscles and subcutaneous tissues.
5. When infected fish are eaten raw or undercooked by the definitive host, the metacercariae excyst in the duodenum and migrate to the bile ducts.
6. Within the biliary tract the larvae become adult worms and begin producing ova.

EPIDEMIOLOGY
- Endemic in the Far East.
- Humans acquire infection by eating raw or undercooked infected fish.
- Fish farming in ponds using "night soil" (untreated human feces) as a fertilizer may result in infection in a large proportion of the fish.
- Dogs are important reservoir hosts.

CONTROL
- Thorough cooking of all fish
- Disuse of human feces as fertilizer in fish farms
- Destruction of the snail host

Fasciola hepatica

Sheep liver fluke

DISEASE. Fascioliasis, "liver rot"

°Enterotest, International Health Services, Mountainview, CA.

CLINICAL LABORATORY DIAGNOSIS. Wet mount of a formalin–ethyl acetate concentrate of a fecal sample stained with D'Antoni's iodine

DIAGNOSTIC MORPHOLOGY. See "Differential Morphology of the Trematode Ova" on p **744.**

LIFE CYCLE

1. Undifferentiated ova are voided with the feces into the external environment by the definitive host (sheep, cattle, and other mammals, including humans).
2. After several weeks, a miracidium develops in each ovum.
3. At maturity, the miracidia escape and swim on the moist vegetation seeking a suitable snail *(Lymnaea)*, which serves as the intermediate host.
4. Within the snail's tissues, each miracidium forms a sporocyst, rediae, and finally cercariae.
5. The cercariae escape from the snail and encyst as metacercariae on vegetation such as grasses and watercress.
6. When vegetation containing the metacercariae are eaten by the definitive host, the larvae excyst in the duodenum, penetrate the intestinal wall, and enter the peritoneal cavity.
7. From the peritoneal cavity the larvae migrate to and enter the liver, where they migrate for several weeks until reaching the biliary tract.
8. The larvae then mature into adults and produce ova.

EPIDEMIOLOGY

- Cosmopolitan in sheep and cattle raising countries.
- Principal definitive hosts are sheep and cattle; the human is an accidental host.
- Humans acquire the infection by eating watercress, lettuce, or radishes or by drinking water infested with the metacercariae.

CONTROL

- Treatment of infected domestic animals
- Destruction of the snail host
- Cooking of edible vegetation in endemic areas before consumption

Paragonimus westermani

Lung fluke

DISEASE. Paragonimiasis, pulmonary distomiasis, lung fluke disease

CLINICAL LABORATORY DIAGNOSIS

- Direct wet mount of sputum and/or a wet mount of sputum that has been treated with an equal volume of 3% sodium hydroxide followed after 30 minutes at room temperature by centrifugation
- Wet mount of a formalin–ethyl acetate concentrate of a fecal sample stained with D'Antoni's iodine

DIAGNOSTIC MORPHOLOGY. See "Differential Morphology of the Trematode Ova" on p **744.**

LIFE CYCLE

1. Unembryonated ova are passed into the external environment by the definitive host (humans and a variety of mammalian carnivores) admixed with sputa or feces.

2. After several weeks, a miracidium develops and matures within each ovum and is spontaneously released.

3. If the free swimming miracidium encounters a suitable fresh water snail (family *Thieridae*), the first intermediate host, it enters the snail and produces a sporocyst, rediae, and finally cercariae.

4. The cercariae leave the snail and seek their second intermediate host, the fresh water crab (*Eriocheir, Patamon, Sesarma, Parathelphusa*) or crayfish (*Cambarus, Astacus*).

5. After penetrating the crab or crayfish, the cercariae encyst as metacercariae in the host's gills, muscles, and viscera.

6. When infected crabs or crayfish are eaten by the definitive host, the metacercariae excyst in the duodenum and penetrate into the abdominal cavity.

7. The larvae then penetrate the diaphragm and enter the pleural cavity.

8. After reaching the lungs, they enter the bronchioles, mature, and produce ova.

EPIDEMIOLOGY

▐ Cosmopolitan among the reservoir hosts (carnivorous mammals); found in humans mainly in the Far East.

▐ The consumption of raw or undercooked infected freshwater crustaceans is the primary route of infection in the human.

CONTROL

▐ Cook all fresh water crustaceans.

▐ Wash hands and utensils after preparing crabs or crayfish to avoid transferring metacercariae to salads and other uncooked foods.

Fasciolopsis buski

Large or giant intestinal fluke

DISEASE. Fasciolopsiasis

CLINICAL LABORATORY DIAGNOSIS. Wet mount of a formalin–ethyl acetate concentrate of a fecal sample stained with D'Antoni's iodine

DIAGNOSTIC MORPHOLOGY. See "Differential Morphology of the Trematode Ova" on p **745.**

LIFE CYCLE

1. Unembryonated ova are passed with the fecal material into the external environment by the definitive host (pig and human).

2. After several weeks, the miracidium develops and matures within the ova and is spontaneously released.

3. The miracidium actively swims, seeking a suitable snail (*Segmentina, Hippeutis*), which serves as the intermediate host.

4. After penetrating the snail, the miracidium metamorphoses into a sporocyst, rediae, and lastly cercariae.

5. The cercariae leave the snail and swim to an aquatic plant, such as water chestnut and lotus, where they encyst as metacercariae.

6. When uncooked plants with encysted metacercariae are consumed by the definitive host, the larvae excyst in the duodenum and mature in the small intestine.

7. After several weeks, the adult worm begins producing ova.

INTESTINAL TREMATODES

EPIDEMIOLOGY

▌ Endemic in the Far East and Southeast Asia.

▌ Humans acquire the infection by consuming raw aquatic plants infested with metacercariae.

▌ Pigs are an important reservoir host.

CONTROL

▌ Thorough cooking of edible aquatic plants.

▌ Disuse of human feces as fertilizer in ponds.

▌ Keeping pig fecal waste from ponds where aquatic plants are harvested for human consumption.

Heterophyes heterophyes

DISEASE. Heterophyiasis

CLINICAL LABORATORY DIAGNOSIS. Wet mount of a formalin–ethyl acetate concentrate of a fecal sample stained with D'Antoni's iodine

DIAGNOSTIC MORPHOLOGY. See "Differential Characteristics of Trematode Ova" on p **745.**

LIFE CYCLE

1. Ova with fully developed miracidia are passed with the stool into the external environment by the definitive host (human, cat, dog, and other fish eating mammals).
2. Ova are ingested by the first intermediate host, brackish water snails (*Pirenella, Cerithidea*).
3. Within the snail's tissues, the miracidium is released and metamorphoses into a sporocyst, then rediae, and finally cercariae.
4. The cercariae emerge from the snail and encyst as metacercariae on the scales, fins, tail, and gills, sometimes in muscle of the second intermediate host, various species of brackish water fish, principally *Mugil* (mullet), *Tilapia,* and *Acanthogobius.*
6. When infected fish are eaten raw or undercooked by the definitive host, the metacercariae excyst in the small intestine and reside within the lumen or between the villi.
7. The larvae mature into the adult within 1 week and begin producing ova.

EPIDEMIOLOGY

▌ Principally found in the Middle East (especially Egypt), southern Europe, and Asia.

▌ Infection is acquired by eating raw or undercooked infected fish and by consuming infected fish that has been pickled for less than 2 weeks.

CONTROL. Thorough cooking of fish

Metagonimus yokogawai

DISEASE. Metagonimiasis

CLINICAL LABORATORY DIAGNOSIS. Wet mount of a formalin–ethyl acetate concentrate of a fecal sample stained with D'Antoni's iodine

DIAGNOSTIC MORPHOLOGY. See "Differential Morphology of the Trematode Ova" on p **745.**

LIFE CYCLE

1. Ova with fully developed miracidia are passed with the stool of the definitive host (humans, dogs, cats, hogs, pelicans, and perhaps other fish eating birds) into the external environment.
2. Ova are ingested by the first intermediate snail host *(Semisulcospira, Thiara,* and *Hua).*
3. Within the snail, the miracidium is released from the ovum and metamorphoses into a sporocyst, then rediae, and lastly cercariae.
4. The cercariae leave the snail and swim until encountering the second intermediate host, a susceptible fresh water fish (salmonoids and cyprinoids).
5. The cercariae encyst as metacercariae on the scales, fins, tail, gills, and sometimes in muscle.
6. When infected fish are eaten raw or undercooked by the definitive host, the metacercariae excyst and develop in the small intestine.
7. In 7 to 10 days the larvae mature into adults and produce ova.

EPIDEMIOLOGY

▌ Endemic in Asia.
▌ Infection is acquired by consuming raw or undercooked infected fish.
▌ Fecal debris from infected humans and other definitive hosts contaminate snail and fish laden waters, thus continuing the infectious cycle.

CONTROL. Thorough cooking of fish

Schistosoma mansoni

DISEASE. Schistosomiasis, intestinal schistosomiasis, bilharziasis, "snail fever"

CLINICAL LABORATORY DIAGNOSIS. Wet mount of a formalin–ethyl acetate concentrate of a fecal sample stained with D'Antoni's iodine

DIAGNOSTIC MORPHOLOGY. See "Differential Morphology of the Trematode Ova" on p **746.**

LIFE CYCLE

1. Ova are passed in the feces of the definitive host (humans, baboons, and rodents) into the environment.
2. On contact with fresh water, the fully formed miracidium hatches out of the egg.
3. The miracidium swims about looking for its appropriate intermediate snail host *(Biomphalaria* species and *Tropicorbis* species).
4. On penetrating the snail host, the miracidium undergoes asexual reproduction (two generations) producing daughter sporocysts.
5. Forked tailed cercariae erupt from the secondary sporocyst, penetrate the tissue of the snail, and enter the water.
6. The cercariae, stimulated to activity by water agitation, attach themselves to the skin of the definitive host by their ventral or oral suckers. This is followed by release of their hold and their penetration of the skin.
7. During penetration of the skin, the cercariae lose their forked tails and are transformed into schistosomulae inside the host tissues.

INTESTINAL TREMATODES

8. Within 24 hours the parasites enter the cutaneous capillaries, then pass into the systemic circulation and thence to the portal circulation.
9. After a period of time in the intrahepatic portal system, they migrate to the mesenteric veins (usually the veins that drain the large intestine).
10. In the mesenteric veins, the adult female is fertilized by the adult male. Thereafter, ova are produced and deposited in the venules of the intestine and rectum.
11. The ova, aided by the action of proteolytic enzymes released from the eggs and the tearing effect of the spines, penetrate the venules, enter the intestine, and are released into the external environment in the feces.

EPIDEMIOLOGY
▌ Geographically distributed in Africa, South America, and the West Indies.
▌ Infection is acquired by contact of the bare skin with cercariae infested waters.

CONTROL
▌ Proper sanitary disposal of fecal material and urine
▌ Control of the snail host by using molluscacides, snail eating fish or birds, removal of vegetation, and drainage of snail infested waters
▌ Avoiding waters infested with cercariae
▌ Mass chemotherapy

Schistosoma haematobium

DISEASE. Urinary schistosomiasis, schistosomal hematuria, urinary bilharziasis

CLINICAL LABORATORY DIAGNOSIS. Microscopic examination of the sediment of a centrifuged urine sample

DIAGNOSTIC MORPHOLOGY. See "Differential Morphology of the Trematode Ova" on p **746.**

LIFE CYCLE. The life cycle of *S. haematobium* is similar to that of *S. mansoni* with the following exceptions:

▌ Definitive host: primarily humans; monkeys and baboons are also infected.
▌ Snail intermediate hosts: *Bulinus*, *Physopsis*, and *Biomphalaria.*
▌ Adult worms live principally in the veins of the urinary bladder plexus.

EPIDEMIOLOGY
▌ Principally found in Africa
▌ Infection acquired by direct contact with cercariae infested waters.

CONTROL. See *"Schistosoma mansoni"* on p **741.**

Schistosoma japonicum

Oriental blood fluke

DISEASE. Schistosomiasis, Katayama fever

CLINICAL LABORATORY DIAGNOSIS. Wet mount of a formalin–ethyl acetate concentrate of a fecal sample stained with D'Anotoni's iodine

DIAGNOSTIC MORPHOLOGY. See "Differential Morphology of Trematode Ova" on p **746.**

LIFE CYCLE. The life cycle of S. *japonicum* is very similar to that of S. *mansoni* with the following exceptions:

- Definitive hosts: humans, dogs, cats, horses, pigs, cattle, deer, caribou, and rodents.
- Snail intermediate host: *Oncomelania.*
- Adult worms live primarily in the veins of the small intestine.

EPIDEMIOLOGY

- Principally found in the Far East
- Infection acquired through direct contact with cercariae infested waters

CONTROL. Same as that of S. *mansoni* except that the control of the intermediate host is impractical because of its amphibious nature (only goes to the water to deposit its eggs).

INTESTINAL TREMATODES

Differential Morphology of the Trematode Ova

ORGANISM	AVERAGE SIZE (μm)	SHAPE	IMPORTANT FEATURES	MICROSCOPIC VIEW
Clonorchis sinensis	29 × 16	Ovoid or elongate; narrow anterior and wide posterior; lightbulb shaped	Distinct operculum at anterior end that fits into broad rim of ovum shell, producing shoulder-like bulge just below operculum; comma shaped process at posterior end	*
Fasciola hepatica	140 × 80	Ellipsoid	Large with indistinct operculum; yolk granules amassed around nuclei of cell	*
Paragonimus westermani	95 × 55	Ovoid	Thick shelled ovum with distinct flattened operculum and unpronounced opercular "shoulders" at wider anterior end; shell thickened at narrower posterior end	*

Continued ▶

▶ Continued **Differential Morphology of the Trematode Ova**

ORGANISM	AVERAGE SIZE (μm)	SHAPE	IMPORTANT FEATURES	MICROSCOPIC VIEW
Fasciolopsis buski	138 × 82	Ellipsoid	Large with indistinct operculum; yolk granules are evenly distributed in yolk cells; almost indistinguishable from *F. hepatica*	✳
Heterophyes heterophyes	29 × 16	Ovoid and shaped like light-bulb	Distinct operculum with unpronounced "shoulders" at narrow end; no comma shaped process at wider end. Similar to *C. senensis* and indistinguishable from *M. yokogawai*	◆
Metagonimus yokogawai	27 × 16	Ovoid and shaped like light-bulb	Same as *H. heterophyes*	◆

Continued ▶

INTESTINAL TREMATODES

▶ Continued **Differential Morphology of the Trematode Ova**

ORGANISM	AVERAGE SIZE (μm)	SHAPE	IMPORTANT FEATURES	MICROSCOPIC VIEW
Schistosoma mansoni	155 × 65	Ovoid to elongate with anterior end and sometimes asymmetric	Nonoperculate with long lateral spine	*
Schistosoma haematobium	150 × 60	Elongate with rounded anterior and cone shaped posterior	Nonoperculate with conspicuous terminal spine	*
Schistosoma japonicum	85 × 60	Oval to rounded	Nonoperculate with minute hooked or knoblike lateral spine that may not be visible	*

* Photomicrographs from Markell EK, Voge M: Medical Parasitology (a slide presentation). Philadelphia, WB Saunders, 1976.
◆ Photomicrographs from Smith JW, ed: Diagnostic Medical Parasitology: Intestinal Helminths. Chicago, American Society of Clinical Pathologists, 1976.

TISSUE NEMATODES AND CESTODES

Trichinella spiralis

DISEASE. Trichinosis, trichiniasis, trichinelliasis

CLINICAL LABORATORY DIAGNOSIS
- Biopsied muscle tissue compressed between two glass slides, followed by microscopic study for encysted larvae
- Serologic tests: the slide flocculation and ELISA tests

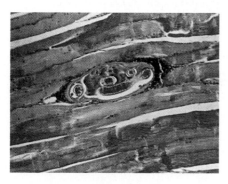

From Markell EK, Voge M: Medical Parasitology (a slide presentation). Philadelphia, WB Saunders, 1976.

DIAGNOSTIC MORPHOLOGY
The encysted larval stage

- Size of larva: 1 mm in length
- Appearance in muscle tissue: encapsulated and coiled in a spiral (0.25 to 0.5 mm long)

LIFE CYCLE
1. Infection begins when a definitive host (human, pig, bear, and other carnivorous or omnivorous animals) consumes raw or undercooked meat containing the encysted larvae.
2. The capsules surrounding the larvae dissolve in the small intestine.
3. The released larvae immediately invade the intestinal mucosa and mature into adult worms.
4. After mating, the males die and the females burrow into the mucosa of the intestinal villi and begin to deposit larvae into the mucosa and occasionally directly into the lymphatics.
5. Most larvae pass into the hepatic portal system through the liver, then to the heart, to the lungs, and finally into the bloodstream.
6. The larvae are carried throughout the body. When reaching the skeletal muscles, they penetrate, grow, spiral, and eventually become encapsulated.

NOTE The same animal serves as the intermediate host.

EPIDEMIOLOGY
- Cosmopolitan, but prevalence rates are highest in temperate and arctic regions.
- *Trichinella* infection is acquired principally by consuming raw or undercooked infected pork, and in the Arctic, raw or undercooked infected bear.

CONTROL
- Thorough cooking of all meat
- Sterilization of food fed to pigs

TISSUE NEMATODES AND CESTODES

Echinococcus granulosus

DISEASE. Echinococcosis, hydatid disease, hydatid cyst

CLINICAL LABORATORY DIAGNOSIS

▌ Microscopic examination of aspirated hydatid cyst fluid for the presence of free protoscolices (hydatid sand)
Note: This is a dangerous procedure, since spillage of cyst fluid into the host during aspiration may result in anaphylaxis and/or dissemination of released protoscolices.

▌ Radiographic, sonographic, and computed tomography (CT) examinations demonstrating a cyst, followed by confirmatory serologic tests such hemagglutination and immunofluorescent antibody tests

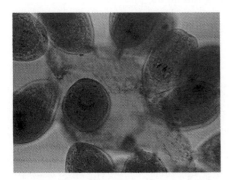

From Markell EK, Voge M: Medical Parasitology (a slide presentation). Philadelphia, WB Saunders, 1976.

DIAGNOSTIC MORPHOLOGY

Protoscolex (invaginated scolex of hydatid cyst)

▌ Size: 140×85 μm
▌ Shape and structure: spherical with an invagination at one pole and a stalk at the opposite pole. The scolex has two suckers and a double crown of hooks.

LIFE CYCLE

1. Ova are passed in the feces of the definitive host (dogs, wolves, and other *Canidae*) into the external environment.
2. The ova are accidentally ingested by an intermediate host (sheep, cattle, hogs, goats, and other grazing herbivores; also humans where the disease is prevalent among the herbivores).
3. In the duodenum, the onchosphere (hexacanth embryo) hatches out and penetrates the intestinal wall to enter the blood circulation.
4. The organism is carried to different parts of the body and lodges principally in the liver and lung.
5. In the liver (or other organ), the onchosphere develops within several hours into a hydatid cyst (a large saclike structure with an outer laminated membrane and an inner germinal layer that bears brood capsules containing many protoscolices; within the cyst are also daughter cysts, which are miniature hydatid-like cysts, free protoscolices, all bathed in proteinaceous fluid).
6. The hydatid cyst grows slowly over several years and may reach a diameter of 20 cm.
7. When a definitive host eats an infected animal (intermediate host), the protoscolices are liberated from the cyst.
8. When the protoscolices reach the intestine, they evaginate, attach to the intestinal wall, and grow.
9. The gravid proglottid of the adult worm fills with ova and eventually ruptures, releasing them into the intestinal tract.

EPIDEMIOLOGY

- *E. granulosus* is found worldwide.
- Human infection occurs primarily when infected domestic herbivores are in close association with dogs. The dogs eat scraps of the butchered infected animals, become infected, and pass the ova into the soil, where humans may accidentally ingest them.
- Herbivores become infected in the same manner as humans.
- Children have a higher prevalence of infection due to their poor hygienic habits.

PREVENTION

- Teaching of hygienic practices regarding the handling of dogs to prevent the ingestion of ova
- Treatment of dogs in endemic areas with taenifuges to rid them of the adult worm
- Sanitary disposal of offal to prevent infection in dogs

Echinococcus multilocularis

DISEASE. Alveolar echinococcosis

CLINICAL LABORATORY DIAGNOSIS. Serologic tests including ELISA, latex agglutination, and indirect hemagglutination tests

DIAGNOSTIC MORPHOLOGY. The alveolar hydatid cyst is difficult to locate with either CT scan or radiographs. In addition, the contents of the cyst are usually sterile. For these reasons, specimens for parasitologic analysis are not received in the clinical microbiology laboratory.

LIFE CYCLE. The life cycle is similar to that of *E. granulosis* with the following exceptions:

- Definitive host: foxes, cats, dogs, and other carnivores.
- Intermediate host: mouse, vole, and lemming; the human is an accidental host.
- The hydatid cyst of *E. multilocularis* (primarily located in the liver) differs from the cyst of *E. granulosus* in that it has a thin outer membrane allowing the germinal epithelium to bud externally, infiltrate surrounding tissues, and even to metastasize (usually to the brain and lung) like a cancer; the cyst has an irregular outline and within consists of small, irregular cavities filled with a jelly-like matrix that are separated from each other by connective tissue; in humans, the cyst is usually sterile.

EPIDEMIOLOGY

- *E. multilocularis* is found in Europe, Asia, and North America. Cases have been reported from South America and New Zealand.
- Transmission to humans occurs by direct hand to mouth ingestion of the ova from infected dogs or cats; eating of raw plants contaminated with the feces of infected animals; and handling of infected foxes or wolves by hunters or trappers.

CONTROL

- Killing of the rodent intermediate host
- Destruction of foxes and/or preventing their access to areas where humans reside

■ Education of trappers and hunters of the danger of acquiring infection while skinning a potentially infected animal

Spirometra Species

DISEASE. Sparganosis

CLINICAL LABORATORY DIAGNOSIS. Surgically remove the plerocercoid larva (sparganum) from the lesion and study macroscopically.

DIAGNOSTIC MORPHOLOGY
Plerocercoid larva:

■ Size: 3 to 9 cm long by a few millimeters wide
■ Shape and color: wrinkled, white, unsegmented, thread or ribbon-like

LIFE CYCLE
1. Ova are passed with the feces of the definitive host (dog, cat, and wild carnivores) into fresh water, where the coracidia are released.
2. The coracidium is ingested by the first intermediate host, the water flea (*Cyclops*).
3. Within the water flea, the coracidium develops into a procercoid larva.
4. After the infected water flea is ingested by the second intermediate host (frogs, snakes, rats, and occasionally humans), the larva migrates to various organs of the body and develops into a plerocercoid larva. In humans, the larva migrates and encysts in subcutaneous tissues, conjunctiva, lymph nodes, and various organs.
5. When the definitive host ingests an infected intermediate host, the cycle is completed.

EPIDEMIOLOGY
■ Cosmopolitan, but most common in Asia.
■ Humans acquire infection by ingesting infected water fleas, eating infected raw snake or frog, or placing poultices of infected frog or snake flesh on open lesions or on the eye.

CONTROL
■ Avoid drinking untreated water from ponds and other water sources where infected water fleas may be found.
■ Discourage the use of poultices from potentially infected animals.

MICROFILARIAE

Wuchereria bancrofti

DISEASE. Bancroftian filariasis, wuchereriasis

CLINICAL LABORATORY DIAGNOSIS. Giemsa stained thick blood smears.

NOTE The optimal time to draw the blood sample is between 10 PM and 2 AM for the periodic form (nocturnal) and between 2 and 5 PM for the subperiodic form.

DIAGNOSTIC MORPHOLOGY. See "Differential Characteristics of the Microfilariae" on p **756.**

LIFE CYCLE

1. When an infected mosquito (*Culex quinquefasciatus [fatigans], Aedes polynesiensis, Anopheles* species) bites a human (definitive host), the third stage infective larvae emerge from its proboscis and creep onto the host's moist skin and penetrate through either the puncture wound made by the mosquito or other abrasions that may be present.
2. The larvae migrate into the peripheral lymphatics and thence to regional lymph nodes and larger lymph vessels (note: the adult worms tend to establish themselves in the varices of the lymphatic vessels of the lower extremities, the groin glands and epididymis of the male, and the labial glands of the female). Here they molt twice before they mature.
3. After mating, the female produce microfilariae (it takes approximately a year from larvae penetration to microfilariae production).
4. The microfilariae migrate from the parent through the wall of the lymphatics to the neighboring blood vessels or are transported by the lymphatic circulation to the bloodstream.
5. A mosquito (intermediate host) bites an infected human and ingests the microfilariae.
6. They migrate to the mosquito's muscles and molt twice and become infective.
7. The infective larvae then leave the muscles and migrate to the proboscis.

EPIDEMIOLOGY

▮ Worldwide range in tropical and subtropical countries.
▮ Occurs in the Far East, Southeast Asia, East Asia, parts of the Middle East, most of Africa, and South and Central America.

Western Hemisphere:

Caribbean Islands

Atlantic coast of Costa Rica

northern South America

▮ The subperiodic form occurs in the South Pacific islands of Fiji, Samoa, the Cook Islands, and French Polynesia.

CONTROL

NOTE Since there is no reservoir host, control lies in interrupting the life cycle between the mosquito and humans.

▮ Spraying of houses with residual insecticides and larvicides. This procedure is effective in controlling domestic mosquitoes such as *C. quinquefasciatus.* It is ineffective in controlling sylvan mosquitoes such as *A. polynesiensis* (subperiodic form).
▮ Mass treatment with diethylcarbamazine (DEC).
▮ Elimination of standing water in the environment.
▮ Latrines fitted with traps to prevent the escape of adult mosquitoes.
▮ Protection by use of screening, bed nets, mosquito repellents, and protective clothing.

MICROFILARIAE

Brugia malayi

DISEASE. Malayan filariasis

CLINICAL LABORATORY DIAGNOSIS. Giemsa stained thick blood smears

> **NOTE** The optimal time to draw the blood sample is between 10 PM and 2 AM for the periodic form (nocturnal) and between 9 and 11 PM for the subperiodic form.

DIAGNOSTIC MORPHOLOGY. See "Differential Characteristics of the Microfilariae" on p **756.**

LIFE CYCLE. The life cycle of *B. malayi* is very similar to that of *W. bancofti* with the following exceptions:

- Definitive hosts: human, monkey, and cat
- Intermediate hosts: *Mansonia, Aedes,* and *Anopheles*

EPIDEMIOLOGY

- Found in Southeast Asia and the eastern territories of the Indian subcontinent.
- In western Malaysia infections are periodic; in eastern Malaysia infections are subperiodic.
- *Mansonia* is usually a vector in rural areas, whereas the *Anopheles* is usually a vector in urban areas. *Aedis* is probably the main vector in Japan.

CONTROL

- Mosquito eradication
- Destruction of water plants necessary for the breeding of *Mansonia*
- Mass treatment of infected individuals

Loa loa

DISEASE. Loiasis, eye worm, fugitive swellings, Calabar swellings

CLINICAL LABORATORY DIAGNOSIS. Giemsa stained thick blood smears

> **NOTE** The optimal time for drawing a blood sample is between 11 AM and 1 PM (diurnal).

DIAGNOSTIC MORPHOLOGY. See "Differential Characteristics of the Microfilariae" on p **756.**

LIFE CYCLE

1. When an infected biting fly (*Chrysops* species) bites a definitive host (human and monkey), third stage infective larvae escape from the fly's mouth and enter the wound.
2. The larvae then penetrate the subcutaneous and muscular tissues, where they mature into adult worms.
3. The adults migrate through subcutaneous and deeper tissues, including the conjunctiva of the eye; thus the name *eye worm.*
4. After mating, the adult female produces microfilariae, which are found in the peripheral blood during the day (diurnal periodicity) and in the lungs at night.

5. A biting fly (intermediate host) bites an infected definitive host and ingests the microfilariae.
6. The microfilariae penetrate the intestinal wall and develop in the fat body of the fly.
7. After developing to the third stage larvae, they migrate to the fly's mouthparts.

EPIDEMIOLOGY

▌ Endemic in the rain forests of tropical Africa.
▌ The biting fly prefers shaded areas such as forests and swamps to breed and to vector the infective larvae of *Loa loa* to its definitive hosts.

CONTROL

▌ Use of larvicides to control the intermediate host
▌ Protection by the use of nets, screens, and insect repellents
▌ Treatment of infected individuals

Mansonella ozzardi

DISEASE. Ozzardi filariasis, Mansonella ozzardi

CLINICAL LABORATORY DIAGNOSIS. Giemsa stained thick blood smear

DIAGNOSTIC MORPHOLOGY. See "Differential Characteristics of the Microfilariae" on p **756.**

LIFE CYCLE

1. When an infected midge° bites a host, third stage infective larvae enter the puncture wound.
2. The larvae find their way to the mesenteries and the visceral fat, where they mature.
3. After mating, unsheathed microfilariae make their way to the peripheral circulation.
4. When a midge (the intermediate host) bites an infected definitive host, microfilariae are taken in with the blood meal and penetrate the insect's stomach and then the thoracic musculature.
5. After two molts and within 6 days, the third stage infective larvae are formed.
6. By the eighth day the infective larvae migrate to the head and proboscis of the midge.

EPIDEMIOLOGY

▌ This parasite is found only in the New World.
▌ It is indigenous in parts of Central and northern South America and some of the islands of the West Indies.

CONTROL. Control depends on elimination of the vectors and the protection of persons from bites (i.e., insect repellents).

NOTE The vectors, *Culicoides* and *Simulium,* are both very small and can pass through screening and mosquito nets.

°*Culicoides* species; in the Amazon Basin both *Culicoides* and *Simulium* species serve as vectors.

MICROFILARIAE

Mansonella perstans

DISEASE. Perstan filariasis

CLINICAL LABORATORY DIAGNOSIS. Giemsa stained thick blood smear

DIAGNOSTIC MORPHOLOGY. See "Differential Characteristics of the Microfilariae" on p **757.**

LIFE CYCLE
1. When a biting midge (*Culicoides* species) bites a definitive host (humans and apes), mature infective larvae leave the midge's mouthparts, are deposited on the skin, and then enter the host.
2. The larvae migrate to the peritoneal, pleural, and pericardial cavities. Here they mature into adults, mate and produce microfilariae.
3. The microfilariae migrate into the peripheral blood and capillaries of the lungs.
4. A biting midge (intermediate host) bites an infected definitive host and ingests the microfilariae.
5. The microfilariae penetrate the stomach and enter the thoracic muscles, where they mature.
6. After developing into mature infective larvae, they migrate to the midge's mouthparts.

EPIDEMIOLOGY
- Endemic in tropical Africa and in South America.
- The biting midge is a night feeder and usually bites after 10 PM.
- The midges breed in the damp forest, swamps, and jungle.

CONTROL
- Drainage of the breeding grounds of the intermediate host
- Protection by the use of nets, lighted rooms, and insecticides

Mansonella streptocerca

DISEASE. Streptocercal filariasis

CLINICAL LABORATORY DIAGNOSIS. Skin snips teased in normal saline, followed by staining with Giemsa stain

DIAGNOSTIC MORPHOLOGY. See "Differential Characteristics of the Microfilariae" on p **757.**

LIFE CYCLE. The life cycle is similar to that of *M. perstans* with the notable exception that the microfilariae appear in the skin. Humans and chimpanzees are the definitive hosts, and the biting midge of the genus *Culicoides* is the intermediate host.

EPIDEMIOLOGY. Endemic in West and Central Africa

CONTROL. Avoid contact with the midge in endemic areas by the use of nets and repellents.

Onchocerca volvulus

DISEASE. Onchocerciasis, onchocercosis, river blindness, "Sowda"

CLINICAL LABORATORY DIAGNOSIS. Skin snips teased in normal saline, followed by staining with Giemsa stain

DIAGNOSTIC MORPHOLOGY. See "Differential Characteristics of the Microfilariae" on p **757.**

LIFE CYCLE

1. When an infected black fly° bites the definitive host, a human, third stage infective larvae enter the puncture wound and wander through the subcutaneous tissues.
2. When they finally come to rest, an inflammatory reaction takes place, resulting in the formation of fibrous cysts. Usually the developing worms are encapsulated into the cysts in groups of two or more.
3. The nodules, produced by the worm's encapsulation, may range from a few millimeters to several centimeters in diameter and may be few to numerous. In Venezuela and Africa they are found mainly on the patient's trunk or limbs, whereas in Guatemala and Mexico they are found principally on the scalp.
4. After mating, unsheathed microfilariae make their way out of the nodules and into the dermis and connective tissue.
5. When a black fly (intermediate host) bites an infected definitive host, its salivary secretions attract microfilariae from adjacent areas of the skin so that numerous microfilariae may be ingested.
6. The microfilariae penetrate the gut and thence move to the flight muscles. Here they molt twice.
7. The third stage larvae then find their way to the head region and finally to the proboscis.

EPIDEMIOLOGY

- The disease is confined to the highlands, where the vector is abundant.
- The black flies bite in the early morning, in shady areas during the afternoon, and in the evening.
- Endemic in Africa.
- Endemic in the Americas; specifically in Guatemala, Mexico, Colombia, Brazil, and northeastern Venezuela.

CONTROL

NOTE   Since there is no reservoir host, control lies in interrupting the life cycle between the black fly and humans.

- Control of the vector by use of larvicides. Spraying of riparian vegetation with insecticides.
- Mass treatment with ivermectin.
- Use of flyproof clothing, head nets, and repellents.

°Principally *Simulium damnosum* in Africa, *S. ochraceum* in Mexico and Guatemala, and *S. metallicum* in Venezuela.

MICROFILARIAE

Differential Characteristics of the Microfilariae

ORGANISM	AVERAGE LENGTH (μm)	SHEATH	TAIL NUCLEI	OTHER FEATURES	MICROSCOPIC VIEW
Wuchereria bancrofti	260	Present	Nuclei do not extend to tip of tail.	Sheath stains slightly with Giemsa stain. Microfilariae found in blood. Periodicity: usually nocturnal.	
Brugia malayi	220	Present	Nuclei extend to tip of tail with two separated and swollen terminal nuclei.	Sheath stains intensely with Giemsa stain. Microfilariae found in blood. Periodicity: nocturnal.	
Loa loa	275	Present	Nuclei extend to tip of tail.	Sheath almost colorless with Giemsa stain. Microfilariae found in blood. Periodicity: diurnal.	
Mansonella ozzardi	200	Absent	Nuclei do not extend to tip of tail.	Microfilariae found in blood. No periodicity.	

Continued ▶

▶ Continued **Differential Characteristics of the Microfilariae**

ORGANISM	AVERAGE LENGTH (μm)	SHEATH	TAIL NUCLEI	OTHER FEATURES	MICROSCOPIC VIEW
Mansonella perstans	195	Absent	Nuclei extend to tip of tail.	Microfilariae found in blood. No periodicity.	*
Mansonella streptocerca	210	Absent	Nuclei extend to tip of tail.	Curved or hooked tail. Microfilariae found in skin. No periodicity.	+
Onchocerca volvulus	290	Absent	Nuclei do not extend to tip of tail.	Microfilariae found in skin. No periodicity.	*

* Photomicrographs from Markell EK, Voge M: Medical Parasitology (a slide presentation). Philadelphia, WB Saunders, 1976.
◆ Photomicrograph courtesy of Edward K. Markell, PhD, MD, Berkeley, CA.
+ Photomicrograph from Smith JW, ed: Diagnostic Medical Parasitology: Blood and Tissue Parasites. Chicago, American Society of Clinical Pathologists, 1976, pp 57–59.

MICROFILARIAE

DRACUNCULUS MEDINENSIS, THE GUINEA WORM

DISEASE. Dracontiasis, dracunculosis, guinea worm disease

CLINICAL LABORATORY DIAGNOSIS. Immerse the blister formed by the female worm in a small amount of water, which will cause the blister to burst. Centrifuge the water and examine the sediment microscopically for free swimming larvae.

DIAGNOSTIC MORPHOLOGY

Free swimming larval stage:

- Size: average 625 μm in length × 20 μm in width
- Shape: slender, and rod shaped (rhabditiform) with a long, threadlike tail that terminates in a pointed tip.
- Internal morphology: a well developed digestive tract

LIFE CYCLE

1. The gravid female worm migrates to the dermis of the definitive host (human, and domesticated and wild fur bearing animals), where a papule forms.
2. A blister develops and ulcerates, and when it is in contact with water, thousands of free swimming first stage larvae are released.
3. The larvae are ingested by the intermediate host, *Cyclops* (a water flea).
4. The larvae penetrate into the body cavity and molt twice to form third stage infective larvae.
5. When the definitive host ingests water containing infected *Cyclops*, the larvae are released and penetrate the wall of the small intestine.
6. They migrate to the subcutaneous connective tissues, where they mature into adult worms and mate.
7. When the female has become gravid, she migrates to the dermis.

EPIDEMIOLOGY

- Endemic in central Africa, and Asia.
- The intermediate host breeds in still waters such as ponds and open wells. These are the primary sources of drinking water in rural areas, resulting in a high infection rate of the populace.

CONTROL

- Avoid drinking from water sources suspected of harboring infected intermediate hosts.
- Boil suspected water before ingestion.
- Chemically treat ponds, open wells, and other suspected sources to eradicate the intermediate host.

SELECTED ECTOPARASITES

PARASITIC LICE OF HUMANS

Pediculus humanus

Pediculus humanus var. *corporis*, *Pediculus humanus* var. *capitis*, and *Phthirus pubis*

DISEASE. Pediculosis

NOTE   *P. humanus* var. *corporis* can act as a vector in the transmission of relapsing fever, epidemic typhus, and trench fever.

CLINICAL LABORATORY DIAGNOSIS. Using a dissecting microscope, examine microscopically for the adult and/or ova in the material from the seams of clothing for *P. humanus* var. *corporis*, on the hairs of the head for *P. humanus* var. *capitis*, and on the pubic hairs for *P. pubis*.

DIAGNOSTIC MORPHOLOGY. See "Differential Characteristics of the Parasitic Lice of Humans" on p **760.**

LIFE CYCLE
1. Ova ("nits") are deposited by the female louse and are cemented to the hairs or clothing (see "Differential Characteristics of the Parasitic Lice of Humans" on p **761.**
2. The nymph develops in the ovum and after approximately a week escapes through the opened operculum.
3. The lice begin to feed immediately and after three molts transform into adults.
4. After several days the female begins to lay her ova.

EPIDEMIOLOGY
▌ Cosmopolitan.
▌ All three lice are exclusively human parasites.
▌ *P. humanus* var. *corporis* is found in individuals who have unhygienic habits and in climates where heavy clothing is worn.
▌ *P. humanus* var. *capitis* is transferred either by direct contact or by exchanging brushes, combs, or hats. It is prevalent in schoolchildren.
▌ *P. pubis* is primarily transmitted by sexual intercourse.

CONTROL
▌ Mass delousing
▌ Use of repellents on clothing

PARASITIC LICE OF HUMANS

Differential Characteristics of the Parasitic Lice of Humans

SPECIES	SIZE RANGE (mm)	SHAPE	HEAD	SHAPE OF ABDOMEN	ABDOMINAL SEGMENTS	SIZE OF CLAWS	MICROSCOPIC VIEW (ADULT)
Pediculus humanus var. *corporis* (body louse)	2.0–4.0	Flattened and elongate	Diamond shaped	Elongate; broader than thorax	Well defined	Medium	*
Pediculus humanus var. *capitis* (head louse)	1.0–2.0	Flattened and elongate	Diamond shaped	Elongate; broader than thorax	Well defined	Medium	*
Phthirus pubis (crab louse)	0.8–1.2	Flattened, oblong, turtle shaped	Rectangular; neck not constricted	Short	Indistinct	Large and heavy	

Continued ▶

▶ Continued **Differential Characteristics of the Parasitic Lice of Humans**

SPECIES	OVUM: LENGTH; SHAPE; LOCATION ON HOST	PRINCIPAL LOCATION ON HOST	MICROSCOPIC VIEW (OVA)
***Pediculus humanus* var. *corporis* (body louse)**	0.8 mm; ellipsoid and operculated; clothing, sometimes hairs	Body	
***Pediculus humanus* var. *capitis* (head louse)**	0.6 mm; ellipsoid and operculated; hairs	Head	
***Phthirus pubis* (crab louse)**	0.8 mm; conical and operculated; hairs	Pubic area	

✻ Photomicrographs by Eugene Wienke, MD, Pathology Laboratory, Deaconess Hospital Systems–Central Campus, St Louis, MO. Adapted from Belding DL: Textbook of Parasitology. Englewood Cliffs, NJ, Prentice Hall [Appleton-Century-Crofts], 1965.

TICKS COMMONLY SEEN IN THE CLINICAL LABORATORY

Ixodes, Dermacentor, and *Amblyomma*

DISEASE. Tick paralysis: *Dermacentor* species and *Amblyomma* species

Vectored Disease
- Babesiosis: *I. scapularis (dammini)*
- Lyme disease: *I. scapularis (dammini), pacificus,* and *ricinus*
- Rocky Mountain spotted fever: *D. andersoni,* and *variabilis*
- Colorado tick fever: *D. andersoni*
- Tularemia: *A. americanum, Dermacentor* species, *I. ricinus*
- Q fever: *D. andersoni* and *Amblyomma* species

CLINICAL LABORATORY DIAGNOSIS. Examine the tick using a dissecting microscope.

DIAGNOSTIC MORPHOLOGY
- *General:* The adult "hard ticks" (Ixodidae) have four pairs of legs and an undivided body. They have a dorsal shield, the scutum, that almost completely covers the back in males but covers only the anterior part of the back in females. The mouthparts are visible from above.
- *Differential Characteristics:* See "Selected Differential Characteristics of the Ticks Most Commonly Seen in the Clinical Laboratory" on p **763.**

LIFE CYCLE
1. After mating and a blood meal, the female tick deposits her eggs on or near the ground.
2. After several weeks, a six legged larva ("seed" tick) hatches out of the egg.
3. After finding a host, the larva attaches and feeds.
4. After a resting period of a few days to several weeks, the larva molts into an eight legged nymph.
5. The nymph climbs on vegetation and when encountering a host, attaches and takes a blood meal.
6. The nymph drops to the ground and after several weeks to up to 3 months molts into an adult.

EPIDEMIOLOGY
- *I. scapularis (dammini),* the deer tick: common tick infesting humans in the eastern United States
- *I. pacificus:* commonly found on the west coast of the United States
- *I. ricinus:* found in Europe, North Africa, Asia, and North America
- *D. andersoni,* the wood tick: endemic to the Rocky Mountain region, northward from New Mexico to western Canada
- *D. variabilis,* the American dog tick: endemic to regions east of the Rocky Mountains, and the west coast of the United States; also in Mexico and Canada
- *A. americanum,* the Lone Star tick: endemic to southern and eastern United States and South America

CONTROL
- Destroy rodents.
- Keep vegetation cut low.

■ Use insecticides on pets and areas surrounding habitation.
■ When in tick infested areas use tick repellents and wear clothing that covers the body. On removing the clothing, carefully search for ticks on the body.

Selected Differential Characteristics of the Ticks Most Commonly Seen in the Clinical Laboratory

SPECIES	SCUTUM	ANAL GROOVE	PALPI	MICROSCOPIC VIEW
Ixodes	Inornate	Anterior to anus, horseshoe shaped	Longer than width of capitulum	✳
Dermacentor	Ornate	Posterior to anus and distinct	Shorter than width of capitulum	✳
Amblyomma	Ornate	Posterior to anus	Longer than width of capitulum	✳

✳ Photomicrographs by Eugene Wienke, MD, Pathology Laboratory, Deaconess Hospital Systems–Central Campus, St Louis, MO.

TICKS COMMONLY SEEN IN THE CLINICAL LABORATORY

SARCOPTES SCABIEI, THE ITCH MITE

DISEASE. Scabies in humans and mange in animals

CLINICAL LABORATORY DIAGNOSIS. Place a drop of mineral oil over the cutaneous serpentine burrow. Either tease out the mite from the distal portion of the burrow with a sterile needle or scrape the burrow with the tip of a sterile scalpel. Place the specimen on a slide and examine microscopically for the mite and its eggs.

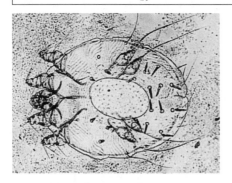

From Markell EK, Voge M, John DT: Medical Parasitology, 7th ed. Philadelphia, WB Saunders, 1992.

DIAGNOSTIC MORPHOLOGY
Adult
▌ Size: male, 200 to 250 μm; female, 330 to 450 μm.
▌ Color: dirty white.
▌ General characteristics: oval and eyeless with the body divided into an anterior portion bearing two pairs of stumpy legs and a posterior portion with another two pairs of stumpy legs. The dorsal outer surface bears cones, scales, and bristles. The mouthparts are visible from above or below.

Egg
▌ Size: 150 μm by 100 μm
▌ Form: transparent and oval

Reproduced with permission from Reeves JRT, Maibach HI: Clinical Dermatology Illustrated, 3rd ed. Sydney, MacLennan & Petty, 1997.

LIFE CYCLE
1. The adult mites burrow into the skin, forming tortuous channels.
2. The impregnated female deposits her eggs as she tunnels within the skin.
3. Larvae hatch out of the eggs in several days and either burrow laterally or form a new tunnel.
4. Within a few days, the larvae transform into nymphs.
5. The male nymph molts into the adult male, whereas the female has a second nymphal stage and then molts into the adult female.
6. Copulation occurs and the cycle is repeated.

EPIDEMIOLOGY
▌ Cosmopolitan, especially in poor and urban populations.
▌ Transmission occurs primarily by direct contact, rarely from clothing or bedding.

CONTROL
▌ Avoid direct contact with infected individuals.
▌ Treat infected individuals.
▌ Sterilize clothing and bedding of those infected with *S. scabiei*.

SELECTED DIAGNOSTIC PROCEDURES

STOOL EXAMINATION

Wet Mount Procedure

● Place a drop of a 0.85% saline suspended fecal sample (direct wet mount) or a drop of stool concentrate in the center of a clean microscope slide.

● Add 1 to 2 drops of modified D'Antoni's iodine solution (alternatives are Dobell and O'Connor iodine solution or diluted Lugol's iodine solution).

● Mix the iodine solution and sample with the edge of a coverslip.

● Examine microscopically under 100× and 400× magnifications. Measure the size of the observed parasite(s) using the ocular micrometer.

Limitations of Procedure

Do not use the iodine stain to study trophozoite stages. Perform the above procedure without the addition of the iodine stain when searching for this form.

Chromatoidal bars seen in the cyst of *E. histolytica* are indistinct when stained with iodine. When amebic forms are observed with four or fewer nuclei, a wet mount without iodine should be prepared and examined for the presence of chromatoidal bars.

Expected Results With the Iodine Wet Mount

Cytoplasm appears yellow.
Chromatin material stains brown or black.
Glycogen appears reddish-brown.

Formalin–Ethyl Acetate Concentration Procedure

● Mix 2 to 5 g (2 to 5 mL) of stool specimen thoroughly in 10 to 12 mL of 10% formalin.

● Filter an aliquot of the suspension through two layers of gauze or a wire screen until 3 mL is in a 15 mL centrifuge tube.

● Add 10 mL of 0.85% saline to the tube and centrifuge for 2 minutes at 2000 RRM.

● Decant the supernatant fluid and resuspend the sediment in 9 mL of 10% formalin.

● Add 3 mL of ethyl acetate.

● Cap the tube with a rubber or cork stopper and shake for 30 seconds.

● While pointing the centrifuge tube away from you, carefully remove the stopper.

NOTE The tube contents should be divided into four layers. From top to bottom: ethyl acetate layer, plug of fecal debris, discolored aqueous layer, and sediment containing the parasites.

● While holding the tube in a vertical position, free the debris by ringing it with a wooden applicator stick. Decant the upper layers, leaving the sediment. Do not turn the tube upright until the sides of the tube have been cleaned with a swab.

STOOL EXAMINATION

● Prepare a wet mount of the sediment and examine microscopically.

Limitations of Procedure

This method is recommended for the detection of cyst forms, ova, and larvae. It is not recommended for the detection of trophozoite forms (see the discussion of the trichrome staining technique).

This procedure is not recommended as the sole procedure for loose stools that may contain trophozoites (see the discussion of the trichrome staining technique).

Other Concentration Procedures

Gravity sedimentation, merthiolate-iodine-formaldehyde concentration, zinc sulfate centrifugal flotation, Sheather's sugar flotation (for *Cryptosporidium*)

Gomori's Trichrome Stain (Wheatley's Modification) Technique

● Fix a portion of the stool sample in polyvinyl alcohol (PVA) (approximately 1 part stool to 3 parts fixative in a screw capped container). The sample must be thoroughly mixed with the fixative.

NOTE Gastric aspirates, duodenal washings, and material from the "string test" may be fixed by placing 1 drop of the specimen onto a slide and mixing it with 3 drops of PVA and then spreading it evenly on the slide.

● Pour a portion of the fixed stool onto several layers of paper toweling and allow to stand for 3 minutes.

● Spread a portion of the specimen from the paper towel onto a clean slide with a wooden applicator stick.

● Dry the specimen overnight at room temperature.

● Immerse the PVA fixed smear in 70% ethanol-iodine for 20 minutes.

● Immerse in 70% ethanol for 5 minutes.

● Immerse in 70% ethanol for 5 minutes.

● Immerse in 90% alcohol with 1% acetic acid, and dip in and out until the stain stops running off.

● Rinse immediately in 100% ethanol.

● Immerse in 100% ethanol for 2 to 5 minutes.

● Immerse in 100% ethanol for 2 to 5 minutes.

● Immerse in xylene for 2 to 5 minutes.

● Immerse in xylene for 2 to 5 minutes.

● Allow slide(s) to air dry and coverslip with mounting medium (Protexx) diluted as follows: 1 part xylene to 2 parts mounting medium.

● Examine the smear(s) under 1000× (oil immersion lens). Measure the size of the observed parasite(s) using the ocular micrometer.

Expected Results

Cytoplasm of trophozoites and cysts stains blue-green tinged with purple.
Nuclear chromatin and chromatoidal bars stain red.
Erythrocytes stain red.
Yeasts and molds usually stain green.
Helminth ova and larvae usually stain red with a green background.

NOTE Tissue cells and histiocytes may stain similar to amebae. Caution must be exercised not to confuse these cells with *E. histolytica.*

Limitations

Incompletely fixed cells may stain predominately red.
Organisms that have degenerated before fixation often stain pale green.
Poor fixation due to inadequate mixing of specimen in the fixative may result in atypical staining reactions and poor preservation of the organisms' morphology.

NOTE The trichrome stain (different formulation) and procedure are different for microsporidia.

Other Permanent Staining Procedure

Schaudinn's or PVA fixed stool sample stained with Heidenhain's iron hematoxylin.

Modified Acid Fast Stain Technique

● Concentrate the stool by the formalin–ethyl acetate procedure* with the following modifications:

  After adding 0.85% saline to the tube (step 3*), centrifuge at 1800 to 2000 rpm for 10 minutes.

  For loose stools, make smears from the saline washed sediment.

  Semisolid or formed stools should undergo the complete concentration procedure.

● Prepare the smear and air dry.

● Fix the smear by placing it in absolute methanol for 1 minute.

● Flood the slide with the Kinyoun carbolfuchsin stain for 5 minutes.

● Wash the slide with 50% ethanol and immediately rinse with tap water.

● Destain the smear with 1% sulfuric acid for 2 minutes or until no color runs off the slide. Wash the slide with tap water.

● Counterstain with brilliant green for 1 minute. Wash the slide with tap water, dry, and examine microscopically at 1000× magnification (oil immersion).

Expected Results

Cryptosporidium, Cyclospora, and *Isospora* stain red.

Other Staining Procedure

Rhodamine-auramine O fluorescent stain

Cellophane Tape Technique for *Enterobius vermicularis* (Pinworm)

● Specimens for pinworm are obtained by pressing clear cellophane tape against the perianal area of the patient.

● The cellophane tape is then pressed, sticky side down, on a microscope slide.

● The slide is examined at 100× magnification.

● If no pinworm ova are seen, lift the tape and apply a drop of xylene or toluene to the slide. Smooth the tape back over the toluene or xylene and re-examine the preparation without delay (over time xylene or toluene cause the ova to collapse).

BLOOD EXAMINATION

Giemsa Stained Thin and Thick Smear Technique

● *Thin Smear:* Place a drop of blood, obtained either from a finger stick or from an EDTA blood sample, on one end of a slide. Using a second slide, draw the drop across the slide to obtain a feathered edge. Air dry for 15 minutes. Fix in methanol for 1 minute and air dry for 3 minutes.

● *Thick Smear:* Place a drop of blood obtained either from a finger stick or from an EDTA blood sample onto the center of a clean slide. With the edge of another side, spread the drop into an area 1 cm in diameter; continue stirring for 30 seconds if the blood is from a finger stick. Air dry for at least 6 hours. Do *not* place in methanol.

● Place both thin and thick smears in Giemsa's stain (1 part Giemsa's stain stock solution to 50 parts phosphate buffered water, pH 7.2) for 45 minutes.

● Rinse the smears in phosphate buffered water, pH 7.2.

● Drain the excess stain off the smears and air dry.

● Examine microscopically under 100× (to scan for microfilariae) and 1000× (oil immersion).

Expected Results for the Malarial Parasite

Nuclear chromatin, red; cytoplasm, blue

BIBLIOGRAPHY

Baird JK et al: North American Brugian filariasis: report of nine infections in humans. Am J Trop Med Hyg 35:1205–1209, 1986.

Beaver PC: Intraocular filariasis: a brief review. Am J Trop Med Hyg 40:40–45, 1989.

Beck JW, Davies JE: Medical Parasitology. St Louis, CV Mosby, 1981.

Belding DL: Textbook of Parasitology, 3rd ed. New York, Appleton-Century-Crofts, 1965.

Bottone EJ: Diagnosis of acute pulmonary toxoplasmosis by visualization of invasive and intracellular tachyzoites in Giemsa stained smears of a bronchoalveolar lavage. J Clin Microbiol 29:2626–2627, 1991.

Burkhart CG: Scabies: an epidemiologic reassessment. Ann Intern Med 98:498–503, 1983.

Cahill KM: Tropical Diseases in Temperate Climates. Philadelphia, JB Lippincott, 1964.

Capo V, Despommier DD: Clinical aspects of infection with *Trichinella* spp. Clin Microbiol Rev 9(1):47–54, 1996.

Chandler AC, Read CP: Introduction to Parasitology, 10th ed. New York, John Wiley, 1955.

Christophersen J: Epidemiology of scabies. Parasitol Today 2:247–248, 1986.

Cohen EJ et al: Diagnosis and management of *Acanthamoeba* keratitis. Am J Ophthalmol 100:389–395, 1985.

Collins RC et al: Parasitological diagnosis of onchocerciasis: comparison of incubation times for skin snips. Am J Trop Med Hyg 29:35–41, 1980.

Cross JH: Intestinal capillariasis. Clin Microbiol Rev 5:120–129, 1992.

Current WL: Human enteric coccidia. II. *Isospora belli* and *Sarcocystis* spp. Clin Microbiol Newslett 7:175–178, 1985.

Current WL: Cryptosporidiosis. Clin Microbiol Rev 4(3):325–358, 1991.

Departments of the Air Force and the Army: Clinical Laboratory Procedures—Parasitology. Washington, DC, US Government Printing Office, 1974.

Desowitz RS: Ova and Parasites. Hagerstown, Harper & Row, 1980.

Garcia LS, Shimizu RY: Diagnostic parasitology: an overview of topics. Lab Med 24(1):13–18, 1993.

Garcia LS, Shimizu RY, Bruckner DA: Detection of microsporidial spores in fecal specimens from patients diagnosed with cryptosporidiosis. J Clin Microbiol 32:1739–1741, 1994.

Grimaldi G Jr, Tesh RB: Leishmaniasis of the New World: current concepts and implications for future research. Clin Microbiol Rev 6(3):230–250, 1993.

Healy GR: Babesiosis. Clin Microbiol Newslett 4(5):33–35, 1992.

Healy GR, Ruebush TK: Morphology of *Babesia microti* in human blood smears. Am J Clin Pathol 73:107–109, 1980.

Herwaldt BL, Stokes SL, Juranek DD: American cutaneous leishmaniasis in United States travelers. Ann Intern Med 118:779–784, 1993.

Holodniy MJ et al: Cerebral sparganosis: case report and review. Rev Infect Dis 13:155–159, 1991.

Hopkins D: Dracunculiasis: an eradicable scourge. Epidemiol Rev 5:208–219, 1983.

Jeffrey HC, Leach RM: Atlas of Medical Helminthology and Protozoology. Baltimore, Williams & Wilkins, 1966.

John DT: Primary amebic meningoencephalitis and the biology of *Naegleria fowleri.* Annu Rev Microbiol 36:101–123, 1982.

Krieger JN et al: Diagnosis of trichomoniasis. Comparison of conventional wet-mount examination with cytologic studies, cultures, and monoclonal antibody staining of direct specimens. JAMA 259:1223–1227, 1988.

Lalitha MK et al: Isolation of *Acanthamoeba castellani* from a patient with meningitis. J Clin Microbiol 21:666–667, 1985.

Laurence BR: The global dispersal of bancroftian filariasis. Parasitol Today 5:260–264, 1989.

Lopez-Antunano FJ, Schmunis GA: Plasmodia of humans. In Kreier JP, ed: Parasitic Protozoa, 2nd ed. San Diego, Academic Press, 1993.

Markell EK, Voge M, John DT: Medical Parasitology, 7th ed. Philadelphia, WB Saunders, 1992.

Muller R, Baker JR: Medical Parasitology. Philadelphia, JB Lippincott, 1990.

Murray PR et al, eds: Manual of Clinical Microbiology, 6th ed. Washington, DC, ASM Press, 1995.

Nanduri J, Kazura JW: Clinical and laboratory aspects of filariasis. Clin Microbiol Rev 2(1):39–50, 1989.

Negesse Y et al: Loiasis: "Calabar" swellings and involvement of deep organs. Am J Trop Med Hyg 34:537–546, 1985.

Neva FA, Brown HW: Basic Clinical Parasitology, 6th ed. Norwalk, Appleton & Lange, 1994.

Ng E et al: Demonstration of *Isospora belli* by acid-fast stain in a patient with acquired immune deficiency syndrome. J Clin Microbiol 20:384–386, 1984.

Orihel TC, Beaver PC: Zoonotic *Brugia* infections in North and South America. Am J Med Hyg 40:638–647, 1989.

Orihel TC, Eberhard ML: *Mansonella ozzardi:* a redescription with comments on its taxonomic relations. Am J Med Hyg 31:1142–1147, 1982.

Ortega Y et al: *Cyclospora* species: a new protozoan pathogen of humans. N Engl J Med 328:1308–1312, 1993.

BLOOD EXAMINATION

Schmidt GD, Roberts LS: Foundations of Parasitology. St Louis, CV Mosby, 1977.

Shadduck JA, Greeley E: Microsporidia and human infection. Clin Microbiol Rev 2(2):158–165, 1989.

Spencer MJ et al: *Dientamoeba fragilis.* A gastrointestinal protozoan infection in adults. Am J Gastroenterol 77:565–569, 1982.

Tanowitz HB et al: Chagas' disease. Clin Microbiol Rev 5:400–419, 1992.

Tortora GT et al: Rhodamine-auramine O versus Kinyoun carbolfuchsin acid fast stains for detection of *Cryptosporidium* oocysts. Clin Lab Science 5(6):358–359, 1992.

U.S. Medical Naval School: Medical Protozoology and Helminthology. Washington, DC, US Government Printing Office, 1965.

Visvesvara GS, Stehr-Green JK: Epidemiology of free-living ameba infections. J Protozool 37:25S–33S, 1990.

Weber R et al: Human microsporidial infections. Clin Microbiol Rev 7(4):426–461, 1994.

Weber R et al: Improved light-microscopical detection of microsporidia spores in stool and duodenal aspirates. N Engl J Med 326(3):161–166, 1992.

Zaman V, Keong LA: Handbook of Medical Parasitology. Sydney, Australia, ADIS Health Science Press, 1982.

Zierdt C: *Blastocystis hominis:* past and future. Clin Microbiol Rev 4:61–79, 1991.

Section V

URINALYSIS AND BODY FLUIDS

Chapter **33**

ROUTINE URINALYSIS

Kathleen Finnegan, MS, MT(ASCP)SH

QUICK CONTENTS

INTRODUCTION

Urine is a fluid that is composed of waste products from the blood. It is formed in the kidney and is eliminated from the body by the urinary system. The kidneys play a very important role in water balance, acid-base balance, and electrolyte balance. The kidney is also involved with the production of erythropoietin, a hormone that stimulates red blood cell (RBC) production, and renin, an enzyme for the control of blood pressure. Urine is more than 95% water by weight. The principal solutes present are urea, sodium, chloride, potassium, creatinine, uric acid, and ammonia.

Routine urinalysis consists of three parts: (1) physical analysis, (2) chemical analysis, and (3) microscopic analysis. All this testing provides information on the function of the kidney and the urinary system to rule out systemic and metabolic disorders.

ANATOMY AND PHYSIOLOGY OF THE KIDNEY

The urinary system consists of two bilateral paired kidneys, which are bean shaped organs; two ureters, which carry the urine to the bladder; a urinary bladder, which is a hollow muscular sac that collects and stores the urine; and the urethra, which extends from the bladder to outside the body.

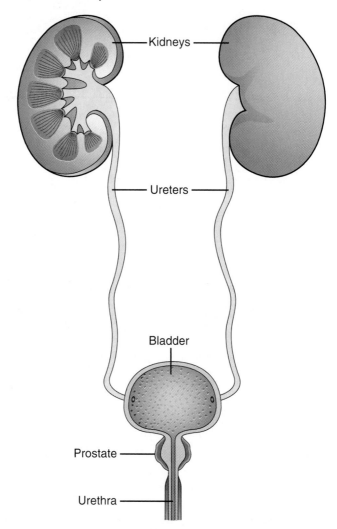

The functional unit of the kidney is the nephron. There are more than 1 million nephrons in each kidney. The nephron consists of a capillary network called the *glomerulus*, which essentially is a filtering system; the proximal convoluted tubule, the function of which is mainly the conservation of substances needed; the loop of Henle with a descending and ascending limb; the distal tubule; and a collecting duct for final concentration and pH balance.

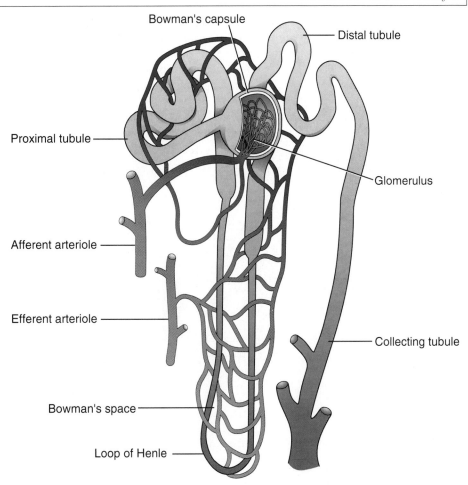

Formation of Urine

Formation of urine involves the process of plasma filtration, tubular reabsorption, and tubular secretion. When blood flows into the capillaries of the glomerulus, blood cells, high molecular weight proteins, and other large molecules are unable to pass through the glomerular membrane. Blood constituents that do pass through the membrane are termed the *glomerular filtrate.* These substances include glucose, uric acid, urea, water, and low molecular weight substances (less than 70,000 Da). The glomerular filtration rate in the average adult is 125 mL/min. Most of the glomerular filtrate is reabsorbed in the renal tubules of the nephron. By the time the filtrate enters the proximal tubule, 80% is reabsorbed. When the plasma concentration of a substance that is normally reabsorbed reaches the maximal concentration of tubular reabsorption, the substance appears in the urine. This is termed *renal threshold.*

In the loop of Henle, the descending portion loses both water and sodium and the ascending portion loses sodium and chloride without water. The distal tubule and collecting duct are responsible for the adjustment of pH, osmolarity, and electrolyte balance. The remainder of the sodium is reabsorbed, influenced by the hormone aldosterone. Aldosterone is secreted by the adrenal cortex in response to a decrease in the serum sodium and an increase in the potassium level.

Final concentration of the filtrate takes place in the late distal tubules and collecting duct. This is dependent on antidiuretic hormone (ADH), which is secreted by the pituitary gland. When the body is hydrated, less ADH is needed, the walls become less permeable, and water will not be reabsorbed. If the body is dehydrated, ADH levels increase, the walls become more permeable to water, and water is reabsorbed.

Tubular secretion eliminates waste products not filtered and regulates acid-base balance through the secretion of hydrogen ions. Hydrogen ions are secreted in both the proximal and distal tubules.

The glomerular filtrate becomes urine after it leaves the distal convoluted tubule and enters the collecting system. In 24 hours the body excretes approximately 60 g of dissolved material, half of which is urea. For an adult the average daily output of urine is 1200 to 1500 mL.

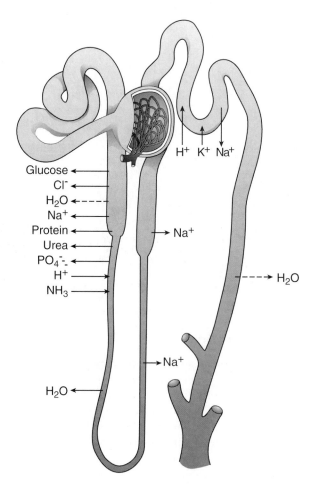

URINE COLLECTION

The care that goes into handling, collecting, and storing the urine specimen is of great importance. The type of specimen and the collection procedure used are determined by the types of tests that are going to be performed. The best urine specimen for urinalysis testing should be a fresh and concentrated for the detection of analytes and formed elements. Another consideration is the dehydration status of the patient.

Summary of Urine Collection

TYPE	PATIENT PREPARATION	AMOUNT NEEDED (mL)	SPECIMEN PREPARATION	USE	SPECIMEN STORAGE
First Morning	Free midstream voided specimen on rising from sleep Specimen that has remained in bladder for 8 hr.	20	Clean, dry container Specimen should be fresh and properly labeled	More concentrated specimen, more likely to find pathologic elements, nitrite, and protein.	Decomposition of urine begins within 30 min at room temperature and 4 hours at refrigeration For long term, boric acid can be used for preservative
Random	Collected anytime during day or night Depends on hydration status of patient	20	Clean, dry container Specimen should be fresh and properly labeled	Most common and convenient, collected anytime, good for chemical and microscopic screen	Decomposition of urine begins within 30 min at room temperature and 4 hr at refrigeration For long term, boric acid can be used for preservative
Fractional	Collected at specific timed intervals On rising first specimen is discarded; second specimen is fasting; others are then followed Can be: Fasting 2 hr	20	Clean, dry container Specimen should be fresh and properly labeled with time of collection	Glucose tolerance Diabetic screening Renal threshold	Decomposition of urine begins within 30 min at room temperature and 4 hr at refrigeration For long term, preservative can be added depending on analyte testing
Postprandial 2 hr	Specimen collected 2 hr after meal Patient is instructed to eat meal high in carbohydrates 2 hr later specimen is collected	20	Clean, dry container Specimen should be fresh and properly labeled with time of collection	Glucose and protein monitoring	Decomposition of urine begins within 30 min at room temperature and 4 hr at refrigeration For long term, preservative can be added depending on analyte testing.
2 hr	Timed specimen for analyte to be maximally excreted	20	Clean, dry container Specimen should be fresh and properly labeled with time of collection	Quantitative determination of urobilinogen between 2 and 4 PM	Decomposition of urine begins within 30 min at room temperature and 4 hr at refrigeration For long term, preservative can be added depending on analyte testing

Continued ▲

URINE COLLECTION

▶ Continued **Summary of Urine Collection**

TYPE	PATIENT PREPARATION	AMOUNT NEEDED (mL)	SPECIMEN PREPARATION	USE	SPECIMEN STORAGE
12 hr	First urine voided at beginning of collection discarded and all others saved for 12 hr	Total volume needs to be recorded for calculation	Clean, dry container Specimen should be fresh and properly labeled with time of collection	Addis count for WBC, RBC, and casts per 12 hr	Formalin preservative and refrigeration
24 hr	First urine voided at beginning of collection is discarded and all others saved for 24 hr	Total volume needs to be recorded for calculation	Total volume of specimen is measured and recorded	For chemical analysis, quantitative results	Preservative needed and depends on analyte testing Refrigeration required
Midstream Clean Catch	Genital area is cleansed, patient passes some urine into toilet, stops urination, proceeds to urinate into container	20	Sterile, dry container Very important that interior of container doesn't come into contact with patient's hands or perineal area.	Culture and sensitivity	Promptly refrigerated Refrigeration prevents bacterial growth for 24 hr

Changes in Unpreserved Urine

Urinalysis should be performed immediately or up until 2 hours at room temperature or 4 hours at refrigeration. Many changes can occur that can affect the results and integrity of the sample.

ANALYSIS	CHANGE	CAUSE
Physical Changes		
Color	Becomes darker on standing	Oxidation or reduction of metabolites
Turbidity	Increases	Bacterial growth and crystal precipitation
Odor	Foul smelling	Bacterial decomposition of urea to ammonia
Chemical Changes		
pH	Increases	Bacterial decomposition of urea to ammonia
Glucose	Decreases	Cellular and bacterial glycolysis
Ketones	Decrease	Volatilization
Bilirubin	Decreases	Exposure to light
Urobilinogen	Decreases	Oxidation of urobilin
Nitrite	Increases	Bacterial production
Microscopic Changes		
Red Blood Cells	Lyse	Standing especially in dilute alkaline urine
White Blood Cells	Disintegrate	Standing especially in dilute alkaline urine
Casts	Disintegrate	Standing especially in dilute alkaline urine
Bacteria	Increase	Bacterial proliferation

URINE COLLECTION

ROUTINE URINALYSIS

Urinalysis is performed to aid in screening, diagnosis, and prognosis and to monitor the treatment of disease. It is a specimen that is easy to obtain, and the testing is simple and quick to perform.

PHYSICAL ANALYSIS

The first step of a routine urinalysis is the assessment of the physical properties, which include color, appearance, odor, and sometimes specific gravity. Specific gravity can be measured by chemical analysis also. These physical properties or findings can be correlated with other chemical and microscopic findings.

Physical Findings

SUBSTANCE	PATHOLOGIC	NONPATHOLOGIC	DRUGS
Color (Freshly voided urine may range from pale yellow to amber depending on concentration. Yellow color comes from pigment urochrome.)			
Orange	Bilirubin	Rhubarb Carrots	Phenazopyridine
Dark Yellow	Bilirubin Urobilin	Carrots Concentrated	Fluorescein
Green	Oxidized bilirubin Biliverdin *Pseudomonas*	Vitamin B complex Clorets	Dithiazanine Nitrofurans Phenol
Red or Pink	RBCs Hemoglobin Myoglobin Porphyrins	Beets	Benzene Acetophenetidin Phenindione
Brown or Black	Biliary pigments Melanin Homogentisic acid	Rhubarb	Phenol derivatives Methyldopa Levodopa
Pale Yellow	Diabetes mellitus Diabetes insipidus	Large fluid intake	Diuretics
Appearance (Freshly voided urine is clear but becomes turbid on standing.)			
Cloudy	White blood cells Bacteria Epithelial cells	Amorphous urate (pink: acid pH) Amorphous phosphates (white: alkaline pH)	
Smoky	RBCs	Radiographic media	
Milky	Fat		
Odor (Freshly voided urine has aromatic odor due to presence of volatile acids.)			
Ammonia	Urinary tract infection	Old urine	
Sweet	Diabetes mellitus	Starvation Dieting Strenuous exercise Vomiting or diarrhea	
Mousy	Phenylketonuria		
Maple Syrup	Maple syrup disease		
Distinctive		Garlic, onions, asparagus	

Continued ▶

▶ Continued **Physical Findings**

SUBSTANCE	PATHOLOGIC	NONPATHOLOGIC	DRUGS
Foam (When urine is shaken, foam at top can be white to indicate presence of protein or yellow to indicate bilirubin.)			
Specific Gravity (Measurement of amount of dissolved substances in solution. It is used to measure ability of kidney to concentrate. Sometimes done as physical property. Refractometer measures specific gravity by using refractive index to indirectly measure dissolved particles.)			
Low SG	Diabetes insipidus Glomerulonephritis Tubular damage		
High SG	Diabetes mellitus Adrenal insufficiency Hepatic disease	Radiographic dye Dehydration Vomiting Diarrhea	

Volume

Also part of the physical characteristics of urine is volume. It is not measured for routine urinalysis but is very important in timed or 24 hour specimens. The average 24 hour volume for an adult is 1200 to 1500 mL but can range from 600 to 2000 mL depending on fluid intake. There is a direct relationship between fluid intake and urine volume.

ABNORMAL URINE VOLUME

TERM	DESCRIPTION	AMOUNT	PATHOLOGIC	NONPATHOLOGIC
Polyuria	Consistent elimination of large amounts of urine	Exceeds 2000 mL/24 hr	Diabetes mellitus Diabetes insipidus	Large fluid intake Diuretic medications
Oliguria	Excretion of small amounts of urine	Less than 500 mL/24hr	Renal tubular dysfunction End stage kidney disease Obstruction Edema	Dehydration Shock Vomiting Diarrhea
Anuria	Complete absence of urine formation	None	Acute renal failure Acute glomerulonephritis Obstruction Heart failure	Shock

CHEMICAL ANALYSIS

Substances present in excess amounts are filtered through the kidney and appear in urine. The chemical testing of urine is an excellent screening for detecting abnormal constituents in the urine. This type of testing is done as a screening or semiquantitative

PHYSICAL ANALYSIS

method using reagent strips. The reagent strips are composed of a plastic strip with colored pads that have been impregnated with various chemicals for testing. When the chemically treated pads come in contact with urine, a reaction that involves a color change takes place. This color change is compared visually to a color chart provided by the manufacturer of the reagent strip or can be read by an automated method. Automation measures the intensity of the light that is provided by the chemical reaction between the substances in the urine and the reagent pad.

General directions for the use of reagent strips, better known as *dipsticks,* for routine urinalysis are that the specimen be fresh, well mixed, and at room temperature. The plastic strip is dipped into the urine so that all the test areas are adequately moistened. The strip must not be left in contact with the urine for a long period of time because the chemicals on the reagent areas will run into each other and become contaminated. Timing is a crucial step in the reading of these strips. The strips must always be read at the times stated by the manufacturer. Ames reagent strips are read during the kinetic phase of the chemical reaction. Chemstrip reagent strips are read at the end point of the chemical reaction. The final reading is based on color comparison.

For quality control the strips should be kept in a tightly capped container at room temperature. The reagent areas deteriorate rapidly when exposed to direct light, heat, and moisture. Each container is marked with a lot and expiration date. The strips should not be used after their expiration date. When the strips are read, they should be held in a horizontal position and read in good light. Individual interpretation can be a source of error. The use of automation has eliminated individual differences.

Chemical Testing

SUBSTANCE	NORMAL VALUES	CLINICAL SIGNIFICANCE	PRINCIPLE OF MEASUREMENT	CLINICAL IMPLICATIONS	FALSE POSITIVE	FALSE NEGATIVE
Glucose	Negative	Primary energy source for body cells	Glucose oxidase Double enzyme Specific for glucose	Diabetes Large amounts of carbohydrate intake	Strong oxidizing reagents Bleach	Ascorbic acid Large amounts of ketones Aspirin Metabolized quickly by microorganisms
Bilirubin	Negative	Breakdown of hemoglobin by the reticuloendothelial system	Diazo reaction Only conjugated bilirubin is excreted into urine.	Biliary obstruction Hepatic or liver disease	Metabolites of drugs (phenazopyridine [Pyridium])	Ascorbic acid Elevated nitrites Light sensitive
Ketone	Negative	Formed during incomplete fat metabolism	Sodium nitroprusside	Decreased intake of carbohydrates Starvation Prolonged vomiting Dehydration Fever Diabetes insipidus	Highly pigmented urine Levodopa	Ascorbic acid Ketone bodies are volatile
Specific Gravity	1.002–1.030	Concentrating or diluting ability of kidney	pK change of polyelectrolyte reaction Ionic concentration	**Low SG:** Diabetes insipidus Tubular damage **High SG:** Diabetes mellitus Dehydration Fever Congestive heart failure	Protein	Alkaline urine

Continued ▶

CHEMICAL ANALYSIS

▶ Continued **Chemical Testing**

SUBSTANCE	NORMAL VALUES	CLINICAL SIGNIFICANCE	PRINCIPLE OF MEASUREMENT	CLINICAL IMPLICATIONS	FALSE POSITIVE	FALSE NEGATIVE
Blood	Negative	Hematuria indicates bleeding within the urinary system. Hemoglobinuria (presence of free hemoglobin) indicates intravascular hemolysis.	Peroxidase activity of hemoglobin	Renal disease Trauma Renal stones Infection Strenuous exercise Hemolytic anemia Transfusion reaction	Urinary myoglobin Oxidizing contaminant Vegetable peroxidase Bacterial enzymes	Ascorbic acid pH <5.0 inhibits hemolysis on reagent pad Nitrite High specific gravity Protein

pH	4.5–7.5	Regulates acid-base balance	Double indicator system
			Methyl red
			Bromthymol blue
				Acid:
				  Diabetes
				  Starvation
				  High protein diet
				Alkaline:
				  After meals
				  Bacterial infections
				  Chronic renal failure
					Production of ammonia	None

Protein	Negative	Proteinuria is increase in protein in urine. First indication of renal disease. Protein should be reabsorbed by kidney.	Protein error of indicators
			Colorimetric method in which proteins have ability to alter color of acid-base indicator without altering pH
			Sensitive to albumin
				Increased:
				  Renal abnormality
				  Glomerular, tubular damage or excess overflow
				Nondisease:
				  Strenuous exercise
				  Exposure to cold
				  Fever
					Highly alkaline pH	High salt concentration

Urobilinogen	0.2–1.0 mg/dL	Byproduct of RBC degradation Highest excretion between 2 and 4 PM	Ehrlich's reaction	Increased amounts in hemolytic anemia and liver damage Negative in biliary obstruction	Indols Porphobilinogen	Rapidly oxidized to urobilin Nitrite Formaldehyde

Continued ▶

▶ Continued **Chemical Testing**

SUBSTANCE	NORMAL VALUES	CLINICAL SIGNIFICANCE	PRINCIPLE OF MEASUREMENT	CLINICAL IMPLICATIONS	FALSE POSITIVE	FALSE NEGATIVE
Nitrite	Negative	For detection of significant bacteriuria Bacterial organisms reduce nitrate to nitrite. Urine should remain in bladder for 4 hr.	Griess's reaction Diazo reaction	Indicator of urinary tract infection (UTI) *Escherichia coli* *Proteus* *Klebsiella* *Enterobacter* *Pseudomonas*	Specimen not fresh Medication color	Ascorbic acid Antibiotic therapy Not in bladder for 4 hr for conversion Organisms do not reduce nitrate to nitrite Diet lacking vegetables to allow nitrates to be formed
Leukocyte Esterase	Negative	Neutrophil contains esterase enzymes that react with reagent area.	Granulocyte esterase reaction	Increased white blood cells indication of inflammation, UTI	Oxidizing reagents Vaginal discharge	Ascorbic acid Increased glucose, protein, specific gravity

CHEMICAL ANALYSIS

Confirmation Testing

The sensitivity and specificity of reagents strips has improved over the years, so there is some discussion about whether confirmation tests are needed. Clinitest should be used to screen for nonglucose reducing substances such as lactose or galactose and should be required for infants and small children under 2 years of age. If the physician suspects a increased amount of abnormal immunoglobulin or Bence-Jones protein, the protein should be confirmed with sulfosalicylic acid (SSA). The Acetest and Ictotest are sometimes a little easier to read and are more specific.

SUBSTANCE	NORMAL VALUES	PRINCIPLE OF MEASUREMENT	CLINICAL IMPLICATIONS	FALSE POSITIVE	FALSE NEGATIVE
Precipitation SSA	Negative	Protein precipitated with strong acid	Detects all proteins, albumins, globulins and Bence-Jones protein	Turbidity Mucin Radiographic dye	Highly buffered alkaline urine
Clinitest	Negative	Copper reduction Cupric ions to cuprous ions in presence of heat	Detects all reducing substances Not as sensitive to glucose as strip	Ascorbic acid	Radiographic dye
Acetest	Negative	Sodium nitroprusside	Detects acetone and acetoacetic acid	Pigments Phenylketones	Conversion of acetoacetic acid
Ictotest	Negative	Diaxonium salt	More sensitive to bilirubin than strip. Special pad is used to absorb urine and leave bilirubin at surface.	Pigmented urine	Ascorbic acid

MICROSCOPIC ANALYSIS

Urine sediment helps clarify the results of the physical and chemical findings. The urine specimen is prepared by centrifuging approximately 10 to 15 mL of well mixed urine for 5 minutes. The supernatant is discarded and the sediment is resuspended, with the remaining urine coating the tube walls. A drop of this resuspended sediment is placed on a clean slide and covered with a cover slip. The sediment is first examined under low power with low light to observe for casts. Then high power is used to identify specific types of cells, casts, bacteria, and crystals. Ten to 15 fields should be examined. Casts are recorded as the average number per low power field (LPF). RBCs, white blood cells (WBCs), and epithelial cells are recorded as a number per high power field (HPF). Bacteria, crystals, and yeasts are recorded as small, moderate, or large per HPF.

Urine sediment or structures that may be found microscopically are described in the following charts.

Cells

Cells that can be present in urinary sediment include WBCs, RBCs, and epithelial cells. These cells can be anywhere in the urinary tract from the tubules to the urethra. They also can be contaminants.

Cells

TYPE	DESCRIPTION	NORMAL VALUES	CLINICAL IMPLICATIONS	OTHER	MICROSCOPIC VIEW
Red Blood Cell	Uniform colorless smooth biconcave disks 7 μm. Hypotonic urine (dilute): RBCs swell and lyse, referred to as ghost cells. Hypertonic urine (concentrated): RBCs crenate.	0–3 RBCs/HPF	Can originate from any part of urinary tract Glomerulonephritis Trauma Systemic and renal disease	Can be confused with yeast, oil droplets, air bubbles, and round calcium oxalate.	*
White Blood Cell	Spherical with dull gray color. Tend to be neutrophils 10–12 μm. Hypotonic: swell and lyse, referred to as glitter cells. Hypertonic: tend to shrink.	0–5 WBCs/HPF	Acute infection of kidney (pyelonephritis) Cystitis (bladder) Urethritis (urethra) Urinary tract infections	Lymphocytes indicate transplant rejection. Monocytes and macrophages indicate tissue damage. Eosinophils can indicate acute interstitial nephritis.	*
Squamous Epithelial	Large, flat, irregularly shaped cells that contain small central nucleus Abundant cytoplasm Cell size: 23–40 μm	Few	Occur in urethra and vagina Vaginal contamination	No diagnostic significance.	*
Renal Epithelial	Slightly larger than WBC with round central nucleus Cell size: 20 μm	Occasional	Originate in convoluted and collecting tubules Increased numbers indicate tubular injury and damage to epithelial basement membrane	When found alone, no diagnostic significance. When found in cast matrix, tubular origin is inferred.	*

Continued ▲

MICROSCOPIC ANALYSIS

▶ Continued **Cells**

TYPE	DESCRIPTION	NORMAL VALUES	CLINICAL IMPLICATIONS	OTHER	MICROSCOPIC VIEW
Transitional Epithelial	Can be round or pear shaped with tail-like projections	Rare	Line urinary tract from urinary pelvis to upper portion of urethra. Increased amounts indicate disease of bladder or renal pelvis.	Increased numbers are seen with catherization.	*
Oval Fat Bodies	Renal epithelial cells filled with lipid that are highly refractive, coarse droplets in various sizes	Negative	Result from tubular epithelial degeneration of nephron Are associated with large amounts of protein Nephrotic syndrome	Polarized light is used for identification of cholesterol (Maltese cross.) For triglycerides, Sudan black B is used.	*
Fat Droplets	Not cellular constituent but can be found free Highly refractive droplets of various sizes	Negative	Can be contaminant or can indicate severe renal dysfunction	Found with oval fat bodies and fatty casts. Polarized light is used for identification of cholesterol (Maltese cross.) For triglycerides Sudan black B is used.	†

* Photomicrographs courtesy of Bayer Corporation, Elkhart, IN.
† Photomicrograph from ASCP Workshop 9275, "Urinalysis," presented by Janice M. Hundley and James K. Fleming. © 1995 American Society of Clinical Pathologists.

Casts

Casts are cylindric structures that form in the lumen of the distal convoluted tubule and collecting ducts. The renal tubules secrete an abnormal mucoprotein called *Tamm-Horsefall mucoprotein*, which is the basic structure of all casts. There are four main factors involved in cast formation: (1) urinary stasis, (2) increased acidity, (3) high solute concentration, and (4) the presence of abnormal protein constituents.

Casts are important clinically. They can contain RBCs, WBCs, fat, and epithelial cells. These are inclusions not normally found in the tubules. Casts are renal in origin and indicate renal disease.

Identification of casts is difficult. They should be observed and enumerated under a low light and the low power objective. They are classified on the basis of their appearance and cellular components. Casts have nearly parallel sides and round or blunt ends and vary in size and width due to the tubule in which they were formed. Casts dissolve in alkaline urine.

MICROSCOPIC ANALYSIS

Casts

TYPE	DESCRIPTION	NORMAL VALUES	SIGNIFICANCE	MICROSCOPIC VIEW
Hyaline	Colorless, homogeneous, semitransparent Low refractive index Difficult to see; use very low light	0–2/LPF	When seen in numbers can indicate mild to severe renal disease Can be found in healthy individuals after strenuous exercise	*
Red Blood Cell	RBCs in hyaline matrix Yellow to red-brown Extremely fragile, degenerate to granular casts	Negative	Intrinsic renal disease Acute glomerulonephritis Acute interstitial nephritis Severe nephritis	*
White Cell	WBCs in hyaline matrix Usually neutrophils High refractive index	Negative	Renal inflammation Renal infection Pyelonephritis Chronic renal disease Acute glomerulonephritis	*
Renal Tubular Epithelial Cell	Renal tubular epithelial cells in hyaline matrix High refractive index	Negative	Interstitial tubular disease Vascular disease Toxins Glomerulonephritis	◆

Continued ▶

▶ Continued **Casts**

TYPE	DESCRIPTION	NORMAL VALUES	SIGNIFICANCE	MICROSCOPIC VIEW
Mixed Cell	Cast with one or more cell types incorporated in matrix Enumerated as cellular casts	Negative	Indicates two parts of nephron are involved	＊
Granular	Variety of granular textures from fine to coarse granules within hyaline matrix Highly refractive All sizes and shapes Colorless to yellow Degeneration of cellular casts	0–2/LPF	Can be found in healthy individual after prolonged exercise Renal disease Heavy proteinuria Acute and chronic renal disease Nephrotic syndrome	＊
Broad	Indicate cast formation in dilated convoluted tubules or collecting ducts May be of any type, usually granular or waxy	Negative	Significant urinary stasis with obstruction or disease Acute tubular necrosis Severe chronic renal disease End stage kidney disease Urinary tract obstruction	＊
Fatty	Fat globules, free fat or oval fat bodies in transparent matrix Vary in size Highly refractive Can use polarized light and Sudan black B for identification	Negative	Nephrotic syndrome Diabetes mellitus Mercury poisoning Crushing injury with disruption of body fat	◆

Continued ▲

▶ Continued **Casts**

TYPE	DESCRIPTION	NORMAL VALUES	SIGNIFICANCE	MICROSCOPIC VIEW
Waxy	High refractive index Homogeneous with well defined edges that are sharp and blunt irregular ends Cracks on lateral edges Colorless or gray to yellow	Negative	Tubular obstruction with prolonged stasis Called *renal failure casts* Severe chronic renal failure Malignant hypertension Acute renal disease Diabetes mellitus	*
Cylindroid	Resemble casts but have one end that tapers to a tail	0–2/LPF	Found in conjunction with casts and have same significance	*
Mucous Strands	Long thin wavy threads, very transparent	Occasional	Can be found in small numbers in normal urine Increased numbers indicate inflammation or irritation of urinary tract	◆

* Photomicrographs courtesy of Bayer Corporation, Elkhart, IN.
◆ Photomicrographs from Henry JB: Clinical Diagnosis and Management by Laboratory Methods. 19th ed. Philadelphia, WB Saunders, 1996.

Crystals

Crystalline forms are usually not found in fresh urine but appear if urine is allowed to stand. The formation of crystals depends on the saturation of a particular crystalline compound or a change in the solubility properties of the crystal. The pH of the urine plays a role in the type of crystal that is found. Many of the crystals have little clinical significance except in stone formation, metabolic disorders, and regulation of medication.

Crystals are identified by their appearance, solubility, and pH.

Crystals

TYPE	DESCRIPTION	PH	SOLUBILITY PROPERTIES	SIGNIFICANCE	MICROSCOPIC VIEW
Uric Acid	*Color:* Yellow to brown *Shape:* Many different shapes, most common are diamond or rhombic plates in clusters, lemon shape Polarize into variety of colors	Acid	Soluble in alkaline solutions, sodium hydroxide Insoluble in acid, alcohol, acetic acid	Associated with renal stones, gout, high purine metabolism, acute febrile conditions, chronic nephritis Can be normal occurrence	*
Calcium Oxalate	*Color:* Colorless *Shape:* Envelope with intersecting diagonal lines, octahedral Can be found in dumbbell or elliptical Birefringent	Acid Neutral	Soluble in hydrochloric acid Insoluble in acetic acid	Associated with renal stones, ethylene glycol poisoning, diabetes mellitus, liver disease, and chronic renal disease Can be found in normal individuals after ingestion of oxalate rich foods and large doses of vitamin C	*
Hippuric Acid	*Color:* Yellow-brown to colorless *Shape:* Elongated prisms or plates with pyramidal ends Can be found in thin needles Birefringent	Acid Neutral	Soluble in H$_2$O, alkali Insoluble in acetic acid	Associated with diets high in fruits and vegetables containing large quantities of benzoic acid	
Sodium Urates	*Color:* Yellow to colorless *Shape:* Needle or slender prisms in sheaves or clusters	Acid	Soluble at 60°C Slightly soluble in acetic acid	Reported as urate crystals No clinical significance	◆

Continued ▶

▶ Continued **Crystals**

TYPE	DESCRIPTION	PH	SOLUBILITY PROPERTIES	SIGNIFICANCE	MICROSCOPIC VIEW
Amorphous Urates	*Color:* Yellow or red *Shape:* Small granular Pink precipitate at refrigeration Salts of sodium, potassium, magnesium, and calcium	Acid Neutral	Soluble at 60°C and alkali Insoluble in acetic acid	No clinical significance	*
Triple Phosphate (ammonium-magnesium-phosphate)	*Color:* Colorless *Shape:* Three to six sided prisms described as coffin covers Feathery form can be found	Alkaline Neutral	Soluble in dilute acetic acid	Associated with renal calculi, chronic pyelitis, enlarged prostate, urinary tract infections Found in normal urine	*
Calcium Carbonate	*Color:* Colorless *Shape:* Small, dumbbells, or spherical forms; can be found in granular masses or in pairs	Alkaline	Soluble in acetic acid	No clinical significance	◆
Calcium Phosphate	*Color:* Colorless *Shape:* Long, thin prisms with one pointed end arranged as rosettes or clusters of needles Thin irregular plates that float on surface of urine	Alkaline	Soluble in acetic acid	Associated with renal calculi Can be found in normal urine	✚

Continued ▶

MICROSCOPIC ANALYSIS

► Continued **Crystals**

TYPE	DESCRIPTION	PH	SOLUBILITY PROPERTIES	SIGNIFICANCE	MICROSCOPIC VIEW
Ammonium Biurate	*Color:* Yellow to brown *Shape:* Spherical bodies with long irregular spicules Thorn apple	Alkaline Neutral	Soluble in acetic acid and warming	Usually indicates old urine	✳
Amorphous Phosphates	*Color:* colorless *Shape:* granular patches with no definite shape White precipitate when refrigerated	Alkaline	Soluble in acetic acid Insoluble at 60°C	No clinical significance	✚

✳ Photomicrographs courtesy of Bayer Corporation, Elkhart, IN.
◆ Photomicrographs from Brunzel NA: Fundamentals of Urine and Body Fluid Analysis. Philadelphia, WB Saunders, 1994.
✚ Photomicrographs from Henry JB: Clinical Diagnosis and Management by Laboratory Methods, 19th ed. Philadelphia, WB Saunders, 1996.

ABNORMAL CRYSTALS

TYPE	DESCRIPTION	PH	SOLUBILITY PROPERTIES	CLINICAL SIGNIFICANCE	MICROSCOPIC VIEW
Cystine	*Color:* Colorless and refractile *Shape:* Hexagonal with equal and unequal sides Appear single or clusters	Acid	Soluble in HCL, alkali, and ammonia Insoluble in acetic acid, alcohol, ether, and acetone	Amino acid crystal, inherited as a metabolic defect that prevents reabsorption of cystine Associated with congenital cystinosis and cystinuria Renal stones	*
Leucine	*Color:* Yellow or brown *Shape:* Spheroids with radial and concentric striations Highly refractile with oil-like appearance	Acid	Soluble in hot acetic acid, hot alcohol, and alkali Insoluble in HCl	Maple syrup disease Severe liver disease Terminal cirrhosis of the liver Viral hepatitis Leucine and tyrosine frequently found together in patients with liver disease.	*
Tyrosine	*Color:* Black or yellow with presence of bilirubin *Shape:* Highly refractile needles occurring in sheaves or clusters	Acid	Soluble in HCl, NH₄OH, dilute mineral oil Insoluble in acetic acid, alcohol, ether	Severe liver disease and tyrosinosis	*
Cholesterol	*Color:* Transparent *Shape:* Regular to irregular flat plates with one corner notched out; may be single or in large numbers Most often found after refrigeration	Acid Neutral	Soluble in chloroform, ether, hot alcohol Insoluble in alcohol	Excessive tissue breakdown Seen in nephritis and nephrotic syndrome Lipiduria, lipiderma, and lymphatic obstruction due to neoplasms	*

Continued ▲

MICROSCOPIC ANALYSIS

▶ Continued **ABNORMAL CRYSTALS**

TYPE	DESCRIPTION	PH	SOLUBILITY PROPERTIES	CLINICAL SIGNIFICANCE	MICROSCOPIC VIEW
Bilirubin	*Color:* Yellow to brown to reddish *Shape:* Granules or clusters	Acid	Soluble in chloroform, acetone, acid, and alkali Insoluble in alcohol and ether	Obstructive jaundice Bilirubin must be present in urine.	＊
Sulfa	*Color:* Brown to yellow *Shape:* Needle-like shapes seen in bundles or sheaves Stacks of wheat	Acid	Soluble in acetone	Most sulfonamide drugs are more soluble than older types.	＊
Ampicillin	*Color:* Colorless *Shape:* Elongated long thin needles	Acid		Administration of large parenteral doses	◆

＊ Photomicrographs courtesy of Bayer Corporation, Elkhart, IN.
◆ Photomicrograph from Henry JB: Clinical Diagnosis and Management by Laboratory Methods, 19th ed. Philadelphia, WB Saunders, 1996.

MISCELLANEOUS CRYSTALS

TYPE	DESCRIPTION	PH	SOLUBILITY	CLINICAL SIGNIFICANCE	MICROSCOPIC VIEW
Radiographic Media	*Color:* Hypaque, appear dark and thick *Shape:* Pleomorphic needles, single or sheaves	Acid	Soluble in 10% NaOH	Intravenous injection for radiography Can appear up to 3 days after injection SG >1.050	*
Hemosiderin	*Color:* Yellow to brown to red *Shape:* Heavy large granules Prussian blue stain for iron	Acid Alkaline	Insoluble granules	Associated with anemia and destruction of RBC Form of ferritin denaturation Severe hemolytic episode	*

* Photomicrographs courtesy of Bayer Corporation, Elkhart, IN.

MICROORGANISMS AND PARASITES

TYPE	DESCRIPTION	NORMAL VALUES	SIGNIFICANCE	MICROSCOPIC VIEW
Bacteria	*Color:* Colorless *Shape:* Rods or cocci may be found singly or chains	Free of bacteria in kidney and bladder	Can be contamination from external sources Rapidly multiply in improperly stored specimen When collected properly and many WBCs are seen, usually indicative of urinary tract infection	*
Yeast	*Color:* Colorless cells *Shape:* Ovid, smooth cells with doubly refractile walls Often show budding and pseudohyphae Sometimes mistaken for RBCs	Negative	Found in urinary tract infections, especially from diabetic patients Immunosuppressed patient Skin or vaginal contamination *Candida albicans* is most common	*
Spermatozoa	Oval heads with long thin tails	Can be found in both male and female urine	Male: Nocturnal emission, ejaculation, and disease of the genital organs Female: After coitus	*
Trichomonas vaginalis	Turnip shaped flagellates, with three anterior flagella and one posterior flagellum Confused with WBCs Needs to be mobile for identification	Negative	Transmitted sexually, frequently infection of vagina and vulva in females. In males, the organism infects urethra.	*

Continued ▶

▶ Continued **MICROORGANISMS AND PARASITES**

TYPE	DESCRIPTION	NORMAL VALUES	SIGNIFICANCE	MICROSCOPIC VIEW
Enterobius vermicularis (Pinworm)	Ova have one flat and one round side with transparent shell. Developing larvae can be seen.	Negative	Usually found in children and in fecal contamination Female worm lays her eggs in perirectal region, and during collection they can be carried into urine specimen.	*
Schistosoma haematobium	Ovum measures 50–150 µm. Clear and colorless with characteristic terminal spine.	Negative	Inhibits veins in urinary bladder Endemic in Africa, Nile Valley, and Middle East	*

* Photomicrographs courtesy of Bayer Corporation, Elkhart, IN.

MICROSCOPIC ANALYSIS

Artifacts

Foreign objects can find their way into the urine specimen during the collection and transportation of the specimen. They are usually considered a contaminant.

TYPE	DESCRIPTION	SIGNIFICANCE	MICROSCOPIC VIEW
Fibers	Large with distinct edges that are highly refractile Flat and thick at margins Do not mistake for casts	Cloth is most frequent, occurring from clothing, diapers, and toilet paper. Other fibers found as contaminants are vegetable.	*
Hair	Long with refractile edges Tend to be dark and large	Contaminant	
Starch or Talcum Powder	Vary in size, not perfectly round with Y in center When polarized, look like Maltese cross	Frequently found because of gloves worn by health care workers Considered contaminant and not reported out	*

✳ Photomicrographs courtesy of Bayer Corporation, Elkhart, IN.

DISEASES OF THE KIDNEY

Diseases of the kidney are classified into four types: glomerular, which is immunologically mediated; tubular, which involves infections or toxic substances affecting the tubules; interstitial, which involves infections of the upper and lower urinary tract; and vascular, which involves any disruption in the blood supply that will affect renal function.

SUMMARY OF SELECTED RENAL DISEASE

DISEASE	CAUSE	CLINICAL FINDINGS	PHYSICAL FINDINGS	CHEMICAL FINDINGS	MICROSCOPIC FINDINGS
Acute Glomerulonephritis	Anti-basement membrane antibodies associated with streptococcal infection, variety of infectious agents, toxins, allergens Inflammation of glomeruli by which they become abnormally permeable and leak plasma proteins and blood into renal tubules	Rapid appearance of hematuria, proteinuria, and casts Varied degree of hypertension, renal insufficiency, and edema Frequently seen in children and young adults	Gross hematuria, turbid, smoky	Protein <1.0 g/dL Blood positive	Increased RBCs, WBCs, renal tubular epithelial Casts: RBCs, granular, occasionally WBCs and renal
Chronic Glomerulonephritis	Represents end stage result of persistent glomerular damage with continuing and irreversible loss of renal function Progress to end stage renal disease	Symptoms include edema, hypertension, anemia, metabolic acidosis, oliguria progressing to anuria	Hematuria	Protein >2.5 g/dL Blood, small amount SG low and fixed	Increased RBCs, WBCs, renal epithelial Casts: Granular, waxy, broad
Nephrotic Syndrome	Glomeruli whose basement membrane have become highly permeable to plasma proteins of large molecular weight and lipids allowing them to pass in tubules	Massive protein, edema, high levels of serum lipids, and low levels of serum albumin	Cloudy	Protein >3.5 g/dL Blood, small amount	Increased RBCs, oval fat bodies, free fat, renal epithelial, RBCs Casts: Fatty, waxy, renal

Continued ▲

▶ Continued **SUMMARY OF SELECTED RENAL DISEASE**

DISEASE	CAUSE	CLINICAL FINDINGS	PHYSICAL FINDINGS	CHEMICAL FINDINGS	MICROSCOPIC FINDINGS
Acute Tubular Necrosis	Destruction of renal tubular epithelial cells Usually following hypotensive event (shock), toxic element, or drugs and heavy metals	Oliguria and complete renal failure	Slightly cloudy	Protein <1.0 g/dL Blood positive SG low	Increased RBCs, WBCs, renal epithelial Casts: Renal, granular, waxy, broad
Cystinuria or Cystinosis	Inability of renal tubules to reabsorb cystine Inborn error of metabolism of cystine	Intracellular deposition of cystine in tissues	Slightly cloudy	Protein positive	Increased RBCs Cystine crystals
Cystitis (Lower Urinary) **Urethritis (Urethra in Males)**	Infection of bladder most commonly caused by bacterium *E. coli* (85%)	Frequent and painful urination	Cloudy, foul smelling	Protein <0.5 g/dL Blood small amount Nitrite positive (usually) Leukocyte esterase positive (usually)	Increased WBCs, bacteria, RBCs, Transitional epithelial
Acute Pyelonephritis (Upper Urinary)	Infection of kidney or renal pelvis. Caused by infectious organism that has traveled through urinary tract and invaded kidney tissue	More frequent in women with repeated urinary tract infections	Turbid, foul smelling	Protein <1.0 g/dL Blood positive Nitrite positive (usually) Leukocyte esterase positive (usually)	Increased WBCs (clumps), bacteria, renal epithelial Casts: WBCs, granular, renal occasionally waxy
Chronic Pyelonephritis	Permanent scarring of renal tissue	Polyuria and nocturia develop as tubular function is lost. With disease progression there is hypertension and altered renal and glomerular flow.	Cloudy	Protein <2.5 g/dL Nitrite positive (usually) Leukocyte esterase positive (usually) SG low	Increased WBCs Casts: Granular, waxy, broad

BIBLIOGRAPHY

Brunzel NA: Fundamentals of Urine and Body Fluid Analysis. Philadelphia, WB Saunders, 1993.

Focus on Urinalysis. Elkhart, IN, Miles Inc., Diagnostics Division, 1991.

Free H, ed: Modern Urine Chemistry Manual. Elkhart, IN, Miles Inc., Diagnostics Division, 1991.

Graff SL: A Handbook of Routine Urinalysis. Philadelphia, JB Lippincott, 1983.

Harber M: Urine. In McClatchey K, ed: Clinical Laboratory Medicine. Philadelphia, Williams & Wilkins, 1994, pp 513–548.

Henry JB, Launzon RB, Schumann GB: Basic urine examination. In Henry JB, ed: Clinical Diagnosis and Management by Laboratory Methods, 19th ed. Philadelphia, WB Saunders, 1996, pp 411–456.

Hundley J, Fleming J: Urine Analysis Workshop. American Society of Clinical Pathologists, Associate Member Section, 1993.

Strasinger SK: Urinalysis and Body Fluids, 3rd ed. Philadelphia, FA Davis, 1994.

Chapter **34**

ROUTINE ANALYSIS OF BODY FLUIDS

Kathleen Finnegan, MS, MT (ASCP)SH

Q U I C K C O N T E N T S

INTRODUCTION

The examination of body fluids is a very important tool with valuable diagnostic information for various medical conditions. The various fluids vary in formation, function, and complexity. These fluids include cerebrospinal fluid (CSF), synovial or joint fluid, and serous fluids, which include pleural (lung), peritoneal (abdomen), and pericardial (heart). Other miscellaneous body fluids that are examined are amniotic fluid and seminal fluid.

Several general observations are made for all body fluids. Gross examination, cell counts, morphologic examination, and chemical analysis are usually done. There are many specialized tests for each fluid. All fluids should be analyzed immediately and should be handled with extreme care.

SUMMARY OF BODY FLUID COLLECTION

FLUID	SOURCE	PATIENT PREPARATION	SPECIMEN COLLECTION	AMOUNT REMOVED (mL)	SPECIMEN PREPARATION	SPECIMEN STORAGE
Cerebrospinal	Brain and spinal cord	Local anesthetic; thoroughly clean area.	Spinal tap: lumbar puncture in third or fourth lumbar interspace	1–2	Four labeled sterile collection tubes: Tube 1: chemical Tube 2: microbial Tube 3: cell counts Tube 4: cytologic studies	Perform examination as soon as possible. Delays can cause cells to lyse, chemical composition to change, and growth in microbial organisms to increase.
Synovial	Joint	If possible, patient should fast for 6–8 hr. Blood specimen should be collected at same time.	Arthrocentesis	3–10	Three labeled sterile tubes: Tube 1: microbiology Tube 2: heparinized cell counts Tube 3: Plain red chemistry	Perform examination as soon as possible. Delays causes cells to lyse, chemical composition to change, and growth in microbial organisms to increase.
Pleural	Thoracic cavity (around lung)	Invasive surgical procedure. Serum samples should be drawn for chemical comparison.	Thoracentesis	Cell count: 5–8 Cytology: 25–50 Chemical: 3–10 Microbiology: 10–20	EDTA tube: cell count and differential Heparin: cytology and microbiology Plain red: chemistry	Transported as soon as possible
Peritoneal	Abdomen	Invasive surgical procedure. Serum samples should be drawn for chemical comparison.	Peritoneocentesis	Same as pleural	Same as pleural	Same as pleural
Pericardial	Around heart	Invasive surgical procedure. Serum samples should be drawn for chemical comparison.	Pericardiocentesis	Same as pleural	Same as pleural	Same as pleural

Continued ▲

▶ Continued **SUMMARY OF BODY FLUID COLLECTION**

FLUID	SOURCE	PATIENT PREPARATION	SPECIMEN COLLECTION	AMOUNT REMOVED (mL)	SPECIMEN PREPARATION	SPECIMEN STORAGE
Amniotic	In membranous sac surrounding fetus	Needle aspiration into sac, transabdominal.	Amniocentesis	10–20	Carefully transferred to sterile plastic containers as soon as possible. Culture and chromosome analysis must be at body or room temperature and done immediately Phospholipid analysis on ice.	For chemical analysis only should be centrifuged and frozen if not examined within 24 hr For bilirubin protect from light
Seminal	Secretions from testes and seminal vesicles	Sexual abstinence for at least 48 hr. Use of condoms is not recommended.	Masturbation: entire ejaculate is collected into sterile container at room temperature. Plastic containers not recommended.	2–5	Specimen must be received within 1 hr of collection. Avoid extreme temperatures. Only complete collections are acceptable for analysis. Analysis should be done within 4 hr and after liquefaction	Fresh specimen is clotted and should liquefy within 30 min of collection. Specimens awaiting motility should be kept at 37°C.

CEREBROSPINAL FLUID

The CSF provides nutrients and the removal of metabolic wastes from the nervous system. It also provides the brain and spinal cord with a cushion and lubrication against injury. CSF fluid is produced at a rate of 21 mL/hr. The total volume of CSF is 140 to 170 mL in adults and 10 to 60 mL in neonates. Formation of CSF is by ultrafiltration under hydrostatic pressure. CSF is present in the space between the arachnoid and the pia mater. The passage of substances into the CSF from the blood is regulated by the blood-brain barrier. This blood-brain barrier accounts for the filtration of blood components to the CSF.

The routine examination of CSF includes appearance, cell count, differential, chemical analysis, and Gram stain. Examination should be performed immediately (within 1 hour of collection) before deterioration takes place. Collection tubes analysis order is as follows: tube 1 for chemical and serologic analysis, tube 2 for microbiologic studies, tube 3 for cell counting, tube 4 for cytologic studies. Differentiating a traumatic collection from a intracranial hemorrhage is a very important step in CSF analysis.

Characteristics of Cerebrospinal Fluid

CSF	NORMAL	ABNORMAL	CAUSE AND CLINICAL IMPLICATIONS	IMPORTANT INFORMATION
Appearance	Clear and colorless	Cloudy	>200 WBC/μL: infection >400 RBC/μL: hemorrhage or traumatic tap Microorganisms: meningitis Very high protein	Appearance is graded 0 for clear to 4+ for turbid. Gross blood source needs to be differentiated between traumatic tap or intracranial hemorrhage:
		Oily	Radiographic contrast media	
		Bloody	>600 RBC/μL: hemorrhage or traumatic tap	
		Xanthrochromic	Color of supernant of centrifuged CSF	Traumatic tap: uneven distribution of blood with decreasing amount of blood from tube 1 to tube 3 with clot formation
		Yellow	Jaundice, elevated bilirubin	
		Brown	Methemoglobin	
		Pink	Oxyhemoglobin	
		Orange	Carotene	
		Clotted	Increased fibrinogen Seen with traumatic tap and not subarachnoid hemorrhage	Hemorrhage: blood evenly in all tubes with no clot formation

Continued ▶

▶ Continued **Characteristics of Cerebrospinal Fluid**

CSF	NORMAL	ABNORMAL	CAUSE AND CLINICAL IMPLICATIONS	IMPORTANT INFORMATION

Cell Count	WBC adult: $<5/\mu L$
	WBC neonate:
	  $0–30/\mu L$
	RBC adult: 0
	RBC neonate: variable
		WBC adult: $>1000/\mu L$
		WBC neonate:
		  $>100/\mu L$
		RBC: $>400/\mu L$
			Bacterial or fungal meningitis
			Viral meningitis
			Hemorrhage or traumatic tap
				WBCs lyse within 1 hr. When doing counts the fluid should be well mixed and used undiluted. If overcrowded, dilute. To enhance WBCs, glacial acetic acid with crystal violet can be used. Hemacytometer count: no. of cells counted × dilution Divided by no. of squares counted × volume of square

Differential	**Adults:**
	  Lymph: 60%
	  Monocyte: 30%
	  Neutrophil: 2%
	
	Neonate:
	  Lymph: 20%
	  Monocyte: 70%
	  Neutrophil: 4%
		Increased neutrophils	Bacterial meningitis, mycotic meningitis, early tuberculosis hemorrhage, cerebral abscess, tumors	To perform differential count specimen should be concentrated by use of cytospin technique. Smear should be prepared and stained with Wright's stain.
				
				Never do differential count from chamber count.

		Increased lymphocytes	Viral meningitis, tuberculosis meningitis, multiple sclerosis, leukemia, lymphoma, drug abuse, Guillain-Barré syndrome, chronic alcoholism	
		Increased monocytes	Chronic bacterial meningitis, partial treatment of meningitis, tumors	
		Macrophages	Tuberculosis and fungal meningitis, blood contamination, and after hemorrhage	
		Eosinophil	Parasitic and fungal meningitis, allergic reactions to shunts, medications, and dyes	
		Tumor cells	Metastatic carcinoma	
		Ependymal or choroid cells	Lining cells usually seen clumps, sometimes from trauma or spinal tap	

CEREBROSPINAL FLUID

Continued ▶

▶ Continued **Characteristics of Cerebrospinal Fluid**

CSF	NORMAL	ABNORMAL	CAUSE AND CLINICAL IMPLICATIONS	IMPORTANT INFORMATION
Chemical Analysis	**Protein:** 15–45 mg/dL	Can be increased or decreased	*Increased:* bacterial or viral meningitis, cerebral hemorrhage, trauma, contamination with peripheral blood, decreased absorption due to an obstruction, and increased synthesis of immunoglobins *Decreased:* increased reabsorption with increased intercranial pressure or a loss of fluid due to trauma	CSF total protein is to determine integrity of blood-brain barrier.
	Glucose: 50–80 mg/dL	Can be increased or decreased	*Increased:* hyperglycemia, traumatic puncture, peripheral blood contamination *Decreased:* hypoglycemia, meningitis, inflammation, and tumors	Blood for glucose determination should be drawn 30–60 min preceding lumbar puncture.

Clinical Considerations

Indications for a spinal puncture include the diagnosis of meningitis (bacterial, viral, fungal), a intercranial hemorrhage, neurologic disorder, or malignancy.

Increase in neutrophils indicate an acute bacterial infection. Lymphocytes and monocytes occur in viral infections, fungal infections, and multiple sclerosis. Plasma cells indicate a humoral response to foreign antigens. Occasionally eosinophils are seen, and this indicates a parasitic infestation.

Malignant cells can be found in spinal fluids. Most common sites to metastasize to the brain are breast, lung, and gastric carcinoma. Acute lymphoblastic leukemia has a high rate of involvement to the central nervous system. Large cell lymphoma also can involve the central nervous system.

Cerebrospinal Fluid Findings in Meningitis

MENINGITIS	CELL COUNT (μL)	CELL TYPE	PROTEIN (mg/dL)	GLUCOSE (mg/dL)	OTHER TESTS	MICROSCOPIC VIEW
Normal CSF	<5 0	WBC mononuclear RBC	15–45	50–80		*
Acute bacterial	1,000–10,000	Neutrophils	100–500	<40	Gram stain	*
Viral	5–300 Some 1000	Lymphocytes	<100	Normal	Normal lactate	*

Continued ▲

CEREBROSPINAL FLUID

▶ Continued **Cerebrospinal Fluid Findings in Meningitis**

MENINGITIS	CELL COUNT (μL)	CELL TYPE	PROTEIN (mg/dL)	GLUCOSE (mg/dL)	OTHER TESTS	MICROSCOPIC VIEW
Fungal	40–400	Lymphocytes, mono-cytes	50–300	Normal to decreased	India ink	
Tuberculous	100–600	Neutrophils early fol-lowed by lympho-cytes	50–300	Decreased <45	Pellicle formation	

＊ Photomicrographs from Rodak BF: Diagnostic Hematology. Philadelphia, WB Saunders, 1995.

SYNOVIAL FLUID

Synovial or joint fluid, which consists of a very viscous fluid, supplies nutrients to the cartilage and also acts as a lubricant to the joint. Synovial membranes line the joints, bursae, and tendon sheaths. This fluid is an ultrafiltrate that has essentially the same chemical composition as plasma. It also contains a mucopolysaccharide called *hyaluronic acid* that is responsible for the viscosity of the fluid and lubricates the joints. Hyaluronate is secreted by the synovial fluid cells that line the joint cavity. Synovial fluid is formed in all joints and contain only a small amount of fluid.

Characteristics of Synovial Fluid

SYNOVIAL FLUID	NORMAL	ABNORMAL	CAUSE AND CLINICAL IMPLICATIONS	IMPORTANT INFORMATION
Appearance	Transparent, clear to pale yellow	Cloudy	Increase in cellular or protein components	Uneven distribution of blood can indicate traumatic tap. Dark red or dark brown supernate is evidence of joint bleeding.
		Dark yellow	Presence of inflammation	
		Dark red	Traumatic tap or bleeding into joints	
Viscosity	Viscous because of high concentration of hyaluronate Will stretch to a string of 1–2 in.	Watery consistency or low viscosity Hyaluronate is degraded	Associated with inflammation	Estimate of viscosity can be made by watching fluid string by suspending drop of fluid from syringe needle. Mucin clot test is used to estimate degree of hyaluronic acid. Quality of clot is rated as good, fair, or poor.
Cell Count	WBC/μL = <150–200 RBC/μL = 0–2000	WBC 200–2000 WBC 2000–15,000 WBC 15,000–100,000 WBC 10,000–30,000 WBC 5000	Type I Noninflammatory Type II Inflammatory Type III Septic Type IV Crystal induced Type V Hemorrhagic	Perform chamber count. When diluting use normal saline. WBC diluting fluids contain acetic acid, which precipitates hyaluronic acid
Differential	<25%neutrophils; 60%monocytes, lymphocytes, macrophages	Reiter cells (vacuolated macrophages) Ragocyte (neutrophils with precipitated rheumatic factor) LE cells	Increased neutrophils indicate septic condition Predominance of lymphocytes suggests nonseptic inflammation	Cytocentrifuged preparations Performed on Wright stained concentrated specimen

SYNOVIAL FLUID

Continued ▶

▶ Continued **Characteristics of Synovial Fluid**

SYNOVIAL FLUID	NORMAL	ABNORMAL	CAUSE AND CLINICAL IMPLICATIONS	IMPORTANT INFORMATION
Chemical Analysis	Glucose 10 mg/dL lower than blood level	Glucose significantly decreased	Infection of joint	Serum glucose should be obtained at same time for result to be valid
	Protein 1–3 g/dL	Protein increased	Gout, infectious arthritis, rheumatoid arthritis	
Microbiologic Examination	None	Bacterial Fungi Mycobacteria Virus	Septic Infection	Incidence: First: staphylococcal Second: gram negative Third: gonococcal
Crystal Identification	None	See table "Crystal Identification"	See table "Crystal Identification"	Ordinary bright field and polarized light

Clinical Considerations

Synovial fluid is present in small amounts. Any increase in fluid enough to aspirate indicates a disease process. Pathologic synovial fluids are classified by the chemical and physical changes that occur in the joint in a disease process. They have been grouped into five types. The results of various laboratory tests associated with each group are shown in the chart on the facing page.

Classification of Synovial Fluid Joint Disorders

TYPES	CAUSE	VOLUME (mL)	APPEARANCE	VISCOSITY	CELL COUNT	GLUCOSE	PROTEIN	OTHER
Noninflammatory Type I	Degenerative joint disorder	>3.5	Clear Yellow	Good	2000–5000/μL Neutrophils: <30%	Normal	Normal	No clotting
Inflammatory Type II	Immunologic including rheumatoid and lupus	>3.5	Cloudy Yellow	Poor Hyaluronidase breaks down	2000–50,000/μL Neutrophils: >50%	Decreased	5–7 g/dL May include fibrinogen	May contain antibodies and autoantibodies
Septic Type III	Microbial infection: *Staphylococcus aureus, Haemophilus influenzae, Neisseria,* beta hemolytic streptococcus, pneumococci	>3.5	Cloudy Yellow-green	Poor	10,000–200,000/μL Neutrophils: >90%	Decreased	5–7 g/dL May include fibrinogen	Positive culture and Gram stain
Crystal Induced Type IV	Gout, pseudogout	>3.5	Cloudy Milky	Poor	500–50,000/μL Neutrophils: <90%	Decreased	5–7 g/dL	Monosodium urate Calcium pyrophosphate
Hemorrhagic Type V	Traumatic injury, coagulation deficiencies, anticoagulant therapy	>3.5	Cloudy Red-brown	Poor	<5000/μL Neutrophils: <50%	Normal	5–7 g/dL	Red blood cells present

SYNOVIAL FLUID

Crystal Identification

Microscopic examination of synovial fluid for crystals is performed with a wet mount, unstained sediment using both direct and compensated polarized light for better identification. Birefringent crystals have the ability to split light into two different rays. The ray of low frequency light appears yellow when compensated, and high frequency light appears blue. A crystal is strongly birefringent when the light appears to be bright.

A small amount of heparin should be used when identifying crystals. Ethylenediaminetetraacetic acid (EDTA) and calcium oxalate (anticoagulants) can be confused with other crystals. This examination should be done as soon as possible because temperature and pH can affect crystal formation and solubility. Always correlate laboratory findings with clinical history to interpret the findings properly.

Crystal Identification

TYPE	DESCRIPTION	SHAPE	OPTICAL CHARACTERISTICS	CLINICAL CONDITION	MICROSCOPIC VIEW
Monosodium Urate (MSU)	Fine needles, with pointed ends appearing extracellularly and within the cytoplasm of neutrophils	Needle	Strong negative birefringence Red compensator: yellow parallel to axis, blue when perpendicular	Gout, arthritis	◆
Calcium Pyrophosphate (CPPD)	Small rod-like needles with blunt ends that are seen as intracellular inclusions	Rhomboid	Weak positive birefringence Red compensator: blue parallel to axis, yellow when perpendicular	Pseudogout	✳
Cholesterol	Large flat plates with notched corners, found extracellularly	Square plates	Strong birefringence but varies with thickness of crystal	Chronic arthritis Rheumatoid arthritis	◆

Continued ▲

SYNOVIAL FLUID

▶ Continued **Crystal Identification**

TYPE	DESCRIPTION	SHAPE	OPTICAL CHARACTERISTICS	CLINICAL CONDITION	MICROSCOPIC VIEW
Hydroxyapatite (HA)	Extremely small needle-like; require electron microscopy to be seen	Globular or small needle	Are not birefringent	Apatite Degenerative joint disease	
Corticosteroid	Rectangular needles with ragged edges. May be found after intra-articular steroid injection	Needle	Negative birefringence	Intra-articular injection	

* Photomicrographs from Henry JB: Clinical Diagnosis and Management by Laboratory Methods, 19th ed. Philadelphia, WB Saunders, 1996.
◆ Photomicrographs from Kjeldsberg CR, Knight JA: Body Fluids: Laboratory Examination of Amniotic Cerebrospinal, Seminal, Serous, and Synovial Fluids, 3rd ed. Chicago, American Society of Clinical Pathologists, 1993.

SEROUS FLUID

Serous fluids include pleural (thoracic fluid), pericardial (chest fluid), and peritoneal (ascitic fluid). These are fluids that are contained within the closed cavities of the body. The word *serous* is defined as having the same characteristics as serum.

These cavities are lined by a thin membrane that covers both the body wall and organs. A small amount of fluid fills the space, lubricates the surfaces of these membranes, and cushions the organs. The formation of these fluids depends on capillary hydrostatic pressure, plasma osmotic pressure, and capillary permeability. These fluids are ultrafiltrates of plasma. They are continuously formed and reabsorbed. Normally the rate of fluid formation equals that of the rate of reabsorption, with a constant amount of fluid surrounding the sacs. Their volume is very small; any increase in or accumulation of the volume of these fluids is termed an *effusion*. An increase in serous fluid (effusion) can occur in many conditions. It must be determined if the effusion is a transudate or a exudate. A transudate is a result of a systemic disease, and an exudate is the result of conditions that directly affect the membrane linings, including inflammation or malignancies.

SEROUS FLUID

Characteristics of Transudate and Exudate

DESCRIPTION	TRANSUDATE	EXUDATE
Cause	Congestive heart failure Liver cirrhosis Portal hypertension Mechanical blockage Nephrotic syndrome	Tuberculosis Decreased lymphocyte drainage Tumor Malignancy Inflammation Infection
Appearance	Color: pale yellow Turbidity: clear	Color: yellow (inflammation), red (hemorrhage), brown (bilirubin) Turbidity; vicious, cloudy
Specific Gravity	<1.015	>1.015
Protein (g/dL)	<3.0	>3.0
Fluid Protein/Serum Protein (F/S)	<0.5	>0.5
Glucose (mg/dL)	Equal to serum levels	Less than or equal to serum level
Lactic Dehydrogenase (LD) (IU/L)	<200	>200
Fluid LD/Serum LD	<0.6	>0.6
Fibrinogen	No clots	Clots
Cell Count	300–1000/μL	>1000/μL
Differential	Mononuclear predominate <25% neutrophils	>25% neutrophils

Pleural Fluid

The pleural cavity is formed by the visceral pleural membrane and the parietal membrane. Pleural fluid surrounds the lungs and lines the walls of the thoracic cavity. This fluid functions as a lubricant for the movement of the lungs. Pleural effusion can be caused by congestive heart failure, hepatic cirrhosis, infections, tuberculosis, malignancy, and pulmonary infarct.

Pericardial Fluid

The pericardial cavity is formed by two thin membranes that surround the heart. The pericardial fluid allows the heart to move easily during contraction and relaxation. Accumulation of fluid in the pericardial cavity is most frequently caused by damage to the lining of the cavity with an increase in capillary permeability. Pericardial effusions can be caused by inflammation, malignancy, bacterial pericarditis, myocardial infarct, trauma, or hemorrhage.

Peritoneal Fluid

Peritoneum is a serous membrane that covers the walls and viscera of the abdomen and pelvis area. Accumulation of fluid in the peritoneal cavity is also referred to as *ascitic fluid*. A patient with a peritoneal effusion is said to have ascites. Peritoneal effusion can be caused by congestive heart failure, hepatic cirrhosis, infections (primary bacterial peritonitis), malignancy, trauma, or a ruptured gallbladder.

Peritoneal lavage is a procedure useful for the diagnosis of intra-abdominal bleeding from trauma or a ruptured organ. Peritoneal dialysis is a treatment for renal failure or renal disease. Dialysis fluids are examined for evidence of infection.

SEROUS FLUID

Characteristics of Serous Fluid

DESCRIPTION	TOTAL VOLUME (mL)	APPEARANCE	CELL COUNT	DIFFERENTIAL
Pleural	10	*Normal:* Clear to pale yellow *Abnormal:* Turbid: the presence of WBCs, indication of infection Bloody: the presence of RBCs, indication of a hemothorax or traumatic injury or malignancy Milky: the presence of chylous indication of thoracic duct rupture	*Normal:* WBC <1000/μL RBC <10,000/μL *Abnormal:* WBC >1000/μL RBC >10,000/μL	*Normal:* lymphocytes, mesothelial cells, macrophages *Abnormal:* Increased neutrophils: bacterial infection, pneumonia Increased lymphocytes: tubercular effusions, malignancy, and viral pneumonia Increased eosinophils: pneumothorax, parasites, and Hodgkin's disease
Pericardial	10–50	*Normal:* Clear to pale yellow *Abnormal:* Turbid: increased WBCs, indication of infection or malignancy Bloody: myocardial infarct, aneurysm, trauma, or pericarditis Milky: lymphatic drainage	*Normal:* WBC <1000/μL RBC <10,000/μL *Abnormal:* WBC >1000/μL RBC >10,000/μL	*Normal:* lymphocytes, mesothelial cells, macrophages *Abnormal:* Increased neutrophils: bacterial endocarditis, malignancy Increased lymphocytes: tuberculosis, lymphoproliferative disorders, viral pericarditis Increased eosinophils: eosinophilic gastroenteritis
Peritoneal	50	*Normal:* Clear to pale yellow *Abnormal:* Turbid: increased WBCs, indication of infection or malignancy Bloody: trauma, hemorrhage Milky: chylous fluid Green: bile	*Normal:* WBC <500/μL RBC <10,000/μL *Abnormal:* WBC >500/μL RBC >10,000/μL	*Normal:* lymphocytes, mesothelial cells, macrophages *Abnormal:* Increased neutrophils: peritonitis

CHEMICAL ANALYSIS	SEROLOGIC TESTING	MICROBIOLOGIC EXAMINATION	MICROSCOPIC VIEW
Glucose: 　Normal: parallels serum level 　Decreased glucose: tuberculosis, malignancy, rheumatoid inflammation *pH:* 　Normal: 7.4 < 6.0 indicates esophageal rupture 　>7.4 indicates malignancies *Amylase:* 　Elevated levels are associated with pancreatic disorders.	CEA: elevated in malignancy	Gram stain Aerobic and anaerobic cultures Acid fast stain	 ＊
Glucose: 　Normal: parallels serum level 　Decreased glucose: bacterial infections and malignancy *pH:* 　<7.1: rheumatic conditions 　7.2–7.4: malignancy, uremia tuberculosis *Adenosine deaminase:* 　Useful for tuberculosis pericarditis	CEA: elevated in malignancy	Gram stain Aerobic and anaerobic cultures Acid fast stain	
Glucose: 　Decreased in tubercular peritonitis, malignancy *Amylase:* 　Increased in pancreatitis, GI perforation *Alkaline Phosphatase:* 　Increased in intestinal perforation	CEA: elevated in malignancy	Gram stain Aerobic and anaerobic cultures Acid fast stain	 ＊

＊ Photomicrographs from Rodak BF: Diagnostic Hematology. Philadelphia, WB Saunders, 1995.

SEROUS FLUID

SEMINAL FLUID

Seminal fluid is routinely analyzed to evaluate cases of infertility or to follow up a post-vasectomy procedure. Other applications for analysis include forensic studies. Seminal fluid, which is also called *semen,* is a body fluid that furnishes fructose and other nutrients to maintain spermatozoa and to transports spermatozoa to the female cervical mucus.

Seminal fluid is composed of secretions from the testes, the epididymis, the seminal vesicles, and the prostate gland. Spermatozoa are produced in the testes and mature in the epididymis. Spermatozoa account for a small amount of the total volume of the fluid.

Specimen collection is very important for analysis. The patient should receive explicit instructions. A 3-day period of abstinence is recommended. A condom with spermicidal agents should not be used. The specimen should be kept at room temperature and should be examined within 4 hours. Liquefaction must be complete before testing.

Characteristics of Seminal Fluid

DESCRIPTION	NORMAL	ABNORMAL	CAUSE AND CLINICAL SIGNIFICANCE	IMPORTANT INFORMATION
Appearance	Gray to white Opalescent	Brown to red	Presence of blood	Color of semen may also be altered by length of abstinence
		Yellow	Certain drugs	
		Turbid	Increased leukocytes	Shorter more transparent
		Clear	Low concentration of sperm	Longer more yellow
Coagulation / Liquefaction	Immediately after ejaculation Within 10–30 min	>60 min	May contain mucus	Time when specimen was collected
Volume	2–5 mL	<2 or >5 mL	Infertility	Sometimes varies with how often patient has had relations
Viscosity	Pours in droplets	String or thread-like	Increased viscosity will interfere with sperm mobility to be able to fertilize ovum	Rated from 0 (watery) to 4 (gel-like)
pH	7.2–7.8	<7.2	Abnormalities of vas deferens, epididymis, or seminal vesicles	Specimens not tested within 1 hr have pH changes
		>7.8	Infection	
Sperm Count	20–250 million/mL	<20 million/mL	Infertility	Manual count using hemacytometer with 1:20 dilution with diluent (saline)
Motility	1 hr after collection >50% show moderate to strong forward motion	<50% after 2 hr	If motility is poor, sperm will not travel through fallopian tubes to reach ovum	Rated on scale 0–4 on their forward motion, 4 being strong and forward progression, 0 no movement
Viability	>65% do not take up stain and are alive	Percentage of dead sperm cells exceeds percentage of immobile sperm cells	Dead sperm have damaged plasma membranes. Evaluated along with motility to decide if sperm are dead or have structural abnormalities.	Eosin or eosin-nigrosin stain is used. Only dead sperm pick up stain.

SEMINAL FLUID

Continued ▶

► Continued **Characteristics of Seminal Fluid**

DESCRIPTION	NORMAL	ABNORMAL	CAUSE AND CLINICAL SIGNIFICANCE	IMPORTANT INFORMATION
Morphology	Normal forms: >70% Immature forms: <4%	>30% abnormal forms	Abnormal head, mid-section, or tail can account for sper-matozoa not being able to penetrate ovum.	Stained specimen exam-ined under oil immer-sion Classified into six cate-gories: normal, pin head, large head, ta-pering head, double head, and amorphous forms
Leukocyte Count	0–2000/mL	Increased white cells	Infection	Seminal fluid should be free of red blood cells and bacteria
Fructose	150–600 mg/dL	Decreased level	Azoospermia (ab-sence of sperm) Obstruction of ejacu-latory duct	Chemical test based on development of or-ange-red color pro-duced in presence of fructose

AMNIOTIC FLUID

Amniotic fluid is found in the membranous sac called the *amnion* that surrounds the em-bryo or fetus. The fluid is formed from the metabolism of fetal cells. Amniotic fluid has several functions that include the protection of the fetus, allowing fetal movement and growth, maintaining an even temperature, and the participation in fetal biochemical homeostasis. Indications for the analysis of amniotic fluid are for chromosomal abnor-mality, metabolic disorder, or neural tube defect at the 16th week of gestation, isoimmu-nization between the 20th and 28th week, fetal lung maturity between the 34th and 42nd week, and chorioamnionitis between the 34th and 42nd week of gestation.

Characteristics of Amniotic Fluid

DESCRIPTION	NORMAL	ABNORMAL	CAUSE AND CLINICAL SIGNIFICANCE
Appearance	Colorless to pale yellow	Yellow	Erythroblastosis
		Green (meconium)	Fetal hypoxia
		Red-brown	Fetal death
		Amber	Presence of bilirubin
		Pink-red	Blood contamination
Volume	Increases steadily throughout pregnancy	Hydramnios	Abnormal increase associated with congenital fetal malformations
	Maximal volume 1100–1500 mL at 36 weeks' gestation	Oligohydramnios	Decrease in fluid associated with ruptured membranes and congenital malformation
Microscopic Analysis	Fetal squamous cells: originate from fetal skin, oral mucosa, and vagina		Diagnosis of ruptured membranes Fetal maturity
	Amnion epithelial cells: originate from lining of sac	Nucleus containing X chromatin mass	Sex prenatally
		Long bipolar cells, cells with multiple filamentous pseudopodia, and large vacuolated cells with inclusions	Neural tube defect
Chemical Analysis			
Bilirubin	28 wk <0.075 mg/dL 40 wk <0.025 mg/dL	28 wk >0.075 40 wk >0.025	Erythroblastosis Hepatitis Infection (maternal) Sickle cell crisis
Lecithin/Sphingomyelin (L/S) Ratio	Mature >2.0 Mature, diabetic mother >3.5	Transitional 1.5–1.9 Immature <1.5	Respiratory distress syndrome
(SPC) Saturated Phosphatidylcholine	>500 μg/L Diabetic mother 1000 μg/L	<500 μg/L	Respiratory distress syndrome
Alpha-Fetoprotein	<2.5 MoM (MoM = multiples of median)	>2.5 MoM	Open spine defects and anencephaly
Creatinine	>2.0 mg/dL after 37th wk	>2.0 mg/dL	Indicates fetal maturity when mother's creatinine levels are normal and fetus's levels are >2.0 mg/dL

AMNIOTIC FLUID

BIBLIOGRAPHY

Brunzel NA: Fundamentals of Urine and Body Fluid Analysis. Philadelphia, WB Saunders, 1993, pp 331–412.

Cavagnaro MJ: An Introduction to Body Fluids Analysis—Basic Techniques and Cellular Morphology Workshop. American Society of Clinical Pathologists, Associate Member Section, 1996.

Collins L: Body fluids—cerebrospinal, serous, synovial fluid. In Rodak B, ed: Diagnostic Hematology, Philadelphia, WB Saunders, 1995, pp 633–648.

Cornbleet J, Sherwood N, Judkins S: Microscopy of CSF and Body Fluids Workshop, American Society of Clinical Pathologists, Associate Member Section, 1992.

Glass L: Extravascular biological fluids. In Kaplan LA, Pesce AJ, eds: Clinical Chemistry: Theory, Analysis and Correlation. St. Louis, CV Mosby, 1995.

Kjeldsberg CR, Knight JA: Body Fluids: Laboratory Examination of Amniotic, Cerebrospinal, Seminal, Serous and Synovial Fluids, 3rd ed. Chicago, American Society of Clinical Pathologists Press, 1993.

Nanji A: Body Fluids. In Howanitz J, ed: Laboratory Medicine Test Selection and Interpretation. New York, Churchill Livingstone, 1991, pp 107–126.

Smith G, Kjeldsberg CR: Cerebrospinal, synovial, and serous fluids. In Henry JB, ed: Clinical Diagnosis and Management by Laboratory Methods, 19th ed. Philadelphia, WB Saunders, 1996, pp 457–482.

Strasinger SK: Urinalysis and Body Fluids, 3rd ed. Philadelphia, FA Davis, 1994, pp 135–186.

Tietz NW: Clinical Guide to Laboratory Tests, 3rd ed. Philadelphia, WB Saunders, 1995.

Theil KS: Body Fluid Analysis. In McClatchey K, ed: Clinical Laboratory Medicine. Philadelphia, Williams & Wilkins, 1994, pp 549–570.

Section VI

HEMATOLOGY

Chapter **35**

HEMATOPOIESIS

Kathleen Finnegan, MS, MT(ASCP)SH

Q U I C K   C O N T E N T S

INTRODUCTION

Hematology is the study of blood and its formed elements. It includes the study of the concentration, structure, and function of erythrocytes, or red blood cells (RBCs); leukocytes, or white blood cells (WBCs); and thrombocytes, or platelets.

The normal adult has approximately 6 L of fluid per kg of body wt. The plasma portion encompasses 55% of the total blood volume, and the formed elements compose about 45% of the total blood volume. The erythrocytes account for about 44% of the total blood volume, and the leukocytes and thrombocytes account for 1% per kg of body wt.

The RBCs contain the protein hemoglobin the function of which is to transport oxygen and carbon dioxide to and from all body tissues. The WBCs defend against bacteria, viruses, and foreign antigens. The thrombocytes' main function is hemostasis or the initiation of the coagulation process.

Variation in the concentration of the blood elements occurs according to age, sex, geographic location, disease, or tissue injury.

HEMATOPOIESIS

Hematopoiesis is defined as the cellular formation, proliferation, differentiation, and maturation of blood cells. The hematopoietic system includes tissues and organs involved in this proliferation, maturation, and the destruction of blood cells. These include the spleen, lymph nodes, thymus, bone marrow, liver, and reticuloendothelial system (RES). Cellular proliferation, differentiation, and maturation take place primarily in the bone marrow. Normally only the mature cells are released into the peripheral blood.

Hematopoiesis has been divided into three phases of blood cell production: the mesoblastic, hepatic, and myeloid stages.

Stages of Hematopoiesis

MESOBLASTIC. Hematopoiesis begins as early as the 19th day of gestation in the blood islands of the yolk sac of the human embryo. These blood islands remain active for 8 to 12 weeks. Most hematopoietic activity is confined to erythropoiesis. These early cells are megaloblastic (large) in morphologic appearance. Early hemoglobin production is limited to embryonic varieties called Portland, Gower-1, and Gower-2.

HEPATIC. By the 3rd month the yolk sac discontinues its role and the fetal liver becomes active. Both erythrocytes and granulocytes are in production. By the end of the 4th month the primitive cells are disappearing, with an increase in the more definitive erythroblasts, granulocytes, monocytes, lymphocytes, and megakaryocytes. Hemoglobin production consists of hemoglobins F, A, and A_2. Also active in hematopoiesis are the spleen, thymus, and lymph nodes.

MYELOID. Between the 5th and 6th month of gestation the bone marrow becomes the primary site of hematopoiesis. At birth the bone marrow is the primary source of blood cell production. There are various stages of cell maturation of all cell lines. Hematopoiesis occurs in most bones but primarily in the flat bones of the sternum, ribs, vertebrae, skull, and pelvis. In the adult the principal source of production is the sternum and other flat bones.

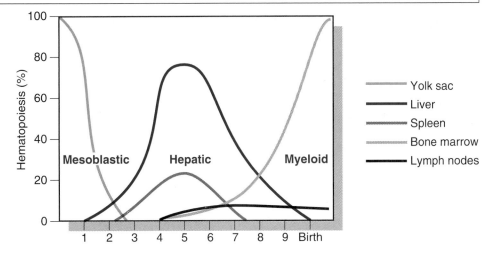

Origin of Marrow Cells

The bone marrow contains a hematopoietic, or pluripotential, stem cell. These stem cells appear morphologically indistinct. They have the capacity to differentiate, proliferate, and renew into the mature blood cell. Under the influence of certain stimuli called *cytokines*, the pluripotential stem cell becomes a committed cell that undergoes cellular division and differentiation. When a stem cell divides, one daughter cell reverts to the stage of stem cell and the other daughter cell becomes a colony forming unit (CFU). This CFU can be stimulated by *erythropoietin*, a glycoprotein produced by the kidney for RBC production; *leukopoietin* for WBC production; and *thrombopoietin*, a glycoprotein also produced by the kidney for thrombocyte production. Other protein molecules or cytokines that stimulate cell lines to proliferate and differentiate are collectively called the *interleukins*. Cytokines are low molecular weight glycoproteins that are signaling molecules that stimulate hematopoiesis, regulate lymphocyte production, and mediate natural immunity. These cytokines include the interleukins (ILs), interferons (IFs), and colony stimulating factors (CSFs; [G-CSF] granulocyte-colony stimulating factor, [GM-CSF] granulocyte-monocyte colony stimulating factor, [M-CSF] monocyte colony stimulating factor).

HEMATOPOIESIS

Scheme for Hematopoiesis

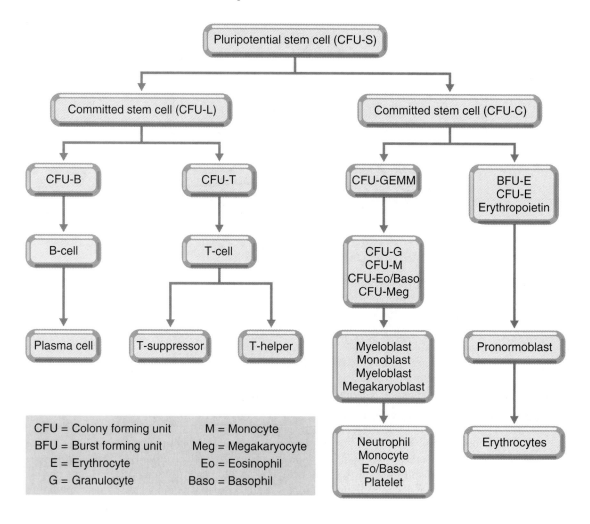

CFU = Colony forming unit   M = Monocyte
BFU = Burst forming unit   Meg = Megakaryocyte
E = Erythrocyte   Eo = Eosinophil
G = Granulocyte   Baso = Basophil

BONE MARROW

Myeloid to Erythroid Ratio

The myeloid to erythroid (M:E) ratio is a numeric expression comparing the relative number of granulocytic precursors, which include the neutrophil, eosinophil, and basophil, with the relative number of erythroid precursors in the bone marrow. This ratio is obtained by counting a minimal number of 200 cells at 100× magnification. The normal M:E ratio in adults ranges from 2:1 to 4:1. Examples of various M:E ratios are infection, 6:1; and leukemia, 25:1. The bone marrow aspirate evaluates the M:E ratio.

Bone Marrow Cellularity

The bone marrow cellularity is the percentage of marrow space occupied by hematopoietic cells compared with fat. A normocellular marrow for a mature adult is 10% to 50% fat, 40% to 60% hematopoietic elements. A child under 2 years of age has 100% red marrow, which is active in hematopoiesis. The bone marrow biopsy evaluates cellular production under low power magnification. In the bone marrow biopsy the placement of cells is preserved. Bone marrow cellularity is age dependent.

TERMS ASSOCIATED WITH THE BONE MARROW

Hypercellular or *hyperplasia* refers to an increase in one or more cell lines usually due to compensation.

Hypocellular or *hypoplasia* refers to a loss of cellularity or incomplete development in one or more cell lines.

Hematopoietic Cell Distribution

CELL TYPE	PERCENTAGE BONE MARROW, ADULT	PERCENTAGE PERIPHERAL, ADULT	ABSOLUTE NUMBER × 10^3/uL, ADULT	PERCENTAGE BONE MARROW, CHILD	PERCENTAGE PERIPHERAL, CHILD	ABSOLUTE NUMBER × 10^3/uL, CHILD
Myeloblast	0–1	0	NA	0–2	0	NA
Promyelocyte	1–5	0	NA	0–4	0	NA
Myelocyte	2–10	0	NA	5–15	0	NA
Metamyelocyte	5–15	0	NA	5–15	0	NA
Band	10–40	5–10	NA	10–20	0–5	NA
Segmented Neutrophil	10–30	40–70	1.5–7.5	5–15	30–60	1.5–7.5
Eosinophil	0–3	1–4	0–0.5	1–8	1–4	0–1
Basophil	0–1	0–1	0–0.2	0–1	0–2	0–0.2
Lymphocyte	5–15	20–40	1–4.5	5–35	30–60	1.5–8.5
Monocyte	0–3	2–10	0–1	0–4	2–11	0–1
Plasma Cells	0–3	0	NA	0–2	0	NA
Pronormoblast	0–3	0	NA	0–2	0	NA
Basophilic Normoblast	0–5	0	NA	0–5	0	NA
Polychromatophilic Normoblast	5–20	0	NA	5–11	0	NA
Orthochromic Normoblast	0–8	0	NA	5–35	0	NA
Megakaryocyte	0–2	0	NA	0–2	0	NA

NA, not applicable.

BONE MARROW

ERYTHROPOIESIS

Erythropoiesis is a process by which early erythroid precursor cells differentiate to become the mature RBCs. The primary regulator of this process is erythropoietin. The cell line undergoes three divisions, which take about 72 hours. As the cells mature, hemoglobin synthesis takes place and is complete by the reticulocyte stage. It normally takes 3 to 5 days for the production of reticulocytes from pronormoblasts. The reticulocytes remain in the bone marrow for 1 to 2 days before being released into the circulation. In peripheral circulation the reticulocyte continues to mature for one more day.

Stages of Red Cell Maturation

PRONORMOBLAST. The pronormoblast is the earliest recognizable and largest cell of the erythrocytic series. This cell undergoes mitosis that produces two daughter cells. This cell produces between 8 and 32 mature erythrocytes.

BASOPHILIC NORMOBLAST. Hemoglobin synthesis begins at this stage. The cell undergoes mitosis and divides twice, giving rise to four polychromatic normoblasts.

POLYCHROMATIC NORMOBLAST. At this stage there is increased production of hemoglobin pigmentation and decreasing amounts of RNA. This is the last stage in which the cell is capable of mitosis.

ORTHOCHROMATIC NORMOBLAST. This is the last nucleated stage. The nucleus is usually ejected from the cell. Hemoglobin production is almost complete at this stage. This group of cells cannot synthesize DNA and cannot undergo cellular division. This cell is the nucleated red blood cell (NRBC) sometimes seen in peripheral circulation.

RETICULOCYTE. This is a slightly larger cell than the mature RBC with residual amounts of RNA. This residual RNA is a violet tinting, with fine basophilic stippling, which is called polychromasia. A special stain, new methylene blue, precipitates the RNA in a network of clear visible strands or a clump that can be observed under the microscope. The reticulocyte continues to mature for 1 or 2 more days in the peripheral blood. The reticulocyte count is an index of bone marrow activity or effective erythropoiesis.

ERYTHROCYTE. The RBC is a biconcave 6 to 8 μm disc. The life span is 120 days. The cell's main function is to transport hemoglobin, a protein that delivers oxygen from the lungs to tissue and cells. The erythrocyte contains 90% hemoglobin and 10% water. Erythrocytes are flexible and deformable, which is necessary for passage through the microcirculation. The RBC lacks cellular organelles and enzymes to synthesize new lipids or proteins, so metabolism is limited. It is essential for RBC function and survival that it have a normal and intact membrane. RBC stability requires ATP from glycolysis as an energy source. This involves four pathways: (1) the Embden-Meyerhof pathway, which provides 90% of anaerobic glycolysis; (2) the hexose monophosphate shunt, which protects the RBC from accumulation of hydrogen peroxide, which denatures hemoglobin; (3) the methemoglobin reductase pathway, which maintains iron in the ferric state, which is required for oxygen transport; and (4) the Luebering-Rapaport shunt, which regulates oxygen delivery to the tissues.

The normal concentration of RBCs varies with age, sex, and geographic location.

Erythrocyte Cell Maturation Morphology

CELL TYPE	CELL SIZE (μM)	NUCLEUS	NUCLEOLI	CYTOPLASM	N/C RATIO	BM (%)	MICROSCOPIC VIEW
Pronormoblast (Rubriblast)	12–20	Large round, oval, dark violet Chromatin: fine	1–2	Deep blue spotty Basophilic with a perinuclear halo	8:1	1	✳
Basophilic Normoblast (Prorubriblast)	10–15	Large round to slightly oval Chromatin: condensed, coarse	0–1	Deeply basophilic Clusters of free ribosomes	6:1	1–4	✳
Polychromatic Normoblast (Rubricyte)	10–15	Round nucleus, deep staining, may be centrally or eccentrically located Chromatin: coarse and clumped	0	Abundant blue-gray (RNA) to pink-gray cytoplasm (hemoglobin)	4:1	10–20	✳
Orthochromic Normoblast (Metarubricyte)	8–10	Small pyknotic nucleus Chromatin: dense	0	Abundant red-orange cytoplasm uniform in color	1:2	5–10	✳

Continued ▶

ERYTHROPOIESIS

▶ Continued **Erythrocyte Cell Maturation Morphology**

CELL TYPE	CELL SIZE (μM)	NUCLEUS	NUCLEOLI	CYTOPLASM	N/C RATIO	BM (%)	MICROSCOPIC VIEW
Reticulocyte	8–10	Anucleate cell containing small amount of basophilic reticulum (RNA)	0	Large amount of blue-pink staining hemoglobin cytoplasm. New methylene blue stains RNA.	NA		*
Erythrocyte	7–8	Anucleated cell	0	Pink staining, zone of central pallor is ⅓ of cell diameter devoid of hemoglobin	NA		*

* Photomicrographs from Carr J, Rodak BF: Atlas of Clinical Hematology. Philadelphia, WB Saunders, 1998.
N/C, Nuclear-to-cytoplasmic; BM, bone marrow.

RED CELL MORPHOLOGY: Red Blood Cell Size

RED CELL TYPE	MORPHOLOGIC APPEARANCE	DEFECT OR CHANGE	ASSOCIATED CONDITIONS	OTHER	MICROSCOPIC VIEW
Anisocytes	Variation in size	Two cell populations Small and large	Anemia	RDW increased	*
Normocytic	Normal sized biconcave disc RBCs 7–8 μm	NA	NA	Normal MCV	◆
Microcytic	Smaller RBCs less than 6 μm MCV <80 fL	Abnormal size due to the failure of hemoglobin synthesis	Iron deficiency anemia Thalassemia Chronic disease	Defective globin synthesis Ineffective iron utilization, absorption, and release	◆
Macrocytic	Larger RBCs greater than 9 μm MCV >90 fL	Impaired DNA synthesis Stress erythropoiesis Excess surface membrane	Megaloblastic anemia Liver disease MDS Alcoholism Malaria	Inherited or acquired	+

* Photomicrograph from Rodak BF: Diagnostic Hematology. Philadelphia, WB Saunders, 1995.
◆ Photomicrographs from Carr J, Rodak BF: Atlas of Clinical Hematology. Philadelphia, WB Saunders, 1998.
+ Photomicrograph from Henry JB: Clinical Diagnosis and Management by Laboratory Methods. 19th ed. Philadelphia, WB Saunders, 1996.
RDW, red cell distribution width; MCV, mean cell volume; MDS, myelodysplastic syndrome; NA, not applicable.

Red Cell Hemoglobin Content

RED CELL TYPE	MORPHOLOGIC APPEARANCE	DEFECT OR CHANGE	ASSOCIATED CONDITIONS	OTHER	MICROSCOPIC VIEW
Normochromic	Normal in color. Pale central area occupies less than ⅓.	Normal amount of hemoglobin	NA	Normal indices	*
"Hyperchromia"	No central pallor	Greater than normal MCHC	Spherocytosis	A misnomer, more because of shape of cell than color	◆
Hypochromic	Central pallor exceeds ⅓ of diameter of cell.	Reduced hemoglobin content (↓MCHC)	Iron deficiency anemia Thalassemia	Associated with microcytosis	◆
Polychromasia	Blue-gray coloration	Presence of RNA RBCs delivered prematurely to circulation	Increased erythropoietic activity Hemorrhage Hemolysis	Indicates young red blood cell	◆

* Photomicrograph courtesy of Bernadette Rodak and Jacqueline Carr, Medical Technology Program, Indiana University, Indianapolis, IN.
◆ Photomicrographs from Carr J, Rodak BF: Atlas of Clinical Hematology. Philadelphia, WB Saunders, 1998.
MCHC, mean cell hemoglobin concentration.

Red Cell Shape

Continued ▶

RED CELL TYPE	MORPHOLOGIC APPEARANCE	DEFECT OR CHANGE	ASSOCIATED CONDITIONS	OTHER	MICROSCOPIC VIEW
Poikilocyte	Variation in shape	Irreversible alteration of membrane	Anemia Hemolytic states	Extramedullary hematopoiesis	*
Acanthocyte	Spheroid with 3–12 irregular spike spicules Decreased cell volume	Increased ratio of cholesterol to lecithin	End stage liver disease Pyruvate kinase deficiency Hemolytic anemia Abetalipoproteinemia	Spur cell Thorn cell Nonreversible	*
Blister	Contains one or more vacuoles Thinned periphery	Formed by removal of Heinz's bodies	Hemolytic episodes G6PD deficiency Hemoglobinopathies	Bite cell Helmet cell	*
Codocyte	Peripheral rim of hemoglobin surrounded by clear area and central hemoglobinized area (bull's eye)	Excess of surface membrane to volume ratio	Hemoglobinopathies Thalassemia Liver disease Postsplenectomy	Target cells Leptocytes Sometimes artifact in drying and excess EDTA	*

RED CELL MORPHOLOGY

▶ Continued **Red Cell Shape**

RED CELL TYPE	MORPHOLOGIC APPEARANCE	DEFECT OR CHANGE	ASSOCIATED CONDITIONS	OTHER	MICROSCOPIC VIEW
Discocyte	Normal biconcave erythrocyte 6–8 μm diameter, 0–2 μm thickness	NA	NA	Normocyte	*
Dacryocyte	Teardrop or pear shape with single elongated point or tail	Squeezing and fragmentation during splenic passage	Myeloid metaplasia Thalassemia Megaloblastic anemia Hypersplenism	Tear drop cell	*
Drepanocyte	Crescent shaped cell that lacks zone of central pallor	Polymerization of de-oxygenated hemoglobin	Sickle cell anemia SC disease S-thalassemia	Sickle cell Shape reversible with re-oxygenation	*

Continued ▶

▲ Continued **Red Cell Shape**

RED CELL TYPE	MORPHOLOGIC APPEARANCE	DEFECT OR CHANGE	ASSOCIATED CONDITIONS	OTHER	MICROSCOPIC VIEW
Echinocyte	Regular 10–30 scalloped short projections evenly distributed Spiny-like	Depletion of ATP Exposure to hypertonic solution Artifact in air drying	Uremia Cirrhosis Hepatitis Chronic renal disease	Burr's cell Crenated RBC Usually reversible	◆
Elliptocyte	Rod or cigar shape, generally narrower than ovalocytes	Polarization of hemoglobin	Thalassemia Iron deficiency Hereditary elliptocytosis	Can be hypochromic and dense	✳
Ovalocyte	Egglike or oval shaped cell Wider than elliptocytes	Hemoglobin has bipolar arrangement Reduction in membrane cholesterol	Megaloblastic bone marrow Myelodysplasia Sickle cell anemia	Varies in hemoglobin concentration	✳

Continued ▲

RED CELL MORPHOLOGY

▶ Continued **Red Cell Shape**

RED CELL TYPE	MORPHOLOGIC APPEARANCE	DEFECT OR CHANGE	ASSOCIATED CONDITIONS	OTHER	MICROSCOPIC VIEW
Schistocyte	Fragments of RBCs varying in size and shape	Extreme fragmentation produced by damage of RBC by fibrin, altered vessel walls, prosthetic heart valves	Disseminated intravascular coagulation (DIC) Thrombotic thrombocytopenia purpura (TTP) Burns Microangiopathic hemolytic anemia	Keratocyte Helmet Bite	◆
Spherocyte	Smaller in diameter than normal RBC with concentrated hemoglobin content No visible central pallor	Lowest surface area to volume ratio Defect of loss of membrane	Hereditary spherocytosis Isoimmune and autoimmune hemolytic anemia Severe burns Hemoglobinopathies	Shape is irreversible Usually trapped by spleen	*
Stomatocyte	Normal sized cell with slitlike area in center	Occurs as artifact of slow drying Known to have increased permeability to sodium	Hereditary stomatocytosis Acute alcoholism Liver disease	More often artifactual than true manifestation	◆

* Photomicrographs from Carr J, Rodak BF: Atlas of Clinical Hematology. Philadelphia, WB Saunders, 1998.
◆ Photomicrographs from Rodak BF: Diagnostic Hematology. Philadelphia, WB Saunders, 1995.
G6PD, glucose-6-phosphate dehydrogenase; SC, sickle cell trait; S, sickle.

Red Cell Inclusions

RED CELL TYPE	MORPHOLOGIC APPEARANCE	DEFECT OR CHANGE	ASSOCIATED CONDITIONS	OTHER	MICROSCOPIC VIEW
Basophilic Stippling	Fine: thin round dark blue granules uniformly distributed Coarse: medium sized, uniformly distributed	Fine: represents poly-chromasia (reticulo-cyte) Coarse: represents im-paired erythro-poiesis	Thalassemia Heavy metal Lead poisoning Increased reticulocyto-sis	Artificial precipitation of ribosomes and RNA during staining	*
Babesia	Ring-shaped para-sites, minute chro-matin dot, and minimal amount of cytoplasm Can find more than one ring	Protozoan inclusion (*Babesia microti*) transmitted from deer to humans by tick bite	Causes hemolytic disor-der	Rings can be found out-side RBC	◆
Cabot Ring	Rings, loops, or fig-ure eights red to purple	Remnants of micro-tubules of mitotic spindle	Megaloblastic anemia Dyserythropoiesis	Occurs in both nucleated and non-nucleated RBCs	*
Heinz Bodies	Deep purple irregu-larly shaped inclu-sions 2 to 3 μm Found on RBC inner surface of mem-brane	Represent precipi-tated, denatured he-moglobin due to ox-idative injury	Hereditary defects in hexose monophos-phate shunt G6PD deficiency Unstable hemoglobins Splenectomized pa-tients Thalassemia	Cannot be seen with Wright's stain. Must use supravital stain (methylene blue or crystal violet)	+

Continued ▶

RED CELL MORPHOLOGY

▲ Continued **Red Cell Inclusions**

RED CELL TYPE	MORPHOLOGIC APPEARANCE	DEFECT OR CHANGE	ASSOCIATED CONDITIONS	OTHER	MICROSCOPIC VIEW
Hemoglobin C Crystals	Tetragonal, rectangular rod shaped; dense staining crystals formed	In HbC lysine replaces glutamic acid at sixth position of beta chain	Hemoglobin C disease Hemoglobin SC disease	Bar of gold Clam shell	*
Howell-Jolly Bodies	Coarse round densely stained purple 1–2 μm granules eccentrically located on periphery of membrane. May be single or double	Nuclear remnants contain DNA	Megaloblastic anemia Severe hemolytic process Thalassemia Accelerated erythropoiesis	Spleen pits these bodies from cell	*
Malaria	Protozoan found in ring and many other forms within RBC	Protozoan transmitted by bite of female *Anopheles* mosquito	*Plasmodium vivax* *Plasmodium ovale* *Plasmodium malariae* *Plasmodium falciparum*	See Chapter 32 for life cycles and stages	◆

Continued ▲

▶ Continued **Red Cell Inclusions**

RED CELL TYPE	MORPHOLOGIC APPEARANCE	DEFECT OR CHANGE	ASSOCIATED CONDITIONS	OTHER	MICROSCOPIC VIEW
Pappenheimer Bodies	Small 2–3 μm irregular basophilic inclusions that aggregate in small clusters near periphery with Wright's stain	Unused iron (nonheme) deposits	Sideroblastic anemia MDS Thalassemia Hemolytic anemia Defective erythropoiesis	Siderotic granules with Prussian blue stain See siderocyte, sideroblast, and ringed sideroblast	*
Ringed Sideroblast	Nucleated RBC that contains nonheme iron particles (siderotic granules) arranged in ring form	Excessive iron overload in mitochondria of normoblasts Due to defective heme synthesis Ringed sideroblast Pathologic	Sideroblastic anemia MDS	Ringed sideroblast Prussian blue stain needed for identification Found in bone marrow	✚
Siderocyte	Non-nucleated cell containing iron granules	Same as above	Same as above	Iron granules are called Pappenheimer bodies with Wright's stain	See photomicrograph above

* Photomicrographs from Carr J, Rodak BF: Atlas of Clinical Hematology. Philadelphia, WB Saunders, 1998.
◆ Photomicrographs from Rodak BF: Diagnostic Hematology. Philadelphia, WB Saunders, 1995.
✚ Photomicrographs courtesy of Bernadette Rodak and Jacqueline Carr, Medical Technology Program, Indiana University, Indianapolis, IN.
MDS, myelodysplastic syndrome.

RED CELL MORPHOLOGY

Miscellaneous Red Cell Morphology

RED CELL TYPE	MORPHOLOGIC APPEARANCE	DEFECT OR CHANGE	ASSOCIATED CONDITIONS	OTHER	MICROSCOPIC VIEW
Autoagglutination	Clumping of RBCs	Presence of antibody	Cold agglutinin Autoimmune Hemolytic anemia	Can be eliminated by warming	*
Rouleaux	Alignment of RBCs linear appearing as stack of coins	Caused by concentration of fibrinogen and immunoglobin	Multiple myeloma Waldenström's macroglobulinemia	Encountered as artifact at thick area of slide	*

* Photomicrographs from Carr J, Rodak BF: Atlas of Clinical Hematology. Philadelphia, WB Saunders, 1998.

LEUKOPOIESIS

Leukopoiesis is a process by which the WBCs differentiate and proliferate. The development of the WBC occurs primarily in the bone marrow with the exception of the lymphocyte, the development of which takes place in the bone marrow and thymus. The leukocytes can be divided into categories according to function, site of origin, and morphology. These include the neutrophil, lymphocyte, monocyte, eosinophil, and basophil.

Granulocyte

Granulopoiesis is the orderly production of mature granulocytes (neutrophils, eosinophils, and basophils), which begins in the bone marrow under the influence of growth hormone. It takes about 14 days from the blast stage to the release of the mature granulocyte into the peripheral blood. The neutrophil undergoes six different morphologic stages from blast to mature cell. The neutrophil, eosinophil, and basophil undergo the same maturation sequence.

Granulocytes are cells that contain visible granules. They are further subdivided by the types of granules they contain. The granules found in the neutrophil contain acid phosphatase, acid hydrolase, peroxidase, muramidase, and lactoferrin, which are essential for the phagocytic function of the cell. The eosinophil granules contain peroxidase, acid phosphatase, and other proteolytic enzymes but do not contain alkaline phosphatase. The function of the eosinophil is important in allergy, drug reactions, and parasitic infections. The eosinophil is primarily a tissue cell and spends very little time in the peripheral blood. The basophil granules contain histamine, heparin, and chondroitin sulfates, which function with immediate hypersensitivity reactions.

Function of the Granulocytes

CELL TYPE	FUNCTION
Neutrophil	Protects body from infection by phagocytosis of bacteria and other foreign organisms. Defense reactions against microorganisms, removal of damaged or dead cells, and removal of cellular debris.
Eosinophil	Protects body by ingestion of parasites and limiting allergic reactions.
Basophil	Involved with immediate hypersensitivity reaction by release of histamine and heparin from basophilic granule.

NEUTROPHIL

Kinetics of Neutrophils

The life span of the neutrophil from myeloblast to mature neutrophil is approximately 10 to 14 days. There are several pools associated with neutrophil kinetics. The *mitotic pool,* or proliferating pool, involves cells that are capable of mitotic divisions. The *postmitotic pool,* or maturation pool, consists of cells that do not undergo mitosis. The *storage pool* is subdivided into the *marginal pool* and the *circulating pool.* The marginal pool neutrophils adhere to the vessel endothelium, and when demand for neutrophils in the peripheral blood increases, they enter the circulating pool. The circulating pool constitutes the neutrophils that are counted in a WBC count. There is a freedom of movement of neutrophils from the marginal pool and the circulating pool. Within hours the neutrophil can enter the tissues by diapedesis (a passing through the vessel wall). Once it enters the tissue its life span is short and the neutrophil cannot re-enter circulation.

SCHEME FOR NEUTROPHIL KINETICS

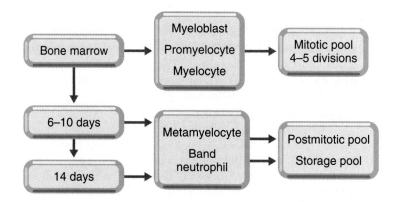

White Blood Cell Maturation Morphology

GRANULOCYTE MATURATION

CELL TYPE	CELL SIZE (μM)	NUCLEUS	NUCLEOLI	CYTOPLASM	N/C RATIO	BM (%)	MICROSCOPIC VIEW
Myeloblast	10–20	Shape: large round to oval, indented on one side Color: dark blue Chromatin: fine strands with no clumping, open reticulum	1–5 Round and blue	Amount: scant Color: basophilic Granulation: none to less than 20 Distinct parachromatin	5:1–7:1	1–2	*
Promyelocyte	12–21	Shape: large round to oval, often flattened Color: dark blue Chromatin: fine with some thickening	2–3 Often visible	Amount: increasing Color: medium blue Granulation: nonspecific or primary granules (red)	5:1	2–5	◆
Myelocyte	10–18	Shape: central to eccentric, large, round, oval Color: blue Chromatin: coarse	Rarely visible	Amount: moderate Color: bluish pink or light pink, becoming light May be light area under nucleus Granulation: specific or secondary granules (violet)	4:1	10–20	◆
Metamyelocyte	10–16	Shape: kidney or bean, indented Color: blue-purple Chromatin: coarse and compact	None	Amount: abundant Color: pink Granulation: full complement of secondary granules	4:1	15–30	◆

NEUTROPHIL

Continued ▶

▲ Continued **GRANULOCYTE MATURATION**

CELL TYPE	CELL SIZE (μM)	NUCLEUS	NUCLEOLI	CYTOPLASM	N/C RATIO	BM (%)	MICROSCOPIC VIEW
Band	10–15	Shape: C or S Color: dark purple Chromatin: dense and clumpy (leopard skin)	None	Amount: abundant Color: pink to violet Granulation: large amount of secondary granules	1:3	10–40	◆
Neutrophil	10–15	Shape: segmented or lobulated (2–5 lobes) Color: dark purple Chromatin: coarse and clumped	None	Amount: abundant Color: pink Granulation: abundant secondary granules	1:3	10–30	◆
Eosinophil	10–15	Shape: segmented or lobed with 1–3 lobes Color: dark purple and obscured by granules Chromatin: coarse and clumped	None	Amount: abundant Color: pink Granulation: large orange granules (eosinophilic)	1:3	0–3	*
Basophil	10–15	Shape: segmented or lobed with 1–3 lobes Color: dark purple Chromatin: coarse and clumped	None	Amount: abundant Color: pale blue Granulation: heavy with black-blue granules	1:3	0–1	*

* Photomicrographs from Rodak BF: Diagnostic Hematology. Philadelphia, WB Saunders, 1995.

◆ Photomicrographs from Carr J, Rodak BF: Atlas of Clinical Hematology. Philadelphia, WB Saunders, 1998.

MORPHOLOGIC ABNORMALITIES ASSOCIATED WITH GRANULOCYTES

DESCRIPTION	MORPHOLOGIC APPEARANCE	DEFECT OR CHANGE	ASSOCIATED CONDITIONS	OTHER	MICROSCOPIC VIEW
Alder-Reilly Granules	Large purple-black coarse cytoplasmic granules	Accumulation of degraded mucopolysaccharides	Adler-Reilly anomaly Mucopolysaccharides Hunter's syndrome	May be found in all leukocytes	*
Auer Rods	Pink or red rod shaped cytoplasmic structures 0.1–2 μm	Fused primary granules Lysosomal in nature	AML AMML Found in myeloid and monocytic series only	Peroxidase positive	◆
Chédiak-Higashi Granules	Giant red, blue to grayish round inclusions in cytoplasm	Large cytoplasmic inclusions of fused primary granules that are deficient in enzymes for phagocytosis	Chédiak-Higashi syndrome Recurrent infections Albinism	Peroxidase and sudan black positive Seen in lymphocyte, neutrophil, monocyte	▶
Döhle Bodies	Single or multiple blue cytoplasmic (0.1–2.0 μm) inclusions in neutrophil	Aggregates of free ribosomes of rough endoplasmic reticulum	Severe infections Burns Toxic states	Confused with May-Hegglin	▶

Continued ▶

AML, acute myelocytic leukemia: AMML, acute myelomonocytic leukemia; CML, chronic myelocytic leukemia.

NEUTROPHIL

▲ Continued **MORPHOLOGIC ABNORMALITIES ASSOCIATED WITH GRANULOCYTES**

DESCRIPTION	MORPHOLOGIC APPEARANCE	DEFECT OR CHANGE	ASSOCIATED CONDITIONS	OTHER	MICROSCOPIC VIEW
Hypersegmented Neutrophil	>5 lobes	Abnormal DNA synthesis	Megaloblastic anemia	Right shift	▶
LE Cell	Neutrophil with large purple homogeneous round inclusion with nucleus wrapped around	Three factors needed to produce cell: antinuclear antibodies, cell nuclei, phagocytes with ingested material	Lupus erythematosus	Several LE cells must be seen for positive test	✚
Pelger-Huët	Single or bilobed nucleus	Decreased segmentation	Pelger-Huët Pseudo-Pelger-Huët CML MDS Chemotherapy	Hyposegmentation	◆

Continued ▲

▲ Continued **MORPHOLOGIC ABNORMALITIES ASSOCIATED WITH GRANULOCYTES**

DESCRIPTION	MORPHOLOGIC APPEARANCE	DEFECT OR CHANGE	ASSOCIATED CONDITIONS	OTHER	MICROSCOPIC VIEW
Pyknotic Nucleus	Condensed round nuclei or nuclear fragments	Usually due to cells' prolonged contact in the anticoagulant EDTA	Artifact Bacteria infections	Fresh smear should be evaluated	◆
Toxic Granules	Large purple to black azurophilic granules	Primary granules	Infections, toxic states Burns Malignancy Chemical poisoning	Seen with Döhle bodies and toxic vacuoles	▶
Toxic Vacuoles	Large empty white areas within cytoplasm	Represent end stage phagocytosis	Septicemia Severe infections Toxic states	Associated with toxic granules	▶

* Photomicrographs from Henry JB: Clinical Diagnosis and Management by Laboratory Methods, 19th ed. Philadelphia, WB Saunders, 1996.
◆ Photomicrographs from Rodak BF: Diagnostic Hematology. Philadelphia, WB Saunders, 1995.
✚ Photomicrographs from Stevens ML: Fundamentals of Clinical Hematology. Philadelphia, WB Saunders, 1997.
▶ Photomicrographs from Carr J, Rodak BF: Atlas of Clinical Hematology. Philadelphia, WB Saunders, 1998.
AML, acute myelocytic leukemia; AMML, acute myelomonocytic leukemia; CML, chronic myelocytic leukemia.

NEUTROPHIL

MONOCYTE

Kinetics of the Monocyte

The monocyte arises from the same cell as the neutrophil. The monocyte maturation takes place in the bone marrow under the influence of granulocyte-macrophage colony stimulating factor (GM-CSF). The cell matures in the bone marrow in about 60 hours and then moves into the peripheral blood. There is no reserve or storage pool of monocytes in the bone marrow. Most are released within a day. In circulation there is a marginal pool and a circulating pool. The marginal pool is about three times the size of the circulating pool. Monocytes remain in peripheral blood for about 12 to 14 hours, and they then enter the tissues. Once they enter the tissues, the monocytes become tissue macrophages and can live months to years. Monocytes and differentiated macrophages are part of the mononuclear phagocytic system (MPS). Macrophages are scattered throughout the body. They line the sinusoids of the spleen and bone marrow. When found in the liver they are called *Kupffer's cells*.

Function of the Monocyte

The monocyte has several functions:

1. It protects the body by phagocytosis of varied material. Monocytes can ingest dead or dying cells, bacteria, fungi, and viruses. They help the neutrophil. In infection the monocyte numbers tend to rise after neutrophil numbers increase.
2. Monocytes play a role in processing specific antigens for the lymphocyte to recognize and transform for future reactions.
3. Monocytes also function as antitumor agents for surveillance or self or nonself recognition.
4. Monocytes produce and secrete various substances: lysosomes, colony stimulating factor (CSF), thromboplastin, platelet activating substances, and complement.

Monocyte Maturation

CELL TYPE	CELL SIZE (μM)	NUCLEUS	NUCLEOLI	CYTOPLASM	N/C RATIO	BM (%)	MICROSCOPIC VIEW
Monoblast	12–20	Shape: round to oval with slight indentation centrally located Color: pale blue to red-purple Chromatin: fine and lacy	0–3	Amount moderate with regular border Color: basophilic and homogeneous Granulation: none	4:1–6:1	0–3	✱
Promonocyte	14–18	Shape: large indentation, folding more distinct, centrally located Color: pale red-purple Chromatin: slightly clumped	0–2	Amount: moderate with pseudopod at border Color: gray-blue opaque Granulation: with or without fine red dustlike particles	4:1–3:1	0–3	
Monocyte	12–20	Shape: increased folding, often horseshoe Color: blue-purple Chromatin: moderately clumped	None	Amount: abundant, equally proportioned around nucleus Color: pale gray-blue Granulation: fine red dustlike particles and vacuoles	4:1–2:1	0–3	◆
Macrophage	20–50	Shape: round to oval indented eccentric Color: blue-purple Chromatin: spongy reticulum	1–2	Amount: abundant and usually vacuolated and irregular Color: sky blue Granulation: coarse azure granules			✱

✱ Photomicrographs from Rodak BF: Diagnostic Hematology. Philadelphia, WB Saunders, 1995.
◆ Photomicrograph from Carr J, Rodak BF: Atlas of Clinical Hematology. Philadelphia, WB Saunders, 1998.

MONOCYTE

LYMPHOCYTE

Kinetics of the Lymphocyte

Lymphocytes play an important role in antigen recognition and the development of an immune response. Lymphocytes are divided into two groups, the T cell lymphocytes and the B cell lymphocytes.

Lymphocyte precursors undergo maturation in the bone marrow before they migrate to extramedullary sites. The T lymphocytes migrate to the thymus, where they proliferate and differentiate to produce T helper cells and T suppressor cells. From the thymus the mature lymphocytes migrate to the peripheral lymphoid tissue. T lymphocytes make up 60% to 80% of the lymphoid cells in the lymphoid pool. The B lymphocytes differentiate to maturity within the bone marrow and are released into circulation to be distributed to lymph nodes, spleen, and other lymphoid tissue. The final maturation of the B lymphocyte is the plasma cell. The B lymphocyte accounts for 10% to 20% of lymphocytes. A third population of lymphocytes lacks the characteristics of both B and T and is called the *null lymphocyte,* which accounts for less than 10% of the lymphoid population.

Both T and B lymphocytes develop under the control of their respective humoral factors and microenvironment. As the lymphocyte matures the characteristics of the B and T lymphocyte surface markers change according to maturation and differentiation. The majority of lymphocytes are long lived with a life span of about 4 years and may live as long as 10 years. The short lived lymphocytes last about 3 to 4 days.

Function of the Lymphocyte

The primary function of the lymphocyte is to provide recognition and elimination of foreign stimuli. This includes the synthesis and secretion of antibodies. The B lymphocyte is responsible for humoral immunity and the synthesis of antibodies in response to antigen. The T lymphocytes are responsible for the development of cellular immunity, which includes tumor suppression, graft rejection, protection from intracellular organisms, and delayed hypersensitivity. Other functions of the T lymphocyte are regulation of humoral immune reactions by helping or suppressing the B lymphocyte and the regulation of hematopoiesis by producing colony stimulating factors.

Lymphocyte Maturation

CELL TYPE	CELL SIZE (μM)	NUCLEUS	NUCLEOLI	CYTOPLASM	N/C RATIO	BM (%)	MICROSCOPIC VIEW
Lymphoblast	10–20	Shape: round or oval with definite nuclear membrane Color: blue-purple Chromatin: not as fine as myeloblast	0–3	Amount: scant Color: moderately basophilic, lighter near nucleus, and darker at periphery Granulation: none	4:1	0–2	*
Prolymphocyte	9–18	Shape: ovoid, round, or slightly indented Color: blue-purple to red-purple Chromatin: clumped and coarse	0–1 Less distinct	Amount: moderate Color: clear basophilic Granulation: none	4:1	0–1	
Small Lymphocyte	7–10	Shape: round to oval with slight indentation Color: blue-purple Chromatin: coarse and clumpy	Not visible	Amount: scant Color: moderate to dark blue Granulation: usually absent, occasional azurophilic granules	4:1	5–15	*

Continued ▶

LYMPHOCYTE

▶ Continued **Lymphocyte Maturation**

CELL TYPE	CELL SIZE (μM)	NUCLEUS	NUCLEOLI	CYTOPLASM	N/C RATIO	BM (%)	MICROSCOPIC VIEW
Large Lymphocyte	12–16	Shape: round to oval with slight indentation Color: blue-purple Chromatin: coarse and clumpy	Not visible	Amount: abundant Color: clear and pale blue Granulation: may contain few azurophilic granules	3:1–2:1	5–15	◆
Reactive Lymphocyte	10–20	Shape: round, ovoid, or irregular, or central or eccentric indentation Color: red-purple Chromatin: fine, medium, and coarse	0–1	Amount: abundant, may surround the adjacent RBCs Color: blue, often darker at periphery Granulation: may or may not be present	Varies	NA	*
Plasma Cell	10–20	Shape: round to oval, eccentrically located Color: dark blue-purple Chromatin: dense, coarse, and clumpy (cartwheel)	None	Amount: moderate Color: basophilic with perinuclear clear zone Granulation: none	2:1–1:1	0–3	+

* Photomicrographs from Rodak BF: Diagnostic Hematology. Philadelphia, WB Saunders, 1995.

◆ Photomicrograph courtesy of Bernadette Rodak and Jacqueline Carr, Medical Technology Program, Indiana University, Indianapolis, IN.

+ Photomicrograph from Carr J, Rodak BF: Atlas of Clinical Hematology. Philadelphia, WB Saunders, 1998.

Miscellaneous Lymphocyte Morphology

DESCRIPTION	MORPHOLOGIC APPEARANCE	DEFECT OR CHANGE	ASSOCIATED CONDITIONS	OTHER	MICROSCOPIC VIEW
Basket Cell	Degenerated nucleus or ruptured cell in form of smudge or basket	Lymphocytes that are fragile and break upon smearing	Chronic lymphocytic leukemia Small numbers are arti-fact	Smudge cell	*
Flame Cell	Plasma cell with red to pink cytoplasm	Associated with in-crease in IgA	Multiple myeloma of IgA in nature		
Grape Cell	Plasma cell that con-tains small colorless vacuoles	Large protein globules giving appearance of grapes	Multiple myeloma Reactive states	Mott cell Russell bodies when vacuoles are blue	◆

Continued ▶

LYMPHOCYTE

▶ Continued **Miscellaneous Lymphocyte Morphology**

DESCRIPTION	MORPHOLOGIC APPEARANCE	DEFECT OR CHANGE	ASSOCIATED CONDITIONS	OTHER	MICROSCOPIC VIEW
Hairy Cell	Lymphocyte with hair-like cytoplasmic projections surrounding nucleus	Thought to be of B cell origin	Hairy cell leukemia	Stains positive with tartrate resistant acid phosphatase (TRAP)	✛
Sézary Cell	Round lymph cell with nucleus that is grooved or convoluted	Represents leukemic phase of mycosis fungoides T-cell characteristics	Sézary syndrome Mycosis fungoides Malignant lymphoma	Cutaneous T-cell lymphoma	✛

✳ Photomicrograph from Stevens ML: Fundamentals of Clinical Hematology. Philadelphia, WB Saunders, 1997.
◆ Photomicrograph from Carr J, Rodak BF: Atlas of Clinical Hematology. Philadelphia, WB Saunders, 1998.
✛ Photomicrographs from Rodak BF: Diagnostic Hematology. Philadelphia, WB Saunders, 1995.

THROMBOCYTE OR PLATELET

Kinetics of the Platelet

Platelet production begins with the differentiation of the pluripotential stem cell in the bone marrow. Along with colony stimulating factor and thrombopoietin the megakaryoblast is the first cell to be recognized. The megakaryocytes are very large cells that are derived from a process of *endomitosis*, which is nuclear division without cell or cytoplasm division. Continued endomitotic divisions of the megakaryoblast give rise to a multinucleated giant cell with 8 to 16 nuclei. The maturation sequence of the megakaryoblast takes about 5 days. Platelets are produced directly from the megakaryocyte cytoplasm. As the megakaryocyte matures, clusters of granules aggregate to form platelets. Once platelets are released into the sinuses, they survive for 8 to 10 days in circulation. Each megakaryocyte produces 2000 to 4000 platelets. The circulating platelets represent two thirds, and the remaining one third are stored in the spleen. The platelets in the spleen are the splenic platelet pool and are interchangeable with those in the blood.

Function of the Platelet

Platelets' essential role is in primary hemostasis and in maintaining vascular integrity. At the site of injury a platelet plug is formed by platelet adhesion to exposed subendothelial tissue; platelet activation then takes place: the platelets undergo a shape change and release the internal platelet contents resulting in platelet aggregation. Platelet aggregation is the interaction of platelets, which stick to each other to form a platelet plug. With the formation of a temporary plug, secondary hemostasis is activated and fibrin is deposited to reinforce the plug until the site of injury is repaired.

Platelet Maturation

CELL TYPE	CELL SIZE (μM)	NUCLEUS	NUCLEOLI	CYTOPLASM	N/C RATIO	BM (%)	MICROSCOPIC VIEW
Megakaryoblast	15–35	Shape: round, oval, sometimes indented and lobed Color: red-purple Chromatin: variable density	0–6	Amount: small to moderate with pseudopod projections Color: blue, basophilic Granulation: usually absent	8:1–10:1	0–1	✳
Promegakaryocyte	30–60	Shape: round, oval, indented, 2–4 lobes Color: red-purple Chromatin: coarse	0–2	Amount: abundant Color: blue Granulation: fine azurophilic granules	6:1	0–1	◆
Granular Megakaryocyte	40–90	Shape: small in comparison to cell, multilobed Color: red-purple	None visible	Amount: abundant Color: pink to blue Granulation: numerous and diffuse granules	2:1	0–1	✚

Continued ▶

▶ Continued **Platelet Maturation**

CELL TYPE	CELL SIZE (μM)	NUCLEUS	NUCLEOLI	CYTOPLASM	N/C RATIO	BM (%)	MICROSCOPIC VIEW
Mature Megakaryocyte	40–100	Shape: multinucleated Color: red-purple Chromatin: coarse	0	Amount: Abundant Color: light blue to pink Granulation: coarse clumps of granules aggregating into bundles from which platelets bud off	2:1–1:1	0–1	◆
Platelet	1–4	NA	NA	Amount: small Color: pale blue or colorless Granulation: evenly distributed fine red-purple granules	NA	NA	◆

* Photomicrograph from Rodak BF: Diagnostic Hematology. Philadelphia, WB Saunders, 1995.
◆ Photomicrograph courtesy of Bernadette Rodak and Jacqueline Carr, Medical Technology Program, Indiana University, Indianapolis, IN.
✦ Photomicrographs from Carr J, Rodak BF: Atlas of Clinical Hematology. Philadelphia, WB Saunders, 1998.

THROMBOCYTE OR PLATELET

Miscellaneous Platelet Morphology

DESCRIPTION	MORPHOTIC APPEARANCE	ASSOCIATED CONDITIONS
Bizarre Platelet	Many different, irregular shapes with pseudopod projections	Myeloproliferative disorders
Dysplastic Megakaryocyte	Tend to be smaller than normal with maturation abnormality Separate nucleus	MDS
Giant Platelet	7–8 μm	Thrombocytopenia Myeloproliferative disorders
Gray Platelet Agranular	Pale blue staining, lacking granules	Gray platelet syndrome MDS Myeloproliferative disorders
Small Platelet	<2 μm	Wiskott-Aldrich syndrome
Platelet Satellitism	Rosette of platelets surrounding the neutrophil	In vitro phenomenon associated with EDTA Decreased platelet count with automation

HEMATOLOGY NORMAL REFERENCE VALUES

TEST	ADULT MALE	ADULT FEMALE	NEWBORN (1–3 DAYS)	1–2 YR
White Blood Cell (WBC) ($\times 10^3/\mu$L)	3.9–10.6	3.5–11.0	18.0–22.0	10.6–11.4
Red Blood Cell (RBC) ($\times 10^6/\mu$L)	4.4–5.9	3.8–5.2	4.7–6.1	3.5–5.2
Hemoglobin (Hb) (g/dL)	13.3–17.7	11.7–15.7	16.5–21.5	9.6–15.6
Hematocrit (Hct) (%)	40–52	35–47	48–68	34–48
Mean Cell Volume (MCV) (fL)	80–100	80–100	95–125	76–92
Mean Cell Hemoglobin (MCH) (pg)	27–34	27–34	30–42	23–31
Mean Cell Hemoglobin Concentration (MCHC) (g/dL)	31–36	31–36	30–42	32–36
Red Cell Distribution Width (RDW) (%)	11.5–14.5	11.5–14.5	11.5–14.5	11.5–14.5
Platelet ($\times 10^3/\mu$L)	150–400	150–400	150–400	150–400
Mean Platelet Volume (MPV) (fL)	7.4–10.4	7.4–10.4	7.4–10.4	7.4–10.4
Band (%)	0–5	0–5	4–14	0–5
Neutrophil (%)	54–62	55–62	37–67	30–60
Lymphocyte (%)	20–40	20–40	18–38	29–65
Monocyte (%)	4–10	4–10	1–2	2–11
Eosinophil (%)	1–3	1–3	1–4	1–4
Basophil (%)	0–1	0–1	0–1	0–1

BIBLIOGRAPHY

Brown B: Hematology: Principles and Procedures, 6th ed, Philadelphia, Lea & Febiger, 1993.

Brown KA: Hematology M & M's Workshop, New York, American Society of Clinical Pathologists, Associate Member Section, 1996.

Diggs LW, Sturm D, Bell A: The Morphology of Human Blood Cells, 3rd ed. North Chicago, Abbott Laboratories, 1975.

Dutcher T: Hematology Morphology Workshop, American Society of Clinical Pathologists, Associate Member Section, 1992.

Hanson C: Hematology Section VII. In McClatchey K, ed: Clinical Laboratory Medicine. Baltimore, Williams & Wilkins, 1994, pp 817–1040.

Harmening D: Clinical Hematology and Fundamentals of Hemostasis, 3rd ed. Philadelphia, FA Davis, 1997.

Harrison-Godwin J, Godwin T: Bone Marrow Examination and Interpretation Workshop, American Society of Clinical Pathologists, Associate Member Section, June 1996.

Heckner F, Lehmann HP, Kao YS: Practical Microscopic Hematology, 3rd ed. Baltimore, Urban & Schwarzenberg, 1988.

Hutchison R, Davey F: Hematopoiesis. In Henry JB: Clinical Diagnosis and Management by Laboratory Methods, 19 ed. Philadelphia, WB Saunders, 1996, pp 594–616.

Hyun BH, Gulati G, Ashton JK: Hematopoiesis and Blood Cell Morphology. In Howanitz J, ed: Laboratory Medicine Test Selection and Interpretation. New York, Churchill Livingstone, 1991, pp 425–446.

Kjeldsberg C, Foucar K, et al: Practical Diagnosis of Hematologic Disorders, 2nd ed. Chicago, American Society of Clinical Pathologists Press, 1995.

Lopspeich-Steininger C: Clinical Hematology. Philadelphia, JB Lippincott, 1992.

McKenzie S: Textbook of Hematology, 2nd ed. Baltimore, Williams & Wilkins, 1996.

O'Connor B: A Color Atlas and Instruction Manual of Peripheral Blood Cell Morphology. Baltimore, Williams & Wilkins, 1984.

Pereira I: Peripheral Smears: The Primary Diagnostic Tool I and II Workshop, American Society of Clinical Pathologists, Associate Member Section, Philadelphia, October 1995.

Rodak B: Diagnostic Hematology. Philadelphia, WB Saunders, 1995.

Chapter **36**

ERYTHROCYTE DISORDERS

Bruce T. Kube, BS, MT(ASCP)H

Kathleen Finnegan, MS, MT(ASCP)SH

QUICK CONTENTS

INTRODUCTION

The purpose of this chapter is to outline and provide some insight into erythrocytic disorders. These disorders include both quantitative and qualitative changes in the ability of the erythrocyte to perform its proper functions. There are essentially two types of erythrocytic disorders. These include erythrocytosis, an increase in circulating erythrocytes, and anemia, with an associated decrease in circulating erythrocytes or the ability of the erythrocyte to transport oxygen.

SAMPLE COLLECTION. Samples for hematologic testing should be drawn optimally by venipuncture into lavender top tubes (sodium edetate [EDTA]) or by free flowing capillary stick into a lavender micro sample container, such as the Becton-Dickinson Microtainer, which contains EDTA. Samples should be well mixed to avoid clotting.

DESCRIPTION OF TERMS

Size Descriptors

NORMOCYTIC. This is a term used to describe a red blood cell (RBC) that has a mean cell volume (MCV) between 80 and 100 fL. There is normally a small degree of variation in the size of the RBC, and this variation should not be described as anisocytosis. A normal appearance of RBCs does not preclude the diagnosis of anemia or other RBC disorders.

MICROCYTIC. This is a term to describe an RBC population with an MCV of less than 80 fL. RBCs of this type are encountered in iron deficiency, thalassemias, and secondary anemias.

MACROCYTIC. This term is used to describe RBCs that have an MCV greater than 100 fL. These RBCs can appear round or oval. Round macrocytes are often seen in hepatic disease, whereas oval macrocytes are seen in vitamin B_{12} and folate deficiency.

ANISOCYTOSIS. This term is used to describe the variation in the size of RBCs due to a pathologic condition. One must be careful not to mistake the normal variation in the size of the RBC for anisocytosis. The parameter of the CBC used to measure the degree of variation in RBC size is the RDW (red cell *d*istribution *w*idth). Anisocytosis is a nonspecific finding and generally indicates a change in marrow function.

Chromicity Descriptors

NORMOCHROMIC. This is the term used to describe RBCs that have a darker pink outer rim that gradually fades to a lighter central pallor. The normal RBC has an apparent biconcavity. The mean cell hemoglobin (MCH) is between 27.0 and 34.0 pg, and the mean cell hemoglobin concentration (MCHC) from 31.0 to 36.0 g/dL.

HYPOCHROMIC. This term is used to describe an RBC that has a decreased hemoglobin complement. The hypochromic RBC appears pale compared with a normal RBC. The central pallor of these types of RBC has an extremely light pink color or appears to be totally devoid of color. This condition is usually caused by iron deficiency; however, other disorders such as hemoglobinopathies can cause a similar picture.

"HYPERCHROMIC." This refers to cells that appear to have an oversaturation of hemoglobin; however, oversaturation is not possible, as indicated by the fact that the upper limit of the MCHC is 36.0 g/dL. This phenomenon is caused by an increase in the mean cell thickness as in spherocytosis.

POLYCHROMIC. This refers to RBCs that appear slightly basophilic with a Romanowsky stain. The amount of basophilia is related to the maturity of the cell. Since polychromatophilic RBCs are less mature RBCs, they are slightly larger than their mature counterparts.

Shape Descriptors

POIKILOCYTOSIS. This describes the variation in the shape of the RBC. It is a general term and should be followed by the types of different cells seen. It should be noted, however, that it is normal for the shape of the RBC to change to a small degree during its normal life span. Following is a list of common "poikilocytes" and their primary causes:

POIKILOCYTES

TYPE OF CELL	APPEARANCE	CAUSE IN ORDER OF PREVALENCE	MICROSCOPIC VIEW
Acanthocyte	Crenated RBC with very spiny, irregular projections	Membrane defect, congenital or acquired abetalipoproteinemia	
Burr Cell	Similar to crenated RBC, but projections are pointier than crenated RBC and more regular than those of acanthocyte	Primarily renal failure; can be seen in other disorders	
Codocyte (Target Cell)	RBCs have bull's-eye appearance	Hepatic disease, absence of spleen, hemoglobinopathy	
Crenated RBC	Regular projections all around cell	Artifact, severe anemia, severe dehydration	
Dacryocyte (Teardrop)	Round cell with elongated tail or point; resembles teardrop	Myelofibrosis, thalassemia, hemolytic anemia, pernicious anemia	
Drepanocyte (Sickle Cell)	Usually thin crescent shaped cell	Hemoglobinopathy, usually S/S, could occur in S/A if other variants are present	

Continued ▶

DESCRIPTION OF TERMS

▶ Continued **POIKILOCYTES**

TYPE OF CELL	APPEARANCE	CAUSE IN ORDER OF PREVALENCE	MICROSCOPIC VIEW
Elliptocytes	RBCs oval or elliptic	Congenital disorder, dis-erythropoiesis	
Ovalocyte	Oval cell, wider than el-liptocyte; central pal-lor not oval	Megaloblastic anemia	
Schistocyte	Pieces of RBC that can have vast variety of shapes and sizes	Mechanical destruction of RBC due to DIC or TTP; heart valve re-placement	
Spherocyte	Cells appear perfectly round and have no central pallor. They are often smaller than normal RBCs.	Hereditary spherocyto-sis, post-transfusion, immune induced he-molytic anemia	
Stomatocytes	RBCs appear to have slot in center instead of round central pal-lor.	Artifactual; can occur in liver disease due to membrane defect	

S/S, sickle disease; S/A, sickle trait; DIC, disseminated intravascular coagulation; TTP, thrombotic throm-bocytopenic purpura.

ERYTHROCYTIC INCLUSIONS*

INCLUSION	APPEARANCE	CAUSE	MICROSCOPIC VIEW
Basophilic Stippling	Small or large blue-black dots uniformly throughout erythrocyte	Heavy metal poisoning	
Cabot Rings	Red-violet staining ring, partial ring or figure eight	Severe anemia	
Heinz Bodies	Intensely purple staining round inclusion when stained with vital stain; not seen with Wright's stain	Denatured or unstable hemoglobin; G6PD deficiency	
Hemoglobin H Bodies	Multiple blue green spherical inclusions; stained with brilliant cresyl blue	Tetramer of beta chains; Hgb H disease is form of α thalassemia	
Howell-Jolly Bodies	Large singular dark purple inclusion	Splenectomy, diserythropoiesis (B_{12} deficiency, etc)	
Pappenheimer Bodies	Small dark blue-purple staining hemoglobin iron granules. Stained with Romanowsky's stain	Hemolytic anemia, post-splenectomy	

ERYTHROCYTIC INCLUSIONS

Continued ▶

► Continued **ERYTHROCYTIC INCLUSIONS***

INCLUSION	APPEARANCE	CAUSE	MICROSCOPIC VIEW
Parasites	Pink-purple staining inclusion, either rings or other forms depending on species	Malaria, *Babesia*	
Reticulocytes	Dark blue granules or strands stained supravitally with new methylene blue or brilliant cresyl blue	Immature RBCs, increased bone marrow response to anemia, increased erythropoietin levels	
Siderotic Granules	Bright blue staining non-hemoglobin iron granules stained with Prussian blue	Hemolytic anemia, post-splenectomy	

*See Chapter 35 for photomicrographs and more descriptions.
G6PD, glucose-6-phosphate dehydrogenase.

ANEMIA

DEFINITION. When defining anemia, you must approach it with a broad outlook. Ordinarily, anemia is defined as a decrease in circulating RBCs, a decrease in hemoglobin concentration, or a decrease in the hematocrit compared with a normal population. However, the normal group must be representative. For example, hemoglobin levels are lower at sea level than at high altitudes since the oxygen concentration at high altitudes is less than that at sea level and more hemoglobin is necessary to supply tissues with oxygen. The hematocrit can also be a deceptive parameter, because in hypovolemia, the RBC mass is decreased, but so is the plasma volume, thus producing a normal hematocrit. In hypervolemia, the blood volume is increased and the hematocrit decreased but the RBC mass is actually increased. Therefore, in order to accurately define anemia you must take into account the functional ability of blood to supply oxygen to tissues.

CLASSIFICATION. Anemias can be classified in several ways, the two most popular being based on RBC morphology and by the pathophysiologic mechanism that caused the RBC deficit.

Red Blood Cell Morphology. This classification is useful because it follows from initial laboratory data in respect to a patient's RBC size and chromicity and leads to a consideration of underlying disease states most likely responsible. The indices used are (where Hct is hematocrit and Hgb is hemoglobin):

$$MCV = \frac{\text{Vol. of packed RBCs (Hct)} \times 10}{\text{RBCs } (\times 10^{12}/L)}$$

$$MCHC = \frac{\text{Hgb (g/dL)} \times 100}{\text{Hct}}$$

MCH is less often used in classifying anemias:

$$MCH = \frac{\text{Hgb (g/dL)} \times 10}{\text{RBCs } (\times 10^{12}/L)}$$

RDW. RDW is a statistical analysis of the variation in size of a population of RBCs and is used to gauge the degree of anisocytosis in a blood sample. RDW is calculated based on the standard deviation of the MCVs of the RBC.

Microcytic Anemia

In this group of anemias, the MCV is less than 80 fL. Generally microcytic anemias are associated with iron deficiency or a defect in hemoglobin synthesis such as thalassemia.

Iron Deficiency

This is a condition that can cause a microcytic hypochromic anemia. There are several mechanisms by which an individual can become iron deficient.

1. *Dietary Deficiency.* The amount of iron taken in is not sufficient to meet the demand of the body. This is may be seen in infants who have been too long on a milk-only diet and in elderly persons with poor diets. Deficiency of this type can also be encountered in certain parasitic infections.
2. *Insufficient Absorption.* This is often seen postoperatively, especially in gastrectomy patients. Defective absorption can also occur in chronic malabsorption syndromes such as sprue or celiac disease.
3. *Insufficient Transport.* This occurs in transferrin deficiency, which can happen in certain inflammatory conditions such as chronic rheumatoid arthritis.
4. *Abnormal Iron Loss.* This is very often caused by the loss of red cell mass due to hemorrhage or menstruation; it presents first as a normochromic/normocytic anemia. In men this iron loss is usually due to pathologic means such as occult bowel carcinoma.
5. *Increased Requirement.* This occurs primarily in children and pregnant woman.

ANEMIA

MORPHOLOGY AND IRON PROFILE IN MICROCYTIC HYPOCHROMIC ANEMIAS

CAUSE	ANISOCYTOSIS/ POIKILOCYTOSIS	BASOPHILIC STIPPLING PRESENT	IRON	TIBC	IRON SATURATION	MARROW STORES
Iron Deficiency	Yes	No	↓	↓	↓	↓
Thalassemia	No	Yes	↑ or normal	↓ or normal	↑ or normal	↑ or normal
Hereditary Sideroblastic Anemia	Yes	Yes	↑	↓ or normal	↑	↑
Acquired Sideroblastic Anemia	Yes or no	Yes	↑	↓ or normal	↑	↑
Chronic Disease	No	No	↓	↓	↓	↑

TIBC, total iron-binding capacity.

Sideroblastic Anemia

Sideroblastic anemia is an anemic state that resembles anemia of chronic disease. This particular anemic state can be associated with a wide variety of conditions both congenital and acquired. One item is consistent throughout, however: these types of anemia respond to pyroxidine, suggesting that it may play a role it the pathogenesis. This role, however, is not fully understood. The peripheral blood picture is variable; however, ringed sideroblasts are diagnostic in bone marrow.

Anemia of Chronic Disease

Anemia of chronic disease is generally a mild nonprogressive condition that may be seen in long term hospital patients, patients with rheumatoid arthritis, and patients with collagen vascular diseases. In these cases the serum iron level appears to be directly correlated with the albumin level and varies inversely with the erythrocyte sedimentation rate.

Aplastic Anemia

Aplastic anemia is an anemia of nonproduction. The bone marrow is markedly hypocellular, and there is a decrease in all cell lines (pancytopenia). The severity of anemia varies from patient to patient.

Macrocytic Anemia

Macrocytic anemia can be of two types: those that occur with megaloblastic changes in the bone marrow and those that do not. In a macrocytic anemia, the MCV is greater than 100 fL. Macrocytic anemias that occur without megaloblastic changes in the bone marrow can be caused by alcoholism and some hemolytic anemias

Megaloblastic Anemia

Megaloblastic anemia is a term used to describe a group of disorders in which blood and bone marrow hematopoietic cells display changes. These changes are generally caused by asynchrony in cell maturation due to impaired DNA synthesis. Megaloblastic anemias can be divided into groups: anemia caused by folate deficiency, that caused by vitamin B_{12} deficiency, and those anemias nonresponsive to either therapy. Another method of determining the cause of a macrocytic/megaloblastic anemia is by following the reticulocyte count. The figure below offers a schematic view of this approach.

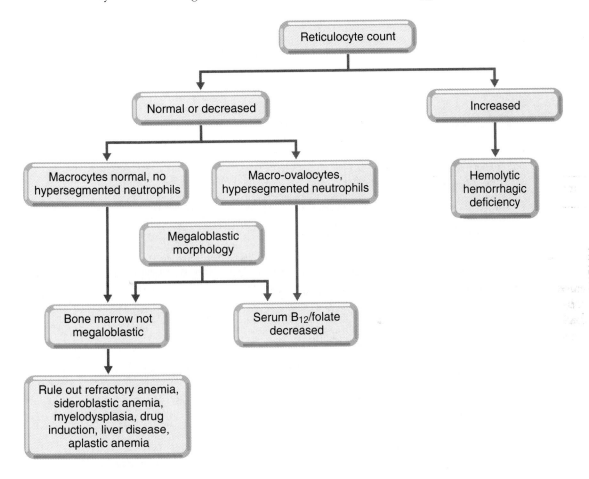

ANEMIA

CAUSES OF MACROCYTIC/MEGALOBLASTIC ANEMIAS

TYPE OF ANEMIA	CAUSATIVE MECHANISM
B$_{12}$ Deficiency	
Decreased Intake	Poor diet Strict vegetarianism Malabsorption: Pernicious anemia; gastrectomy (partial or total); destruction of gastric mucosa due to caustics; antibodies to intrinsic factor (IF) in gastric juice; abnormal IF molecule; Imerslund syndrome; ileal resection; ileitis; sprue; celiac disease; infiltrative intestinal disease (lymphoma, sclero-derma); drug induced malabsorption; parasitic infections (fish tape-worm); chronic pancreatic disease
Increased Requirement	Pregnancy Malignancy Hyperthyroidism
Impaired Utilization	Enzyme deficiencies Abnormal serum B$_{12}$ binding protein
Folate Deficiency	
Decreased Intake	Poor diet Insufficient vegetable intake Alcoholism Infancy Hemodialysis Malabsorption: Intestinal disorders, steatorrhea, sprue, celiac disease, intrinsic intestinal disease, phenytoin, oral contraceptives, other drugs
Increased Requirement	Pregnancy Infancy Hyperthyroidism Hyperactive hematopoiesis Malignancy
Impaired Utilization	Folic acid antagonists (trimethoprim, triamterene) Enzyme deficiencies
Unresponsive to B$_{12}$ or Folate Therapy (Enzyme, Congenital Disorders)	
Metabolic Inhibition	Purine synthesis: 6-mercaptopurine, 6-thioguanine, azathioprine Pyrimidine synthesis: 6-azauridine Thymidylate synthesis: 5-fluorouracil Deoxyribonucleotide synthesis: Hydroxyurea, cytosine arabinoside, severe iron deficiency
Congenital Errors	Lesch-Nyhan syndrome Hereditary orotic aciduria Deficiency of formimino transferase Deficiency of methyltransferase
Miscellaneous	Pyroxidine responsive megaloblastic anemia Thiamine responsive megaloblastic anemia Di Guglielmo's syndrome

PERIPHERAL BLOOD FINDINGS

WBCs	Normal or decreased
RBCs	Decreased
Hgb	Decreased
MCV	Increased (usually >100 fL)
MCH	Increased
MCHC	Normal or slightly decreased
Platelet Count	Normal or decreased
Reticulocyte Count	Decreased

SMEAR FINDINGS. Generally the peripheral smear of an individual with a megaloblastic anemia presents with an oval macrocytosis. The RBCs appear decreased and well hemoglobinized. Generally a degree of other poikilocytes, i.e., dacryocytes, schistocytes is displayed, as well as characteristic hypersegmented neutrophils (macropolycytes).

BONE MARROW. The cells in a megaloblastic bone marrow are larger than their normal counterparts. The nuclear chromatin of these cells is finer and stains a lighter lilac color. A common feature is the lack of the tendency to form dark chromatin clumps. The stages of maturation are promegaloblast, basophilic megaloblast, polychromatophilic megaloblast, late megaloblast, and macrocyte. If the condition is slight to moderate, normal and megaloblastic cells are present.

Usually there is significant maturation arrest, with 50% or greater of the erythroid cells being promegaloblasts or early megaloblasts. Howell-Jolly bodies are prominent, and the degree of hemoglobinization is increased compared with nuclear maturation. A megaloblastic marrow is characterized by several criteria: the ease and abundance with which the marrow is aspirated, the presence and numbers of megaloblastic precursors, and the presence and extent of granulocytic maturation arrest, as well as the presence of giant metamyelocyte and giant band forms.

ANEMIA

PATHOPHYSIOLOGIC DESCRIPTIONS OF ANEMIA

DISORDER	LABORATORY MORPHOLOGY	MECHANISM OR CAUSE OF DEFICIT	INDICES	RETICULOCYTE COUNT	ADDITIONAL LABORATORY TESTING	MICROSCOPIC VIEW
Acute Blood Loss	PB: Platelet count increases at time of bleed Neutrophilic leukocytosis 2–5 hr after bleed Polychromatic RBCs BM: Normal	Depends on severity of bleeding Associated with traumatic conditions	Normocytic-normochromic	Elevated in 2–3 days Peaks in 6–10 days		*
Iron Deficiency	PB: Anisocytosis Poikilocytosis Target cells Microcytes Hypochromic cells BM: Erythroid hyperplasia Decreased myeloid: erythroid (M:E) ratio Poorly hemoglobinized rubricytes with scanty cytoplasm Prussian blue stain for iron negative	Iron need exceeding supply Dietary malabsorption Increased iron loss Chronic blood loss	Microcytic-hypochromic ↑RDW	Decreased	Iron studies ↓iron ↓ferritin ↑TIBC	* *

Continued ▶

▶ Continued **PATHOPHYSIOLOGIC DESCRIPTIONS OF ANEMIA**

DISORDER	LABORATORY MORPHOLOGY	MECHANISM OR CAUSE OF DEFICIT	INDICES	RETICULOCYTE COUNT	ADDITIONAL LABORATORY TESTING	MICROSCOPIC VIEW
Megaloblastic Anemia	PB: Pancytopenia Macro-ovalocytes Hypersegmented neutrophils Howell-Jolly bodies NRBCs	Defect in DNA synthesis B₁₂ deficiency Folic acid deficiency Pernicious anemia (lack of IF or antibodies to IF)	Macrocytic- Normochromic ↑ RDW	Decreased	↑ LDH ↑ indirect bilirubin ↑ iron ↑ ferritin ↓ B₁₂ (B₁₂ deficiency)	
	BM: Hypercellular Low M:E ratio Megaloblasts Giant bands and metamyelocytes	Dietary, malabsorption, drugs			↓ Folic acid (FA deficiency) Antibody testing to IF	
Nonmegaloblastic Anemia	PB: RBCs large and round not oval BM: Normoblastic	Chronic liver disease Alcoholism Acute hemorrhage	MCV > 100 < 120 fL	Normal	Liver enzymes ↑ ↑ LDH ↑ bilirubin	

Continued ▶

▶ Continued **PATHOPHYSIOLOGIC DESCRIPTIONS OF ANEMIA**

DISORDER	LABORATORY MORPHOLOGY	MECHANISM OR CAUSE OF DEFICIT	INDICES	RETICULOCYTE COUNT	ADDITIONAL LABORATORY TESTING	MICROSCOPIC VIEW
Chronic Disease	PB: Mild anemia Anisocytosis Poikilocytosis BM: Macrophages show increased hemosiderin	Block in release of iron from macrophages or inaccessibility of storage iron	Normocytic-normochromic to microcytic-hypochromic Normal RDW	Decreased	Iron studies: ↓ iron N to ↑ ferritin ↓ TIBC	✻
Sideroblastic Anemia	PB: Dimorphic anemia Anisocytosis Poikilocytosis Pappenheimer bodies Basophilic stippling BM: Erythroid hyperplasia Increase in stored iron Ringed sideroblasts with Prussian blue stain	Hereditary or acquired Block in the incorporation of iron into protoporphyrin ring Iron accumulation in mitochondria	Normocytic-normochromic Microcytic-hypochromic ↑ RDW	Decreased	↑ iron ↑ ferritin N to ↓ TIBC ↑ transferrin saturation	✻ ✻

Continued ▶

▶ Continued **PATHOPHYSIOLOGIC DESCRIPTIONS OF ANEMIA**

DISORDER	LABORATORY MORPHOLOGY	MECHANISM OR CAUSE OF DEFICIT	INDICES	RETICULOCYTE COUNT	ADDITIONAL LABORATORY TESTING	MICROSCOPIC VIEW
Lead Poisoning	PB: Microcytes Hypochromic cells Basophilic stippling	Lead intoxication interferes with iron storage in mitochondria and a damaging effect on the activity of enzymes for heme synthesis.	Microcytic-hypochromic	Normal to increased	Hemoglobin A$_2$ or F may be elevated.	*
Aplastic Anemia	PB: pancytopenia Hgb <7.0 g/dL Hct <20% WBCs <1.5 × 10^9/L Platelets 20–60 × 10^9/L BM: Hypocellular or dry tap Reduction in all three cell lines	Acquired or hereditary basic defect is failure in production of RBCs, WBCs, and platelets.	Normocytic-normochromic	Normal to decreased	Bone marrow must be performed to confirm.	*

PB, peripheral blood; BM, bone marrow; NRBC, nucleated red blood cells; M:E, myeloid erythroid ratio; MCV, mean cell volume; LDH, lactate dehydrogenase hormone; RDW, red cell distribution width; TIBC, total iron-binding capacity; N, normal.

* Photomicrographs from Carr J, Rodak BF: Atlas of Clinical Hematology. Philadelphia, WB Saunders, 1998.
◆ Photomicrograph courtesy of Bernadette Rodak and Jacqueline Carr, Medical Technology Program, Indiana University, Indianapolis, IN.

PATHOPHYSIOLOGIC DESCRIPTIONS OF ANEMIA

HEMOLYTIC ANEMIAS

Hemolytic anemias are a group of disorders that can be inherited, acquired, or drug induced. This group of anemias is characterized by increased destruction or shortened survival of the RBC. Patients with inherited disease have a defect within the RBC. That defect can be a membrane defect, an enzyme defect, or abnormal hemoglobin structure or production. Patients with acquired anemias have normal RBCs that are destroyed by outside forces. These anemias can range from mild to severe.

Hemolytic anemias are characterized by increased bone marrow activity, polychromasia, nucleated RBCs, and an increased reticulocyte count with stress reticulocytes.

Inherited Hemolytic Anemias

DISORDER	CAUSE	INHERITANCE	CLINICAL FEATURES	LABORATORY FINDINGS	MORPHOLOGIC FINDINGS	ADDITIONAL TESTING	MICROSCOPIC VIEW
Hereditary Spherocytosis	Defect in RBC membrane protein composition Hyperpermeability to sodium	Autosomal dominant	Anemia Splenomegaly Jaundice	Mild to moderate anemia MCV 77–87 fL ↑ MCHC ↑ RDW Reticulocyte count 5%–20% ↑ Bilirubin	Spherocytes Nucleated RBCs Polychromasia	Osmotic fragility increased Autohemolysis increased; correction with glucose	*
Hereditary Elliptocytosis	Defect in membrane cytoskeleton	Autosomal dominant	90% of patients show no signs of hemolysis.	Normocytic-normochromic Reticulocyte count <4%	Elliptocytes Ovalocytes Polychromasia	Osmotic fragility normal Autohemolysis normal	*
Hereditary Stomatocytosis	RBC membrane abnormally permeable to sodium and potassium	Autosomal dominant	Anemia Slight jaundice	↑ MCV ↓ MCHC ↑ Reticulocyte count ↑ Bilirubin	10%–50% stomatocytes	Osmotic fragility increased Autohemolysis increased	◆

Continued ▲

HEMOLYTIC ANEMIAS

▶ Continued **Inherited Hemolytic Anemias**

DISORDER	CAUSE	INHERITANCE	CLINICAL FEATURES	LABORATORY FINDINGS	MORPHOLOGIC FINDINGS	ADDITIONAL TESTING	MICROSCOPIC VIEW
Hereditary Pyropoikilocytosis	Membrane defect with very unstable spectrin. Membrane loss and rigidity Cells very sensitive to heat	Autosomal recessive	Presents early in childhood and tend to be severe	MCV 55 fL	Marked poikilocytosis, anisocytosis Fragmented and bizarre shaped RBCs Polychromasia	Osmotic fragility increased Autohemolysis increased; no correction with glucose	◆
G6PD Deficiency	Defect in hexose monophosphate shunt. Enzyme deficiencies of this pathway result in denatured hemoglobin. Usually related to drug intake or oxidant stress.	Sex linked recessive	Usually asymptomatic Varies with degree of oxidant stress	Normocytic-normochromic Reticulocyte count elevated 4–5 days after onset of hemolysis	Polychromasia Poikilocytosis Occasional spherocyte	Heinz body preparation (supravital stain) Heinz bodies represent denatured hemoglobin Enzyme testing	✚
Pyruvate Kinase Deficiency	Enzyme deficiency in Embden-Meyerhof pathway Inability of RBC to maintain normal ATP levels	Autosomal recessive		Normocytic-normochromic ↑Reticulocyte count	Polychromasia Poikilocytosis Nucleated RBCs	Enzyme testing	✚

※ Photomicrographs from Carr J, Rodak BF: Atlas of Clinical Hematology. Philadelphia, WB Saunders, 1998.
◆ Photomicrographs from Rodak BF: Diagnostic Hematology. Philadelphia, WB Saunders, 1995.
✚ Photomicrographs from Henry JB: Clinical Diagnosis and Management by Laboratory Methods, 19th ed. Philadelphia, WB Saunders, 1996.

Acquired Hemolytic Anemias

DISORDER	CAUSE	LABORATORY FINDINGS	ANTIBODIES	ADDITIONAL NOTES	MICROSCOPIC VIEW
Autoimmune Hemolytic Anemia	Warm type: usually acute extra vascular hemolysis Cold type: occurs primarily in old age; associated with *Mycoplasma* pneumonia	Warm type: sphero-cytosis+, poly-chromasia+, schistocytes± Cold type: DAT+ Hemoglobinuria± Haptoglobin de-crease	Warm type: usually IgG Cold type: IgM with anti-I specificity	Warm type: of-ten accom-panies other autoimmune diseases	*
Infectious Hemolysis	Infection by various microorganisms such as *Clostridium perfringens, Bartonella baciliformis,* and malarial parasites	Recovery of mi-croorganisms or serologic demon-stration Intracellular para-sites on periph-eral smear			◆
Microangiopathic Hemolytic Anemia	Mechanical trauma to RBCs (cardiac valve re-placement) Microcirculatory damage (thrombotic thrombocy-topenic purpura) Intravascular fibrin (DIC)	Increased FDP/FSP Increased D-dimer Thrombocytopenia Peripheral blood smear consistent with hemolysis			*

Continued ▶

▶ Continued **Acquired Hemolytic Anemias**

DISORDER	CAUSE	LABORATORY FINDINGS	ANTIBODIES	ADDITIONAL NOTES	MICROSCOPIC VIEW
Paroxysmal Nocturnal Hemoglobinuria (PNH)	Acquired; RBC becomes sensitive to complement mediated hemolysis.	Hemosiderinuria; mild reticulocytosis; peripheral blood picture looks like iron deficiency. Increased hemolysis with iron therapy.		LAP score increased Sugar water or Ham's testing for confirmation Positive urine hemosiderin	✳
Paroxysmal Cold Hemoglobinuria (PCH)	Autohemolysin that is attached to RBC in cold and hemolyzes when warmed; common in syphilis; associated with viral disorders in children such as measles, mumps, chickenpox.	↑ Gamma globulin, ± cryoglobulin, DAT+ during attack	IgG with anti-P specificity	Donath-Landsteiner antibody	✳
Toxic Chemicals and Drugs (Immune)	Drug-RBC complex forms hapten-like substance (penicillin). Drug-antibody complex forms that binds complement and attaches to RBC activating complement and causing hemolysis (quinidine). Drug induces IgG autoantibody, which often has specificity to Rh antigen on RBC seen with some hypertensive drugs.	DAT+	Complement dependent	Nonimmune hemolysis caused by heavy metal poisoning (lead)	◆

DAT, direct antiglobulin test; FDP, fibrin (ogen) degradation products; FSP, fibrin (ogen) split products; DIC, disseminated intravascular coagulation; LAP, leukocyte alkaline phosphatase.

✳ Photomicrographs from Carr J, Rodak BF: Atlas of Clinical Hematology. Philadelphia, WB Saunders, 1998.
◆ Photomicrographs from Rodak BF: Diagnostic Hematology. Philadelphia, WB Saunders, 1995.

EVALUATION OF HEMOLYTIC ANEMIA

Hematology Testing

▌ Complete blood count: check for spherocytes, shistocytes, sickle cells, target cells, evidence of infection or leukemias, malarial parasites.

▌ Reticulocyte count: increased production of RBCs

Urine Testing

▌ Urobilinogen

▌ Urobilin

▌ Urine hemosiderin

Special Testing

▌ Plasma hemoglobin

▌ Bilirubin fractionation (direct, indirect)

▌ Direct antiglobulin test (DAT)

If Hereditary or Congenital Anemia Is Suspected

▌ Osmotic fragility

▌ Autohemolysis test

▌ Glucose-6-phosphate dehydrogenase (G6PD)

▌ Glutathione stability

▌ Hemoglobin electrophoresis and hemoglobin F

▌ Heat stability

▌ Heinz body stain

Suggested Testing if Autoimmune Process is Suspected

▌ Direct and indirect Coombs' test using polyvalent IgG and C′ sera

▌ Cold agglutinins and hemolysins

▌ Antibody elutions from patient's cells

▌ Donath-Landsteiner test for paroxysmal cold hemoglobinuria (PCH)

▌ Ham's test, sucrose hemolysis test for paroxysmal nocturnal hemoglobinuria (PNH)

▌ Serum protein electrophoresis and immunoelectrophoresis or immunofixation

▌ Rapid plasma reagin (RPR) or Venereal Disease Research Laboratory (VDRL) test to rule out syphilis

HEMOLYTIC ANEMIAS

HEMOGLOBINOPATHIES

In normal circumstances the hemoglobin molecule is composed of a tetramer of globin chains. Normal hemoglobin, hemoglobin A (HgbA$_1$), is composed of two α chains and two β chains (α$_2$β$_2$), and this constitutes over 90% of normal hemoglobin. The remainder is composed of approximately 5% HgbA$_{2c}$ and usually less than 1% HgbF. There are many hemoglobin variants, some of which can cause severe anemias. Originally when hemoglobin variants were discovered, they were given the next letter in sequence; however, when Q was reached, it was decided that any additional variants would be named for the place in which they were discovered, such as Hgb Kansas.

Normal Hemoglobin

HEMOGLOBIN TYPE	STRUCTURE	HEMOGLOBIN PRESENT
Adult		
A$_1$	α$_2$β$_2$	>95%
A$_2$	α$_2$δ$_2$	<3.5%
F	α$_2$γ$_2$	<1%–2%
Birth		
F	α$_2$γ$_2$	60%–90%
A	α$_2$β$_2$	10%–40%

Summary of Hemoglobinopathies

Hgb TYPE	STRUCTURE	HEMOGLOBIN ELECTROPHORESIS	CLINICAL MANIFESTATIONS	LABORATORY FINDINGS
Sickle Cell Trait (S/A)	$\alpha_2\beta^A\beta^S$	A: >50% S: <50% A_2: varies F: N	Can develop severe hematuria; otherwise normal Can develop fixed urine SG of 1.010 due to renal damage	N RBCs, Hgb, Hct N MCV, MCHC N reticulocytes Normal morphology Sickle screen positive (dithionite)
Sickle Cell Disease (S/S)	$\alpha_2\beta^S\beta^S$	A: 0% S: 80%–90% A_2: variable F: variable	Severe hemolytic anemia throughout life. Vascular occlusive crises due to blockage. Organ damage, cerebral vascular accidents, acute chest syndrome. In older patients organ damage becomes apparent, variable organs affected.	Dec RBCs, Hgb, Hct N MCV, MCHC Inc reticulocytes Peripheral blood shows marked drepanocytes; NRBCs; RBC inclusions; Howell-Jolly bodies; Pappenheimer bodies
SC Disease	$\alpha_2\beta^S\beta^C$	A: 0% S: 47% C: 47% F: variable	Vascular occlusive crises, increased risk of ischemic attacks marked splenomegaly	Dec RBCs, Hgb, Hct N MCV, MCHC Inc reticulocytes
Sickle-β^0 Thalassemia	$\alpha_2\beta^S\beta^0$	A: 0% S: 70%–90% F: 1%–30% A_2: 4%	Milder manifestation than sickle cell disease	Dec RBCs, Hgb, Hct N–Inc MCV, MCHC Inc reticulocytes Drepanocytes, target cells, microcytes
Sickle-β^+ Thalassemia	$\alpha_2\beta^S\beta^+$	A: <50% S: >50% A_2: variable F: variable	Mild anemia	Dec RBCs, Hgb, Hct Dec MCV, MCHC Dec reticulocytes Drepanocytes, microcytes
Hgb C Disease	$\alpha_2\beta^C\beta^C$	A: 0% C: >90% A_2: varies F: N	Homozygous condition relatively mild disorder	Dec RBCs, Hgb, Hct N MCV, MCHC Inc reticulocytes Target cells, small distorted folded cells, Hgb C crystals
Hgb C Trait	$\alpha_2\beta^A\beta^C$	A: >50% C: <40% F: N	No clinical manifestations in heterozygote	N RBCs, Hgb, Hct N MCV, MCHC N reticulocytes Peripheral blood normal; may be a rare target cell

HEMOGLOBINOPATHIES

Continued ▶

► Continued **Summary of Hemoglobinopathies**

Hgb TYPE	STRUCTURE	HEMOGLOBIN ELECTROPHORESIS	CLINICAL MANIFESTATIONS	LABORATORY FINDINGS
Hgb D	$\alpha_2\beta^D_2$	D: 95% Trait: equal amount of A and D	Asymptomatic	N–Dec RBCs, Hgb, Hct N MCV, MCHC N–Inc reticulocytes Peripheral blood normal with a few target cells
Hgb E	$\alpha_2\beta^E_2$	E: 90%–95% Trait: equal amount of A and E	Asymptomatic	N–Inc RBCs, Hgb, Hct Dec MCV, MCHC N reticulocytes Target cells, microcytes, hypochromic cells
Thalassemia Major	$\alpha_2\beta^0\beta^0$ $\alpha_2\beta^+\beta^+$	A: 0% F: ↑ A_2: ↑ A_2: <F	Presents in 1st year of life with severe anemia, jaundice, and failure to thrive Survival dependent on transfusion	Dec RBCs, Hgb, Hct Dec MCV, MCHC Reticulocytes vary Marked anisocytosis, poikilocytosis, target cells, schistocytes, ovalocytes, NRBCs, basophilic stippling
Thalassemia Minor	$\alpha_2\beta\beta^0$ $\alpha_2\beta\beta^+$	A: ↓ F: N to ↑ A_2: ↑ A_2: >F	Mild microcytic-hypochromic anemia Usually asymptomatic except during pregnancy and infection	Inc RBCs N–Dec Hgb, Hct Dec MCV, MCHC Inc reticulocytes Microcytes, target cells, hypochromic cells, basophilic stippling
Hgb H Disease	$--/+\alpha$	Newborn: Bart's >5% Adult: Hgb H 40%–50%	Mild to moderate anemia that becomes worse with infections and pregnancy. Hemolytic crisis may occur.	Dec RBCs, Hgb, Hct Dec MCV, MCHC Inc reticulocytes Microcytes, hypochromic cells, target cells, basophilic stippling
α Thalassemia Trait	$-\alpha/-\alpha$ $--/\alpha\alpha$	Newborn: Hgb Bart's Adult: N or rarely Hgb H	Minimal amount of anemia	N–Dec RBCs, Hgb, Hct Dec MCV, MCHC N–Inc reticulocytes Normal to slight microcytic cells, some hypochromic cells, basophilic stippling

N, normal; Inc, increased; Dec, decreased; NRBC, nucleated red blood cell; SG, specific gravity.

MORPHOLOGIC MANIFESTATIONS OF THE HEMOGLOBINOPATHIES

DISORDER	SICKLE CELL DISEASE	Hgb C
Microscopic View		
	SC DISEASE	**THALASSEMIA MAJOR**
Microscopic View		
	THALASSEMIA MINOR	
Microscopic View		

Photomicrographs from Carr J, Rodak BF: Atlas of Clinical Hematology. Philadelphia, WB Saunders, 1998.

HEMOGLOBINOPATHIES

Thalassemia Syndromes

Thalassemia syndromes appear primarily in individuals of Mediterranean descent. These syndromes result from varied degrees of impairment of the synthesis of the polypeptide chains that form the hemoglobin molecule. Characteristics of all thalassemia syndromes are:

1. *Impaired Hemoglobin Synthesis.* This results in the characteristic morphology, codocytes, microcytes, ovalocytes, and basophilic stippling.
2. *Imbalance in the Production of Globin Chains.* This results in the formation of tetramers of single chains either in solution (Hgb Bart's, HgbH) or as α_4 precipitates causing rapid RBC destruction. It also leads to elevated levels of $HgbA_2$, HgbF, or both in β thalassemia syndromes.

α **THALASSEMIAS.** For the most part, α thalassemias result from an α gene deletion. Normal cells contain four genes; deletion of a single gene produces no clinical manifestations, and deletion of all four produces a stillbirth (hydrops fetalis syndrome). This is due to a α_4 tetramer that has a great avidity for O_2 and thus does not act as an effective transport medium. The thalassemia syndromes seen in living individuals are as follows.

α **Thalassemia Trait.** This is due to the deletion of two genes either on the same gene or on two genes. Clinically this produces a slightly reduced hemoglobin level and a slight increase in RBCs. Microcytes are also found. There are no other measurable manifestations; hemoglobin is present, however not in demonstrable quantities.

β **THALASSEMIAS.** β Thalassemia is a condition caused by the deletion or mutation of the gene(s) that code for the β chain of the hemoglobin molecule. The deletion or mutation can occur in the β gene only or in β gene and the δ gene or in the β, δ, and $^A\gamma$ genes. Most of the β thalassemias are the result of a single nucleotide deletion or substitution that causes either faulty transcription, processing, or transport of the β chain mRNA. The mutation may impair or totally supress β chain synthesis (β^+ thalassemia or $\beta^\emptyset$ thalassemia)

POLYCYTHEMIA

The term *polycythemia* means an increase in erythropoiesis. The number of RBCs, the hemoglobin level, and the hematocrit are increased. There are three groups of polycythemia, which include polycythemia vera, or primary; absolute polycythemia, or secondary; and relative.

Polycythemia rubra vera (primary erythrocytosis) is an absolute increase in all cell types, RBCs, white blood cells (WBCs), and platelets. This condition occurs primarily in middle age and is characterized by erythrocytosis and an elevated hemoglobin level, sometimes greater than 20 g/dL. This erythrocytosis is not dependent on erythropoietin levels. The bone marrow is hyperplastic with all cell lines showing hyperplasia. The disease is chronic, and many of the victims die of cardiac and thrombotic disease. Those who survive often develop myelofibrosis with myeloid metaplasia or granulocytic leukemia.

Secondary erythrocytosis is an erythropoietin mediated increase in RBCs and hemoglobin due primarily to a hypoxic situation. This condition is remedied by solving the reason for the hypoxia. Disorders that can effect secondary erythrocytosis are various tumors, anabolic steroids, and renal disorders such as cystic disease, hydronephrosis, and adrenal cortical hypersecretion.

Relative polycythemia is caused by a decrease in plasma volume while the RBC mass remains unchanged. Most often this condition is caused by dehydration or hemoconcentration or a condition known as Gaisböck's syndrome (pseudopolycythemia or stress erythrocytosis).

Summary of Polycythemia

DISORDER	CAUSE	CLINICAL FEATURES	LABORATORY FINDINGS	BONE MARROW	ADDITIONAL TESTING
Polycythemia Vera (Primary)	Myeloproliferative disorder in which all three cellular elements are increased	40–60 yr age group Splenomegaly Cerebral circulatory disturbances Vascular complications Thrombotic complications	Inc RBC, Hgb, Hct Normal MCV, MCH Neutrophilia Platelets normal to increased	All three cell lines increased Panhyperplasia	Red cell mass increased pO_2 normal Erythropoietin normal LAP increased
Absolute Polycythemia (Secondary)	Physiologic response to need for more production of RBCs due to increased need for oxygen, pulmonary disorder, or inappropriate increase in erythropoietin	Cyanosis Heart or lung disease Normal spleen size	Inc RBC, Hgb, Hct Normal MCV, MCH WBCs normal Platelets normal	Erythroid hyperplasia	Red cell mass increased pO_2 decreased Erythropoietin increased LAP normal
Relative Polycythemia	Caused by dehydration, decrease in plasma volume	Benign course Nonspecific symptoms such as headache, nausea, and dyspepsia	Inc RBC, Hgb, Hct WBCs normal Platelets normal	Normal	Red cell mass decreased Plasma volume decreased

POLYCYTHEMIA

QUICK REFERENCE TO ERYTHROCYTE DISORDERS

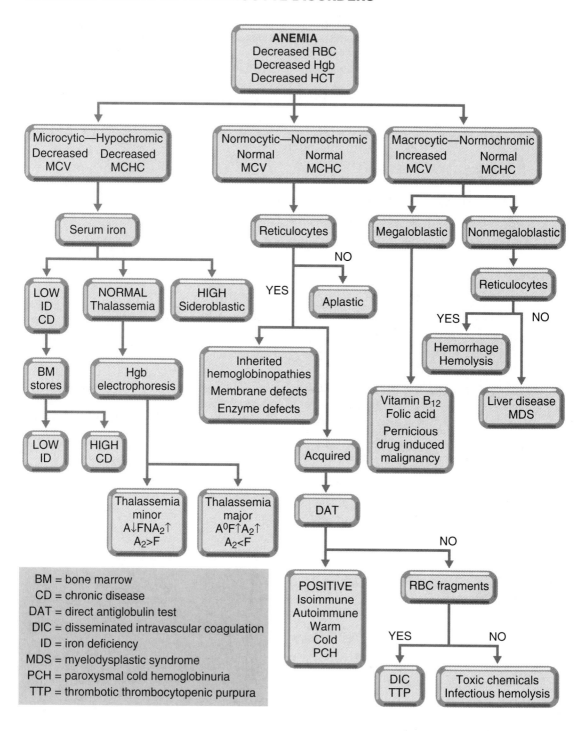

QUICK REFERENCE TO ERYTHROCYTE DISORDERS

DISORDER	LABORATORY FINDINGS	INDICES	ETIOLOGY	SMEAR MORPHOLOGY	DIAGNOSTIC TESTS
Normocytic–Normochromic Anemia	Hgb ↓, Hct normal	MCV 85–100 fL MCHC 31–35 g/dL RDW < 14.5%	Acute blood loss	Normal	CBC, peripheral smear
Hemolytic Anemia	Hgb ↓, Haptoglobin ↓, bilirubin ↑	MCV ↑ MCHC N or ↑ RDW ↑	Extrinsic: burn transfusion reaction, parasitemia	Microspherocytes, spherocytes, schistocytes	CBC, peripheral smear, haptoglobin, liver profile
			Intrinsic: hemoglobinopathy, enzyme deficiency, membrane defects, autoimmune	Elliptocytes, spherocytes, stomatocytes, codocytes, depranocytes,	Hgb electrophoresis, HgbF, HgbA₂, HgbH inclusions, Hgb s solubility, Heinz body stain, unstable Hgb screen, G6PD screen, osmotic fragility, Ham's test
Macrocytic Anemia	↑ MCV, ↑ MCH, normal or ↓ MCHC	MCV >100 fL MCH >32 pg MCHC 32–36 g/dL	B₁₂, folate deficiency; enzyme abnormality, etc.	Oval macrocytes, hypersegmented neutrophils	B₁₂, folate, bone marrow, metabolic assays
Microcytic–Hypochromic Anemia	↓ MCV, ↓ or normal MCH, ↓ or normal MCHC	MCV <76 fL	Iron deficiency, thalassemia	Microcytic hypochromic RBCs, cigar shaped cells, occasional target cell	CBC, peripheral smear, iron, TIBC, ferritin, Hgb electrophoresis, bone marrow iron
Sideroblastic Anemia	MCV variable, RDW ↑		Congenital or drug induced, malabsorption, hematopoietic malignancies	Normocytic as well as microcytic hypochromic RBCs, occasional macrocyte	Bone marrow aspirate, iron, TIBC
Anemia of Chronic Disease	Hgb ↓, MCV normal		Rheumatoid arthritis, Collagen vascular diseases, generalized inflammatory conditions	Normal or microcytic hypochromic RBCs	Iron, ESR, TIBC, bone marrow iron

Continued ▲

▶ Continued **QUICK REFERENCE TO ERYTHROCYTE DISORDERS**

DISORDER	LABORATORY FINDINGS	INDICES	ETIOLOGY	SMEAR MORPHOLOGY	DIAGNOSTIC TESTS
Aplastic Anemia	All ↓	MCV ↑, MCH normal, MCHC normal	Exposure to chemicals, ionizing radiation, idiopathic (no known cause), viral hepatitis	Normal or slightly macrocytic	CBC, reticulocyte count, bone marrow aspiration
α Thalassemia Trait	Hgb ↓ or normal, MCV ↓, slight RBC ↑	↓ MCV	Double gene deletion	Microcytes, hypochromia	CBC, Hgb electrophoresis
α Thalassemia Disease (HgbH Disease)	↓ Hgb, ↓MCV, ↑ bilirubin, ↑ HgbH	↓ MCV	Three gene deletion	Target cells, ovalocytes, microcytes, HgbH inclusions in RBCs	Hgb electrophoresis
β Thalassemia in Heterozygotes	↓ Hgb, ↓ MCV, sl ↑ RBC, ↑ HgbA$_2$, sl ↑ HgbF	↓ MCV	β Gene deletion, either alone or in conjunction with δ gene or the δ and ^{A}γ gene	Microcytes, target cells, elliptocytes, basophilic stippling	CBC, Hgb electrophoresis, ferritin, serum iron, TIBC
β Thalassemia in Homozygotes	↓ Hgb (to 3 g/dL), ↓ MCV, ↑ HgbF, sl ↑ HgbA$_2$, ↑ Fe, ↓ TIBC	↓ MCV	β Gene deletion, either alone or in conjunction with δ gene or the δ and ^{A}γ gene	Marked hypochromia with polychromatic rims, bizarre morphology, target cells, ovalocytes, basophilic stippling, HgbH crystals	CBC, Hgb electrophoresis, ferritin, serum iron, TIBC
Polycythemia Rubra Vera	↑ Hgb, ↑ RBC, ↑ LAP, ↑ WBC, ↑ platelets	Normal	Bone marrow hyperplasia due possibly to chemical or radiation exposure	Normal, increased cellularity	CBC, bone marrow biopsy, ^{51}Cr RBC survival, LAP

BIBLIOGRAPHY

Beck WS: Hematopoiesis and Introduction to Anemia, Hematology, 4th ed. Cambridge, MIT Press, 1987.

Brown B: Hematology: Principles and Procedures, 6th ed. Philadelphia, Lea & Febiger, 1993.

Dutcher T: Hematology Morphology Workshop, American Society of Clinical Pathologists, Associate Member Section, 1992.

Elghetant M, Davey F: Erythrocytic disorders. In Henry JB, ed: Clinical Diagnosis and Management by Laboratory Methods, 19th ed. Philadelphia, WB Saunders, 1996.

Harmening D: Clinical Hematology and Fundamentals of Hemostasis, 3rd ed. Philadelphia, FA Davis, 1997.

Heckner F, Lehmann HP, Kao YS: Practical Microscopic Hematology, 3rd ed. Baltimore, Urban & Schwarzenberg, 1988.

Kjeldsberg C: Anemias, Hematologic Disorders. Chicago, American Society of Clinical Pathologists Press, 1989.

Kjeldsberg C, Foucar K, et al: Practical Diagnosis of Hematologic Disorders, 2nd ed. Chicago, American Society of Clinical Pathologists Press, 1995.

Lopspeich-Steininger C: Clinical Hematology. Philadelphia, JB Lippincott, 1992.

McGhee D, Payne M: Hemoglobinopathies and hemoglobin defects. In Rodak BF, ed: Diagnostic Hematology. Philadelphia, WB Saunders, 1995.

McKenzie S: Textbook of Hematology, 2nd ed. Baltimore, Williams & Wilkins, 1996.

O'Connor B: A Color Atlas and Instruction Manual of Peripheral Blood Cell Morphology. Baltimore, Williams & Wilkins, 1984.

Pereira I: Peripheral Smears: The Primary Diagnostic Tool I and II Workshop. American Society of Clinical Pathologists, Associate Member Section, Philadelphia, 1995.

Raphael SS: Principles of Hematology, Lynch's Medical Laboratory Technology, 4th ed. Philadelphia, WB Saunders, 1983.

Rodak B, ed: Diagnostic Hematology. Philadelphia, WB Saunders, 1995.

Sommer SR, Maedel L: Red Cell Disorders: A Review and Update Workshop. American Society of Clinical Pathologists, Associate Member Section, 1994.

Chapter *37*

LEUKOCYTE DISORDERS

Kathleen Finnegan, MS, MT(ASCP)SH

QUICK CONTENTS

INTRODUCTION

The white blood cells, or leukocytes, play a very important role in the defense against infection; they defend by phagocytosis or by the production of antibodies for the immune response. Various types of leukocytes serve many different functions as previously discussed (Chapter 35). A decrease or increase in either number or function can cause a change in the body's ability to combat infection and disease.

The total white count, or *WBC*, and *differential* are very important tests in diagnosis, treatment, and prognosis of disease. The total normal white cell count ranges from 4.0 to 11.0 × 10^9/L but varies with age, race, and geographic location. Many things can cause a variation in the white cell count. Examples of conditions resulting in an increase in WBC are infections, prolonged exercise, stress, drugs, or a malignant disorder. Examples of conditions resulting in a decrease in WBC are viral infections, drugs, bone marrow depression, radiation, and malignant disorders. The total white cell count of the peripheral blood cells is differentiated into five types of cells, which include the neutrophil, eosinophil, basophil, monocyte, and lymphocyte. The differential count when expressed as a percentage of the total white cell count is referred to as the *relative number*. The *absolute number* is obtained by multiplying the percentage by the total white cell count. For accurate interpretation of an increase or decrease in a particular cell line, the absolute concentration should be determined.

NON-NEOPLASTIC DISORDERS

Non-neoplastic disorders can be acquired or inherited. These disorders do not have characteristics of malignancy. Acquired disorders are associated with different conditions that mostly are quantitative, involving an increase or decrease in white cell numbers but with normal function and morphology. The inherited abnormalities are more often qualitative disorders with abnormal nuclear and cytoplasmic morphologic characteristics.

Quantitative disorders of the leukocyte are termed *leukocytosis*, an increase in the number of white blood cells greater than 11,000/μL, or *leukopenia*, a decrease in the number of cells to less than 4000/μL. Primary factors affecting a white cell count are the rate of flow of cells from the bone marrow, the proportion of cells in the marginal and circulating pools, the rate of cells leaving the peripheral blood, and/or increased cell loss.

Qualitative disorders of white blood cells include functional, structural, or morphologic abnormalities in the cytoplasm and nucleus. These disorders tend to be less common than the acquired disorders.

QUANTITATIVE LEUKOCYTE DISORDERS

Terms Associated with Quantitative White Blood Cell Disorders

TERM	LABORATORY CORRELATIONS
Neutrophilia	Absolute concentration of neutrophils is $>7.0 \times 10^9$/L.
Leukemoid Reaction	Extreme neutrophilic reaction to severe stimulation of the neutrophil. For example, severe infection. White cell count is $>30.0 \times 10^9$/L with shift to left (increase of younger cells). It is temporary and sometimes confused with chronic myelogenous leukemia.
Neutropenia	Absolute concentration of neutrophil count is $<2.0 \times 10^9$/L in whites and 1.3×10^9/L in blacks.
Agranulocytosis	Severe neutropenia with eosinopenia and basopenia. Neutrophil count is $<0.5 \times 10^9$/L. It is a decrease of all granulocytes.
Eosinophilia	Absolute concentration of eosinophil is $>0.45 \times 10^9$/L. Usually associated with allergic or parasitic reaction.
Eosinopenia	Decrease in eosinophil, difficult to establish because of low numbers normally found.
Basophilia	Absolute concentration of basophils is $>0.5 \times 10^9$/L.
Basopenia	Decrease in basophils; difficult to establish because of low numbers normally found.
Monocytosis	Absolute monocyte count is $>0.8 \times 10^9$/L.
Monocytopenia	Absolute monocyte count is $<0.2 \times 10^9$/L.
Lymphocytosis	Absolute lymphocyte count is $>4.0 \times 10^9$/L in adults and 9.0×10^9/L in children.
Lymphocytopenia	Absolute lymphocyte count is $<1.5 \times 10^9$/L in adults and $<2.0 \times 10^9$/L in children.

There are many causes of an increase or decrease in the number of white blood cells. The following chart is a summary of these causes.

Causes of an Increase or Decrease in Leukocytes

NEUTROPHILIA

Cause	Example
Infection	Bacterial, fungal, viral
Inflammation	Tissue damage, MI, trauma, surgery, hypersensitivity, stress, pregnancy
Physiologic	Exercise
Drug	Corticosteroids, toxins
Hematologic	Hemorrhage, myeloproliferative

NEUTROPENIA

Cause	Example
Infection	Bacterial, viral, rickettsial, protozoan
Physical Agents	Radiation, chemicals, drugs, antibiotics
Hematologic	Aplastic anemia, pernicious anemia, MDS, bone marrow replacement
Immune Mediated	Lupus erythematosus, rheumatoid arthritis

EOSINOPHILIA

Cause	Example
Allergic Reactions	Hay fever, asthma, drugs
Parasites	Tapeworm, intestinal, malaria, toxins
Skin Disease	Dermatitis
Hematologic Malignancies	Myeloproliferative, lymphoma, leukemia
Infection	Tuberculosis, recovery phase from acute infection

BASOPHILIA

Cause	Example
Inflammation	Infection, varicella, variola
Hematologic	CML, myeloproliferative, Hodgkin's
Allergic Reactions	Hypersensitivity reactions
Hypothyroidism	Antithyroid therapy

MONOCYTOSIS

Cause	Example
Infections	Tuberculosis, subacute bacterial endocarditis, rickettsia
Hematologic Disease	Chronic myeloproliferative, MDS, Hodgkin's, lymphoma, histiocytosis
Miscellaneous	Recovery from acute infection, radiation therapy, lipid storage disorders, malignancies, collagen vascular disorders

MONOCYTOPENIA

Cause	Example
Hematologic Disease	Hairy cell leukemia
Therapy Related	Corticosteroids

LYMPHOCYTOSIS

Cause	Example
Acute Viral Infections	Infectious mononucleosis, CMV, hepatitis, infectious lymphocytosis, viral hepatitis
Chronic Infection	Brucellosis, tuberculosis, syphilis
Hematologic Disorders	ALL, CLL, lymphoma, hairy cell, Sézary
Miscellaneous	Toxins, drug sensitivity, autoimmune, dermatitis, graft rejection

LYMPHOCYTOPENIA

Cause	Example
Inherited Immunodeficiencies	SCID, DiGeorge's Burton's, Wiskott-Aldrich
Acquired Immunodeficiency	AIDS
Increased Destruction	Corticosteroids radiation therapy, cytotoxic agents
Miscellaneous	Bone marrow aplasia, renal failure, sarcoidosis, collagen vascular disorders

MI, myocardial infarction; MDS, myelodysplastic syndrome; CML, chronic myelogenous leukemia; CMV, cytomegalovirus; ALL, acute lymphocytic leukemia: CLL, chronic lymphocytic leukemia: AIDS, acquired immunodeficiency syndrome; SCID, severe combined immunodeficiency syndrome.

INHERITED QUALITATIVE DISORDERS

The inherited disorders of white blood cells can have functional or morphologic abnormalities. The abnormalities of the neutrophil can be seen in the cytoplasm, the granules, or the nucleus. Most are rare, and the patients suffer from recurrent infection, delayed wound healing, and/or abscess.

Inherited Abnormalities of the Neutrophil

DISORDER	MORPHOLOGY	OTHER BLOOD ABNORMALITIES	INHERITANCE	DEFECT	OTHER FINDINGS	MICROSCOPIC VIEW
Alder-Reilly	Large azurophilic granulation in cytoplasm	Also found in eosinophil, lymphocyte, basophil, and monocyte	Autosomal recessive	Incomplete breakdown of mucopolysaccharides due to enzyme deficiency	May be associated with mucopolysaccharide disorders, Hurler's and Hunter's syndrome	✳
Chédiak-Higashi	Giant lysosomes that stain gray–green in neutrophils and monocytes Pink in lymphocytes	Neutropenia Thrombocytopenia Inclusions also seen in lymphocytes	Autosomal recessive	Defective locomotion and chemotaxis Fusion of primary and secondary granules	Frequent pyogenic infections Death at early age Albinism, silver hair, photophobia Bleeding tendencies Abnormal platelet aggregation	◆
Chronic Granulomatous Disease	Appear normal	Monocytosis may be present	Sex linked or autosomal recessive	Defective enzyme activation of membrane oxidase for killing bacteria	Recurrent infections with low grade pathogens NBT test useful	
Leukocyte Adhesion Deficiency	Appear normal	Increased leukocytosis due to stimulation of bone marrow	Autosomal recessive	Absence of leukocyte adhesion proteins for proper adhesion for chemotaxis	Frequent bacterial and fungal infections Lack of pus formation and poor wound healing	

Continued ▲

▶ Continued **Inherited Abnormalities of the Neutrophil**

DISORDER	MORPHOLOGY	OTHER BLOOD ABNORMALITIES	INHERITANCE	DEFECT	OTHER FINDINGS	MICROSCOPIC VIEW
May-Hegglin	Large blue cytoplasmic granules (resemble Döhle bodies)	Thrombocytopenia, large platelets Neutropenia variable	Autosomal dominant	Alterations in amount of RNA	Tend to have bleeding problems	◆
Myeloperoxidase Deficiency	Appear normal	NA	Autosomal recessive	Absence of myeloperoxidase	Increased bacterial and fungal infection due to lack of killing mobility	
Pelger-Huët	Bilobed or hyposegmented nucleus	NA	Autosomal dominant	Nucleus does not segment Cell function of neutrophils normal	Confused with bands *Note:* Pseudo–Pelger-Huët associated with some leukemias and MDS	◆

* Photomicrographs from Henry JB: Clinical Diagnosis and Management by Laboratory Methods, 19th ed. Philadelphia, WB Saunders, 1996.
◆ Photomicrographs from Carr J, Rodak BF: Atlas of Clinical Hematology. Philadelphia, WB Saunders, 1998.
NBT, nitroblue tetrazolium; NA, not applicable; RNA, ribonucleic acid; MDS, myelodysplastic syndrome.

INHERITED QUALITATIVE DISORDERS

QUALITATIVE MONOCYTE OR MACROPHAGE DISORDERS

The macrophage function is the breakdown of cellular debris by enzymatic degradation. When the macrophage is unable to digest the phagocytic material because of a particular enzyme deficiency for this process, the undigested material accumulates within the cell. These disorders are also called the *lipid storage disorders.* Some of these disorders have a distinct looking macrophage that may be found in the bone marrow.

Abnormalities of the Macrophage

DISORDER	MORPHOLOGY	OTHER ABNORMAL BLOOD FINDINGS	DEFECT	INHERITANCE	GENERAL COMMENTS	MICROSCOPIC VIEW
Gaucher	Gaucher cells: irregular shape round to oval 20–70 μm Cytoplasm large with fine folding wrinkles PAS and Sudan black positive	N/N anemia Thrombocytopenia Leukopenia Look for Gaucher cell in bone marrow. Other organs involved: spleen, liver, and lymph nodes	Deficiency in β-glucocerebrosidase with accumulation of unmetabolized glucocerebroside	Autosomal recessive	Ashkenazi Jews Hepatosplenomegaly Skin pigmentations Bone lesions Mental retardation Three types	*
Niemann-Pick	Foam cell: 20–90 μm with small nucleus often eccentrically placed Cytoplasm: foamy vacuoles Sudan black and oil red O positive, PAS negative	Microcytic anemia Thrombocytopenia Leukocyte count variable Cells found in bone marrow and lymph tissue	Deficiency of sphingomyelinase with accumulation of unmetabolized lipid and sphingomyelin	Autosomal recessive	Ashkenazi Jews Hepatosplenomegaly Skin pigmentations Bone lesions Mental retardation	*
Tay-Sachs	Foam cells may be seen in peripheral blood; not diagnostic Bone marrow negative Oil red O and Sudan black positive	Vacuolated lymphocytes Spleen liver and lymph nodes not enlarged	Deficiency of β-hexosamidase with accumulation of gangliosides (GM2), glycolipids, mucopolysaccharides	Autosomal recessive	Ashkenazi Jews Central nervous system involvement Cherry red macula in eye Mental retardation	*
Sea Blue Histiocyte	Large cells 10–60 μm with densely stained nucleus Cytoplasm contains granules, stains blue-green with Wright's stain, Sudan black and PAS positive	Can be found in liver, spleen, and bone marrow	Enzyme unknown but accumulation of lipids containing cerebroside, and carbohydrates	Autosomal recessive	Hepatomegaly Neurologic abnormalities Skin pigmentation	*

* Photomicrographs from Carr J, Rodak BF: Atlas of Clinical Hematology. Philadelphia, WB Saunders, 1998.
PAS, periodic acid–Schiff; N/N, normocytic/normochromic.

QUALITATIVE MONOCYTE OR MACROPHAGE DISORDERS

NONMALIGNANT LYMPHOCYTE DISORDERS

Nonmalignant lymphocyte disorders can be acquired, which involve a reactive change in the lymphocyte, or congenital, which affect either the B or T lymphocyte or both. In the acquired disorders the disease is self-limiting with an increase in the relative and absolute lymphocyte count and with striking lymphocyte morphology known as the *reactive lymphocyte*. The congenital disorders involve a low to normal lymphocyte count with normal morphology.

Acquired Quantitative Disorders

DISORDER	ETIOLOGY	CLINICAL FINDINGS	PERIPHERAL FINDINGS	BONE MARROW	LABORATORY TESTS	MICROSCOPIC VIEW
Infectious Mononucleosis	Epstein-Barr virus Transmission: oral through saliva most common method	Age: young adult (14–24 yr) Symptoms: malaise, sore throat, fever, chills, headache, lymphadenopathy Splenomegaly 50%–75% Hepatomegaly 25%	Leukocytosis 12,000–25,000/µL Relative and absolute lymphocytosis Variety of reactive lymphocytes Platelet count mild decrease	Not indicated	Serologic testing Heterophil antibody positive Monospot positive Antibody to EBV positive EBNA positive	 *
Toxoplasmosis	*Toxoplasma gondii* Transmission: cat feces or poorly cooked meat Can pass through placenta	Acquired or congenital Can multiply in all body cells except RBCs Symptoms: asymptomatic or symptoms similar to those of IM	Leukocytosis Relative and absolute lymphocytosis Reactive lymphocytes	Not indicated	Heterophil titer negative Confirmation of rising titer of toxoplasmosis antibodies	 *
Cytomegalovirus	Herpes group virus Transmission: venereal Can pass through placenta	Acquired or congenital Symptoms: fever and malaise No pharyngitis Occasionally splenomegaly	Leukocytosis and absolute lymphocytosis Reactive lymphocytes	Not indicated	Heterophil titer negative Disease confirmed by rise in titer of cytomegalovirus titer	 *
Infectious Lymphocytosis	Unknown	Occurs in young children Symptoms: diarrhea, gastrointestinal distress, respiratory infection, and fever	Leukocyte count: 40,000–50,000/µL 60%–70% small normal lymphocytes Primarily T lymphocytes small with scant cytoplasm Eosinophilia	Not indicated	Antibody and viral studies	 †

NONMALIGNANT LYMPHOCYTE DISORDERS

Continued ▶

▶ Continued **Acquired Quantitative Disorders**

DISORDER	ETIOLOGY	CLINICAL FINDINGS	PERIPHERAL FINDINGS	BONE MARROW	LABORATORY TESTS	MICROSCOPIC VIEW
Bordetella Pertussis (Whooping Cough)	*Bordetella* pertussis	Age: young children who have not been immunized. Symptoms: severe coughing. Respiratory tract involvement	Leukocyte count: 25,000–50,000/µL. Lymphs are small with folded nuclei with less condensed chromatin	Not indicated	Culture of nasal swab, identification for bacteria	
Lymphocytic Leukemoid Reaction	Associated with whooping cough, chickenpox, TB	Age: young. Splenomegaly absent	High WBC with increase in lymphocyte count. Reactive or immature looking lymphocytes	Minimal if any increase in lymphocytes		
Plasmacytosis	Stimulation of immune system. Seen in intense viral or bacterial infections	Seen in chronic infections, allergic reactions, viral, and bacterial	Increased plasma cells peripherally along with increase of monocytes, eosinophils, and lymphocytes	1%–2% normal amount found; increased beyond 4% is significant		

* Photomicrographs from Carr J, Rodak BF: Atlas of Clinical Hematology. Philadelphia, WB Saunders, 1998.
† Photomicrograph from Rodak BF: Diagnostic Hematology. Philadelphia, W.B. Saunders. 1995
◆ Photomicrograph from Henry JB: Clinical Diagnosis and Management by Laboratory Methods, 19th ed. Philadelphia, WB Saunders, 1996.
IM, infectious mononucleosis; EBV, Epstein-Barr virus; EBNA, Epstein-Barr nuclear antigen; TB, tuberculosis; RBC, red blood cells.

Acquired Qualitative Disorders

Acquired defects in either T or B lymphocyte can result in serious clinical manifestations. Acquired immunodeficiency syndrome (AIDS) is a progressively fatal infectious disorder. The cause of the disorder is the direct cytopathic effect of the human immunodeficiency virus (HIV) or the retrovirus HIV-1. This disorder involves the T lymphocyte. There is a rapid decrease in the number of T helper (CD4) cells that creates an imbalance in T suppressor (CD8) and cytotoxic cells in the blood. Because of this imbalance, a cellular immune depression occurs and these patients are prone to infections with various opportunistic organisms such as *Pneumocystis carinii*. Malignancies (Kaposi's sarcoma), autoimmune disease, and neurologic disorders also occur.

The most common hematologic abnormality seen in AIDS is anemia of chronic disease (which is normochromic-normocytic), leukopenia, lymphocytopenia with a decrease in the CD4/CD8 ratio and with thrombocytopenia. Neutropenia occurs in about 40% of the cases. The peripheral blood smear typically shows reactive lymphocytes. These lymphocytes sometimes have a plasmacytoid appearance.

Congenital Qualitative Disorders

Immunodeficiency disorders can result from defects of function that is required for proper immune response. Depending on the cells or organs affected, many disorders result from defective T or B cell function. These disorders are characterized by a decrease in lymphocytes and impairment of T cell lymphocytes responsible for cell mediated immunity and B cell lymphocytes responsible for humoral immunity. Their clinical features are variable, but all patients suffer from recurrent and persistent infections. Congenital disorders are apparent at birth, and these children usually die of overwhelming infections.

NONMALIGNANT LYMPHOCYTE DISORDERS

CONGENITAL QUALITATIVE DISORDERS

DISORDER	CLINICAL FINDINGS	LABORATORY FINDINGS	IMMUNOGLOBINS	B LYMPHOCYTE	T LYMPHOCYTE	INHERITANCE
SCID	Repeated infection, skin rashes, diarrhea, and failure to thrive	Decreased lymphocyte count Lymph nodes lack plasma cells, B and T lymphocytes Both T and B lymph systems are deficient.	Decreased IgG, IgM, IgA	Decreased or normal	Absence of mature T cells	X-linked, autosomal recessive
Wiskott-Aldrich	Repeated bacterial, viral, and fungal infections, bleeding tendencies	Decreased platelet count Decreased platelet size Increased bleeding time PT and APTT normal Progressive decrease in T lymphocytes	Decreased IgM Increased IgA, IgE Normal IgG	Normal	Progressive decrease	X-linked
DiGeorge's	Repeated yeast, fungal, and viral infections Hypoplasia or nonfunctional thymus	Decreased lymphocyte count Hypocalcemia Decrease in peripheral T lymphocytes	Normal	Normal	Decreased	
X-Linked Agammaglobulinemia	Frequent respiratory and skin infections	Decrease or absence of all immunoglobins Decrease in B lymphocytes and absence of plasma cells in lymph nodes	Decreased IgG, IgM, IgA	Decreased	Normal	X-linked

SCID, severe combined immunodeficiency syndrome; Ig, immunoglobulin; PT, prothrombin time; APTT, activated partial thromboplastin time.

MALIGNANT DISORDERS

Hematopoiesis is a regulated process by which new cells in the bone marrow proliferate and differentiate. When the bone marrow is replaced by mutated hematopoietic stem cells, the control for proliferation and differentiation is compromised, and the result is an unregulated production of cells. Disorders of the hematopoietic bone marrow stem cells are divided into three main categories: (1) myelodysplastic syndrome (MDS), (2) acute leukemia, and (3) myeloproliferative disorders (MPDs). All disorders have an unregulated proliferation of one or more hematopoietic precursors.

MYELODYSPLASTIC SYNDROME

MDSs are a group of hematopoietic stem cell bone marrow disorders with *dysplastic* (abnormal maturation) changes in one or more cell lines. The disease manifests by peripheral blood cytopenias that are refractory to therapy. There are morphologic abnormalities of both peripheral and bone marrow cells. MDS characteristics are peripheral cytopenias, hypercellular marrow with less than 30% blasts, ineffective hematopoiesis, dysplastic red blood cells, and myeloid cells with a decrease in platelets. The platelets are bizarre in size and shape. The diseases may progress to acute leukemia, so they were historically called the *preleukemias* or *smoldering leukemia*. MDS can occur as a primary, secondary, or therapy related disorder. It occurs primarily in men over the age of 50 years.

Presenting symptoms are bone marrow failure, fatigue due to anemia that does not respond to therapy, increased infection due to the decrease in the WBC, and easy bruising and bleeding from the decreased platelet count.

The French-American-British (FAB) classification has subdivided this group of disorders into five groups. This classification is based on the number of blasts in the bone marrow, which is less than 30%, in conjunction with morphologic dysplasia in one or all of three cell lines. They include refractory anemia (RA), refractory anemia with ringed sideroblasts (RARS), refractory anemia with excess blasts (RAEB), refractory anemia with excess blasts in transformation (RAEB-t), and chronic myelomonocytic leukemia (CMML).

FAB Classification of Myelodysplastic Syndrome

DISORDERS	SUBTYPE	PERIPHERAL BLOOD	BONE MARROW	CYTOGENETICS	LEUKEMIC PROGRESSION (%)	MICROSCOPIC VIEW
Refractory Anemia	RA	Mild to severe anemia often macrocytic MCV and RDW increased Macro-ovalocytes Decreased reticulocyte count WBC low to normal <1% blasts Platelets normal to low	Cellularity normal to hypercellular Erythrocytic hyperplasia <5% blasts <15% ringed sideroblasts	5q— +8	12	*
Refractory Anemia with Ringed Sideroblasts	RARS	Dimorphic anemia MCV increased Siderotic granules <1% blasts WBC normal to low Platelets normal to low	Hypercellular <5% blasts >15% ringed sideroblasts	5q— +8	8	*
Refractory Anemia with Excess Blasts	RAEB	Dimorphic anemia Morphologic abnormalities of WBC, RBCs, and platelets Increased monocytes Decreased reticulocyte count Neutropenia Thrombocytopenia	Hypercellular <25% blasts Micromegakaryocytes Morphologic abnormalities of WBCs, RBCs, and platelets	5q— −7 +8	44	*

Continued ▶

▶ Continued **FAB Classification of Myelodysplastic Syndrome**

DISORDERS	SUBTYPE	PERIPHERAL BLOOD	BONE MARROW	CYTOGENETICS	LEUKEMIC PROGRESSION (%)	MICROSCOPIC VIEW
Refractory Anemia with Excess Blasts in Transformation	RAEB-t	The same as RAEB with >5% blasts Cytopenias Auer rods	20%–30% blasts Auer rods	5q— —7 +8	60	*
Chronic Myelomonocytic Leukemia	CMML	Dimorphic anemia WBC variable, usually elevated Increased monocytes (absolute monocytosis) <5% blasts	Hypercellular Granulocytic hyperplasia Increased immature monocytes 5%–10% blasts Abnormalities of all cell lines	12q— —7 +8	14	*

* Photomicrographs courtesy of Bernadette Rodak and Jacqueline Carr, Medical Technology Program, Indiana University, Indianapolis, IN.
MCV, mean cell volume; RDW, red cell distribution width; WBC, white blood cell; RBC, red blood cell.

MYELODYSPLASTIC SYNDROME

LEUKEMIA

Leukemia is a progressive malignant disease of the bone marrow. It is characterized by unregulated proliferation of cells with the replacement of normal bone marrow with malignant leukemic cells. The disease is subdivided into two major groups: acute leukemia and chronic leukemia. This classification depends on the aggressiveness of the disease, the degree of differentiation of the neoplastic cell, and the cell origin.

Each of these groups is further subdivided according to the predominant cell involved. When granulocytes are predominant, the leukemia is termed *myelocytic* or *non-lymphocytic leukemia*. When the lymphocyte is involved, the leukemia is termed *lymphocytic leukemia*.

In 1976 (modified in 1985), the FAB Cooperative Group defined the classification of leukemia based on the morphology of cells using Wright's stain in peripheral and bone marrow slides, the degree of differentiation, and cytochemical staining.

Classification of Leukemia

AML	Acute myelocytic leukemia
ANLL	Acute nonlymphocytic leukemia
CML	Chronic myelocytic leukemia
ALL	Acute lymphocytic leukemia
CLL	Chronic lymphocytic leukemia

Comparison of Acute and Chronic Leukemia

PRESENTATION	ACUTE LEUKEMIA	CHRONIC LEUKEMIA
Frequency (%)	50	50
Onset	Rapid	Insidious
Duration	Short	Long
Survival	Usually short	Longer
Age	All	Usually older adults
WBC Count	Elevated or low or normal	Elevated
Morphology of Cells	Immature	Mostly mature
Percentage of Blasts in Bone Marrow	>30	<30
Neutropenia	Present	Absent
Anemia	N/N	N/N
Platelet Count	Usually decreased	Normal or increased

Continued ▶

► Continued **Comparison of Acute and Chronic Leukemia**

PRESENTATION	ACUTE LEUKEMIA	CHRONIC LEUKEMIA
Clinical Findings	Fever, weakness, anemia, thrombocytope-nia, bone pain, occasional splenomegaly and hepatomegaly	Usually found for unrelated complaint or complaints of fatigue and weakness Occasional enlarged lymph nodes Nonspecific complaints
Organomegaly	Occasional	Usually

N/N, normocytic-normochromic anemia.

ACUTE LEUKEMIA

The acute leukemias are a group of stem cell disorders with unregulated proliferation and accumulation of the immature cells. These cells have little or no maturation, being primarily blast cells. An important criterion in the diagnosis of leukemia is the percentage of blasts found in the bone marrow. Thirty percent or greater blasts in the bone marrow are needed to classify the disorder as an acute leukemia.

The disease appears suddenly with weakness, fatigue, low grade fevers, bruising, mild bleeding from the gums, and bone pain due to the expansion of the marrow. Patients present with a normochromic-normocytic anemia, nucleated red blood cells, and thrombocytopenia. The leukocyte count is variable, ranging from less than 1.0×10^9/L to 100.0×10^9/L with the presence of blasts on the blood smear (15% to 95%). Dysplastic neutrophils are common along with an increase in monocytes.

Acute Myelocytic Leukemia

AML results from an uncontrolled proliferation of the myeloblast and immature cells of the myeloid series. When the bone marrow's normal cells are replaced with the immature cells, they then spill into the peripheral blood and other tissues such as the lymph nodes, liver, and spleen. AML is seen during the first few months of life and during the middle to later years. During childhood and adolescence it is rare.

With the exception of erythroleukemia (M6), the diagnosis of AML is established when 30% or more of the nucleated cells of the bone marrow are blasts.

ACUTE LEUKEMIA

CLASSIFICATION OF ACUTE MYELOCYTIC LEUKEMIA

DISORDER	INCIDENCE (%)	BONE MARROW MORPHOLOGY	CYTOCHEMISTRY	IMMUNOPHENOTYPE	CYTOGENETICS	CLINICAL FINDINGS	MICROSCOPIC VIEW
M0 AML Undifferentiated	<5	>30% blasts Blasts nondescript with no granules in cytoplasm	<3% reactive for MPO, SBB, NSE	HLA-DR, CD13, CD14, CD33, CD34 ± Negative for lymphocyte antigens		With new techniques for identification this subtype is rare.	*
M1 AML Without Maturation	18	>30% blasts (types I and II) <10% granulocytic <10% monocytic Nucleus: one or more nucleoli, fine chromatin Cytoplasm: few azurophilic granules, Auer rods (50%)	>3% reactive for MPO Positive for SBB, CAE Negative for NSE, PAS	HLA-DR, CD34, CD13, CD33, CD11B	t(9:22) occ t(8:21) occ	Usually accompanied by anemia and thrombocytopenia Median age 45–50 yr	*
M2 AML with Maturation	28	>30% blasts >10% promyelocytes <50% erythroid >10% granulocytic <20% monocytic Nucleus: one or more nucleoli, fine chromatin Cytoplasm: various amounts with numerous granules and Auer rods	Positive: MPO, SBB, CAE Negative: NSE, PAS	HLA-DR, CD13, CD33, CD11B±	t(8:21)	Maturation beyond myeloblast 70% of cases are positive for Auer rods Median age 45–50 yr Organomegaly common	*
M3 Acute Promyelocytic	8	>30% blasts <50% promyelocytes <50% erythroblasts >10% granulocytes <20% monocytes Nucleus: reniform or bilobed Cytoplasm: heavy granulation, bundles of Auer rods and Fagot cells	Positive: MPO, SBB, CAE Negative: NSE, PAS	CD13, CD33, HLA-DR negative	t(15:17)	Common in young adults (35–40 yr) High frequency of DIC; elevated PT and APTT; decreased fibrinogen; and positive FDP 90% positive for Auer rods	*

Continued ▶

DISORDER	INCIDENCE (%)	BONE MARROW MORPHOLOGY	CYTOCHEMISTRY	IMMUNOPHENOTYPE	CYTOGENETICS	CLINICAL FINDINGS	MICROSCOPIC VIEW
M3v Micro-granular Variant		Same as M3, except granules are fine or absent and nuclear shape is irregular	Same as M3	Same as M3	Same as M3	WBC markedly increased compared with hypergranular M3 Remission usually brief	*
M4 Acute Myelomonocytic	27	>30% blasts >20% granulocytic >20% promyelocytes >20%–<80% monocytes Blasts appear as in M1	Positive: MPO, SBB, CAE, NSE Negative: PAS	Negative: HLA-DR, CD34 Positive: CD13, CD33, CD11b, CD14	t(6;9) 5q−, 7q−	Tissue infiltrated, CNS involvement Increased lysosome Both children and adults Organomegaly	◆
M4E M4 with Eosinophilia	7	30% of marrow cells are eosinophils Cytoplasmic granules are large basophilic granules.	Positive: CAE, PAS		t(16;16) del(16q) inv(16)		◆
M5a Acute Monoblastic Poorly Differentiated	10	>80% monocytic Nucleus: lacy chromatin with nucleoli Cytoplasm: basophilic with pseudopods, some granulation	Positive: NSE and PAS Negative: CAE Weakly positive: MPO, SBB	Positive: HLA-DR, CD33, CD11b, CD14 CD13±	t(9;11) t(8;16) Abnormalities of long arm of chromosome 11 with deletions and translocations	Tissue infiltrates Gum involvement CNS involvement Increased lysozyme Usually younger patient with poor prognosis	*

Continued ▶

ACUTE LEUKEMIA

▶ Continued CLASSIFICATION OF ACUTE MYELOCYTIC LEUKEMIA

DISORDER	INCIDENCE (%)	BONE MARROW MORPHOLOGY	CYTOCHEMISTRY	IMMUNOPHENOTYPE	CYTOGENETICS	CLINICAL FINDINGS	MICROSCOPIC VIEW
M5b Acute Monoblastic with Differentiation		>80% monocytic cells <80% monoblasts Promonocytes predominate Nucleus: cerebriform with nucleoli Cytoplasm: gray with ground glass appearance with fine azurophilic granules	Positive: NSE	Positive: CD11b, CD13, CD14, CD15, CD33, CD36		Skin and gum involvement Adults 50 yr of age	✱
M6 Acute Erythroleukemia	4	>50% erythroid cells in all stages of maturation >30% myeloblasts Nucleus: megaloblastic features, multiple nuclear lobes, multiple nuclei, and nuclear fragments Cytoplasm: vacuolization	Positive: PAS, NSE	Myeloblasts express myeloid antigens Erythroid precursors positive CD36	5q— 7q— +8	Significant peripheral normoblasts Bizarre megaloblastic erythropoiesis Primary adults with advanced age Pancytopenia Tissue infiltration	◆
M7 Acute Megakaryoblastic	1	>30% blasts >30% megakaryocytic cells Nucleus: dense chromatin or fine with nucleoli Cytoplasm: scant, blebs, vacuoles Platelets may be shedding from cytoplasm	Platelet peroxidase positive Acid phosphatase ± PAS ±	Platelet glycoproteins CD41 and CD61	+21 t(21)	May be hard to aspirate bone marrow due to myelofibrosis Electron microscopy confirmation Pancytopenia and myelofibrosis Short clinical course Poor response to chemotherapy	◆

✱ Photomicrographs from Carr J, Rodak BF: Atlas of Clinical Hematology. Philadelphia, WB Saunders, 1998.
◆ Photomicrographs courtesy of Bernadette Rodak and Jacqueline Carr, Medical Technology Program, Indiana University, Indianapolis, IN.
MPO, myeloperoxidase; SBB, Sudan black B; NSE, nonspecific esterase; CAE, chloracetate esterase; PAS, periodic acid–Schiff; OCC, occasional; DIC, disseminated intravascular coagulation; FDP, fibrin degradation product; PT, prothrombin time; APTT, activated partial thromboplastin time; CNS, central nervous system.

Cytochemical Stains

Cytochemistry is defined as the identification of chemical constituents within the cell. The cell morphology is not changed in the staining process. Cytochemical stains along with cell surface markers are used in the differentiation of the acute leukemias. Cytochemical stains are either enzymatic, which include myeloperoxidase, esterase, acid and alkaline phosphatase, or nonenzymatic, which include Sudan black B, periodic acid–Schiff, and terminal deoxynucleotidyl transferase.

ACUTE LEUKEMIA

Special Stains

NAME	TYPE	CONSTITUENTS STAINED	INTERPRETATION	IMPORTANT INFORMATION	MICROSCOPIC VIEW
Myeloperoxidase	Enzyme	Marker for primary granules and Auer rods	Peroxidase activity produces dark brown granules in cytoplasm of granulocytes and monocytes. Neutrophil and precursors Monocyte weak positive	Myeloperoxidase enzyme deteriorates. Stain should be done only on fresh specimens.	*
Sudan Black B (SBB)	Nonenzyme	Marker for phospholipids and lipids	Dark purple-black granules in neutrophil precursors Lymphoblasts are negative.	Can be done on stored specimens Parallels myeloperoxidase for interpretation	*
Naphthol AS-D Chloroacetate Esterase	Enzyme	Marker of mature and immature neutrophils and mast cells	Enzyme activity results in bright red granules in cytoplasm of neutrophils, neutrophil precursors, and mast cells.	Known as specific esterase Stable enzyme that lasts for months Monocytes are weakly positive.	*
α-Naphthyl Acetate Esterase	Enzyme	Marker for monocytes, megakaryocytes, and plasma cells	Monocytes stain red-brown.	Known as nonspecific esterase (NSE)	*

Continued ▶

▲ Continued Special Stains

NAME	TYPE	CONSTITUENTS STAINED	INTERPRETATION	IMPORTANT INFORMATION	MICROSCOPIC VIEW
α-Naphthyl Butyrate Esterase	Enzyme	Identifying monocytes, promonocytes, and monoblasts	Enzyme activity results in dark red precipitates in cytoplasm.	Known as nonspecific esterase (NSE)	∗
Acid Phosphatase	Enzyme	Present in all hematopoietic cells and found in lysosomes	Activity is indicated by purple to red granules.	Cannot be stored	
Tartrate Resistant Acid Phosphatase	Enzyme	Marker for hairy cell leukemia	Activity is indicated by purple to dark red granules in cytoplasm.	Excellent marker for hairy cell leukemia	∗
Leukocyte Alkaline Phosphatase (LAP)	Enzyme	Neutrophil is the only leukocyte that contains this activity.	100 cell count is done. Neutrophils are scored from 0 with no activity to 4 with a large amount of activity.	Used to differentiate CML from a leukemoid reaction. CML has decreased activity.	†

Continued ▲

ACUTE LEUKEMIA

▲ Continued **Special Stains**

NAME	TYPE	CONSTITUENTS STAINED	INTERPRETATION	IMPORTANT INFORMATION	MICROSCOPIC VIEW
Periodic Acid–Schiff (PAS)	Nonenzyme	Marker for glycogen, glycoproteins, mucoproteins, and high molecular weight carbohydrates	Activity results in bright fuchsia pink. Pattern of staining varies with each cell type.	Lymphoblastic leukemias show blocky or chunky pattern. L1 and L2, blocky pattern L3 negative Erythroblasts in M6 Leukemia also positive	\n\n*
Terminal Deoxynucleotidyl Transferase (TdT)	Enzyme	DNA polymerase immunoperoxidase	Is present in 90% cases of ALL	Used to differentiate AML from ALL	
Toluidine Blue	Nonenzyme	Binds with acid mucopolysaccharides in blood cells	Strongly metachromatic	Useful for recognition of mast cells and basophils	

* Photomicrographs from Rodak BF: Diagnostic Hematology. Philadelphia, WB Saunders, 1995.
◆ Photomicrograph from Anne Stiene-Martin, Ph.D., Division of Clinical Laboratory Science, University of Kentucky, Chandler Medical Center, Lexington, KY.
ALL, acute lymphocytic leukemia; AML, acute myelocytic leukemia.

Cytochemistry Flow Sheet in Acute Leukemia

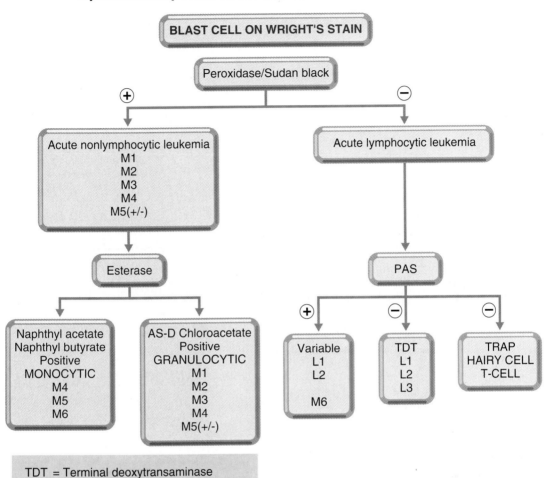

TDT = Terminal deoxytransaminase
TRAP = Tartrate resistant acid phosphatase

Bone Marrow Analysis

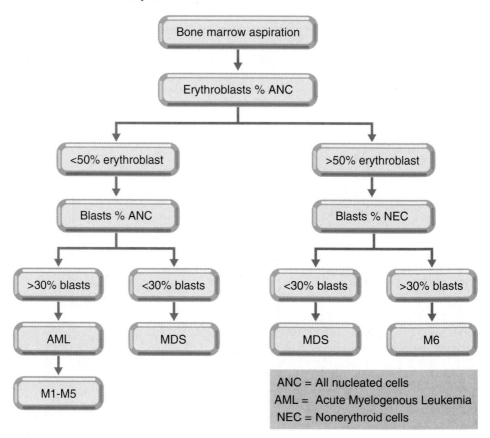

Acute Lymphocytic Leukemia

ALL is a proliferation of lymphoblasts. ALL is divided into three subgroups, L1, L2, and L3, by the FAB classification. This disorder occurs in all age groups with a peak occurrence in children between the ages of 2 and 10 years. The second peak occurs in the middle-aged to older adult. Clinical features of these disorders are fatigue, fever, bleeding, infection, lymphadenopathy, splenomegaly, hepatomegaly, and sometimes central nervous system involvement. Bone pain often results from the infiltration of leukemic cells. Acute lymphocytic leukemia presents with a variation in the WBC from high to low. Cytochemical staining is used to exclude a diagnosis of AML. ALL shows a chunky or block pattern with periodic acid–Schiff (PAS); other stains are usually negative. The method for the classification of ALL consists of cell and surface markers.

CLASSIFICATION OF ACUTE LYMPHOCYTIC LEUKEMIA

DISORDER	INCIDENCE (%)	BONE MARROW MORPHOLOGY	PHENOTYPE	TdT ACTIVITY	CLINICAL FINDINGS	MICROSCOPIC VIEW
L1	65	Cell size: small cells Nucleus: regular with occasional clefting Chromatin: homogeneous Nucleoli: usually not visible Cytoplasm: very small amount may be basophilic	B or T	Positive	Most common ALL found in children Patients 2–10 yr have best prognosis Those <1 yr do poorly	*
L2	30	Cell size: large Nucleus: irregular with clefting Chromatin: heterogeneous Nucleoli: one or more, often large Cytoplasm: moderately abundant and basophilic	B or T	Positive	Frequent ALL found in adults This blast tends to vary in size.	*
L3	5	Cell size: large Nucleus: round to oval Chromatin: fine and stippled Nucleoli: Prominent usually one to three Cytoplasm: moderate amount deep basophilia with prominent cytoplasmic vacuoles	B	Lacks reactivity	Rarest form that occurs in children and adults L3 blasts resemble morphology of Burkitt's type lymphoma.	*

* Photomicrographs from Rodak BF: Diagnostic Hematology. Philadelphia, WB Saunders, 1995.
TdT, terminal deoxynucleotidyl transferase.

ACUTE LEUKEMIA

IMMUNOLOGIC PHENOTYPE OF ACUTE LYMPHOCYTIC LEUKEMIA

Research with surface markers and intracellular markers has shown that lymphoblasts in ALL vary considerably in immunologic maturation. Treatment protocols and prognosis are proving to be more effective and accurate when the leukemic cell is immunologically classified.

COMMON CELL MARKERS FOR ACUTE LYMPHOCYTIC LEUKEMIA

SUBGROUP	TdT	CYTOPLASMIC μ (Cμ)	MEMBRANE Ig (SIg)	CD10	CD19	CD24	CD20	CD7
Early B Precursor	+	−	−	−	+	−	−	−
Common B (CALLA)	+	−	−	+	+	+	−	−
Pre-B	+	+	−	+	+	+	+	−
B Cell ALL	−	−	+	±	+	+	+	−
Early T Precursor	+	−	−	−	−	−	−	+
T Cell ALL	+	−	−	−	−	−	−	+

CALLA, common ALL antigen; CD, cluster designation; SIg, surface immunoglobulin; ALL, acute lymphocytic leukemia.

MYELOPROLIFERATIVE DISORDERS

These are a group of blood disorders with a common characteristic of an abnormal stem cell that leads to an increased or unchecked autonomous proliferation of one or more cell lines. The peripheral blood shows an increase in the number of red blood cells, white blood cells, and/or platelets. These cells tend to be mature, but at later stages of the disease they can terminate in an acute leukemia. These disorders include chronic myelocytic leukemia, myelofibrosis with myeloid metaplasia (MMM), polycythemia vera (PV), and essential thrombocythemia (ET).

General characteristics of these disorders are that the age of onset is middle-aged to elderly. The disorder typically manifests as a normochromic-normocytic anemia; usually all three cellular lines are involved. The bone marrow is hypercellular, often becoming fibrotic at later stages of the disease.

Differentiation of Myeloproliferative Disorders

LABORATORY FINDINGS	CML	MMM	PV	ET
Hematocrit	Normal or decreased	Decreased	Markedly increased	Normal or decreased
WBC	Marked neutrophilia with shift to left Basophilia and eosinophilia	Increased Left shift with myeloblasts (occ), basophilia, and eosinophilia	Normal or increased Leukocytosis with neutrophilia and basophilia	Normal or increased Leukocytosis usually mild
RBC	Normal to slight decrease Few NRBCs	Dacryocytes (teardrop) Reticulocytosis NRBCs	Normal morphology; as disease progresses, iron deficiency anemia (microcytic-hypochromic) morphology	Normal morphology and maturation
Platelets	Normal or increased Enlarged size and fragments	Normal or decreased or increased giant and abnormal platelets present Micromegakaryocytes in peripheral blood Abnormal platelet aggregation	Increased	Increased platelet count >600,000/μL Giant size Bizarre shapes Micromegakaryocytes and megakaryocytic fragments in peripheral blood
Immature Granulocytes	Increased	Increased	Absence or increase of bands	Rare
LAP	Decreased	Normal or increased	Increased	Normal
Ph Chromosome	Present	Absent	Absent	Absent
Spleen	Normal or increased	Increased	Increased	Normal or increased
Bone Marrow	Hypercellular Predominantly granulocytic Decreased iron stores M:E ratio 10:1–50:1	Increased fibrosis Megakaryocytic hyperplasia RBCs and WBC usually normal Bone marrow aspirate Dry tap	Hypercellular moderate to severe All three lines increased with normal maturation Deceased iron stores	Hypercellular mild to moderate Megakaryocytic hyperplasia Clusters and sheets of megakaryocytes Some marrow fibrosis

Continued ▶

◄ Continued **Differentiation of Myeloproliferative Disorders**

LABORATORY FINDINGS	CML	MMM	PV	ET
Diagnostic Criteria	Complete rainbow of all stages of neutrophil maturation Less than 5% blasts in peripheral blood Ph chromosome present in 90%–95% of cases Three clinical phases: Chronic Accelerated Blast crisis	Leukoerythroblastic picture with dacryocytes Fibrotic marrow as disease progresses Enlarged spleen	Excessive RBC production Increased red cell volume, normal O_2 saturation, all three lines increased Enlarged spleen	Platelet count >600,000/µL with no known cause for reactive thrombocytosis Complications of thrombosis and hemorrhage
Microscopic View *Peripheral Blood Smear*				
Bone Marrow Biopsy				

All photomicrographs except bone marrow biopsy of MMM from Rodak BF: Diagnostic Hematology. Philadelphia, WB Saunders, 1995. Bone marrow biopsy of MMM from Henry JB: Clinical Diagnosis and Management by Laboratory Methods. 19th ed. Philadelphia, WB Saunders, 1996.
NRBC, nucleated red blood cell; LAP, leukocyte alkaline phosphatase; occ, occasional; M:E, ratio: myeloid: erythroid; Ph, Philadelphia.

Differentiating a Neutrophilic Leukemoid Reaction and Chronic Myelocytic Leukemia

CRITERION	CML	LEUKEMOID REACTION
Neutrophil	Whole spectrum of cells mature to blast	Shift to the left, more bands, metamyelocytes, blast very rare
Eosinophils	Increased	Normal
Basophils	Increased	Normal
Platelets	Increased with abnormal forms	Normal
Anemia	Usually present	Not typical
LAP Score	Decreased	Increased
Chromosome	Present	Absent
Toxic Granulation	Absent	Increased
Döhle Bodies	Absent	Increased
Duration	Permanent	Transient

LAP, leukocyte alkaline phosphatase.

CHRONIC LEUKEMIA

The chronic leukemias are a group of bone marrow disorders that are often diagnosed on a routine physical examination. Patients have symptoms of long duration, frequently being asymptomatic. In chronic leukemia there is organ involvement, anemia develops later in the disease, and the platelet count is normal to increased.

CLL is an acquired disorder usually of B cell lineage. The most outstanding feature is the absolute lymphocytosis in the bone marrow and peripheral blood. The cells are mature in nature. Other disorders that are classified as chronic leukemias are prolymphocytic leukemia (PLL), hairy cell leukemia, and Sézary syndrome. CML is considered to be one of the chronic myeloproliferative disorders and was discussed previously.

MYELOPROLIFERATIVE DISEASES

Classification of Chronic Leukemia

DISORDER	HEMATOLOGIC FINDINGS AND MORPHOLOGY	CYTOCHEMICAL	PHENOTYPE	CYTOGENETICS	CLINICAL FINDINGS	MICROSCOPIC VIEW
Chronic Lymphocytic Leukemia (CLL)	PB: Extreme lymphocytosis, small to medium, mature condensed lymphocytes usually ruptured or smudged. Occasional prolymphocyte. Normochromic-normocytic anemia BM: Hypercellular, >40% mature lymphocytes, morphology as in PB	NA	Pan B cell surface antigens CD19, CD20, CD24 Weak SIg (IgM and IgD) CD5 positive	Trisomy 12 13q14	Over the age of 50 yr Male predominance with 2:1 ratio Asymptomatic Lymphadenopathy Hepatomegaly or splenomegaly less common Patients develop hypogammaglobulinemia because of impaired B cell function	†
Prolymphocytic Leukemia (PLL)	PB: Often WBC is >100,000/μL. Medium to large prolymphocytes with eccentric nucleus, moderate condensed chromatin, prominent nucleoli, and moderate rims of basophilic cytoplasm Anemia, thrombocytopenia, and neutropenia BM: Moderate to heavy infiltration	NA	Pan B cell CD19, Cd20, CD22 CD5 negative	14q+	Rare variant usually seen in older men Prominent splenomegaly Marked hepatomegaly Aggressive clinical course with short survival time	◆
Hairy Cell Leukemia (HCL)	PB: Pancytopenia; lymphocytes are two or three times size of small lymphocytes with round to oval kidney shaped nucleus, stippled chromatin, with single small inconspicuous nucleolus. Cytoplasm moderately pale blue with poorly defined borders with hairlike projections. BM: Heavy infiltration of mononuclear cells, often hard to aspirate because of reticulum fibrosis or dry tap	Tartrate resistant acid phosphatase (TRAP)	Pan B cell CD19, CD20, CD22, CD25		Onset middle age with male predominance Minimal lymphadenopathy Marked splenomegaly Progressive disease Abdominal discomfort Recurrent infections due to pancytopenia	†
Sézary Syndrome Mycosis Fungoides T Cell Lymphoma of Skin	PB: Lymphocytosis with small or large lymphocytes. Nucleus has marked convolution or cerebriform shape, nucleoli absent, small to moderate amount of cytoplasm. BM: Usually not involved; minimal infiltration.	PAS positive	Pan T cell Mature helper T CD3, CD4, CD8		Onset late adult with male predominance Initially plaques of skin that progress to exfoliative erythroderma with Sézary's cell in peripheral blood Lymphadenopathy and hepatosplenomegaly Chronic course	*

CLASSIFICATION OF THE LYMPHOMAS

The lymphomas are a group of malignant disorders that originate from unregulated growth of the lymphoid tissue. Lymphomas have been subdivided into two groups that include Hodgkin's and the non-Hodgkin's lymphomas. Diagnosis and classification of lymphomas are based on histologic examination of the lymph node tissue and the staging of the enlarged nodes for the extent of the disease. As the disease progresses, proliferation spreads to other lymph tissue. Enlarged lymph nodes are often the presenting feature, but frequently involvement of the liver, spleen, and bone marrow is seen. Peripheral blood is involved at later stages of the disease.

Hodgkin's disease requires the Reed-Sternberg (R-S) cell for diagnosis. This is a very distinct cell that is 20 to 50 μm and has a bilobed nucleus and contains a large nucleolus in the center. Cytoplasm is abundant. These cells are found in the lymph nodes and bone marrow but not in the peripheral blood.

Clinical Staging for Hodgkin's and Non-Hodgkin's (Ann Arbor)

STAGE	EXTENT OF DISEASE
I	Disease confined to one or more lymph node sites
II	Disease confined to lymph tissue in more than one site but only one side of the diaphragm
III	Disease confined to lymph tissue or spleen but on both sides of the diaphragm
IV	Other organ involvement: bone marrow and liver

The principles of classification of non-Hodgkin's lymphoma are based on morphology or pattern, cytologic appearance or size, nuclear contour, chromatin pattern, nucleoli, and biologic behavior. A number of different classifications are currently used to describe the diversity of the lymphomas. In 1966 Rappaport described the morphology of the cells, size of infiltrates, and presence or absence of nodularity. Lukes and Collins based their classification on T and B subsets and their function. The Working Formulation of non-Hodgkin's correlated the tumor aggressiveness with the histologic appearance. More recent is the Revised European American Lymphoma Classification, which uses a practical approach based on the ability to identify clinically distinctive entities regardless of the stage of differentiation or function.

◄ * Photomicrographs from Rodak BF: Diagnostic Hematology. Philadelphia, WB Saunders, 1995.
♦ Photomicrographs from Henry JB: Clinical Diagnosis and Management by Laboratory Methods, 19th ed. Philadelphia, WB Saunders, 1996.
† Photomicrographs from Rodak BF, Carr J: Medical Technology Program, Indiana University, Indianapolis, IN.
PB, peripheral blood; BM, bone marrow; SIg, surface immunoglobulin; PAS, periodic acid–Schiff; NA, not applicable.

International Working Classification of Malignant Lymphomas

TYPE	DESCRIPTION
Low Grade	Small lymphocyte Follicular Mixed
Intermediate Grade	Follicular Diffuse Diffuse mixed Diffuse large
High Grade	Large cell Lymphoblastic Burkitt's

Comparison of Malignant Lymphomas

CHARACTERISTIC	HODGKIN'S	NON-HODGKIN'S
Age (yr)	Bimodal: 14–30; >50	20–40 Increased incidence with age
Site of Origin	Enlarged lymph node usually cervical	Nodal or extranodal Variable
Involvement	Usually localized	Rarely localized
Mode of Spread	Orderly manner Ann Arbor staging	Noncontiguous spread Variable
Clinical Findings	Painless enlarged lymph node usually in the neck, night sweats, low grade fever, weight loss	Painless enlarged lymph node, most commonly in the cervical region Extranodal: GI, skin, lung
Diagnosis	Biopsy of lymph node Reed-Sternberg cell	Biopsy of lymph node Histologic interpretation
Staging	Ann Arbor	National Cancer modified
Pathology	RYE CLASSIFICATION: Lymphocyte predominant Mixed cellularity Lymphocyte depleted Nodular sclerosis	WORKING: Low grade Intermediate High
Peripheral Blood	Neutrophilia, monocytosis Mild eosinophilia	Normal blood counts Anemia may develop
Bone Marrow	Unusual involvement (10%) Mononuclear cells with nuclear features of Reed-Sternberg cells	Overall involvement 30%–50% Nodular rather than diffuse
Other Involvements	Mediastinal GI, skin, CNS rare	GI and skin common CNS occasionally

GI, gastrointestinal; CNS, central nervous system.

IMMUNOPROLIFERATIVE DISORDERS OR PLASMA CELL DYSCRASIAS

These disorders are a clonal proliferation of immunoglobulin producing cells that are the plasma cells or the B lymphocyte. In these disorders there is a malignant or uncontrolled production of monoclonal serum proteins. Another name for these disorders is *monoclonal gammopathies* because a single class of immunoglobulin is secreted. These disorders include multiple myeloma (MM), Waldenström's macroglobulinemia, heavy chain disease (HCD), and monoclonal gammopathy of undetermined significance (MGUS).

Comparison of the Plasma Cell Dyscrasias

CRITERION	MULTIPLE MYELOMA (MM)	WALDENSTRÖM'S MACROGLOBULINEMIA	HEAVY CHAIN DISEASE	MGUS
Description	Neoplastic proliferation of plasma cells in bone marrow that presents with oste-olytic bone lesions. Increase in produc-tion of single im-munoglobulin.	Plasma dyscrasia that is low grade lympho-plasmacytoid lym-phoma with in-creased production of single immuno-globulin	Characterized by overproduction of abnormal heavy chains of immunoglobulin molecule Rare	Presence of mono-clonal immuno-globulin in serum, urine, with no evi-dence of MM or other related dis-eases
Age (yr)	50–70	Median age 60 Male predominance	Median age 60	Rare before age 40 but increases with each suc-ceeding decade Median age 64
Presentation	Pallor, fatigue, bone pain with bone lesion and compression frac-tures	Weakness, fatigue, and bleeding	Weakness, fatigue, and fever	No related specific symptoms or physical findings
Course	Proliferation of plasma cells Aggressive disease Chemotherapy dimin-ishes organ damage due to immunoglobu-lin deposition	Low grade malignant lymphoma Median survival 5 yr	Ranges from rapid downhill to sta-ble	Stable benign dis-ease 25% of patients de-velop multiple myeloma.
Clinical Findings	Bone pain and lesions Hypercalcemia Minimal hepatospleno-megaly	Lymphadenopathy Hepatosplenomegaly Hyperviscosity Bone lesion absent	Hepatomegaly Splenomegaly Lymphadenopathy	Usually no symp-toms of plasma dyscrasia
Peripheral Blood	Normocytic-normochromic anemia Rouleaux Occasional plasma cells	Normocytic-normochromic anemia Rouleaux Plasmacytoid lympho-cytes	Normocytic-normochromic anemia, leukopenia, and thrombocytope-nia	Normal No anemia Rouleaux may be present
Bone Marrow	Minimum of 10% plasma cells 20%–40% of plasma cells mature appear-ing with cytoplasmic inclusions Sheets of plasma cells may be seen	Increased number of well differentiated lymphocytes and plasmacytoid lym-phocytes	Some involvement	<10% plasma cells Mild plasmacytosis

Continued ▶

▶ Continued **Comparison of the Plasma Cell Dyscrasias**

CRITERION	MULTIPLE MYELOMA (MM)	WALDENSTRÖM'S MACROGLOBULINEMIA	HEAVY CHAIN DIEASE	MGUS
Laboratory Tests	Serum calcium increased Renal function tests increased Proteinuria present ESR elevated Bence Jones protein present	ESR elevated Positive DAT Serum viscosity elevated	Serum electrophoresis Urine electrophoresis	Serum calcium normal Renal function normal ESR may be elevated Bence Jones protein negative Proteinuria negative
Monoclonal Immunoglobulin	>3 g/dL IgG, 55% IgA, 22% IgD, 2% Light chain only, 18%	>3g/dL IgM, 100%	γHC fragment 25% αHC fragment 75% μHC fragment 5%	<3 g/dL
Other Tests	β₂ Macroglobulin elevated Bone radiograph lytic lesions	Cold agglutinin present		Bone radiograph negative

ESR, erythrocyte sedimentation rate; DAT, direct antiglobulin test; MGUS, monoclonal gammopathy of undetermined significance; IG, immunoglobulin.

Plasma Cell Leukemia

Plasma cell leukemia is a very rare type of plasma cell dyscrasia. Diagnostic criteria for plasma cell leukemia are based on an absolute peripheral blood cell count of $2000/mm^3$, or 20% of peripheral blood leukocytes are plasma cells in circulation. This leukemia is accompanied by marked cytopenias. The plasma cell morphology has blastlike features. Patients with this leukemia tend to have tissue infiltration and have a poor prognosis.

IMMUNOPROLIFERATIVE DISORDERS OR PLASMA CELL DYSCRASIAS

BIBLIOGRAPHY

Brown B: Hematology: Principles and Procedures, 6th ed. Philadelphia, Lea & Febiger, 1993.

Brown KA: Hematology M & M's Workshop, American Society of Clinical Pathologists, Associate Member Section, New York (June), 1996.

Cornbleet PJ, Astarita R, Wolf PL: White Blood Cells and Platelet Disorders. In Howanitz J, ed; Laboratory Medicine Test Selection and Interpretation. New York, Churchill Livingstone, 1991.

Davey F, Hutchison R: Leukocytic Disorders. In Henry JB, ed: Clinical Diagnosis and Management by Laboratory Methods, 19th ed. Philadelphia, WB Saunders, 1996.

Dutcher T: Hematology Morphology Workshop, American Society of Clinical Pathologists, Associate Member Section, 1992.

Hanson C: Hematology Section VII. In McClatchey K, ed: Clinical Laboratory Medicine. Baltimore, Williams & Wilkins, 1994.

Harmening D: Clinical Hematology and Fundamentals of Hemostasis, 3rd ed. Philadelphia, FA Davis, 1997.

Harrison-Godwin J, Godwin T: Bone Marrow Examination and Interpretation Workshop, American Society of Clinical Pathologists, Associate Member Section, New Jersey (June), 1996.

Heckner F, Lehmann HP, Kao YS: Practical Microscopic Hematology, 3rd ed. Baltimore, Urban & Schwarzenberg, 1988.

Kjeldsberg C, Foucar K, et al: Practical Diagnosis of Hematologic Disorders, 2nd ed. Chicago, American Society of Clinical Pathologists Press, 1995.

Lopspeich-Steininger C: Clinical Hematology. Philadelphia, JB Lippincott, 1992.

McKenna R, Hanson C: Diagnosis and Classification of Acute Leukemias and Myelodysplastic Syndromes Workshop, American Society of Clinical Pathologists, Associate Member Section, 1994.

McKenzie S: Textbook of Hematology, 2nd ed. Baltimore, Williams & Wilkins, 1996.

O'Connor B: A Color Atlas and Instruction Manual of Peripheral Blood Cell Morphology. Baltimore, Williams & Wilkins, 1984.

Pereira I: Peripheral Smears: The Primary Diagnostic Tool I and II Workshop, American Society of Clinical Pathologists, Associate Member Section, Philadelphia (October), 1995.

Rodak B: Diagnostic Hematology. Philadelphia, WB Saunders, 1995.

Variakojis D, Vardiman J: Myeloproliferative Disorders Workshop, American Society of Clinical Pathologists, Associate Member Section, 1994.

Chapter **38**

HEMATOLOGY PROCEDURES

Bruce T. Kube, BS, MT(ASCP)H

Q U I C K   C O N T E N T S

INTRODUCTION

This section attempts to provide some insight into the principles and purposes behind hematologic tests. Hematologic testing can be used for a wide variety of reasons, which range from determining the presence of an infection to the diagnosis of leukemia and anemias. Some of the testing is specific and other testing is very general, and an abnormal result in and of itself is insignificant unless correlated with other related results.

QUALITY CONTROL AND QUALITY ASSURANCE

Quality control (QC) and quality assurance are programs that implemented in a laboratory environment that enable the laboratorian to release results that can be assumed to be reliable based on all internal influences.

QC can include such things as performing analyses on materials of known concentrations or quantities, and running repeat analyses on samples that have been deemed to have yielded accurate results. Participation in proficiency testing is administered by various accrediting agencies such as the College of American Pathologists (CAP) or state and local accrediting agencies. XB analysis (see later) is also a method of QC used in many laboratories that have a high volume of samples.

Quality assurance measures are checks that are put into place in the laboratory to ensure that the data released from the laboratory is true and accurate to the best ability of the laboratory. This can involve the obvious steps of verifying the patient's identity to performing a delta check analysis between samples.

Quality Control Methods

ASSAYED MATERIAL

Assayed stabilized blood products can be purchased from various sources and used in the laboratory. There are a couple of methods in which these materials can be used:

1. Internal determination of values can be done. The material can be analyzed for the necessary parameters in the laboratory using an analyzer that has been deemed to be in control according to the current lot of control material. In other words the two lots will be run coincidentally for a period of 5 to 7 days before the expiration of the current lot in use. At the end of this period the mean ($\overline{X}$) and standard deviation (SD) of each parameter is determined and used to establish control for the given parameter.
   The formulas for the $\overline{X}$ and SD are as follows:

$$\overline{X} = \frac{\Sigma X}{n} \quad \text{where } n \text{ is the value obtained from analysis}$$

$$SD = \frac{\sqrt{\Sigma(X - \overline{X})^2}}{n-1}$$

2. Manufacturer provided values and ranges can be used, and the data generated can be compared with that of a group using the same lot of control material and similar instrumentation and reagent systems. The recovered values are analyzed and a comprehensive report returned to the submitting agency.

REPLICATE TESTING

A sample can be chosen that has been processed just subsequent to the QC procedure and deemed to be accurate. The sample is then processed at intervals during the course of the day and the differences monitored for acceptability.

PROFICIENCY TESTING

Blind samples are sent from an outside agency, the samples are analyzed, and the results are returned to the agency for evaluation. Most laboratory facilities participate in this type of program as a matter of regulatory compliance. Failure to complete this testing accurately usually results in some sort of punitive action. Programs of this type are usually administered quarterly.

$\overline{\text{XB}}$ ANALYSIS

$\overline{\text{XB}}$ analysis is an internal QC mechanism by which parameters that generally remain stable in a given population are monitored for a given number of analyses (batches) and the mean and variance of the samples are analyzed to determine the functionality and accuracy of instrumentation. The indicators most commonly used are mean cell volume (MCV), mean cell hemoglobin (MCH), and mean cell hemoglobin concentration (MCHC). Variance from the established mean could represent a potential problem with an analyzer or subsystem and should be handled accordingly.

Quality Assurance

Quality assurance is simply a group of steps that are implemented to assure the physician that the laboratory is generating the best possible result and that the patient is not being compromised. Steps that can be taken during the preanalytic process include verification of patient identity at phlebotomy; defining delta checks; and implementing laboratory action limits and protocols for use during the analytic process and postanalytically.

PREANALYTIC STEPS

The primary tool necessary to ensure accurate results is good phlebotomy. The phlebotomist should be experienced and knowlegeable. The phlebotomist must also ascertain at the time of the blood drawing that blood from the correct patient is being drawn and the samples are being collected in the proper order.

DELTA CHECKS

Ranges are established for parameters that are relatively stable on a day to day basis, and these parameters are monitored on samples from patients who have repetitive samples drawn over the duration of a hospital stay. The parameters, ranges, and stability should be ascertained at the site performing the delta check analysis. Various actions can be taken in the event of a delta failure: these actions can include repeating the offending sample, repeating the previous sample, or possibly manual verification of results.

LABORATORY ACTION LIMITS

Laboratory action limits are limits determined by the analytic site that are established to provide the most accuracy. These take into account the ability of instrumentation to accurately process abnormal samples, the needs of the clinical staff, and labor constraints.

QUALITY CONTROL AND QUALITY ASSURANCE

ROUTINE HEMATOLOGY METHODS

ANALYTE	METHOD	RESULT UNITS	PROCEDURE	LIMITATIONS
White Blood Cells (WBCs)	Hemocytometer	$\times 10^3/\mu L$	1:100 dilution of whole blood in ammonium oxalate. Incubate 15 min. Charge chamber (see procedure for calculating manual count).	Counting chamber must be clean and dry to minimize debris on counting grid.
	Automated analyzer	$\times 10^3/\mu L$	Blood sampled directly from tube and mixed with lysing reagent, which removes RBCs from solution and strips WBCs of cell membrane. WBC nuclei counted.	1. Linearity of instrumentation. 2. Platelet clumps cause spuriously high values. 3. Cryoglobulins cause spuriously high values. 4. WBC aggregates can cause spuriously low values.
Red Blood Cells (RBCs)	Automated analyzer	$\times 10^6/\mu L$	Blood sampled directly from tube is diluted and cells counted without further manipulation of sample.	1. Linearity of instrumentation. 2. RBC aggregates can cause spuriously low values. 3. Microcytic cells can cause spuriously low values. 4. Giant platelets can cause spuriously high values. 5. Extremely macrocytic or microcytic RBC can cause spuriously low results.
Hemoglobin (Hgb)	Automated analyzer	g/dL	Blood is sampled directly from tube. Reagent is added to lyse the RBCs and to form cyanmethemoglobin, and sample is read colorimetrically at 540 nm.	1. Lipemic samples will yield falsely elevated results. 2. Insufficient lysing will cause falsely elevated results.
	Manual method	g/dL	20 μL of blood is diluted into 5 mL of potassium ferricyanide and potassium cyanide. After 10 min colorimetric reading is taken at 540 nm with H_2O as blank. Value is then read from standard curve, which is made using known standards.	1. Gross lipemia can elevate results. 2. Results can be elevated in samples with extremely high WBC levels. 3. RBCs that resist lysis can cause false elevation. This can be compensated by increasing the incubation.

Continued ▶

▶ Continued **ROUTINE HEMATOLOGY METHODS**

ANALYTE	METHOD	RESULT UNITS	PROCEDURE	LIMITATIONS
Hematocrit (Hct)	Automated analyzer	%	Calculated parameter, based on RBC and MCV values: Hct = MCV × RBC/10	1. Extremely microcytic or macrocytic specimens can cause spuriously low results as can an-toagglutinins.
	Manual, microcentrifuge	%	Small volume of blood is placed into capillary tube and spun at 10,000 G for 5 min, and percentage of packed cells read from graduated Hct reading device.	1. Incomplete packing of cells due to improper centrifugation. 2. Hemolysis. 3. Clotted samples. 4. Unclear plasma-RBC interface.
Mean Cell Volume (MCV)	Automated analyzer	fL	Directly measured. Magnitude of the electronic pulses generated by RBCs is converted to cell volume	1. Severely microcytic cells can be counted as platelets and falsely elevate MCV. 2. Severely macrocytic cells may not be counted and falsely decrease MCV.
	Calculated	fL	$MCV = \dfrac{Hgb \times 10}{RBC \times 10^6/\mu L}$	1. Hct and RBC values must be accurate.
Mean Cell Hemoglobin (MCH)	Calculated	pg	$MCH = \dfrac{Hgb \times 10}{RBC \times 10^6/\mu L}$	1. MCH may be increased in macrocytic anemia due to increased cell volume. 2. In microcytic anemias MCH is decreased. If anemia is also hypochromic it can be further decreased.
Mean Cell Hemoglobin Concentration (MCHC)	Calculated	g/dL	$MCHC = \dfrac{Hgb \times 100}{Hct}$	1. Decreased values are found in iron deficiency. 2. Values in macrocytic anemias can be slightly decreased or normal.

Continued ▶

▶ Continued **ROUTINE HEMATOLOGY METHODS**

ANALYTE	METHOD	RESULT UNITS	PROCEDURE	LIMITATIONS
Platelets	Hemocytometer	$\times 10^3$/mL	Blood is diluted 1:100 in ammonium oxalate and incubated for 15 min to lyse RBCs. Chamber is charged and center boxes are counted.	1. Chamber must be clean and free of dirt and dust. 2. Platelets must be allowed to settle before analysis. 3. Error in recognition of platelets.
Platelets	Automated analyzer	$\times 10^3$/mL	Blood is sampled directly from tube. Platelets counted from RBC dilution.	1. Linearity of instrumentation 2. Giant platelets cause spuriously low results. 3. Clumps cause spuriously low results. 4. Microcytic RBCs can cause spuriously high values. 5. Cryoglobulins can cause spuriously high values.
Reticulocytes	Manual	%	Equal volumes of blood and supravital stain are incubated together 10–15 min. Prepare slide and count number of reticulocytes/1000 RBCs.	1. Insufficient cells counted. 2. RBC inclusions that can be mistaken for reticulocytes, i.e., Pappenheimer bodies or basophilic stippling, Heinz bodies.
	Semiautomated	% and/or $\times 10^9$/L	Blood is mixed with supravital stain and incubated for 15 min. Second dilution is made of previous dilution of 2 mL of blood-stain mixture into 2 mL of dilute sulfuric acid solution. Incubated for 30 sec and sampled by analyzer, which provides final count.	1. RBC inclusions can cause false elevation. 2. Some hemoglobinopathies can cause false elevation of results.
Erythrocyte Sedimentation Rate	Modified Westergren method	mm/hr	0.8 mL of blood is added to reservoir containing 0.2 mL of saline solution and graduated tube placed into reservoir with blood filling tube to 0 mark. Tube-reservoir is allowed to stand vertically undisturbed for 1 hr, and reading is taken at RBC-plasma interface.	1. Testing should be performed within 2 hrs of obtaining specimen. 2. Clotted samples. 3. Susceptible to outside influences, i.e., temperature, vibration. 4. Nonspecific.
Erythrocyte Sedimentation Rate	Wintrobe method	mm/hr	1 mL of blood is placed into Wintrobe Hct tube from bottom up to 100 mm mark. Tube is placed into vertical support and distance cells have fallen measured after 1 hr.	1. Very susceptible to blood/anticoagulant ratio. 2. Not as sensitive as Westergren method. 3. Clotted samples. 4. Susceptible to outside influences, i.e., temperature, vibration. 5. Nonspecific.

Additional Notes Regarding the Erythrocyte Sedimentation Rate

GENERAL USE. The erythrocyte sedimentation rate (ESR) is used as a nonspecific indicator of infection.

PRINCIPLE. RBCs with anticoagulant added sediment until a packed column is formed. The rate at which the cells fall is dependent on rouleaux formation, the concentration of fibrinogen in plasma, and the concentrations of α and β globulins in plasma.

FACTORS AFFECTING ROULEAUX FORMATION. Increased plasma viscosity due to increased fibrinogen or α and β globulin concentrations increases the rate of rouleaux formation. Decreased RBC mass as seen in anemia also enhances rouleaux formation, and increased RBC mass as in polycythemia tends to deter rouleaux formation.

α AND β GLOBULINS IN PLASMA. Plasma albumin tends slow the rate of RBC sedimentation in the ESR; however in acute infection the plasma albumin level is decreased and the level of α and β globulins in plasma is generally increased. In liver disease and nephrosis, the decreased albumin and increased globulin levels (both relative and absolute) are responsible for the elevation of the ESR. The increase in plasma proteins in multiple myeloma greatly enhances the rate of rouleaux formation and creates a greatly elevated ESR.

THREE STAGES OF THE ERYTHROCYTE SEDIMENTATION RATE. The initial stage is a period of a few minutes in which rouleaux formation occurs. In the second stage, the primary sedimentation occurs at a constant rate lasting 30 minutes to 2 hours, and in the final stage the sedimented cells fall at a slower rate, forming a packed column of cells that will sediment no further.

ROUTINE HEMATOLOGY METHODS

Notes on the Hemocytometer

Currently the most common hemocytometer in use is the Neubauer hemocytometer. Following are a few guidelines for performing calculations using this hemocytometer. The hemocytometer consists of a glass slide etched with a 3 mm square. This square is then etched into nine smaller 1 mm squares. These squares are then further subdivided (see below).

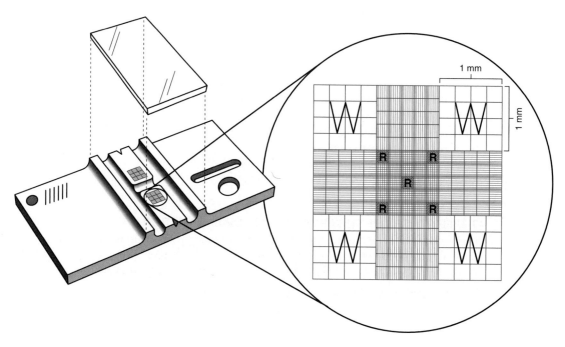

From Rodak BF: Diagnostic Hematology. Philadelphia, WB Saunders, 1995.

When the coverslip is correctly placed, the depth of the chamber is 0.1 mm. Thus the total volume of the chamber is 3 mm × 3 mm × 0.1 mm, or 0.9 mm³. This equates to 0.9 mL, and to calculate a number from a count obtained on the hemocytomer you must take into account the total number of cells counted, the number of squares counted, and the total volume of those squares:

Cells counted × dilution factor × number of squares counted × depth

PRINCIPLES OF AUTOMATED CELL COUNTING

IMPEDANCE. Cells are placed into an isotonic solution and passed through an aperture across which there is a voltage potential. Each cell that is drawn through the aperture creates a decrease in the voltage across the aperture, and each drop in voltage is counted. The volume of the cell is directly proportional to the magnitude of the voltage drop.

RADIO FREQUENCY. As cells are passed through a flow cell they are subjected to high frequency radio waves, which examine the nuclear components of analyzed cells. The radio waves pass through the cytoplasm of the cell undisturbed; however, the density of the nuclear material inhibits the radio waves, and this inhibition is analyzed by being passed through predefined algorithms to determine the nature of the cell.

LASER LIGHT SCATTER. As cells are passed through a flow cell, they are subjected to the beam of a laser; on striking the cell some of the light is either defracted, reflected, or refracted. Depending on the quantities of these three items, each of which is measured, the complexity of the cell being analyzed can be determined. Information about cell structure and cytoplasmic components can be obtained in this manner. The different types of light scatter are as follows:

> *Forward light scatter* (0°): This refers to light that is defracted. This is related to the volume of the cell being analyzed.
> *Forward low angle scatter* (2° to 3°): This is also related to cell size or volume.
> *Forward high angle scatter* (5° to 15°): This correlates with the refractive index of the cellular components, the complexity of the cell.
> *Orthagonal light scatter* (90°): Also called *side scatter.* This is the result of reflection and refraction of the light from the larger internal components of the cell and as such correlates with the internal complexity of the cell.

Conditions That Cause Interference on Most Hematology Analyzers

The hematology analyzers available on the market utilize some or all of these principles in obtaining the data they supply. It is important to realize, however, that this technology has its limitations, and the technologist should be familiar with these limitations. On the following page is a table of potential pitfalls as well as some corrective actions.

PRINCIPLES OF AUTOMATED CELL COUNTING

CONDITIONS THAT CAUSE INTERFERENCE ON MOST HEMATOLOGY ANALYZERS

CONDITION	PARAMETER(S) AFFECTED	CAUSE	INSTRUMENT INDICATORS	CORRECTIVE ACTION
Cold Agglutinins	RBC↓, MCV↑, MCHC↑, grainy appearance	Agglutination of RBCs	Dual RBC population on RBC map or right shift on RBC histogram	Warm sample to 37°C and rerun.
Lipemia, Icterus, or Chylomicrons	Hgb↑, MCH↑	↑Turbidity affects spectrophotometric reading	Hgb × 3 ≠ Hct ± 3, abnormal histogram or cytogram*	Plasma replacement‡
Hemolysis	RBC↓, Hct↓	RBCs lysed and not counted	Hgb × 3 ≠ Hct ± 3, may show lipemia pattern on histogram or cytogram*	Request new sample.
Lysis Resistant RBCs with Abnormal Hemoglobins	WBC↑, Hgb↑	RBCs with Hgb S, C, or F may fail to lyse and be counted as WBCs.	Interference at noise/WBC interface on histogram or cytogram	Manual dilutions, allowing incubation time for lysis
Microcytosis or Schistocytes	RBC↓	Size of RBCs or RBC fragments < lower RBC threshold	Left shift on RBC histogram, MCV flagged if below limits	Smear review
NRBCs, Megakaryocyte Fragments, or Micro Megakaryoblasts	WBC↑	NRBCs or micromegakaryoblasts counted as WBCs	NRBC/N‡ flag resulting from interference at noise lymphocyte interface on histogram/cytogram	Count NRBCs or micromegakaryoblasts per 100 WBCs and correct§.
Platelet Clumps	PLT↓, spurious WBC↑	Large clumps counted as WBCs	Platelet clumps or N flag interference at noise-lymphocyte interface on histogram or cytogram	Redraw specimen in sodium citrate.
WBCs >50,000/μL	Hgb↑, RBC↑, Hct incorrect, abnormal indices	↑Turbidity on Hgb, WBCs counted with RBC count	Hgb × 3 ≠ Hct ± 3 If WBC > 100,000/μL, count may be above linearity and may not be reported	Spun microhematocrit, manual Hgb (spin or read supernatant)†, correct RBC count, recalculate indices; if above linearity dilute for correct WBC.

Continued ▲

Continued **CONDITIONS THAT CAUSE INTERFERENCE ON MOST HEMATOLOGY ANALYZERS**

CONDITION	PARAMETER(S) AFFECTED	CAUSE	INSTRUMENT INDICATORS	CORRECTIVE ACTION
Leukemia, Especially with Chemotherapy	Spurious WBC↓, spurious PLT↑	Fragile WBCs, fragments counted as platelets	Inconsistent PLT count with previous results	Smear review, phase PLT count
Old Specimen	MCV↑, MPV↑, PLT↓, automated differential may be incorrect	RBCs swell as sample ages, platelets swell and degenerate, WBCs affected by prolonged exposure to EDTA.	Abnormal clustering on WBC histogram or cytogram	Establish stability and sample rejection criteria.

EDTA, ethylenediaminetetraacetic acid; MPV, mean platelet volume; NRBC, nucleated red blood cell; PLT, platelet.
*Lipemia shows signature pattern on Technicon H cytogram.
†Hgb can be back-calculated from directly measured CHCM on Technicon H Systems.
‡N flag is specific for Technicon H systems; indicates interference at noise-lymphocyte valley; possible NRBCs, platelet clumps, lipids, excess noise.
§Correct WBCB on Technicon H systems. Small NRBCs thresholded out of WBC count on Sysmex NE-8000 and Cell-Dyn 3000/3500; correction for NRBCs may not be necessary. Semiautomated Sysmex instruments have adjustable lower thresholds to allow inclusion of all nucleated cells in the WBC count.
For other analyzers, alternate WBC counts may be necessary before correction.

PRINCIPLES OF AUTOMATED CELL COUNTING

SPECIAL HEMATOLOGIC TESTING

TEST NAME	NORMAL		RESULT UNITS	PROCEDURE	LIMITATIONS
Osmotic RBC Fragility	Saline (%)	Hemolysis (%)	% hemolysis	Oxygenated blood is added to series of tubes containing saline dilutions and incubated for 30 min. Tubes are then mixed and centrifuged at 1000 G for 10 min. Absorbance of supernatant is then measured at 540 nm. Tube 12 is used as blank.	1. Sample must be obtained with minimum of trauma. 2. Test must be set up as soon as possible after obtaining sample. 3. Samples should be drawn in heparinized tubes. 4. Sample must be introduced directly into saline to avoid getting blood on dry sides of tube and thus increasing hemolysis.
	0.30	97–100			
	0.35	90–99			
	0.40	50–90			
	0.45	5–45			
	0.50	0–5			
	0.55	0			
Heinz Body Test	30% or less containing 5 or more Heinz bodies			Freshly drawn blood is mixed with solution of acetylphenylhydrazine and incubated at 37°C for 4 hr. After incubation, mix on slide 1 drop of crystal violet and the mixture; place coverslip and examine microscopically. Count percentage of RBCs having 5 or more Heinz bodies.	1. Splenectomy can increase number of Heinz bodies. 2. Normal control should be run in parallel.
Cresyl Blue Decolorization Test	Complete decolorization in 100 min		Qualitative complete, partial, or no decolorization	Volume of packed RBCs is lysed and mixed with known amounts of glucose 6-phosphate (G-6-P) and NADP. If glucose-6-phosphate dehydrogenase is present it will remove H^+ from G-6-P; brilliant cresyl blue accepts H^+, and it becomes colorless.	1. Qualitative. 2. All abnormal tests should be repeated.
Donath-Landsteiner Test for Paroxysmal Cold Hemoglobinuria	Negative		Positive or negative	Blood is placed into 2 prewarmed tubes. One tube (W) is incubated at 37°C and other (C) placed in ice block for 30 min. After 30 min., tube is placed in 37°C bath. Both tubes remain until clot has retracted. If test is positive, serum of tube C will show obvious hemolytic discoloration.	
Ham's Test	No hemolysis		Hemolysis or no hemolysis	Patient cells are washed and 40%–50% solution prepared. 0.1 mL of 5 N HCl is added to 1 mL of normal serum and mixed. 2 drops of cell suspension are added to acidified serum. As controls, use patients cells in nonacidified serum (1) and normal cells in acidified serum. (2) Incubate 1 hr at 37°C. Centrifuge and inspect supernatant for hemolysis.	1. Severe spherocytosis will yield false positive result.

TESTS FOR ABNORMAL HEMOGLOBINS

ASSAY	NORMAL	END RESULT	PROCEDURE	LIMITATIONS
Alkali Denaturization (Quantitative)	<2.0%	% hemoglobin F present	Patient cells are washed with normal saline. Add equal volumes of distilled H_2O and 0.4 of volume of CCl_4. Stopper and shake until hemolysis is complete. Centrifuge at 2000 G for 10 min.	Sensitive to low levels of Hgb F; however, levels are underestimated at higher levels (above 10%).
Column Chromatography	Normal: 1.5%–3.5% β-thalessemia: >3.5%–8.0%	% Hgb A_2 present	Hgb A_2 is separated using column of DEAE cellulose as ion exchange resin. Hgb solution is applied to column and Hgb A adheres to resin and Hgb A_2 passes through and is measured colorimetrically.	Other Hgb variants are also extracted by this method, including Hgb C, E, O, D, and S. If values are above 8.0%, presence of another variant should be suspected.
Isopropanol Stability Test	Precipitation after 30–40 min	Presence or absence of unstable Hgb's	Whole blood is hemolysed and hemolysate added to buffered isopropanol solution and incubated at 37°C. Preparation is observed for precipitation at 5 min intervals. Unstable Hgbs usually precipitate out in 5–10 min.	Hgb S, F, and methemoglobin can cause false positive results
Test for Hgb H Inclusions	<50% of cells showing precipitated Hgb H after 1 hr incubation		Whole blood is incubated with brilliant cresyl blue at ratio of 4 drops to 0.5 mL for 4 hr. Smears are made and examined at 10 min, 1 hr, and 4 hr.	10 min slide shows degree of reticulocytes. Other unstable Hgbs also precipitate, but usually after longer periods.
Sickle Solubility Test	Hgb soluble	Presence or absence of insoluble Hgb	Whole blood is added to solution of KH_2PO_4/K_2HPO_4 containing saponin, to lyse the RBCs, and dithionite to reduce the Hgb. Solution is then observed for turbidity by noting ability to read black lines placed behind tubes.	In samples with low Hgb (<7.0 g/dL) sample size should be doubled in order to provide sufficient Hgb to cause turbidity. Lipemic samples may yield false positive results.
Cellulose Acetate Hgb Electrophoresis	Absence of abnormal Hgb patterns	Relative % of Hgb isotypes present	Washed RBCs are lysed and hemolysate placed onto cellulose acetate at pH of 8.4–8.8 and electrophoresed for 15–30 min. Control is run concurrently. Controls commonly contain Hgb A, F, A_2, S, and C. After electrophoresis, gel is stained and Hgbs identified by their positions. Hgbs can be quantitated by reading film on densitometer.	Hgbs that contain amino acid substitutions that do not change net charge of molecule can't be detected by this method. Included in this group are some unstable Hgbs and those associated with altered O_2 affinity.
Citrate Agar Hgb Electrophoresis	Absence of abnormal Hgb patterns	Relative % of Hgb isotypes present	Same as above only citrate agar is used as medium. pH is 6.2. Electrophoresis is required for period of 45–90 min.	Used in conjunction with above method. When prominent band is found in Hgb S region, this method can be used to determine composition.

Notes on Hemoglobin Electrophoresis

MOBILITY OF HEMOGLOBIN

▌ Hemoglobin (Hgb) at an alkaline pH normally posesses a negative charge and migrates toward the anode, or positive pole.

▌ The speed at which Hgb migrates toward the anode is proportional to its net negative charge.

▌ At acid pH, Hgb is positively charged and its mobility is the reverse of that seen at alkaline pH.

▌ Amino acid substitutions affect the net charge of the Hgb molecule and thus its mobility.

INTERPRETATION

▌ Hgbs are generally categorized based on their anodal electrophoretic mobility

Slow Hgbs: C, E, A_2, and O

Intermediate Hgbs: D, G, S, and Lepore's

Fast moving Hgbs: H, I, and Bart's

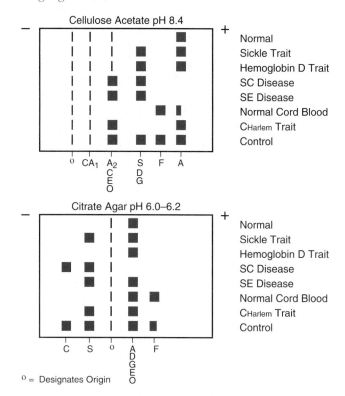

From Schmidt RM, Brosious EF: Basic Laboratory Methods of Hemoglobinopathy Detection, 6th ed. HEW publication no. (CDC)77-8266. Atlanta, U.S. Department of Health, Education and Welfare, Centers for Disease Control, 1976.

EVALUATION OF LABORATORY DATA

TEST PARAMETER	INCREASED	DECREASED
WBCs	Infections parasitic and bacterial; inflammatory conditions; leukemia; leukocytosis; viral infection (rubeola, varicella, smallpox, Epstein-Barr); drug induced	Acquired immune deficiency syndrome, agranulocytosis, alcoholism, anemia (aplastic, pernicious), arsenic poisoning, infection (severe bacterial, viral), hepatitis, leukopenia, mononucleosis, measles, lymphoma, preleukemia, rheumatic fever, immunosuppressive therapy, drug induced
RBCs	Polycythemia, burns, cardiovascular disease, increased erythropoietin production, Hgb concentration, hemoglobinopathy, hereditary spherocytosis, shock, sickle cell disease, Cushing's disease	Addison's disease, anemia, bone marrow suppression, hemodilution, Hodgkin's disease, chronic infection, leukemia, malaria, multiple myeloma, systemic lupus erythematosus, vitamin deficiency, drug induced
Hgb	Burns, chronic obstructive pulmonary disease (COPD), congestive heart failure, dehydration, diarrhea, hemoconcentration, polycythemia, drug induced	Anemia, cirrhosis, fluid retention, hemorrhage, hemolysis, pregnancy, hyperthyroidism, leukemia, lymphoma, drug induced
Hct	Addison's disease, burns, COPD, congestive heart failure, dehydration, diarrhea, hemoconcentration, polycythemia, drug induced	Fluid overload, anemia, cirrhosis, fluid retention, hemorrhage, hemolysis, pregnancy, hyperthyroidism, leukemia, lymphoma, drug induced
MCV	Alcoholism, anemia (immune and acquired hemolytic, aplastic, pernicious, other megaloblastic), liver disease, chronic lymphocytic leukemia (CLL), infants, methanol poisoning, myelodysplastic syndrome, reticulocytosis	Anemia (iron deficiency, microcytic, sickle cell, pyroxidine responsive), thalassemia, chronic disease, glucose-6-phosphate dehydrogenase deficiency, gangrene, hemoglobin H, marked leukocytosis, warm autoantibodies
MCH	Anemia (pernicious, macrocytic), cold agglutinins, newborns, dysproteinemia, monoclonal blood proteins, heparin induced	Anemia (iron deficiency, microcytic)
MCHC	Anemia (pernicious, macrocytic), cold agglutinins, hereditary spherocytosis, infants, intravascular hemolysis, lipemia, heparin induced	Anemia (iron deficiency, microcytic, normocytic)
Platelets	Anemia (hemolytic, iron deficiency), asphyxia, trauma, infection, leukemia (CML), malignancy, polycythemia vera, rheumatoid arthritis, surgery, pregnancy	Anemia (aplastic, pernicious, megaloblastic), hypoplastic bone marrow, metastatic cancer, disseminated intravascular coagulation (DIC), hemolytic disease of the newborn, May-Hegglin anomaly, irradiation, idiopathic thrombocytopenic purpura (ITP), lymphoproliferative disorders, hypersplenism, acute leukemia, myelofibrosis, multiple myeloma, myelodysplastic syndrome
Reticulocytes	Autoimmune anemia, Di Guglielmo disease, erythremic myelosis, hemoglobin C disease, hemorrhage, hereditary spherocytosis, sickle cell disease, hemoglobinuria, thrombotic thrombocytopenic purpura (TTP), thalassemia, malaria, paroxysmal nocturnal hemoglobinuria (PNH)	Anemia (aplastic, iron deficiency, megaloblastic, pernicious), alcoholism, chronic infection, radiation therapy, drug induced

EVALUATION OF LABORATORY DATA

BIBLIOGRAPHY

Beck WS: Hematopoiesis and introduction to anemia. In Beck WS, ed: Hematology, 4th ed. Cambridge, MIT Press, 1987.

Chernecky CC, Krech RL, Berger BJ: Laboratory Tests and Diagnostic Procedures. Philadelphia, WB Saunders, 1993.

Kjeldsberg C: Anemias. In Kjeldsberg C, ed: Hematologic Disorders. Chicago, ASCP Press, 1989.

McGhee D, Payne M: Hemoglobinopathies and hemoglobin defects. In Rodak BF, ed: Diagnostic Hematology. Philadelphia, WB Saunders, 1995.

Raphael S: Principles of hematology. In Raphael SS, ed: Lynch's Medical Laboratory Technology, 4th ed. Philadelphia, WB Saunders, 1983.

Section VII

HEMOSTASIS

Chapter *39*

THE MECHANISM OF BLOOD COAGULATION

Donna D. Castellone, MS, MT(ASCP)SH

QUICK CONTENTS

INTRODUCTION

Hemostasis is defined as the process by which blood is kept in a fluid state within the vascular system despite trauma to the vessel wall. The arrest of bleeding from a site is facilitated by a series of interactions between three inter-related events. The first is vasoconstriction. This is followed by blood platelet aggregation and blood coagulation. The effectiveness of hemostatic mechanisms depends on several conditions:

1. The type and degree of injury and the ability of vasoconstriction to occur
2. The availability of platelets and their activity
3. Blood factors and their relation to function as enzymes or cofactors and antigenic concentrations
4. The absence of inhibitors, circulating anticoagulants, and antagonists

Once the clot has been formed and stabilized, tissue repair occurs and the process of dissolution of the clot begins. This is known as *fibrinolysis.*

Hemostasis depends on a system of checks and balances utilizing many activators and inhibitors. This system must remain in check or will result in either hemorrhage or thrombosis. Hemorrhage may be due to disease, blood vessel rupture, or an abnormality within the blood itself. This can be due to a factor deficiency, a platelet dysfunction, inhibitors that can be inherited or acquired, drugs that inhibit function, or liver disease. Thrombosis is the activation of the hemostatic system at an inappropriate time in an inappropriate blood vessel. This can be caused by an inhibitor, or a hypercoagulable state due to deficiencies of certain anticoagulants that are inherited or acquired states. Many causes still remain unknown.

Vascular Injury and Hemostasis—An Overview

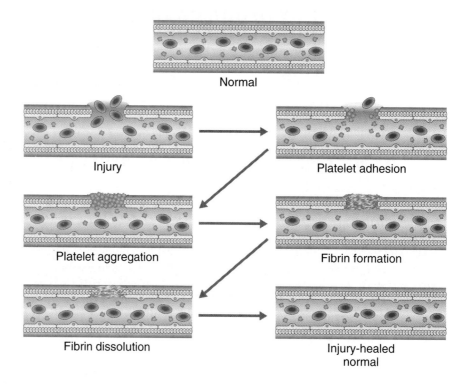

Normal

Injury

Platelet adhesion

Platelet aggregation

Fibrin formation

Fibrin dissolution

Injury-healed normal

PRIMARY HEMOSTASIS

Primary hemostasis involves the functioning of two systems and their response:

1. The vascular system
2. The platelets

Vascular System

Blood normally flows through the system without any adherence to the walls of the vessels. A thin layer of endothelial cells maintains a thromboresistant surface. When responding to vascular damage, blood clots to try to seal this damage. Vascular damage prompts the initiation of a major event in coagulation. This reflex, called *vascular constriction*, results in immediate reduced blood flow to the site. It is believed to be initiated by vasoactive substances like serotonin and thromboxane A_2 released from platelets, and also from endothelin released from endothelial cells themselves. In addition during injury these endothelial cells can rapidly express thrombotic tendencies. This is due to the function of tissue factor activity and the formation of phospholipid sites that become available as binding sites for coagulation factors.

Platelets

Platelets measure about 2 to 4 μm in diameter. They are produced in the bone marrow from a megakaryocyte, which produces about 2000 platelets; 70% to 80% circulate in the blood, whereas the remaining 20% to 30% pool in the spleen. Their life span is 7 to 10 days. Normally, platelets circulate throughout the blood as a round disc shaped form. In response to vessel wall injury the platelets begin to adhere to the vessel surface. The most important function of the platelets is the formation of a plug, which is used as an all important primary barrier to prevent further blood loss. In turn, this contact with subendothelial tissue initiates a series of reactions.

PLATELET NUMBER VERSUS FUNCTION

To maintain effectiveness in hemostasis, platelet function is more relevant than platelet numbers. In conditions in which patients have normal platelet counts (150 to 400×10^9/L) or elevated counts ($>450 \times 10^9$/L—thrombocytosis) and exhibit bleeding disorders, the condition can be caused by dysfunctional platelets. When counts fall below 50×10^9/L (thrombocytopenic), patients often do not bleed but may not maintain vascular integrity in a compromised situation such as stress, trauma, or surgery. Spontaneous bleeding may occur when platelet counts are below 10×10^9/L, but young platelets can have increased functional activity that will correct for the defect in numbers.

PLATELET KINETICS

REACTION 1 (ADHESION). Platelets adhere to collagen and undergo a shape change from discs to spiny spheres. This is primary aggregation and is reversible.

REACTION 2 (RELEASE). Platelets release the contents of their dense granules (ADP, ATP, ionized calcium, magnesium, epinephrine, phosphate, and serotonin) and alpha granules (fibrinogen, platelet derived growth factor, plasminogen activator inhibitor, fibrinonectin, albumin, β thromboglobulin, and factor V absorbed from plasma). The release of these granules constitute secondary aggregation, which is irreversible.

REACTION 3 (AGGREGATION). In response to chemical changes, these events lead to platelet aggregation in which platelets cohere to other platelets.

PRIMARY HEMOSTASIS

REACTION 4 (STABILIZATION OF THE CLOT). This reaction is responsible for thrombus formation. The adherent and aggregated platelets release factor V and expose platelet factor 3 to accelerate the coagulation cascade and promote activation of clotting factors and ultimately will stabilize the platelet plug with a fibrin clot.

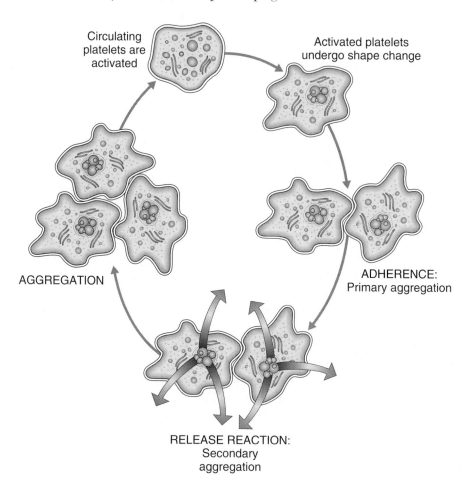

Circulating platelets are activated

Activated platelets undergo shape change

AGGREGATION

ADHERENCE: Primary aggregation

RELEASE REACTION: Secondary aggregation

ACTIVATION OF HEMOSTASIS

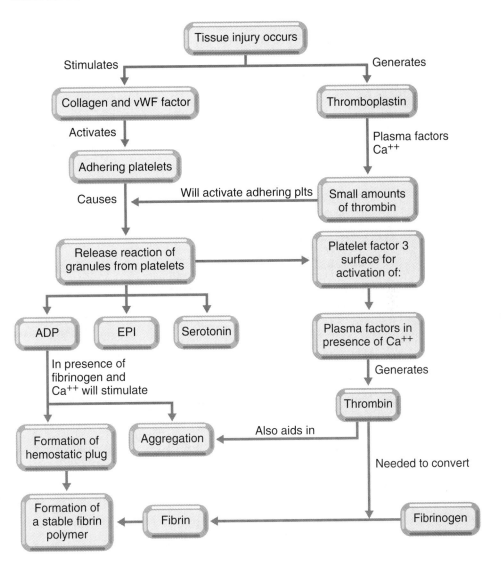

SECONDARY HEMOSTASIS

SECONDARY HEMOSTASIS

Secondary hemostasis involves a series of blood protein reactions through a cascade-like process that occurs in a series of four reactions:

1. Initiation
2. Activation of X
3. Formation of thrombin
4. Formation of an insoluble fibrin clot

In primary hemostasis the initial vasoconstriction is a short lived process; this occurrence allows a second event of platelet aggregation. This results in the production of a platelet mass that plugs the vessel. Prolonged hemostasis depends on the formation of a fibrin clot that is formed promptly and confined to the damaged portion of the vessel. The balance between coagulation proteins and anticoagulants progresses to coagulation. This secondary phase of hemostasis is the process in which fibrinogen (a soluble plasma protein) is converted to an insoluble fibrin clot. This occurs through a cascade type process that involves cofactors, and multiple enzymes that are converted from a precursor (zymogen) to an active enzyme (protease).

Coagulation Cascade

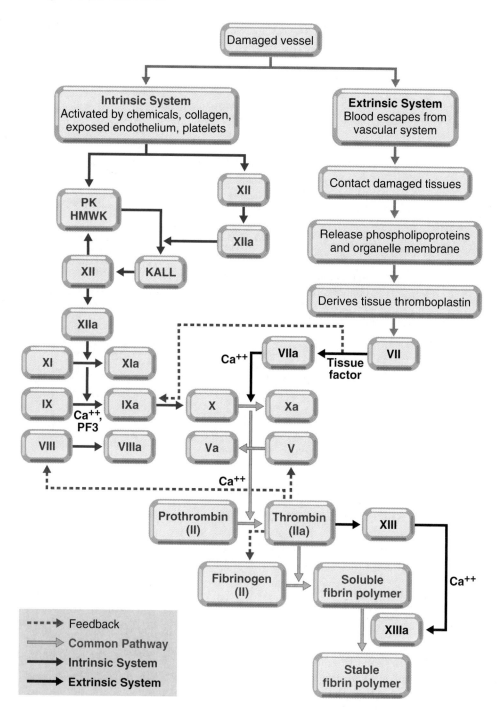

Initiation

The initiation of clotting begins with the activation of two enzymatic pathways that ultimately lead to fibrin formation: the *intrinsic* and *extrinsic* pathways. The pathway that is activated depends on the source of activators. Intrinsic activation occurs by trauma within the vascular system, such as exposed endothelium. This system is slower and yet more important compared with the extrinsic pathway, which is initiated by an external trauma, such as a clot, and occurs quickly.

EXTRINSIC INITIATION

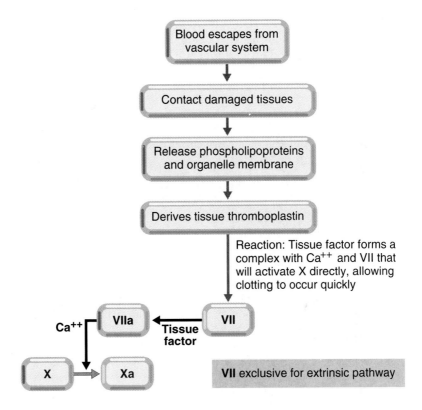

SECONDARY HEMOSTASIS

PROTHROMBIN TIME. Prothrombin time (PT) measures the *extrinsic* system of coagulation. It is dependent on the addition of calcium chloride and tissue factor and uses a lipoprotein extract from rabbit brain and lung. The PT will detect low levels of activity of factors I, II, V, VII, and X. It is used to monitor oral anticoagulation therapy (warfarin [Coumadin]). To monitor oral anticoagulation you need to consider several problems. The response to oral anticoagulation is variable and unpredictable. If the level is inadequate it increases the risk of thrombosis; if it is excessive there is an increased risk of bleeding. The goal is to maintain a narrow therapeutic range. It is important to understand the pharmacology of oral anticoagulation.

Oral Anticoagulation Therapy

Warfarin is a drug used to prevent thrombosis. It works by inhibiting the synthesis of vitamin K dependent factors (II, VII, IX, and X). Warfarin renders them nonfunctional by affecting the liver's ability to carboxylate the glutamic acid residues of these factors, the end result being impaired fibrin formation. Factors lose their function in order of their half-life, factor VII being the first to go, with a half-life of 6 hours, and factor II being the last to go, with a half-life of 2 to 3 days. If a patient is at risk of bleeding due to overanticoagulation, the patient is treated with vitamin K as long as there are no bleeding symptoms. However, if active bleeding occurs, fresh frozen plasma or prothrombin complex should be considered. The recommended dosage for oral anticoagulation is 1.5 to 2.5 times the normal range. There are many variations in the composition and responses of reagents due to the species and source of tissue factor.

Standardization of the Prothrombin Time

This mechanism for standardization is a representation of the PT that would have been obtained if the International Reference Method has been performed. This method uses a tilt tube method for performing PTs. It utilizes a preparation of human brain thromboplastin called the *Manchester reagent*. This is the most sensitive of reagents and is therefore given an International Sensitivity Index (ISI) of 1. The following formula was derived:

$$\text{INR (International Normalized Ratio)} = \left(\frac{\text{patient's PT}}{\text{PT of normal range (mean)}} \right) \text{ISI}$$

Reagents are given an ISI by the manufacturer. This is derived by comparing the value of the PT obtained using the Manchester reagent with the PT obtained with their reagent. This is graphed: X = value of PT with test reagent versus Y = value of PT with Manchester reagent. The slope is calculated and an ISI value is assigned. The closer the ISI is to 1, the *more* sensitive the reagent is; the higher the ISI, the less sensitive the reagent. The purpose of this standardization is to be able to monitor a *stable dose* of warfarin, regardless of the reagent, instrument, or place the sample was taken. The normal range of the INR is 2.0 to 3.0. This range is used in prophylaxis to prevent embolism, venous thrombosis, pulmonary embolism, and myocardial infarction. A high dose range, 2.5 to 3.5, is used in the patients with mechanical heart valves.

INTRINSIC INITIATION

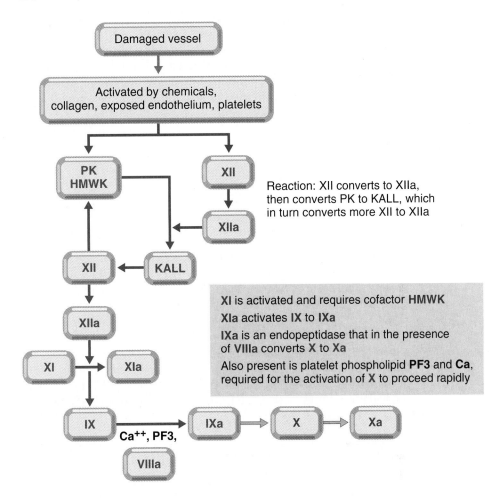

Reaction: XII converts to XIIa, then converts PK to KALL, which in turn converts more XII to XIIa

XI is activated and requires cofactor **HMWK**

XIa activates **IX** to **IXa**

IXa is an endopeptidase that in the presence of **VIIIa** converts **X** to **Xa**

Also present is platelet phospholipid **PF3** and **Ca**, required for the activation of **X** to proceed rapidly

Activation of X

The activation of factor X is crucial for blood clotting; once the activation of factor X to Xa occurs via the intrinsic or extrinsic pathway, coagulation enters the common pathway.

COMMON PATHWAY

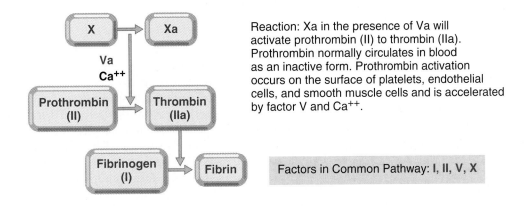

Reaction: Xa in the presence of Va will activate prothrombin (II) to thrombin (IIa). Prothrombin normally circulates in blood as an inactive form. Prothrombin activation occurs on the surface of platelets, endothelial cells, and smooth muscle cells and is accelerated by factor V and Ca^{++}.

Factors in Common Pathway: **I, II, V, X**

ACTIVATED PARTIAL THROMBOPLASTIN TIME

The activated partial thromboplastin time (APTT) measures the intrinsic system of coagulation. The reaction is dependent on adding plasma to an activator of factor X (for example, ellagic acid) and phospholipid (to provide a platelet-like substitute). This accelerates the reactions involving factors VIII and V. Coagulation is then initiated by adding calcium. When an APTT is performed it detects functioning of factors XII, XI, X, IX, VIII, V, II, and I. This test is used to monitor heparin therapy and to evaluate patients with a bleeding or thrombotic history or acquired inhibitors.

Heparin

Heparin is a heterogeneous polysaccharide chain that is found in organ systems including the heart, kidney, lung, and mast cells. It is used clinically for two reasons:

1. To treat established venous thromboembolism
2. To prevent postoperative venous thromboembolism

Heparin contains a specific pentasaccharide chain that is used as a binding site for antithrombin III (ATIII), which regulates the generation of thrombin. Heparin accelerates the inhibition of thrombin, preventing the formation of a clot. The therapeutic range of heparin is 0.2 to 0.4μ/ml, which is usually achieved at 1.5 to 2.5 times the normal range of the APTT. If there is a failed response to heparin, several variables should be considered. Obesity affects the anticoagulant to blood ratio, thereby decreasing the APTT. An increase in acute phase reactive proteins (I, VIII—elevated in stress, pregnancy, and infections) to greater than 300% will result in a shortened APTT. In addition, if there is a decreased amount of ATIII, there may be a shortened APTT due to the deficiency of the binding site capacity of the ATIII, which is needed to allow the heparin to function to prevent clotting.

Low Molecular Weight Heparin

This type of heparin is prepared by chemical degradation of standard heparin by reducing the molecular weight from the range of 5000 to 30,000 to a low molecular weight of 2000 to 10,000. The advantage to this preparation is that it binds less to endothelial cells and circulating proteins. It does not bind to platelets. Due to its low molecular weight it is better absorbed. Its effect is very predictable and doesn't need to be monitored. It cannot be monitored by an APTT because of the absence of the long chain and the ability of heparin to bind with ATIII to inhibit thrombin. This can be measured by testing for the inactivation of factor Xa. Low molecular weight heparin is not widely used in the United States except in hip replacement surgery.

Thrombin Formation

When plasma fibrinogen is activated by thrombin, this conversion results in a stable fibrin clot. This clot is visible proof that the action of the protease enzyme thrombin has achieved fibrin formation. This conversion of protransglutaminase to transglutaminase is the final step of clot formation. Thrombin is also involved in the factor XIII to factor XIIIa activation in which thrombin cleaves a peptide bond from each of two alpha chains; inactive factor XIII along with Ca^{2+} ions enables factor XIII to dissociate into factor XIIIa. If thrombin were allowed to circulate in its active form (IIa), uncontrollable clotting would occur; as a result it circulates in its inactive form, prothrombin (II).

REACTION. Thrombin, a protease enzyme, cleaves fibrinogen (factor I), which results in a fibrin monomer, fibrinogen peptides A and B. These initial monomers polymerize end to end due to hydrogen bonding.

Fibrin Formation

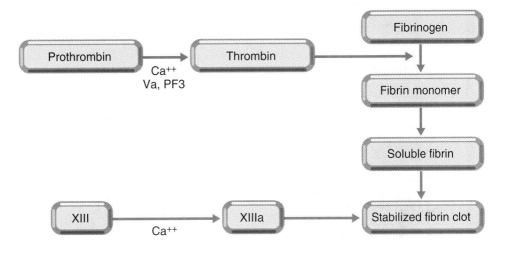

FORMATION OF FIBRIN OCCURS IN THREE PHASES:

1. *Proteolysis:* Protease enzyme thrombin cleaves fibrinogen, resulting in a fibrin monomer, A and B fibrinopeptide.
2. *Polymerization:* This occurs spontaneously due to fibrin monomer that polymerizes end to end by hydrogen bonding.
3. *Stabilization:* This occurs when the fibrin monomers are linked covalently by factor XIIIa into fibrin polymers, forming an insoluble fibrin clot.

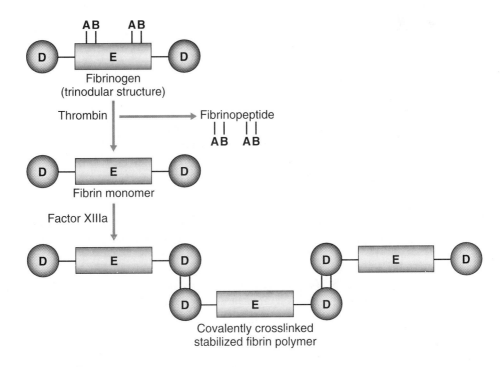

Covalently crosslinked
stabilized fibrin polymer

FIBRINOLYSIS

Dissolution of clotting begins almost as soon as the clot is formed. Fibrin clots are not intended to be permanent; their purpose is to stop the flow of blood until the damaged vessel can be repaired. Fibrinolysis is the process by which the hydrolytic enzyme plasmin digests fibrin and fibrinogen, resulting in progressively reduced clots. Normal plasma contains the inactive form of plasmin in a precursor called *plasminogen*. This precursor remains dormant until it is activated by proteolytic enzymes, the kinases, or plasminogen activators. These are found in tissues, urine, plasma, lysosomal granules, and vascular endothelium. This activator, tissue plasminogen activator (t-PA), results in the activation of plasminogen to plasmin, resulting in the degradation of fibrin. This system is in turn controlled by inhibitors to t-PA and plasmin-plasminogen activator inhibitor (PAI-1) and α_2-antiplasmin.

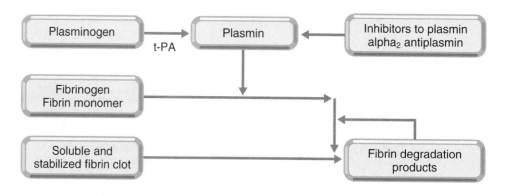

COAGULATION FACTORS

Blood factors can be classified as:

1. *Substrate*, the substance on which an enzyme acts
2. *Zymogen*, an enzyme precursor
3. *Cofactor*, a component that aids in the activation of zymogen to active enzyme
4. *Calcium*

In the conversion of zymogens to enzymes, either they are serine proteases (factors II, VII, IX, X, XI, XII), which use serine as the active site and cleave peptide bonds, or they create covalent bonds as transaminases. Blood factors are produced mostly in the liver and circulate in an inactive precursor form.

Characteristics of Factor Functions

FACTOR I: FIBRINOGEN. Substrate for thrombin and precursor of fibrin, it is a large globulin protein; when it is exposed to thrombin, two peptides split from the fibrinogen molecule, leaving a fibrin monomer to form a polymerized clot.

FACTOR II: PROTHROMBIN. In the presence of Ca^{2+}, prothrombin is converted to thrombin (IIa), which in turn stimulates platelet aggregation and activates cofactors, protein C, and factor XIII.

FACTOR III: THROMBOPLASTIN. This tissue factor activates factor VII when blood is exposed to tissue fluids.

FACTOR IV: IONIZED CALCIUM. This active form of calcium is needed for the activation of thromboplastin and for the conversion of prothrombin to thrombin, factor XIII to its active form factor XIIIa, and factor X to factor Xa, its active form.

FACTOR V: PROACCELERIN. This is consumed during clotting and accelerates the transformation of prothrombin to thrombin.

FACTOR VI: This is nonexistent

FACTOR VII: PROCONVERTIN. This is activated by tissue thromboplastin, which in turn activates factor X.

FACTOR VIII: ANTIHEMOPHILIC. This has several functions. Factor VIIIc/vWF (von Willebrand's factor) makes up the total factor. VIII:c, the active portion, is measured by clotting and vWF:Ag measures antigen that binds to endothelium for platelet function. Factor VIIIc is deficient in hemophilia A.

FACTOR IX: PLASMA THROMBOPLASTIN COMPONENT. This is a component of the thromboplastin generating system; it influences amount as opposed to rate and is deficient in hemophilia B.

FACTOR X: STUART-PROWER. The final common pathway merges to convert prothrombin to thrombin; activity is also related to factor VII.

FACTOR XI: PLASMA THROMBOPLASTIN ANTECEDENT. This is essential to intrinsic thromboplastin generating of the cascade.

FACTOR XII: HAGEMAN'S FACTOR. This is a surface contact factor that is activated by collagen.

FACTOR XIII: FIBRIN STABILIZING FACTOR. In the presence of calcium, this transaminase stabilizes polymerized fibrin monomers in the initial clot.

COAGULATION FACTORS

BIBLIOGRAPHY

American Dade: Coagulation Education. American Hospital Supply Corporation of Florida, 1983.
Antiano-Green D: Reporting PT results with INR values. Advance, 6:10–12, 1994.
Hudson JL, Bunting RF: A Study Guide of Clinical Hematology: Theory and Practice. Philadelphia, FA Davis, 1994.
Jensen R: Heparin therapy and monitoring. Clin Hemostasis Rev Aug, pp 9–10, 1995.
Kjeldsberg CR: *Practical Diagnosis of Hematologic Disorders,* 2nd ed. Chicago, ASCP Press, 1995.
Lemery L: Understanding the theory behind anticoagulant therapy. Advance, 7:6–8, 1995.
National Committee for Clinical Laboratory Standards: One Stage Prothrombin Time Test (PT): Tentative Guidelines H28-T 1992. Activated Partial Thromboplastin Time (APTT) Test: H29-T 1992. Villanova, PA, 1992.
Palkuti H: INR, Clinical Significance and Applications. Horsham, PA, BioData Corporation, 1995, pp 2–11.
Rodak B: Diagnostic Hematology. Philadelphia, WB Saunders, 1995.
Turgeon ML: Clinical Hematology. Boston, Little, Brown, 1993.

Chapter

40

EVALUATION OF BLEEDING DISORDERS

Donna D. Castellone, MS, MT(ASCP)SH

Q U I C K   C O N T E N T S

INTRODUCTION

Abnormalities that may cause a hemorrhage/bleed can be found in three major components of coagulation:

1. Vascular endothelium
2. Platelet function
3. Coagulation factors

The family history is an important tool in distinguishing if the condition is acquired or inherited. An *inherited* defect shows a positive family history with bleeding manifested during childhood. In addition, bleeding may occur before hemostatic stress. An *acquired* defect shows an absence of family history, occurs in adulthood, and shows a tolerance under hemostatic stress. It is important to rule out drug interactions and underlying disease states that predispose the patient. These include abnormalities such as cancer, myeloproliferative disorders, leukemias, liver failure, and vitamin K deficiency. Many drugs, most commonly aspirin, interfere with platelet functions of adherence, release, and aggregation.

EVALUATION OF BLEEDING IN PRIMARY HEMOSTASIS

Abnormalities of the Vascular Endothelium

Normal vessel walls provide three functions. These are:

1. To provide a surface resistant to the formation of thrombi
2. If disrupted, to react by providing the initial stimuli for thrombus formation
3. To provide inhibitors for platelet activity as well as activators for clearance of a thrombus through fibrinolysis

HEREDITARY VASCULAR DISORDERS

SYNDROME	GENETIC PATTERN	CLINICAL CHARACTERISTICS	LABORATORY FINDINGS
Hereditary Telangiectasia Rendu-Osler-Weber	Autosomal dominant	Thinning of vessel walls Telangiectasia seen on lips, tongue, face, and hands; frequent nose bleeds in childhood; anemia	Normal bleeding time Tourniquet test may show increased capillary resistance, depleted Fe stores, hypochromia, microcytic anemia.
Hemangioma-Thrombocytopenia Kasabach-Merritt	Unknown	Giant vascular tumor, thrombocytopenia and bleeding. External hemangiomas may become engorged with blood and resemble hematomas.	Low platelet count Low fibrinogen levels Acute or chronic disseminated intravascular coagulation Microangiopathic hemolytic anemia
Ehlers-Danlos	Autosomal dominant	Severity of bleeding ranges from easy bruises to arterial rupture.	Positive tourniquet test Prolonged bleeding time
Homocystinuria	Autosomal recessive	Increased in patients with cobalamin and folate deficiency	Decreased levels of B_6, cobalamin, folate Increased homocystine level

ACQUIRED VASCULAR DISORDERS

SYNDROME	MODE ACQUIRED	CLINICAL CHARACTERISTICS	LAB FINDINGS
Allergic Purpura Henoch-Schönlein Purpura	Allergies to food, drugs, cold, insect bites, and vaccinations	Skin rash, edema, joint pain, abdominal colic, urticaria, possible petechiae	Platelet count normal Bleeding time normal White blood cells, erythrocyte sedimentation rate elevated
Amyloidosis	Deposit of amyloid on endothelium	Vascular disease with hemorrhage and thrombosis	Platelet function may be abnormal. In rare cases patients have thrombocytopenia.
Vitamin C Deficiency Scurvy	Insufficient dietary intake of ascorbic acid, resulting in decreased synthesis of collagen and weakening of capillary walls	Tendency to bruise, ecchymosis, bleeding gums	Positive tourniquet test, low plasma levels of vitamin C, decreased ascorbic acid levels

Evaluation of Platelet Abnormalities

THROMBOCYTOPENIA. This condition occurs most frequently. Platelets are low in number but normal in function; bleeding time may be prolonged with poor clot retraction. Lack of marrow megakaryocyte precursors results in low platelet counts, or low counts due to platelet destruction.

1. Immunologic, idiopathic thrombocytopenic purpura (ITP), no known cause
2. Result of diseases or viral
3. Drugs, especially aspirin

THROMBOCYTOPATHIA. One sees poor platelet factor 3 (PF3) activity; platelet count normal, poor in function; bleeding time prolonged; poor clot retraction; decreased serum prothrombin. The condition can be caused by:

1. Too little PF3, due to systemic disease—uremia, scurvy, and hepatic disease
2. Failure to release PF3, due to abnormal protein coating platelets, or immunoglobulins
3. Deficiency of plasma factor necessary for normal platelet function— von Willebrand's factor (vWF)

THROMBOCYTOSIS. Platelets are increased in number, normal in function, and can be just a transient rise. The condition is seen in:

1. Acute hemorrhage
2. Hemolysis
3. Postsplenectomy

THROMBOCYTHEMIA. One finds platelets increased in number, large and bizarre forms, bleeding time prolonged, poor clot retraction, defective adhesiveness, abnormal release of PF3. The condition can cause simultaneous clotting and hemorrhage and is seen in:

1. Myeloproliferative disorders

Tests to Evaluate a Bleeding Disorder of Primary Hemostasis

EVALUATION OF BLEEDING IN PRIMARY HEMOSTASIS

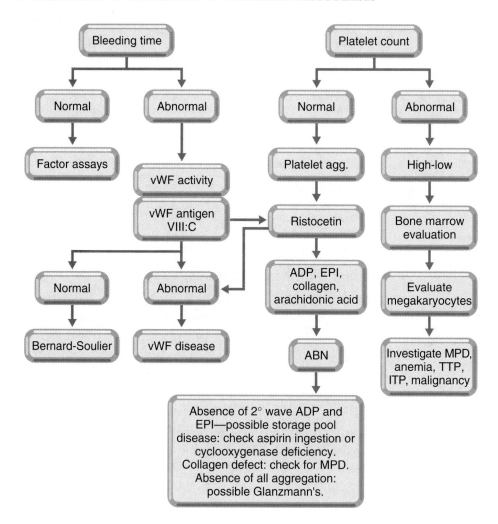

BLEEDING TIME. Most common is the Ivy method, which uses an instrument called *Surgicutt,* which ensures a precise surgical incision depth of 1 mm and enhances reproducibility. A blood pressure cuff is pumped up to 40 mm Hg and held at this pressure for the entire test. With filter paper the incision is "wicked," not blotted, every 30 seconds, with care taken to wick in the direction of the flow of blood. The time for bleeding to cease is recorded. The normal range is less than 8 minutes. This detects the formation of the initial hemostatic plug, which forms as a result of the platelets' adhesion to the severed vessel and subsequent platelet aggregation at the wound site. A prolonged bleeding time requires further analysis and suggests a disorder of primary hemostasis that can be acquired, hereditary, or drug induced. It is very important that the patient not take aspirin and other nonsteroidal anti-inflammatory drugs for at least 10 days before this test or the results will be falsely prolonged. In addition, the patient should have a platelet count greater than 100,000 to ensure the accuracy of the test.

CLOT RETRACTION. This test is used as a tool to gain information, following fibrin formation, from the inspection of the clot. Clot retraction occurs by the interaction between platelet pseudopods and fibrin strands. This occurs within 60 minutes, and the clot occupies 50% of total volume of blood. Clot retraction results in a stabilized mass of platelets and fibrin that seals off a wounded vessel to prevent further blood loss. Thrombocytopenia is a quantitative platelet defect, and thrombasthenia is a qualitative platelet defect.

SERUM PROTHROMBIN TIME. If thromboplastin is formed at the proper rate, prothrombin is converted to thrombin, fibrinogen is converted to fibrin, and 80% to 90% of the prothrombin is consumed in clotting. If PF3 is abnormal, thromboplastin is formed more slowly, leaving unconsumed prothrombin in the serum.

PLATELET AGGREGATION STUDIES. The purpose of this test is to detect abnormal aggregation that is associated with the diagnosis of platelet functional disorders. The principle of this test is that when platelet rich plasma is used, there will be a change in optical density of the sample as various reagents are added; this is measured on an aggregometer. Aggregation of platelets can be induced by the addition of various reagents such as ADP, EPI (epinephrine), collagen, ristocetin, thrombin, and arachidonic acid. The results correspond to certain disease states. Aggregation occurs in two phases: phase 1 is indicative of platelet adherence and shape change; this is reversible and represents the primary wave. Phase 2 represents the release of granules, and aggregation is secondary and irreversible.

Interpretation of Aggregating Agents

1. *Normal Response:* This is a biphasic pattern of response to ADP, EPI, ristocetin, and arachidonic acid. Thrombin is measured by release with ATP, and a slope is measured for collagen. These are compared with an established normal range.

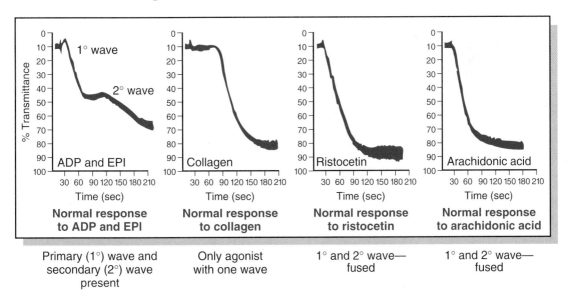

Normal response to ADP and EPI	Normal response to collagen	Normal response to ristocetin	Normal response to arachidonic acid
Primary (1°) wave and secondary (2°) wave present	Only agonist with one wave	1° and 2° wave— fused	1° and 2° wave— fused

2. *Abnormal Response to ADP and EPI:* There is a slow release of nucleotides that begins after the secondary wave of aggregation is under way. Lack of a secondary wave is indicative of defective prostaglandin production and a defective release of nucleotides.

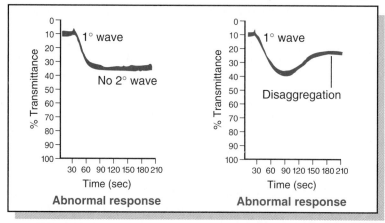

Primary (1°) wave—present
Secondary (2°) wave—absent

Primary (1°) wave—present
No secondary (2°) wave—
disaggregation present

3. *Abnormal Response to Collagen:* This indicates if prostaglandin formation or the release mechanism is deficient. Aggregation is slower and less complete, resulting in a decreased response to collagen.

4. *Abnormal Response to Arachidonic Acid:* Arachidonic acid is converted by the platelets into prostaglandin endoperoxides and thromboxanes; if cyclo-oxygenase is deficient or if the enzyme is inhibited by a drug, there will be no aggregation, or release will be absent.

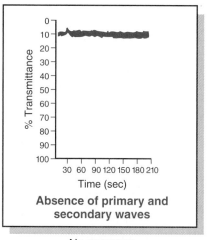

No response

5. *Abnormal Response to Ristocetin:* This response is impaired in patients that have platelets that are unable to adhere to subendothelial surfaces due to a decrease in the von Willebrand factor (vWF) on the surface of the platelet.

6. *Abnormal Response to Thrombin:* Thrombin is measured by Lumi aggregation, which demonstrates both the aggregation and the secretion of the dense granules of ATP by utilizing luciferin. Thrombin induces full secretion independent of the prostaglandin or cyclo-oxygenase pathway.

PLATELET DISORDERS

PLATELET DISORDER	MODE OF TRANSMISSION	BIOCHEMISTRY	CLINICAL FINDINGS	AGGREGATION RESULTS	OTHER LABORATORY TESTS
von Willebrand's	Autosomal dominant; can be acquired; IgG inhibitor, or in disease states; myelo- or lymphoproliferative	Defect is a decreased vWF factor on platelet membrane, which is needed to bind with glycoprotein Ib	Bleeding varies from mild to severe; depends on multimeric type*	ADP, EPI, AA, thrombin, collagen all normal; ristocetin decreased; will correct by adding normal plasma	Abnormal BT; normal platelet count; abnormal ristocetin cofactor; decreased antigen; factor VIII activity, low normal
Bernard-Soulier	Autosomal recessive	Lacks glycoprotein Ib on surface of cell and can't adhere to platelets	Severe bleeding tendencies	ADP, EPI, AA, thrombin, collagen all normal; ristocetin decreased; will not correct by adding normal plasma	Platelet count decreased; giant platelets, large as lymphocytes; BT abnormal
Glanzmann's Thrombasthenia	Autosomal recessive; seen in consanguinity	Lacks glycoprotein IIb/IIIa, which impairs ability of platelets to bind fibrinogen	Hemorrhagic findings may vary; seen in infancy, may cause severe mucous membrane bleeding	ADP, EPI, AA, thrombin, collagen, no response; ristocetin not diagnostic	Platelet count normal; size normal; BT prolonged; abnormal clot retraction
Storage Pool Disease	Autosomal dominant; also variable; can be acquired with disease states	Dense granule deficiency, resulting in no release reaction	Various mild to severe bleeding tendencies	ADP, EPI, primary wave present; no secondary EPI; collagen decreased	Platelet count normal, or decreased; BT prolonged
Hermansky-Pudlak	Autosomal recessive; rare	Lipid metabolism disorder; abnormal platelet morphology associated with deficient release reaction	Albinism; mild bleeding problems; Swiss cheese platelets	Primary wave ADP; no secondary; EPI and collagen decreased	Platelet count normal; size normal; BT slightly prolonged
Wiskott-Aldrich	Sex linked recessive; primarily in boys	Platelets structurally abnormal; micro-thrombocytes, number of alpha and dense granules decreased	Severe eczema; recurrent infections; thrombocytopenia	Primary wave ADP + EPI—no secondary wave; collagen decreased; thrombin normal	Platelet count decreased; size decreased; BT prolonged

Continued ▲

▲ Continued **PLATELET DISORDERS**

PLATELET DISORDER	MODE OF TRANSMISSION	BIOCHEMISTRY	CLINICAL FINDINGS	AGGREGATION RESULTS	OTHER LABORATORY TESTS
Chédiak-Higashi	Rare autosomal recessive	Defective platelet function; lack normal dense bodies and ADP	Pancytopenia, albinism, infections, hemorrhage	Decreased ADP, EPI, and collagen	Platelet count low; large lysosomal granules in WBCs
Chronic Liver Disease	Various etiologies	Decreased coagulation factor production; fibrinolysis; thrombocytopenia	Thrombocytopenia from hypersplenism, DIC, severe bleeding in end stage liver disease	Abnormal platelet aggregation to ADP, EPI, thrombin	Mild–moderate thrombocytopenia; BT prolonged; abnormal PF3 availability
Uremia	Renal failure; disturbances of body fluid balance; results in azotemia	Inhibition of platelet function; altered prostaglandin metabolism	Bleeding occurs when drugs that inhibit platelet function are given; nausea; hemorrhagic lesions; intestinal tract bleeding; heart failure	Patterns not uniform; lack of primary ADP induced aggregation; collagen defective	Platelet count normal or decreased; platelet size normal; BT prolonged; abnormal PF3 activity
Gray Platelet Syndrome	Hereditary, probably autosomal	Marked deficiency of platelet alpha granules releasing PF4, VIII R:ag, acid hydrolases	Lifelong mild bleeding; reticulum fibrosis of marrow	Normal platelet aggregation with ADP, EPI, collagen	Platelet count low; platelet size large; appear gray on Wright stained smear; BT increased
Afibrinogenemia	Rare autosomal recessive	Platelet dysfunction poorly understood; supports theory fibrinogen is necessary for normal platelet aggregation	Hematomas, bruising, epistaxis, defective wound healing	Deficient platelet aggregation with ADP and collagen	Platelet count normal; platelet size normal; BT normal or prolonged; PT, APTT, TT, all prolonged
Cyclo-oxygenase Deficiency	Rare autosomal dominant	Inability to form thromboxane A_2, but still form less potent cyclic endoperoxides	Mild to moderate defect in hemostasis	Abnormal response to ADP, EPI; diminished response to AA; thrombin normal	Platelet count normal; platelet size normal; BT prolonged

Continued ▲

▶ Continued **PLATELET DISORDERS**

PLATELET DISORDER	MODE OF TRANSMISSION	BIOCHEMISTRY	CLINICAL FINDINGS	AGGREGATION RESULTS	OTHER LABORATORY TESTS
Defects of Platelet Adhesion	Acquired or autoimmune disorders	DIC or fibrinolysis may induce platelet dysfunction.	SLE, ITP Scleroderma; rheumatoid arthritis	Acquired platelet defects do not show typical platelet aggregation abnormalities.	Platelet count normal; platelet size normal
Drug Inhibition of Prostaglandin	Acetylsalicylic acid; ibuprofen; naproxen; furosemide; prolonged exposure to alcohol, cyclosporine, dextran, hydrocortisone	Drugs irreversibly acetylate prostaglandin producing enzyme cyclo-oxygenase and inhibit its activity for life of the platelet, 7–10 days.	Gastrointestinal irritation; capillary damage; decreased utilization of vitamin K by liver; antifibrinogenic action	Primary wave ADP+ EPI; no secondary wave; collagen defective; AA, no response	Platelet count normal; platelet size normal; PT and APTT normal; BT prolonged
Drug Induced Membrane Defects	Elavil, Tofranil, Thorazine, cocaine, lidocaine, ampicillin, Benadryl, Aventyl, alcohol	Drugs can interfere with platelet membrane or receptor sites; interference with prostaglandin pathway or phosphodiesterase activity	Clinically significant platelet defects and hemorrhage; mucous membrane bleeding, hemarthroses	Primary wave ADP+ EPI; no secondary wave; AA no response	Platelet count normal; platelet size normal; PT and APTT normal; BT prolonged
Myelo- and Lymphoproliferative Disorders	Chronic myeloproliferative disorders	Defect due to loss of platelet surface membrane receptors for alpha adrenergic receptors and prostaglandin D₂; depletion of dense granules, secretion of ADP, and impaired oxidation of AA	Differ according to disorder; chronic myelogenous leukemia; polycythemia vera; myelofibrosis; essential thrombocythemia	Decreased response to ADP, EPI, collagen, and thrombin	WBCs vary; platelet size varies; normochromic anemia; abnormal platelet shapes; decreased procoagulant activity
Antiplatelet Antibodies	ITP, SLE, and platelet alloimmunization	Immunoglobulins bind to platelet membrane and interfere with its function	Thrombocytopenia, bruises, epistaxis, petechiae, hemorrhage	Will not supply clinically useful information; normal aggregation	Platelet count low; platelet size varies; BT prolonged; PT, PTT normal

*Refer to multimeric chart on p 984.
BT, bleeding time; TT, thrombin time; ADP, adenosine diphosphate; EPI, epinephrine; AA, arachidonic acid; SLE, systemic lupus erythematosus; ITP, idiopathic thrombocytopenic purpura; PT, prothrombin time; APTT, activated partial thromboplastin time.

EVALUATION OF BLEEDING IN PRIMARY HEMOSTASIS

VON WILLEBRAND'S DISEASE—CLASSIFICATION AND MULTIMERIC STRUCTURE

There are several variant forms of von Willebrand's disease (vWD); they are characterized by the results of certain laboratory tests. These variations are due to the range of multimers that are present. The bleeding time is prolonged in all variant types. It is important to know the type of multimer when treating the patient with the drug 1-deamino-8-d-arginine vasopressin (DDAVP). DDAVP induces the release of stored vWF, resulting in a temporary increase of vWF and thus enabling procedures to be performed that might otherwise result in bleeding. In type IIB vWD, this drug may cause hyperaggregability of platelets. All types are autosomal dominant with the exception of type IIC, which is autosomal recessive, and type III, which can be variable.

CHARACTERISTIC	TYPE I	TYPE IIA	TYPE IIB	TYPE IIC	TYPE III
Multimer	Normal	Absence of large and intermediate multimers	Absence of large multimers	Absence of large multimers; aberrant triplet structure	Variable
Factor VIII	Decreased	Decreased or normal	Decreased or normal	Normal	Markedly decreased
Ristocetin Cofactor	Decreased	Markedly decreased	Decreased or normal	Decreased	Absent
vWF Antigen	Decreased	Decreased or normal	Increased	Decreased	Absent
Ristocetin Induced Platelet Aggregation	Decreased or normal	Absent or decreased	Increased	Decreased	Absent
Response to DDAVP	Normal	Does not correct vW multimers, will increase vWF	Bleeding time may correct due to transient correction of multimers		

Conclusions

In beginning to evaluate a patient for a bleeding disorder of primary hemostasis, it is important to assess all the information that a good patient history can provide. The next line of testing is to evaluate the patient's coagulation factors and their effect in diagnosis and patient management.

EVALUATION OF BLEEDING IN SECONDARY HEMOSTASIS

In coagulation disorders, a bleed due to a factor abnormality can be for several reasons:

1. A decreased production of factors, inherited, or acquired due to disease states or drug interference
2. Abnormal molecular production of the factor that interferes with its role in the coagulation cascade
3. The loss of factors through nephrotic syndromes or liver disease or their consumption as in disseminated intravascular coagulation (DIC)
4. Inactivation of factors by antibodies or inhibitors that can occur spontaneously with any factor or in response to drugs

The screening tests that give the most information are the prothrombin time (PT), the activated partial thromboplastin time (APTT), the thrombin time (TT), and fibrinogen. From the results of these tests, additional studies can be determined to aid in patient diagnosis.

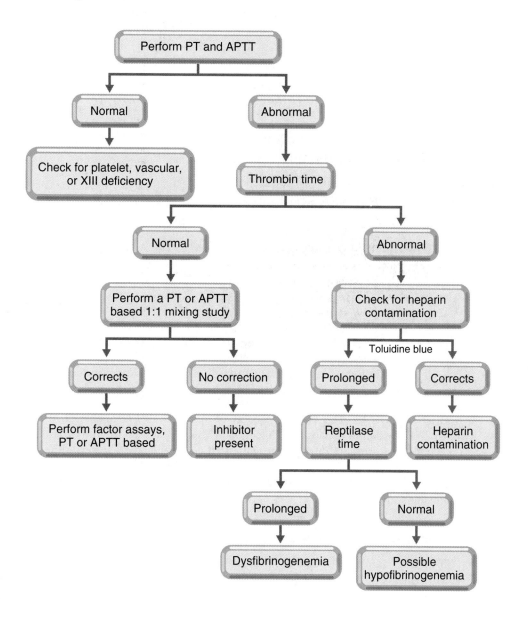

EVALUATION OF BLEEDING IN SECONDARY HEMOSTASIS

INTERPRETATIONS OF THE PROTHROMBIN TIME AND ACTIVATED PARTIAL THROMBOPLASTIN TIME RESULTS

1. *PT and APTT are normal:* Hemostatic abnormalities can be due to a platelet deficiency, a vascular defect, or a factor XIII abnormality.
2. *PT or APTT are prolonged:* The most common cause of a prolonged test is that the patient is taking oral anticoagulation medication. The goal of oral anticoagulation therapy is to prevent the formation of a thrombus.
3. *PT is prolonged and APTT is normal:* The PT test is exclusive for factor VII. This abnormality usually indicates a factor VII deficiency.
4. *PT is normal and APTT is prolonged:* This indicates a problem within the intrinsic pathway and suggests a deficiency of prekallikrein, HMWK (high molecular weight kininogen), or factor VIII, IX, XI, or XII.
5. *PT and APTT are prolonged:* This indicates an abnormality of the common pathway, that is, factors I, II, V, and X, or a possibility of multiple factor deficiencies.

> **Note** It is important that the specimen—including specimens drawn through a line—not be contaminated with heparin; this will falsely prolong results. A repeat sample will verify contamination and possibly eliminate an expensive work-up.

Tests for Disorders of Secondary Hemostasis

SCREENING TESTS

PROTHROMBIN TIME. This screening is used to detect coagulation factor deficiencies within the extrinsic pathway. It measures factors I, II, V, VII, and X. It is used to measure oral anticoagulant therapy such as warfarin (Coumadin).

ACTIVATED PARTIAL THROMBOPLASTIN TIME. The APTT is used to measure coagulation deficiencies within the intrinsic pathway. This will detect deficiencies of factors I, II, V, VIII, IX, X, XI, XII, HMWK, and prekallikrein. It is used to monitor heparin therapy.

FIBRINOGEN. A functional assay used to test the quantity of fibrinogen is called the *Clauss method.* The patient's plasma is diluted with buffer, a high concentration of thrombin is added, and the clotting time is measured. This is read off a standard curve and tests the amount of available fibrinogen. The test is affected by heparin. Fibrinogen can also be tested antigenically to help distinguish between hereditary fibrinogen deficiencies.

THROMBIN TIME. This tests the quality of the functional fibrinogen. It uses a weak amount of thrombin to allow the detection of abnormalities in the thrombin-fibrinogen reaction that a stronger thrombin may mask. It is also the best test for residual heparin. If the test is repeated using toluidine blue for the buffer, this neutralizes any heparin that may be present and corrects the result into the normal range, confirming heparin contamination.

CONFIRMATORY TESTS

MIXING STUDIES. The patient's plasma is mixed with an equal volume of pooled normal plasma (PNP). A PT or an APTT is then performed on the patient's plasma, the PNP, and the 1:1 mix. If the addition of the PNP has corrected the patient's sample into the normal range, that PNP has replaced a factor the patient was missing. This indicates that a factor deficiency is present. If the sample does not correct or partially corrects, this indicates that an inhibitor is present, such as a lupus anticoagulant or a specific factor inhibitor.

FACTOR ASSAYS. These are specific assays to determine the cause of a prolonged PT or APTT. PT based factors are II, V, VII, and X; APTT based factors are VIII, IX, XI, XII, HMWK, and prekallikrein. The PT or APTT is performed on dilutions of the patient's plasma with a substrate that is *deficient* only in the factor being tested. These are then read off a standard curve prepared by plotting times of dilutions with a standard that contains a *known* concentration of the factor being assayed; the result will be the percentage of activity of the factor tested.

Interpretation by Choice of Substrate

SUBSTRATE	FACTORS CONTAINED	FACTORS LACKING
Normal Plasma	All factors	None
Absorbed Plasma	HMWK, prekallikrein, XII, XI, VIII, V, and I	Vitamin K dependent II, VII, IX, and X
Serum	HMWK, prekallikrein, XII, XI, X, IX, and VII	I, V, and VIII

FACTOR XIII. Fibrin stabilizing factor does not circulate in plasma and is therefore not detected by a mixing study, or specific factor assays. Factor XIII is tested by adding the patient's plasma to 5 molar urea and allowing a clot to form. This is incubated for 24 hours at 37°C. If factor XIII is deficient, a clot will form but will lyse after 24 hours. This confirms a deficiency of factor XIII. It confirms that enough fibrin has been formed to initiate a clot, but there is not enough factor XIII to stabilize the clot. These patients do not bleed right away, but ooze a day or a few days after an invasive procedure has been performed.

FIBRIN/FIBRINOGEN DEGRADATION PRODUCTS. This test detects plasmin cleaved fibrin or fibrinogen. It utilizes nonspecific polyclonal antibodies to human fibrinogen fragments X and Y. It tests for both fibrinolysis and fibrinogenolysis and is therefore more sensitive for DIC.

D-DIMER. The D-dimer addresses both thrombin and plasmin by testing thrombin-cleaved fibrinogen that will form soluble fibrin by factor XIIIa and plasmin. D-Dimer is a specific marker for fibrinolysis; its presence indicates plasmin degradation of crosslinked fibrin. The test uses specific monoclonal antibodies that are not further digestible by plasma and will not crossreact with fibrinogen. D-Dimers are found in disseminated intravascular coagulation (DIC), pulmonary embolism, deep vein thrombosis, and arterial thrombosis.

REPTILASE TIME. This test is used as a qualitative test for fibrinogen function when heparin is present and is also used to detect dysfibrinogenemia. It is used in studies of fibrin formation and disturbances of fibrin formation. The test uses snake venom added to plasma to see how long it takes for clot formation. This test is not affected by heparin. It is prolonged when there is dysfibrinogenemia, hypofibrinogenemia, afibrinogenemia, and high levels of FDPs.

EVALUATION OF BLEEDING IN SECONDARY HEMOSTASIS

Classification

A bleeding disorder can be classified as either hereditary or acquired. In a hereditary abnormality a positive family history or genetic pattern will be evident with bleeding manifesting itself during early childhood. These problems arise from a deficiency or functional abnormality of a single factor. In contrast, an acquired disorder can arise at any time. There may be mild bleeding, or acute bleeding may arise in a compromised situation in which factors are destroyed or consumed. This occurs in DIC or in defective synthesis of factors resulting from liver disease or an abnormality of vitamin K synthesis. In addition, spontaneous antibodies and inhibitors may occur and cause a factor to be ineffective in the coagulation cascade. Massive transfusions may also cause bleeding because of the dilution of the factors.

HEREDITARY DISORDERS OF SECONDARY HEMOSTASIS

When diagnosing and classifying hereditary disorders of secondary hemostasis, one must note that several tests will be normal regardless of the percentage of the factor present. The platelet count, bleeding time, FDP, and D-dimer levels will all be unaffected by a hereditary disorder.

HEREDITARY DISORDERS OF SECONDARY HEMOSTASIS

FACTOR DEFICIENCY	SITE OF PRODUCTION	GENETIC PATTERN	HALF-LIFE	COAGULATION PATHWAY	CLINICAL SYMPTOMS AND CAUSE	SCREENING TESTS OR CLINICAL FINDINGS	OTHER LABORATORY TESTS	TREATMENT, MODE OF ACTION, AND NORMAL RANGE
Factor I: Hypofibrinogenemia	Liver	Autosomal recessive	3–4 days	Common	Mild tendency to bleed due to low amount of fibrinogen Cause: Liver disease	PT, APTT, TT all increased	Factor I assay is low; qualitative and quantitative and reptilase prolonged	Replacement with infusion of cryoprecipitate, Substrate NR = 200–400 mg/dL
Factor I: Dysfibrinogenemias	Liver	Autosomal dominant	3–4 days	Common	Asymptomatic Cause: Qualitatively abnormal, functionally defective fibrinogen/GI-GU tract bleed, umbilical cord, postoperative, trauma	PT, APTT, TT all increased	Factor I functional assay is low, quantitative is normal, reptilase is prolonged	Cryoprecipitate used in patients requiring surgery Substrate NR = 200–400 mg/dL
Factor I: Afibrinogenemia	Liver	Autosomal recessive, rare	3–4 days	Common	Mild Symptoms: Hematomas, bruising, epistaxis, defective wound healing Cause: No measurable fibrinogen	PT, APTT, TT all increased	Factor I functional assay is low, quantitative is low, reptilase is prolonged	Replacement of fibrinogen in form of cryoprecipitate Can use fibrinogen concentrates but may initiate a thrombotic episode

Continued ▲

► Continued **HEREDITARY DISORDERS OF SECONDARY HEMOSTASIS**

FACTOR DEFICIENCY	SITE OF PRODUCTION	GENETIC PATTERN	HALF-LIFE	COAGULATION PATHWAY	CLINICAL SYMPTOMS AND CAUSE	SCREENING TESTS OR CLINICAL FINDINGS	OTHER LABORATORY TESTS	TREATMENT, MODE OF ACTION, AND NORMAL RANGE
FACTOR II: Prothrombin	Liver	Autosomal recessive, rare	2–3 days	Common Vitamin K dependent	Mild to moderate bleeding caused by decreased synthesis of normal functioning factor II, or synthesis of abnormal factor II molecule Liver disease Coumadin therapy Vitamin K deficiency DIC	Prolonged PT and APTT Clinical Findings: Bleed mucous membrane-liver disease, excessive bruising, can be acquired due to lupus anticoagulant (LA) or excessive antibiotics	1:1 mix will correct for PT and APTT, test for I, II, V, X; II will be abnormal.	Treat with infused plasma, or prothrombin complex. NR = 50%–150% Proenzyme I→Ia
FACTOR III: Thromboplastin	Liver, kidney, brain, lungs	—	—	Extrinsic				Activates factor VII when exposed to tissue fluids
FACTOR IV: Ionized Calcium	—	—	—	Required in all	Deficiency occurs only in massive transfusions.			Cofactor Activation of thromboplastin converts II→IIa.

Continued ►

▶ Continued **HEREDITARY DISORDERS OF SECONDARY HEMOSTASIS**

FACTOR DEFICIENCY	SITE OF PRODUCTION	GENETIC PATTERN	HALF-LIFE	COAGULATION PATHWAY	CLINICAL SYMPTOMS AND CAUSE	SCREENING TESTS OR CLINICAL FINDINGS	OTHER LABORATORY TESTS	TREATMENT, MODE OF ACTION, AND NORMAL RANGE
FACTOR V: Parahemophilia Proaccelerin	Liver	Autosomal recessive	12–36 hr	Common	Mild to moderate bleeding. Caused by: Lack of factor present or antibodies to Factor V Liver disease Vitamin K deficiency Coumadin therapy	Increased PT and APTT Post-traumatic bruising, epistaxis and mucous membrane GI bleeding	1:1 mix will correct for both PT and APTT, test for I, II, V, X; V will be abnormal.	Use fresh frozen plasma; factor V is labile and will keep under most conditions. NR = 50%–150% Cofactor
Factor VI		Nonexistent						
FACTOR VII: Proconvertin	Liver	Autosomal recessive	6 hr	Extrinsic Vitamin K dependent	Type of bleed varies, hemorrhage after tooth extraction Defect caused by lack of factor VII antigens that interact with heterologous antibodies. Liver disease Vitamin K deficiency Coumadin therapy	PT increased, APTT and TT normal, some hemarthroses, fatal cerebral hemorrhage	1:1 mix for PT will correct; prolonged PT is exclusive for factor VII deficiency; factor VII assay is prolonged; 50% of VII are heterozygous; 0%–20% of VII are homozygous.	Replacement with prothrombin complex, every 12–24 hr. Short half-life will ensure hemostasis. NR = 50%–150% Enzyme/proenzyme

Continued ▲

▶ Continued **HEREDITARY DISORDERS OF SECONDARY HEMOSTASIS**

FACTOR DEFICIENCY	SITE OF PRODUCTION	GENETIC PATTERN	HALF-LIFE	COAGULATION PATHWAY	CLINICAL SYMPTOMS AND CAUSE	SCREENING TESTS OR CLINICAL FINDINGS	OTHER LABORATORY TESTS	TREATMENT, MODE OF ACTION, AND NORMAL RANGE
FACTOR VIII:C: Antihemophilic Factor	Site not known; not produced in liver	Sex linked recessive	12 hr	Intrinsic Acute phase reactant Factor VIII will be elevated in infections, stress	Hemophilia A deficiency of VIII:c <3% is severe–will have hemarthrosis or CNS bleeding; VIII:C between 5 and 10% is moderate, will result in serious posttraumatic bleed; VIII:C between 10 and 50% is mild hemophilia, manifested during major surgery or compromised situation	APTT is increased, PT and TT are normal. Test for factors VIII, IX, XI, XII	1:1 mix will correct for APTT. BT is upper limit of normal range. Factor VIII assay is prolonged.	Cryoprecipitate Purified factor VIII DDAVP can elevate VIII:c NR = 50%–150% Cofactor Conversion of X→Xa, measures activity portion of macromolecule
FACTOR VIII:AG: von Willebrand's	Megakaryocyte, endothelial cells	Sex linked recessive	36 hr	Intrinsic	Mucosal, postop, epistaxis, GI bleed, cutaneous easy bruising	BT long, PT normal, APTT may be high 1:1 APTT-corrects	Factor VIII:c slightly low Abnormal ristocetin, Abnormal vWF antigen	Treatment same as factor VIII: C Platelet adhesion carrier of factor VIII NR = 50%–150%

Continued ▶

▶ Continued **HEREDITARY DISORDERS OF SECONDARY HEMOSTASIS**

FACTOR DEFICIENCY	SITE OF PRODUCTION	GENETIC PATTERN	HALF-LIFE	COAGULATION PATHWAY	CLINICAL SYMPTOMS AND CAUSE	SCREENING TESTS OR CLINICAL FINDINGS	OTHER LABORATORY TESTS	TREATMENT, MODE OF ACTION, AND NORMAL RANGE
FACTOR IX: Antihemophilia B Christmas Disease		Sex linked recessive	24 hr	Intrinsic Vitamin K dependent	Clinically, cannot distinguish from factor VIII	BT normal, PT normal, APTT prolonged, TT normal	1:1 mix for APTT corrects. Test for VIII, IX, XI, and XII. IX will be abnormal.	In major bleed, vitamin K concentrate Minor bleed, FFP NR = 50%–150% Enzyme X→Xa
FACTOR X: Stuart-Prower	Liver	Autosomal recessive	1–2 days	Common Vitamin K dependent	Reduced or abnormal synthesis of X <1% X severe bleeding 10% X mild bleeding Liver disease Vitamin K deficiency	PT and APTT are prolonged. TT is normal. May also be seen in amyloidosis. Easy bruising, epistaxis, GI, hematomas, mucous membrane bleed, intracranial bleed	Test for factors I, II, V, and X. X assay is prolonged, 6%–9% X in homozygotes, 50% X in heterozygotes	Bleeding can be managed with FFP, because of long half-life of X. For major bleeds, prothrombin complex is used. NR = 50%–150% Enzyme X→Xa

Continued ▶

▲ Continued **HEREDITARY DISORDERS OF SECONDARY HEMOSTASIS**

FACTOR DEFICIENCY	SITE OF PRODUCTION	GENETIC PATTERN	HALF-LIFE	COAGULATION PATHWAY	CLINICAL SYMPTOMS AND CAUSE	SCREENING TESTS OR CLINICAL FINDINGS	OTHER LABORATORY TESTS	TREATMENT, MODE OF ACTION, AND NORMAL RANGE
FACTOR XI: Plasma Thromboplastin antecedent	Liver	Autosomal recessive Frequently occurs in Ashkenazi Jews	2–3 days	Intrinsic Contact factors	Reduced synthesis of protein, delayed bleeding, seen in Rosenthal's syndrome	PT is normal, APTT is prolonged, TT is normal. Epistaxis, hematuria, menorrhagia	1:1 mix for APTT will correct. Test for factors VIII, IX, XI. Factor XI is abnormal.	Treatment is rare, XI is labile, can use FFP, half-life is several days. NR = 50%–150% Enzyme X→Xa
FACTOR XII: Hageman's Factor	Liver	Autosomal recessive	2–3 days	Intrinsic Contact factors	Hageman's factor deficiency, does not cause bleeding, is surface contact factor, in vivo role not fully understood	PT is normal, APTT is prolonged, TT is normal.	1:1 mix for APTT will correct. Test for factors VIII, IX, XI, and XII. XII will be decreased.	Patients do not bleed, and no treatment is required; however, patients may be predisposed to thrombosis. Enzyme

Continued ▲

▶ Continued **HEREDITARY DISORDERS OF SECONDARY HEMOSTASIS**

FACTOR DEFICIENCY	SITE OF PRODUCTION	GENETIC PATTERN	HALF-LIFE	COAGULATION PATHWAY	CLINICAL SYMPTOMS AND CAUSE	SCREENING TESTS OR CLINICAL FINDINGS	OTHER LABORATORY TESTS	TREATMENT, MODE OF ACTION, AND NORMAL RANGE
FACTOR XIII: Fibrin Stabilizing Factor	Liver	Autosomal recessive	3–5 days	Factor XIII not found in circulation	Qualitative and quantitative abnormality of factor XIII, manifested in early childhood.	PT, APTT, TT are all normal. Slow wound healing and abnormal scar formation	Factor XIII assay in 5 M urea will demonstrate lysis of clot after 24 hr.	Small doses of plasma Enzyme Covalently binds fibrin monomers
PREKALLIKREIN: Fletcher's Factor	Liver	Autosomal recessive	—	Intrinsic Contact factors	No bleeding symptoms, yet patients suffer from myocardial infarction (MI), possible lack of protection from thrombosis. Incidence is unknown.	PT is normal, APTT is prolonged, TT is normal	1:1 APTT corrects with prolonged incubation. Prekallikrein assay decreased.	No treatment Enzyme XII→XIIa Activates kinin system and complement system
HIGH MOLECULAR WEIGHT KININOGEN (HMWK): Fitzgerald's Factor	Liver	Autosomal recessive	5–6 days	Intrinsic Contact factors	Deficient in HMWK, clinically asymptomatic in terms of bleeding	PT is normal, APTT is abnormal, TT is normal.	1:1 mix for APTT corrects with prolonged incubation, HMWK assay will be abnormal	No treatment Cofactor XI→XIa XII→XIIa

ACQUIRED DISORDERS OF SECONDARY HEMOSTASIS

DISSEMINATED INTRAVASCULAR COAGULATION. This condition arises from a major tissue injury and results in the formation of thrombin and plasmin simultaneously. The degree is dependent on the etiology and the acuteness. In normal hemostasis, thrombin cleaves fibrinogen and activates factors V, VIII, and XIII and protein C. It also activates platelets to aggregate and secrete. In DIC, coagulation is activated; platelets will not function normally and will aggregate, resulting in thrombocytopenia and a prolonged bleeding time. Plasmin is activated in the fibrinolytic system by the direct conversion of plasminogen to plasmin by tissue plasminogen activator (t-PA), or by activation of the contact phase—Hageman's factor or kallikrein. It proteolyses factors V, VIII, and IX, and high molecular weight kininogen (HMWK) and interferes with the adhesive function of platelets. The major mechanism of the coagulation system is activated—factor VIIa/tissue factor (TF) activates factors X and IX; normally factor Xa quenches the activity of factor VIIa/TF. In DIC this system is reduced. DIC is also seen in acute promyelocytic leukemia; the granules of the promyelocytes release a thromboplastin-like substance, and this causes DIC. There are two types of DIC:

1. Acute hemorrhagic DIC
2. Subacute chronic DIC

Acute. Acute DIC develops rapidly from a few hours to days. It has a high mortality rate, about 54% to 87% and is seen in infections, obstetric complications, malignancy, tissue injury, liver disease, and tissue necrosis.

Chronic. Treat the disease and not the DIC; as the disease improves, DIC will lessen. Chronic DIC is seen in malignancy, incomplete abortions, connective tissue disorders, and renal disease.

Laboratory Diagnosis. In acute cases, tests are diagnostic, whereas in chronic cases, tests are usually normal or slightly abnormal.

LABORATORY TESTS	ACUTE DIC	CHRONIC DIC
Screening Tests		
PT and APTT	Usually prolonged	Normal
Fibrinogen	Usually decreased May be normal Is acute phase reactive May be in normal range but previously very high; monitor carefully	Usually normal
Confirmatory Tests		
FDP	Positive >40 µg/mL	Positive <40 µg/ml
D-Dimer	Positive	Positive

LIVER DISEASE. The liver produces most of the clotting factors, activators, and inhibitors. If the liver is dysfunctional, the production of these hemostatic proteins will be affected. Complications arise when the liver is unable to adequately synthesize factors. Factor VIII is not produced in the liver and as a result will be elevated to compensate for the other decreased factors. In addition, an accumulation of metabolic waste will affect the bone marrow and the immune system, and vascular changes will occur. This results in serious, complex, and extensive bleeding problems.

COAGULATION PROFILE—LIVER DISEASE	PANIC VALUES	
CBC	Hct <25%	
Platelet Count (/mm³)	<100,000	NR = 150–450,000
Prothrombin Time (sec)	>15	NR = 10–12
Activated Partial Thromboplastin Time (sec)	>40	NR = 27–33
Fibrinogen (mg/dL)	<100	NR = 200–400
Factor V (%)	<35	NR = 50–150
Factor VII (%)	<10	NR = 50–150
Factor VIII (%)	<100, should be > 160, since it is not made in liver, and is an acute phase reactive	NR = 50–150
Factor IX (%)	<30	NR = 50–150
Plasminogen (%)	<75	NR = 80–120
Antithrombin III (%)	<65	NR = 80–120
Euglobulin Clot Lysis	<30 min, >24 hr	NR = >1 hr, <24 hr

In obstructive liver disease, only vitamin K dependent factors are affected. This is due to the absorption of liquid soluble vitamin K and its need for bile salts in the gastrointestinal (GI) lumen. Hepatocellular disease impairs the synthesis of all factors except ristocetin cofactor VIII R:vWF. Deficiencies of antithrombin III and plasminogen are common in liver disease. The PT is a sensitive test of liver function and can serve as an early marker for liver disease. Deficiency of fibrinogen indicates severe liver disease. Thrombocytopenia is a cause of bleeding in liver disease as a result of splenomegaly and sequestration.

Treatment of liver disease is difficult. If patients are not bleeding, no course of therapy is required. Administration of factors, or fresh frozen plasma (FFP), provides limited results, rarely leading to remission. A large volume of fresh frozen plasma can cause circulatory overload, and concentrates should only be used in an emergency situation.

VITAMIN K DEFICIENCY. Vitamin K is present in green leafy vegetables, fish, and liver. Decreased levels of factors II, VII, IX, and X will be corrected with the administration of vitamin K. These levels are decreased in oral anticoagulant therapy; severe liver disease; impaired dietary intake of vitamin K due to: malabsorption syndrome, obstructive jaundice, prolonged antibiotic syndrome, and hemorrhagic disease of the newborn.

RENAL DISEASE. In renal disease the bleeding tendency is manifested by mucosal bleeding, epistaxis, GI bleeding, and hematuria. In nephrotic syndrome, factors are lost because of production defects of synthesis. In addition many factors can be lost through the urine. There is indication that urine degradation products of fibrinogen or fibrin are present in the urine and absent in the blood; this indicates that consumption has occurred in the kidneys.

PRIMARY FIBRINOLYSIS. This is caused by gross activation of fibrinolytic and coagulation factor consumption and an excess of plasminogen activators—t-PA, streptokinase, or urokinase. These are activated without simultaneous coagulation. The release of activators can be caused by malignancies of the prostate or, lungs, liver disease, or obstetric complications. Plasmin acts on fibrinogen, fibrin, and factors II, V, and VIII (see Figure on facing page). Clot formation does not occur because of large amounts of circulating plasminogen activator, which also interferes with platelet aggregation. The PT, APTT, TT, and fibrinogen are all increased. Primary fibrinolysis can be treated with antiplasmins.

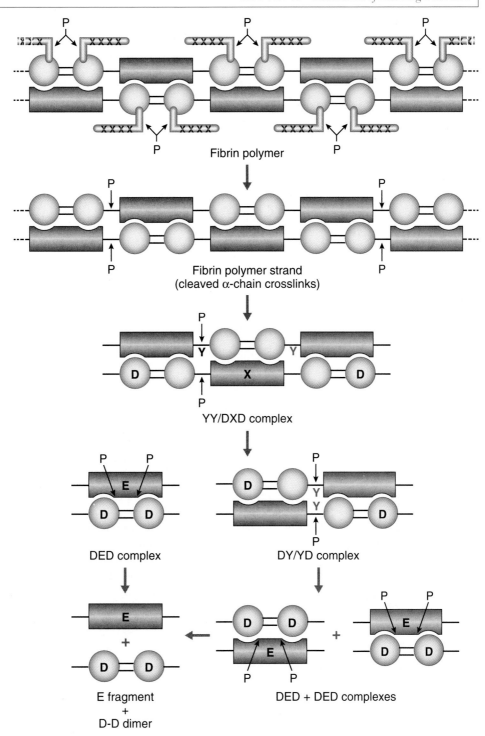

(Modified from Thompson AR, Harker LA: Manual of Hemostasis and Thrombosis. Philadelphia, FA Davis, 1983.)

ACQUIRED CIRCULATING ANTICOAGULANTS. These inhibitors or antibodies may be directed against single or multiple coagulation factors. Many are associated with certain diseases or intake of drugs. There several types. The most common type is immunoglobulins of the IgG type. These acquired inhibitors are reversible and inactivate

EVALUATION OF BLEEDING IN SECONDARY HEMOSTASIS

individual coagulation factors. Other inhibitors are immediate in action and occur in patients with multiple myeloma, DIC, and liver disease. The antibodies are treated with steroids or chemotherapy to reduce production of the antibody.

Specific Factor Inhibitors and Causes

FACTOR INHIBITOR	CAUSE
I	Transfusions, autoimmune disorders, chronic inflammatory disease
II	Systemic lupus erythematosus (SLE)
V	Plasma transfusion, postsurgical streptomycin, topical bovine thrombin
VII	Cancer of the lung, IgG
VIII:c	Hemophilia; may develop spontaneously in postpartum patients or elderly patients, collagen vascular disease, drug reactions
VIII R:vWF	Autoimmune disorders; lymphoma; myeloproliferative, myelodysplastic syndromes
IX	Rheumatic fever, postpartum, SLE
X	Leprosy, systemic amyloidosis
XI	Autoimmune disorders, IgG type
XII	SLE, Waldenström's macroglobulinemia, glomerulonephritis
XIII	Drug induced—isoniazid, phenytoin, penicillin

In contrast, nonspecific inhibitors are not specific for any single coagulation protein, but rather they interfere with the interactions of clotting factors on a phospholipid surface. As a result the APTT is affected more than the PT, showing the prolongation is the result of an inhibitor rather than deficiencies. These nonspecific inhibitors are demonstrated by the failure to correct in a mixing study and the presence of the inhibitor in several dilutions of the plasma into the normal range. The most common of these acquired inhibitors is antiphospholipid syndrome. This is discussed in detail in Chapter 41.

BIBLIOGRAPHY

Beeler MF, Catroou PG: Interpretations in Clinical Chemistry. Chicago, ASCP Press, 1988.

Caruana C: Review and Update in Coagulation: Workshops in Medical Technology. ASCP seminar, Philadelphia, Sept.1993.

Comprehensive Medical Technology Review Course, Hemostasis. Atlanta, Department of Medical Technology, June 1994.

Davidson I, Henry JB: Clinical Diagnosis. Philadelphia, WB Saunders, 1974.

Keldsberg C: Practical Diagnosis of Hematologic Disorders. Chicago, ASCP Press, 1995.

Rodak BF: Diagnostic Hematology. Philadelphia, WB Saunders, 1995.

Chapter *41*

EVALUATION OF THROMBOSIS

Donna D. Castellone, MS, MT(ASCP)SH

Q U I C K   C O N T E N T S

INTRODUCTION

Thrombosis is the development of blood clots within the vascular system. *Thromboembolism* is the joint term for deep vein thrombosis (DVT) and pulmonary embolism (PE). These account for 300,000 to 600,000 hospitalizations per year and 50,000 deaths in the United States; 1 out of every 10,000 people will have a thrombotic event. Thrombotic events are on the rise due to an increase in people's life spans and their sedentary habits.

THROMBOPHILIA. Thrombophilia is the familial or acquired disorders of the hemostatic mechanism that are likely to predispose someone to thrombosis. A complete family history is essential in evaluating thrombophilia. Evaluation should take place *several weeks after a thrombotic event and after anticoagulant therapy has been discontinued.* This is due to the possibility that thrombosis will induce an acute phase response that will obscure the true basal level. If it is not possible to delay evaluation, several methods can be used, regardless of the patient's anticoagulation state, but it is still simpler and more cost effective to avoid this problem.

PATIENTS TO EVALUATE
    ▌ Patients younger than 45 years with a spontaneous venous event
    ▌ Patients younger than 30 years with arterial thrombosis
    ▌ Patients with a family history with recurrent thrombosis

■ Patients with recurrent fetal loss
■ Neonates with unexplained thrombosis

A major consideration in evaluating thrombosis is cost. The appropriate utilization of tests can prove cost effective and is important in the therapeutic management for long and short term. If your anticoagulants have decreased or abnormal function, you are prone to thrombosis. The tests performed most frequently are quantitative and qualitative deficiencies of Protein C (PC), Protein S (PS), and Antithrombin III (ATIII), and the newest test, Activated Protein C Resistance (APCR). Each is discussed in detail. Their frequency of occurrence is:

APCR	20%–40%
Factor XII deficiency	10%
PC	2%–5%
PS	2%–5%
Plasminogen	1%–2%
Fibrinolysis	10%–15%
Fibrinogen	1%
Antiphospholipid syndrome	2%–3%

In testing for hypercoagulability there is no one single screening test:

1. You need a panel of tests.
2. You must evaluate selectively.
3. You must screen with function tests.
4. It is not cost effective or necessary to perform all tests simultaneously

Functional assays are used in the first line of assessment for thrombosis; this type of testing will determine all types of deficiencies:

Type I: decreased antigenic levels, protein missing
Type II: protein present at a normal level, but dysfunctional

Use antigenic levels for characterization of typing of patients with a deficiency. Type I will have abnormal functional and antigenic levels. Type II will show a low functional level and a normal or high antigenic level.

ANTICOAGULATION DEFICIENCIES

Antiphospholipid Syndrome

The antiphospholipid syndrome includes both the lupus anticoagulant (LA) and the anticardolipin antibodies (ACAs).

ACAs. These are autoantibodies of the IgG or IgM type that are directed specifically against cardiolipin and other negatively charges phospholipids. They are five times more common than the LA.

LAs. These are polyclonal IgG, IgM, or IgA types. The antibody has activity against a phospholipid, and it cannot serve as a surface on which various coagulation enzymes can sequentially interact to form fibrin in the test system.

CLINICAL MANIFESTATIONS

Patients do not bleed and are predisposed to thrombosis. Other problems occur concurrently:

1. Thrombocytopenia
2. Isolated deficiency of prothrombin
3. Qualitative platelet defects
4. Acquired von Willebrand's disease (vWD)
5. Antibodies to factor VIII
6. Recurrent spontaneous abortions

LABORATORY DIAGNOSIS

Testing is difficult because of the variability of reagent sensitivity and because of interfering substances that alter test specificity. Specimen collection is critical. The sample *must* be platelet poor plasma (PPP), that is, a platelet count less than 10,000. A baseline activated partial thromboplastin time (APTT) is essential before heparin administration, or an LA could be missed. The prothrombin time (PT) is not usually elevated because of a high amount of phosphilipid that neutralizes the antibody.

In 1995 the Scientific Subcommittee Criteria for the Lupus Anticoagulant established the following protocol for identifying an LA:

1. Prolongation of at least one phospholipid dependent clotting test.
2. Evidence of inhibitory activity shown by the effect of patient plasma on pooled normal plasma.
3. Evidence that the inhibitory activity is dependent on phospholipid. This may be achieved by alteration of the phospholipid, platelets, or platelet vesicles in the test system.
4. LA disorders must be carefully distinguished from other coagulopathies, which may give similar lab results or may occur concurrently with the LA.

NOTE One must clarify screening versus confirmation.

SCREENING TEST. This is an assay with a single concentration of phospholipid.

CONFIRMATORY TEST. This is an assay based on the principle of adding or altering the phospholipid content.

NOTE In the diagnosis of the LA it is important that the confirmatory study correspond to the screening test that is abnormal.

ANTICOAGULATION DEFICIENCIES

For example, if the APTT (clot based assay) is normal and the dilute Russel viper venom (DRVV) test is abnormal, the confirmatory test should be based on a DRVV test rather than an APTT system.

Studies for the Lupus Anticoagulant

TYPE OF TEST	SCREEN	CONFIRM
Clot Based Assay	APTT	Platelet neutralization Hexagonal phase
Adjusted Phospholipid	DRVV Tissue thromboplastin inhibitor (TTI)	DRVV confirm Phospholipid dilutions

Principles of Tests

ACTIVATED PARTIAL THROMBOPLASTIN TIME. This clot based assay measures the intrinsic system. It depends on adding plasma to an activator of factor XII, such as ellagic acid and phospholipid, and accelerates the reactions involved in factor VIII and V activation. In the presence of an LA or an ACA, this activation will be prolonged, due to the utilization of a reagent that has a low concentration of phospholipid.

TISSUE THROMBOPLASTIN INHIBITOR. The tissue thromboplastin inhibitor (TTI) test uses the lipoprotein extract of rabbit brain and lung that is used in the PT. It uses a low and high concentration of phospholipid. This test is not very specific for the LA and contains many interfering substances.

DILUTE RUSSELL VIPER VENOM. The DRVV test uses viper (snake) venom to activate the cascade at factor X. It screens by using a low dilution of phospholipid, allowing the reaction to be prolonged. It is confirmed by bringing the phospholipid to a high concentration, resulting in a shorter time. This assay is not affected by any deficiencies or inhibitors to any of the factors since it initiates activation at factor X. Only if factor X or V is less than 40% will the assay be affected.

PLATELET NEUTRALIZATION PROCEDURE. The platelet neutralization procedure (PNP) is a clot based assay that utilizes a high concentration of platelets as the source of phospholipid. As a result the clotting time will be shorter, because of neutralization of the antibody.

HEXAGONAL PHASE NEUTRALIZATION. The hexagonal phase neutralization (HPN), a clot based assay, is based on the theory that LAs have a higher affinity for (and react exclusively with) phospholipids in a hexagonal configuration than for phospholipids in a bilayer configuration, which ACAs have a greater affinity for. Plasma is tested with and without hexagonal phase phosphatidylethanolamine (HPE). If a LA is present it will be neutralized in the tube with HPE, resulting in a shortening of the clotting time. Comparison of the two results with greater than an 8 second difference is considered positive.

Flow Chart

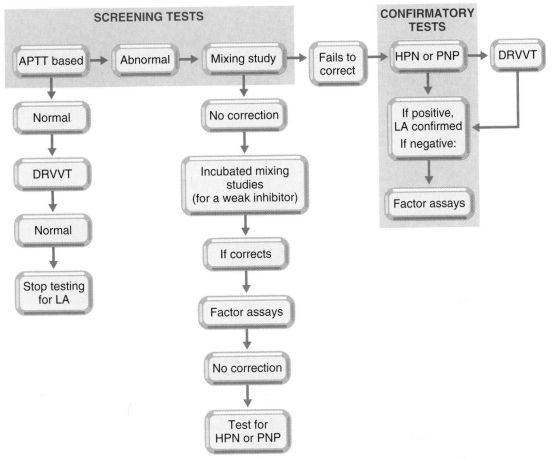

Begin with one or more screening assay based on different properties,
before eliminating the possibility of LA

Antithrombin III

ATIII is a naturally occurring anticoagulant protein, produced in the liver. It is the most important of the serine proteases—thrombin and factors XIIa, IXa, XIa, and Xa. ATIII neutralizes by covalently binding at its active site the enzyme to be inhibited and can no longer activate its substrate. Thrombin is the most powerful coagulant and must be kept in check. ATIII action is enhanced 1000-fold in the presence of heparin, allowing heparin to function as an anticoagulant. In order for heparin to function properly to prevent clot formation, ATIII must be present in sufficient amounts and must have a functional enzyme binding site and a heparin binding site.

Decreased levels of ATIII lead to thrombosis. A decreased level may be caused by a hereditary or an acquired disorder. The occurrence of ATIII deficiency is 1 per 2000, and 70% have a thrombotic episode before they are 35 years old. Clinically a patient will display normal routine blood tests but will show a decreased response to heparin and may require an unusually high dose for treatment. If ATIII levels are less than 30% (normal range, 80% to 125%), one can administer fresh frozen plasma (FFP) or ATIII concentrate to provide a substrate on which heparin can function as an anticoagulant. FFP contains 1 unit of ATIII activity per milliliter.

ANTICOAGULATION DEFICIENCIES

ACQUIRED ANTITHROMBIN III DEFICIENCY. ATIII deficiency is found in disseminated intravascular coagulation (DIC) (consumed), nephrotic syndrome (lost through the urine), and liver disease (decreased production). Amounts are decreased in estrogen and oral contraceptive therapy.

INHERITED ANTITHROMBIN III DEFICIENCY. This condition is autosomal dominant. In heterozygotes, 30% to 60% plasma levels of ATIII types I and II are found; however, a homozygous type I (decreased activity and antigen) has not been found and may be lethal in utero.

TESTING

ATIII can be tested antigenically or functionally. ATIII activity is measured chromogenically. The test relies on the addition of either thrombin or factor Xa in excess and a chromogenic substrate to detect the activity. The amount of ATIII is related to the amount of enzyme remaining:

$$\underset{\text{(amount being tested)}}{\text{ATIII}} + \underset{\text{(excess)}}{\text{thrombin}} \rightarrow \underset{\text{(presence)}}{\text{heparin}} \rightarrow \underset{\text{(chromogenic)}}{\text{ATIII-thrombin}} + \underset{\text{(measured)}}{\text{thrombin}}$$

Protein C

Protein C (PC) a vitamin K dependent enzyme that is synthesized in the liver, with a half-life of about 7 to 9 hours. The PC system includes PC, its cofactor PS, activated PC inhibitor (APC), and thrombomodulin, a cell surface receptor. PC has a dual function in that it is an inhibitor of coagulation and a stimulator of fibrinolysis. PC is converted to its active form by thrombomodulin, and it inhibits the clotting cascade by enzymatically degrading activation of factors V and VIII, preventing further fibrin formation. It also enhances fibrinolytic activity by inhibiting PAI-1 (Plasminogen activating inhibitor 1).

CLINICAL

PC deficiency is seen in about 1% to 3% of patients and is manifested as venous thromboembolism. The normal range is 70% to 130%, and deficiencies can be acquired or hereditary. Heterozygotes—values about 50%—are about 1 in 200, yet their risk for thrombosis is about 1 in 10,000 the great majority of these individuals appear to be asymptomatic. A homozygous newborn may have purpura fulminans neonatalis. This results in excessive skin necrosis; PC levels are hard to determine, since newborn levels are about 30% lower. In addition many homozygous newborns never experience skin necrosis.

PC deficiency is acquired in liver disease (site of production), DIC (consumed), oral anticoagulant therapy (vitamin K dependent), and postoperative conditions.

One can treat the deficiency with FFP or purified PC concentrates. In addition, due to warfarin (Coumadin) induced skin necrosis, it is advisable to begin heparin therapy and have the patient achieve anticoagulation and then administer warfarin in small doses.

TESTING

PC is a vitamin K dependent factor and is affected by warfarin therapy. It is essential that a patient not be tested while being treated with warfarin; PC function will be greatly affected.

An antigenic level can be tested and is usually not affected by anticoagulant therapy. This can be monitored by running a factor X antigen test simultaneously. If X antigen level is decreased, then the Protein C antigen has been affected by warfarin.

A first line of testing is by a clotting assay, using snake venom activator; this measures all functions of the PC molecule. A chromogenic test will measure some but not all of the functions of the PC molecule, since a chromogenic assay only determines the function of the active site.

Protein S

PS is a vitamin K dependent factor that is synthesized in the liver, endothelial cells, and platelet alpha granules. It is not an enzyme but a cofactor of PC, which in turn acts as an anticoagulant by inhibiting factors Va and VIIIa. PS potentiates PC anticoagulation function by increasing PC affinity for phospholipid membranes. PS circulates in two forms: *total* (bound), with no anticoagulant activity, and *free* (unbound), which acts as the cofactor for the activated PC and carries the anticoagulant activity. Sixty percent of PS is bound in a reversible complex with C4b binding protein, which is a regulatory protein of the complement system. C4b is an acute phase reactive protein, and it responds to inflammation by shifting the free PS to the bound PS. If the free PS level is decreased, the C4b binding protein level should be tested. If the C4b binding protein level is normal, the patient is truly deficient in PS; if the C4b binding protein level is elevated, it is because of an acute phase reactant.

CLINICAL

PS occurs in about 2% to 5% of patients and is manifested as venous thromboembolism, usually occurring after puberty; 70% of these patients have DVT and PE in their early 20s. This condition can be acquired or hereditary. A hereditary deficiency is autosomal dominant. Homozygous PS deficiencies have been identified in several newborns. Many patients previously thought to have been PS deficient are actually deficient in APC, since PS acts as the cofactor in the PC system. The condition can be acquired in liver failure (decreased production), DIC (consumed), diabetes, nephrotic syndrome, pregnancy, and warfarin therapy.

TESTING

One can test for PS activity or antigen; since it is vitamin K dependent, activity cannot be tested while the patient is receiving warfarin therapy. It is still ideal to test after the patient has ceased to receive oral anticoagulant therapy for 2 weeks. Activity is tested by using a clot based assay that measures the patient's PS in the presence of APC, factor V, and PS depleted plasma. This measures the ability of PS to function as a cofactor for PC. Antigenic assays will measure the amount of protein that is available. This can be done by immunologic methods in which the free PS is separated from the total PS by polyethylene glycol (PEG) precipitation.

FIBRINOLYTIC DEFECTS

Problems that occur in the fibrinolytic system may also result in thrombosis. They may be caused by:

1. A decreased level of tissue plasminogen activator (t-PA). As a result, not enough will be available for the conversion of plasminogen to plasmin, and fibrinolysis will not occur.
2. An increased level of alpha 2 antiplasmin. This is an inhibitor that inhibits the formation of plasmin.
3. Decreased plasminogen levels. As a result, not enough will be available for its conversion to plasmin.

These activators and inhibitors can be tested and their levels reviewed for possible causes of thrombosis.

HOMOCYSTINEMIA

Homocysteine is an amino acid involved in the enzymatic reaction of cobalamin and folate. This is associated with an increased risk of vascular disease, including venous thromboembolism. Elevated levels of homocysteine seem to have a direct toxic effect on the endothelium. It may promote thrombosis by:

1. Down regulating the activation of protein C
2. Increasing endothelial cell factor V activity
3. Inducing tissue factor
4. Promoting platelet adhesion
5. Suppressing heparin sulfate expression
6. Accentuating t-PA activity

Studies have shown that hyperhomocystinemia can be reversed with increased intake of vitamin B_{12} and folate.

ACTIVATED PROTEIN C RESISTANCE

In 1993 Dahlback looked at patients with thrombolytic disease. Their plasma showed poor in vitro response with APC. PC is a key element that circulates in plasma as an inactive precursor that is rapidly converted to APC when thrombin binds to thrombomodulin receptors on endothelial cells. Once generated, APC in the presence of cofactor PS inactivates two cofactors, Va and VIIIa, by limited proteolysis. This was exhibited in 20% to 60% of patients with "idiopathic thrombosis."

This disorder, known as activated Protein C resistance (APCR), is a result of a molecular defect in factor V, which results in amino acid substitution of arginine to glutamine. This inherited single base pair mutation in the factor V gene is known as factor V Leiden, or FV:Q506. The regulation of factor V is affected, but APCR does not interfere with factor V's procoagulant activity, and factor V continues to contribute to thrombin formation. The site of mutation of arginine 506 to glutamine is the site at which APC cleaves factor Va and renders it resistant to APC. This is a hereditary disorder and increases the risk of thrombosis fivefold to 10-fold in heterozygous patients and 50- to 100-fold in homozygotes. From 20% to 60% of patients are heterozygous; 1% to 5% are homozygous. In the general population in Sweden, 0% to 15% are heterozygous; in the United States, 6% to 7%, and in Japan, the incidence is 0% to 1%.

Testing

To diagnose APCR, two methods may be used:

1. An APTT is performed and compared with an APTT performed with APC. Normal patients produce a twofold increase in the APTT when APC is added. If a patient is positive, the time shortens in the APTT when APC is added. The results are reported as a ratio; anything less than 2 is usually positive. This test can be a problem if the initial APTT is prolonged because of the presence of heparin or abnormal factor levels. But this problem can be eliminated by performing the assay with mixing the patient's plasma with factor V deficient plasma. This will correct any abnormal factor deficiencies, without any interference by additional factor V that would be found if pooled normal plasma were used. The sensitivity of this method is 100%.

2. To diagnosis a factor V Leiden mutation, one analyzes genomic DNA in peripheral blood mononuclear cells by polymerase chain reaction (PCR). The cleaved product is analyzed on ethidium bromide stained agarose gels after restriction enzyme digestion. This unequivocally determines whether the patient has the mutation. The sensitivity and specificity of the test is 100%. The problem is that the test is laborious, requires experience, and may be costly.

Clinical

If this APCR is so prevalent, why aren't people thrombosing left and right? There is a "two hit hypothesis." That is, when this condition is present, it will most likely not cause thrombosis by itself, but thrombosis will occur with an additional event or when the hemostasis system is challenged. With an efficient regulatory system one would not expect a thrombotic event to occur unless a significant compromise occurred in one of these systems.

Acute thrombotic events often occur when in addition to an underlying hereditary disorder there is a superimposed condition or event such as:

1. Pregnancy
2. Stasis
3. Air travel
4. Malignancies
5. Obesity
6. Postoperative conditions
7. Nephrotic syndrome
8. Myeloproliferative disorders

ACTIVATED PROTEIN C RESISTANCE

INHERITED THROMBOSIS

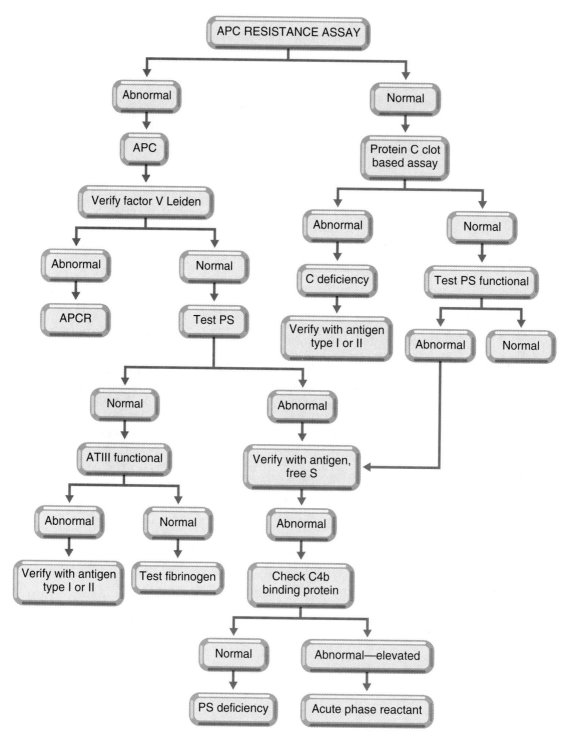

If, in hypercoagulability and thrombosis, limited testing is available, one should use functional assays. These are good, cost effective screening tests that will provide a substantial amount of information. This will allow verification with antigens to proceed and will enable timely patient care and management.

BIBLIOGRAPHY

Abrams C: Knowing assay limitation helpful in detecting thrombotic disorders. Advance, 7:18–19, 1995.

Adcock DM, Marlar RA: Hereditary Hypercoagulability. San Diego, CA, ASCP Commission on Continuing Education Council on Hematology, 1996.

Bauer KA: Resistance to activated protein C. Clin Hemostasis Rev 9(8), Aug 1995.

Bick RL, Ancypa D, McIntyre K: Understanding the antiphospholipid thrombosis syndromes. Lab Med 226(2):124–130, 1995.

Bick RL, Baker WF:, Antiphospholipid and thrombosis syndromes. Semin Thromb Hemost, 20(1):3–15, 1994.

Bick RL, Kunkel L: Hypercoagulability and thrombosis. Lab Med 23(4):233–238, 1992.

Brandt JT, Triplett DA, Alving B, Scharrer I: Criteria for the diagnosis of lupus anticoagulant: an update. Thromb Haemost 74(4):1185–1190, 1995.

Brandt JT, Triplett DA, Roch WA, et al: Effects of lupus anticoagulant on the activated partial thromboplastin time. Arch Pathol Lab Med 115:109–114, 1991.

Campbell JB, Matthews SG, Hendersen KR: Antiphospholipid syndrome. American Clinical Laboratory, 7-8, 1995.

Chromogenix-Pharmacia Hepar: Coatest APC resistance: methodological update. Franklin, Ohio, Sept 1995.

Chromogenix-Pharmacia Hepar: Thrombophilia 1995—Major steps toward understanding. Franklin, Ohio, Sept 1995.

Dahlback B: Resistance to activated Protein C; the ARG506 to Gin mutation in the factor V gene and venous thrombosis. Thromb haemost 73(5):739–742, 1995.

DiGuiseppe JA, Kroll MH: Laboratory evaluation of hypercoagulable states. Clin Lab News Am Assoc Clin Chem 21(10):8–13, 1995.

Ens GE: Cost effective diagnosis of thrombotic disorders. Clin Hemostasis Rev 9(8):2–4, 1995.

Exner T, Papdopoulos G, Koutts J: Use of a simplified DRVVT to confirm heterogeneity among lupus anticoagulants. Blood Coagul Fibrinol 1:259–66, 1990.

Harris N: The anti-cardiolipin ELISA test. American Clinical Laboratory, 18, 1995.

Harrison RL, Alperin JB, Kumar D: Concurrent lupus anticoagulant and prothrombin deficiency due to phenytoin use. Arch Pathol Lab Med 3:719–722, 1987.

Horner A: Advancement in the diagnosis of lupus anticoagulant: Staclot LA hexagonal phospholipid neutralization procedure. Clin Hemostasis Rev 1–4, 1993.

Kampe CE: Clinical syndromes associated with lupus anticoagulant. Semin Thromb Hemost 20(1):16–26, 1994.

Lopez LR, Santos ME, Espinoza LR, LaRosa F: Clinical significance of immunoglobulin A versus immunoglobulin G and M anticardiolipin antibodies with SLE. Coagul Trans Med 99(4):449–454, 1992.

Reyes H, Dreary L, Shoenfeld Y, Peter J: Antiphospholipid antibodies: a critique of their heterogeneity and hegemony. Semin Thromb Hemost 20(1):89–100, 1994.

Rogers GM, Garr SB: An Approach to the Laboratory Diagnosis of Inherited Thrombotic Disorders and Practical Aspects of Monitoring Anticoagulation. New Orleans, ASCP Commission on Continuing Education Council on Hematology, 1995.

Triplett DA: Activated Protein C resistance and thrombophilia. New Orleans, ASCP Commission on Continuing Education Council on Hematology, 1995.

Triplett DA, Barna LK, Unger GA: A hexagonal phase phospholipid neutralization assay for lupus anticoagulant identification. Thromb Haemost 70(5):787–793, 1993.

Triplett Da, Samama MM, Exner T: The clinical and laboratory spectrum of lupus anticoagulants. American Bioproducts Company, Parsippany, NJ, 1–25.

Section

VIII

SPECIALTY AREAS

Chapter **42**

CLINICAL MYCOLOGY

Ronald Malowitz, PhD, MT(ASCP)

QUICK CONTENTS

INTRODUCTION

The vast majority of the fungi are nonpathogenic to humans. Most fungal diseases are opportunistic and require some predisposing factor in the host for mycotic infection to occur. Recent advances in medicine such as chemotherapy and radiation treatment for malignancies, the widespread use of antibiotic therapy, and diseases such as acquired immunodeficiency syndrome (AIDS) that attack the immune system predispose people to mycotic infection.

The fungi are eukaryotic organisms that are divided broadly into the yeasts and the molds. These two groups of fungi differ significantly from each other. In the clinical laboratory these dissimilarities are reflected in their differing microscopic and macroscopic morphologies.

The yeasts are a diverse group of fungi that in the clinical laboratory setting appear similar. Most of the yeasts isolated in the laboratory have been termed *yeastlike* (imperfect yeasts), in that only the asexual reproductive form (anamorph), i.e., budding cells, has been observed. The principal genera belonging to this group are *Candida, Torulopsis,* and *Cryptococcus.* The true yeasts (perfect yeasts), however, are those in which the sexual state (teleomorph), i.e., ascospores, has been described. The most common true yeasts isolated in the microbiology laboratory belong to the genera *Saccharomyces* and *Hansenula.* For practical purposes in this chapter, the term *yeast* will include both the imperfect and the perfect forms.

The molds are known as the *filamentous fungi* because they are composed of branching tubular structures known as *hyphae.* These protoplasmic structures may be either septate, in which the hyphal elements are divided by cross-walls known as *septa* into regularly spaced compartments, or aseptate, in which there is an absence or sparcity of these partitions. The colony that results from the intertwining of the hyphae is known as a *thallus, mycelium,* or *mold.* The fungal mycelium serves two basic functions. The vegetative mycelium penetrates into the medium and absorbs nutrients, whereas the aerial mycelium bear reproductive structures for the mold's dissemination. It is these reproductive structures that are necessary to identify these organisms.

YEASTS

Of the numerous yeasts found in nature, six genera, namely, *Candida, Cryptococcus, Torulopsis, Trichosporon, Malassezia,* and *Rhodotorula,* are responsible for the majority of infections in the human host. The vast majority of these yeasts have low pathogenic potential and are part of the human microflora. Infection occurs when the normal host defenses are abrogated. The clinical manifestations that result from yeast infections encompass the entire spectrum of pathology. *C. albicans,* the most common cause of yeast infection, and to a lesser extent other *Candida* species produce superficial, cutaneous, mucocutaneous, and systemic disease. *Cryptococcus neoformans* may cause multisystem disease with a predilection for the central nervous system. *Torulopsis* is usually involved in urinary tract infections as well as fungemia. The remaining three genera are seen infrequently in the clinical setting with *Trichosporon beigelii* being the cause of white piedra, *Malassezia furfur* being the etiologic agent of tinea versicolor, and *Rhodotorula* causing disease at various sites in the severely debilitated host.

YEASTS

LABORATORY DIAGNOSIS

Flow Chart for the More Commonly Isolated Yeasts

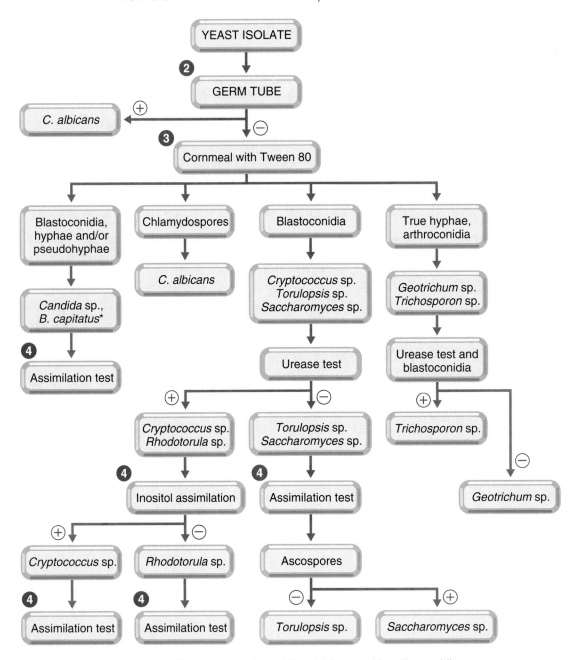

*Does not produce blastoconidia; forms annelloconidia, which resemble arthroconidia

Procedure

● Confirm purity of yeast isolate.

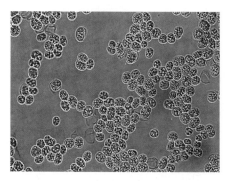

(Courtesy of Dr. Michael McGinnis, Department of Pathology, University of Texas Medical Branch, Galveston, TX.)

A. Suspend a small portion of the yeast colony in 0.5 mL of sterile distilled water, mix thoroughly, and streak onto a Sabouraud dextrose agar plate (SDA). Place a drop of the suspension on a slide, add a coverslip (wet preparation), and study microscopically under 40× magnification. Look for typical yeast cells, ascospores, or sporangia of the yeastlike alga *Prototheca wickerhamii* (see left).

Incubate the SDA plate at 30°C for 48 to 72 hours.

a. If bacterial contamination is suspected, streak the yeast isolate onto either two brain heart infusion blood agar plates or two sheep blood agar plates. Incubate one plate at 35° to 37°C and the other at 30°C.

b. If the yeast is contaminated with a mold, pick the top of the yeast colony with a loop and suspend it into 1.0 mL of sterile distilled water, mix, and streak onto an SDA plate and either a Mycobiotic or Mycosel agar plate. Incubate at 30°C for 72 hours.

● Perform germ tube test.

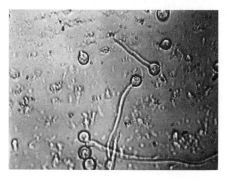

(From Mahon CR, Manuselis G: Textbook of Diagnostic Microbiology. Philadelphia, WB Saunders, 1995.)

A. Inoculate 0.5 mL of rabbit (coagulase) plasma with a *light* inoculum of the 24 to 48 hour yeast isolate.

B. Incubate at 35° to 37°C for 2.5 to 3 hours.

C. Make a wet preparation and under 40× magnification search for germ tubes (see left).

● If no germ tubes are seen, inoculate the isolate onto cornmeal polysorbate 80 (Tween 80) agar by the Dalmau technique.

A. With a sterile inoculating loop or needle, touch the yeast colony and make three close parallel streak lines, slightly longer than a 22 by 22 mm coverslip, on the agar plate. After sterilizing the loop, streak over the original three lines.

B. After sterilizing a 22 by 22 mm coverslip (dip coverslip in alcohol, flame, and cool), place it over the three parallel streak lines.

°To decrease turnaround time, step 3 is often performed in conjunction with assimilation studies, step 4.

YEASTS—LABORATORY DIAGNOSIS

C. Incubate at 22° to 26°C for 48 to 72 hours and look for the characteristic morphology of the yeast isolate. See "Morphologic Characteristics of Commonly Isolated Yeasts" on p 1022.

● If no chlamydospores are seen, additional biochemical studies such as carbohydrate and nitrate assimilation tests are required for final identification (see "Differential Characteristics of Yeasts Isolated in the Clinical Laboratory" on p 1025). These studies are laborious and time consuming and have largely been replaced with commercial identification systems. Three commonly used systems are discussed briefly below.

API-20C (bioMerieux Vitek, Inc., Hazelwood, MO)

This system is a miniaturized version of the sugar assimilation test discussed previously. Basically, the system consists of a strip containing 20 microcupules, 19 of which contain dehydrated substrates. Each of the cupules is inoculated with melted agar containing the yeast isolate. The strips are placed in a plastic humidity chamber and incubated at 30°C for 72 hours. The turbidity of the substrate containing cupules is compared with that of the 0 cupule, which serves as a negative control. The reactions are converted to a 7 digit biotype profile number, and the identification is made from a profile register supplied by the manufacturer.

Uni-Yeast-Tek System (Remel Laboratories, Lexena, KS)

This system consists of a plate containing 11 peripheral wells in which are incorporated agar based media used to detect carbohydrate, urea, and nitrate utilization. In addition, there is a center well containing cornmeal agar, and this well is used to determine microscopic morphology. Each of the peripheral wells is inoculated with a drop of the yeast suspension. The cornmeal agar well is inoculated with a small amount of yeast inoculum by streaking a small amount of the yeast colony across the surface and then placing a sterile coverslip over the well. Substrate utilization is characterized by color changes in the peripheral wells. An identification scheme is supplied by the manufacturer.

Vitek Yeast Biochemical Card (bioMerieux Vitek, Inc.)

The yeast biochemical card (YBC) contains 26 biochemical substrates and four negative control broths. The card is used with the Fully Automated Bacteriology Identification System (Vitek), which consists of a card filling module–sealing unit, a reader-incubator module, a computer, a printer, and terminal. In brief, the procedure involves filling the card with a suspension of the yeast isolate and incubating the card at 30°C for 24 to 48 hours. After incubation, the card is placed in the reader module, where the biochemical reactions are read and thence transmitted to the computer for final identification.

OTHER TESTS AND TECHNIQUES USED IN YEAST IDENTIFICATION

Urease Test

CONVENTIONAL METHOD

● Inoculate with a sterile inoculating needle the entire slant of a Christensen urea agar slant (Difco) with yeast isolate that is 24 to 48 hours old.

● Incubate the slant at 30°C for 48 to 72 hours.

A positive result is a pink-red color on slant.

RAPID METHOD

● Add 3 mL of sterile distilled water to a vial of dehydrated urea broth (Difco).

● Add four drops of rehydrated urea broth to a small volume receptacle, i.e., a microtiter tray.

NOTE   Once rehydrated, the broth must be used that day or frozen at −20°C.

● Inoculate the broth with a large inoculum of a 24 to 48 hour yeast isolate.

● Seal the well(s) with cellophane tape.

● Incubate at 35° to 37°C for 4 hours.

A positive result is the production of a pink color.

Sugar Fermentation Reactions

This test is seldom needed. It is occasionally useful in aiding in the identification of *Candida* species (see "Differential Characteristics of Yeasts Isolated in the Clinical Laboratory" on p 1025.)

Ascospore Production and Detection

There are several genera of yeasts that are routinely isolated in the teleomorphic state. In order to stimulate ascospore production, it is often necessary to subculture the organism onto special media. Kleyn's acetate medium is an excellent medium for this purpose.

● Make a wet preparation of the yeast colony and observe microscopically for ascospores. Alternatively, prepare a smear of the yeast, dry, heat fix, and then stain with a modified Kinyoun acid fast stain.

Ascospores will stain red.

● If no ascospores are seen, streak a slant of Kleyn's acetate agar with the yeast isolate and incubate at 25°C for 5 to 7 days.

● Prepare a smear from the slant and procede as in step 1.

Phenol oxidase test for *Cryptococcus neoformans*

● Streak a birdseed agar or caffeic acid agar plate with yeast isolate.

● Incubate at 30°C for 2 to 5 days.

C. neoformans *colonies will turn dark brown.*

MORPHOLOGIC CHARACTERISTICS OF COMMONLY ISOLATED YEASTS

ORGANISM	COLONIAL MORPHOLOGY ON SDA, 72 H	MICROSCOPIC MORPHOLOGY, SDA	*DIFFERENTIAL MORPHOLOGY, CORNMEAL AGAR, 3–5 DAYS	MICROSCOPIC VIEW
Candida albicans (*C. stellatoidea*)	Raised, creamy, smooth	Ovoid cells, 2.5 × 6–10 μm	Pseudohyphae with clusters of blastoconidia internodally (4 μm, *d*); chlamydospores (8–12 μm, *d*)	*
C. tropicalis	see *C. albicans*	Ovoid to globose cells, 4–8 × 5–11 μm	Branching pseudohyphae bearing blastoconidia singly or in clusters	*
C. guilliermondii	Flat, cream to pink	Ovoid cells, 2–5 × 3–7 μm	Slender, curved pseudohyphae with tear shaped blastoconidia in whorls	*
C. parapsilosis	Small, raised, smooth to lacy and off-white	Ovoid cells, 4 × 2.5–9 μm	Very thin pseudohyphae bearing a few blastoconidia in whorls giant hyphal elements	*

Continued ▶

▶ Continued **MORPHOLOGIC CHARACTERISTICS OF COMMONLY ISOLATED YEASTS**

ORGANISM	COLONIAL MORPHOLOGY ON SDA, 72 H	MICROSCOPIC MORPHOLOGY, SDA	*DIFFERENTIAL MORPHOLOGY, CORNMEAL AGAR, 3–5 DAYS	MICROSCOPIC VIEW
C. kefyr (*C. pseudotropicalis*)	Smooth and cream colored	Short to ovoid cells; 2.5–5 × 5–10 μm; longer cells may occur.	Branched pseudohyphae bearing blastoconidia in verticils; pseudohyphae disintegrate with cells remaining linear, resembling "logs in a stream."	*
C. krusei	Cream colored, flat, dull, and dry	Ovoid and cylindric cells, 3–5 × 6–20 μm	Elongate pseudohyphae in "treelike" or "matchstick" arrangement; verticils of blastoconidia	*
Torulopsis glabrata	Cream colored, smooth, soft, and shiny	Ovoid cells, 2.5–4.5 × 4–6 μm	Compacted cells; no pseudohyphae or blastoconidia	*
Cryptococcus neoformans	White, granular or wrinkled at first, becoming moist, shiny, and mucoid	Sherical cells with thick walls, 3.5–7 × 3.7–8 μm; capsules are apparent in most strains.	Compacted cells, no or rarely rudimentary mycelium formed	*

Continued ▶

▶ Continued **MORPHOLOGIC CHARACTERISTICS OF COMMONLY ISOLATED YEASTS**

ORGANISM	COLONIAL MORPHOLOGY ON SDA, 72 H	MICROSCOPIC MORPHOLOGY, SDA	*DIFFERENTIAL MORPHOLOGY, CORNMEAL AGAR, 3–5 DAYS	MICROSCOPIC VIEW
Trichosporon spp.	Dry and wrinkled, off-white to tan	Arthroconidia	Pseudohyphae, true hyphae, arthroconidia, and blastoconidia	*
**Geotrichum candidum*	White to buff colored, moist or dry, mealy texture	True hyphae, arthroconidia	True hyphae fragmenting into arthroconidia	*
Saccharomyces cerevisiae	Cream colored	Spherical to ovoid to elliptic cells; size: up to 7 × 10 μm. Presence of ascospores	Compact cells, no blastoconidia, rudimentary pseudohyphae may occur.	

* *G. candidum* is actually a mold that resembles a yeast.

DIFFERENTIAL CHARACTERISTICS OF YEASTS ISOLATED IN THE CLINICAL LABORATORY

ORGANISM	Growth at 37°C	Ascospore	Pseudohyphae	Chlamydospores	Germ tubes	Capsule, India ink	ASSIM. Glucose	Maltose	Sucrose	Lactose	Galactose	Melibiose	Cellobiose	Inositol	Xylose	Raffinose	Trehalose	Dulcitol	FERM. Glucose	Maltose	Sucrose	Lactose	Galactose	Trehalose	Urease	KNO₃ utilization
Candida albicans	+	–	+	+	+	–	+	+	+	–	+	–	–	–	+	–	+	+	G	G	–	–	G	G	–	–
C. stellatoidea	+	–	+	+	+	–	+	+	–	–	+	–	–	–	+	–	+	–	G	G	–	–	G	G	–	–
C. guilliermondii	+	–	+	–	–	–	+	+	+	–	+	+	+	–	+	+	+	+	G	G	G	–	G	G	–	–
C. kefyr	+	–	+	–	–	–	+	–	+	+	+	–	+	–	+	–	–*	+	G	–	G	G	–	–	–	–
C. krusei	+*	–	+	–	–	–	+	–	–	–	–	–	–	–	–	–	–	–	G	–	–	–	–	–	+*	–
C. lambica	+	–	+	–	–	–	+	–	–	–	–	–	–	–	+	–	+	–	–	–	–	–	–	–	+	–
C. lipolytica	+	–	+	–	–	–	+	–	–	–	–	–	–	–	–	–	–	–	–	–	–	–	–	–	+	–
C. lusitaniae	+	–	+	–	–	–	+	+	+	–	+	–	+	–	+	–	+	–	G	G	G	–	G	G	–	–
C. parapsilosis	+	–	+	–	–	–	+	+	+	–	+	–	–	–	+	–	+	–	G	–	–	–	G	–	–	–
C. rugosa	+	–	+	–	–	–	+	–	–	–	+	–	–	–	+	–	–	–	–	–	–	–	–	–	–	–
C. tropicalis	+	–	+	–	–	–	+	+	+	–	+	–	+	–	+	–	+	–	G	G	G	–	G	G	–	–
Torulopsis glabrata	+	–	–	–	–	–	+	–	–	–	+	–	–	–	+	–	+	–	G	G	–	–	G	G	–	–
T. candida	+	–	–	–	–	–	+	+	+	–	+	+	+	–	+	+	+	+	WK	–	WK	–	–	WK	+	–
Cryptococcus neoformans	+	–	–	–	–	+	+	+	+	–	+	+	+	+	+	+	+	–	–	–	–	–	–	–	+	–
C. albidus	–*	–	–	–	–	+	+	+	+	+	+	+	+	+	+	+	+	+	–	–	–	–	–	–	+	+
C. laurentii	–*	–	–	–	–	+	+	+	+	+	+	+	+	+	+	+	+	*	–	–	–	–	–	–	+	+
C. luteolus	–	–	–	–	–	+	+	+	+	*	+	+	+	+	+	+	+	–	–	–	–	–	–	–	+	+
C. terreus	–*	–	–	–	–	+	+	+	+	+	+	+	+	+	+	*	+	+	–	–	–	–	–	–	+	+
C. uniguttulatus	–	–	–	–	–	+*	+	+	+	–	*	–	+	–	+	–	+	*	–	–	–	–	–	–	+	+
Rhodotorula glutinis	+	–	–	–	–	–*	+	+	+	+	+	+	+	–	+	+	+	–	–	–	–	–	–	–	+	+
R. rubra	–*	–	–	–	–	–	+	+	+	*	+	*	*	–	+	*	+	*	–	–	–	–	–	–	+	+
Saccharomyces cerevisiae	+	+	+	–	–	–	+	+	+	–	+	+	–	–	–	+	+	–	G	G	G	–	G	G	–	–
Hansenula anomala	+*	+	*	–	–	–	+	*	+	–	*	+	+	*	*	+	*	*	G	G	G	–	G	G	–	+
Trichosporon beigelii	+*	–	+	–	–	–	+	+	+	+	+	+	+	–	+	+	+	+	–	–	–	–	–	–	+	+
Trichosporon pullulans	–*	–	+	–	–	–	+	+	+	–	+	–	+	–	+	+	+	+	–	–	–	–	–	–	+	+
Geotrichum candidum	–	–	+	–	–	–	+	–	–	–	+	–	–	–	+	–	–	–	–	–	–	–	–	–	–	+
Blastoschizomyces capitatus	+	–	+	–	–	–	+	+	–	–	+	+	+	–	+	*	+	–	G	G	G	–	G	G	+	+
Prototheca wickerhamii	+	–	–	–	–	–	+	–	–	–	–	–	–	–	–	–	+	–	–	–	–	–	–	–	–	–

*, strain variation; G, gas production; WK, weak reaction.

Modified from Dixon DM, Fromting RA: Candida, Cryptococcus and other yeasts of medical importance. In Murray PR, Barron EJ, Pfaller MA, et al, eds: Manual of Clinical Microbiology, 6th ed. Washington, DC, ASM Press, 1995, p. 725.

DIFFERENTIAL CHARACTERISTICS OF YEASTS ISOLATED IN CLINICAL LAB

AEROBIC ACTINOMYCETES

The aerobic actinomycetes are slow growing filamentous and branched bacteria that superficially resemble the fungi. Traditionally, these bacteria have been processed in the mycology laboratory and therefore are discussed with the fungi. Among the aerobic actinomycetes, it is the genera *Nocardia, Actinomadura, Streptomyces,* and *Nocardiopsis* that are the principal causative agents of human disease. *Nocardia* causes two main clinical syndromes: nocardiosis and mycetoma. *Actinomadura, Streptomyces,* and *Nocardiopsis* are principally etiologic agents of mycetoma.

LABORATORY DIAGNOSIS

Flow Chart of the More Common Aerobic Actinomycetes

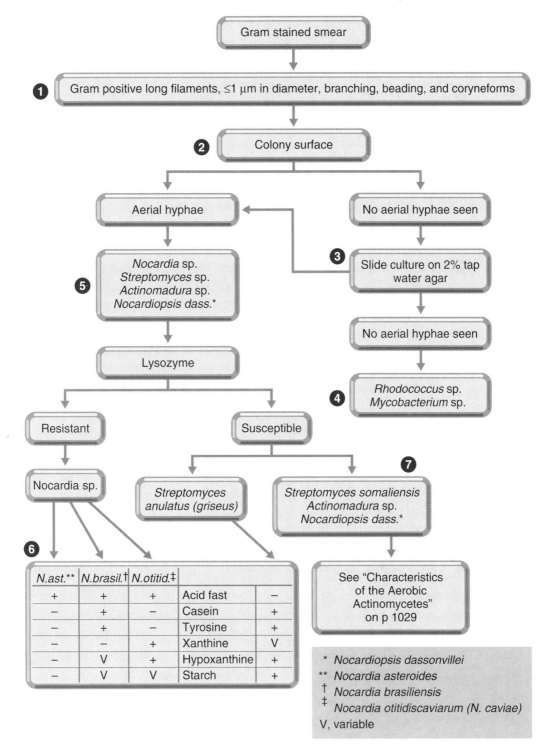

Procedure

● Perform Gram's stain of the isolate and look for gram positive thin, long filaments that may fragment into bacillary forms.

● Observe the colony surface for the presence of aerial hyphae.

● If no aerial hyphae are seen, prepare a slide culture of the organism using 2% tap water agar. Incubate the slide culture at its optimal temperature (usually 30°C) until adequate growth is observed. Study microscopically for aerial hyphae.

● If no aerial hyphae are seen, the genera *Rhodococcus* and *Mycobacterium* should be suspected.

● If aerial hyphae are observed, perform the lysozyme resistance test.

   A. Add several fragments of the culture into a tube of glycerol broth with lysozyme and to a second tube of glycerol broth without lysozyme.

   B. Incubate both tubes at 30°C until the tube without lysozyme shows good growth.

   Growth in both tubes indicates lysozyme resistance. Growth only in the broth without lysozyme indicates lysozyme susceptibility.

● The six tests described usually identify the majority of suspected aerobic actimomycetes routinely isolated in the clinical laboratory.

   A. If the organism is resistant to lysozyme, make a smear and perform the modified Kinyoun acid fast stain.

      a. If the organism is non–acid fast, subculture the isolate into a milk based medium such as litmus milk broth, incubate at optimal temperature for several days, and redo the acid fast stain procedure.

   B. Inoculate casein,* tyrosine,* xanthine,* hypoxanthine, and starch* agars by making a single heavy streak of the isolate, approximately 1.5 cm in length, across the center of each of the agars. Incubate at optimal temperature for up to 4 weeks.

EXPECTED RESULTS

Partial acid fast organisms (*Nocardia* species are partially acid fast) show both red filaments (acid fast) and blue filaments (non–acid fast).

Utilization of casein, tyrosine, xanthine, and hypoxanthine is indicated by a clearing of the medium around the inoculum.

Utilization of starch is demonstrated by observing a clear area around the inoculum after flooding the plate with Gram's iodine.

● If the described tests are insufficient to identify the suspected aerobic actinomycte, refer to "Characteristics of the Aerobic Actinomycetes" on p 1029.

---

*Agars may be obtained from Becton Dickinson, Cockeysville, MD.

CHARACTERISTICS OF THE AEROBIC ACTINOMYCETES

ORGANISM	ACID FAST	CASEIN	TYROSINE	XANTHINE	HYPOXANTHINE	UREA	LYSOZYME	CONIDIA	AERIAL HYPHAE	STARCH	GELATIN	BCP MILK	LACTOSE	XYLOSE
Nocardia asteroides	+	–	–	–	–	+	R	–	+	–	–	–	–	–
Nocardia brasiliensis	+	+	+	–	+|	+	R	–	+	–	+	+	–	–
Nocardia otitidiscaviarum	+	–	–	+	+	+	R	–	+	–	–	–	–	–
Actinomadura madurae	–	+	+	–	+|	–	S	–	+	+	+	+|	+|	+
Streptomyces anulatus	–	+	+	+	+	+	S	+	+	+	+	+	+	+
Actinomadura pelletieri	–	+	+	–	+|	–		–	+	–	+	+|	–	–
Nocardiopsis dassonvillei	–	+	+	+	–	+|		+|	+	+	+	+	–	–
Streptomyces somaliensis	–	+	+	–	–	–		–	+	+|	+	+	–	+
Dermatophilus congolensis	–	+	–	–	–	+		–		+	+	+	–	–
Streptomyces paraguayensis	–	+	+	+	–	+		–		+		+		

R, lysozyme resistant; S, lysozyme susceptible; BCP, bromcresol purple.

Adapted from Berd B: Laboratory identification of clinically important aerobic actinomycetes. Appl Microbiol, 25(4):665–691, 1973; and Gordon MA: Aerobic pathogenic actinomycetaceae. In Lennette EW, Balows A, Hausler Jr WJ, Truant JP, eds: Manual of Clinical Microbiology, 3rd ed. Washington, DC, ASM Press, 1980, p 181.

SUPERFICIAL AND CUTANEOUS MYCOSES

The superficial mycotic agents invade the outermost layers of the skin (stratum corneum) and the hair. They have very low virulence, and their principal effect is cosmetic. The cutaneous mycotic agents (agents of dematophytoses, tinea, ringworm) attack the keratinized tissue of the skin, hair, and nails. Dermatophytic fungal infection provokes a host response that includes both cell mediated and humoral components.

SUPERFICIAL MYCOTIC AGENTS

The superficial mycotic agents are often identified by a combination of the host response (clinical picture) and the direct smear. Rarely is the culturing of the organism necessary.

Disease and Organism: Black piedra and *Piedraia hortae*

CLINICAL PICTURE. Patients have firm, hard, and black irregular nodules along the scalp hair shafts.

LABORATORY DIAGNOSIS

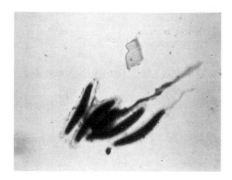

Direct Examination. Place infected hairs with their nodules on a slide in 10% to 25% KOH. Heat slightly, place a coverslip over the hair, and press down. Examine microscopically for oval asci containing slightly curved fusiform ascospores with a polar filament at each end (see left).

(From Dolan CT et al: Atlas of Clinical Mycology. VI: Systemic Mycoses: Saprobic Fungi (a slide set). Chicago, American Society of Clinical Pathologists, Educational Products Division, 1975.)

Disease and Organism: White Piedra and *Trichosporon beigelii*

CLINICAL PICTURE. Patients have soft, white to tan nodules found principally on the hairs of the beard, mustache, axilla, and genital area, less often on the hairs of the scalp.

LABORATORY DIAGNOSIS

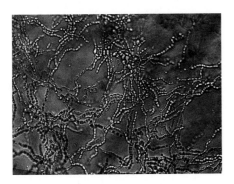

(Courtesy of Connie R. Mahon, Department of Clinical Laboratory Sciences, University of Texas Health Science Center at San Antonio, San Antonio, TX.; and Lee Sadarowski, Department of Microbiology, Audie Murphy VA Medical Center, San Antonio, TX.)

Direct Examination. For procedure, see under black piedra. Examine microscopically for septate hyphae fragmenting into round or oval arthroconidia. Blastoconidia may also be seen (see left).

Confirmation of Etiologic Agent. See "Flow Chart for the More Commonly Isolated Yeasts" on p 1018 and "Differential Characteristics of Yeasts Isolated in the Clinical Laboratory" on p 1025.

Disease and Organism: Tinea Nigra and *Phaeoannellomyces (Exophiala) werneckii*

CLINICAL PICTURE. Patients have brown to black, nonscaly, sharply marginated macules, usually on the palms of the hands. The appearance is similar to that of a KNO_3 skin stain.

LABORATORY DIAGNOSIS

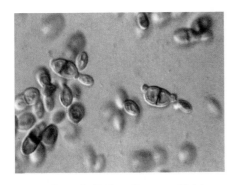

(Courtesy of Dr. Michael McGinnis, Department of Pathology, University of Texas Medical Branch, Galveston, TX.)

Direct Examination. Perform a microscopic examination of skin scrapings in a coverslipped 10% KOH preparation. A positive finding demonstrates brownish septate hyphae and elongated budding cells (see left).

SUPERFICIAL MYCOTIC AGENTS

Disease and Organism: Tinea Versicolor (Pityriasis Versicolor) and *Malassezia furfur*

CLINICAL PICTURE. Patients have white, tan, or brown, sharply marginated, noninflammatory lesions. Lesions fluoresce bright gold under Wood's lamp.

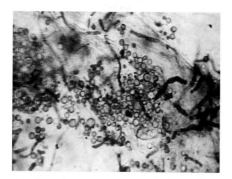

(From Dolan CT et al: Atlas of Clinical Mycology. VI: Systemic Mycoses (a slide set). Chicago, American Society of Clinical Pathologists, Educational Products Division, 1975.)

LABORATORY DIAGNOSIS. For procedure, see under tinea nigra. A positive finding demonstrates septate hyphae with oval yeast cells (resembles "spaghetti and meatballs") (see left).

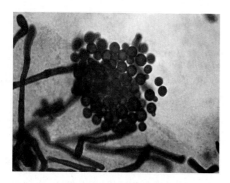

(Courtesy of Dr. Michael McGinnis, Department of Pathology, University of Texas Medical Branch, Galveston, TX.)

NOTE *M. furfur* has been associated with systemic infections in patients receiving intralipid therapy. For culture of this lipophilic organism, fungal media such as modified SDA must be overlaid with a thin film of sterile olive oil and incubated at 30° to 37°C. Microscopic examination of the growth will show yeastlike cells that are bottle-like (phialidic) (see left).

CUTANEOUS MYCOTIC AGENTS

The cutaneous mycotic agents are primarily identified by their macroscopic as well as their microscopic morphologies. Physiologic and biochemical tests are limited and are discussed briefly.

Laboratory Diagnosis

Flow Chart of the Commonly Isolated Dermatophytes

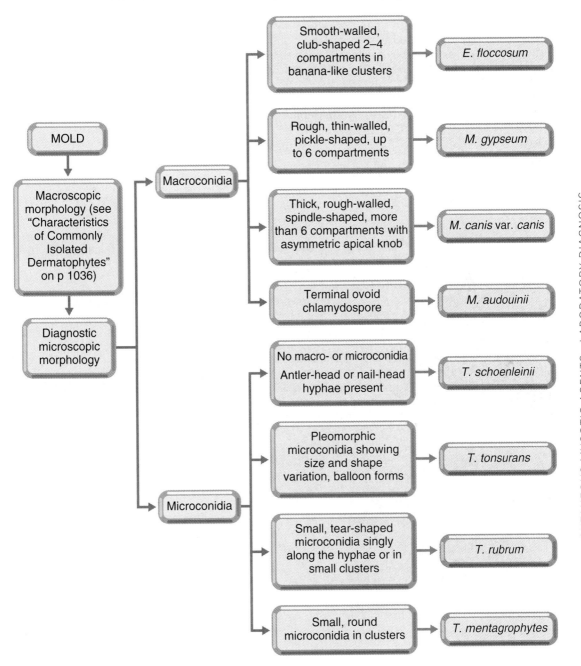

Procedure

● After the fungal isolate has reached maturity, usually in 7 to 10 days, study its obverse as well as its reverse characteristics. Refer to "Flow Chart of the Commonly Isolated Dermatophytes" above.

● Make a teased or cellophane tape lactophenol cotton blue wet mount of the outer growing edge of the mold and study it microscopically at 400×. Refer to "Flow Chart of the Commonly Isolated Dermatophytes" on p 1033 and "Characteristics of Commonly Isolated Dermatophytes" on p 1036.

● If the conidial arrangement on the conidiophore is necessary for speciation and is disrupted by the teased and cellophane tape preparations, a slide culture using potato dextrose agar (PDA) should be performed.

● Confirmatory tests:

Growth on Rice Grain Media

Inoculate a flask containing rice grain medium by placing several small pieces of the fungal isolate on the rice grains. Incubate at 30°C for 7 to 10 days.

EXPECTED RESULTS

Microsporum canis shows luxuriant growth.
M. audouinii shows no growth with or without browning of the rice grains.

Urease Test

Place a small portion of the fungal isolate on the surface of a Christensen's urea agar slant (Difco). Incubate at 30°C for 7 days.

EXPECTED RESULTS

Trichophyton mentagrophytes produces a red color on the urea agar slant.
T. rubrum produces no color change on the urea agar slant.

In Vitro Hair Perforation Test

Place several autoclaved, untreated hair strands in a sterile petri dish containing 25 mL of sterile distilled water to which has been added 2 to 3 drops of sterile 10% yeast extract. Incubate at 30°C for up to 4 weeks. Remove, at weekly intervals, a single strand of hair and place it on a slide in a drop of lactophenol cotton blue and coverslip. Examine microscopically at 100× or 400× for perforating organs.

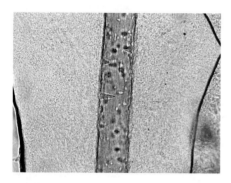

EXPECTED RESULTS

T. mentagrophytes perforates hair (see left).
T. rubrum does not perforate hair.

(Courtesy of Connie R. Mahon, Department of Clinical Laboratory Sciences, University of Texas Health Science Center at San Antonio, San Antonio, TX.; and Lee Sadarowski, Department of Microbiology, Audie Murphy VA Medical Center, San Antonio, TX.)

Pigment Production on Cornmeal Agar Containing 1% Dextrose

Place a small portion of the fungal isolate on the cornmeal with 1% dextrose agar plate. Incubate at 30°C for 7 to 10 days.

EXPECTED RESULTS

T. mentagrophytes produces no pigment.
T. rubrum produces red pigment.

Trichophyton Agars (T-Agars) Nutritional Test

Seven T-agar slants, numbered 1 through 7, are available from Difco. Their content may be summarized as follows: T-agar 1: casein agar basal medium; T-agar 2: T-agar 1 + inositol; T-agar 3: T-agar 1 + inositol plus thiamine; T-agar 4: T-agar 1 + thiamine; T-agar 5: T-agar 1 + nicotinic acid; T-agar 6: ammonium nitrate agar basal medium; T-agar 7: T-agar 6 + histidine.

Place a small portion of the fungal isolate with no adhering agar onto the center of the T-agar slants. Incubate at 30°C for 7 to 14 days.

EXPECTED RESULTS

See—Laboratory Diagnosis "Characteristics of Commonly Isolated Dermatophytes" below.

Characteristics of Commonly Isolated Dermatophytes

ORGANISM	MACROSCOPIC MORPHOLOGY	MICROSCOPIC MORPHOLOGY	COMMENTS	MICROSCOPIC VIEW
Microsporum audouinii	Flat, spreading, grayish or tannish white	See "Flow Chart of Commonly Isolated Dermatophytes" on p 1033.	Poor growth on polished rice grains	✳
M. canis var. *canis*	White, spreading, yellow periphery after few days	See "Flow Chart of Commonly Isolated Dermatophytes" on p 1033.	Good growth on polished rice grains	◆
M. gypseum	Flat, powdery, cinnamon-buff	See "Flow Chart of Commonly Isolated Dermatophytes" on p 1033.	—	◆
M. canis var. *distortum*	Flat, fuzzy to powdery, white to buff	Macroconidia similar those of to *M. canis* var. *canis* but distorted and bent in shape	—	✛

Continued ▶

▶ Continued **Characteristics of Commonly Isolated Dermatophytes**

ORGANISM	MACROSCOPIC MORPHOLOGY	MICROSCOPIC MORPHOLOGY	COMMENTS	MICROSCOPIC VIEW
M. nanum	Spreading, powdery, buff	Rough, thin walled, egg shaped macroconidia, one to three compartments; microconidia present	a. Distinguish from *Chysosporium* species (no microconidia). b. Distinguish from *Trichothecium* species (no microconidia, colonial morphology).	✛
M. cookei	Spreading, powdery, deep grape-red pigment	Thick, rough walled, oval macroconidia; clavate microconidia	—	✛
M. vanbreuseghemii	Spreading, fluffy to cottony, lavender-pink to buff	Long, tapered, rough, thick walled macroconidia with usually eight or more compartments	—	▶
Epidermophyton floccosum	Heaped, lumpy, olive-gray to khaki	See "Flow Chart of Commonly Isolated Dermatophytes" on p 1033.	—	◆

Continued ▲

CHARACTERISTICS OF COMMONLY ISOLATED DERMATOPHYTES

▶ Continued **Characteristics of Commonly Isolated Dermatophytes**

ORGANISM	MACROSCOPIC MORPHOLOGY	MICROSCOPIC MORPHOLOGY	COMMENTS	MICROSCOPIC VIEW
Trichophyton mentagrophytes	White, flat and powdery or white, flat, densely downy	See "Flow Chart of Commonly Isolated Dermatophytes" on p 1033.	a. Grows at 35°–37°C (see *T. terrestre*) b. Uses urea in 5 days; perforates hair (see *T. rubrum*) c. No red pigment on cornmeal agar with 1% dextrose (see *T. rubrum*)	◆
T. rubrum	White, fluffy to downy; reverse is blood-red	See "Flow Chart of Commonly Isolated Dermatophytes" on p 1033.	a. Does not use urea within 7 days b. Does not perforate hair c. Red pigment maintained on cornmeal agar with 1% dextrose	◆
T. tonsurans	Flat, powdery, white to yellowish to brownish; mahogony red or yellow reverse	See "Flow Chart of Commonly Isolated Dermatophytes" on p 1033.	Growth enhanced by thiamin: grows poorly on T-agar 1 and luxuriantly on T-agars 3 and 4	+
T. terrestre	White to yellow; gray reverse	Pear shaped, truncated microconidia	No growth at 35°–37°C	

Continued ▶

▶ Continued **Characteristics of Commonly Isolated Dermatophytes**

ORGANISM	MACROSCOPIC MORPHOLOGY	MICROSCOPIC MORPHOLOGY	COMMENTS	MICROSCOPIC VIEW
T. schoenleinii	White, glabrous to slightly downy; later heaped and convoluted	See "Flow Chart of Commonly Isolated Dermatophytes" on p 1033.	—	+
T. verrucosum	Yellow to gray-white, glabrous and heaped or flat and slightly downy	On SDA, hyphae suggestive of *T. schoenleinii;* on enriched media with thiamin, tear shaped microconidia and rarely macroconidia shaped like string beans or rat tails	a. Grows better at 37°C b. 84% require thiamin and inositol (4+ growth on T-agar 3), whereas 16% only require thiamin (4+ growth on T-agars 3 and 4)	●
T. violaceum	Glabrous, wrinkled, heaped up with a deep purplish-red color at maturation	Tangled branched hyphae containing cytoplasmic granules. No conidia on SDA. On enriched media micro and occasionally macroconidia are formed.	Enhanced growth in presence of thiamine (4+ growth on T-agars 3 and 4)	

* Courtesy of the Centers for Disease Control and Prevention, Atlanta, GA.
◆ Courtesy of Connie R. Mahon, Department of Clinical Laboratory Sciences, University of Texas Health Science Center at San Antonio, San Antonio, TX; and Lee Sadarowski, Department of Microbiology, Audie Murphy VA Medical Center, San Antonio, TX.
✚ Courtesy of Dr. Michael McGinnis, Department of Pathology, University of Texas Medical Branch, Galveston, TX.
▶ From Dolan CT et al: Atlas of Clinical Mycology. VI: Systemic Mycoses (a slide set). Chicago, American Society of Clinical Pathologists, Educational Products Division, 1975.
● From Fisher F, Cook NB: Fundamentals of Diagnostic Mycology. Philadelphia, WB Saunders, 1998.

SUBCUTANEOUS MYCOSES

The subcutaneous mycoses are caused by a variety of fungal agents, most of which are soil microbes, that gain access to the host by traumatic implantation. The resulting infection involves principally subcutaneous tissue, usually without dissemination. There are six major categories of fungal disease within the subcutaneous mycoses.

CHROMOBLASTOMYCOSIS

Chromboblastomycosis is caused by a variety of soil inhabiting dematiaceous fungi that produce verrucoid lesions, later generating vegetative growths resembling cauliflower florets. The principal etiologic agents responsible for this fungal infection are *Phialophora verrucosa*, *Cladosporium carrionii*, and *Fonsecaea pedrosoi*.

Laboratory Diagnosis

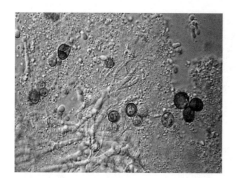

(Courtesy of Dr. Michael McGinnis, Department of Pathology, University of Texas Medical Branch, Galveston, TX.)

DIRECT EXAMINATION. A 10% KOH (with dimethylsulfoxide) preparation of lesions containing "black dots" will show microscopically fungal elements and planate dividing, 4 to 12 μm, thick walled, brown yeastlike bodies termed *sclerotic cells* or commonly referred to as "Medlar bodies," "muriform cells," or "copper pennies" (see left).

CULTURE
Macroscopic Morphology. The etiologic agents of chromoblastomycosis are slow growing, with a velvety surface that may be heaped, folded, or flat. The colonies range in color from gray to black to olive-black to olive-gray.

Microscopic Morphology. The etiologic agents are principally identified on the basis of their type of conidiation.

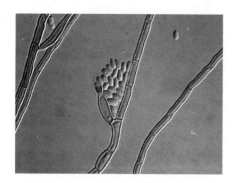

(Courtesy of Dr. Michael McGinnis, Department of Pathology, University of Texas Medical Branch, Galveston, TX.)

Phialophora verrucosa. Along the brown, septate, branching hyphae arise vase or flask shaped phialides, each having a distinct, flared collarette around its opening. Small elliptic or ovoid conidia collect at the top of the phialide, appearing as a vase of flowers (see left).

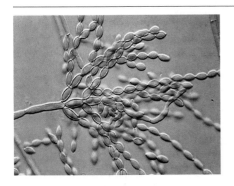

(Courtesy of Dr. Michael McGinnis, Department of Pathology,
University of Texas Medical Branch, Galveston, TX.)

Cladosporium Carrionii. Dark and septate hyphae give rise to lateral and terminal simple conidiophores with long and branched chains of pigmented, smooth walled oval or elliptic conidia. These conida are easily detached and show thickenings or scars, known as *disjunctors,* at their former points of attachment (see left).

Characteristics Differentiating Between the Morphologically Similar Nonpathogenic Cladosporium *species,* C. carrionii, *and* Xylohypha bantiana:

ORGANISM	PRESENCE OF DISJUNCTORS	MAXIMAL GROWTH TEMPERATURE (°C)	GROWTH IN 15% NACL	GELATIN LIQUIFACTION	PATHOLOGIC
C. carrionii	+	35–36	–	–	+
X. bantiana	–	42–43	–	–	+
Cladosporium species	+	Usually <37	+	Usually +	–

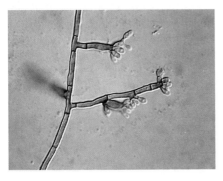

(Courtesy of Dr. Michael McGinnis, Department of Pathology,
University of Texas Medical Branch, Galveston, TX.)

Fonsecaea pedrosoi. Dark, septate hyphae may give rise to several types of conidiophores. The rhinocladiella type conidiophore is characteristic of this organism. The upper zone of this type of conidiophore is slightly swollen or club shaped and bears elliptic conidia at its top or irregularly on its sides. These primary conidia can give rise to secondary and even tertiary conidia, thus resembling a short chained cladosporium type sporulation. In addition to the rhinocladiella type sporulation, cladosporium type and rarely phialophora type sporulation may occur in the same isolate (see left).

CHROMOBLASTOMYCOSIS

SPOROTRICHOSIS

The etiologic agent of sporotrichosis, the dimorphic fungus *Sporothrix schenckii,* is commonly found in the soil and on decaying vegetation. The most common manifestation of sporotrichosis is a chronic subcutaneous infection that later involves the lymphatic system.

Laboratory Diagnosis

CULTURE

Macroscopic Morphology at 25° to 30°C. *S. schenckii* is a moderately slow growing organism that, at first, appears yeastlike with a white or grayish-white color. On prolonged incubation, the colony becomes leathery and brown to black. Variations in colonial appearance do occur.

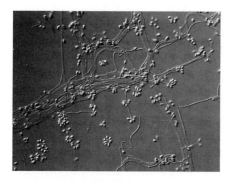

Microscopic Morphology at 25° to 30°C. The organism has septate hyphae bearing erect, slender conidiophores narrowing at its apex. Pyriform to spherical conidia arise on thin denticles and forms a "daisy head" or "rosette-like" aggregate at the tip of the conidiophore (see left).

S. schenckii is a thermally dimorphic fungus. Conversion to the yeast phase is required for final identification.

(Courtesy of Dr. Michael McGinnis, Department of Pathology, University of Texas Medical Branch, Galveston, TX.)

Conversion of Mycelial Form to Yeast Form. Subculture a small piece of mold to a brain-heart infusion agar with blood. Incubate at 35° to 37°C for several days.

Macroscopic Morphology at 35° to 37°C. The mycelial character of the colony transforms, over time, into a white or gray-white yeastlike colony.

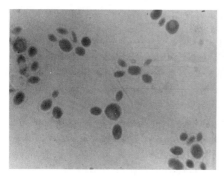

Microscopic Morphology at 35° to 37°C. The organism has spherical to oval to cigar shaped yeasts cells (see left).

NOTE: Any presence of yeast forms is indicative of conversion.

(Courtesy of the Centers for Disease Control and Prevention, Atlanta, GA.)

RHINOSPORIDIOSIS

Rhinosporidiosis is a chronic infection of the mucocutaneous tissue that usually involves the nose, with the production of polyps, tumors, papillomas, or wartlike lesions; less often the conjunctiva is involved. The etiologic agent, *Rhinosporidium seeberi*, is believed to be a saprobe, although its natural habitat is unclear.

Laboratory Diagnosis

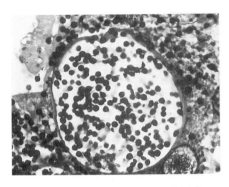

DIRECT EXAMINATION. Microscopic examination of a 10% KOH preparation of slightly macerated tissue or nasal discharge reveals sporangia (reaching 350 μm in diameter) containing many endospores (see left).

> **NOTE** The sporangia of *R. seeberi* resemble the spherules of *Coccidiodes immitis,* the important difference being the considerably larger size of the sporangia.

(Courtesy of Dr. Michael McGinnis, Department of Pathology, University of Texas Medical Branch, Galveston, TX.)

CULTURE. This organism has not been cultured using routine fungal culture techniques. It has been grown in an epithelial culture line.

LOBOMYCOSIS

Lobomycosis is a chronic disease characterized by subcutaneous nodules that may become verrucoid and may occasionally ulcerate. The etiologic agent, *Loboa loboi* has not been cultured, and its ecology is unknown.

Laboratory Diagnosis

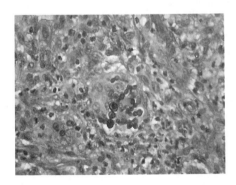

DIRECT EXAMINATION. Microscopic study of a 10% KOH preparation of macerated infected tissue shows chains of large yeast cells of similar size that are connected to each other by a narrow neck (see left).

(Courtesy of Dr. Michael McGinnis, Department of Pathology, University of Texas Medical Branch, Galveston, TX.)

RHINOSPORIDIOSIS

PHAEOHYPHOMYCOSIS

Phaeohyphomycosis is a mixture of diseases caused by a diverse group of dematiaceous filamentous fungi. These fungi are pigmented, brown to black because of the presence of melanin in their hyphal walls. Phaeohyphomycotic infection may be superficial, subcutaneous, or systemic. Phaeohyphomycosis includes all clinical entities caused by dematiaceous fungi, other than chromoblastomycosis.

The principal dematiaceous fungi associated with subcutaneous infection are *Exophiala jeanselmei* and *Wangiella dermatitidis*.

Laboratory Diagnosis

CULTURE

Macroscopic Morphology. *E. jeanselmei* and *W. dermatitidis* resemble each other in colonial appearance. They initially grow as a shiny black yeast that on continued incubation develop a velvety gray-black to black mycelium.

Microscopic Morphology

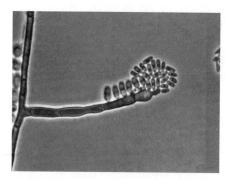

(Courtesy of Dr. Michael McGinnis, Department of Pathology, University of Texas Medical Branch, Galveston, TX.)

E. jeanselmei. Microscopic examination of the early, black yeast colony shows black yeastlike cells. Microscopic study of the mycelial form reveals brownish septate hyphae that form slender tublelike conidiophores (annelophores) with tapered tips. Oval conidia cluster at the conidiophore tip and along its sides (see left).

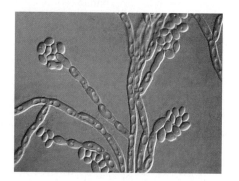

(Courtesy of Dr. Michael McGinnis, Department of Pathology, University of Texas Medical Branch, Galveston, TX.)

W. dermatitidis. The yeast form is microscopically indistinguishable from *E. jeanselmei*. The mycelial form also closely resembles *E. jeanselmei* under the light microscope. It forms light brown septate hyphae that bear slender and tapered conidiopores (phialophores). Ovoid conidia cluster at the tip and often appear to fall down the sides of the conidiophore (see left).

Characteristics Differentiating Between the Morphologically Similar
E. jeanselmei, W. dermatitidis, *and the Superficial Mycotic Agent* P.
werneckii.

| ORGANISM | DECOMPOSITION OF | | MAXIMAL GROWTH TEMPERATURE (°C) | KNO$_3$ UTILIZATION | GROWTH IN 15% NACL |
	CASEIN	TYROSINE			
W. dermatitidis	−	+	40	−	−
E. jeanselmei	−	+	37	+	−
P. werneckii	+	−		+	+

NOTE   Selected dematiaceous fungi causing phaeohyphomycosis may be found in the section dealing with the dematiaceous fungi.

The clinical syndrome mycetoma is the sixth major category within the subcutaneous mycoses and is discussed in the next section.

MYCETOMA

Mycetoma is a chronic, suppurative, granulomatus disease involving subcutaneous tissues, fascia, and bone. The etiologic agents are predominately soil organisms that gain entry into the host by traumatic implantation. The disease is characterized by tumefaction, draining sinuses, and the presence of granules or grains.

The causative agents of mycetoma are both bacterial and fungal. The actinomycetes, chiefly the aerobic actinomycetes, account for approximately half the cases of mycetoma, and the other half are caused by the true fungi.

LABORATORY DIAGNOSIS

Direct Examination

Specimens submitted to the laboratory should be examined for the presence of granules (size range: 0.2 to 2 mm). The granules should be washed in sterile normal saline, crushed, spread on a slide, and cultured in appropriate media. The slide is Gram stained and studied microscopically. The presence of thin filaments, less than or equal to 1.0 μm in diameter, is indicative of aerobic actinomycotic organisms, whereas hyphal elements ranging from 2 to 5 μm in diameter indicate a fungal etiology.

Aerobic Actinomycotic Mycetoma

The organisms within this group that most commonly cause mycetoma are *Nocardia brasiliensis*, *Actinomadura madurae*, *Actinomadura pelletieri*, and *Streptomyces somaliensis*.

PHAEOHYPHOMYCOSIS

CULTURAL CHARACTERISTICS AND DIAGNOSTIC TESTS. See the section on the aerobic actinomycetes.

Eumycotic Mycetoma

At least 23 different filamentous fungi have been reported to cause mycetoma. Of these, two fungi, *Pseudallescheria boydii* and *Madurella mycetomatis,* are common etiologic agents of this disease.

CULTURE

PSEUDALLESCHERIA BOYDII
Macroscopic Morphology
Teleomorph: *P. boydii.* This organism shows fluffy, white mycelium becoming mousy gray or brown. Reverse is initially white, later becoming gray, sometimes showing concentric rings. The teleomorphic stage is inhibited on media containing cycloheximide.

Anamorph: *Scedosporium apiospermum.* The macroscopic morphology is the same as that of *P. boydii.* The anamorphic stage will grow on media containing cycloheximide.

Microscopic Morphology

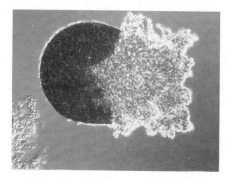

(Courtesy of Dr. Michael McGinnis, Department of Pathology, University of Texas Medical Branch, Galveston, TX.)

P. boydii. This organism has septate hyphae with brownish to black cleistothecia, 100 to 300 μm in diameter, which form just below the agar surface. The cleistothecia contain asci in which eight ascospores are contained (see left).

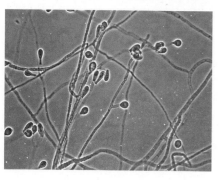

(Courtesy of Dr. Michael McGinnis, Department of Pathology, University of Texas Medical Branch, Galveston, TX.)

S. apiospermum. This organism has oval and truncated conidia borne singly, occasionally in groups, from the tips of conidiophores or laterally along the septate hyphae (see left).

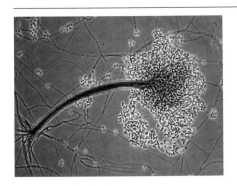

NOTE On occasion, a synanamorph of *P. boydii* showing *Graphium* type of asexual reproduction may be isolated. Microscopically, erect conidiophores cemented together and bearing groups of truncated conidia at their apex are seen (see left).

(Courtesy of Dr. Michael McGinnis, Department of Pathology, University of Texas Medical Branch, Galveston, TX.)

MADURELLA MYCETOMATIS

Macroscopic Morphology. Colonies vary, being cottony to leathery, white initially, later becoming olivaceous, yellow, or brown. A brown diffusible pigment is produced in the agar medium. Optimal temperature is 37°C.

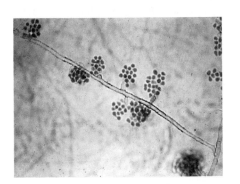

Microscopic Morphology. On SDA, the mycelia are sterile, composed of only septate hyphae and chlamydospores. On nutritionally deficient media such as cornmeal agar, phialides bearing round conidia are seen. Black sclerotia, 750 μm in diameter, may also be produced on this type of medium (see left).

(Courtesy of Dr. Michael McGinnis, Department of Pathology, University of Texas Medical Branch, Galveston, TX.)

AGENTS OF SYSTEMIC MYCOSES— THE DIMORPHIC FUNGI

The dimorphic fungi, which include *Blastomyces dermatitidis*, *Histoplasma capsulatum*, *Coccidioides immitis*, and *Paracoccidioides brasiliensis*, are primary pathogens causing infections that range from asymptomatic and self-limiting to those that are progressive and disseminating. In the natural environment these fungi exist in their infectious filamentous form, whereas in tissue they exist as the parasitic or invasive yeast or spherule form.

BLASTOMYCOSIS

Inhalation of the etiologic agent, *B. dermatitidis*, most often results in a primary subclinical infection. Several subsequent clinical courses may occur, including self-resolving pulmonary infection, primary pulmonary disease, chronic cutaneous disease with or without bone involvement, single or multiple organ involvement, or generalized disseminated disease. Traumatic implantation of the infecting agent, a rare occurrence, results in a self-limited primary infection.

Laboratory Diagnosis

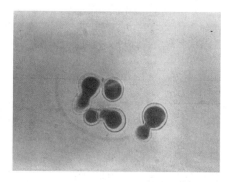

(Courtesy of the Centers for Disease Control and Prevention, Atlanta, GA.)

DIRECT EXAMINATION. Wet mounts of specimens treated with 10% KOH with or without Calcofluor white can reveal large, up to 20 μm, thick walled single budding yeast cells, the parent yeast cell connected by a broad base to its daughter cell (see left).

CULTURE

Macroscoscopic Morphology at 25° to 30°C. *B. dermatitidis* is usually a moderately slow growing organism forming a smooth, white yeastlike colony that after several days becomes tan to brown. On extended incubation, hyphal projections form in the center of the colony, giving it a prickly appearance.

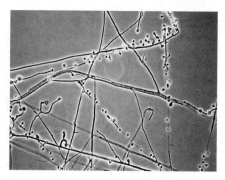

(Courtesy of Dr. Michael McGinnis, Department of Pathology, University of Texas Medical Branch, Galveston, TX.)

Microscopic Morphology at 25° to 35°C. Ovoid conidia are borne on slender conidiophores or directly on septate hyphae (see left).

B. dermatitidis is a thermally dimorphic fungus.° Conversion to the yeast phase is required for final identification (see *Sporothrix schenckii* for technique).

°The exoantigen test (Immunoimycologics, Meridian Diagnostics, Gibson Laboratories) or a nucleic acid probe (the Gen-probe Accuprobe System) may be substituted for thermal conversion.

Macroscopic Morphology at 35° to 37°C. Within several days, the filamentous phase transforms into a waxy, white to tan, wrinkled yeast phase (see left).

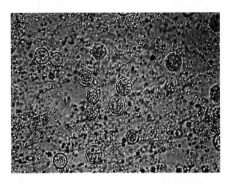

Microscopic Morphology at 35° to 37°C. At this temperature range the organism appears as large yeast cells with broad base buds (see left).

(Courtesy of Dr. Michael McGinnis, Department of Pathology, University of Texas Medical Branch, Galveston, TX.)

MORPHOLOGICALLY SIMILAR FUNGI. *Chrysosporium* species and *Scedosporium apiospermum* are morphologically similar.

HISTOPLASMOSIS

Histoplasmosis is a cosmopolitan disease caused by *Histoplasma capsulatum.* Infection occurs due to the inhalation of infectious conidia, which are abundant in areas where there is an accumulation of guano of birds and bats. The majority of humans exposed to the fungus develop a benign primary pulmonary infection. Chronic pulmonary or disseminated disease, principally of the reticuloendothelial system, may occur in cases of heavy exposure to the infecting agent and/or a compromised immune status of the patient.

Laboratory Diagnosis

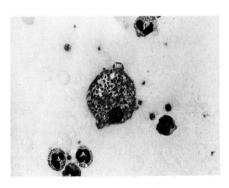

DIRECT EXAMINATION. Smears of specimens such as the buffy coat of peripheral blood, bone marrow aspirates, and biopsy material should be stained by the Giemsa method. Small, oval budding yeasts are seen within macrophages (see left).

(From Mahon CR, Manuselis G: Textbook of Diagnostic Microbiology. Philadelphia, WB Saunders, 1995.)

CULTURE
Macroscopic Morphology at 25° to 30°C. *H. capsulatum* is a slow growing mold that appears on fungal media within 2 to 4 weeks. The colonies may range from fluffy to glabrous and from white to brown.

BLASTOMYCOSIS

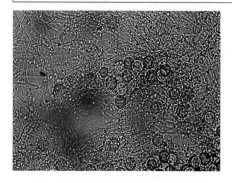

Microscopic Morphology at 25° to 30°C. Slender, branching, septate hyphae give rise to small microconidia. Smooth and/or the distinctive tuberculate macroconidia as well as microconidia are borne on narrow, tubular conidiophores (see left).

H. *capsulatum* is a thermally dimorphic fungus.° Conversion to the yeast phase is required for final identification (see *Sporothrix schenckii* for technique).

(Courtesy of Connie R. Mahon, Department of Clinical Laboratory Sciences, University of Texas Health Science Center at San Antonio, San Antonio, TX.; and Lee Sadarowski, Department of Microbiology, Audie Murphy VA Medical Center, San Antonio, TX.)

Macroscopic Morphology at 35° to 37°C. After several days and often requiring several transfers to enriched media, white, moist to dry yeastlike colonies form.

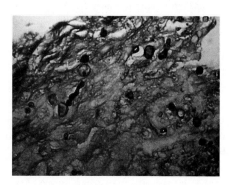

Microscopic Morphology at 35° to 39°C. Small, spherical to oval budding yeast cells (see left).

(From Mahon CR, Manuselis G: Textbook of Diagnostic Microbiology. Philadelphia, WB Saunders, 1995.)

MORPHOLOGICALLY SIMILAR FUNGI. *Sepedonium* species are morphologically similar. In young cultures where the macroconidia may be smooth (nontuberculate), *Chrysosporium* species and *B. dermatitidis* are morphologically similar.

PARACOCCIDIOIDOMYCOSIS

The etiologic agent of paracoccidioidomycosis, *Paracoccidioides brasiliensis*, causes a chronic granulomatous disease that begins as a primary, frequently inapparent pulmonary infection, often with subsequent dissemination to many visceral organs. Conspicuous oropharyngeal lesions are often the most evident clinical manifestation of the disease.

°The exoantigen test or the nucleic acid probe is recommended in lieu of thermal conversion due to this organism's resistance to conversion by the latter in vitro technique.

Laboratory Diagnosis

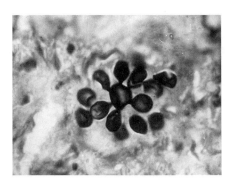

(Courtesy of Dr. Michael McGinnis, Department of Pathology, University of Texas Medical Branch, Galveston, TX.)

DIRECT EXAMINATION. Wet mounts of specimens treated with 10% KOH with or without Calcofluor white can reveal thick walled yeast cells ranging in size from 10 to 60 μm bearing multiple buds connected to the mother cell by narrow necks (see left).

CULTURE

Macroscopic Morphology at 25° to 30°C. *P. brasiliensis* is a very slow growing fungus, first appearing white, and later becoming beige, with a texture varying from glabrous to floccose.

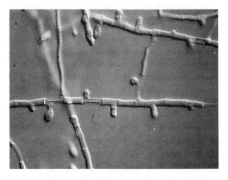

(Courtesy of Dr. Michael McGinnis, Department of Pathology, University of Texas Medical Branch, Galveston, TX.)

Microscopic Morphology at 25° to 30°C. Fine septate hyphae with intercalary and terminal chlamydospores are seen. Certain strains, after prolonged incubation, produce small globose to pyriform conidia along the hyphae (see left).

  P. brasiliensis is a thermally dimorphic fungus.° Conversion to the yeast phase is required for final identification (see *Sporothrix schenckii* for technique).

———————

°The exoantigen test may be substituted for thermal conversion.

PARACOCCIDIODOMYCOSIS

Macroscopic Morphology at 35° to 37°C. Within 1 to 2 weeks, smooth to wrinkled, white to tan yeast colonies appear.

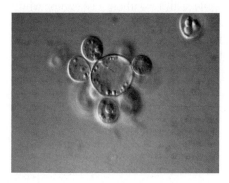

(From Mahon CR, Manuselis G: Textbook of Diagnostic Microbiology. Philadelphia, W.B. Saunders, 1995.)

Microscopic Morphology at 35° to 37°C. Multiply budding yeast cells intermixed with hyphal elements are seen (see left).

MORPHOLOGICALLY SIMILAR FUNGI. Some isolates of *P. brasiliensis* may form conidia typical of *B. dermatitidis* and *Chrysosporium* species. In the yeast phase, single budding cells of *P. brasiliensis* resemble the yeast phase of *B. dermatitidis*, whereas multiple budding cells of *P. brasiliensis* resemble the yeast phase of *Cokeromyces recurvatus*.

COCCIDIOIDOMYCOSIS

Coccidioidomycosis is a highly infectious disease limited to areas with semiarid climates. Infection is acquired by the inhalation of the airborne infective arthroconidia of *Coccidioides immitis*. The majority of individuals exposed to the arthroconidia develop a benign, often inapparent and self-limiting pulmonary disease. However, a small percentage of those exposed develop a progressive and disseminated disease that may involve multiple organ systems.

Laboratory Diagnosis

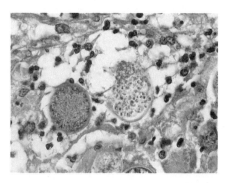

(Courtesy of Connie R. Mahon, Department of Clinical Laboratory Sciences, University of Texas Health Science Center at San Antonio, San Antonio, TX.; and Lee Sadarowski, Department of Microbiology, Audie Murphy VA Medical Center, San Antonio, TX.)

DIRECT EXAMINATION. Wet mounts of specimens treated with 10% KOH with or without Calcofluor white may reveal round spherules that range in diameter from 30 to 60 μm and are filled with endospores whose average diameter is 3.5 μm (see left).

CULTURE

 This organism is highly infectious and potentially extremely virulent. Agar slants or bottles instead of Petri dishes should be used when culturing samples suspected of containing *C. immitis*. All work should be performed under a class II biologic safety cabinet. Wetting down the fungal growth with a 0.5% aqueous solution of polysorbate 80 should precede any transfer of the fungus.

Macroscopic Morphology at 25° to 30°C. *C. immitis* is a fast growing fungus appearing usually within 3 to 5 days. Initially the growth is moist, glabrous, and gray, later developing a white to gray cottony aerial mycelium that often turns tan with age.

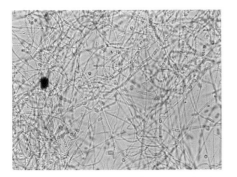

Microscopic Morphology at 25° to 30°C. One sees thin, branching septate hyphae that when mature develop thick walled, barrel shaped arthroconidia, alternating with thin walled, empty disjunctor cells. When the arthroconidia fragment and separate, they commonly have attached to each end a portion of the disjunctor cell, giving it a frilled appearance (see left).

(Courtesy of Connie R. Mahon, Department of Clinical Laboratory Sciences, University of Texas Health Science Center at San Antonio, San Antonio, TX; and Lee Sadarowski, Department of Microbiology, Audie Murphy VA Medical Center, San Antonio, TX.)

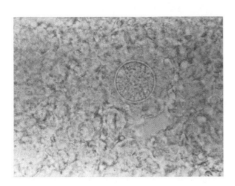

Microscopic Morphology at 37° to 40°C. *C. immitis* does not have a yeast phase. However, with special media such as Breslau's modification of Converse medium together with an increased CO_2 concentration and temperature, the arthroconidia transform into spherules (see left). *This conversion is required for final identification.*°

(Courtesy of the Centers for Disease Control and Prevention, Atlanta, GA.)

MORPHOLOGICALLY SIMILAR FUNGI. In the mycelial form, morphologically similar fungi are *Malbranchea* species, *Sporendonema* species, and *Geotrichum* species. In the tissue form a morphologically similar fungus is *Rhinosporidium seeberi*.

°The exoantigen test or the nucleic acid probe may be substituted for and is preferred to thermal conversion.

COCCIDIOIDOMYCOSIS

OPPORTUNISTIC MYCOTIC AGENTS

ASPERGILLOSIS

Aspergillosis is a collection of diseases caused, in large part, by a few of the numerous species within the genus *Aspergillus;* these include *A. fumigatus, A. flavus, A. glaucus* group, *A. niger, A. terreus,* and *A. nidulans.* The principal clinical types of mycotic disease caused by *Aspergillus* species are (1) pulmonary, including allergic and colonizing (fungus ball); (2) superficial, including skin, sinus, and ear; and (3) systemic.

Laboratory Diagnosis

DIRECT EXAMINATION. Wet mounts of specimens such as sputum, bronchial washings, body fluids, and skin scrapings may be studied as wet mounts prepared with 10% KOH with or without Calcofluor. Tissue samples are best studied by staining with Gridley's and Grocott-Gomori methenamine silver stain.

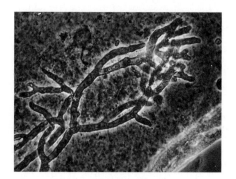

Aspergilli appear in patients' samples as septated hyphal elements, 2.5 to 4.5 μm in diameter, characteristically showing dichotomous branching with several branches oriented in the same direction, giving an extended finger-like appearance (see left).

(Courtesy of Dr. Michael McGinnis, Department of Pathology, University of Texas Medical Branch, Galveston, TX.)

CULTURE
A. fumigatus
Macroscopic Morphology. This is a rapidly growing mold, flat and smooth, at first white, later with the production of conidia becoming gray-green to blue-green.

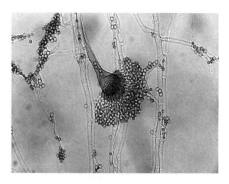

Microscopic Morphology. The conidiophore is short and smooth walled, enlarging at its tip to form a flask shaped vesicle that bears a single row of phialides (uniserate) on its upper half only. Green, spherical, and echinulate conidia arise from the phialides (see left).

(Courtesy of Connie R. Mahon, Department of Clinical Laboratory Sciences, University of Texas Health Science Center at San Antonio, San Antonio, TX; and Lee Sadarowski, Department of Microbiology, Audie Murphy VA Medical Center, San Antonio, TX.)

Other Characteristics. *A. fumigatus* will grow at 45°C or higher.

A. flavus

Macroscopic Morphology. This is a rapidly growing cottony mold, at first yellow but quickly becoming yellow-green.

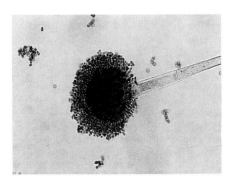

Microscopic Morphology. The conidiophore has a rough wall, enlarging at its apex into a vesicle that is at first elongate, later becoming spherical. The phialides, which cover the entire vesicle, may either arise directly from it (uniserate) or arise from intermediate cells, the metulae (biserate); rarely both biserate and uniserate conditions can occur on the same vesicle. Conidia may at first be elliptic, later becoming spherical, and are noticeably echinulate (see left).

(Courtesy of Connie R. Mahon, Department of Clinical Laboratory Sciences, University of Texas Health Science Center at San Antonio, San Antonio, TX; and Lee Sadarowski, Department of Microbiology, Audie Murphy VA Medical Center, San Antonio, TX.)

A. glaucus Group

Macroscopic Morphology. This is a rapidly growing feltlike, green to yellow-green fungus.

Microscopic Morphology. Conidiophores are smooth walled, terminating in a dome-like vesicle. Phialides arise from the entire vesicle in a single series (uniserate) bearing elliptic to spherical and usually echinulated conidia. Cleistothecia are usually present.

A. niger

Macroscopic Morphology. This is a rapidly growing cottony mold, white at first, becoming heavily speckled with black dots as conidia are produced.

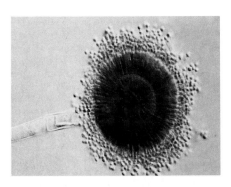

Microscopic Morphology. Smooth walled conidiophores enlarge to spherical vesicles at their apices. Phialides are in two series (biserate) over the entire vesicle and give rise to spherical, rough, black conidia (see left).

(Courtesy of Dr. Michael McGinnis, Department of Pathology, University of Texas Medical Branch, Galveston, TX.)

A. terreus

Macroscopic Morphology. This is a rapidly growing velvety to cottony fungus, cinnamon-buff to brown, rarely bright orange-brown.

ASPERGILLOSIS

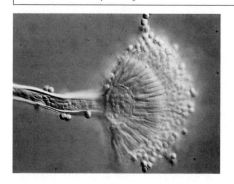

Microscopic Morphology. Smooth walled conidiophores subtly terminate in domelike vesicles. Phialides are arranged in a biserate pattern and bear spherical to slightly elliptic, smooth walled conidia. Round to oval translucent cells are produced either singly or in clusters on the submerged vegetative mycelium (see left).

(Courtesy of Dr. Michael McGinnis, Department of Pathology, University of Texas Medical Branch, Galveston, TX.)

A. nidulans

Macroscopic Morphology. This is a rapidly growing, velvety, dark green mold; when cleistothecia are present, the fungus appears buff to yellow. The colony reverse is purplish red.

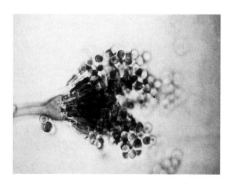

Microscopic Appearance. Conidiophores are smooth walled, forming hemispheric vesicles at their apices. Phialides have a biserate arrangement that bears spherical, finely wrinkled green conidia. Cleistothecia are usually present and are associated with elliptic to spherical thick walled cells known as *Hulle cells* (see left).

(Courtesy of Dr. Michael McGinnis, Department of Pathology, University of Texas Medical Branch, Galveston, TX.)

ZYGOMYCOSIS

Zygomycosis can be divided into two broad categories: (1) mucormycosis, which is often an acute infection that occurs throughout the world in the immunocompromised and particularly in the debilitated patient with uncontrolled diabetes, and (2) entomophthoromycosis, a chronic infection occurring in the immunocompetent and geographically limited to certain tropical regions of the world.

In the clinical laboratory, of the zygomycetes, the following mucormycotic agents are routinely isolated: *Rhizopus* species, *Mucor* species, *Absidia* species, *Rhizomucor* species, *Syncephalastrum* species, and *Cunninghamella* species.

Laboratory Diagnosis

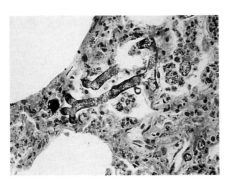

DIRECT EXAMINATION. 10% KOH (with or without Calcofluor) wet mounts of sputum, bronchial brushing, sinus aspirates, scrapings, and biopsy material from infected sites reveal microscopically aseptate, broad hyphal elements, 10 to 20 μm in diameter, which branch irregularly. Rare septa may occasionally be observed. When a zygomycotic infection is suspected, tissue specimens should not be ground with a tissue grinder, since this will often render the organism nonviable; rather one can mince the tissue aseptically with a scalpel (see left).

(Courtesy of Dr. Michael McGinnis, Department of Pathology, University of Texas Medical Branch, Galveston, TX.)

CULTURE
Macroscopic Morphology. The routinely isolated mucormycotic agents are indistinguishable macroscopically. They are rapidly growing, cottony, white at first, later becoming gray and filling the Petri dish within 3 to 4 days.

Microscopic Morphology

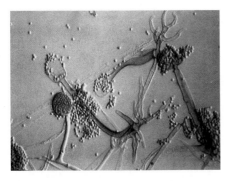

***Rhizopus* Species.** One sees broad, aseptate, usually unbranched hyphae that produce runners (horizontal hyphae), known as *stolons*. Where the stolons make contact with the medium, rootlike structures called *rhizoids* form. An erect specialized hyphal branch, known as a *sporangiophore*, arises opposite the rhizoid (nodal area) and enlarges at its apex to form a hemispheric columella. At the base of the columella is formed a round, closed ball-like structure, known as a *sporangium,* which encloses numerous sporangiospores (see left).

(Courtesy of Dr. Michael McGinnis, Department of Pathology, University of Texas Medical Branch, Galveston, TX.)

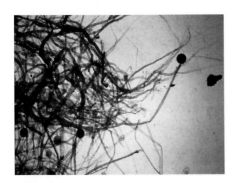

***Mucor* Species.** Erect sporangiophores, branched or unbranched, arise directly from broad aseptate hyphae. Each sporangiophore terminates in a spherical columella that is enclosed in a round sporangium. There are no stolons or rhizoids (see left).

(Courtesy of Dr. Michael McGinnis, Department of Pathology, University of Texas Medical Branch, Galveston, TX.)

ZYGOMYCOSIS

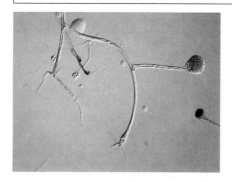

(Courtesy of Dr. Michael McGinnis, Department of Pathology, University of Texas Medical Branch, Galveston, TX.)

***Absidia* Species.** Branched sporangiophores originate from stolons between rhizoids (internodal). The sporangiophore swells at its apex (apophysis), merging into a hemispheric columella that is encircled by a pear shaped sporangium (see left).

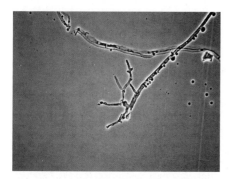

(Courtesy of Dr. Michael McGinnis, Department of Pathology, University of Texas Medical Branch, Galveston, TX.)

***Rhizomucor* Species.** Branched sporangiophores arise from aerial hyphae or stolons. The sporangiophore terminates in a columella that is enclosed within a round sporangium. Few and poorly developed rhizoids occur lateral to the sporangiophore base.

Other characteristics include a maximal growth temperature of 60°C (see left).

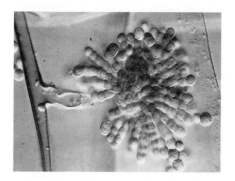

(Courtesy of Dr. Michael McGinnis, Department of Pathology, University of Texas Medical Branch, Galveston, TX.)

***Syncephalastrum* Species.** Hyphae are nonseptate but may form irregular septa with age. Arising from the hyphae are short sporangiophores, each of which terminates in a spherical vesicle. Cylindrical merosporangia originate from the vesicle in a finger-like pattern; each is filled with a single row of sporangiospores (see left).

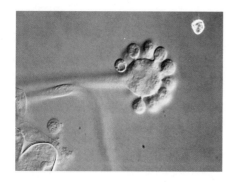

(Courtesy of Dr. Michael McGinnis, Department of Pathology, University of Texas Medical Branch, Galveston, TX.)

***Cunninghamella* Species.** Hyphae are sparsely septate and bear usually branched sporangiophores. The sporangiophore terminates in a spherical vesicle that is covered by round, single celled sporangiola, each of which is attached to the vesicle by peglike projections (denticles) (see left).

PNEUMOCYSTOSIS

The fungus *Pneumocystis carinii* is an opportunistic pathogen whose primary site of invasion is the lung alveoli. If these pulmonary vesicles are not adequately protected by the host immune system, blockage of the alveoli occurs, resulting in an interstitial pneumonia.

Laboratory Diagnosis

DIRECT EXAMINATION. Infection with *P. carinii* is proved by visualizing the organism microscopically in patient samples. Specimens such as lung tissue, induced sputum, bronchial brushings, and bronchopulmonary lavage are treated with stains that either stain the wall of the cyst or the intracystic bodies within the cyst form of *P. carinii*. Examples are given below.

STAIN	MICROSCOPIC APPEARANCE OF CYST (6–8 μM DIAMETER)
Methenamine Silver	Cyst wall stains brown or black; cyst may appear spherical or crescent shaped.
Toluidine Blue O	Cyst wall stains purplish.
Calcofluor White	Cyst wall fluoresces.
Giemsa	Unstained spheres containing four to eight red-purple intracystic bodies

DEMATIACEOUS FUNGI

The dematiaceous fungi are a group of organisms that produce brown, black, gray, or olive pigmentation. These fungi are found in the environment and may be encountered as laboratory contaminants as well as disease producing agents.

Several genera that are included within the dematiaceous fungi have already been discussed, namely *Piedraia*, *Phaeoannellomyces*, *Scedosporium* (*Pseudallescheria*), *Madurella*, *Phialophora*, *Cladosporium*, *Fonsecaea*, *Sporothrix*, *Exophiala*, and *Wangiella*. This section discusses those dematiaceous mycotic agents that are more commonly isolated in the clinical laboratory.

Xylohypha

PATHOGENICITY. *X. bantiana* causes cerebral phaeohyphomycosis.

MACROSCOPIC MORPHOLOGY. This is a moderately fast growing mold, with a velvety, folded surface. Colonies may range in color from olive-gray to olive-brown with a black reverse.

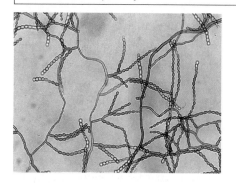

(Courtesy of Connie R. Mahon, Department of Clinical Laboratory Sciences, University of Texas Health Science Center at San Antonio, San Antonio, TX; and Lee Sadarowski, Department of Microbiology, Audie Murphy VA Medical Center, San Antonio, TX.)

MICROSCOPIC MORPHOLOGY. Hyphae and conidiophores are septate, darkly pigmented, and structurally similar; conidiophores bear long, branched, and bending chains of oval conidia. Disconnected conidia do not display distinct pigmented scars (hila) at their former point(s) of attachment (see left).

OTHER CHARACTERISTICS. see "Subcutaneous Mycoses" on p 1040.

Curvularia

PATHOGENICITY. *Curvularia* is a rare cause of mycetoma and phaeohyphomycosis.

MACROSCOPIC MORPHOLOGY. This organism is rapidly growing, at first gray, later becoming a brown to black woolly colony. The reverse is black.

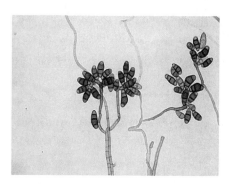

(Courtesy of Connie R. Mahon, Department of Clinical Laboratory Sciences, University of Texas Health Science Center at San Antonio, San Antonio, TX; and Lee Sadarowski, Department of Microbiology, Audie Murphy VA Medical Center, San Antonio, TX.)

MICROSCOPIC MORPHOLOGY. The septate hyphae are either hyaline or brown. Brown, septate, and geniculate (like a bent knee) conidiophores, simple or branched, bear dark, 3 to 5 celled boomerang shaped conidia measuring 8×15 μm. The conidial central cell is usually larger and darker than the distal cells; a dark hilum (dotlike) is present at the end of the conidium that is attached to the conidiophore (see left).

Alternaria

PATHOGENICITY. *Alternaria* is a rare cause of phaeohyphomycosis; it may be involved in allergic disease.

MACROSCOPIC MORPHOLOGY. This is a rapid growing woolly mold, with young colonies usually gray, later becoming gray-brown, green to black. The reverse is black.

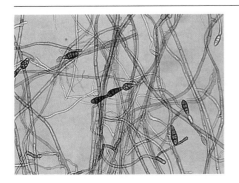

MICROSCOPIC MORPHOLOGY. One finds brown septate hyphae with chains of muriform (arranged like bricks in a wall, with both transverse and longitudinal septa) drumstick shaped conidia arising from simple or branched septated brown conidiophores. The conidial chain arrangement is such that the rounded distal end of one conidium is attached to the tapered apex of the adjacent conidium (see left).

(Courtesy of Connie R. Mahon, Department of Clinical Laboratory Sciences, University of Texas Health Science Center at San Antonio, San Antonio, TX; and Lee Sadarowski, Department of Microbiology, Audie Murphy VA Medical Center, San Antonio, TX.)

Aureobasidium

PATHOGENICITY. *Aureobasidium* is a rare cause of phaeohyphomycosis.

MACROSCOPIC MORPHOLOGY. This is a moderately fast growing fungus. Early growth appears as a white to tan yeastlike colony; at maturation, the colony becomes dark brown to black, pasty, and often with a fringe of white encircling the outer periphery. Older colonies become darker, folded, and leathery. The reverse is black.

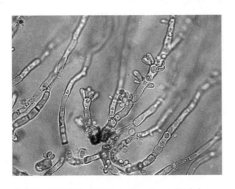

MICROSCOPIC MORPHOLOGY. The septate hyphae and the conidiophore are morphologically similar. Young hyphae are hyaline and thin walled, later becoming dark brown and thick walled. Small oval conidia are produced directly from the hyphae or from small peglike projections. These initial conidia may further bud and form secondary and tertiary conidia (see left).

(Courtesy of Dr. Michael McGinnis, Department of Pathology, University of Texas Medical Branch, Galveston, TX.)

Drechslera

PATHOGENICITY. *Drechslera* is a rare cause of cutaneous and systemic infection in immunocompromised hosts.

MACROSCOPIC MORPHOLOGY. This is a rapid growing fluffy, brown to gray to black mold. The reverse is black.

DEMATIACEOUS FUNGI

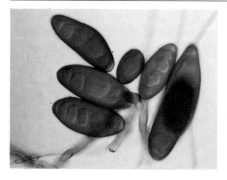

MICROSCOPIC MORPHOLOGY. One sees septate, brown hyphae, and brown pigmented conidiophores having, where conidia are produced, a twisted or zigzag appearance. The pigmented conidia are cylindric and multiseptate, arising successively on either side of the conidiophore. The conidium has a nonprotruding hilum, and, when the conidium is incubated in sterile water, a germ tube is formed perpendicular to its long axis (see left).

(Courtesy of Dr. Michael McGinnis, Department of Pathology, University of Texas Medical Branch, Galveston, TX.)

Bipolaris

PATHOGENICITY. *Bipolaris* is a rare cause of mycotic infection at various sites.

MACROSCOPIC MORPHOLOGY. This is a rapid growing woolly, dark brown, gray or gray-green to black mold. The reverse is black.

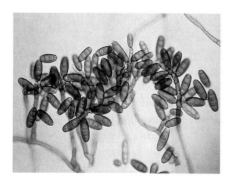

MICROSCOPIC MORPHOLOGY. One sees septate, pigmented hyphae. Conidiophores are dematacious and geniculate where conidia are formed; they are 3 to 5 celled, brown, and ellipsoid. The conidium has a slightly protruding and truncated hilum. When the conidium is incubated in sterile water, germ tubes are formed at one or both ends along its long axis (see left).

(Courtesy of Dr. Michael McGinnis, Department of Pathology, University of Texas Medical Branch, Galveston, TX.)

Exserohilum

PATHOGENICITY. *Exserohilum* is a rare cause of mycetoma and other phaeohyphomycotic infections.

MACROSCOPIC MORPHOLOGY. See *"Bipolaris"* above.

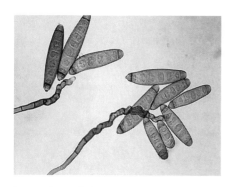

MICROSCOPIC APPEARANCE. One sees septate and pigmented hyphae. Conidiophores are dematacious and geniculate where conidia are produced. The conidia are brown and ellipsoid and have 7 to 11 compartments and a pronounced hilum. Conidial germ tube formation resembles that of *Bipolaris* (see left).

(Courtesy of Dr. Michael McGinnis, Department of Pathology, University of Texas Medical Branch, Galveston, TX.)

Helminthosporium

PATHOGENICITY. *Helminthosporium* is not pathogenic.

MACROSCOPIC MORPHOLOGY. One sees a rapid growing cottony, gray to black mold. The reverse is black.

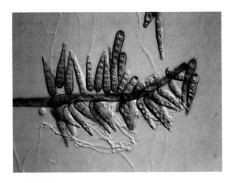

MICROSCOPIC MORPHOLOGY. One sees septate pigmented hyphae. Conidiophores are dark brown and laterally bear club shaped multicelled conidia whose wider end is contiguous with the conidiophore (see left).

(Courtesy of Dr. Michael McGinnis, Department of Pathology, University of Texas Medical Branch, Galveston, TX.)

Stachybotrys

PATHOGENICITY. *Stachybotrys* causes mycotoxicosis.

MACROSCOPIC MORPHOLOGY. This organism is rapidly growing, at first white, becoming black with age. The reverse is black at maturity.

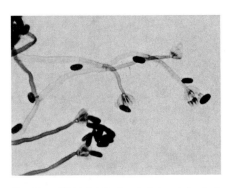

MICROSCOPIC MORPHOLOGY. One sees septate hyaline to pigmented hyphae. Septate conidiophores, at first colorless and smooth, later becoming rough and brown, arise from the vegetative hyphae. At the apex of the conidiophore are borne a group of egg shaped phialides bearing brown, single celled, smooth to rough conidia (see left).

(From Rippon JW: Medical Mycology: the Pathogenic Fungi and the Pathogenic Actinomycetes, 3rd ed. Philadelphia, WB Saunders, 1988.)

Ulocladium

PATHOGENICITY. *Ulocladium* is a rare cause of phaeohyphomycosis.

MACROSCOPIC MORPHOLOGY. This is a rapidly growing cottony, brown to black mold. The reverse is black.

DEMATIACEOUS FUNGI

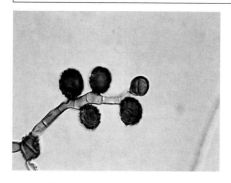

MICROSCOPIC MORPHOLOGY. Pigmented septate hyphae bear brown conidiophores. Brown to black, smooth to rough muriform conidia are formed on either side of zigzag shaped conidiophores (see left).

(Courtesy of Dr. Michael McGinnis, Department of Pathology, University of Texas Medical Branch, Galveston, TX.)

Stemphylium

PATHOGENICITY. *Stemphylium* is not pathogenic.

MACROSCOPIC MORPHOLOGY. This is a rapidly growing cottony, brown to black mold. The reverse is black.

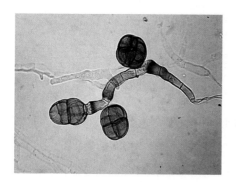

MICROSCOPIC MORPHOLOGY. One sees septate, brown hyphae and conidiophores. Brown, spherical, muriform conidia with a noticeable constriction in their middle arise from the swollen tips of the conidiophores (see left).

(Courtesy of Dr. Michael McGinnis, Department of Pathology, University of Texas Medical Branch, Galveston, TX.)

Nigrospora

PATHOGENICITY. *Nigrospora* is not pathogenic.

MACROSCOPIC MORPHOLOGY. This is a rapidly growing mold, woolly, at first white and later becoming gray and then black. The reverse is black.

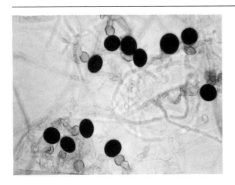

MICROSCOPIC MORPHOLOGY. Septate hyphae bear short conidiophores that flare at their tips and then narrow at the attachment points of the conidia. The conidia are oval, single celled, horizontally flattened and jet black (see left).

(Courtesy of Dr. Michael McGinnis, Department of Pathology, University of Texas Medical Branch, Galveston, TX.)

HYALINE FUNGI

The hyaline fungi include those filamentous organisms that have colorless, septate hyphae and colorless or pigmented conidia. These organisms produce colonies ranging from white to shades of green, red, yellow, orange, and tan. They may act as primary or secondary pathogens such as the dermatophytes, the dimorphic fungi, and the aspergilli. They may also act as opportunists causing disease in the immunocompromised patient and may occur as laboratory fungal contaminants as well.

This section discusses those hyaline fungi that are more commonly isolated in the clinical laboratory.

Penicillium

PATHOGENICITY. *Penicillium* is a rare cause of mycotic infection.

MACROSCOPIC MORPHOLOGY. This is a rapidly growing flat and velvety mold, white at first, later typically becoming green with a white border. Colonies may also occur in a variety of colors such as brown, red, or yellow.

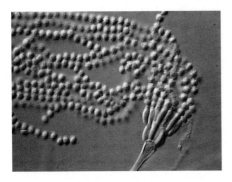

MICROSCOPIC MORPHOLOGY. One sees septate hyphae with hyaline or pigmented septate conidiophores. The conidiophores branch and give rise to secondary, cylindric metulae from which flask shaped phialides arise. Each phialide, from its tuncated apex, bears chains of hyaline or pigmented conidia. The overall structural appearance resembles that of a brush or broom (penicillate head) (see left).

(Courtesy of Dr. Michael McGinnis, Department of Pathology, University of Texas Medical Branch, Galveston, TX.)

HYALINE FUNGI

P. MARNEFFEI

This species of *Penicillium* is unique in being thermally dimorphic and a true pathogen.

Pathogenicity. *P. marneffei* causes systemic and disseminated fungal disease.

Macroscopic Morphology at 25° to 30°C. This is a rapidly growing, flat, grayish green mold, later becoming reddish and producing a deep red pigment that diffuses throughout the medium.

Macroscopic Morphology at 35° to 37°C. One sees a white to tan yeastlike colony.

Microscopic Morphology at 25° to 30°C. See *"Penicillium"* on p 1065.

Microscopic Morphology at 35° to 37°C. One sees oval yeastlike cells having a central septum.

NOTE The tissue phase of this fungus is the planate dividing yeastlike cells.

Paecilomyces

PATHOGENICITY. *Paecilomyces* is a rare cause of mycotic infection, primarily of the eye and endocardium.

MACROSCOPIC MORPHOLOGY. This is a rapidly growing, flat, tan mold; other colors such as purple, pink, or red occur.

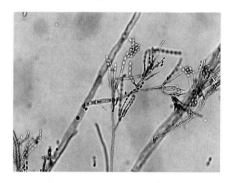

MICROSCOPIC MORPHOLOGY. The microscopic morphology is similar to that of *Penicillium.* One sees colorless or pigmented, septate hyphae. Septate, usually branching conidiophores bear long tubular phialides in the shape of bowling pins. The phialides, which often bend away from the conidiophore, produce long chains of ovate or ellipsoid conidia. Phialides may also occur singly along the hyphae without the typical penicillate head (see left).

(Courtesy of Connie R. Mahon, Department of Clinical Laboratory Sciences, University of Texas Health Science Center at San Antonio, San Antonio, TX; and Lee Sadarowski, Department of Microbiology, Audie Murphy VA Medical Center, San Antonio, TX.)

Scopulariopsis

PATHOGENICITY. *Scopulariopsis* may cause onychomycosis and rarely deep seated infection.

MACROSCOPIC MORPHOLOGY. This is a moderate to rapidly growing mold, at first smooth surfaced and white, later becoming tan and powdery resembling *Microsporum gypseum.*

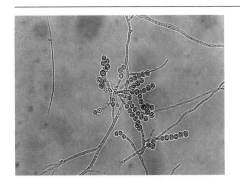

MICROSCOPIC MORPHOLOGY. One sees septate hyphae with conidiophores in a penicillate arrangement. Chains of hyaline to pigmented thick walled, smooth to rough and prickly, round to lemon shaped conidia arise from the conidiophores. The conidium has a truncated base and is twice to 2½ times the size of the *Penicillium* conidium (see left).

(Courtesy of Connie R. Mahon, Department of Clinical Laboratory Sciences, University of Texas Health Science Center at San Antonio, San Antonio, TX; and Lee Sadarowski, Department of Microbiology, Audie Murphy VA Medical Center, San Antonio, TX.)

Acremonium

PATHOGENICITY. *Acremonium* is principally a causative agent of mycetoma, onychomycosis, and mycotic keratitis, rarely an etiologic agent of systemic disease.

MACROSCOPIC MORPHOLOGY. The organism is rapidly growing, flat, at first white and moist, later producing a loose, cottony mycelium. Mature colonies may vary from white to gray to pink.

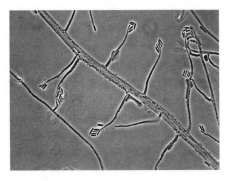

MICROSCOPIC MORPHOLOGY. One sees hyaline, septate hyphae and erect, solitary, slender conidiophores bearing at their tips hyaline, elliptic, predominately single celled conidia, usually in clusters (see left).

HYALINE FUNGI

(Courtesy of Dr. Michael McGinnis, Department of Pathology, University of Texas Medical Branch, Galveston, TX.)

Fusarium

PATHOGENICITY. *Fusarium* is a common etiologic agent of mycotic keratitis; it also causes mycetoma, onychomycosis, cutaneous infections, and systemic disease in immunocompromised hosts.

MACROSCOPIC MORPHOLOGY. This is a rapidly growing, white cottony mold, often becoming pink to purple with age.

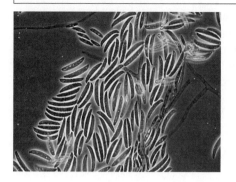

MICROSCOPIC MORPHOLOGY. One sees hyaline, septate hyphae with single or clustered conidiophores bearing two types of conidia: (1) the diagnostic macroconidia: multiseptate, sickle or canoe shaped and produced in banana-like clusters, and (2) the microconidia: ovoid, one or two celled, formed singly or in clusters at the tip of the conidiophore. The microconidia are very similar to those produced by *Acremonium* (see left).

(Courtesy of Dr. Michael McGinnis, Department of Pathology, University of Texas Medical Branch, Galveston, TX.)

Trichoderma

PATHOGENICITY. *Trichoderma* is a rare cause of mycotic infection in the immunocompromised host.

MACROSCOPIC MORPHOLOGY. This is a rapidly growing, cottony to wooly mold, at first white, later becoming yellow-green to green, often in small clusters throughout the mycelium.

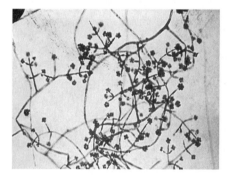

MICROSCOPIC MORPHOLOGY. Hyaline, septate hyphae give rise to branched conidiophores that are often formed at wide angles to each other. Flask shaped phialides, singly or in clusters, are produced at wide angles to the conidiophore and give rise, at its tapered apex, to unicellular, round to elliptic clusters of hyaline to green conidia (see left).

(Courtesy of Dr. Michael McGinnis, Department of Pathology, University of Texas Medical Branch, Galveston, TX.)

Gliocladium

PATHOGENICITY. *Gliocladium* is not pathogenic.

MACROSCOPIC MORPHOLOGY. This is a rapidly growing cottony mold, white initially, becoming green, first in the center and then throughout the colony.

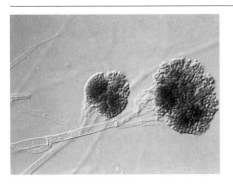

MICROSCOPIC MORPHOLOGY. Structurally, *Gliocladium* is very similar to *Penicillium* except for the arrangement of its conidia. The hyaline to green unicellular, ovoid conidia are produced at the tips of the phialide, where they fuse with conidia on adjacent phialides, forming "balls" of conidia that are held together by a mucilagenous material (see left).

(Courtesy of Dr. Michael McGinnis, Department of Pathology, University of Texas Medical Branch, Galveston, TX.)

Trichothecium

PATHOGENICITY. *Trichothecium* is not pathogenic.

MACROSCOPIC APPEARANCE. This is a rapidly growing mold, at first white, thin, and cottony, later becoming pink to peach and wooly.

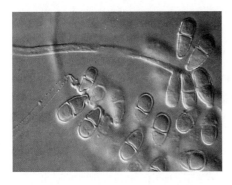

MICROSCOPIC MORPHOLOGY. One sees hyaline, septate and branching hyphae. Thin, hyaline septate conidiophores bear alternating two celled, smooth walled, ovoid to pyriform conidia resembling those produced by *Microsporum nanum* (see left).

(Courtesy of Dr. Michael McGinnis, Department of Pathology, University of Texas Medical Branch, Galveston, TX.)

Sepedonium

PATHOGENICITY. *Sepedonium* is not pathogenic.

MACROSCOPIC MORPHOLOGY. This is a fast growing mold, at first white, becoming tan or yellow.

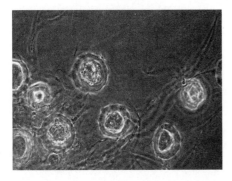

MICROSCOPIC MORPHOLOGY. One sees hyaline, septate hyphae with conidiophores similar to the vegetative mycelium. Large, tuberculate macroconidia resembling those of *H. capsulatum* are produced either singly or in clusters. Microconidia are sparsely produced and are often not seen (see left).

(Courtesy of Dr. Michael McGinnis, Department of Pathology, University of Texas Medical Branch, Galveston, TX.)

HYALINE FUNGI

Chrysosporium

PATHOGENICITY. *Chrysosporium* is not pathogenic.

MACROSCOPIC MORPHOLOGY. This is a moderately fast growing powdery, granular, or fluffy mold. Pigmentation may vary from white to tan, with other colors possible.

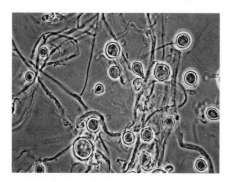

MICROSCOPIC MORPHOLOGY. One sees hyaline, septate hyphae with conidiophores that bear hyaline or pigmented one celled round, oval, or pyriform conidia, either singly or in chains. The conidia may resemble those of *Blastomyces* or *Histoplasma* (see left).

(Courtesy of Dr. Michael McGinnis, Department of Pathology, University of Texas Medical Branch, Galveston, TX.)

APPENDIX: SELECTED TECHNIQUES, MEDIA, AND STAINS

SELECTED TECHNIQUES FOR EXAMINING THE FUNGAL CULTURE

Teased Preparation

● With a pair of sterile teasing needles, remove a fragment of a mature fungal colony approximately 4 to 5 mm from the periphery and a fragment 8 to 10 mm from the periphery.

● Place the fragments into 1 to 2 drops of lactophenol cotton blue that has been placed onto the center of a microscope slide.

● Tease the fragments apart gently.

● Gently lower a coverslip over the teased preparation.

● Study microscopically under 100× and 400×.

Cellophane Tape Preparation

● Place a 4 to 5 cm strip of *clear* cellophane tape onto the actively growing border of the mature mold.

● Remove the strip slowly and place it gently, sticky side down, onto a microscope slide containing several drops of lactophenol cotton blue.

● Study microscopically under 100× and 400×.

Slide Culture Method*

- Place a sterile microscope slide onto a sterile bent glass rod or several sterile applicator sticks in a sterile Petri dish containing sterile filter paper.

- Place a 1.5 × 1.5 cm block of potato dextrose agar medium or other media that will stimulate sporulation onto the center of the slide.

- Inoculate the agar block on all four sides.

- Place a sterile coverslip on the block of agar.

- Moisten the filter paper thoroughly with sterile distilled water.

- When the fungus has matured, remove the coverslip and place it face downward onto a drop of lactophenol cotton blue that has been placed onto the center of a microscope slide.

- Study microscopically under 100× and 400×.

---

*Do not make slide cultures of the systemic dimorphic molds.

SELECTED FUNGAL MEDIA

MEDIUM	PRINCIPAL USE	COMMENTS
Classic Sabouraud's Dextrose Agar	Primary recovery of dermatophytes; subculture and identification	Inhibits most bacteria; not recommended for routine fungal culture except skin, hair, and nails
Emmons's Modification of Sabouraud's Dextrose Agar	Primary fungal culture; subculture and identification	Less inhibitory to bacteria than unmodified Sabouraud's dextrose agar
Inhibitory Mold Agar	Primary fungal culture; subculture	Inhibits bacteria
Mycosel or Mycobiotic Agar	Primary fungal culture; subculture	Inhibits bacteria and saprophytic fungi; inhibits some pathogenic fungi
Brain-Heart Infusion Agar with 5%–10% Sheep Blood	Primary fungal culture; conversion of thermally dimorphic fungi to yeast phase	Supports both fungi and bacteria
Potato Dextrose Agar	Fungal identification	Excellent sporulating medium; pigment production by *T. rubrum*
Birdseed Agar/Niger Seed Agar, or Caffeic Acid Agar	Isolation and presumptive identification of *C. neoformans*	—
Cornmeal Agar with 1% Polysorbate 80 (Tween 80)	Fungal identification	Yeast morphology; sporulating medium for agents of chromoblastomycosis and other pathogenic dematiaceous molds

SELECTED FUNGAL STAINS

MOUNTING STAIN OR FLUID	PRINCIPAL USE	COMMENTS
10% KOH	Direct wet mount of clinical specimens	Fungal structures appear hyaline.
10% KOH–Calcofluor White	Direct wet mount of clinical specimens	With fluoresence microscope, fungal structures fluoresce a brilliant green-yellow; capsules of *C. neoformans* will not fluoresce; debris may fluoresce.
Modified Kinyoun Stain for (1) *Nocardia*	(1) Demonstration of partially acid fast character of filaments of *Nocardia*	(1) Some of filaments appear red; growth of organism in milk based (litmus milk) medium enhances acid fastness.
(2) Ascospores	(2) Visualization of ascospore	(2) Ascospores stain red.
Lactophenol cotton blue	Mounting medium and stain for visualizing fungal structures	Fungal structures appear blue.
India Ink	Direct wet mount of cerebrospinal fluid	Capsule of *C. neoformans* and other encapsulated yeasts excludes ink particles and appears as a clear halo around cell; less than 50% sensitive (cryptococcal latex antigen test considerably more sensitive).

BIBLIOGRAPHY

Ajello L: Coccidioidomycosis and histoplasmosis. A review of their epidemiology and geographic distribution. Mycopathologia 45:221–230, 1971.

Al-Doory Y: Laboratory Medical Mycology. Philadelphia, Lea & Febiger, 1980.

Barnett JA, Payne RW, Yarrow D: Yeasts: Characteristics and Identification. Cambridge, Cambridge University Press, 1983.

Baselski VS et al: Rapid detection of *Pneumocystis carinii* in bronchoalveolar lavage samples by using Calcofluor staining. J Clin Microbiol 28:393–394, 1990.

Beneke EL, Rogers AL: Medical Mycology Manual, 3rd ed. Minneapolis, Burgess Publishing, 1970.

Berd B: Laboratory identification of clinically important aerobic actinomycetes. Appl Microbiol 25(4):665–681, 1973.

Butz WC, Ajello L: Black grain mycetoma. Arch Dermatol 104:197–201, 1971.

Carrion AL, Silva-Hunter M: Taxonomic criteria for fungi of chromoblastomycosis with reference to *Fonsecaea pedrosoi*. Int J Dermatol 10:34–43, 1971.

Chong KC et al: Morphology of *Piedraia hortae*. Sabouraudia 9:157–160, 1975.

Cole GT, Kendrick B: Taxonomic study of *Phialophora*. Mycologia 65:661–668, 1973.

Department of the Army: Laboratory Procedures in Clinical Mycology. Washington, DC, U.S. Government Printing Office, 1964.

Dixon DM et al: Infections due to *Xylohypha bantiana* (*Cladosporium trichoides*). Rev Infect Dis 11:515–525, 1989.

Dixon DM et al: Isolation and characterization of *Sporothrix schenckii* from clinical and environmental sources associated with the largest U.S. epidemic of sporotrichosis. J Clin Microbiol 29:1106–1113, 1991.

Dixon DM, Pollack-Wyss A: The medically important dematiaceous fungi and their identification. Mycoses 34:1–18, 1991.

Dixon DM, Shadomy HJ: Taxonomy and morphology of dematiaceous fungi isolated from nature. Mycopathologia 70:139–144, 1980.

Emmons CW, Binford CH, Utz JP: Medical Mycology, 2nd ed. Philadelphia, Lea & Febiger, 1970.

Fader RC, McGinnis MR: Infections caused by dematiaceous fungi: chromoblastomycosis and phaeohyphomycosis. Infect Dis Clin North Am 2:925–938, 1988.

Georg KL, Camp LB: Routine nutritional tests for the identification of dermatophytes. J Bacteriol 74:477–490, 1957.

Grover S: *Rhinosporidium seeberi:* a preliminary study of morphology and life cycle. Sabouraudia 7:249–251, 1970.

Gueho E, de Hoog GS: Taxonomy of the medical species of *Pseudallescheria* and *Scedosporium.* J Med Mycol 118:3–9, 1991.

Haley LD, Callaway CS: Laboratory Methods in Medical Mycology, 4th ed. Washington, DC, U.S. Government Printing Office, 1978.

Hazen EL, Gordon MA, Reed FC: Laboratory Identification of Pathogenic Fungi Simplified, 3rd ed. Springfield, IL, Charles C Thomas, 1973.

Hazen KC: New and emerging yeast pathogens. Clin Microbiol Rev 8(4):462–478, 1995.

Hoy J et al: *Trichosporon beigelii* infection: a review. Rev Infect Dis 8:959–967, 1986.

Huppert M et al: Rapid methods for identification of yeasts. J Clin Microbiol 2:21–34, 1975.

Ingham E, Cunningham AC: *Malassezia furfur.* J Med Vet Mycol 31:265–288, 1993.

Jayanetra PP et al: *Penicillium marneffei* in Thailand: report of five human cases. Am J Trop Hyg 33:637–644, 1984.

Koneman EW, Roberts GD: Practical Laboratory Mycology. Baltimore, Williams & Wilkins, 1985.

Lambrechts N et al: Black grain eumycetoma *(Madurella mycetomatis)* in the abdominal cavity of a dog. J Med Vet Mycol 29:211–214, 1991.

Larone DH: Medically Important Fungi, 3rd ed. Washington, DC, ASM Press, 1995.

Mahan CT, Sale GE: Rapid methenamine silver stain for pneumocystis and fungi. Arch Pathol Lab Med 102:351–352, 1978.

Matsumoto TA et al: Critical review of human isolates of *Wangiella dermatitidis.* Mycologia 76:232–249, 1984.

Matsumoto T et al: Clinical and mycological spectrum of *Wangiella dermatitidis* infections. Mycoses 36:145–155, 1993.

McGinnis MR: Laboratory Handbook of Medical Mycology. New York, Academic Press, 1980.

McGinnis MR: Chromoblastomycosis and phaeohyphomycosis: new concepts, diagnosis and mycology. J Am Acad Dermatol 8:1–16, 1983.

McGinnis MR et al: *Phaeoannellomyces* and *Phaeococcomycetaceas,* new dematiaceous blastomycete taxa. J Med Vet Mycol 23:179–188, 1985.

McGinnis MR et al: Emerging agents of phaeohyphomycosis: pathogenic species of *Bipolaris* and *Exserohilum.* J Clin Microbiol 24:250–259, 1986.

McNeil MM, Brown JM: The medically important aerobic actinomycetes: epidemiology and microbiology. Clin Microbiol Rev 7(3):357–417, 1994.

Mohr JA, Muchmore HG: Maduromycosis due to *Allescheria boydii.* J Am Med Assoc 204:335–336, 1986.

Murray PR et al, eds: Manual of Clinical Microbiology, 6th ed. Washington, DC, ASM Press, 1995.

Padhye AA et al: Thermotolerance of *Wangiella dermatitidis.* J Clin Microbiol 8:424–426, 1978.

Pautler KB et al: Imported *Penicillium marneffei* in the United States. Report of a second human infection. Sabouraudia 22:433–438, 1984.

Raper KB, Fennell DI: The Genus *Aspergillus.* Huntington, Robert E Krieger, 1973.

Rebell G, Taplin D: Dermatophytes: Their Recognition and Identification, rev ed. Coral Gables, University of Miami Press, 1974.

Redline RW et al: Systemic *Malassezia furfur* infections in patients receiving intralipid therapy. Hum Pathol 16:815–822, 1985.

Rippon JW: Dimorphism in pathogenic fungi. CRC Crit Rev Microbiol 8:49–79, 1980.

Rippon JW: Medical Mycology. Philadelphia, WB Saunders, 1988.

Sekhon AS et al: Evaluation of commercial reagents to identify the exoantigens of *Blastomyces dermatitidis, Coccidioides immitis,* and *Histoplasma* species cultures. Am J Clin Pathol 82:206–208, 1984.

Stanford JL: A simple review of nocardial taxonomy. J Hyg 91:369–376, 1983.

Weitzman I, Summerbell RC: The dermatophytes. Clin Microbiol Rev 8(2):240–259, 1995.

Wheat J: Endemic mycoses in AIDS: a clinical review. Clin Microbiol Rev 8(1):146–159, 1995.

Chapter **43**

VIROLOGY

Stuart Chaskes, MS, M(ASCP)

Q U I C K   C O N T E N T S

INTRODUCTION

Viruses that cause human disease range from 20 to 300 nm. Viruses are obligate intracellular parasites that have deoxyribonucleic acid (DNA) or ribonucleic acid (RNA) as their genetic material. The virus particle, or virion, consists of a capsid, or protein coat, that encloses the genetic material (RNA or DNA). The capsid contains many identical repeating subunits known as *capsomeres.* Viruses that exhibit icosahedral symmetry contain a unique number of capsomeres. The icosahedral capsid always has 20 equilateral triangular faces, 12 vertices, and 20 edges. Capsomeres may also assemble in a helical fashion to form a cylindric capsid (see figure below). A loose membrane may surround a helical or icosahedral nucleocapsid. In contrast a naked nucleocapsid is a virus that has only a protein coat without the outer membrane (envelope). Viruses that contain an envelope are highly pleomorphic since the outer membrane is not rigid. In contrast the nonenveloped viruses have a consistent and highly repetitious appearance. The enveloped viruses contain a lipid bilayer with matrix proteins and glycoproteins. The glycoproteins have a spikelike appearance that allows the virus to attach to host cells. The matrix proteins connect the envelope to the capsid. Viruses with an outer membrane (high lipid content) are susceptible to inactivation by lipid solvents including chloroform and ether. Viruses without the outer membrane are more heat resistant than enveloped viruses.

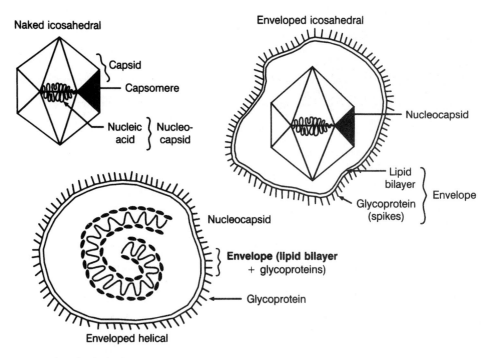

From Howard BJ: Clinical and Pathogenic Microbiology, 2nd ed. St Louis, CV Mosby, 1994; as modified from Freeman BA: Burrows Textbook of Microbiology, 2nd ed. Philadelphia, WB Saunders, 1979.

The schematic representation of enveloped (DNA and RNA) viruses and nonenveloped (DNA and RNA) viruses is illustrated by the figure below.

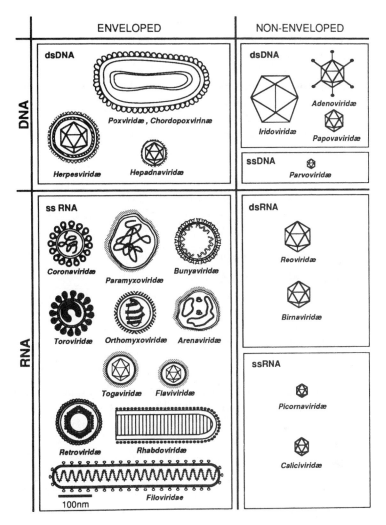

From Fauquet C, Mayo MA: Arch Virol Suppl 2:61, 1991.

VIROLOGY–INTRODUCTION

VIRAL REPLICATION

Viruses are unable to reproduce in an independent fashion and must take over the host cells' cellular control. The viral agents act as pirates and are able to control routine cellular functions so that nucleic acid transcripts and translation of mRNA become viral directed. Viral cell replication always includes the following sequence of events:

1. *Attachment and Adsorption.* The initial step is the attachment and the adsorption of the virus to the host receptor site. Enveloped viruses have specific specialized structures such as glycoprotein spikes for attachment, whereas nonenveloped viruses probably have attachment sites over all of their surface components.

2. *Penetration.* The next step is penetration and occurs via fusion or phagocytosis into the host cell.
3. *Uncoating.* The virus sheds its capsid in a process that is known as *uncoating*. The viral nucleic acids are released into the cytoplasm.
4. *Eclipse (Biosynthesis of Viral Nucleic Acids and Proteins).* During the eclipse stage, the viral genome acts as a template for the production of messenger RNA that directs the synthesis of viral proteins. Capsid production can occur in the nucleus or the cytoplasm of the host cells, whereas other viral proteins are synthesized in the cytoplasm.
5. *Assembly of the Virus.* DNA viruses generally are assembled in the nucleus of the host cell, whereas RNA viruses are synthesized in the cytoplasm. The envelope of some viruses is acquired via budding past the nuclear or cytoplasmic membranes.
6. *Release.* Viruses are released either by budding through the membrane (most RNA viruses) or via the production of enzymes that lyse the cell and cause a cytopathic effect (many nonenveloped viruses).

VIRAL INFECTIONS

Viruses are responsible for causing many human diseases (see chart below). Many human viruses are associated with multiple disease states, especially the adenoviruses and enteroviruses. Some viruses have the ability to cross the placenta and infect the developing fetus. The acronym *TORCH* (*t*oxoplasmosis, *o*ther infections, *r*ubella, *c*ytomegalovirus, and *h*erpes simplex virus) indicates the agents that are most likely to cause transplacental infection. Childhood diseases associated with rash include chickenpox (varicella), measles (rubeola), German measles (rubella), 5th disease (parvovirus B19), 6th disease (roseola), and the bacterial disease scarlet fever.

Disease or Syndrome Associated with Common Viruses

DISEASE OR SYNDROME	Respiratory, croup, bronchiolitis, and pharyngitis	Common cold	Gastroenteritis	Hepatitis	Infectious mononu-cleosis*
VIRUSES	Adenovirus, cytomegalovirus, enterovirus, herpes simplex virus, influenza virus, mumps virus, parainfluenza virus, respiratory syncytial virus	Rhinovirus, coronavirus, enterovirus, influenza virus, respiratory syncytial virus	Adenovirus, rotavirus, calicivirus, astrovirus, coronavirus	Hepatitis A, B, C, D, E, and G viruses	Epstein-Barr virus, cytomegalovirus, and herpes virus 6; occasionally hepatitis A, B, and C viruses
DISEASE OR SYNDROME	Genital infections	Eye infections	Myocarditis and pericarditis	Central nervous system	Parotitis
VIRUSES	Herpes simplex virus, human papilloma virus, molluscum contagiosum virus	Herpes simplex virus, adenovirus, varicella zoster virus, cytomegalovirus (retinitis in AIDS patients)	Coxsackie B virus and echovirus	Enterovirus, herpes simplex virus, arbovirus, rabies virus, measles virus, mumps virus, Eastern and Western encephalitis virus, St. Louis encephalitis virus, and lymphocytic choriomeningitis virus	Mumps virus and parainfluenza virus
DISEASE OR SYNDROME	Congenital and perinatal	Post-Transplantation	Immunodeficiency	Dermatologic and mucous membrane	
VIRUSES	Cytomegalovirus, herpes simplex virus, rubella virus, varicella-zoster virus, enterovirus, hepatitis B virus, human immunodeficiency virus, adenovirus, and parvovirus B19	Herpes simplex virus, cytomegalovirus, Epstein-Barr virus, human herpes virus 6	Human immunodeficiency virus	Vesicular Enterovirus, herpes simplex virus, varicella-zoster virus Exanthematous Enterovirus, rubeola virus, rubella virus, parvovirus B19, human herpes virus 6	

*Human immunodeficiency virus infection initially causes a mononucleosis-like disease.

VIRAL INFECTIONS

Antiviral Therapy

The accessibility of specific antiviral therapeutic drugs has enhanced the urgency for the laboratory to rapidly diagnose viral infections. Accurate diagnosis of the exact viral agent is required to justify the use of the usually expensive and often toxic agents. The patient often must be closely monitored to detect the emergence of resistant viral agents. A summary of viral therapeutic agents and their mechanism of action is described in the chart below.

ANTIVIRAL AGENTS

THERAPEUTIC AGENT	MECHANISM OF ACTION	SUSCEPTIBLE VIRUS
Acyclovir	Acyclovir causes termination of viral DNA synthesis.	Herpes simplex virus Varicella-zoster virus
Amantadine or Rimantadine	Amantadine and rimantadine prevent viral uncoating and release of viral RNA into cytoplasm.	Influenza A
Foscarnet	Foscarnet serves as noncompetitive inhibitor of viral DNA polymerase and of reverse transcriptase (human immunodeficiency virus [HIV]).	Acyclovir resistant herpes simplex virus and varicella-zoster virus; cytomegalovirus (CMV) infections in immunocompromised patients; and ganciclovir resistant CMV infections
Ganciclovir	Ganciclovir is phosphorylated to produce ganciclovir triphosphate, which acts as competitive inhibitor of viral DNA polymerase. However, it does not initiate DNA chain termination.	CMV infections in immunocompromised patients
Ribavirin	Ribavirin inhibits several steps in viral replication including elongation of viral mRNA and capping of viral mRNA.	Severe respiratory syncytial fever
Nucleoside Analog *Zidovudine (AZT)* *Didanosine (ddI)* *Zalcitabine (ddC)* *Lamivudine (3tC)* *Stavudine (d4T)*	Nucleoside analogs block ability of HIV to make copies of itself by inhibiting enzyme reverse transcriptase.	HIV
Non-Nucleoside Analog *Nevirapine* *Delavirdine*	Non-nucleoside analogs carry out same function as nucleoside analogs but do so without mimicking viral genetic material.	HIV
Protease Inhibitors *Saquinavir* *Ritonavir* *Indinavir* *Nelfinar*	Protease inhibitors block viral protease enzyme of HIV, which is needed for packaging and release of new viruses.	HIV
Interferon Alfa	Interferon alfa induces biochemical changes in noninfected cells that render these cells resistant to subsequent viral infection.	Chronic hepatitis B and C and genital warts, which are caused by the papillomavirus
Idoxuridine and Trifluridine	Nucleoside analogs interfere with synthesis of viral DNA.	Keratitis caused by herpes simplex virus

Hematologic Changes Associated with Human Viruses

The classic virus that is associated with hematologic changes is the Epstein-Barr virus (EBV). During EBV mononucleosis, lymphocytosis, including at least 10% large atypical lymphocytes, is commonly observed. The chart below summarizes hematologic changes that are associated with viral infection.

VIRUS	HEMATOLOGIC CHANGE
Epstein-Barr Virus	Lymphocytosis with atypical lymphocytes.
Cytomegalovirus	Atypical lymphocytes. Rare complications include thrombocytopenia and hemolytic anemia.
Hepatitis A Virus	Atypical lymphocytes.
Hepatitis C Virus	A few cases of aplastic anemia.
Human Immunodeficiency Virus	An asymptomatic thrombocytopenia may occur during the initial mononucleosis-like illness. Atypical lymphocytes and depressed T4 lymphocyte counts occur later in the disease.
Human T Lymphotrophic Virus	T cell leukemia-lymphoma with nearly all leukemic cells expressing the CD4 antigen. Acute patients exhibit leukocytosis and often eosinophilia and/or granulocytosis.
Measles Virus	Leukopenia is common.
Human Herpes Virus 6 (HHV-6)	Leukopenia is associated with reactivation or reinfection of HHV-6 in bone marrow transplant patients.
Parvovirus B19	Aplastic crisis may occur in patients with sickle cell anemia. Chronic anemia may occur in immunosuppressed patients. In the fetus, parvovirus B19 lyses erythroid precursor cells, and severe anemia and death may follow.
Rubella Virus	Rare cases of thrombocytopenia occur. In congenital rubella a transient hemolytic anemia occurs.

VIRAL INFECTIONS

THE VIRUSES

EPSTEIN-BARR VIRUS

Family	Herpesviridae
Common Name(s)	Herpesvirus disease: mononucleosis
Collection of Specimen	Viral isolation not attempted
Direct Examination	Early antigen (EA) and Epstein-Barr viral antigen (EBVA) can be demonstrated by using anti-complement indirect immunofluorescent staining technique.
Description of Agent *Diameter* *Capsid symmetry* *Envelope* *Type of Nucleic Acid*	120 nm 162 capsomeres in icosahedral arrangement Yes Double stranded DNA
General Disease Categories	Infectious mononucleosis (IM) and progressive lymphoreticular disease
Population Infected	Childhood infections with IM are mostly asymptomatic; 50%–75% of young adults have mild to severe cases of IM.
Incubation Period	10–50 days
Primary Symptoms	Fever, pharyngitis, and cervical lymphadenopathy lasting 1–4 weeks. Occasionally splenomegaly, pericarditis, hepatitis, or central nervous system involvement.
Transmission	Close contact with saliva for IM.
Treatment	Supportive
Prevention	Avoid contact. Vaccine not available for IM.
Serologic Diagnosis	Paul-Bunnell heterophile antibody and viral antibodies (anti-IgM early antigen, anti-IgM capsid antigen, anti-IgG viral capsid antigen, and anti–Epstein-Barr nuclear antigen).
Cell Cultures for Detection of Viruses from Clinical Specimen	Cell cultures generally not used clinically, but fetal B lymphocytes can be used for isolation.
Oncogenic Potential	Burkitt's lymphoma, nasopharyngeal carcinoma

GENERAL INFORMATION. EBV is the causative agent of infectious mononucleosis (IM), which infects both children and young adults. Approximately 90% of the population will become infected with EBV. Childhood infections are either subclinical or mild, whereas young adults with primary infection exhibit symptoms that range from mild to severe. EBV enters the patient's body through the oropharynx, and dissemination occurs via the B lympocyte. EBV can cause cell lysis or it can become latent. A small percentage of the latently infected cells can spontaneously enter the lytic cycle, and therefore low levels of the virus are periodically produced during a person's life span. Reactivation of the latent virus has been implicated in a chronic illness as the EBV associated fatigue syndrome. However, this interpretation is not universally accepted.

CLINICAL SYMPTOMS. IM can be diagnosed from the clinical symptoms, which include fever, sore throat, lymphadenopathy, and sometimes splenomegaly. Patients often exhibit mild liver disease with elevated liver enzyme levels. Severe complications include pericarditis, hepatitis, and central nervous system involvement. Neurologic complications include Guillain-Barré syndrome, Bell's palsy, myelitis, cranial nerve neuritis, and meningoencephalitis. Finally, fatal primary infections can occur in immunologically incompetent patients, such as transplant recipients.

LYMPHOCYTOSIS. Lymphocytosis, including at least 10% large atypical lymphocytes, is commonly observed. Atypical lymphocytes appear 3 or 4 days after the onset of symptoms and reach a maximum by the 5th to 10th day. The high leukocyte count may persist for 3 months but usually decreases to normal by the end of week 3.

LABORATORY DIAGNOSIS. Laboratory diagnosis is also based on a positive Paul-Bunnel heterophile test that is observed in 80% to 90% of the patients. False positive heterophile tests may occur in 2% to 3% of the patients. The EBV specific serologic tests are helpful in differentiating the 10% to 15% of the heterophile negative EBV infections from the mononucleosis caused by other microorganisms, such as adenovirus, rubella virus, cytomegalovirus, and *Toxoplasma gondii* infections.

LYMPHOPROLIFERATIVE DISORDERS. EBV is also associated with Burkitt's lymphoma (BL), a childhood cancer of the head and neck commonly seen in Africa and New Guinea. In addition, EBV is linked to nasopharyngeal carcinoma (NPC) in China. EBV lymphoproliferative disorder sometimes is seen after immunosuppressive therapies during organ transplantation. The lymphoproliferative disorders range from benign to malignant. The viral genomes can be detected in these tumors as well as in BL and NPC. EBV is also detected in the Reed-Sternberg cells of Hodgkin's lymphoma and in B cell lymphomas of patients with acquired and inherited immunodeficiencies. Finally, in in vitro testing, EBV is able to transform and immortalize human B lymphocytes.

EPSTEIN-BARR VIRUS

CYTOMEGALOVIRUS

Family	Herpesviridae
Common Name(s)	Herpesvirus, salivary gland virus
Collection of Specimen	Urine, throat swabs, sometimes sputum, blood (buffy coat), or bronchoalveolar lavage
Direct Examination	Molecular dot blot hybridization techniques can detect CMV genome in urine. Electron microscopy can detect CMV in urine or oral specimens of congenitally infected newborns. CMV antigens can be detected by using immunofluorescence tests (monoclonal antibody) on tissues obtained by biopsy. Cytomegalic cells have "owl's eye" appearance with hematoxylin and eosin stain. Exfoliative cytologic techniques are used on urine specimens.
Description of Agent	
Diameter	120–200 nm
Capsid Symmetry	Icosahedral arrangement
Envelope	Yes
Type of Nucleic Acid	Double stranded DNA
General Disease Categories	Clinical disease that resembles mononucleosis occurs in 7%–8% of the immunologically normal population. Majority of cases are asymptomatic. Morbidity due to systemic CMV can occur in every organ system in immunosuppressed patient.

Continued ▶

► Continued **CYTOMEGALOVIRUS**

Population Infected	Developing fetus, newborn, children, and adults as well as immunocompromised hosts
Incubation Period	4–8 wk for primary infection
Primary Symptoms *Congenital*	Neurologic symptoms, neuromuscular disorders, jaundice, and hepatosplenomegaly as well as petechiae (50% of infants). Hearing impairments may develop in infants who lacked early symptoms.
Perinatal	Most newborns are asymptomatic even though they excrete the virus at 3–12 wk of age.
Childhood and Adult Infection	7%–8% have mononucleosis-like syndrome generally without pharyngitis, lymphadenopathy, or splenomegaly. AIDS patients and organ and bone marrow transplant recipients often experience prolonged leukopenia, hepatitis, pneumonitis, encephalitis, and gastrointestinal disease. In AIDS patients retinitis can result in blindness.
Transmission	Intimate contact with secretions or excretions, including urine, respiratory or genital secretions, tears, or feces. Can also be spread by blood transfusions (white blood cells), organ transplants, and transplacental transmission.
Treatment	Supportive; decrease immune suppression; ganciclovir. Vistide is used to treat CMV retinitis in AIDS patients.
Prevention	Transfusions and transplantation should utilize CMV negative tissue.
Serologic Diagnosis	Enzyme immunoassays (EIAs), passive latex agglutination (PLA), complement fixation (CF), anticomplement immunofluorescence (ACIF), and indirect fluorescent antibody (IFA)
Cell Cultures for Detection of Viruses from Clinical Specimen	Human fibroblast cells (WI-38, MRC-5, or IMR-90). MRC-5 cells can be employed in a spin amplification shell vial assay.
Oncogenic Potential	Not reported

GENERAL INFORMATION. Cytomegalovirus (CMV) infections are mostly asymptomatic from childhood to early adult years. Some patients exhibit very mild nonspecific clinical disease, and up to 8% have a clinical picture that resembles mononucleosis. The illness is characterized by peripheral lymphocytosis, fever, and malaise. However, pharyngitis, lymphadenopathy, or splenomegaly are not usually observed.

RARE COMPLICATIONS. Rare complications of CMV infection include thrombocytopenia, hemolytic anemia, hepatitis, interstitial pneumonitis, myocardia, meningoencephalitis, and Guillain-Barré syndrome.

SEROCONVERSION AND TRANSMISSION. Seroconversion generally occurs in immunocompetent individuals who are infected with CMV. Transmission of the virus may be by oral, respiratory, or venereal routes. Generally, intimate contact with secretions or excretions is required for the transmission of CMV. The virus may be sporadically excreted for months or years in urine.

CYTOMEGALOVIRUS AND IMMUNOCOMPROMISED HOSTS. Active infections with CMV may develop in immunocompromised hosts after organ and bone marrow transplantation as well as in patients with acquired immunodeficiency syndrome (AIDS). Seronegative immunosuppressed patients carry a significant risk of developing a CMV infection. Additionally, CMV itself can suppress the host's immune system and thus decrease a patient's ability to localize and control infections. The immunosuppressed patients often exhibit prolonged fever, encephalitis, hepatitis, pneumonitis, esophagitis, gastrointestinal disease, and leukopenia. AIDS patients often experience retinitis, which can lead to blindness. Transmission of CMV via transfusion of blood products is a major concern for immunosuppressed patients. Their risk can be lowered by careful donor screenings and by administering immune globulin containing antibodies to CMV. CMV infections in immunosuppressed children can be treated with a combination of ganciclovir and intravenous IgG. Additionally, the mortality rate due to CMV pneumonia following bone marrow transplantation can be greatly reduced by using the same treatment.

CONGENITAL CYTOMEGALOVIRUS INFECTIONS. A commonly identified source of congenital infection in newborn infants is CMV. The rate is between 0.4% and 2.5% in newborn infants. Approximately 95% of the infected newborns are asymptomatic. The asymptomatic infants may, however, later develop learning disabilities or have learning defects. Five percent have severe manifestations that include intrauterine growth retardation, petechiae, central nervous system abnormalities, jaundice, hepatosplenomegaly, and retinitis. Most of the symptomatic newborns survive but are neurologically damaged. CMV infections acquired perinatally are usually asymptomatic. Finally, low birth weight neonates that require blood products must receive CMV seronegative blood.

VARICELLA-ZOSTER VIRUS

Family	Herpesviridae
Common Name(s)	Herpesvirus diseases: chickenpox, shingles
Collection of Specimen	Primarily skin scraping, vesicular lesions, or tissues obtained at autopsy
Direct Examination	Direct immunofluorescence (IF) staining from lesions. Vesicular fluids can be used for electron microscopic studies but not for IF. Cytologic examination of cellular material from vesicular lesions with buffered Giemsa's stain reveals multinucleated giant epithelial cells. Polymerase chain reaction (PCR) is currently research tool.
Description of Agent *Diameter* *Capsid Symmetry* *Envelope* *Type of Nucleic Acid*	 150–200 nm Icosahedral capsid consisting of 162 capsomeres Yes Double stranded DNA
General Disease Categories	Chickenpox (varicella) as primary infection and shingles (zoster) when reactivated.
Population Infected	Chickenpox occurs primarily in children under 10 years of age. Shingles occurs in adults after reactivation of latent virus. Both manifestations may cause severe dissemination resulting in fatal infections in immunocompromised patient.
Incubation Period	Incubation period is 2–3 wk, and period of contagion lasts about 2 wk; beginning 2 days before rash starts.

CYTOMEGALOVIRUS

Continued ▶

▶ Continued **VARICELLA-ZOSTER VIRUS**

Primary Symptoms	Prodromal symptoms include slight fever, headache, backache, and loss of appetite. Simultaneously or within 2 days, small red spots erupt, often on back and chest. Spots enlarge and vesicle filled with clear fluid follows. Later fluid turns yellow and crust forms, which peels off in 5–20 days.
Transmission	Virus is spread by respiratory secretions.
Treatment	Supportive care, such as bed rest and forcing liquids during fever state, is helpful. Newborn infants are placed on isolation precautions if their mothers have active varicella infection. The administration of varicella immunoglobulin can prevent severe cases of chickenpox in newborns whose mother acquired varicella-zoster virus (VZV) infection shortly before or after delivery. Acyclovir reduces morbidity in immunocompromised children who have VZV infection. New vaccine is available.
Prevention	Live attenuated vaccine (oka/Merck strain) is currently recommended for routine childhood vaccination.
Serologic Diagnosis	Serologic tests may be difficult to interpret since VZV and herpes simplex virus 1 have some common antigenic determinants. Currently serologic tests are not method of choice to determine VZV infections.
Cell Cultures for Detection of Viruses from Clinical Specimen	Human fetal diploid cells such as fetal diploid kidney or fetal diploid lung are satisfactory for primary isolation. Shell vial technique using human fetal diploid lung cells is convenient means of identifying VZV.
Oncogenic Potential	Not observed

GENERAL INFORMATION. Varicella-zoster virus (VZV) is responsible for most frequently causing chickenpox in children (fever and generalized vesicular exanthem) and shingles (reactivation of the latent virus) in adults and immunocompromised patients. In adults primary infection is rare, but severe complications such as encephalitis and disseminated disease can occur. Reactivation of or reinfection with VZV can sometimes be asymptomatic. Severe disseminated and sometimes fatal infections in immunocompromised patients (including those with AIDS) can occur with both manifestations of VZV. Winter and spring are the peak seasons for epidemic-like outbreaks of chickenpox, whereas shingles is not associated with a seasonal pattern. Both the severity and the incidence of shingles is greater in patients with AIDS, Hodgkin's disease, lymphoma, and leukemia and in transplant recipients. Mortality is generally low even if the disease becomes disseminated.

CONGENITAL INFECTIONS. VZV has the ability to cross the placenta and cause severe infections to the fetus, especially if the mother contracts VZV during the first trimester. Also, severe manifestations occur if the newborn contracts VZV from the mother within 5 to 10 days after the delivery. Cases of congenital varicella are rare, but severe symptoms, such as microencephaly and mental retardation, can occur. A live attenuated vaccine for VZV is currently available, and it should prove useful in preventing fatal infections in immunocompromised children as well as for routine childhood immunization. Acyclovir is also helpful for immunocompromised children.

HERPES SIMPLEX VIRUSES

Family	Herpesviridae
Common Name(s)	Oral herpes (herpes simplex virus 1 [HSV-1]), genital herpes (herpes simplex virus 2) (HSV-2)
Collection of Specimen	Vesicular fluid or scraping from lesions, conjunctival scrapings, throat swabs, spinal fluid, and tissues (lungs, liver, or brain).
Direct Examination	Lesions and scrapings are examined via direct immunofluorescence or immunoperoxidase staining. Because both false positive and false negative results can be obtained, viral cultures should also be made from the lesions. Cytologic changes can often be observed with Tzanck's test or Papanicolaou (Pap) stain.
Description of Agent *Diameter* *Capsid Symmetry* *Envelope* *Type of Nucleic Acid*	 110–120 nm 162 capsomeres in icosahedral arrangement Yes Double stranded DNA
General Disease Categories	HSV-1 causes gingivostomatitis, conjunctivitis, keratitis, and herpetic whitlow (HSV-1 infection of terminal segment of finger). HSV-2 causes 85% of genital herpes, and HSV-1 remaining 15%. Neonates can become infected with HIV-2.
Population Infected	HSV-1 infections increase slowly from childhood through adult years and can infect as much as 70%–80% of population. HSV-2, which is sexually transmitted, begins during adolescence and affects between 15% and 50% of adult population.
Incubation Period	Primary infections have incubation period of 2–11 days.
Primary Symptoms	At least 60% of patients experience prodromal symptoms of tingling, burning, or itching with HSV-1. Symptoms can involve rhinitis, pharyngitis, and tonsillitis including painful oral mucosa vesicular lesions associated with high temperature. Initial infection may be followed by recurrent episodes of cold sores. Symptoms of HSV-2 include fever, lesions in genital area, and inguinal lymphadenopathy.
Transmission	Direct contact with infected secretions
Treatment	Acyclovir
Prevention	Avoid contact.
Serologic Diagnosis	Serologic diagnosis is limited to primary infections since recurrent HSV infections are often not associated with rise of antibody titer. Some cross-reactivity occurs between HSV and VZV. Furthermore, past HSV-1 and HSV-2 infections cannot be differentiated from each other because of cross-reactivity. Major serologic tests for HSV include enzyme linked immunosorbent assay (ELISA) or latex agglutination procedures. Use of HSV specific monoclonal antibody can also separate HSV-1 from HSV-2.
Cell Cultures for Detection of Viruses from Clinical Specimen	Most sensitive method for laboratory diagnosis of HSV is viral culture. Most commonly used cell lines are MRC-5, human embryonic lung fibroblast cells, mink lung, or primary rabbit kidney.
Oncogenic Potential	Not observed

HERPES SIMPLEX VIRUSES

GENERAL INFORMATION. Herpes simplex viruses (HSVs) have two distinct serotypes, type 1 (HSV-1) and type 2 (HSV-2). Type 1 is usually transmitted by oral and respiratory secretions, whereas type 2 is most often transmitted sexually. Primary infection by HSV-1 involves the oral mucosa and is accompanied by painful vesicular lesions, a high fever, and submandibular lymphadenopathy. A latent infection of the neuronal cells in the dorsal root ganglia follows primary infection. Reactivation of HSV can be symptomatic or asymptomatic. In contrast, HSV-2 causes infection of the genitalia and the skin below the waist. After the primary infection, the virus ascends through nerves to the sacral ganglia and latency is established. If reactivation occurs, viral replication is initiated in the ganglia and the virus travels back to the skin and genitals and may cause recurrent infections. Whether the infection with HSV is oral or genital, most patients will not experience symptomatic recurrences. However, the virus may be shed while the patient is asymptomatic. Finally, even the primary infection involving HSV-2 may be asymptomatic.

IMMUNOSUPPRESSED PATIENTS. Patients with immunodeficiencies or malignancies or immunosuppressed patients can have severe infections caused by HSV. The infection can be primary or reactivation. Viremia can occur in these patients, and dissemination to the brain, lung, and liver can occur. Generally, disseminated disease is fatal. Acyclovir can be used to treat some HSV infections in immunocompromised patients as well as patients with genital herpes.

NEONATES AND HERPES SIMPLEX VIRUS 2. Neonates may acquire HSV-2 infections at birth. The virus may cause an infection of the skin, mouth, eyes, or central nervous system (CNS) or be disseminated to multiple organs. Mortality rates are very rare for the localized mucosal infections but are high for the disseminated form (57%), as well as the CNS form (15%). Mortality rates are even higher for untreated infants.

HUMAN HERPES VIRUS 6

Family	Herpesviridae
Common Name(s)	Herpesvirus disease: roseola, sixth disease, exanthem subitum
Collection of Specimen	HHV-6 can be isolated from peripheral blood lymphocytes (PBLs), especially if PBLs are obtained before rash appears.
Direct Examination	PCR and Southern blot assays have been used.
Description of Agent *Diameter* *Capsid Symmetry* *Envelope* *Type of Nucleic Acid*	160–200 nm 162 capsomeres in icosahedral arrangement Yes Double stranded DNA
Population Infected	Roseola occurs in children; heterophile negative mononucleosis and hepatitis occur in adults.
Incubation Period	Several days
Primary Symptoms	Roseola is mild disease of children (usually under age of 3 years) that is associated with high fever as well as skin rash that starts out on neck and back. Initial infection with HHV-6 is unusual in adults, and patients often exhibit short febrile illness with elevated liver enzymes and mild cervical lymphadenopathy.

Continued ▶

▶ Continued **HUMAN HERPES VIRUS 6**

Transmission	Respiratory, close contact
Treatment	Supportive
Prevention	Avoid contact. Vaccine not available.
Serologic Diagnosis	Confirmation of HHV-6 infection is based on at least fourfold titer increase using IFA or ACIF methods. Significant increase in EIA values between acute and convalescent phase sera is also diagnostic for HHV-6.
Cell Cultures for Detection of Viruses from Clinical Specimen	Best results are obtained by cultivation of peripheral blood mononuclear cells from patient or phytohemagglutinin stimulated cord blood lymphocytes (CBLs). Cells are observed for cytopathic effects on biweekly basis. ACIF or IFA test is used to detect viral antigen after 7–10 days.
Oncogenic Potential	Not reported

GENERAL INFORMATION. Roseola (exanthem subitum) is a childhood disease with a duration of 2 to 7 days. The disease generally affects children under the age of 3 years and is characterized by an abrupt high temperature up to 40°C. When the temperature drops toward normal an erythematous maculopapular rash appears first on the neck and may spread to the scalp, chest, abdomen, and thighs. The disease is mild, and children, despite the high fever, do not appear to be very sick. Approximately 90% of the children are infected by HHV-6 before the age of 2 years.

PRIMARY INFECTION IN CHILDREN. Primary infection takes the form of roseola in 30% of the cases. Primary infection can also result in fever without a rash and a rash without fever. CNS disorders including seizures and encephalitis have occasionally been reported.

ADULT INFECTION WITH HHV-6. Adults infected with HHV-6 may experience a heterophile negative mononucleosis as well as a non-A, non-B form of hepatitis. Primary infection with HHV-6 is a rare occurrence for adults because of the very high rate of infection in children. HHV-6 has also been detected in transplant patients (especially if they were previously HHV-6 seropositive). Symptoms such as malaise, fever, and leukopenia are associated with reactivation or reinfection of HHV-6 in bone marrow transplant patients.

STRAINS OF HHV-6. At least two different strains of HHV-6 exist. Currently HHV-6B has been associated with nearly all cases of roseola and febrile illness. In contrast, HHV-6A has not been associated with primary infection. Both types have been isolated from immunocompromised hosts.

HUMAN HERPES VIRUS 6

PARVOVIRUS B19

Family	Parvoviridae
Common Name(s)	Parvovirus, fifth disease, slapped cheek disease, erythema infectiosum
Collection of Specimen	Laboratory diagnosis of B19 infections is based on collection of serum.
Direct Examination	Electron microscopy is used to detect virus in serum. DNA detection in serum is by dot blot hybridization. PCR methods have also been employed on serum samples.
Description of Agent *Diameter* *Capsid Symmetry* *Envelope* *Type of Nucleic Acid*	20–25 nm 32 capsomeres in icosahedral arrangement No Single stranded DNA
General Disease Categories	Fifth disease (or erythema infectiosum) is common childhood disease that starts with intense rash of cheeks. In normal adults polyarthralgic syndrome may occur. B19 also causes aplastic crisis in sickle cell anemia patients and chronic anemia in immunosuppressed patients. Intrauterine fetal death may occur if there is maternal B19 infection.
Population Infected	Primarily young children and occasionally developing fetus.
Incubation Period	6–14 days for fifth disease
Primary Symptoms	Fifth disease is associated with cheek rash that often spreads to trunk and limbs. There may also be joint involvement and/or lymphadenopathy.
Transmission	Close contact, probably respiratory. Placental transfer may occur between mother and fetus.
Treatment	Supportive
Prevention	Avoid contact; vaccine not currently available.
Serologic Diagnosis	Counterimmunoelectrophoresis (CIE) renders results within 1 hr but is insensitive since it is positive in about 30% of cases. More sensitive but time consuming methods include immunoassays, dot blot hybridization, and PCR.
Cell Cultures for Detection of Viruses from Clinical Specimen	Cell cultures are not clinically used to isolate B19.
Oncogenic Potential	Not reported

GENERAL INFORMATION. Parvovirus B19 is the cause of the childhood disease known as *erythema infectiosum,* which is often called fifth disease. Initially the erythematous rash gives the appearance of slapped cheeks, but later a lacy reticular rash may occur on the trunk and extremities. The disease is generally benign, and the children (4 to 11 years of age) recover within a few days.

B19 INFECTIONS IN OLDER PATIENTS. B19 occasionally infects patients older than 11 years, and the result is often a nonspecific illness that is associated with fever, chills, myalgia, and malaise. Some patients can have an influenza-like illness. The nonspecific illness is rarely accompanied by a rash. Some patients are completely asymptomatic when infected with B19. Normal adult patients may experience a polyarthralgic syndrome in which the arthritis affects the hands, wrists, knees, and ankles. The symptoms usually resolve within a few weeks.

HEMATOLOGIC COMPLICATIONS. Parvovirus B19 invades and lyses erythroid precursor cells. The viremia that is associated with B19 infection give the virus the opportunity to cross the placenta and invade the fetus. The virus can damage the hematopoietic cells and can cause severe anemia that is followed by death. Fetal infections are not always fatal, and birth defects are not associated with B19. The B19 virus is also responsible for causing transient aplastic crisis (TAC) in patients with hemolytic states, especially sickle cell anemia. TAC is a serious problem for these patients, and death sometimes occurs. Blood transfusions are necessary in the acute phase of the illness since the depressed bone marrow generally requires about 1 week to recover. The B19 virus can also cause chronic anemia in immunodeficient patients such as those with AIDS and acute lymphatic leukemia as well as those with Nezelof's syndrome.

HUMAN PAPILLOMAVIRUS

Family	Papovaviridae
Common Name(s)	Human papillomavirus (HPV), wart virus
Collection of Specimen	Endocervical swab, biopsy tissue
Direct Examination	Virus can be detected in Papanicolaou (Pap) stained cells. Currently best method is detection of HPV DNA by hybridization technology using DNA or RNA probes. PCR technology can also be employed.
Description of Agent *Diameter* *Capsid Symmetry* *Envelope* *Type of Nucleic Acid*	44–55 nm 72 capsomeres in icosahedral arrangement No Double stranded DNA
General Disease Categories	HPV causes warts on feet, hands, arms, forehead, larynx, and genitals. HPV is associated with cervical cancer and has been implicated in head and neck squamous cell cancer.
Population Infected	Warts caused by HPV are generally more common among children and young adults. Older adults are less likely to develop warts.
Incubation Period	Warts develop between 1 and 8 mo after virus lodges on skin or mucosa. Genital warts develop after 1–3 mo of incubation.
Primary Symptoms	When subjected to irritation, warts may become quite tender. Anal warts may cause itching, and plantar warts are very sensitive because of pressure. Symptoms of cervical cancer occur when HPV is responsible for malignancy.
Transmission	Transmission of genital type is thought to be primarily through sexual contact, whereas transmission of cutaneous types is by direct contact or fomites.
Treatment	Warts should be removed only by physician, who may use electrodesiccation, acids, or freezing with liquid nitrogen. Spontaneous disappearance does occur.
Prevention	Avoid contact with HPV.
Serologic Diagnosis	Reliable serologic assay for HPV is not available.

PARVOVIRUS B19

Continued ▶

▶ Continued **HUMAN PAPILLOMAVIRUS**

Cell Cultures for Detection of Viruses from Clinical Specimen	Cell cultures not used
Oncogenic Potential	HPV is the cause of 90% of cervical cancers, with high risk types including 16, 18, 45, and 56. HPV can also cause penile cancer, head and neck squamous cell cancer, and the rare Buschke-Löwenstein tumor (cauliflower-like mass of warts in perianal region).

GENERAL INFORMATION. The two members of the Papovaviridae family are the papillomaviruses and the small polyomavirus. The human papillomavirus (HPV) contains double stranded supercoiled circular DNA. There are at least 70 different types of HPV that are associated with warts as well as epidermal and epithelial lesions. The classification of HPV into types is based on the demonstration of less than 50% DNA homology. HPV is classified as cutaneous when the types infect keratinizing epithelial tissue, or mucosal when the types infect nonkeratinizing epithelium. Cutaneous HPV infection with types 1 to 4 initiate wart formation on the soles of the feet. Type 1 HPV also initiates wart formation on the hand and types 2 to 4 on the arms. The infections are benign and generally self-limited. Type 5 and those with designations above 5 can sometimes cause neoplastic lesions. The mucosal types of HPV can infect the respiratory tract, conjunctiva, oral mucosa, and especially the vulva, vagina, cervix, anus, and penis. HPV is currently known to be the cause of at least 90% of the cervical cancers. Some types of genital warts are low risk since they are rarely associated with malignancy, other types are intermediate, and others that most frequently lead to malignancy are high risk, namely types 16, 18, 45, and 56.

POLYOMAVIRUSES

Family	Papovaviridae
Common Name(s)	Polyomavirus strains JC and BK
Collection of Specimen	Body fluids used for analysis include urine, blood (lymphocytes), and CSF. Urine is generally best source for BK virus. JC virus is isolated from brain tissue, and both viruses can be isolated from kidney tissue.
Direct Examination	When brain tissue biopsy is available, in situ DNA hybridization can reliably detect JC in tissue.
Description of Agent *Diameter* *Capsid Symmetry* *Envelope* *Type of Nucleic Acid*	40 nm 72 capsomeres in icosahedral arrangement No Double stranded DNA
General Disease Categories	JC is associated with progressive multifocal leukoencephalopathy (PML), and BK is associated with Wiskott-Aldrich syndrome and renal infections in both bone marrow and kidney transplant patients.

Continued ▶

▶ Continued **POLYOMAVIRUSES**

Population Infected	Seroconversion occurs in 80% of population by age of 8 years. Effect of primary viral infection with BK and JC is not known. The two viruses appear to be reactivated in immunocompromised adults.
Incubation Period	Primary disease is restricted to latent infection.
Primary Symptoms	Symptoms associated with PML (caused by JC virus) are primarily paralysis on one side of the body or motor dysfunction as well as progressive dementia and visual defects. BK virus symptoms are unclear since presence of virus does not always accompany poor graft survival or illness of host.
Transmission	Possibly direct contact with contaminated respiratory secretion
Treatment	Supportive; decrease immunosuppression if possible.
Prevention	Since mode of transmission is not definitive, prevention is currently unknown.
Serologic Diagnosis	Serologic study is not helpful in diagnosis of acute infection. However, serologic study is important for demonstrating spread of human polyomavirus. Method of choice is hemagglutination inhibition assay.
Cell Cultures for Detection of Viruses from Clinical Specimen	Viral isolation via cell cultures is not routinely performed since DNA probes are available. However, BK can be cultivated in human embryonic kidney cells and JC in human fetal brain cells.
Oncogenic Potential	JC has not been associated with human tumors but is tumorigenic for various animals. BK has been detected in some brain and pancreatic cancers, but it is not known as causative agent.

POLYOMAVIRUSES

GENERAL INFORMATION. The polyomaviruses, like the papillomaviruses, belong to the Papovaviridae family. The polyomaviruses (BK and JC) carry their genetic information on both strands of DNA, whereas the papillomavirus carries its genetic information on one of the two DNA strands. The polyoma animal viruses such as simian virus 40 cause lymphomas and sarcomas in rats and hamsters. The human virus JC also causes various tumors in animals but has not been associated with human neoplasms. A second human virus, BK, has been associated with human cancers of the brain and pancreas. Currently, it is not known whether BK plays a role in the formation of these tumors. Both BK and JC can hemagglutinate human type O red blood cells.

HUMAN INFECTIONS. The majority of humans (80%) contact both BK and JC before the age of 8 years. Many individuals exhibit a serum titer to one or both viruses throughout their life span. Whether the primary human contact with these viruses is symptomatic or associated with a disease process is unknown. However, JC does infect the white matter of the brain in immunocompromised adults and is responsible for causing progressive multifocal leukoencephalopathy (PML). BK is associated with kidney infections in bone marrow and renal transplant patients. The virus has not been identified as the cause of the kidney infection, and the presence of the virus does not necessarily indicate illness or poor graft survival. Both PML and kidney infection are thought to be due to reactivation of latent infection.

ADENOVIRUS

Family	Adenoviridae
Common Name(s)	Adenovirus
Collection of Specimen	Following specimens are collected: stool, rectal swabs, urine, urethral and cervical swabs, nasal and nasopharyngeal swabs or aspirates, and eye swabs, as well as biopsy or autopsy specimens.
Direct Examination	Identification of adenoviruses in clinical material is often performed via electron microscope. Additionally, immunofluorescence assays, radioimmune assay, and enzyme immunoassays can be used.
Description of Agent *Diameter* *Capsid Symmetry* *Envelope* *Type of Nucleic Acid*	70–90 nm 252 capsomeres in icosahedral arrangement No Double stranded DNA
General Disease Categories	Adenoviruses cause large variety of infections including gastroenteritis, hemorrhagic cystitis, pneumonia, pharyngitis, tonsillitis, bronchitis, coryza, keratoconjunctivitis, CNS disease, and venereal disease.
Population Infected	All age groups are affected, but infections are most common for school age children.
Incubation Period	Generally 5–10 days
Primary Symptoms	Multiple symptoms; see general disease categories.
Transmission	Major routes of transmission are fecal, oral, respiratory, and direct contact (eye infections).
Treatment	Supportive
Prevention	Military recruits receive a vaccine for serotypes 4 and 7, which cause severe respiratory disease.
Serologic Diagnosis	Adenovirus infection is diagnosed by complement fixation methods or enzyme immunoassays using both acute and convalescent phase sera. Hemagglutination inhibition or serum neutralizing antibody assays are generally used if serotyping is to be performed. Virus must also be isolated for serotyping to be successful.
Cell Cultures for Detection of Viruses from Clinical Specimen	Most human adenoviruses will replicate in HeLa, KB, A549, Hep-2, or primary human embryonic kidney cells.
Oncogenic Potential	Not reported for humans. Adenoviruses never initiate tumors in their natural hosts but cause tumors when the viruses are transmitted to other species.

GENERAL INFORMATION. Adenoviruses are species specific, and human strains cause infections only in humans. At least 47 serotypes have been described, with approximately 95% of the human infections caused by serotypes 1 to 3, 5, and 7. Adenovirus isolation is age dependent since 22% are recovered from persons less than 1 year old. The recovery rates are 42% for children 1 to 4 years of age, 18% for those 5 to 14 years of age, 10% for those 15 to 24 years of age, 7% for those 25 to 29 years of age, and only 1% for those above 60 years. The 47 human serotypes are divided into six subgenera by sodium dodecyl sulfate (SDS) polyacrylamide gel electrophoresis of virion polypeptides. Classification using SDS polyacrylamide gel electrophoresis coincides with hemagglutination patterns using rat and rhesus monkey erythrocytes. The chart below lists the serotypes of the subgenera A to F. The second chart below lists the disease or syndrome initiated by the major serotypes of the adenoviruses.

Human Adenovirus Serotypes of Subgenera A to F

SUBGENUS	SEROTYPE(S)
A	12, 18, 31
B:1	3, 7, 16, 21
B:2	11, 14, 34, 35
C	1, 2, 5, 6
D	8–10, 13, 15, 17, 19, 20, 22–30, 32, 33, 36–39, 42–47
E	4
F	40, 41

Serotypes and Adenovirus Disease

DISEASE OR SYNDROME	GROUP AFFECTED	MAJOR SEROTYPES
Acute Respiratory Disease with Pneumonia	Military recruits	4, 7, 14, and 21
Pneumonia	Infants, young children	3, 4, 7, and 21
Pertussis-like Syndrome	Infants, young children	5
Pharyngitis	Infants, young children	1–3, 5, and 7
Pharyngoconjunctival Fever	School age children	3 and 7
Follicular Conjunctivitis	All age groups	3, 4, and 11
Epidemic Keratoconjunctivitis	Mostly adults	8, 19, and 37
Acute Hemorrhagic Cystitis	Infants, young children	11 and 21
Diarrhea	Infants, young children	31, 40, and 41
AIDS and Other Immunosuppressive Conditions	Adults including transplant recipients, intravenous drug abusers, homosexuals, and infants with congenital immunodeficiencies including severe combined immunodeficiency (SCID)	1, 2, 5, 11, 34, and 35
CNS	Adults and young children	7 (3 in young children)
Venereal Disease	Adults	7

ADENOVIRUS

MILITARY RECRUITS AND RESPIRATORY DISEASE. Acute respiratory disease in newly enlisted military recruits is associated with adenovirus types 4, 7, 14, and 21. The disease often occurs in the third week of training, and the symptoms include fever, headache, nasal congestion, malaise, sore throat, coughing, and hoarseness. At least 10% may develop pneumonia, which can lead to a fatal outcome. Since the introduction of the vaccine in 1976, virus associated pneumonia is no longer a problem for military recruits. The vaccine cannot be used for children.

CHILDHOOD PNEUMONIA. Pneumonias are often complications of lower respiratory illness that is caused by types 3, 4, 7, and 21. Severe infections may have a fatal outcome in infants and children. Residual lung disease can occur in children infected with these types of adenovirus. Finally, adenovirus 5 is associated with a fatal pneumonia in children who have a pertussis-like infection.

PHARYNGITIS AND TONSILLITIS. Adenoviruses initiate about 5% of the acute respiratory infections seen in young children. The disease can resemble tonsillitis caused by group A streptococci. Major symptoms include pharyngitis, tonsillitis, nasal congestion, coughing, and sometimes conjunctivitis.

PHARYNGOCONJUNCTIVAL FEVER AND FOLLICULAR CONJUNCTIVITIS. Pharyngoconjunctival fever is caused by types 3 and 7 and is often acquired by children who use swimming pools that do not have adequate levels of chlorine. The major symptoms include conjunctivitis, pharyngitis, fever, and adenoiditis. Acute follicular conjunctivitis may appear as a separate entity or can be part of pharyngoconjunctival fever. Follicular conjunctivitis is characterized by engorgement of the bulbar and palpebral conjunctiva as well as a preauricular lymphadenopathy. Some patients also have damage to the cornea.

EPIDEMIC KERATOCONJUNCTIVITIS. Epidemic keratoconjunctivitis is a separate syndrome associated with aggressive conjunctivitis, pain, lymphadenopathy, and photophobia. A superficial punctate keratitis follows the initial symptoms. The disease is sometimes called *the shipyard eye* because large outbreaks have been associated with individuals working at marine shipyards. Epidemic keratoconjunctivitis can be spread by ophthalmic wash solutions, towels, and contaminated hands and medical instruments.

ACUTE HEMORRHAGIC CYSTITIS. Acute hemorrhagic cystitis (AHC) is caused by serotypes 11 and 21. The primary symptoms are hematuria, dysuria, frequency, and urgency in urinating. The disease is more common in males, and careful diagnosis is needed since AHC can be confused with glomerulonephritis.

GASTROENTERITIS. Adenoviruses cause 4% to 15% of the cases of gastroenteritis that are seen in infants and young children. Serotypes 40 and 41 account for approximately two thirds of these cases. The diarrhea is not as severe as observed for rotavirus infections, but the duration is longer. The children may have additional symptoms that include fever, vomiting, dehydration, and respiratory symptoms.

IMMUNOCOMPROMISED PATIENTS. Immunocompromised patients are very susceptible to the adenovirus group. Subgenera A and C are often associated with severe combined immunodeficiency disease. These patients have life threatening infections that include pneumonia and hepatitis. Subgenera B and D are the most common adenovirus isolated from AIDS patients. The B subgenus causes latent kidney infections, whereas subgenus D is associated with the gastrointestinal tract. Bone marrow transplant patients are susceptible to all latent DNA viruses including the adenoviruses. Severe enteric disease caused by these viruses can be fatal.

MENINGITIS. Serotypes 3 and 7 are responsible for two thirds of all adenovirus associated cases of meningitis or meningoencephalitis. Reye's syndrome is sometimes associated with type 3 serotype. However, adenoviruses are infrequently associated with CNS disease.

GENITAL LESIONS. Serotypes 2, 19, and 32 are associated with a herpes-like genital lesion.

MEASLES VIRUS

Family	Paramyxoviridae
Common Name(s)	Measles virus (MV)
Collection of Specimen	Failure to isolate MV from clinical specimens is common. During prodromal and early rash stage, MV can be isolated from nasopharyngeal and conjunctival specimens. Stool and urine specimens are collected during late illness. CSF specimens generally are poor specimens for viral isolation. Samples should be refrigerated after collection and stabilized with bovine serum albumin or fetal calf serum.
Direct Examination	MV can be detected in nasopharyngeal secretion, peripheral blood, and urine sediment by immunofluorescence staining of tissues. Electron microscope can detect MV infected cells that are typically multinucleated and are produced by fusion of infected cells. Presence of multinucleated cells in peripheral blood monoclear cells or in throat washings usually indicates MV infection. Patients with subacute sclerosing panencephalitis (SSPE) have viral neucleocapsid material deposited in cytoplasm or nuclei of infected cells. These eosinophilic inclusions are usually diagnostic in SSPE patients.
Description of Agent *Diameter* *Capsid Symmetry* *Envelope* *Type of Nucleic Acid*	100–250 nm Helical Yes Single stranded RNA
General Disease Categories	Measles; rare complications include acute encephalitis, SSPE, and giant cell pneumonia
Population Infected	Measles is childhood disease in which infection rate in United States has decreased by 99% since introduction of vaccine.
Incubation Period	10–11 days
Primary Symptoms	Early symptoms of measles include fever, rhinorrhea, cough, and conjunctivitis. Four or 5 days later, maculopapular rash starts on head and moves down body. Koplik's spots appear just before rash develops. Koplik's spots are bright red spots with blue-white central area that appear on buccal and labial mucosa. Leukopenia usually occurs because virus infects white blood cells. Occasionally pneumonia and secondary bacterial infections occur.
Transmission	Measles is spread by respiratory secretions and aerosol droplets. Before vaccine, infectious rate in North America tended to increase in winter and spring when low relative humidity favored spread by respiratory secretions.
Treatment	Supportive—immune serum globulin can be given to immunocompromised patients.

MEASLES VIRUS

Continued ▶

▶ Continued **MEASLES VIRUS**

Prevention	Measles vaccine
Serologic Diagnosis	Diagnosis of acute infection is made by significant increase of specific antibody titers in paired serum samples taken at 7–14 day intervals. Specific diagnosis can also be made by demonstrating MV-IgM antibodies in single specimen. Demonstration of specific antibodies in single serum specimen demonstrates past MV vaccination or infection. The hemagglutination inhibition (HI) test, EIAs, and fluorescent antibody techniques have all been used to detect MV.
Cell Cultures for Detection of Viruses from Clinical Specimen	Primary monkey kidney (PMK), human fetal, or infant kidney cells are used. Multinucleate syncytia are formed in PMK cells.
Oncogenic Potential	Not observed

GENERAL INFORMATION. Measles virus (MV) is a member of the Paramyxoviridae family but lacks the neuraminidase enzyme and is therefore classified into a separate genus, the morbillivirus. The canine distemper virus (CDV) that infects dogs has antigenic similarities to the MV. Both viruses can produce chronic neurologic diseases. The MV contains single stranded linear RNA and has an envelope from which two types of viral glycoproteins protrude. The hemagglutinin (H) and fusion (F) glycoproteins generally initiate antibody formation against MV. H glycoprotein causes the production of neutralizing antibodies, and F results in antibodies that inhibit the spread of MV in the tissues. The hemagglutination inhibition test is based on the fact that antibodies against the H protein prevent the virus from aggregating monkey erythrocytes.

MEASLES. Before the vaccine era, measles was a common childhood disease and death from uncomplicated measles was unusual in the developed world, but the fatality rate did approach 15% to 25% in remote regions of the world. The prodromal phase lasts 2 to 4 days, and typical complaints include fever, sneezing, congestion, rhinitis, malaise, cough, and conjunctivitis. The maculopapular rash generally appears about 14 days after exposure and is initially observed on the head, and then the exanthem spreads over several days to the face, neck, trunk, and extremities. Before the appearance of the rash, Koplik's spots appear 11 days after the infection on the mucosa opposite the lower molars.

During the systemic infection, the virus first multiplies in the respiratory tract and reticuloendothelial systems (primary viremia). The lymphoid tissue destruction in this stage results in a pronounced leukopenia. The virus then infects the skin, kidney, bladder, and viscera (secondary viremia). The rash follows the secondary viremia. The appearance of both Koplik's spots and the rash are probably delayed hypersensitivity reactions. Finally, measles infection is unusual since infection is characterized by lymphoid hyperplasia in all infected organs.

MODIFIED MEASLES. This form of measles can occur in infants with residual maternal antibody or in patients who have received immune serum globulin for protection. The illness follows the regular sequence of events but it is usually characterized by reduced or mild symptoms.

ATYPICAL MEASLES. This form of measles occurs when a patient does not complete the vaccination series and later becomes exposed and is infected with the natural MV. In atypical measles, the patient's antibody titer rises to a very high level not seen with patients with typical measles. However, atypical measle patients lack antibodies to the F protein and therefore cannot prevent the spread of MV in the tissues. These patients do not develop Koplik's spots, and the rash starts on the palms and soles and then spreads to the extremities and trunk. These patients also tend to develop a pneumonia that is slow to resolve.

GIANT CELL PNEUMONIA AND MEASLES INCLUSION BODY ENCEPHALITIS. Patients who have immunodeficiencies or who are immunocompromised can encounter a life threatening measles infection that is characterized by a severe pneumonia and the appearance of giant cells. Measles inclusion body encephalitis occurs most often in leukemic children undergoing axial radiation therapy. The disease begins with convulsions, and the seizures are often localized to one site. The CNS disease is rapid, and death occurs within a few months.

ACUTE MEASLES POSTINFECTIOUS ENCEPHALITIS. Approximately 15% of the cases of acute measles postinfectious encephalitis (AMPE) are fatal, and at least 20% who recover have selective brain damage. This complication from measles is relatively rare, with an upper frequency at about 0.1%. The symptoms include headache, fever, cerebellar ataxia, seizures, and coma, which frequently develop while the exanthem is still present.

SUBACUTE SCLEROSING PANENCEPHALITIS. The overall incidence of subacute sclerosing panencephalitis (SSPE) is extremely low (1 case per 1 million cases of measles). Boys are more commonly affected than girls. SSPE is slowly developing neural disease that follows measles after a period of 6 to 8 years. Approximately half the SSPE patients usually contact measles before the age of 2 years. The MV that causes SSPE may be a temperature sensitive mutant. The progression of SSPE is variable, and death occurs between 1 and 3 years after the onset, which is characterized by a general intellectual decline. Neurologic or motor dysfunctions follow, and the virus invades the retina in approximately 75% of the cases.

MEASLES VIRUS

MUMPS VIRUS

Family	Paramyxoviridae
Common Name(s)	Paramyxovirus, mumps virus
Collection of Specimen	Specimens should be collected early in illness when viral titers are at their peak. The mumps virus can be isolated from saliva, urine, the area around Stensen's duct, and cerebrospinal fluid if meningitis is present.
Direct Examination	Mumps infected cells from saliva or urine can be detected by direct or indirect immunofluorescence.
Description of Agent *Diameter* *Capsid Symmetry* *Envelope* *Type of Nucleic Acid*	150–200 nm Helical Yes Single stranded RNA

Continued ▶

► Continued **MUMPS VIRUS**

General Disease Categories	Mumps or classic parotitis
Incubation Period	Average incubation period is 16–18 days, but it can be as short as 14 days or as long as 25.
Primary Symptoms	Prodromal symptoms last for 1 or 2 days and include malaise, myalgia, low grade fever, and headache. In classic mumps one parotid gland becomes swollen and in 75% of cases bilateral enlargement occurs within 1–5 days. Swelling usually subsides after 4–7 days. Complications include meningitis, encephalitis, pancreatitis, polyarthritis, orchitis, and oophoritis.
Transmission	By droplet infection
Treatment	Supportive. Analgesics are given when pain is excessive.
Prevention	Vaccine. The attenuated mumps virus is incorporated into a triple vaccine, MMR (measles, mumps, and rubella).
Serologic Diagnosis	Cross-reactions between mumps and parainfluenza viruses have limited use of serologic testing. Many methods detect significant increase in titer between acute and convalescent sera. ELISA, CF, HI, IF, FIAX (a solid-phase immunofluorescence assay), and hemolysis in gel tests have all been used. Finally, skin testing to assay immunity is not reliable since both false positive and false negative results may occur.
Cell Cultures for Detection of Viruses from Clinical Specimen	Virus isolation in cells susceptible to mumps virus include PMK, HeLa, and HEK. Large granular syncytial cells are observed in PMK culture.
Oncogenic Potential	Not observed

GENERAL INFORMATION. Mumps virus, Newcastle disease virus (NDV), and the parainfluenza viruses belong to the genus *Paramyxovirus.* All the paramyxoviruses have diameters of 150 to 200 nm and contain a helical nucleocapsid with single stranded RNA as the genetic information. The mumps virus has two surface glycoproteins that project from the lipid envelope. The HN molecule has both hemagglutinating and neuraminidase activity that mediate the adsorption of the virus to the host cells. The HN component is able to hemolyze erythrocytes, and antibody to this component neutralizes viral infectivity. The second surface protein or glycoprotein F is probably important in spreading the mumps virus in a cell population. The HN and F protein form the V antigen. The V antigen (HN and F) is responsible for cross-reactivity observed between the mumps virus and the parainfluenza viruses. The M protein is located under the viral envelope and is important in the assembly of the virion during the replication cycle. Additionally, there are three proteins (NP, P, and L) associated with the nucleocapsid. The nucleoprotein (NP) is the most abundant protein of the mumps virus, and it determines the helical structure of the nucleocapsid. The mumps S antigen is composed largely of the NP protein. The current serologic philosophy is that it is necessary to test for both the V and S antigens in order to confirm seroconversions. The phosphorylated protein (P) and the L protein are also associated with the nucleocapsid and probably play a role in the enzymatic function of RNA replication.

MUMPS. Mumps infections are spread by droplets, and the major initial target is the upper respiratory or gastrointestinal tissues or the eyes. The virus then spreads to the local lymphoid tissue, and additional multiplication eventually leads to a primary viremia.

After the primary viremia the virus spreads to the salivary glands, the parotid gland, and often to the pancreas, CNS, testes, or ovaries. Virus multiplication in various organs leads to a secondary viremia. The course of mumps can be very variable, but parotitis (bilateral or unilateral) occurs in 95% of the clinical cases. At least one third of the cases are asymptomatic. The majority of the patients are between 5 and 19 years of age. The MMR trivalent vaccine consists of live attenuated mumps, measles, and rubella viruses and is inoculated into children at 15 months and again at 4 to 6 years. Outbreaks of mumps in both vaccinated and unvaccinated populations still occasionally occur in the United States. Two well known complications of mumps are orchitis and oophoritis, which have a much higher frequency in adolescents and young adults than in children.

COMPLICATIONS WITH THE MUMPS VIRUS. Classic parotitis is so clinically dominating in mumps patients that other clinical features are often described as complications. Aseptic meningitis occurs in about 10% of mumps patients, with the frequency two or three times greater in males than in females. The symptoms of meningitis can start 1 week before parotid swelling or as late as 3 weeks after the parotitis. The more severe clinical picture of encephalitis occurs in 1 in 6000 cases of mumps and may be associated with a polio-like paralysis. Hearing loss associated with mumps has been greatly reduced since the vaccine was introduced. Pancreatitis is confirmed by an elevated serum amylase level and occurs at a rate as high as 5% in mumps patients. Symptoms include vomiting and epigastric pain followed normally by complete recovery. In males and females above the age of puberty, the incidence of orchitis is 20% to 40% in males, and oophoritis occurs at about a 5% rate in females. Orchitis may cause the male testes to enlarge three- or fourfold, and occasionally testicular atrophy occurs and results in male infertility. Infertility has not been reported in female patients with oophoritis.

RUBELLA VIRUS

Family	Togaviridae
Common Name(s)	Togavirus disease: rubella, German measles
Collection of Specimen	Blood, cerebrospinal fluid, urine, nasopharyngeal, or throat specimens can be collected. Rubella virus is difficult to isolate, and nearly all laboratories depend on serologic tests rather than viral isolation.
Direct Examination	Direct examination of tissues for rubella virus is not performed.
Description of Agent *Diameter* *Capsid Symmetry* *Envelope* *Type of Nucleic Acid*	60–70 nm Icosahedral Yes Single stranded RNA
General Disease Categories	Rubella is usually mild childhood disease in which rash is present. Rash may not be present in some cases, making rubella rather difficult to diagnose clinically. Congenitally acquired rubella infections can cause severe abnormalities if virus is acquired early in pregnancy.
Population Infected	Rubella infections occur in young children and adults. MMR vaccine is about 90% effective, and outbreaks occasionally occur in adolescents and adults. Congenital rubella infections still occur.
Incubation Period	Rubella has incubation period of 13–20 days. Congenital rubella infections are most likely if mother is exposed to rubella during 1st month of pregnancy.

Continued ▶

MUMPS VIRUS

▶ Continued **RUBELLA VIRUS**

Primary Symptoms	Postnatally acquired rubella infections feature rash and lymphadenopathy. Rash initially appears on face and spreads quickly to trunk and then to extremities. Rash is present for 3 days or less. Lymphadenopathy may commence as early as 1 wk before rash and may persist for 10–14 days after it has disappeared. In up to one quarter of cases subclinical infection may occur. Congenital rubella infection often causes ophthalmic, cardiac, auditory, and neurologic defects.
Transmission	Rubella virus is transmitted via respiratory route and congenital rubella via transplacental route.
Treatment	Supportive. Early term pregnant women can be given normal or high titered rubella immunoglobulin, which will reduce overt infection rate. It is thought that immunoglobulins may decreases viremia and there will be less damage to fetus. Routine use of immunoglobulin therapy in early pregnancy is not recommended.
Prevention	Rubella vaccine (MMR) produces 95% response but should not be given 3 mo before conception or during pregnancy.
Serologic Diagnosis	The old routine standard for measuring antibody to rubella virus was HI testing. Currently, common tests employed include latex fixation, EIA, IFA, and passive hemagglutination.
Cell Cultures for Detection of Viruses from Clinical Specimen	Primary African green monkey kidney (AGMK) cells are considered to be standard cells used to isolate virus. Rubella virus is indicated in AGMK cells by interference with cytopathic effects of challenge virus such as echovirus type 11 or coxsackievirus A9. RK-13 or Vero cells can also be used to isolate rubella virus.
Oncogenic Potential	Not reported

GENERAL INFORMATION. Rubella is classified as a member of the Togaviridiae family and is the only virus in the genus *Rubivirus*. Rubella virus is related to the genus *Alphavirus* but is not transmitted via arthropod vectors. The virus possesses two glycoproteins (E1 and E2) that are membrane bound and a nonglycosylated nucleocapsid protein C that is found internally. Rubella virus possesses a hemagglutinin that reacts with red blood cells of many animal species including humans and birds. The hemagglutination activity is associated with the E1 glycosylated protein. The E1 protein also appears to be associated with neutralization and hemolysis activity. In contrast the E2 appears more inaccessible to immunoglobulins. Currently only one type of rubella virus has been recognized.

POSTNATAL RUBELLA. The rubella vaccine has ended the epidemic (6 to 9 year cycle) disease that occurred in schoolchildren. The major features are a rash and lymphadenopathy (see the chart above). A prodromal phase including fever or malaise may occur in adults 1 or 2 days ahead of the rash. Transient polyarthritis and polyarthralgia are the most common complication of naturally occurring rubella infection. These complications are more likely to occur in postpubertal adults. Rare complications include thrombocytopenia and encephalitis.

CONGENITALLY ACQUIRED RUBELLA INFECTION. Maternal rubella infection during the first trimester may result in a variety of outcomes including a healthy infant, a minimally damaged infant, a severely malformed infant, or fetal death and spontaneous abortion. Generally, the earlier in the trimester, the more likely the fetus will develop birth defects. Some clinical features associated with congenitally acquired rubella are transient during the first few weeks of life, and permanent sequelae do not occur. The common transient anomalies include low birth weight, hepatosplenomegaly, hemolytic anemia, and thrombocytopenic purpura. Transient bone lesions and meningoencephalitis are less common transient anomalies. The transient anomalies are nearly always found in tandem with permanent birth defects. Developmental defects may develop slowly but will persist for a lifetime. Hearing defects and even deafness may develop after 9 to 12 months. Mental retardation, central language defects, and diabetes mellitus are additional developmental defects. The most common permanent defects include cardiovascular and ocular defects. Heart defects are responsible for the high perinatal mortality observed in these infants. The major ocular defects are retinopathy and cataracts, with glaucoma far less common.

The figure below illustrates an antibody response in an infant congenitally infected with rubella virus. The finding of rubella virus specific IgM antibody at birth is indicative that a congenital rubella infection occurred. Also suggestive of congenital rubella is the persistence of a high hemagglutination inhibition titer during the first 6 months of life.

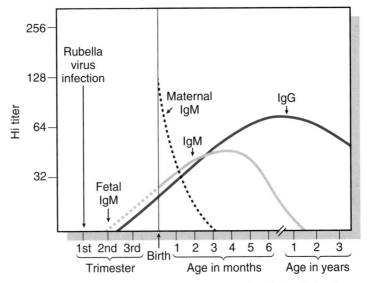

Modified from Murray PR, Baron EJ, Pfaller MA, et al: Manual of Clinical Microbiology, 6th ed. Washington, D.C. ASM Press, 1995.

RUBELLA VIRUS

PARAINFLUENZA VIRUS

Family	Paramyxoviridae
Common Name(s)	Paramyxovirus, parainfluenza virus (PIV) 1–4.
Collection of Specimen	Nasopharyngeal secretion from young children should be collected early in course of illness to ensure efficient isolation of PIV. Throat swabs, although less satisfactory, can be employed when it is not possible to obtain nasopharyngeal suctions or garglings.

Continued ▶

► Continued **PARAINFLUENZA VIRUS**

Direct Examination	Direct examination of nasopharyngeal secretion by combination of electron microscope and immunofluorescence can yield results within 3 hr of collection. Type specific antiserum is required to identify PIV type.
Description of Agent *Diameter* *Capsid Symmetry* *Envelope* *Type of Nucleic Acid*	120–300 nm Helical Yes Single stranded RNA
General Disease Categories	PIV-1 and PIV-2 are major causes of laryngotracheobronchitis (croup). PIV-3 causes bronchiolitis and pneumonia in infants but rarely causes croup. PIV-4 generally causes mild respiratory illness.
Population Infected	Childhood disease with acute respiratory illness is common. PIV infections in adults are relatively uncommon except in patients with AIDS and those receiving organ transplants.
Incubation Period	2–6 days
Primary Symptoms	Typical symptoms of croup (PIV-1 and PIV-2) include hoarse voice, croupy cough, and respiratory difficulty on inspiration. Runny nose often occurs 1–3 days before croup. Epiglottitis may occasionally occur. Recurrent attacks of croup may occur in children younger than 3 years. PIV-3 can cause pneumonia or bronchiolitis since it descends to lower respiratory tract. PIV may initiate coldlike or influenza-like syndrome in adults.
Transmission	Contact with respiratory secretions
Treatment	Supportive. Young children are placed in plastic tents (croupettes) supplied with cooled humidified oxygen. Tracheotomy is sometimes necessary to establish open airway.
Prevention	Avoid contact with virus. Vaccine is not currently available.
Serologic Diagnosis	Serologic diagnosis is difficult because reinfection with PIV is very common in young children. Additionally, young children can be reinfected with same PIV type partly because they produce ineffective antibody. Heterotrophic response involving other PIV types as well as mumps also makes specific serologic diagnosis of PIV difficult. Both acute phase and convalescent phase sera should be examined for antibody to PIV. Conversion from negative to positive status generally requires at least fourfold increase in antibody titer. HI, CF, IF, EIA, and neutralization tests have been used. CF test is more specific than HI or EIA. Advantage of EIA is that it is more sensitive than CF or HI.
Cell Cultures for Detection of Viruses from Clinical Specimen	Most sensitive cell cultures for isolation of PIV are primary monkey kidney and primary human embryonic kidney. PIV can be detected after appearance of cytopathic effect. Care must be taken since other viral types besides PIV may have been in sample and can also replicate in primary monkey kidney cells.
Oncogenic Potential	Not observed

GENERAL INFORMATION. Like the mumps virus, PIV produces six polypeptides. Two glycoproteins form spikes on the outside of the virus. The hemagglutinin neuraminidase (HN) is necessary for the adsorption of the virus to the host cell. The hemagglutinin component causes hemagglutination of mammalian erythrocytes. The F glycoprotein spike mediates virion entry into the cell and is able to initiate cell to cell spread that eventually results in syncytia formation. The additional four proteins include the matrix (M), nucleoprotein (NP), phosphoprotein (P), and L protein and are located inside the virus.

CROUP AND UPPER RESPIRATORY INFECTIONS.   Laryngotracheobronchitis (croup) is initiated commonly by PIV-1 and PIV-2 and occasionally by PIV-3. Severe illness is most likely to occur in children between 2 and 4 years of age. Reinfection with PIV is generally less severe than the primary infection. The typical clinical symptoms of the croup are described in the PIV summary chart above. PIV-1 and PIV-2 cases of the croup tend to occur every other year in the autumn. Bronchiolitis and pneumonia are often severe manifestations caused by PIV-3 in infants less than 1 year of age. However, respiratory syncytial virus is still currently the most common cause of bronchiolitis and pneumonia in infants. PIV-3 is endemic and tends to cause infections in the late spring and early summer. PIV-4 (subtypes 4a and 4b) causes mild illness and occurs sporadically. Adults and older children experience PIV infections that may be asymptomatic or resemble the common cold syndrome or a mild influenza-like syndrome. In contrast adult patients with AIDS or those patients with organ transplants may experience severe respiratory disease.

RESPIRATORY SYNCYTIAL VIRUS

Family	Paramyxoviridae, but different morphologic and antigenic differences place it in *Pneumovirus* genus within Paramyxoviridae family.
Common Name(s)	Paramyxovirus, respiratory syncytial virus (RSV)
Collection of Specimen	Nasopharyngeal secretions are best specimen to collect. Aspirate samples lead to greater recovery of epithelial cells than washes or swabs.
Direct Examination	Indirect and direct immunofluorescence techniques detect RSV in epithelial cells and respiratory secretions within few hours. EIA methods are also frequently employed and are able to yield results in times as short as 15–20 min. One advantage of employing EIA is that intact respiratory cells are not needed.
Description of Agent *Diameter* *Capsid Symmetry* *Envelope* *Type of Nucleic Acid*	100–350 nm Helical Yes Single stranded RNA
General Disease Categories	RSV is most common agent isolated from infants and young children with bronchiolitis and pneumonia. RSV is also associated with mild upper respiratory disease and otitis media.
Population Infected	RSV infects nearly all children by the time they are 3 years of age, with approximately 69% infected during their 1st year of life. RSV causes repeated upper respiratory tract infection in older children and adults. Elderly and immunocompromised patients often experience severe respiratory infections.
Incubation Period	Incubation period is 3–6 days, but range is 2–8 days.
Primary Symptoms	Primary symptoms are generally symptomatic and range from mild to severe lower respiratory tract infections. Severe symptoms include bronchiolitis that is characterized by necrosis and sloughing of bronchial epithelium. Small airways become plugged and obstruct flow of air. Apnea is most common complication observed with RSV infections. Bronchiolitis may coexist with or lead to pneumonia. RSV infection is spread by close contact with respiratory secretions, either via fomites or large particle aerosols. Nosocomial spread of RSV is major problem.

Continued ▶

PARAINFLUENZA VIRUS

▶ Continued **RESPIRATORY SYNCYTIAL VIRUS**

Transmission	Respiratory contact and person to person via contaminated hands
Treatment	Supportive. For hospitalized infants with severe lower respiratory disease, antiviral agent ribavirin is administered by aerosol into oxygen tent.
Prevention	Vaccine is not available. Development of successful vaccine would depend on being administered to infants, and it would have to produce immunity greater than that acquired by natural infection. RSV hyperimmune globulin appears to reduce RSV infections in high risk children. Prevention from contacting RSV early after birth may be feasible.
Serologic Diagnosis	Neutralizing antibody titers do correlate with protection against reinfection with RSV. Serologic response is often poor, especially in young infants, and up to 40% of RSV infections may fail to elicit detectable antibody. Neutralization titers generally peak at 20–30 days after acute infection but can often rise after 10th day. EIA and IF assays can also be used. Currently serologic tests have not achieved widespread acceptance.
Cell Cultures for Detection of Viruses from Clinical Specimen	Cell culture isolation and rapid diagnostic techniques are more sensitive than serologic techniques. Nasopharyngeal aspirates contain RSV and are grown in cell lines such as Hep-2 and HeLa. After incubation of 3–7 days cytopathic effects are observed. Eosinophilic cytoplasmic granules within cytoplasm and large syncytia are generally observed. Subtype A strains develop CPE–cytopathogenic effect quicker than subtype B. Shell vial techniques can also be used to rapidly isolate RSV, often within 16 hr.
Oncogenic Potential	Not reported

GENERAL INFORMATION. The Paramyxoviridae family has the following members: RSV, PIV, MV, and the mumps virus. RSV is assigned to the genus *Pneumovirus*, since it lacks the neuraminidase and hemagglutinin found with the other Paramyxoviridae viruses. RSV also has a smaller nucleocapsid (13 to 14 nm diameter). RSV produces at least 10 protein products, including the two large surface glycoproteins F and G. The fusion (F) and glycoprotein (G) form spikes, and both proteins appear to evoke the production of neutralizing antibody. The F protein initiates the penetration and spread of the virus via fusion, whereas the G spike plays a major rule in the attachment of RSV to the host cell. There are two major strains of RSV (A and B), with the major antigenic difference linked to the G protein. The G protein contains only 55% amino acid homology between strains A and B. The A strain outbreaks of RSV are more common, and outbreaks caused by only the B strain are rare. N, P, and L are nonglycosylated proteins associated with the nucleocapsid, whereas matrix proteins M and M2 are located in the viral envelope. The SH protein is expressed on the surface of RSV infected cells as well as being a small integral membrane protein. The last two proteins are nonstructural and are designated NS-1 and NS-2.

BRONCHIOLITIS, PNEUMONIA, AND OTHER INFECTIONS CAUSED BY RESPIRATORY SYNCYTIAL VIRUS. Nearly everyone is infected with RSV within the first 3 years of life. Severe lower respiratory infection including pneumonia and bronchiolitis occurs in young infants and children. RSV may be responsible for 50% to 90% of all cases of bronchiolitis and as many as 5% to 40% of pneumonias in young children and infants. In contrast, RSV is responsible for only 10% of the cases of the croup since the parainfluenza virus dominates in this disease. Males are hospitalized with RSV more frequently than females despite an equal attack rate. Socioeconomic factors are linked to

RSV hospitalizations: there is a much higher rate for infants who come from industrialized and poor economic background than those raised in a nonurban middle class setting. RSV infections are global in their distribution and are distinctive; the virus produces significant outbreaks of infection that peak between January and March of each year in the United States. Slightly more variation is observed in the southern states (December to March). In contrast, tropical countries observe illness that tends to correspond to the rainy season (December to June). RSV outbreaks tend to precede or follow influenza or parainfluenza infections. Concurrent infections with RSV, influenza, and parainfluenza are unusual.

COMPLICATION OF RESPIRATORY SYNCYTIAL VIRUS INFECTIONS. Infants with congenital heart disease or pulmonary disease and children who are immunosuppressed have a high mortality rate. Apnea is a frequent complication that occurs in 20% of the infants hospitalized with RSV. Apnea rates are common in premature neonates and infants less than 44 weeks postconceptional age. The apnea tends to develop within the first few days of illness.

RHINOVIRUS

Family	Picornaviridae
Common Name(s)	Picornavirus, common cold virus
Collection of Specimen	Nasal wash collected at day 1 or 2 of the illness is best specimen. Combination of nasal or nasopharyngeal swab and throat swab can be used if nasal wash is not available.
Direct Examination	It has been difficult to develop direct examination tests for rhinoviruses since they lack group specific antigen and number of serotypes is approximately 100. IF and EIA methods have been used with limited success.
Description of Agent *Diameter* *Capsid Symmetry* *Envelope* *Type of Nucleic Acid*	24–30 nm Icosahedral No Single stranded RNA
General Disease Categories	Rhinoviruses are etiologic agent of 30%–35% of all common colds.
Population Infected	Normal person has two to five colds per year, and about one third are caused by rhinoviruses.
Incubation Period	Incubation period is approximately 2–3 days.
Primary Symptoms	Major symptoms last for average of 7 days and include profuse watery discharge, sneezing, headache, nasal congestion, mild sore throat, and cough. Nasal discharge and cough can last up to 1 mo. Lower respiratory tract infections including bronchitis and bronchopneumonia can occur.
Transmission	Contact with respiratory secretions
Treatment	Supportive

RESPIRATORY SYNCYTIAL VIRUS

Continued ▶

▶ Continued **RHINOVIRUS**

Prevention	Since there are about 100 serotypes, vaccine development is difficult. Some success in preventing rhinovirus infections has been achieved in volunteers given interferon alfa and beta as well as 3-methoxy-6[4-(3-methylphenyl)-1-piperazynyl] pyridazine via nasal route. Currently, best method of prevention is to avoid contact with rhinoviruses.
Serologic Diagnosis	Because of number of serotypes, routine testing is impractical. Patient's serum can be tested via neutralization test if specific rhinovirus is isolated.
Cell Cultures for Detection of Viruses from Clinical Specimen	Human diploid fibroblasts (HDFs) such as human embryonic lung strains W1-38 and MRC-5 give superior results. Before cytopathic effects are detected passage may be required.
Oncogenic Potential	Not reported

GENERAL INFORMATION.   The Picornaviridae family includes the rhinoviruses and the enteroviruses. At least 100 serotypes of the rhinovirus are known as the result of neutralization tests. Cross-reactions between antigen types have been detected using high titer rabbit and guinea pig antisera. However, no group antigen exists. The icosahedral nucleocapsid has four protein subunits (VP1, VP2, VP3, and VP4). VP4 resides inside the rhinovirus protein shell, whereas VP1, VP2, and VP3 compose the protein coat.

Epidemiologic studies indicate that there are two seasonal peaks for colds initiated by the rhinovirus. Peak infections generally are in early fall when children return to school and in the spring. Generally, only a small amount of virus is needed to infect a susceptible individual assuming that the virus reaches the nasal epithelium. The above summary chart contains a description of the primary symptoms. Bacterial infection in conjunction with the common cold may lead to sinusitis and otitis media. Rhinoviruses may trigger acute asthmatic attacks in both children and adults who have a history of asthmatic disease. Immunity studies have shown that volunteers with high levels of serum IgA and IgG along with high nasal levels of IgA were less likely to develop colds caused by rhinoviruses than those with low levels of these immunoglobulins.

Rhinoviruses, coronaviruses, adenoviruses, enteroviruses, RSV, and the influenza viruses can all cause common cold–like illnesses.

INFLUENZA VIRUSES

Family	Orthomyxoviridae
Common Name(s)	Orthomyxovirus, influenza viruses A, B, and C
Collection of Specimen	Specimens are collected within first 3 days after onset of symptoms. Routine specimens collected for detection of influenza viruses include nasopharyngeal aspirates, nasal washings, nasopharyngeal swabs, and throat and nasal swabs.
Direct Examination	Detection of influenza infected epithelial cells in nasopharyngeal aspirates or swabs is accomplished with either IF or EIA methods.

Continued ▶

► Continued **INFLUENZA VIRUSES**

Description of Agent	
Diameter	80–120 nm
Capsid Symmetry	Helical
Envelope	Yes
Type of Nucleic Acid	Single stranded RNA
General Disease Categories	Influenza and respiratory infections are common manifestations of the influenza viruses. Generally, types B and C cause infections that are milder than those caused by A. Asymptomatic infections caused by type A are common.
Population Infected	Types B and C are responsible for localized cases of mild upper respiratory tract infections in children, whereas type A is more closely associated with adult type influenza.
Incubation Period	Generally 48 hr, but may vary from 24 to 96 hr
Primary Symptoms	In adults common symptoms include fever (classically lasting for 3 days), headache, myalgia, malaise, photophobia, shivering, sore throat, and sometimes cough. Some variations occur for different age groups; sore throats and myalgia are commonly observed in adults but less frequently recorded in children. Vomiting, convulsions, and croup are sometimes observed in infants. Influenza B causes similar symptoms with a higher incidence of nasal symptoms. Influenza C infection is nearly always mild.
Transmission	By respiratory secretions
Treatment	Supportive. Amantadine and rimantadine reduce the duration of fever and illness for influenza type A. Children should not be treated with salicylates since incidence of Reye's syndrome is higher when young children with acute influenza take aspirin.
Prevention	Vaccine for types A and B. Type A can be prevented with amantadine and rimantadine.
Serologic Diagnosis	Serologic diagnosis is complicated by fact that antibody response is directed to original infecting influenza strain as well as to current infecting strain. CF methods are correlated with specific type of influenza virus, but CF antibodies tend to decrease several weeks after infection. Neutralization test (NT) and hemagglutination inhibition test are able to measure antibodies against subtype and strain specific antigens. NT closely predicts whether individual has sufficient antibody to prevent infection with currently circulating viral types. EIA methods may eventually replace CF testing.
Cell Cultures for Detection of Viruses from Clinical Specimen	Influenza A, B, and C viruses can be isolated in embryonated chicken eggs. Madin-Darby canine kidney cell, primary cynomolgus, or rhesus monkey kidney cells are susceptible to influenza viruses.
Oncogenic Potential	Not observed

GENERAL INFORMATION. The influenza viruses belong to the family Orthomyxoviridae, which are RNA viruses that contain eight (A and B types) or seven (C type) segments of single stranded RNA. Influenza C virus also differs from A and B in that it possesses only one surface glycoprotein that exhibits hemagglutinating esterase and fusion activities. In contrast, the most striking feature of both influenza A and B is their two projecting glycoproteins inserted into the viral membrane. The hemagglutinin (HA) spike initiates virus attachment, virus penetration, and membrane fusion. The HA also causes hemagglutination of erythrocytes. The second glycoprotein, or neuraminidase (NA), has a mushroom appearance, and the enzyme probably allows penetration of the virus past the mucous layer to the epithelial cells of the respiratory tract. The develop-

INFLUENZA VIRUSES

ment of antibody to both HA and NA helps determine an individual's immune status. Antibodies to NA can restrict the level of virus replications and are able to attenuate the disease. The more important antibodies to HA can prevent the start of an infection. The M2 or NB protein is also associated with the viral membrane and functions in viral uncoating and maturation. Resistance to the drugs amantadine and rimantadine is linked to a single amino acid change in the M2 protein.

Five internal nonglycosylated proteins (NP, M, and three polymerase proteins) are produced by the influenza viruses. NP plays a structural role in viral ribonucleoprotein formation. The M protein is located under the lipid envelope of the virus and participates in the control of viral RNA polymerase activity. NS1 and NS2 are nonstructural proteins, with NS1 synthesized early in infection and NS2 late in infection. Currently their function is unknown.

NOMENCLATURE OF INFLUENZA VIRUSES. All influenza viruses are either type A, B, or C. The classification of types A and B is followed consecutively by the geographic location of isolation, the laboratory number, the year of isolation, and finally, in parentheses, the subtype designation. A/Hong Kong/1/68 (H_3N_2) and A/Leningrad/360/86 (H_3N_2) are examples of this classification method. The two charts below list the hemagglutinin and neuraminidase subtypes of influenza A virus and the subtypes responsible for the influenza pandemics of the past hundred years.

Hemagglutinin and Neuraminidase: Subtypes of Influenza A

HEMAGGLUTININ		NEURAMINIDASE	
Subtype	Old Terminology	Subtype	Old Terminology
H_1	H_0, H_1, H_{SW}	N_1	N_1
H_2	H_2	N_2	N_2
H_3	H_3, Heq_2, HAV_7	N_3	NAV_2, NAV_3
H_4	HAV_4	N_4	NAV_4
H_5	HAV_5	N_5	NAV_5
H_6	HAV_6	N_6	NAV_6
H_7	Heq_1, HAV_1	N_7	Neq_1
H_8	HAV_8	N_8	Neq_2
H_9	HAV_9	N_9	NAV_6
H_{10}	HAV_2		
H_{11}	HAV_3		
H_{12}	HAV_{10}		
H_{13}	—		
H_{14}	—		
AV, avian; SW, swine; EQ, equine.			

Adapted from Zuckerman AJ, Banatuala JE, Pattison JR, eds: Principles and Practice of Clinical Virology, 3rd ed. New York, John Wiley, p 238.

**Pandemics Initiated by Influenza A
During the Last Hundred Years**

DATE	SUBTYPE
1890	H_2N_8
1900	H_3N_8
1918	H_1N_1
1957	H_2N_2
1968	H_3N_2

The previous chart illustrates that all pandemics are accompanied by a change in the hemagglutinin subunit, and in some pandemics the neuraminidase also underwent a change. Change in the hemagglutinin does not guarantee that a pandemic will follow. For example, in 1977 H_1N_1 reappeared without the initiation of a new pandemic (and was still circulating alone with H_3N_2 in 1997). When pandemics occur a new influenza virus subtype emerges and the population has no immunity against the new subtype.

ANTIGENIC SHIFT AND DRIFT. Antigenic shift is a major change in the subtype of influenza A, whereas antigenic drift is a minor change (point mutation) in the HA or NA of either influenza A or influenza B. The abrupt change, antigenic shift, is usually associated with pandemics, whereas antigenic drift is responsible for periodic epidemics. Two theories exist for explaining genetic shift. The first is called *genetic reassortment,* which occurs when a cell is infected with two different influenza viruses. New serotype(s) emerge due to the reassortment of eight RNA segments that constitute the influenza A viral genome. If the reassortment of the RNA segments results in a viral genome not previously present in a human population, a pandemic could result. The second theory states that a limited number of subtypes exist and they are periodically recycled after being inactive for several generations. It is possible that several mechanisms are responsible for the development of new subtypes.

COMPLICATIONS OF INFLUENZA. The common symptoms of influenza are described in the summary chart on pp 1108 and 1109. Pneumonia complications may be primary or secondary. Primary viral pneumonia is relatively uncommon but tends to be observed during influenza epidemics and is more likely to be seen in patients with preexisting cardiovascular disease. The more common secondary bacterial pneumonia tends to occur late in the disease. Secondary bacterial pneumonia is often observed in elderly persons and those with chronic disease including bronchitis, heart disease, diabetes mellitus, and renal disease and also in pregnant women. *Streptococcus pneumoniae, Haemophilus influenzae* and *Staphylococcus aureus* are the common etiologic agents responsible for the secondary pneumonias. Tracheobronchitis and bronchiolitis are additional respiratory symptoms observed in some patients who have influenza. A few patients develop myositis and myoglobulinuria in which the muscles are painful to touch, and muscle biopsies reveal necrosis of the muscle fibers.

Reye's syndrome (a life threatening illness) has been associated with both influenza A and influenza B as well as with VZV, HSV, adenovirus, CMV, echovirus, and coxsackievirus B5. Reye's syndrome is generally observed in children and rarely observed above the age of 17 years. Reye's syndrome is usually associated with a recent vi-

INFLUENZA VIRUSES

ral infection and is characterized by encephalopathy and fatty liver degeneration. Salicylates are not given to influenza patients as a rule because there is circumstantial evidence that the combination of acute influenza and salicylates increases the chance of Reye's syndrome.

VACCINATION. The vaccine that is currently in use employs inactivated virus that is cultured in eggs. A subunit vaccine has for the most part replaced the earlier whole or split virus vaccines. The current vaccines produce immunity in 60% to 90% of the population and produce relatively few side reactions. In contrast, the swine flu vaccine of 1976 (A/New Jersey/76) was associated with a high incidence of Guillain-Barré syndrome. This vaccine had to be recalled since approximately 350 people suffered from the syndrome. The current influenza vaccine is made from the subtypes of A and B that were prevalent the year before.

ENTEROVIRUSES

Family	Picornaviridae
Common Name(s)	Picornavirus, poliovirus, coxsackievirus A and B, and echovirus
Collection of Specimen	Specimens include throat and rectal swabs, feces, blood, spinal fluid, urine, pericardial fluid, conjunctival swabs, and tissue. Samples are often collected from several sites simultaneously.
Direct Examination	Direct examination is difficult because of large number and diversity of serotypes. PCR technique is currently most promising method for direct detection of enteroviruses (EVs).
Description of Agent *Diameter* *Capsid Symmetry* *Envelope* *Type of Nucleic Acid*	24–30 nm Icosahedral No Single stranded RNA
General Disease Categories	EVs cause wide range of diseases that affect respiratory, cardiovascular, and neurologic systems. See five charts on pp 1113 to 1115.
Population Infected	Neonates, young children, and families. See five charts on pp 1113 to 1115.
Incubation Period	Commonly 5–12 days
Primary Symptoms	See five charts on pp 1113 to 1115.
Transmission	Fecal-oral route
Treatment	Supportive
Prevention	Oral vaccine for polio is effective; otherwise avoid contact with the EVs.
Serologic Diagnosis	Serologic testing is difficult since there are so many EV serotypes and single common antigen is not available for testing.
Cell Cultures for Detection of Viruses from Clinical Specimen	"Gold standard" for diagnosis of EV is tissue culture isolation. Many laboratories employ combination of human diploid fibroblast cells (including W1-38, MRC-5, or HELF) along with continuous monkey kidney cells such as cynomolgus monkey kidney (CMK). Polioviruses, coxsackievirus B, and echoviruses are isolated in monkey kidney cells, whereas coxsackievirus A grows best in HELF.
Oncogenic Potential	Not observed

GENERAL INFORMATION. The enteroviruses (EVs) include 67 serotypes that are among the most important viral agents of human disease. They belong to the Picornaviridae family and have a capsid that contains four proteins (VP1 to VP4). Antigen diversity of the EVs is linked to variations within capsid proteins VP1, VP2, and VP3. In contrast, VP4 is in close association with the RNA core, and destabilization of this protein causes viral uncoding.

ENTEROVIRUS INFECTIONS. The next five charts list the various diseases that are associated with the EVs. Specific clinical syndromes are frequently associated with a few specific serotypes, but overlap occurs among the serotypes and the types of infections that they initiate. For example, paralytic poliomyelitis is usually caused by poliovirus serotypes 1, 2, and 3, but nonpolio EV can also be the etiologic agent (see next five charts). Febrile illness is the most common disease linked to the EVs. Rashes and upper respiratory symptoms (summer colds) may or may not accompany the febrile episode. The rhinoviruses in contrast are usually responsible for winter colds. The EVs may initiate outbreaks of "summer flu," which is sometimes associated with minor gastrointestinal symptoms such as diarrhea. The EVs are rarely associated with major enteric manifestations.

The most common cause of aseptic meningitis in young infants and children in the United States is EV. The outcome is nearly always benign, but many young infants are unnecessarily treated with antibiotics and antiherpes medication because simple criteria are not available to distinguish EV meningitis from the more serious forms of meningitis. The EVs are also responsible for causing many additional acute syndromes including poliomyelitis, encephalitis, myopericarditis, neonatal sepsis, Bornholm's disease (pleurodynia), hemorrhagic conjunctivitis, and exanthema (see next five charts).

The EVs have also been considered as possible etiologic agents in several chronic diseases. The exact role of coxsackievirus B's involvement in juvenile onset insulin dependent (type 1) diabetes mellitus remains unclear. Approximately 30% of type 1 diabetes patients have detectable IgM antibody against the coxsackievirus B. It has still not been determined whether these viruses initiate the events that cause diabetes. The EVs have also been implicated as possibly playing a role in chronic fatigue syndrome, amyotrophic lateral sclerosis, dermatomyositis, polymyositis, and hydrocephalus. The EVs have been linked to these diseases via serologic and nucleic acid hybridization studies. Direct proof has not yet been established.

Enterovirus: Poliovirus Subgroup

SEROTYPES	MAJOR DISEASE	TYPICAL PATIENT	SYMPTOMS
1–3	Polio	Children	Mild febrile illness, aseptic meningitis, or paralytic poliomyelitis may occur. Only 1% of infections end with neurologic involvement.
1–3	Postpolio syndrome	Adults	Additional muscle weakness develops many years after polio.

ENTEROVIRUSES

Enterovirus: Coxsackievirus A Subgroup

SEROTYPES	MAJOR DISEASE	TYPICAL PATIENT	SYMPTOMS
1–22, 24			
2, 4, 7, 9, 10	Aseptic meningitis	Young children	Patients have meningitis symptoms including stiffness of neck and muscle weakness.
1–6, 8, 10, and 22	Herpangina	Young children	Disease is characterized by sore throat, fever, vomiting, abdominal symptoms, and pain on swallowing. Small vesicular lesions are noted on palate, tonsils, fauces, and uvula.
4, 5, 9, and 16, with 16 most common	Exanthema (hand, foot, and mouth disease)	Family outbreaks are common.	Typical symptoms include mild fever and vesicular lesions on hands and feet. Buccal mucosa involvement also occurs. Lesions can be on genitals and buttocks.
24	Conjunctivitis	Family members; can occur in epidemics	Conjunctivitis can be mild, or subconjunctival hemorrhage may occur. Recovery generally occurs in 1 or 2 wk.
Many serotypes	Febrile illness with or without respiratory symptoms	Young children	Mild illness generally observed in summer and autumn.
4, 5, 6, 9, and 16	Rubelliform rashes	Children	Major symptoms are rubella-like maculopapular rash with or without fever, malaise, and cervical lymphadenopathy.
7	Polio-like illness	Children	See "Enterovirus: Poliovirus Subgroup" on p 1113.
4, 6, 9, 10	Bornholm's disease	Families and communities	See "Enterovirus: Coxsackievirus B Subgroup" following.

Enterovirus: Coxsackievirus B Subgroup

SEROTYPES	MAJOR DISEASE	TYPICAL PATIENTS	SYMPTOMS
1–6	Neonatal disease	Neonates	Symptoms range from mild to fulminating to death. Severe symptoms include myocarditis, pneumonia, meningoencephalitis, and sometimes hepatitis and jaundice.
1–6	Myopericarditis	Neonates, adolescents, and adults	Heart is infiltrated by virus and inflammatory cells. Disease is usually acute and severe in neonates but benign in adolescents and adults.
1–5	Bornholm's disease (epidemic pleurodynia)	Families and sometimes communities	Major symptoms are chest pain, abdominal pain, and fever. Some patients experience limb pain. Pain may mimic that of myocardial infarction.
1–6	Encephalitis	Children and young adults	Focal encephalitis with or without aseptic meningitis occurs, with few patients encountering damage to hypothalamus and pituitary endocrine glands.

Continued ▶

► Continued **Enterovirus: Coxsackievirus B Subgroup**

SEROTYPES	MAJOR DISEASE	TYPICAL PATIENTS	SYMPTOMS
1–6	Febrile illness with or without respiratory symptoms	Young children	See "Enterovirus: Coxsackievirus A Subgroup" on p 1114.
5	Rubelliform rash	Children	See "Enterovirus: Coxsackievirus A Subgroup" on p 1114.

Enterovirus: Echovirus Subtype

SEROTYPES	MAJOR DISEASE	TYPICAL PATIENTS	SYMPTOMS
1–9, 11–27, and 29–31			
Many	Febrile illness with or without respiratory symptoms	Young children	See "Enterovirus: Coxsackievirus A Subgroup" on p 1114.
Most	Aseptic meningitis	Young children	See "Enterovirus: Coxsackievirus A Subgroup" on p 1114.
9 and 16	Rubelliform rash	Children	See "Enterovirus: Poliovirus Subgroup" on p 1113.
Many	Paralysis, polio-like disease	Children	See "Enterovirus: Coxsackievirus A Subgroup" on p 1114.
9, 11, and 22	Myopericarditis	Neonates, adolescents, and adults	See "Enterovirus: Coxsackievirus B Subgroup" above.
19	Neonatal disease	Neonates	See "Enterovirus: Coxsackievirus B Subgroup" above.

Enterovirus: Enterovirus Subtype

SEROTYPES	MAJOR DISEASE	TYPICAL PATIENTS	SYMPTOMS
68, 69, and 70	Febrile illness with respiratory symptoms	Young children	See "Enterovirus: Coxsackievirus A Subgroup" on p 1114.
70	Epidemic conjunctivitis	Family members	See "Enterovirus: Coxsackievirus A Subgroup" on p 1114.
71	Polio-like illness	Children	See "Enterovirus: Coxsackievirus A Subgroup" on p 1114.
71	Exanthema (hand, foot, and mouth disease)	Family members	See "Enterovirus: Coxsackievirus A Subgroup" on p 1114.
71	Aseptic meningitis	Young children	See "Enterovirus: Coxsackievirus A Subgroup" on p 1114.

ENTEROVIRUSES

ROTAVIRUSES

Family	Reoviridae
Common Name(s)	Reovirus, rotavirus
Collection of Specimen	Stool specimens are collected during acute phase of illness, which optimally means 3–5 days after illness begins.
Direct Examination	Three different methods are used to detect rotavirus in stool specimens. EIAs, rapid membrane EIA, and latex agglutination (LA) methods have all been successful in detecting rotavirus. Membrane EIA yields results in 7 min, LA test within 30 min, and standard EIA in 75–150 min. Kits for all three methods are commercially available.
Description of Agent *Diameter* *Capsid Symmetry* *Envelope* *Type of Nucleic Acid*	70 nm 32 capsomeres in icosahedral arrangement No Double stranded RNA
General Disease Categories	Rotaviruses are major etiologic agent of viral gastroenteritis in infants and young children.
Population Infected	Infants and young children and occasionally elderly persons
Incubation Period	Approximately 1–2 days
Primary Symptoms	Major symptoms appear suddenly and include fever, vomiting, diarrhea, and dehydration. Occasionally, respiratory symptoms and abdominal pain are present.
Transmission	By fecal-oral route
Treatment	Supportive. Electrolyte and fluid replacement are necessary when severe dehydration occurs.
Prevention	Avoiding contact with virus is essential. Approximately 50% of rotavirus infections in hospitalized patients are nosocomial. Live attenuated vaccines administered by oral route are being evaluated.
Serologic Diagnosis	Serologic testing with serum is not performed. Major approach is to detect rotavirus via stool specimens.
Cell Cultures for Detection of Viruses from Clinical Specimen	Diagnostic laboratories do not attempt to culture rotaviruses. Virus is detected directly from stool specimens.
Oncogenic Potential	Not observed

GENERAL INFORMATION. Rotaviruses acquired their name because of the wheel-like appearance that was detected using the electron microscope. Rotaviruses belong to the Reoviridae family and are unique because the virus has 11 segments of double stranded RNA. Five rotavirus groups (A to E) exist, and types A, B, and C are associated with human disease. Type A is the major pathogen for humans. VP6 is the major inner core structural protein and is responsible for the group specificity (A to E) of the rotaviruses. VP7 is a glycosylated outer capsid protein and is responsible for G serotype specificity of the A rotavirus group. Serotypes 1 to 4 are the major G serotypes, with serotype 1 the most common in causing human gastroenteritis.

ROTAVIRUS GASTROENTERITIS. In the United States, the rotaviruses are commonly associated with endemic infections that usually occur in the winter and occasionally in the autumn or spring. Small epidemics may occur, but large epidemics are uncommon. In the tropics rotavirus infection takes place year-round. Nosocomial infections are common, especially in neonatal nurseries.

The major clinical symptoms are diarrhea, vomiting, fever, and in severe cases dehydration. Patients may also experience abdominal pain and respiratory symptoms. Reinfection with different serotypes of rotavirus does occur, but antibody production tends to reduce the severity of the reinfection. Breast feeding affords some protection to the infant against rotavirus infection. The mechanism of this protection is currently unknown.

ADDITIONAL VIRUSES ASSOCIATED WITH GASTROENTERITIS. The rotavirus and the adenoviruses (especially serotypes 40 and 41) are the two most common etiologic agents associated with gastroenteritis in young patients. The diarrhea symptoms associated with the adenoviruses can last typically for 5 to 12 days and in some cases more than 2 weeks. The diarrhea associated with rotavirus tends to be of shorter duration, but the degree of dehydration can sometimes be life threatening. The chart on p 1118 compares the characteristics of the rotaviruses and adenoviruses along with the other viruses associated with gastroenteritis, namely the caliciviruses, Norwalk, Norwalk-like viruses, and astroviruses. Less detail is known about the caliciviruses and Norwalk-like viruses. Direct electron microscopy on fecal samples is useful in identifying the gastroenteritis viruses. Finally, coronaviruses have been implicated in causing sporadic human cases of gastrointestinal disease. The coronaviruses are unique among the enteric viruses since electron microscopic studies show helical viruses with an envelope.

ROTAVIRUSES

Characteristics of Human Gastroenteritis Viruses

CHARACTERISTIC	CALICIVIRUS*	NORWALK AND NORWALK-LIKE VIRUSES*	ROTAVIRUS	ADENOVIRUS	ASTROVIRUS
Diameter (nm)	35	27–35 (diameter smaller than that of calicivirus)	70	70–90	28–30
Capsid Symmetry	32 capsomeres in icosahedral arrangement	32 capsomeres in icosahedral arrangement	32 capsomeres in icosahedral arrangement	252 capsomeres in icosahedral arrangement	—
Envelope	No	No	No	No	—
Nucleic Acid	Single stranded RNA	Single stranded RNA	Double stranded RNA	Double stranded DNA	Single stranded RNA
Serotypes Associated with Human Disease	5	3	3 (groups A, B, and C)	2	5
Incubation Period	48–72 hr	24 hr	24–48 hr	8–10 days	3–4 days
Typical Age of Patient (yr)	<2†	<6†	0.5–2†	<2†	<7†
Duration of Illness	1–11 days	12–48 hr	2–10 days	2–14 days	Usually 3 days but can be up to 14 days if diarrhea is severe
Occurrence	Year-round (higher in winter months)	Year-round	Winter (occasionally autumn or fall)	Year-round	—
Endemic or Epidemic	Endemic and epidemic	Endemic and epidemic	Endemic and epidemic	Endemic	Endemic

*Calicivirus, Norwalk virus, and Norwalk-like virus are closely related and belong to the Caliciviridae family.
†Gastroenteritis occasionally occurs in adults, especially if they are elderly and/or immunosuppressed.

RABIES VIRUS

Family	Rhabdoviridae
Common Name(s)	Rabies, rhabdovirus
Collection of Specimen	No single tissue sample has been positive in every case of human rabies. Specimens collected generally include skin biopsy, saliva, serum, and occasionally CSF. Postmortem specimens include medulla, cerebellum, and hippocampus. Animals suspected with rabies are killed and their brain tissue is collected.
Direct Examination	Direct IF antibody test is employed to detect viral antigen in brain tissue. Histologic tests that rely on detected Negri bodies are not as sensitive.
Description of Agent *Diameter* *Capsid Symmetry* *Envelope* *Type of Nucleic Acid*	180 by 75 nm (bullet shape) Helical Yes Single stranded RNA
General Disease Categories	Rabies virus affects CNS.
Population Infected	Rabies is infectious disease of warm blooded animals, including humans of any age.
Incubation Period	Varies from 10 days to 1 yr in humans, with average between 1 and 3 mo. Incubation period is shorter in children and shorter if bite is close to brain.
Primary Symptoms	Prodromal period of 2–7 days is characterized by nonspecific complaints. Two basic clinical patterns that can follow are "furious form" or "dumb form." Furious form is characterized by periods of extreme agitation, delirium, and insomnia, with hydrophobia occurring in 50% of cases. These episodes may be accompanied by frothing of mouth. Second form, or dumb rabies, appears in 14%–60% of cases and is characterized by paralysis that often involves initially bitten limb but then rapidly spreads.
Transmission	Rabies is spread by deposition of virus laden saliva into wound via animal bite. It can also be spread by ingestion of infected material. Human to human transmission has been recorded after cornea transplant.
Treatment	Supportive. If wound is superficial, cleaning with benzalkonium chloride may inactivate virus.
Prevention	Rabies immunoglobulins and vaccine (five injections) are given to patients exposed to saliva of rabid animals.
Serologic Diagnosis	ELISA or neutralization assay is used to test for immunity after vaccine is initiated. These assays measure antibody to surface G protein of virus.
Cell Cultures for Detection of Viruses from Clinical Specimen	Murine neuroblastoma cells are sensitive to street rabies strain. Saliva or brain suspensions of medulla, cerebellum, and hippocampus are used as inoculum source.
Oncogenic Potential	Not observed

RABIES VIRUS

GENERAL INFORMATION. The rabies virus is bullet shaped and contains five proteins including the surface glycoprotein (G), a second membrane or matrix (M) protein, a phosphorylated nucleoprotein (N), a nucleocapsid associated phosphoprotein (NS), and a transcriptase protein (L). Only the G and N proteins are important in the diagnosis and treatment of rabies. Vaccines containing only the G protein ensure immunity to infection with the rabies virus. The N protein conveys some host immunity against the rabies virus, but it is not as effective as the G. Serologic tests are performed after the initiation of the vaccine protocol. Neutralization and ELISA tests are directed against the G protein.

The rabies virus is found in the saliva of infected animals. Dogs are a major risk in transferring the virus to humans, especially in Latin America, Asia, and Africa. In contrast, dog rabies cases in the United States have declined to about 200 a year because of the rabies control programs. The major threat in the United States comes from wild animals such as skunks, raccoons, foxes, wolves, and bats. Bats are a perpetual source of the rabies virus, and the disease may debilitate a bat so that it falls to the ground and then is eaten by another animal.

DISEASE. The incubation period for rabies is generally 1 to 3 months, but it can range from 10 days to 1 year. The shorter incubation periods are associated with bites that are close to the brain. Preventive treatment includes a series of five injections (vaccine) and the administration of human rabies immunoglobulin. Patients not receiving the treatments nearly always die. There are only a few recorded cases in which a person survived rabies without receiving the vaccine.

After the rabies virus has entered an animal or a person it travels from the nerve trunks to the CNS. A prodromal syndrome may be followed by early symptoms of tingling or burning, as well as pain at the site of infection. This is followed by the paralysis of the muscles of swallowing and glottal spasms that occur when drinking. The patient also exhibits periods of extreme agitation, delirium, hyperactivity, and insomnia. These are the symptoms of "furious" rabies, which terminates in tetany, respiratory paralysis, and convulsions. A second form of rabies is known as "dumb rabies." Dumb, or paralytic, rabies is also initiated with prodromal symptoms, after which paralysis often begins at the site of the bite and spreads rapidly. Sphincter control is lost and failure of the respiratory muscles is a terminal event. Generally, patients with dumb rabies survive for a longer period than those with the furious type. Survival times are generally less than 2 weeks. Those patients whose survival time is extended by intensive therapy suffer complications including cardiac dysrhythmias, and electrolyte, pH, and blood gas disturbances, as well as CNS complications including diabetes insipidus and abnormal thermoregulation.

HUMAN IMMUNODEFICIENCY VIRUSES

Family	Retroviridae
Common Name(s)	Retrovirus, HIV-1 and HIV-2
Collection of Specimen	Serologic analyses usually depend on blood samples collected by venipuncture. The virus can be collected from peripheral blood mononuclear cells or from other body fluids such as CSF, urine, genital secretions, saliva, tears, and breast milk. Biopsy specimens are occasionally used even though viral load may be low.
Direct Examination	HIV can be detected in serum or cell culture supernatants via sandwich ELISA. Generally P24 protein is detected by this method. IFA method can detect virus from peripheral blood mononuclear cells.

Continued ▶

HUMAN IMMUNODEFICIENCY VIRUSES

Description of Agent	
Diameter	80–130 nm
Capsid Symmetry	Icosahedral
Envelope	Yes
Type of Nucleic Acid	Single stranded RNA
General Disease Categories	HIV induces variety of disease states including acute mononucleosis-like or flulike syndrome, prolonged asymptomatic state, symptomatic state, and finally AIDS. HIV-2 may cause milder disease than HIV-1.
Population Infected	HIV infects primarily adults and occasionally neonates and children.
Incubation Period	Approximately 10 yr are required for 50% of HIV infected individuals to develop full blown AIDS. Another 20%–30% show signs of infections, and 20% are symptom free for more than 10 yr.
Primary Symptoms	Initial acute infection is characterized by headache, fatigue, diarrhea, fever, sore throat, myalgia, arthralgia, lymphadenopathy, macular rash, and neurologic complaints. The most common symptoms when an HIV positive individual develops AIDS include fatigue, night sweats, persistent diarrhea, and sustained weight loss. Increased frequency of infection especially with HSV and *Candida albicans* (thrush and vulvovaginal candidiasis) are commonly observed.
Transmission	HIV can be transmitted sexually or by blood and blood products, and by perinatal exposure.
Treatment	Three classes of drugs have been approved to treat HIV infections. Zidovudine (AZT), didanosine (ddI), zalcitabine (ddC), lamivudine (3TC), and stavudine (d4T) are nucleoside analogs. Protease inhibitors include saquinavir, ritonavir, and indinavir. Non-nucleoside analogs such as nevirapine constitute the 3rd class of antiviral therapy. Treatment of all opportunistic infections in HIV patients is essential.
Prevention	Prevention is achieved by avoiding contact with infected blood, blood products, and body secretions. Blood banks currently screen donors for antibody to HIV. Sexual transmission can be minimized by practicing safe sex.
Serologic Diagnosis	ELISA is used to screen for HIV and Western blot assay is most common test to confirm presence of HIV specific antibodies.
Cell Cultures for Detection of Viruses from Clinical Specimen	Classic method is to grow HIV in human peripheral blood mononuclear cells (PBMCs) that are stimulated with phytohemagglutinin and interleukin 2. Indicator cells are usually cocultured with PBMCs. P24 antigen is detected in culture supernatants.
Oncogenic Potential	Not observed. HIV infection is associated with certain cancers including Kaposi's sarcoma, B cell lymphoma, and anal carcinoma. Increased rate of these cancers in HIV patients awaits clarification. One theory suggests that immune suppression prevents proper immune surveillance.

GENERAL INFORMATION. The retroviruses belong to the family Retroviridae, which is divided into three subfamilies: the Lentivirinae (HIV), the Oncovirinae (the oncogenic viruses including the human T cell leukemia virus types I and II [HTLV-I and HTLV-II]), and the Spumavirinae (the foamy viruses), which are not known to be pathogenic. HIV-1 was the first human immunodeficiency virus isolated from a patient. Three years later (1986) a second subtype of HIV (HIV-2) was isolated from patients from West Africa. Currently, HIV-1 is the predominant virus in the United States with relatively few cases of HIV-2 known. HIV-2 has become common in Europe, South

America, and India. Patients infected with HIV-2 do develop AIDS, but infected patients survive for a longer time than those with HIV-1. HIV-2 also exhibits reduced cytopathic effects in cell culture. The viral load of HIV-2 appears to be less than that of HIV-1 and probably accounts for the longer survival rate of HIV-2 patients.

All retroviruses including HIV have three genes in the order 5′-*gag-pol-env*-3′. The envelope *(env)* gene first produces a glycosylated precursor polypeptide (gp160) that is processed by a cellular protease into the surface glycoprotein (SU, gp120) and the transmembrane glycoprotein (TM, gp41). The gp120 protein forms a spike on the HIV and binds to the CD4 receptor present on host cells such as CD4+ lymphocytes and undifferentiated CD4+ monocytes. The gp41 transmembrane protein allows the virus to fuse with the cell surface and is also responsible for cytopathic changes such as syncytium formation. Neutralizing antibodies that are produced react with the susceptible regions of the gp120 protein. When HIV is recovered over time from the same individuals, studies have shown that their sera fail to neutralize the homologous virus (the strain isolated at the same time the serum was collected) in an effective fashion. The sera are better able to neutralize autologous strains or strains grown in the laboratory. These studies indicate that the virus undergoes a change to avoid immune antiviral responses of the host. The inability of the host to neutralize the current HIV strain is commonly observed in symptomatic patients.

In addition to CD4 receptors, macrophages have a second receptor site (CCR5) that plays a role in allowing HIV to bind to the cell. Eventually a more lethal form of HIV may emerge from the infected macrophage. This enhanced version of HIV can bind to CCR5 as well as to additional receptors such as CXCR4, CCR3, and CCR26.

This expanded range of receptors allows HIV to enter many types of T cell lymphocytes as well as addition cells such as those found in the brain. Recently, a mutant form of the CCR5 gene has been discovered. The mutation makes it more difficult for HIV to enter macrophages. Patients who are heterozygous for the altered CCR5 gene generally develop full blown AIDS more slowly than patients with normal CCR5 receptors. It is believed that patients with a homozygous altered CCR5 gene produce macrophages that are not infected by HIV. Many patients with a homozygous altered CCR5 gene have not become HIV positive even though they have engaged in high-risk behavior. However, protection against HIV infection is not absolute for those with a homozygous altered CCR5 gene, as several cases of HIV infection have been reported for this patient group.

The first two genes, or Gag-Pol precursor protein, are cleaved by the viral protease into seven proteins. The four gag proteins include p17(MA); p24 or p25(CA); p9; and p6. The p25 is the major Gag protein and forms a protein shell around the viral RNA and proteins p9 and p6. P9 is required for packaging of the RNA, whereas the function of p6 is not certain, but its absence blocks infectivity. P17 is a matrix protein and is required for virion formation.

The Gag-Pol precursor protein is cleaved into three components. The protease (PR) is involved in the post-translation processing of viral proteins. In clinical trials a number of protease inhibitors have been able to reduce the patients' viral load. The Pol region also encodes a reverse transcriptase molecule or RNA dependent DNA polymerase. The nucleoside analogs such as AZT work by inhibiting the enzyme reverse transcriptase (RT). The last component of Pol protein is the integrase (IN), which allows the virus to integrate into host DNA. Antiviral drugs have not yet been developed against this protein.

There are at least three regulatory genes *(Tat, Rev,* and *Nef)* associated with HIV, and their functions are described in the chart on p 1123. There are also several accessory HIV viral gene products (ViF, Vpu/Vpx, and Vpr) that affect viral infectivity, assembly, and budding.

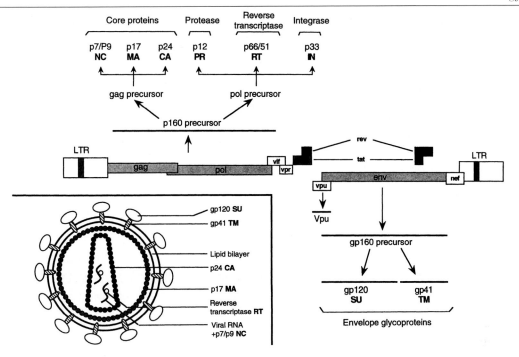

From Bour S, Gelezuwasir R, Wainberger M: The human immunodeficiency virus type 1 (HIV-1) CD4 receptor and its central role in promotion of HIV-1 infection. Microbiol Rev 59(1):69, 1995.

HUMAN IMMUNODEFICIENCY VIRUSES

Human Immunodeficiency Virus Proteins and Their Functions

PROTEIN	SIZE (kDa)	FUNCTION
Gag	p25 (p24)	Capsid (CA) structural protein
	p17	Matrix (MA) protein—myristoylated
	p9	RNA binding protein (?)
	p6	RNA binding protein (?); helps in virus budding
Polymerase (Pol)	p66, p51	Reverse transcriptase (RT); RNAse H—inside core
Protease (PR)	p10	Post-translation processing of viral proteins
Integrase (IN)	p32	Viral cDNA integration
Envelope	gp120	Envelope surface (SU) protein
	gp41 (gp36)	Envelope transmembrane (TM) protein
Tat†	p14	Transactivation
Rev†	p19	Regulation of viral mRNA expression
Nef†	p27	Pleiotropic, including virus suppression; myristoylated
Vif	p23	Increases virus infectivity and cell to cell transmission; helps in proviral DNA synthesis and/or in virion assembly (?)

Continued ▶

▶ Continued **Human Immunodeficiency Virus Proteins and Their Functions**

PROTEIN	SIZE (kDa)	FUNCTION
Vpr	p15	Helps in virus replication; transactivation (?)
Vpu†‡	p16	Helps in virus release; disrupts gp160-CD4 complexes
Vpx§	p15	Helps in infectivity
Tev§	p26	Tat and Rev activities

†Not found associated with the virion.
‡Only present with HIV-1. Expression appears regulated by Vpr.
§Only coded by HIV-2. May be a duplication of Vpr.
From Levy JA: HIV and the Pathogenesis of AIDS. Washington, DC, ASM Press, 1994.

CLINICAL EVENTS IN HUMAN IMMUNODEFICIENCY VIRUS INFECTIONS. The initial mononucleosis-like illness initiated by HIV is well documented (see summary chart above). In addition to the mononucleosis-like syndrome, many patients experience mucocutaneous disease in which ulcers may develop on the buccal mucosa, esophagus, gingiva, palate, and even on the anus and penis. Lymphadenopathy is often seen by the second week of illness and affects up to 70% of the patients. Many patients experience an erythematous maculopapular rash on the face and trunk. Temporary neurologic features including aspectic meningoencephalitis can also occur. The number of CD8 lymphocytes increases, and this helps to reverse the CD4 to CD8 ratio. A temporary drop in CD4 cells is also observed, and an asymptomatic thrombocytopenia may occur during this phase. A viremia occurs but is cleared via the action of cytotoxic T lymphocytes.

An asymptomatic phase or latent phase may last for months or years. The length of this phase is dependent on multiple factors including the dose of the virus, the route of the infection, the genetics of the host, and the immune response generated by the host. The clinical latency described here is not associated with viral latency. The virus still continues to replicate in the lymphoreticular tissue.

The progression of HIV infection to symptomatic disease is associated with signs of an activated immune system. Clinically the patient may experience a generalized lymphadenopathy, and dermatologic signs such as lesions associated with eczema or psoriasis may appear. Laboratory signs that immune activation is occurring include elevated levels of β_2 microglobulin, neopterin, and interleukin 2. The Centers for Disease Control and Prevention (CDC) has listed criteria in which an individual may be classified as having AIDS. Adolescents and adults with HIV are classified as having AIDS if their CD4+ lymphocyte count is under 200/μL and/or if their CD4+ T lymphocyte percentage is less than 14. In addition, HIV infected patients whose CD4+ count is less than 200/μL who acquire certain infectious diseases or malignancies are also classified as having AIDS. A partial list includes Kaposi's sarcoma, Burkitt's or immunoblastic or primary brain lymphoma, invasive cervical cancer, *Pneumocystis carinii* pneumonia, toxoplasmosis of the brain, histoplasmosis, cryptococcosis (extrapulmonary), candidiasis, coccidioidomycosis, CMV retinitis, chronic isosporiasis, chronic intestinal cryptosporidiosis, and various *Mycobacterium* infections. Successful treatment of the infectious diseases is paramount to the long term survival of AIDS patients.

The various organisms that initiate opportunistic infections in AIDS patients can be placed into three categories. The first category includes pathogens that can also invade hosts with normal immune systems. *Mycobacterium tuberculosis*, *Salmonella*, and *Shigella* species are examples of microorganisms that cause widespread severe disease in normal hosts as well as in AIDS patients. The second category is pathogens that usually cause mild disease in normal hosts but may cause life threatening disease in AIDS patients. *Toxoplasma gondii* and herpes simplex virus are examples. Finally, the last category is organisms that do not initiate disease in the normal host. Pneumonias caused by *P. carinii* and *Mycobacterium avium-intracellulare* are examples.

STATUS OF HUMAN IMMUNODEFICIENCY VIRUS PATIENTS. The CD4+ count, viral loads, and the presence of immune activation markers can be used to predict the progression of the disease. An abrupt or gradual decline in the CD4 count usually indicates that clinical disease will follow. Approximately 87% of patients who have a CD4+ count of less than 200/μL develop AIDS within 3 years, whereas patients whose counts are between 200 and 400 convert to AIDS at about a 46% rate within 3 years. Finally those patients with a CD4+ count above 500/μL develop AIDS at a 16% rate for the same time period. The rate of decline of CD4+ cells is also linked to developing AIDS. Patients whose CD4+ count drops by 125/μL per year are much more likely to develop AIDS than those patients who average a CD4+ loss of 60/μL per year.

Plasma viremia has also been directly linked to clinical stages. In acute primary infection the viral load rises to about 5×10^6 virions/mL and then drops back to 8×10^4 virions/mL during the asymptomatic stage. The viral load rises to 3.5×10^5 virions/mL during the early symptomatic stage and continues to climb to about 2.5×10^6 virions/mL when AIDS is diagnosed.

Viral load and CD4+ cell counts are used to monitor the effectiveness of antiviral therapy. Combinations of various drugs including nucleoside analogs, protease inhibitors, and non-nucleoside analogs are administered to the patient. Often the viral load decreases in about 2 weeks, and if the treatment is successful the maximal effect should occur by 6 months. The viral load level at the 6 month point is referred to as the *set point*. The patient should then be monitored for viral load every 3 or 4 months. If the viral load rises above the set point, the patient should be switched to a new combination of drugs.

An indirect method to measure virus production is to monitor immune activation markers. Increases of β_2 microglobulin in plasma or increases in neopterin in the urine correlate with the degree of lymphocyte activation and also indicate progression to disease in HIV patients.

ANTIVIRAL THERAPY. The oldest class of drug, namely the nucleoside analogs, blocks the ability of HIV to make copies of itself by inhibiting the enzyme RT. The non-nucleoside analogs carry out the same function as the nucleoside analogs but do so without mimicking viral genetic material. The protease inhibitors block the protease enzyme of HIV, which is needed for packaging new viruses and releasing them into the bloodstream. Clinical trials have indicated that the protease inhibitors can reduce viral loads especially when multiple combinations of drugs are employed. HIV has been shown to readily mutate to overcome the effects of a potent antiviral drug. It is thought that HIV will find it more difficult to mutate if three or more drugs are used in combination. Theoretically a three drug combination may mean that about a dozen mutations will be required for HIV to become resistant. Preliminary testing indicates that cross-resistance develops in patients taking protease inhibitors. The smallest amount of cross-resistance appears to be induced when saquinavir is employed.

OTHER RETROVIRUSES. HTLV-I is an oncogenic virus that is the etiologic agent for adult T cell leukemia-lymphoma (ATL) and tropical spastic paraparesis (TSP) or HTLV-I associated myelopathy (HAM). The routes of transmission for HTLV-I resemble those described for HIV, except HTLV-I transmission is cell associated. Recipients of HTLV-I cellular component will seroconvert, whereas blood transfusion patients who

Anti-HIV Therapy

CLASS		
Nucleoside Analog	**Non-Nucleoside Analog**	**Protease Inhibitor**
Zidovudine (AZT)	Nevirapine (Viramine, B1-RG-587) Delavirdine (Rescriptor)	Saquinavir (Invirase)
Didanosine (ddl)		Ritonavir (Norvir)
Zalcitabine (ddC)		Indinavir (Crixivan)
Lamivudine (3TC)		Ag1343* (Viracept)
Stavudine (d4t)		Nelfinar* (Viracept)
		141W94*
		DMP-450*
*Experimental, not approved by Food and Drug Administration.		

receive only plasma from infected donors remain seronegative. HTLV-I can also be transmitted via breast milk containing lymphocytes. In the United States asymptomatic blood donors have an infection rate of only 0.025%, whereas a high rate of 7% to 49% is observed in prostitutes and intravenous drug users. Japan (southwestern), Taiwan, parts of Central and South America, sub-Saharan Africa, and the Caribbean basin experience a higher (0.3% to 8%) seropositive population.

Only 5% of HTLV-I carriers will develop leukemia during their life span. The disease has a long latency period of 30 to 40 years. Asymptomatic, preleukemic, smoldering chronic, and acute are the four transitional categories of ATL. Patients with acute ATL generally survive for less than 1 year. The major symptoms include lymphadenopathy, hepatosplenomegaly, and infiltration of leukemic cells, which causes skin lesions. Abnormal chemistry tests such as hypercalcemia associated with bone resorption, hyperbilirubinemia, and elevated serum lactate dehydrogenase levels are observed. Patients also exhibit elevated leukocyte counts and sometimes granulocytosis and eosinophilia.

A second syndrome associated with HTLV-I infection is the neurologic disease HAM/TSP, which may develop within a few years after infection by blood products. The disease is rare and only occurs at a frequency of 0.3% of HTLV-I carriers. The disease begins slowly, often with leg weakness and spastic paraparesis, which results in sphincter malfunction and incontinence. HAM/TSP patients may have atypical lymphocytes resembling ALT cells in the peripheral blood.

A second virus, HTLV-II, was originally isolated from a patient with hairy T cell leukemia. The possible association of HTLV-II with disease is uncertain since nearly all infected patients are asymptomatic and exhibit no significant hematologic or immunologic abnormalities.

A third retrovirus, simian immunodeficiency virus (SIV), can give rise to an AIDS-like disease in certain primate species such as the rhesus macaque but is relatively avirulent for their species of origin, which is the African green monkey. HIV-2 and SIV have glycoproteins that cross-react serologically, and a few investigators have suggested that HIV-2 may be derived from SIV.

HEPATITIS A VIRUS AND HEPATITIS E VIRUS

	HEPATITIS A VIRUS (HAV)	**HEPATITIS E VIRUS (HEV)**
Family	Picornaviridae	Family not currently assigned. Suggested classification is as calicivirus.
Common Name(s)	Infectious hepatitis	Enterically transmitted non-A, non-B hepatitis (ET-NANB)
Collection of Specimen	Feces are collected either before illness or up to several days after symptoms begin. Fecal slurries can be stored at −70°C for several months. Serum can be stored at 4°C for up to 5 days since antibody titers are reasonably stable. Longer term storage for up to 6 mo is acceptable if temperature is reduced to −20 to −70°C.	Feces and serum are collected as early as possible during illness. Acute phase samples are also collected, with serum stored at −70°C until it is tested.
Direct Examination	Immune electron microscopy (IEM) can detect HAV particles in fecal specimens. However, IEM is expensive and time consuming. Radioimmune assays (RIAs) are able to detect HAV particles in serum samples. Clinical specimens can also be processed by PCR or molecular hybridization of HAV RNA with cloned HAV cDNA to detect virus particles. Commonly, serologic methods to detect antibody are method of choice to detect HAV infections.	There are no routine methods for detecting HEV particles in clinical specimens. Both IEM and PCR methods have been able to detect HEV particles in feces, as well as in bile and liver samples.
Description of Agent *Diameter* *Capsid Symmetry* *Envelope* *Type of Nucleic Acid*	27 nm 32 capsomers in icosahedral arrangement No Single stranded RNA	29 nm Icosahedral No Single stranded RNA
General Disease Categories	Gastroenteritis	Gastroenteritis
Population Infected	Asymptomatic infections generally occur in children. Most symptomatic cases involve adults.	HEV is mostly a disease of young adults. Children can have symptomatic disease.
Incubation Period	Average of 28 days	Average of 40 days
Prevalence	Worldwide	Mostly in Africa, Asia, and Mexico
Endemic Infection United States	Yes, estimated at 143,000 cases per year	No; also not observed in northern Europe, Japan, and Australia
Natural Host	Humans and primates. Disease in nonhuman primates is very mild.	Humans are only known hosts.

Continued ▶

▶ Continued **HEPATITIS A VIRUS AND HEPATITIS E VIRUS**

	HEPATITIS A VIRUS (HAV)	**HEPATITIS E VIRUS (HEV)**
Primary Symptoms	Nonspecific prodromal period of fever, chills, fatigue, malaise, and headache is followed a few days later by nausea, vomiting, anorexia, and sometimes abdominal pain associated with right upper quadrant. When jaundice occurs, there is usually rapid improvement of clinical symptoms.	Prodromal symptoms may occur with HEV and are followed by acute phase symptoms of nausea, vomiting, abdominal pain, anorexia, fever, and pruritus. Jaundice may or may not be present.
Cholestasis	Less frequent	More frequent
Mortality Rate	Approximately 0.6%	Generally 1%–2%. 10%–20% during pregnancy, with highest rate occurring in 3rd trimester.
Transmission	Fecal-oral is major route. However, sexual transmission, especially within male homosexual population, has been described. Transmission via blood transfusion and intravenous drug use is rare.	Fecal-oral
Treatment	Supportive	Supportive
Prevention	In Europe inactivated vaccine is available. Vaccine preparation will shortly be available in United States. Passive immunization with immune serum globulin can protect individuals after known exposure to HAV.	Passive immune serum globulin has not prevented HEV. Vaccine is not available. Improvements in sanitation control outbreaks.
Serologic Diagnosis	Acute disease is diagnosed by IgM anti-HAV, and immunity is accessed by total anti-HAV.	Accurate conclusions with particular patient are difficult. However, IgM anti-HEV or IgA-anti HEV are used to identify acute or recent infections. Past infections are indicated by presence of anti-HEV antibody (IgG or total).
Cell Cultures for Detection of Viruses from Clinical Specimen	HAV is difficult to propagate in cell culture. Many human and primate cell lines can be employed.	There are no practical cell lines to propagate HEV.
Oncogenic Potential	Not observed	Not observed

GENERAL INFORMATION ON HEPATITIS VIRUSES (A TO G). Five different viruses known as hepatitis A to E can cause acute hepatitis. A new hepatitis virus provisionally called G could be responsible for disease in 10% to 20% of individuals who have unexplained chronic hepatitis. A few cases of hepatitis F disease have been described. However, the existence of HVF remains very unclear.

The viruses are divided into two groups based on their mechanism of transmission. Hepatitis B (HBV), hepatitis C (HCV), hepatitis D (HDV), and probably hepatitis G (HGV) are transmitted predominantly by the parenteral route, whereas hepatitis A (HAV) and hepatitis E (HEV) are spread predominantly by the fecal-oral route. HAV and HEV usually cause mild, self-limiting infections without adverse sequelae. In contrast, HBV, HCV, and HDV are able to cause more serious disease that can lead to chronic hepatitis, cirrhosis, and hepatocellular carcinoma. HGV (also referred to as GBV-C) appears to be most similar to HCV in terms of the clinical consequences of infection. Approximately 10% to 20% of patients infected with HCV are coinfected with HGV.

The symptoms do not allow the diagnosis of a specific agent. Viral hepatitis can be asymptomatic, symptomatic, acute, or fulminant. The gravity of viral hepatitis varies from individual to individual. If the symptoms of hepatitis persist 6 months or more and if accompanied by abnormal liver enzyme levels, the patient is classified as having chronic hepatitis. Chronic active hepatitis may lead to cirrhosis, hepatic failure, or hepatocellular carcinoma. In contrast, patients with chronic persistent hepatitis often exhibit benign symptoms even though they continue to carry the virus. Their liver enzyme levels often return to normal limits.

HEPATITIS A VIRUS AND HEPATITIS E VIRUS. HAV is a member of the Picornaviridae family and belongs to the genus *Hepatovirus*. The virus produces four major structural proteins (VP1, VP2, VP3, and PX). A fifth truncated protein (VP4) has been predicted. The specific cell receptors for HAV have not been characterized. There is a single serotype that is very stable and resists a temperature of up to 60°C as well as a pH of 3.

The classification of HEV has not reached the point that allows HEV to be assigned a family designation. There are suggested similarities with the caliciviruses. Only one serotype is known, and the proteins associated with HEV are poorly characterized.

Neither HAV nor HEV is associated with chronic liver disease, although complications can occur for either type of hepatitis. A cholestatic form is more common with HEV than with HAV. Fulminant forms of HAV and HEV are unusual except in the case of HEV infecting pregnant women, especially during the third trimester. The mortality rate may then reach between 10% and 20%. Currently HEV cases that occur in the United States result from travel in the known areas of endemicity (see summary chart above). Still most epidemiologists believe that all Americans should be considered at risk for infection with HEV.

HEPATITIS B VIRUS AND HEPATITIS D VIRUS

	HEPATITIS B VIRUS (HBV)	**HEPATITIS D VIRUS (HDV)**
Family	Hepadnaviridae	Unclassified
Common Name(s)	Hepadnavirus, hepatitis B virus (HBV)	Hepatitis D virus (HDV), delta virus
Collection of Specimen	Serum is usually optimal specimen.	Serum is usually optimal specimen.
Direct Examination	Direct examination of liver and other tissue can be performed by utilizing IF, immunohistochemistry, in situ hybridization, biotin-streptavidin system, and thin section electron microscopy. Serologic testing is routinely performed since direct examination techniques are not practical for testing large number of specimens.	Detecting HDV in liver biopsies is restricted to specialized laboratories. Liver biopsies are processed by immunohistochemical staining to demonstrate intrahepatic HD antigen.

Continued ▶

► Continued **HEPATITIS B VIRUS AND HEPATITIS D VIRUS**

	HEPATITIS B VIRUS (HBV)	**HEPATITIS D VIRUS (HDV)**
Description of Agent *Diameter*	42–47 nm is infectious particle; 20 nm spherical particle and filamentous 20 nm by 1 μm particle are noninfectious.	35–37 nm
Capsid Symmetry	Icosahedral	—
Envelope	Yes	Yes
Type of Nucleic Acid	Double stranded DNA; one strand is incomplete.	Single stranded RNA
General Disease Categories	Acute hepatitis, chronic hepatitis, cirrhosis, and hepatocellular carcinoma	Acute hepatitis, chronic hepatitis, cirrhosis, and hepatocellular carcinoma
Population Infected	Primarily young adults	HDV can initiate infections in patients with previous HBV infection or requires HBV in order to co-infect. Population infected is primarily young adults.
Incubation Period	For acute HBV infection, incubation period is generally 6–16 wk. Incubation period is dose dependent.	For acute HDV infection incubation period is about 3–13 wk.
Primary Symptoms	Symptoms range from mild to severe. Slow insidious prodromal period often includes fevers, malaise, myalgia, dulling of gustatory and olfactory senses, nausea, vomiting, and weight loss. Acute or icteric phase lasts about 1 mo, and jaundice as well as presence of dark urine may be detected.	Acute coinfections with HBV and HDV result in acute hepatitis that cannot be distinguished from acute HBV infection except that severity is often greater. Superinfection of HDV in HBV carriers usually causes chronic HDV.
Asymptomatic Patients	Most children and 50% of adults are asymptomatic.	Patients are rarely asymptomatic.
Onset of Symptoms	Insidious	Abrupt
Fulminant Hepatitis Rate	<1.5%	About 5% with coinfection, but can reach 30% in chronic patients
Chronicity	Chronicity of HBV decreases with age: 85% rate is seen in neonates; 25%–50% in children; and 6%–10% in adults.	Chronicity rate is somewhat higher with HDV: adults have 10%–15% rate.
Transmission	HBV is transmitted by parenteral, sexual, and perinatal routes.	HDV is transmitted by parenteral, sexual, and perinatal routes.
Treatment	Liver transplants are treatment for fulminant disease.	Liver transplants are treatment for fulminant disease, and outcome is better than in those patients who have HBV alone. Patients with chronic hepatitis D have in limited fashion responded to interferon alfa, but relapses are frequently observed when therapy is stopped.

Continued ►

► Continued **HEPATITIS B VIRUS AND HEPATITIS D VIRUS**

	HEPATITIS B VIRUS (HBV)	**HEPATITIS D VIRUS (HDV)**
Prevention	HBV vaccine is method of choice. Passive hepatitis B immunoglobulins along with HBV vaccine are administered shortly after birth to infants born to carrier mothers.	HBV vaccination prevents coinfections of HBV and HDV.
Serologic Diagnosis	Acute HBV can be diagnosed by presence of HB$_S$Ag and IgM anti-HB$_c$.	Acute HDV is diagnosed by presence of HD antigen.
Cell Cultures for Detection of Viruses from Clinical Specimen	Serial propagation of HBV in cell cultures has not been accomplished.	See HBV.
Oncogenic Potential	Long term infection with HBV is associated with high risk of developing hepatocellular carcinoma.	See HBV.

GENERAL INFORMATION ON HEPATITIS B VIRUS AND HEPATITIS D VIRUS. HBV is a member of the Hepadnaviridae family and exists in three distinct morphologic entities in human sera. The most common form is a noninfectious 20 nm spherical particle. A second particle is a noninfectious filamentous form of various lengths but also containing the 20 nm diameter particle. The infectious particle, or Dane particle, has a diameter of 42 to 47 nm with an electron dense inner core of 27 nm. Hepatitis B surface antigen (HBsAg) is the complex antigen that is located on the surface of HBV. HBsAg can also be referred to as the *Australian antigen* (Au antigen) or the *hepatitis associated antigen.* The major antigenic determinant of HB$_S$Ag is the group specific antigen a. Protective immunity with the subunit HB$_S$Ag vaccine produces sufficient anti-a antibodies to confer protective immunity. Several subdeterminants (d or y and w or r) exist on the HB$_S$Ag. Therefore, four principal subtypes of HB$_S$Ag exist (Adw, Ayw, Adr, and Ayr). Additional variation on the w determinant increases the major serotypes of HBV to 10. Subtype determination is important in tracing HBV infection from source to source.

The core antigen (HB$_c$Ag) is associated with the nucleocapsid. The third antigen, hepatitis B e antigen (HB$_e$Ag) is soluble and found in HBV positive sera. The HB$_e$Ag antigen is closely related to the core antigen, and its presence in sera indicates that the individual should be considered highly infectious.

HDV is a defective virus that requires a helper virus (HBV) for its own replication and expression. HDV contains an RNA genome that is associated with hepatitis D antigen (HDAg) but is also surrounded by an HB$_S$Ag envelope. The HDAg is detected in serum only when the outer envelope of the virus is removed by using detergent. Two major types of HDV infections may occur. The first type is a co-infection of both HBV and HDV, which often results in a more severe form of hepatitis than HBV. The second type is observed when a chronically infected HBV individual becomes superinfected with HDV. Generally, the presence of IgM anti-HB$_S$Ag indicates that the patient has a co-infection, and its absence indicates that a superinfection is present (see chart below).

Hepatitis D Virus Co-infection and Superinfections

INFECTION TYPE	ANTIGEN	ANTIBODY	
	HB$_s$Ag	Anti-HB$_c$ IgM	Anti-HDAg
Co-infection	+	+	+
Superinfection	+	−	+

The figures below illustrate the appearance and disappearance of serologic markers and liver enzymes in patients with asymptomatic HBV infections (first figure) and acute and chronic hepatitis (second figure). The third figure illustrates HDV (co-infection and superinfection).

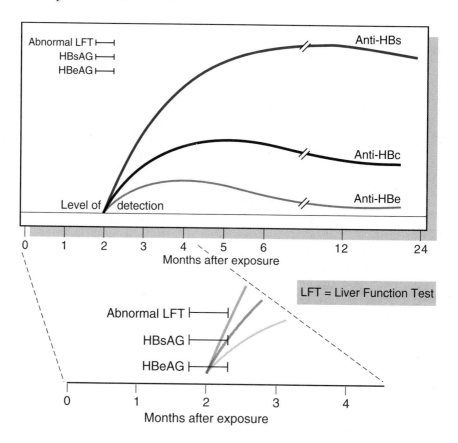

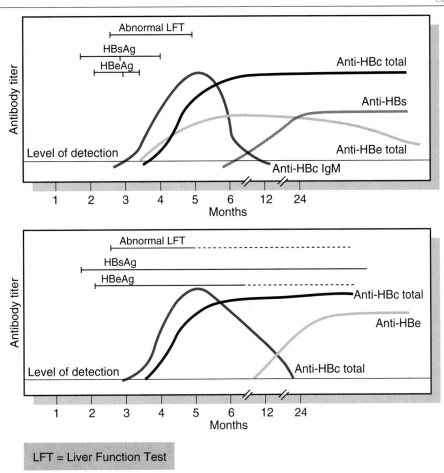

LFT = Liver Function Test

Modified from Mahon CR, Manuselis G: Textbook of Diagnostic Microbiology. Philadelphia, WB Saunders, 1995.

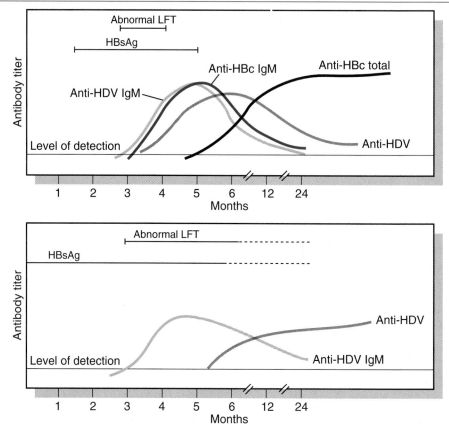

Modified from Mahon CR, Manuselis G: Textbook of Diagnostic Microbiology. Philadelphia, WB Saunders, 1995.

In HBV infection the factors that determine chronicity remain unknown. What is known is that chronicity decreases with age (see summary chart on p 1130), and chronicity is associated with hepatocellular carcinoma. HDV infections do not raise the frequency of chronic HBV infections. However, if an HBV carrier experiences an HDV superinfection, chronic HDV infection is common for those not experiencing fulminant hepatitis.

HEPATITIS C VIRUS

Family	Flaviviridae (probable)
Common Name(s)	Flavivirus, hepatitis C virus (HCV), non-A, non-B hepatitis (NANB)
Collection of Specimen	Serum or plasma is specimen of choice. Serum or plasma is separated from cellular components as rapidly as possible to avoid viral degradation by granulocytes.
Direct Examination	Amplification methods including reverse transcriptase PCR or branched-DNA (bDNA) signal amplification can detect HCV RNA in serum.

Continued ▶

▶ Continued **HEPATITIS C VIRUS**

Description of Agent	
Diameter	—
Capsid Symmetry	—
Envelope	Yes
Type of Nucleic Acid	Single stranded RNA
General Disease Categories	Chronic infection occurs in 50%–80% of cases. Chronic infection is often asymptomatic. Cirrhosis and hepatocellular carcinoma do occur after chronic infection. Acute hepatitis may also occur.
Population Infected	HCV infects primarily young adults, and in many countries it is the most common form of hepatitis occurring after blood transfusions.
Incubation Period	Incubation period is 2–52 mo with average period being 7 or 8 wk.
Primary Symptoms	Disease is usually milder than hepatitis B. Subclinical infections may occur. Chronic liver damage can occur. Small group of hepatitis C patients may develop aplastic anemia.
Onset of Symptoms	Insidious
Fulminant Hepatitis Rate	1%–2%
Chronicity	May be as high as 50%–80% of patients
Transmission	HCV is transmitted by parenteral route, especially in intravenous drug users. Transfusion associated HCV has been reduced by anti-HCV testing of blood donors. Sexual transmission has been reported in few cases as has placental transfer, especially if mother is co-infected with HIV. Currently 50% of HCV infections are without known route of transmission.
Treatment	Interferon alfa gives some benefit to <50% of HCV patients. However, relapse is common after treatment is stopped.
Prevention	Vaccine is not available. Testing for HCV in blood donors has decreased incidence of transfusion-associated hepatitis.
Serologic Diagnosis	Multiple antigen EIAs as well as strip immunoassays (RIBA, Chiron Corp.) detect specific HCV antibody.
Cell Cultures for Detection of Viruses from Clinical Specimen	Routine culture methods are not available.
Oncogenic Potential	HCV chronic infection can lead to hepatocellular carcinoma.

HEPATITIS C VIRUS GENERAL INFORMATION. HCV has not been isolated in cell culture and has not been visualized by the electron microscope. The structure as well as the existence of HCV has been derived from cloning experiments. The genome of HCV resembles the genomes of the flavivirus and pestivirus. The envelope region of HCV appears to be rather variable, and multiple genotypes have been described. Currently it is not known if genotyping of HCV has clinical significance.

The symptoms of HCV hepatitis are usually milder than those of HBV. Fulminant hepatitis or severe cases of hepatitis are unusual. In contrast, persistent infection and chronic hepatitis are often observed. Asymptomatic cases of chronic infection are common even when liver damage is discernible on biopsy. Alanine aminotransferase (ALT) levels fluctuate during chronic HCV infections. Peak levels of ALT are lower than those observed for hepatitis A or hepatitis B. The fluctuating ALT levels are not seen in cases of hepatitis A or B. Chronic infection with HCV may lead to cirrhosis and/or hepatocellular carcinoma.

MISCELLANEOUS VIRUSES

Arbovirus

More than 500 viruses belong to a taxonomically heterogeneous group known as the arboviruses (arthropod-born illness). The majority of arbovirus infections are spread by arthropod vectors, but zoonotic transmission does occur for some arboviruses such as the hantavirus. Many arboviruses cause febrile illness that is characterized by debilitating symptoms such as extreme headache, and lumbar pain. The RNA arboviruses usually have an envelope. The major families include the Togaviridae (alphaviruses) including Western equine encephalitis (WEE) and Eastern equine encephalitis (EEE), the Flaviviridae including St. Louis encephalitis (SLE), the Bunyaviridae including the hantavirus, the Reoviridae, and the Rhabdoviridae.

NEUROTROPIC ARBOVIRUSES

The neurotropic arboviruses (WEE, EEE, and SLE) may cause aseptic meningitis, or encephalitis, but the majority of the infections are often mild (such as a minor headache) or asymptomatic. The mosquito may transmit these viruses to birds, horses, or humans.

RESPIRATORY DISTRESS SYNDROME

A rodent borne (usually a mouse) member of the Bunyaviridae known as the hantavirus causes a fatal adult respiratory distress syndrome in North America. The Muerto Canyon hantavirus was discovered in the American Southwest but is now known to cause infections in 20 states and Canada. The hantavirus can cause epidemic or sporadic infections. The hantaviruses in other countries are associated with hemorrhagic fever as well as with renal disease.

VISCEROTROPIC DISEASE

The clinical manifestations of hepatitis are noticed in yellow fever (YF) and with some cases of dengue fever (DF). Occasionally, DF occurs in the United States. Both DF and YF may initiate a hemorrhagic fever with multisystem organ failure. Both viruses are transmitted by mosquitoes.

NONDESCRIPT FEBRILE ILLNESS

The lymphocytic choriomeningitis (LCM) virus is a member of the arenaviruses and is transmitted by contact with the house mouse. It is a very mild virus compared with the Lassa, Junin, and Machupo viruses. LCM infections are characterized by fever, weakness, anorexia, myalgia, and retro-orbital headaches. A rash may occur with aseptic meningitis or meningoencephalitis. Some LCM infections may be of a subclinical nature.

Slow Viruses

Kuru, Creutzfeldt-Jakob disease (CJD), and the Gerstmann-Sträussler-Scheinker syndrome (GSS) are diseases caused by unconventional agents (spongiform encephalopathies, prion diseases, or infectious amyloids). The agents of kuru, CJD, and GSS await clarification. Some investigators feel that prions are made up of all protein, whereas others feel that they are small nucleic acid genomes associated with protein. Currently, the nature of the infectious agents of spongiform encephalopathies remains uncertain. CJD usually commences with vague sensory complaints, often of a visual nature. The disease causes dementia, with the patients having repetitive myoclonic jerking movements of their extremities. Most patients are at least middle aged adults. In the United States, CJD was recorded as the cause of 3642 deaths between 1979 and 1994. The mean age of death was 67 years. Approximately, 90% of the cases occur in a sporadic fashion, and the exact mode of transmission is unknown. Another 10% are a result of an autosomal dominant inheritance. Less than 1% have been linked to iatrogenic transmission such as contaminated surgical instruments, dural grafts, corneal transplants, cortical electrodes, and human pituitary hormones. Incubation periods as long as 20 years or as short as 14 months can occur after iatrogenic transmission.

GSS, a variant of CJD, is a rare disease with cerebellar ataxia and a late onset of dementia. Kuru, confined to New Guinea and transmitted via cannibalism, has an incubation period of 4 to 35 years and is defined by a loss of coordination. Patients also have shivering tremors and usually die within a year from pneumonia or other infections. The disease has nearly disappeared from New Guinea.

Poxviruses

The poxviruses belong to the family Poxviridae and have a length of 220 to 450 nm with double stranded DNA as the genetic material.

SMALLPOX VIRUS

Transmission of the variola virus between humans is usually by aerosol as well as by fomite contact. Variola major strains were associated with death rates of up to 40% and were associated with fever, prostration, rash, and shock. Variola minor strains produce less severe symptoms with a fatality rate of 1%. The last known naturally occurring case of smallpox was recorded in October 1977 in Somalia.

MOLLUSCUM CONTAGIOSUM VIRUS

Molluscum contagiosum virus (MCV) is transmitted only between humans via direct or indirect skin contact including activities such as swimming or wrestling. The lesions often appear on the trunk, limbs, and face of children and teenagers. A second form, which is transmitted sexually, causes lesions on the genitalia, inner thighs, pubis, and lower abdominal wall. AIDS patients often encounter severe dissemination of MCV.

MISCELLANEOUS VIRUSES

BIBLIOGRAPHY

Arvin AM: Varicella-zoster virus. Clin Microbiol Rev 9(3):361–381, 1996.

Baron EJ, Peterson LR, Fenegold SM: Bailey and Scott's Diagnostic Microbiology, 9th ed. St Louis, Mosby, 1994.

Bean B: Antiviral therapy: current concepts and practices. Clin Microbiol Rev 5(2):146–182, 1992.

Bour S, Gelezlunas R, Wainberg MA: The human immunodeficiency virus type 1 (HIV-1) CD4 receptor and its central role in promotion of HIV-1 infection. Microbiol Rev 59(1):63–93, 1995.

Boyce N: Hepatitis G and the race to develop an assay. Clin Lab News 22(8):1 and 8, 1996.

Cleminti M, Menzo S, Bagnarelli P, et al: Clinical use of quantitative molecular methods in studying human immunodeficiency virus type 1 infection. Clin Microbiol Rev 9(2):135–147, 1996.

DeClereq E: Antiviral therapy for human immunodeficiency virus infections. Clin Microbiol Rev 8(2):200–239, 1995.

Domachowske JB: Pediatric human immunodeficiency virus infection. Clin Microbiol Rev 9(4):448–468, 1996.

Drew WL: Nonpulmonary manifestations of cytomegalovirus infections in immunocompromised patients. Clin Microbiol Rev 5(2):204–210, 1992.

Field AK, Biron KK: "The end of innocence" revisited: resistance of herpesviruses to antiviral drugs. Clin Microbiol Rev 7(1):1–13, 1994.

HCV Learning Guide. Abbott Park, Abbott Diagnostics Educational Services, 1989.

Hemming VG, Prince GA, Grodthuis J, Siber GR: Hyperimmune globulins in prevention and treatment of respiratory syncytial virus infections. Clin Microbiol Rev 8(1):22–33, 1995.

Holman RC, Khan As, Belay ED, Schonberger L: Creutzfeldt-Jakob disease in the United States using national mortality data to assess the possible occurrence of variant cases. Emerg Infect Dis 2(4):333–337, 1996.

Howard JH, Keiser TF, Weissfeld AS, Tilton RC: Clinical and Pathogenic Microbiology, 2nd ed. St Louis, Mosby, 1994.

Levine AJ: Viruses. New York, Scientific American Library, 1992.

Levy JA: HIV and the pathogenesis of AIDS. Washington, DC, American Society for Microbiology, 1994.

Levy JA: Pathogenesis of human immunodeficiency virus infection. Microbiol Rev 57(1):183–289, 1993.

Levy JA, Fraenkel-Conrat H, Owens RA: Virology, 3rd ed. Upper Saddle River, Prentice-Hall, 1994.

Mahon CR, Manuselis Jr G: Textbook of Diagnostic Microbiology. Philadelphia, WB Saunders, 1995.

McNicholl JM, Smith DK, Qari SH, Hodge T: Host genes and HIV: The role of the chemokine receptor gene CCR5 and its allele ($\triangle$32CCR5). Emerg Infect Dis 3(3):261–271, 1997.

Melnick JL: Current status of poliovirus infections. Clin Microbiol Rev 9(3):293–300, 1996.

Midthun K, Kapikian AZ: Rotavirus vaccines: an overview. Clin Microbiol Rev 9(3):423–434, 1996.

Murray PR, Baron EJ, Pfaller MA, et al: Manual of Clinical Microbiology, 6th ed. Washington, DC, American Association of Microbiologists Press, 1995.

Principles in Practice, Testing for Viral Hepatitis—Monograph. Abbott Park, Abbott Diagnostics Educational Services, 1994.

Tsoukas CM, Bernard NF: Markers predicting progression of human immunodeficiency virus–related disease. Clin Microbiol Rev 7(1):14–28, 1994.

Vainionpaa R, Hyypia T: Biology of parainfluenza viruses. Clin Microbiol Rev 7(2):265–275, 1994.

Webster RG, Bean WJ, Gorman OT, et al: Evolution and ecology of influenza A viruses. Microbiol Rev 56(1):152–179, 1992.

Wood DL, Brunell PA: Measles control in the United States: problems of the past and challenges for the future. Clin Microbiol Rev 8(2):260–267, 1195.

Yablonsky T: The mystery of the hantavirus. Lab Med 25(9):557–560, 1994.

Zucherman AJ, Banatvala JE, Pattison Jr: Principles and Practices of Clinical Virology, 3rd ed. West Sussex, England, 1994.

Chapter *44*

MOLECULAR DIAGNOSTICS

Silvia G. Spitzer, PhD
Eric D. Spitzer, MD, PhD

QUICK CONTENTS

INTRODUCTION

The techniques of molecular biology have led to great advances in our understanding of gene expression, DNA replication, and cell growth and development during the past three decades. More recently, tests based on molecular biologic principles have been introduced into clinical laboratories. Nucleic acid based tests can be used in the diagnosis of genetic diseases, characterization of malignancies, forensic studies, paternity testing, and the detection and identification of infectious agents.

Defects in cellular DNA are associated with a broad spectrum of diseases including inherited and acquired disorders. The former include genetic disorders such as cystic fibrosis and sickle cell anemia. The latter are best typified by malignancies including leukemia, lymphoma, and breast cancer.

BASIC TECHNIQUES

Purification of Nucleic Acids

All molecular diagnostic tests begin with the extraction of DNA or RNA from the sample to be tested. DNA and RNA can be isolated from lymphocytes from blood, bone marrow, tissue, cultured cells, body fluids, bacteria, and yeast. The nature of the test to be performed determines the type of nucleic acid to be extracted (DNA or RNA), the amount, the origin of the sample, and the degree of purification.

ISOLATION OF DNA. To obtain genomic DNA, cells are first lysed with detergents to solubilize cellular components; RNA is removed by treatment with RNase, an RNA digesting enzyme; cytoplasmic and nuclear proteins are removed by precipitation or organic extraction; and finally, the DNA is precipitated with alcohol and dissolved in a buffered aqueous solution. Additional cell lysing reagents may be required for particular microorganisms.

ISOLATION OF RNA. Total RNA is obtained by lysing cells in a denaturing solution containing detergents and chaotropic agents, removing proteins and DNA by extraction with phenol-chloroform, and precipitating the RNA in isopropanol. RNA is a very labile molecule that is easily degraded by RNases. Extreme care must be taken when purifying RNA. RNase free labware and solutions and gloves must be used at all times.

Restriction Enzymes

Restriction endonucleases are enzymes that cleave double stranded DNA at specific sequences. The enzymes are obtained from bacteria and are named after the source organism, e.g., *Eco*RI from *Escherichia coli* and *Hind*III from *Haemophilus influenzae* type d. Most restriction enzymes recognize a palindromic sequence (one that reads the same 5′ to 3′, on both strands), typically four or six nucleotides in length, and cleaves both strands of the DNA, producing fragments with either cohesive ends or blunt ends. The enzyme *Eco*RI recognizes the six-base sequence:

$$
\begin{array}{ccc}
5' & \blacktriangledown & 3' \\
\ldots\ldots\text{GAATTC}\ldots\ldots \\
\ldots\ldots\text{CTTAAG}\ldots\ldots \\
3' & \blacktriangle & 5'
\end{array}
$$

and cuts the DNA at the site of the arrowheads to produce two fragments:

$$
\begin{array}{cc}
5' & 3' \\
\ldots\ldots\text{G} \qquad \text{AATTC}\ldots\ldots \\
\ldots\ldots\text{CTTAA} \qquad \text{G}\ldots\ldots \\
3' & 5'
\end{array}
$$

Restriction endonucleases are important tools in the analysis of DNA. The absence of a restriction site can indicate a point mutation in a gene, whereas a change in the length of a DNA fragment may indicate a deletion or insertion of nucleotides within a particular gene.

Because of the complexity of the human genome, there can be millions of recognition sites for a particular enzyme. If restriction endonuclease sites were distributed randomly, an enzyme with a six base pair (bp) recognition site would cleave human DNA once every 4^6 (4096) nucleotides and an enzyme with a four bp recognition site would cut once every 4^4 (256) nucleotides. In actuality restriction sites are located nonrandomly; thus the digestion of genomic DNA with the enzyme *Eco*RI generates approximately 1 million fragments ranging in size from a few base pairs to 10^5 bp. Because the size distribution is nearly continuous, individual fragments cannot be resolved in an agarose gel; as a result, electrophoresis of restriction digested DNA produces a smear. The only way to identify individual fragments is through hybridization.

Hybridization

Hybridization analysis has widespread applications in the molecular diagnosis of leukemias, lymphomas, fragile X syndrome, and other diseases. This sensitive method allows the detection of single copy genes within genomic DNA. The principle of hybridization analysis is that a short fragment of single stranded DNA or RNA of known sequence, called the *probe*, binds to target DNA or RNA sequences that are complementary to the probe [C with G and A with T (or U)].

PRINCIPLES OF DNA HYBRIDIZATION. Double stranded DNA is denatured, and the resulting single stranded DNA is hybridized to a labeled probe. Only one of the DNA fragments contains a sequence complementary to the probe.

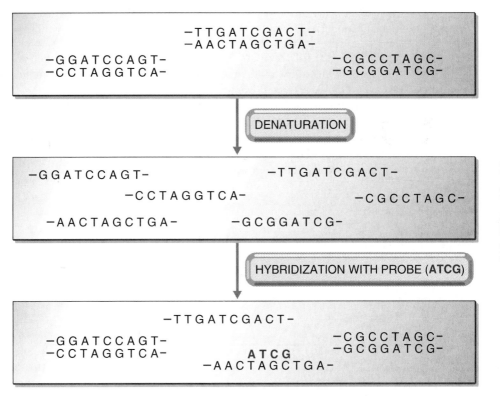

The two components in a hybridization are a labeled probe and the single stranded target DNA that is immobilized on a solid support. The label on the probe can be radioactive (^{32}P) or nonradioactive (biotin, digoxygenin). The latter method of labeling and detection is becoming more popular because of the safety and administrative issues associated with the use of radioisotopes.

HYBRIDIZATION ASSAYS

All hybridization assays are based on the binding of a labeled probe to the target nucleic acid by complementary base pairing. There are different types of hybridization techniques, depending on how the nucleic acid is immobilized. The target nucleic acid can be intact or digested DNA, RNA, or whole cells. In dot blot analysis, the purified nucleic acids are applied directly on a membrane. In the Southern transfer, the DNA is digested with restriction endonucleases and gel fractionated before transfer to the membrane. In a Northern blot, gel fractionated RNA is immobilized on a membrane. In in situ hybridization, intact cells or tissue sections are fixed to a slide. The selection of a particular hybridization technique depends on the type of information that is required.

Southern blot analysis identifies the presence of a particular DNA sequence in a specimen and also provides information about the size of the fragment that hybridized to the probe. This analysis is particularly useful for detecting certain types of mutations and gene rearrangements.

Northern blots are used to detect the presence of specific RNA transcripts and to determine their size. This information is used to assess whether a specific gene is quiescent or is actively expressed.

Dot blot analysis is used to identify the presence or absence of a particular DNA (or RNA) sequence. Although it does not provide information about fragment sizes, it can be adapted to automated methods.

In situ hybridization is used to determine whether individual cells contain a particular sequence. This information can be correlated with histopathologic information.

TYPES OF HYBRIDIZATION ASSAYS. The cells in tube 2 contain a DNA sequence that is complementary to the probe. The cells in tube 1 lack this sequence. In the Southern blot, DNA is extracted from cells, digested with restriction enzymes, fractionated on a gel, and transferred to a membrane. In the dot blot, DNA is extracted from cells and spotted directly onto a membrane. In in situ analysis, intact cells are fixed onto a slide and proteins are then enzymatically digested. Once the nucleic acid is fixed onto a support, the membrane or glass slide is incubated with a labeled probe. The probe binds only to complementary sequences in the DNA samples.

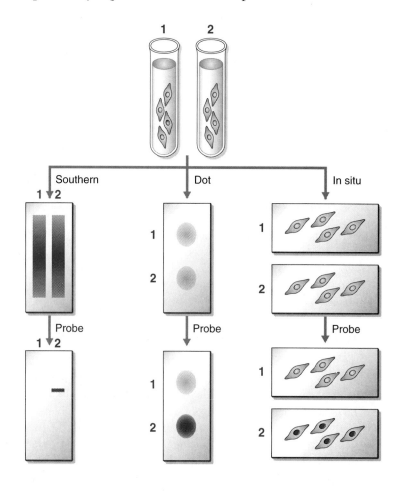

Amplification Techniques

The sensitivity of hybridization methods is limited by the specific activity of the label and the amount of target sequence present in the sample. The development of the polymerase chain reaction (PCR) and other enzymatic amplification techniques allows selective enrichment of target sequences to facilitate detection. Applications for this methodology include identification of disease causing viruses and/or bacteria, forensic studies, paternity testing, and diagnosis of genetic diseases.

In a *PCR reaction* the segment of DNA that is to be amplified is defined by two short DNA sequences termed *primers*. The reaction mixture contains a template of double stranded DNA (the target sequence); two single stranded primers that bracket the DNA fragment to be amplified; deoxynucleotides (A, C, G, T) that are the building blocks of DNA, a heat stable DNA polymerase enzyme, and a buffer. To initiate the reaction, DNA is heat denatured to separate the strands, then the temperature is lowered to allow the primers to anneal to the target sequence by complementary base pairing, and finally a new strand of DNA is synthesized by the DNA polymerase. These three steps constitute one cycle, which takes approximately 3 minutes. Since the DNA is duplicated in each cycle, carrying out 20 successive cycles gives a theoretic amplification of one million–fold. After amplification, the PCR products are analyzed by gel electrophoresis.

PCR AMPLIFICATION. A PCR cycle consists of 3 steps: heat denaturation of double stranded DNA, annealing of primer 1 and primer 2 to single stranded DNA, and synthesis of two new strands of DNA utilizing the pre-existing strands as templates. At the end of each cycle the amount of DNA is duplicated. The deoxyribonucleotides (dNTPs) are dCTP, dATP, dTTP, and dGTP.

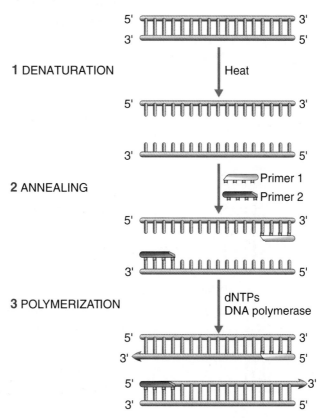

PCR has proved useful in the diagnosis of genetic and infectious diseases and in paternity and/or forensic determinations. This latter is done by analyzing patterns of variable families of repeated DNA sequences, VNTRs.

A technique closely related to PCR, the reverse transcriptase–polymerase chain reaction (RT-PCR) was developed to detect the presence of RNA viruses (e.g., human papillomavirus, human immunodeficiency virus, hepatitis C virus) and mRNAs (e.g., *BCR/abl* in chronic myelogenous leukemia, p53 tumor suppressor gene) in cells. The RNA is first reverse transcribed to complementary DNA (cDNA) by an enzyme called *reverse transcriptase* (RT), after which the cDNA is amplified in the series of cycles described above.

RT-PCR AMPLIFICATION. The enzyme RT synthesizes a cDNA copy of the RNA. In the first cycle of PCR the single stranded DNA is converted to double stranded DNA. This DNA is then amplified as described in the previous figure.

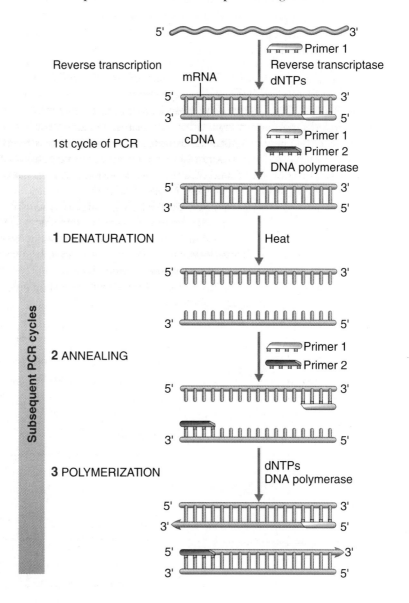

DIAGNOSIS OF GENETIC DISORDERS

Defects in cellular DNA are associated with a broad spectrum of diseases including inherited disorders. The detection of molecular defects in DNA by molecular techniques is crucial in diagnosis and genetic counseling. It can also provide prognostic information.

Types of Mutations

All mutations ultimately affect the structure, function, or expression of the protein that is the product of that particular gene. Mutations can occur in the coding region or in the regulatory domains of the gene. In the first case, the abnormal protein is nonfunctional because the active site of an enzyme is mutated, as in hemophilia B. In the second, although a normal protein is synthesized, its expression is not properly regulated, as in hypofibrinogenemia.

In addition to nucleotide *substitutions, deletions,* and *insertions,* mutations may result from *expansions* of one or more bases. In recent years the molecular basis for 10 genetic disorders including fragile X syndrome, myotonic dystrophy, and Huntington's disease have been established. These diseases are characterized by the expansion of a triplet (CGG, CTG, and CAG, respectively) repeat from a few copies in normal individuals to hundreds of copies in affected individuals.

Although great progress continues to be made in analyzing the human genome, not all genetic diseases are amenable to molecular diagnosis using current techniques. In order for a disease to be diagnosed, the gene that carries the mutation must be identified and sequenced. Also, it is necessary to identify mutations that correlate with the disease. Many base substitutions or deletions occur in introns, untranslated segments of DNA, or lead to changes in amino acids that do not affect the function of a particular protein and thus have no clinical significance. These normal variants are called *polymorphisms.*

PRACTICAL CONSIDERATIONS. Only when the gene responsible for a genetic disease has been identified and sequenced and the most common mutations that produce the disease have been determined can a practical diagnostic test be developed. At present, tests based on linkage analysis, Southern and Northern blots, PCR, RT-PCR, dot blot, and DNA sequencing have been developed for several genetic diseases. DNA testing for cystic fibrosis and fragile X syndrome are discussed as examples of PCR and Southern blot based assays.

Genetic counseling must be offered in conjunction with genetic testing. Appropriate information on a whole family may be necessary to identify a particular mutation. Individuals need to be informed of the implications of the result for the proband and his or her offspring. The knowledge of being a carrier or being affected with a disease that has a late onset in life (e.g., Huntington's disease) may have not only medical but deep psychologic implications for the individual, and the results should be discussed with a trained health care professional.

Cystic Fibrosis

Cystic fibrosis (CF) is one of the most common autosomal recessive disorders among whites. One in 25 persons is an asymptomatic carrier. The gene containing the mutations for CF was cloned in 1989. It is located on chromosome 7 and contains 24 exons. The gene codes for a transmembrane conductance regulator, CFTR, a chloride channel dependent on cyclic AMP (cAMP). In patients with CF, defective chloride transport across membranes causes a lack of water in external secretions. This leads to mucus in the lungs and protein plugs in the pancreas, which causes pulmonary infections and pancreatic insufficiency. More than 300 genetic defects have been identified, including deletions, missense, nonsense, splice site, and frameshift mutations.

ΔF508. One of the most common mutations is ΔF508, which accounts for 70% of the CF alleles. Individuals carrying two copies of this allele are at risk for developing severe pulmonary disease and pancreatic insufficiency. This mutation is localized in exon 10 of the *CFTR* gene, and it is due to the loss of 3 bp's that causes a deletion of the 508th amino acid. To analyze the ΔF508 mutation, a 98 bp fragment from exon 10 is amplified by PCR and the product is analyzed on a polyacrylamide gel. In normal individuals a 98 bp fragment is expected; in homozygous CF patients a 95 bp fragment is obtained, and in heterozygous individuals both fragments, 95 and 98 bp, from the mutated and normal alleles are present at the same time.

PCR Analysis of the Cystic Fibrosis ΔF508 Mutation. PCR was used to amplify a fragment from exon 10 that contains the ΔF508 mutation. Each sample was then analyzed on a 10% acrylamide gel. Lane 1 contains a 98 bp fragment from a normal individual; in lane 2, a heterozygous individual shows two fragments, 98 and 95 bp, that correspond to the normal and mutated alleles, respectively.

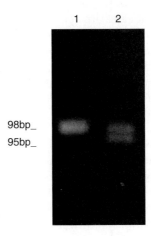

W1282X. Another common mutation associated with pancreatic insufficiency is W1282X. In this case a substitution in the triplet coding for the amino acid tryptophan at position 1282 leads to a stop signal that produces a truncated protein. The substitution is located in exon 20 of the *CFTR* gene. This mutation also disrupts the restriction site for the enzyme *MnlI*, making the PCR fragment refractory to enzyme digestion.

PCR Analysis of the Cystic Fibrosis W1282X Mutation. A. Diagram showing the location of *MnlI* sites in the normal and mutant genes. B. Agarose gel demonstrating normal and mutant genes. A 473 bp fragment from exon 20 was amplified, digested with the restriction enzyme *MnlI*, and electrophoresed on an agarose gel. In lane 1, control DNA produces an unresolved doublet at 185/183 bp and a 105 bp fragment after *MnlI* digestion. In lane 2, DNA from a heterozygous individual yields three bands, an uncut 288 bp fragment from the mutated allele, and the 185/183 and 105 bp fragments from the normal allele. In lane 3, DNA from a normal individual has same pattern as control DNA.

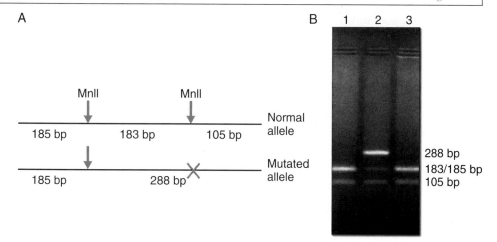

Fragile X Syndrome

Fragile X syndrome is one of many genetic diseases that are detected by Southern blot analysis. The fragile X syndrome is the most common form of inherited mental retardation. Before the availability of a molecular biology based test for fragile X, diagnosis rested on the cytogenetic demonstration of the fragile site at chromosomal band Xq27.3. However, normal male carriers and many female carriers are refractory to cytogenetic analysis. DNA mutation analysis is an excellent diagnostic tool to detect carriers of the fragile X trait.

CLINICAL FEATURES. The phenotype of the fragile X syndrome includes moderate to severe mental retardation, macro-orchidism, large ears, prominent jaw, and high pitched, jocular speech. The molecular basis of this disease is an expansion of CGG repeats that increases the size of a specific DNA fragment of the X chromosome. The number of repeats is proportional to the severity of the condition. Persons with a small increase in the size of this DNA fragment (premutation) have little or no risk of retardation but are at high risk of having affected children or grandchildren. In normal individuals the range of allele sizes varies from a low of 6 to a high of 54 repeats. Premutations showing no phenotypic effect range in size from 52 to more than 200 repeats. Fragile X positive males have much larger fragments, containing more than 300 repeats.

DIAGNOSIS. In the test for fragile X syndrome, high molecular weight DNA is purified from proband individuals, cut with the restriction endonuclease *Pst*I, gel fractionated, transferred to a nylon membrane, and hybridized to a probe that is complementary to a portion of the *Pst*I fragment. Normal individuals have a band corresponding to 1.0 kb; however, in affected individuals there is an increase in size reflecting an increase in the number of CGG repeats.

DIAGNOSIS OF GENETIC DISORDERS

Southern Blot Assay for Fragile X Syndrome. A. Diagram showing the location of the *Pst*I sites and the CGG expansion in the *FRAX* (fragile X) gene. B. Southern blot analysis. Genomic DNA was extracted from peripheral blood and was then digested with *Pst*I, gel fractionated, transferred to a nylon membrane, and hybridized to a ^{32}P labeled fragile X probe. Lane 1 shows a normal individual; lane 2 shows an affected proband; lane 3 shows a normal individual. The larger band in lane 2 results from the presence of an increased number of CGG repeats.

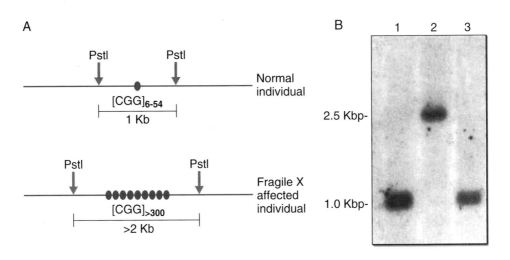

DIAGNOSIS OF NEOPLASTIC DISEASES

Molecular Basis of Malignancy

Cell growth and division are the result of a delicate balance of stimulatory and inhibitory pathways known as the *cell cycle*. Uncontrolled activation of the cell cycle or loss of negative controls is the cause of cancer. There are two classes of genes that play a major role in the regulation of the life cycle of the cell, *proto-oncogenes* and *tumor suppressor genes*.

When proto-oncogenes are altered by mutation, they can become oncogenes and drive the cell to multiply excessively. Under normal conditions the proteins encoded by the *ras* family of oncogenes transmit stimulatory signals from growth factor receptors to other proteins in a regulatory cascade. The proteins coded by mutant *ras* oncogenes are continuously active even when the growth factor receptors are not prompting them. Abnormal *ras* proteins are found in a quarter of human tumors, including carcinomas of the colon, pancreas, and lung. Other oncogenes include *RET*, a growth factor receptor that is associated with thyroid tumors, and the *myc* oncogene family that is associated with leukemias; breast, lung, and stomach cancer; neuroblastoma; and glioblastoma.

Mutations that inactivate tumor suppressor genes deprive the cell of crucial brakes that prevent inappropriate growth. Included in this group are the tumor suppressor genes *RB*, *p53*, and *BRCA1* and *BRCA2*. Mutations in *RB* are associated with retinoblastoma, sarcoma, and bladder and breast cancer. Mutations in *p53* are the most common cancer related genetic changes and are involved in a wide variety of tumors, including breast cancer and sarcomas. *BRCA1* is mutated in breast and ovarian cancers and *BRCA2* in breast and other cancers. Inherited mutations in the BRCA genes confer a high risk of developing cancer in early adulthood.

Clinical Applications

Changes in DNA due to chemical or radiation damage, rearrangements, or replication errors are the primary event in neoplasia. Molecular diagnostic testing plays an important role in patient management from prevention to initial diagnosis to monitoring the response to treatment.

DIAGNOSIS OF LEUKEMIAS AND LYMPHOMAS. Assays that detect rearrangements of immunoglobulins and T cell receptor genes can be used to detect abnormal clonal proliferations of B and T cells. In chronic myelogenous leukemia (CML) there is a cytogenetic abnormality termed the *Philadelphia chromosome* (Ph[1]). This abnormality is the result of a reciprocal translocation between two proto-oncogenes, c-*abl* located in chromosome 9 and *BCR* located in chromosome 22. The malignant transformation affects a pluripotentential hematopoietic stem cell. The translocation produces a novel fused gene known as *BCR/abl* (see "Molecular Basis of Chronic Myelogenous Leukemia" below). Molecular diagnostic testing can detect the *BCR/abl* gene rearrangement in CML patients. The rearrangement can be detected at different levels: DNA detection of the fusion gene by Southern blot, messenger RNA (mRNA) detection of the *BCR/abl* transcripts by RT-PCR, and protein detection of the fusion protein. These tests can be used for initial diagnosis of CML and detection of residual disease after chemotherapy or bone marrow transplantation.

Molecular Basis of Chronic Myelogenous Leukemia. Rearrangement of the *BCR* and c-*abl* genes. A translocation between chromosomes 9 and 22 results in the formation of the *BCR/abl* fusion gene. The *BCR/abl* fusion gene is transcribed into a fusion mRNA and translated into a novel protein known as p210.

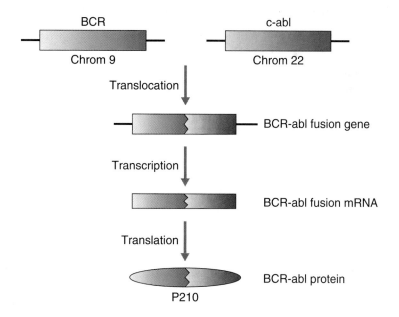

CANCER PREVENTION. Molecular diagnostics can be used to detect individuals at high risk of developing certain tumors. In families that harbor mutations in tumor suppressor genes or oncogenes, various preventive measures have been recommended. Examples include screening for the presence of specific point mutations in the *ras* oncogene in colorectal, bladder, and lung cancer. The type of mutation can be used to predict the tumor's malignant behavior and thus the choice of therapy. In mild cases surgery can be used for early removal of polyps to prevent the cancer from spreading. In more severe cases aggressive combined therapy may be chosen. Women carrying *BRCA1* or *BRCA2* mutations face a high risk of developing breast cancer before the age of 40. Members of a genetically susceptible family may need to schedule screening mammograms as well as counseling.

INFECTIOUS DISEASES

Indications for Molecular Tests

Molecular diagnostic techniques are being increasingly applied to the diagnosis of infectious diseases. Research protocols have been developed for the detection of a large number of infectious agents including bacteria, viruses, fungi, and parasites. Molecular techniques have also been used to discover previously unrecognized pathogens such as the agents of human ehrlichiosis, bacillary angiomatosis, and hantavirus pulmonary syndrome. The detection of microbial nucleic acid is especially useful in three situations: when the infectious agent cannot be cultured in vitro; when isolation of the organism requires specialized techniques; or when growth of the organism in vitro cannot be detected within a clinically useful time frame. Much of the commercial work on molecular assays for infectious diseases has focused on tests for the detection of mycobacteria, *Chlamydia*, hepatitis C virus (HCV), and human immunodeficiency virus (HIV). Prevention of cross-contamination and false positive results has been a particular concern in the development of infectious disease assays.

Commercially Available Tests

The slow growth of *Mycobacterium tuberculosis* precludes rapid detection and identification using traditional methods. Hybridization assays that utilize cDNA probes derived from species specific ribosomal RNA sequences permit rapid identification of *M. tuberculosis* (and other mycobacteria) once growth has been detected on solid or in liquid media. Commercial nucleic acid amplification assays based on PCR or a transcription mediated amplification process can now provide same day identification of *M. tuberculosis* in clinical specimens that are acid fast bacillus (AFB) smear positive. Currently, these assays cannot replace traditional culture owing to a lack of sensitivity on smear negative specimens and the need to obtain isolates for susceptibility testing.

   Chlamydia trachomatis is an obligate intracellular prokaryotic organism that is the leading cause of nongonoccocal urethritis. Subclinical infections are also an important cause of infertility in women. A hybridization assay utilizing cDNA probes directed against ribosomal RNA has been in use for several years and compares favorably with direct antigen detection and cell culture. Recently introduced amplification assays based on PCR or the ligase chain reaction (LCR) offer improved sensitivity over previous assays and simpler specimen requirements.

   HCV is an RNA virus that is highly associated with the development of chronic hepatitis. Patients with persistent HCV infection are at significant risk of developing cirrhosis or hepatocellular carcinoma. HCV cannot be cultured in vitro. The virus was discovered in 1989 by using antibody-containing sera from patients with non-A, non-B hepatitis to screen a cDNA library prepared from plasma capable of transmitting non-A, non-B hepatitis. Cloning and sequencing of the complete virus led to the identification of viral proteins and the development of immunoassays for detecting anti-HCV antibodies. Diagnosis is based on the presence of anti-HCV antibodies and/or the detection of viral RNA in blood. Measurement of the amount of viral RNA in blood (also referred to as the *viral load*) has been used to monitor the effectiveness of interferon alfa (IFN-α) therapy. Two types of quantitative assays are available. Quantitative RT-PCR tests include internal or external standards to control for the variable efficiency of the amplification reactions. Viral load has also been measured with a *branched DNA* (bDNA) assay in which direct hybridization is followed by signal amplification rather than target amplification.

Amplification of HIV proviral DNA has been used to diagnose HIV infection when serologic tests are inconclusive in high risk individuals, and when serologic testing is not practical, as in the case of infants born to HIV positive mothers. Plasma levels of HIV-1 RNA can be quantitated by RT-PCR, isothermal transcription mediated amplification, or bDNA. Clinical trials are in progress to determine the ability of these assays to predict disease progression and response to antiretroviral therapy.

Antibiotic Resistance Genes and Molecular Epidemiology

Detection of antibiotic resistance genes is feasible when these genes represent exogenously acquired sequences that are not present in sensitive strains such as the *mecA* gene in methicillin resistant *Staphylococcus aureus*, or when resistance is due to a restricted number of mutations in an endogenous gene, such as mutations in the *rpoB* gene that confer resistance to rifampin in *M. tuberculosis*.

DNA based strain typing methods have been used to trace the epidemiology of many types of nosocomial and community acquired infections. Typing techniques include restriction fragment length polymorphism (RFLP) analysis, separation of intact chromosomes and macrorestriction fragments by pulsed field gel electrophoresis, and generation of fingerprints by random amplification of polymorphic DNA (RAPD).

INFECTIOUS DISEASES

BIBLIOGRAPHY

Alberts B, Bray D, Lewis J, et al, eds: Molecular Biology of the Cell, 3rd ed. New York, Garland Publishing, 1994.

Arbeit RD: Laboratory procedures for the epidemiologic analysis of microorganisms. In Murray PR, Baron EJ, Pfaller MA, et al, eds: Manual of Clinical Microbiology, 6th ed. Washington, DC, ASM Press, 1995, pp 190–208.

Centers for Disease Control and Prevention: Nucleic acid amplification tests for tuberculosis. Morb Mortal Wkly Rep MMWR 45(43):950, 1996 (available at http://www.cdc.gov).

Cossman J, Uppenkamp M, Sundeen J, et al: Molecular genetics and the diagnosis of lymphoma. Arch Pathol Lab Med 112:117, 1988.

Easton DF, Ford D, Bishop DT, et al: Breast and ovarian cancer incidence in *BRCA1* mutation carriers. Am J Hum Genet 56:265, 1995.

Farkas DH: Clinical applications of molecular techniques. Lab Med 24(10):633, 1994.

Fredericks DN, Relman DA: Sequence-based identification of microbial pathogens: a reconsideration of Koch's postulates. Clin Microbiol Rev 9:18, 1996.

Hamosh A, Rosestein BJ, Nash E, et al: Correlation between genotype and phenotype in patients with cystic fibrosis. N Engl J Med 329(18):1308, 1993.

Innis M, Gelfand D, Sninsky J, White T, eds: PCR Protocols: A Guide to Methods and Applications. San Diego, Academic Press, 1990, p 21.

Leibowitz DS: Molecular diagnosis of chronic myelocytic leukemia (CML). In Cossman J, ed: Molecular Genetics in Cancer Diagnosis. New York, Elsevier, 1990, p 179.

Lerman C, Croyle R: Emotional and behavioral responses to genetic testing for susceptibility to cancer. Oncology 10(2):191, 1996.

Mullis KB, Faloona FA, Scharf SJ, et al: Specific synthesis of DNA in vitro: the polymerase chain reaction. Cold Spring Harbor Symp Quant Biol 51:263, 1986.

Persing DH, Relman DA, Tenover FC: Genotypic detection of antimicrobial resistance. In Persing DH, ed: PCR Protocols for Emerging Infectious Diseases. Washington, DC, ASM Press, 1996, pp 33–57.

Podzorski RP, Persing DH: Molecular detection and identification of microorganisms. In Murray PR, Baron EJ, Pfaller MA, et al, eds: Manual of Clinical Microbiology, 6th ed. Washington, DC, ASM Press, 1995, pp 130–157.

Quinn TC, Welsh L, Lentz A, et al: Diagnosis by AMPLICOR PCR of *Chlamydia trachomatis* infection in urine samples from women and men attending sexually transmitted disease clinics. J Clin Microbiol 34:1401, 1996.

Sharara AI, Hunt CM, Hamilton JD: Hepatitis C. Ann Intern Med 125:658, 1996.

Sidransky D: Advances in cancer detection. Sci Am 275(3):104, 1996.

Snow K, Doud L, Hagerman R, et al: Analysis of a CGG sequence at the *FMR-1* locus in fragile X families and in the general population. Am J Hum Genet 53:1217, 1993.

Van Doornum GJJ, Buimer M, Prins M, et al: Detection of *Chlamydia trachomatis* infection in urine samples from men and women by ligase chain reaction. J Clin Microbiol 33:2042, 1995.

Weinberg RA: How cancer arises. Sci Am 275(3):63, 1996.

Wells R: Molecular basis of genetic instability of triplet repeats. J Biol Chem 271(6):2875, 1996.

Yen-Lieberman B, Brambilla D, Jackson B, et al: Evaluation of a quality assurance program for quantitation of human immunodeficiency virus type 1 RNA in plasma by the AIDS clinical trials group virology laboratories. J Clin Microbiol 34(11):2695, 1996.

Chapter *45*

CYTOGENETICS

Joseph T. Lanman, PhD, FACMG

Q U I C K   C O N T E N T S

INTRODUCTION

Clinical cytogenetics is the identification and description of chromosome abnormalities in humans. Although the actual techniques used by cytogenetics laboratories are quite extensive with regard to cell culture, cell harvesting, and chromosome banding procedures, there are several underlying principles regarding the processing and interpretation of laboratory data.

CHROMOSOME ANALYSIS

The following chart includes the type of analyses commonly performed in a general service cytogenetics laboratory. This list includes the principles; specimen type; specimen handling and processing; and normal reference ranges for each type of analysis. The numbers of cells analyzed and photographed are intended as general guidelines, because these numbers may vary from laboratory to laboratory. In cases where chromosome mosaicism is suspected but not confirmed, additional cells may need to be analyzed.

Chromosome Analysis

SAMPLE	PRINCIPLE	SPECIMEN	SPECIMEN HANDLING	PROCEDURE	REFERENCE RANGE AND RESULTS
Lymphocytes (Peripheral Blood)	Determines constitutional chromosome number and structure of patient when cells are cultured with phytohemagglutinin. Also used to detect acquired chromosome abnormalities in leukemic cells when cells are cultured without phytohemagglutinin. Performed most often on patients who are believed to have constitutional chromosome abnormalities.	Volume: 2–10 mL whole blood. Preparation: Whole blood should be collected aseptically in sodium heparin.	Specimen may be kept at room temperature for up to 24 hrs. If specimen is to be stored for longer than 24 hrs, it should be kept in refrigerator.	Chromosome analysis includes following: 1. Chromosomes are counted and examined in minimum of 20 metaphases. 2. All chromosomes are analyzed in 8 of 20 metaphases. Under certain circumstances, additional metaphases may be partially or completely analyzed (i.e., suspected chromosome mosaicism). 3. Three to five metaphases are photographed or imaged. 4. Two metaphases are karyotyped.	Reference range is normal chromosome number and structure (45,XX female chromosome complement and 46,XY male chromosome complement) to abnormal chromosome number and structure.
Amniotic Fluid Cells	Determines constitutional chromosome number and structure in fetus. Usually performed at midtrimester (14–18 wk gestation), but may be performed anytime in 2nd or 3rd trimester. Performed on women who have increased risk of producing fetus with chromosome abnormality.	Volume: 15–30 mL of amniotic fluid. Preparation: Aspirate 2–4 mL. Discard first aspiration, and place subsequent aspirations in appropriately labeled tubes. Fluid must be collected aseptically.	Transport specimen to laboratory immediately after procedure. Keep specimen at room temperature. Small volumes of amniotic fluid and bloody fluid increase likelihood chromosome analysis will not be completed and increase turnaround times.	Chromosome analysis includes following: 1. Chromosomes are counted and examined in minimum of 15 banded metaphases (clones) or 20 metaphases harvested from two or more cultures. 2. Two to five metaphases are photographed or imaged. 3. Two metaphases are karyotyped.	Reference range is normal chromosome structure and number (46,XX female chromosome complement and 46,XY male chromosome complement) to abnormal chromosome number and structure.

Continued ▲

▶ Continued **Chromosome Analysis**

SAMPLE	PRINCIPLE	SPECIMEN	SPECIMEN HANDLING	PROCEDURE	REFERENCE RANGE AND RESULTS
Bone Marrow	Determines chromosome number and structure in bone marrow cells. Performed on patients who have leukemias and hematologic disorders that are associated with acquired chromosome abnormalities.	Volume: 2–5 mL of bone marrow aspirate. Preparation: Bone marrow should be aspirated aseptically in sodium heparin.	Specimen should be kept at room temperature.	Chromosome analysis includes following: 1. Chromosomes are counted and examined in minimum of 20 metaphases. 2. Two to five metaphases are photographed or imaged. 3. Minimum of two metaphases are karyotyped.	Reference range is normal chromosome number and structure (46,XX female chromosome complement and 46,XY male chromosome complement) to clonal chromosome abnormalities that include abnormal chromosome number and structure.
Solid Tissue	Determines the chromosome number and structure in biopsy specimens of skin, placenta (including chorionic villus samples), and other tissue(s) that can be established in culture for chromosome analysis. Performed on: 1. Patients who are believed to have constitutional chromosome abnormalities when blood lymphocytes are not available for testing (ex: products of conception and placental tissue) 2. Patients believed to be chromosome mosaics 3. Patients with solid tumors	Specimen from skin biopsies, chorionic villus samples, or products of conception (placenta and fetal tissue) should be delivered to laboratory in tissue culture medium or saline.		Chromosome analysis includes following: 1. Chromosomes are counted in minimum of 20 metaphases. 2. Sex chromosomes are analyzed in 12 of 20 metaphases. 3. All chromosomes are analyzed in 8 of 20 metaphases. Under certain circumstances, additional metaphases may be partially or completely analyzed (i.e., suspected chromosome mosaicism). 4. Two to five metaphases are photographed. 5. Two metaphases are karyotyped.	Reference range is normal chromosome number and structure (46,XX female chromosome complement and 46,XY male chromosome complement) to abnormal chromosome number and structure. Abnormal results are reported to referring physician by phone and followed by written report.

CHROMOSOME ANALYSIS

TISSUE CULTURE

The chart below lists the type of tissue culture method or methods that may be used for each type of analysis.

TYPE OF ANALYSIS	CULTURE METHOD
Lymphocytes (Whole Blood Bone Marrow Lymph Node)	Suspension culture with or without phytohemagglutinin stimulation
Amniotic Fluid Cells	Monolayer cultures in flasks or coverslips (in situ harvest)
Solid Tissue	Monolayer cultures or coverslips

CHROMOSOME BANDING TECHNIQUES

Chromosome banding techniques can be divided into groups. One group includes the techniques that produce chromosome bands on all the chromosomes according to the G-banding (Giemsa banding) patterns represented and defined in International System for Human Cytogenetic Nomenclature (ISCN, 1995). These techniques can be further subdivided into categories illustrated below:

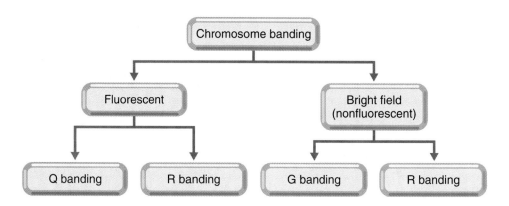

A karyotype of an amniotic fluid cell metaphase that has been CTG banded is shown below:

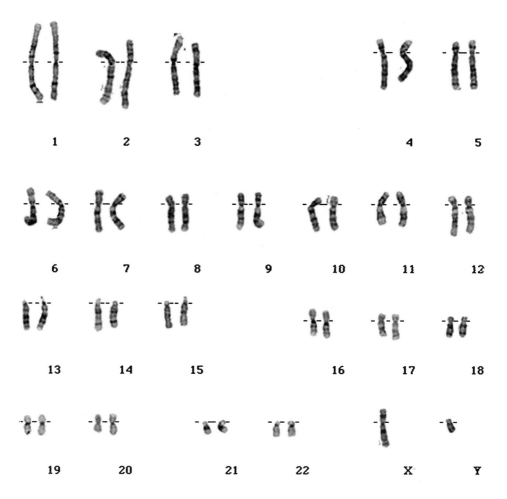

The second group includes techniques that identify special features of individual chromosome regions. These regions may or may not be polymorphic and include staining techniques such as C-banding, G11-banding, AgNOR staining, and T-banding.

The nomenclature and the characteristics of these staining techniques are described in ISCN, 1995.

FLUORESCENT IN SITU HYBRIDIZATION

Fluorescent in situ hybridization has become increasingly important as specific DNA probes have become commercially available. The types of DNA probes include single sequence probes, repetitive DNA sequence probes, and whole chromosome paint probes (WCPs). Single sequence probes are used to detect chromosome deletions or rearrangements that cannot be detected by using conventional chromosome banding techniques. Repetitive DNA sequence and whole chromosome paint problems are useful for identifying cryptic chromosome rearrangements and chromosome segments that cannot be identified by the use of conventional banding techniques.

The figure below shows an example of a patient with a deletion of a DNA sequence in the DiGeorge critical region. The DiGeorge critical region is in the q11.2 region of chromosome 22. This deletion was not identifiable by high resolution chromosome banding analysis.

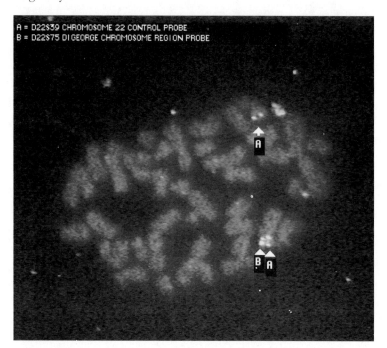

CHROMOSOME MOSAICISM

Chromosome mosaicism is the presence of two or more karyotypically distinct cell lines in the specimen. Chromosome mosaicism is a common feature in neoplastic tissues, and the detection of mosaicism is most problematic in amniotic fluid cell chromosome analyses.

This method for detecting chromosome mosaicism in cells harvested directly (bone marrow and chorionic villi) or from suspension is different from the method used to detect mosaicism in cells harvested from monolayer cultures.

The chart below illustrates the criteria for determining the presence of abnormal cell lines in different types of culture:

TYPE OF CULTURE AND HARVEST	CRITERIA
Suspension Cultures and Direct Harvests	Trisomies and structural abnormalities: two or more cells with same abnormality Monosomy: three or more cells with same monosomy
Monolayer Cultures	Trisomies and structural abnormalities: two or more cells with same abnormality from two or more primary cultures
From Mitelman F, ed: An International System for Human Cytogenic Nomenclature. Basel, S Karger, 1995.	

INTERPRETATION OF RESULTS

Although most chromosome analyses result in normal male or female chromosome complements, additional information should be communicated to the referring physician when abnormal chromosome complements are observed. This information includes additional chromosome analyses on family members in the cases in which constitutional structural abnormalities and extra marker chromosomes are found. Recurrence risks should be stated in cases in which the recurrence risks have been estimated. Patients with abnormal chromosome complements should always be referred to a clinician who can communicate the results and the genetic risks to the patients and their family members.

CHROMOSOME MOSAICISM

BIBLIOGRAPHY

Barch MJ, Knugsen T, Spurbeck JL, eds: The AGT Cytogenics Laboratory Manual, 3rd ed. Philadelphia, Lippincott–Raven, 1997.

Cheung SW, Spitznagel E, Featherstone T, Crane JP: Exclusion of chromosomal mosaicism in amniotic fluid cultures: efficacy of in situ versus flask techniques. Prenat Diagn 10(1):41–57, 1990.

Heim S, Mitelman F: Cancer Cytogenetics. New York, AR Liss, 1987.

Hook EB: Exclusion of chromosomal mosaicism: tables of 90%, 95% and 99% confidence limits and comments on use. Am J Hum Genet 29(1):94–97, 1977.

Mitelman F, ed: ISCN (1995): An International System for Human Cytogenetic Nomenclature. S Karger, Basel, 1995.

Therman E, Susman M: Human Chromosomes: Structure, Behavior, and Effects. New York, Springer-Verlag, 1993.

Verma RS, Babu A: Human Chromosomes: Manual of Basic Techniques. New York, Pergamon Press, 1989.

Vig BK, Sandberg AA, eds: Aneuploidy. New York, AR Liss, 1988.

Section **IX**

APPENDICES

Chapter *46*

LABORATORY INFORMATION SYSTEMS

Stanley D. Cooper, PhD, FCACB

Q U I C K   C O N T E N T S

INTRODUCTION

Laboratory Information Systems Technology in Transition

The late 1990s find laboratory information systems (LISs) in a period of transition. With the increasingly rapid evolution of software technologies combined with the pace of development and deployment of network infrastructure, microprocessor evolution, and Internet and Intranet proliferation, developers and consumers of LISs are faced with a great disparity between the architecture of the existing solutions that are currently installed, the "vaporware" that is presented and marketed as deliverable software, and the true "state of the art" of network, hardware, and software technologies.

There is a substantial gap in the use and deployment of modern tool sets compared with commercial business applications. LISs are incredibly complex pieces of software that handle extremely high volumes of data in a complex environment of instrument interfaces, system to system interfaces, and user interfaces, most typically in distributed networked environments. Very few commercial applications approach the degree of complexity that LISs are typically designed to handle. Given that performance is critical in LISs (response times for users, time-outs for host query interfaces, and the coming automation, online instrumentation, and so forth), system performance has been and is a barrier to many vendors in the deployment of relational databases in high volume multisite laboratories.

By the end of this century, the evolution from the installed base of legacy systems (most of which are still sold and installed by virtually all major LIS vendors) to the next generation of systems can be expected to be well under way. For some consumers of LISs, the evolution to modern technology will have been or will shortly be completed. For most, given the time, cost, and vendor and client resources required to undertake this evolution, the decision to undertake the process is deferred. What is the motivation for this change? The ability to adapt information systems cost effectively and rapidly to the evolving and changing models of the delivery of health care, intense competition, and fewer laboratory dollars.

Laboratory Workflow and Information Management

In simple terms the main functions and objectives of a clinical laboratory are:

▌ Cost effective performance of a variety of accurate and precise qualitative and quantitative analyses on a variety of body fluids, tissues, and excretions in order to aid physicians in the diagnosis, treatment, and resolution of disease. All aspects of quality management should be understood to be a part of this.
▌ Provision for the collection and receipt of the appropriate specimens for these analyses.
▌ The rapid and accurate reporting of the results to the physician.
▌ Consultation to ensure appropriateness of testing and interpretation as required.
▌ Also billing and accumulating workload statistics (although some laboratorians may consider this to be secondary) and management reporting.

Many important factors go into these functions, and this discussion of information management is intended to highlight only one, without diminishing the others.

To achieve the objective of good laboratory management, the management of information is crucial to a number of aspects. Assume that all the analytic requirements of quality testing are met. No matter how valid the result of the test, no matter how quick the performance of the test, no matter how appropriate the test or the interpretation of the result,

> ▌ Reporting of the result to the physician is required before the result becomes useful.

Although this may seem self-evident, the point here is:

> An LIS should not only be able to ensure that this information transfer occurs as expeditiously as possible, it should also be able to validate at each step along the way that all of the other prerequisites have been met far more efficiently and cost effectively than a high quality manual system.

The modern LIS should provide numerous cost effective benefits to laboratory staff and management and to clinicians and their patients.

TECHNOLOGY

New Technology

Almost all the major vendors today offer legacy systems developed in MUMPS, COBOL, FORTRAN, and so forth, that interact with a closed hierarchic database. Some have put "fresh paint" on their systems along with some sort of graphical interface. Others have installed a relational database engine to run beside the old hierarchic database in order to move data into a relational database once the processing of active work has been completed for reporting and query (SQL) purposes. Although most of these legacy systems are very functional (as a result of 10 to 20 elapsed years of development), the fundamentals of the database, languages, and tools used in writing the application are based on software technologies that were state of the art many years ago.

Although functionality and application flexibility should drive the replacement and/or selection process, fundamental software and database design and technology of the prospective LIS will have an impact on both functionality and flexibility.

Although software developers and IT departments have specifics that they look for in terms of the architecture of proposed solutions, the laboratory must be cognizant of technical issues, some of which are touched on here. The use of buzzwords has proliferated in most high tech fields. It is very important that installation and operation of an application be capable of demonstrating "buzzword compliance." If you are buying a *graphical user interface (GUI), client server, open system,* or *relational database* system, this can have dramatic impact on the users, managers, executives, and long term flexibility of any organization. The impact can be very positive or very negative, depending on whether the users got what they were expecting.

Open Systems

An open system is one with a demonstrated ability of the software to run on servers from many different vendors. The procurement of hardware is far more cost effective when the application can run on servers from vendors such as IBM, HP, and SUN/DIGITAL, who can compete on equal footings. The server decision can become much shorter term as performance increases greatly and costs continue to drop.

An application's portability is related to the avoidance of features that are tied to a specific operating system from a specific hardware vendor. Typically, the vendor of the tools that a software developer has chosen to use in the development and deployment of its application provides portability across the chosen servers.

TECHNOLOGY

Fourth Generation Programming Languages

Fourth generation programming languages (4GLs) generate code and screens far more quickly than traditional third generation languages (3GLs), greatly streamlining once onerous and repetitive development tasks. Look for database independence of the development tools and integration with other third party tools.

Client Server

The client (a personal computer, workstation) running local software or a network computer requests services (database, printing, and so forth) through a network type connection from the server. Early models were based on two tier models that resulted in "fat" clients (PCs with beefed up memory, processors, and so forth that did a lot of local processing of information) that put tremendous loads on networks and presented tremendous challenges for desktop management. Look for systems that offer three tier client server models that support "thin" clients (PCs, network computers, Java stations, and so forth that act as terminals only), application servers (for centralized PC application maintenance, software updates, exception event handling, and so forth), and database servers (relational) that service SQL requests.

With the vendors who are releasing their "new" client server and relational database product, check under the hood. Beware of a graphical front end on a hierarchic (nonrelational) database and other flavors of code. In most cases, the upgrade to the new technology results in a new database, new code, new servers, and new operating systems.

Look for integrated tools that assist in the additional overhead associated with the support of client server architecture. Multisite laboratories should require solutions that already offer proven relational engines in high volume multisite environments, 4GLs, and open system servers. Ideal solutions offer the ability to move to full graphical front ends on a gradual basis while continuing to support character based terminals with no change to the back end relational database, application servers, software, or data definition tables setup.

Relational Database Management Systems and Standard Query Language (SQL)

The relational database management system (RDBMS) provides the foundation as the repository and manager of all data. Unify, Oracle, Informix, and Sybase are some of engines that provide utilities to build, monitor, and manage performance, tuning, backup/restore, journaling, transaction logging, security, and so forth, of an RDBMS.

Make sure that the prospective LIS vendor has not modified the generic release of these tools in a way that would render them proprietary. An extremely popular "modern" vendor has done just that. The LIS vendor then gives up the leverage, and the buyer gives up the advantages, that a database and tools vendor can bring in the updates and migration to new tools without starting from scratch! Database support and warranties may also be an issue in such circumstances.

SQL is a powerful but simple American National Standards Institute (ANSI) standard query language that allows very flexible access to any or all of the data in the relational database.

Open Database Connectivity

Open database connectivity (ODBC) allows access to relational databases from popular products such as Microsoft Word, Microsoft Excel, Microsoft Access, Reportsmith, and many popular third party packages that provide "point and click" PC access through the network to the database. These tools allow managers and pathologists to access their data through intuitive, easy to use user interfaces.

Graphical User Interfaces

Graphical user interfaces (GUIs) provide the user with a mouse driven point and click front end. The most popular GUI is Windows, but there are others such as X Windows and Windows NT. Look for those tools that support concurrent development for Internet browsers (Java programming language) and the Windows environment.

Object Oriented Programming

The development tools should incorporate object oriented programming methodologies. This allows the programmer to define both data types and functionality associated with a data structure and to create relationships between data structures. The concept of reusable software objects greatly streamlines the ongoing development and enhancement of software.

The Intranet and the Internet

The network within the enterprise (the intranet) and the Internet present opportunity for modern LISs to seamlessly cater to both central and remote user communities. Look for three (or N) tier client server LIS products that operate under character mode, Microsoft Windows user interface, and standard Internet browsers such as Netscape Navigator using the same source code. The ability for an LIS vendor to compile an application to run under Windows or Java code provides local processing and functionality not available on HTML (hypertext markup language).

Although security may seem to be an issue, the proliferation of on-line banking services should speak volumes about the availability of security for Internet access of confidential laboratory data.

TECHNOLOGY

FEATURE	BENEFITS TO LAB MANAGEMENT	BENEFITS TO LAB STAFF	BENEFITS TO CLINICIAN
Open Systems	Procurement of hardware is far more cost effective when vendors such as IBM, HP, and SUN/DIGITAL, compete on equal footings. Server decision can become much shorter term as performance increases greatly and costs continue to drop. Ability to maintain state of art information systems (ISs) technology without having to change software and all concomitant inconvenience.	Users can be confident that as need for bigger and better hardware approaches, software does not necessarily have to change.	Physicians do not need their lives disrupted needlessly because laboratory is changing LIS system functionality

Continued ▶

▶ Continued

FEATURE	BENEFITS TO LAB MANAGEMENT	BENEFITS TO LAB STAFF	BENEFITS TO CLINICIAN
RDBMS	Relational database and SQL provide laboratory with data that can be accessed and used. Far more powerful for test reporting and management reporting than nonrelational systems.	Relational database and SQL provide laboratory with data that can be accessed and used.	Relational database and SQL provide laboratory with data that can be accessed and used.
4GL, ODBC, Object Oriented Programming	Development tools that allow quick turnaround of new requirements in functionality and reporting.	Development tools that allow quick turnaround of new requirements in functionality and reporting.	Development tools that allow quick turnaround of new requirements in functionality and reporting.
Intranet and Internet	Once confidence in security is achieved, communications capability both inside and outside organization is almost limitless. Can be used for online remote productivity, interfacing of remote analyzers and remote systems, as well as for reporting, inquiry, development, and support.	Remote access with appropriate security protection. High speed communications.	Remote access with appropriate security protection. High speed communications.

LABORATORY WORKFLOW AND INFORMATION MANAGEMENT REQUIREMENTS

Hospital and Independent and Reference Laboratories—Different Needs

There are many features of LISs that on the surface seem much the same but turn out to be very different from one type of laboratory to another.

Some laboratories are very localized single site facilities, and some never need to communicate with another testing site. Others are multisite, and many need to communicate with other laboratories or other health care systems. Some laboratories have absolute (within reason) control of the specimens they collect and/or receive.

FEATURE*	HOSPITAL LAB	INDEPENDENT LAB	REFERENCE LAB
Order Entry (O/E)	Interface from hospital information system (HIS) O/E system and/or direct to LIS	Direct to LIS	Interface from referring lab and/or direct entry to LIS
Specimen Collection and/or Receipt	Inpatient: collection lists Outpatient: Specimen labels or specimen requirement manual, hard copy or on-line	Specimen labels or specimen requirement manual, hard copy or on-line	Provide specimen requirements manual *but* they must take what they get (may or may not perform test based on specimen received)
Patient Type	Inpatient, outpatient, emergency, day surgery, referred in, research, and so forth	Outpatient	Outpatient
Physician Reports	Report by test or profile, serial graphic reports, discharge summary reports, cumulative summary reports	Report by test or profile, complete request report, serial graphic reports	Report by test or profile, complete request report, serial graphic reports

*When features or benefits are common across all table headings, they are not included in the table(s).

Single Site Versus Multiple Site Requirements

Laboratories with multiple testing locations need to ensure that specimens are delivered to the appropriate testing facility. The allocation of the testing facility should occur automatically at the order entry.

Results from multiple locations should be able to be consolidated into a single report, and the report should in some way identify the laboratory that performed each test.

FEATURE	SINGLE SITE LAB	MULTISITE LAB
Specimen Routing	Not required	Different sites may perform different tests. The test menu for each lab location may be permanent or it may vary based on: Time of day Day of week Ordering location Test priority
Ability to Identify Testing Facility on Report	Required only for test referred out to reference lab	Must be done for all sites within organization as well as reference labs
Database	Database designed for single site lab will have difficulty dealing with multiple location testing.	Database designed to handle multisite testing should have no trouble handling single site lab testing.
Ability to Identify Location of User Logged on to System.	Not required	Required by user logon or location of workstation

LABORATORY WORKFLOW AND INFORMATION MANAGEMENT REQUIREMENTS

User Security Access Control and Audit

To control security, a unique user ID or login and password should be established for each user. The system should force the password to be changed after a predetermined time.

Systems must have multiple levels of security that can be assigned based on the level of access that the users need to perform their jobs. Levels need to be defined for those who have only clerical functions of ordering or looking up results. Other users need to have access to enter test results, and supervisors need a level of security that will allow them to modify results that have been reported.

There needs to be a higher level of security for those who must maintain the database. The LIS should allow the system administrator to assign these security restrictions or accesses by user or groups of users in a simple screen driven manner. For example, note in the screen layout below three different sets of options defined for application *vdu* for user groups defined as *all*, *path*, and *systems*.

```
 replace  stored              update          record    1 of     4 records found

 Action [F]    FORMS & FUNCTIONS
 No: | Group       Applic'n   Form             Options

 1    all          vdu        menu             1-9PDUHWFMUXCSEIRQTGN
 2    path         vdu        menu             14678PYD
 3    systems      master     menu             *
 4    systems      vdu        menu             *











 F1-Prev Form F2-Help                                          F10-More Key
 [A]dd, [C]hange, [F]ind, [S]ave, [X]Delete, [D]uplicate.         [F2-Help]
```

Courtesy of Triple G Corporation, Markham, Ontario, Canada.

In this single screen the administrator can define for a group of users defined as *path* that they have access to the *menu* screen for application defined above as *vdu*, and in it they can use options 1, 4, 6, 7, 8, P, Y, and D.

User group *all* has access to a few more options in vdu, and group *systems* has access to every available option (the asterisk indicates all).

Also note that only group *systems* has access to the menu defined as *master*, and they have access to all options available.

On an individual basis, the administrator should be able to set the unique user ID so that access to sensitive or confidential test results must be treated differently than the normal test results. The system must be able to flag a test as secure so only those with proper access can order, result, and review the test and print the result.

The order entry clerk might have access to order the test but not access to the result or review. The technologist would have access to order, result, and review the test, but only a supervisor might have access to release the report. The system must also allow devices to be set up as secure for printing of sensitive patient data.

An example of this type of individual user security control can be seen in the screen below.

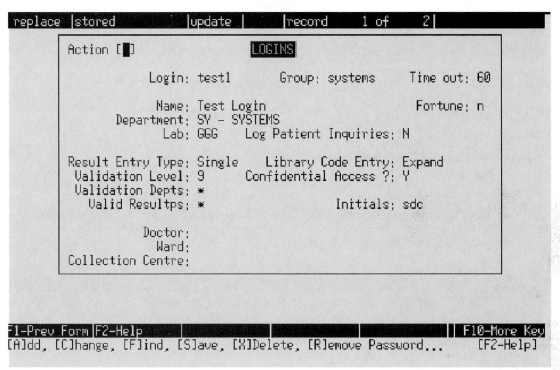

Courtesy of Triple G Corporation, Markham, Ontario, Canada.

LABORATORY WORKFLOW AND INFORMATION MANAGEMENT REQUIREMENTS

In this example user code *test1* has a time out of 60 seconds and has access to confidential data. This screen also defines for the user authority to validate results for release by the department and the result statuses on which the user can inquire.

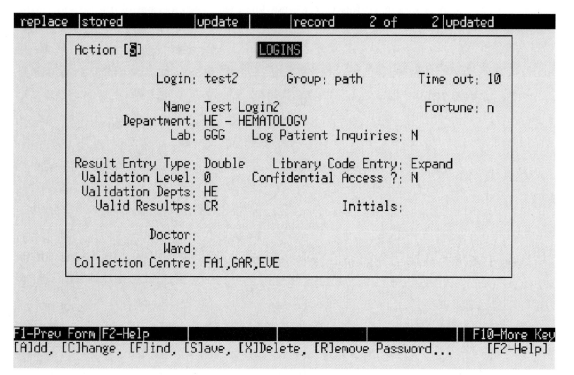

```
 replace  |stored          |update  |      |record     2 of     2|updated

    Action [S]                     LOGINS

              Login: test2         Group: path        Time out: 10

              Name: Test Login2                       Fortune: n
        Department: HE - HEMATOLOGY
              Lab: GGG      Log Patient Inquiries: N

  Result Entry Type: Double    Library Code Entry: Expand
   Validation Level: 0         Confidential Access ?: N
   Validation Depts: HE
     Valid Resultps: CR                    Initials:


            Doctor:
              Ward:
  Collection Centre: FA1,GAR,EVE



 F1-Prev Form|F2-Help    |        |           ||  F10-More Key
 [A]dd, [C]hange, [F]ind, [S]ave, [X]Delete, [R]emove Password...   [F2-Help]
```

Courtesy of Triple G Corporation, Markham, Ontario, Canada.

In the above screen users *test2* have been defined to have more limited restrictions. They have the lowest validation authority, they can validate results only for hematology, they have no access to confidential information, and they can see only completed (verified) or reported results on inquiry. Also note that they have been restricted for inquiry to a set of three collection centers, FA1, GAR, and EVE.

In the same manner they could be restricted to one or a limited group of wards or physician codes. In this way, physicians can be given access to the LIS by dial-up or direct login for review of patient results and have a security code that allows review of only their own patient records.

Another important aspect of LIS security should be that all additions, modifications, or deletions must create an audit of the user who made the modification as well as the date and time the modification was made. This information must be unable to be altered or deleted by anyone.

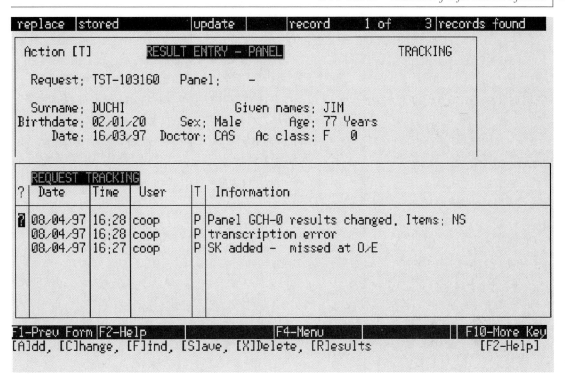

```
replace |stored          |update      |    |record     1 of     3|records found
```
```
 Action [T]          RESULT ENTRY - PANEL              TRACKING

   Request: TST-103160   Panel:    -

   Surname: DUCHI            Given names: JIM
 Birthdate: 02/01/20    Sex: Male      Age: 77 Years
      Date: 16/03/97  Doctor: CAS   Ac class: F   0
```
```
   REQUEST TRACKING
 ?| Date   |Time  |User  |T| Information

 █|08/04/97|16:28 |coop  |P|Panel GCH-0 results changed. Items: NS
  |08/04/97|16:28 |coop  |P|transcription error
  |08/04/97|16:27 |coop  |P|SK added -  missed at O/E
```
```
F1-Prev Form|F2-Help    |       |F4-Menu     |       || F10-More Key
[A]dd, [C]hange, [F]ind, [S]ave, [X]Delete, [R]esults        [F2-Help]
```

Courtesy of Triple G Corporation, Markham, Ontario, Canada.

In the screen above, notice that at 16:27 on April 8, 1997, user *coop* added a test *SK* (serum potassium), which was missed at order entry. The system should automatically log the change with the date and time stamp and user ID. It should also provide the user with an opportunity to comment on why the change was made. Such entries could be free text or codified.

Also note that at 16:28 on the same day, the same user changed the result of a test profile or panel code *GCH* test code *NS* (item within the panel). The original result and the changed result are stored in the database.

Proper security benefits everyone involved in the clinical laboratory.

LABORATORY WORKFLOW AND INFORMATION MANAGEMENT REQUIREMENTS

BENEFITS TO LAB MANAGEMENT	BENEFITS TO LAB STAFF	BENEFITS TO CLINICIAN
Confidence in access of staff to be able to use only permitted functions within system. Difficult to control in manual system.	No need for concern whether they are permitted to perform given task. If not, system won't let them.	Confidence that only qualified individuals (as determined by lab manager or director) are able to access appropriate functions in system.
Error are logged, and positive feedback can be provided to staff to guard against recurrence.	No need to worry that they will be blamed for something done by another user. Receive positive feedback for prevention of recurring errors. Staff learn from their mistakes.	Positive communication should produce reduction in human error in lab.
Appropriate changes are logged as such, in compliance with Clinical Laboratory Improvement Amendments (CLIA), College of American Pathologists (CAP) and various state requirements.	Staff do not need to be concerned about manual documentation to meet these requirements.	Aware that good laboratory practice is being followed.
Routine reporting of tracking information for supervisory review. May be helpful in determining weaknesses in workflow or staff requiring additional training.	Staff requiring remedial training can receive it quickly so that problems do not persist.	Improved quality of staff and service.

Order Entry

The system should allow user definable order entry screens based on the patient type being serviced. Required information fields are determined by each individual ordering entity.

Unique encounter or episode numbers need to be assigned by the system to track each patient encounter separately. User definable billing information needs to be captured for patients at the time of order entry.

The laboratory order entry should accommodate information being passed by a hospital or physician's office or referring laboratory interface system so patient demographic, visit or encounter, and order information can be entered automatically via an order entry system to system interface (O/E S2S).

Standing orders or repetitive orders on the same patient, with start and stop dates, should be entered once into the system. Then at the defined time, labels and/or collection lists are automatically printed.

Additional doctors who require copies of reports should be able to be added at the time of order entry, and those reports then will be generated with the regular reports. The number of additional copies to doctors should be unlimited. The system should also provide a means to add a physician who is not a regular staff physician, or at least a free text name and address, so a report can be generated by the system when results are complete.

The system should allow unlimited numbers of tests with different specimen requirements to be ordered at one time against the same encounter. There should be a system warning if the test being ordered is not appropriate for the patient's age or sex, such as the ordering of a pregnancy test on a male.

In laboratories that receive their work in large batches, that is, reference laboratories, there needs to be a means of a miniorder entry process when very basic information on the patient and request is entered so work can be started. While the work is in progress and before it can be reported out, further ordering and billing information can be added. This means of order entry can also be used to validate that orders and patient information are getting entered correctly.

MANUAL—CENTRAL VERSUS REMOTE ON-LINE

When the majority of the online order entry can be decentralized to remote locations, it may not be necessary to use a two stage order entry system. This depends on workflow and staffing of remote sites.

If the remote locations can be staffed to accommodate on-line ordering and sample processing, then the samples can arrive at the testing facility(s) ready to be tested and already logged in the system. When this is feasible, full entry would make the process much more efficient.

MULTISITE LABORATORIES

The system should support multiple ordering locations and track the location where the order was placed. In addition, multiple testing locations should be supported, and the system should know automatically, based on the test ordered and the ordering location, which testing site should receive the specimen, and if required, which site should receive payment for the testing (if not all paid to one location).

FEATURE	HOSPITAL LAB (HL)	INDEPENDENT LAB (IL)	REFERENCE LAB (RL)
Two Stage Order Entry	Not usually required	Depends on service area and means of specimen acquisition	Usually requires some means of rapid data entry to expedite specimen processing and testing
Remote Order Entry	May be of benefit to all depending on size and nature of service area		
Standing Orders	Requires ability to preenter orders and then, when required, call collection lists and (at some point) specimen labels, or even just have them print automatically. Dependent on workflow and staffing capabilities.	May want to preenter orders but trigger manually as required when patient is available. Compliance may be issue.	Similar to IL.
Add Report Information for Casual Doctor	Most hospital physicians are captive audience. If new one arrives, will usually be repeat referrer. Should be added to database. Depending on data table maintenance, may want to treat as casual until added.	May never see casual physician again (out of jurisdiction). No need to add to database, but need to send report.	Similar to IL.

Continued ▶

LABORATORY WORKFLOW AND INFORMATION MANAGEMENT REQUIREMENTS

▶ Continued

FEATURE	HOSPITAL LAB (HL)	INDEPENDENT LAB (IL)	REFERENCE LAB (RL)
Unique Patient ID	Most hospitals have unique medical record number (MRN). In multifacility group of hospitals, MRN must be unique across all members of group. This may be achieved by having facility code tied to MRN.	May or may not be required based on service requirements	Most often not available
O/E S2S Interface	Physicians or nurses are used to ordering laboratory tests in hospital-wide order entry system. Ability to transfer orders to LIS saves them from having to learn to do this function in LIS. However, O/E would be equally effective if hospital staff were trained to enter the orders directly into LIS.	ILs may wish to automatically transmit orders to RLs. Saves manual documentation of orders sent.	RLs would prefer to have orders from referring laboratories sent electronically to save manual order entry and documentation.

FEATURE	SINGLE SITE LAB	MULTISITE LAB
Remote Order Entry	Requirement depends on service area and relationship with collection locations. Beneficial if large volume with many locations.	Most often beneficial but not always practical. Some may provide terminals or workstations to large volume clients.
Specimen Routing Automatic at O/E	Should not be problem if only one testing facility.	Based on test and O/E location, central or remote, system should automatically route specimen to correct testing site.

FEATURE	BENEFITS TO LAB MANAGEMENT	BENEFITS TO LAB STAFF	BENEFITS TO CLINICIAN
Remote Order Entry	Where feasible, more efficient use of remote staff. More efficient entry of orders and possibly processing of specimens. Specimens arrive at lab entered and processed.	Same	Improved turnaround time (TAT)
Standing Orders	Repeat orders are consistent. No errors from one to next, unless standing order is incorrect.	Same	Better consistency and fewer errors

Continued ▶

► Continued

FEATURE	BENEFITS TO LAB MANAGEMENT	BENEFITS TO LAB STAFF	BENEFITS TO CLINICIAN
Add Report Information for Casual Doctor	More efficient reporting. Do not have to access physician table every time receive order from physician not in system.	Same	Better TAT for casual physicians.
Unique Patient ID	Ability to tie results to individual across multiple orders. This is important for delta checking of results and for finding previous pathology reports, blood bank reports, and for serial or serial/graphic reporting. Also very important for maintaining medical records and cumulative reporting in hospitals.	Same	Much better patient health management if there is linear record of patient laboratory history to go with medical history.
O/E S2S Interface	Ability to have orders entered by physicians or nurses in hospital-wide order entry system, and then transferred to LIS automatically, saves many hours of manual entry by laboratory staff. Equally effective would be for the hospital staff to enter orders directly into LIS.	Lab staff already have orders in LIS when specimens are received and do not need to wait for O/E to begin testing. More efficient front end processing.	Fewer O/E transcription errors and improved TAT.

Specimen Collection—Hospital Versus Independent Versus Reference Laboratory

Specimen collection is usually quite different for the various types of laboratories and often even in similar types from one to another.

Some independent laboratories, for instance, have no remote entry, whereas others attempt to have everything preentered before the specimen arrives at the laboratory. In each of these cases, specimen identification and labeling are quite different. The LIS should be able to allow efficient processing in the majority of circumstances.

For all laboratories there should be a method to track if all specimens have been collected, transported from one location to another, and received, as well as the condition of the specimen and the need for recollection if feasible. If an uncollected specimen is to be canceled or rescheduled, there should be a means of deleting it from the order.

Specimen integrity is or should be a concern for all laboratories; however, the issues may be vastly different for different laboratories. Things like specimen type, temperature of specimen, hours fasting, hemolysis, lipemia, anticoagulant, age of specimen, and preservatives are but a few of the factors that can have relatively major or marginal effects on the analytic outcome of laboratory testing.

The LIS should be able to provide appropriate specimen requirement information to allow the laboratory to collect the appropriate specimen *or* rule out the inappropriate specimen as required.

LABORATORY WORKFLOW AND INFORMATION MANAGEMENT REQUIREMENTS

FEATURE	HOSPITAL LAB (HL)	INDEPENDENT LAB (IL)	REFERENCE LAB (RL)
Specimen Collection	Specimens may be collected by ward staff, phlebotomy staff, or laboratory staff.	Specimens are collected by laboratory phlebotomy staff at laboratory collection location or by physician or physician's office staff.	Specimens are received in large batches all at once. Although RL can publish test directory and specimen requirements, these are very difficult to enforce since they have no direct relationship with collection staff. RL has *very limited* control over what specimens it actually receives. Although HL and IL can define for their phlebotomists what specimens to collect for each order, RL must take what it gets and do with it the best it can.
Collection Lists and Labels	Majority of specimens collected require collection lists. Orders may be entered any time of day for collection as required. Based on institution procedure or policy.	System should be able to provide collection labels at order entry. If two stage system is in use, this must occur at 1st stage.	When specimen collection cannot be directed by LIS, it would be desirable if LIS could at least indicate whether appropriate and sufficient specimen types were available for testing required before printing labels.
	System should be able to print automatically or on demand collection lists for specimens requiring collection. These should be available to print by various sort criteria such as floor, ward, room, or bed, as well as by specimen priority (i.e., stat or fasting specimens) or timed collections. With collection list, system should provide user defined bar code labels to uniquely label and identify each specimen. It is not sufficient to have all specimens identified by same order number (although it is important that this link be available) because automation of testing is much more efficient if analyzers and automation systems can uniquely identify specimen and its required tests from bar code number.	At laboratory collection center labels become collection list for phlebotomists. Specimens that arrive from physicians' offices or other nonlaboratory sites, or from laboratory sites where remote entry is not feasible, can be labeled after order entry when specimens are received. True collection lists may be used by IL for scheduling of house calls at private homes, nursing homes, or patient's offices.	LIS should print labels for specimens received as appropriate. Laboratory may also wish to print labels for those specimens not received, to attach to requisition for documentation.

Continued ▶

► Continued

FEATURE	HOSPITAL LAB (HL)	INDEPENDENT LAB (IL)	REFERENCE LAB (RL)
Specimen Integrity	Specimen integrity in HL for most part relates to collection of proper specimen type (plasma vs. serum), whether or not specimen problems exist (hemolysis, lipemia, and so forth), or appropriate quantity or temperature for test(s) requested. LIS can maintain comprehensive library of specimen requirements and integrity conditions on-line.	Specimen integrity issues in addition to those important for HLs may also include those of concern to the RL depending on scope and area of service.	Specimen integrity is generally much more serious problem here. Because RL receives specimens over large distances, by courier, and by post, specimen integrity may often be issue for reasons other than specimen type. "Out of date" (too old for analysis) or inappropriate temperature (ambient instead of frozen), or for that matter "lost in transport" are serious problems for RL. System should be able to warn user of specimen problem, based on specimen type identifier, or entry date and time vs. collection date and time, or temperature flag.

FEATURE	BENEFITS TO LAB MANAGEMENT	BENEFITS TO LAB STAFF	BENEFITS TO CLINICIAN
Collection Lists and Labels	Specimens required for collection are maintained in standardized database, and system determines appropriate types and number of specimens required for each order. List and labels can then be generated automatically or on demand, and phlebotomist knows exactly what specimens are required.	Phlebotomists do not need to memorize large list of specimen requirements or look them up in large unwieldy manual.	Clinician is confident that appropriate specimen is being used for requested tests.
Specimen Integrity	Inappropriate specimens are kept to minimum and are more easily recognized, kept track of, and resolved.	Same as for management	Same

Specimen Routing, Transportation, Receiving, Rerouting, and Processing

ROUTING

Once a specimen, hopefully an appropriate specimen, has been collected, it is necessary to ensure that it arrives at the appropriate testing facility. If there is only one laboratory, this should not be a problem. Whether it arrives at all may be a problem, but that is a different issue.

For any laboratory with multiple testing facilities of its own (not just send-out laboratories), when an order is sent via interface or entered into the LIS, the system should know based on the test, the ordering location, the day of the week, the time of day, and the priority of the test or order where each and every test is to be tested. This information should all be user definable and table driven.

```
 replace  |stored            |update .|   |record    1 of    4|records found
┌─────────────────────────────────────────────────────────────────────────┐
│ Action [R]              Panels                                            │
│                                                                          │
│   Code: VMA    Lab: TST   Description: VANILLYLMANDELIC ACID              │
│                                                                          │
│ Active From┌──────────────────────────────────────────────────────────┐ │
│ Account aft│Action [ ]          SPECIMEN ROUTING                       │ │
│            │                                                           │ │
│ Single Form│No: │ H/C │ Weekday    │ Start │ End   │ Priority  │ Lab  │ │
│ Report Gro │    │     │            │       │       │           │      │ │
│     Stat Pri│1  │EFK  │            │ ***** │ ***** │           │ SKS  │ │
│ Print Devi │2   │NW   │            │ ***** │ ***** │           │ SKS  │ │
│ Urgent Del │3   │PHC  │            │ ***** │ ***** │           │ SKS  │ │
│ Low Age Lim│4   │RHIN │            │ ***** │ ***** │           │ SKS  │ │
│            │    │     │            │       │       │           │      │ │
│ Format hea │    │     │            │       │       │           │      │ │
│ Format hea │    │     │            │       │       │           │      │ │
│ Underline c│    │     │            │       │       │           │      │ │
│ Label Types│    │     │            │       │       │           │      │ │
│ Info: VMA! │    │     │            │       │       │           │      │ │
└────────────┴────┴─────┴────────────┴───────┴───────┴───────────┴──────┘ │
 F1-Prev Form│F2-Help      │        │        │        │    || F10-More Key
 [A]dd, [C]hange, [F]ind, [S]ave, [X]Delete, [P]rint.        [F2-Help]
```

Courtesy of Triple G Corporation, Markham, Ontario, Canada.

For example, in the screen above the user can define what laboratory should receive the VMA specimen for test VMA by ordering location (H/C), weekday, start and end times (e.g., 4 PM to 6 AM), and test priority (routine, stat), or any combination of these.

TRANSPORTATION

Once the specimen has been designated for a particular laboratory, the actual transportation can be handled many ways—most of them off-line from the LIS.

The LIS cannot transport the specimens, but if it is done properly the LIS should be able to tell you when and if the specimen left the remote site and arrived at its destination.

RECEIVING

Whether a laboratory is a single site or multisite organization the user should have a means to indicate in the LIS that a specimen has been sent from a remote site to the appropriate testing facility. Users at the testing facility should also be able to indicate in the LIS that a specimen has been received at the laboratory. These functions of dispatching and receiving specimens should be available to the user in either a batch mode or specimen by specimen mode.

The user should have the ability to comment on any specimens not received and either delete them or report them as not received.

REROUTING

For some laboratories rerouting of specimens may be required. The simplest case is when a ward or collection center sends a specimen to a single site testing laboratory and that test is not performed by the laboratory. The specimen is referred to a reference laboratory.

For multisite laboratories when different tests may be performed at different sites for cost effective scales of economy, routing can be a nightmare for manual systems. The user should be able to define this in the LIS using the same routing table as the original routing setup.

Information about where the specimen should be routed should be easily available on the specimen label produced by the LIS, or obtainable on inquiry in the LIS by reading the specimen bar code.

PROCESSING

Once received in the appropriate testing facility, the LIS should know whether the specimen is a primary testing container, a master collection container, or an aliquot tube.

Tubes that are ready for testing should be so labeled with the appropriate information, which should include the testing department or section. If specimens require additional processing, i.e., centrifuging, aliquoting, extraction, and so forth, then the label should so indicate.

If specimens are sorted manually this information should be human readable. If sorting is automated, then the LIS should be able to pass the destination information to the automation system by reading the bar code.

It is not necessary for the information to be stored in the bar code. The specimen ID number is sufficient. The less information in the bar code the better. It takes up less label area and is read easier and faster. The LIS has, and can quickly retrieve, all the other required information from the database to pass on to the label printer.

As positive identification technology improves (e.g., two dimensional bar codes), the incorporation of additional information into these systems will no doubt expand and become more useful.

Specimen Tracking

At each of the steps described in the previous section, the LIS should know approximately, if not exactly, where the specimen(s) is for any order, once the order has been entered.

The LIS should know and keep track of when the specimen has been:

- Put on a collection list but not yet been collected
- Collected but not yet transported
- Transported but not yet received
- Received but not yet rerouted (if required)
- Received but not yet tested
- Tested but not yet put into storage
- Stored but not yet discarded
- Discarded

In each case these tracking records should indicate the date and time of the event and the login ID of the user who caused or created the record.

In the screen below, specimens can be found in inquiry, e.g., specimen number 325064 indicates an SST tube sent to laboratory EDM for a sodium (with test code "NA-M").

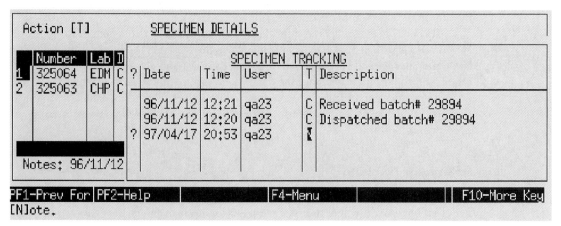

Courtesy of Triple G Corporation, Markham, Ontario, Canada.

Users who inquire about the tracking information for this specimen see (in the screen below) that the specimen was dispatched by user *qa23* on November 12, 1996, at 12:20 in batch 29894. It was received by user *qa23* on the same date at 12:21 in batch 29894.

Courtesy of Triple G Corporation, Markham, Ontario, Canada.

Specimen Storage, Retrieval, and Disposal

When all the testing on a specimen has been completed, the specimen can be placed in storage for a period of time and then disposed of.

The length of storage varies from laboratory to laboratory and may depend on the type and viability of the specimen as well as the remaining quantity of specimen.

The LIS should help keep track of the storage location. This may vary from indicating in what laboratory department the specimen is stored, to a specific cabinet, freezer, or refrigerator, to a shelf in the refrigerator, to a specific rack and position on the shelf.

If specific rack and position are used, this can be designated manually by the user responsible for placement of the specimen indicating to the LIS the position location, or it can be dictated by the LIS.

In any of these possibilities, the user should be able to inquire in the LIS for the position of a stored specimen. In the least case, if a laboratory does not want to fully automate specimen storage, the user should be able to ascertain from the LIS what the last known location of the specimen was, which may provide some clue about where it might be.

FEATURE	SINGLE SITE LAB	MULTISITE LAB
Routing	Required only for send-out tests; this is usually handled separately by the lab from multisite type of routing.	May require complex routing rules based on number of testing sites and tests performed at each site.
Receiving	Whether specimen arrives from ward, collection center, or physician's office, and so forth, it is important for LIS to know when specimen actually arrives at the lab. Only after specimen is received at lab should specimens be available to print on worklist.	It is also important for multisite lab to have LIS keep track of which site has received specimen. It should be able to indicate if lab site attempts to receive specimen that they should not have received.
Rerouting	Not required	If site is used as transportation hub or drop-off center, system should allow site staff to receive specimen and reroute it to next receiving point automatically.
Tracking	Specimen tracking for single site lab may be slightly less complex than that for multisite lab.	All movements of specimen from site to site and within individual site should be traceable. Preferably this should be done automatically by LIS, but at least there should be means of manually inputting this information. This could be very tedious manual process.

FEATURE	HOSPITAL LAB (HL)	INDEPENDENT LAB (IL)	REFERENCE LAB (RL)
Routing, Receiving, Rerouting, Tracking	Each of these features for HL, IL, and RL is more dependent on whether laboratory is single or multisite as in table above.		

FEATURE	BENEFITS TO LAB MANAGEMENT	BENEFITS TO LAB STAFF	BENEFITS TO CLINICIAN
Routing, Receiving, Rerouting, Tracking	All these activities are user defined, but after initial definition, they are prompted, controlled, and/or tracked automatically by LIS. Manager should be confident that tests are targeted for correct testing facility and that all movements of specimen are tracked and can be reported on in management reports.	Can rely on specimen labels and LIS software to indicate where specimen belongs and if errors are made receive reliable reports of such events.	Confidence in specimen management by laboratory.

Laboratory Automation (Robotics) and Laboratory Information Systems

Brief Digression on Laboratory Automation. The evolution of the convergence of the functionality of laboratory automation systems (LASs) and LISs is interesting. As the LASs are deployed and can demonstrate an acceptable return on investment, there is increasing pressure on LISs to provide required functionality (such as unique specimen processing and/or handling) and in some cases a requirement for the LAS vendors to provide additional functionality and workarounds for the existing LIS. Look for talk of standards and the success that has been achieved with instrument interfaces.

Some automation vendors have taken the approach that builds LIS functionality into the automation software management to make up for lack of functionality in many LISs. Where does delta checking logic reside? In the LIS or in the lab automation management software? Are two sets of tables required? What about remote laboratories that are not automated and may do rapid response testing? And what about all the manual testing that still takes place?

These issues have yet to be played out. Nevertheless LAS and LIS integration will more and more play a major role in the cost effectiveness (and survival) of laboratories in the very near future (no offense to those that are already automated). Keep your options open—technological and functional!

Result Entry

AUTOMATED (ANALYZER INTERFACE)

Tests done on analyzers can be downloaded directly from the instrument to the LIS if the instrument has been interfaced. Instrument interfaces can be unidirectional or bidirectional.

A unidirectional interface information flows in only one direction, from the analyzer to the LIS. In these cases it is incumbent on the technologist to use a load list or worklist generated on the LIS to load specimens onto the analyzer in a specific order. The results are then received by the LIS and assumed to be in the correct order.

Although this may seem dangerous, if a properly documented procedure is trained and followed, as long as this load is done correctly it is much more efficient and less prone to error than manually entering results from a high volume analyzer.

There are several types of bidirectional interfaces, but there are three main types:

1. Those in which the LIS transmits patient, order, and test information to the analyzer at the user's request and the analyzer returns the result when ready with appropriate identifying demographics.
2. Those in which the analyzer intermittently requests a list of outstanding requests from the LIS. The LIS transmits the list that is stored in a database on the analyzer. This type of interface is referred to as *host broadcast*. When the instrument then reads the specimen bar code, is searches its own database for the list of tests to be done and transmits results when ready.
3. Those in which the analyzer reads the specimen bar code label ID and queries the host for the tests ordered on that specimen. The LIS responds and the test are run and results transferred. This type of interface is referred to as *host query*.

The results coming from the instruments can be set up to be automatically released to the patient record if user definable criteria have been met, or they can be required to be reviewed by the technologist on-line and then released on a group or individual test or patient basis. The two screens below show examples of a multiple and single order result approval form.

1	101945		COOPER		STAN		O Y	F	DAY	PRL FOL				R

	A202747	202744	202746	202755	202745	202748	202750	202756	202751
T4					L 3.6	L 4.0			
TU						W			
FT4					N 1.2				
T3									
TSH					N 2.18				W N 2.24
FTI						W			
FSH		H 61.2						L 3.5	
LH		H 34.3						N 6.4	
PROLAC	N 6.8							7.4	
B12			!>>>	N 398.			N 400.		
FOLATE	H 75.0		N 13.9	N 7.9					
FERRIT				N 92.					
DIG	H 7.6		N 1.0	H 12.0					
GLU	L 2.0		L 2.0	N 13.0					
NA	N 13.0		L 3.0	N 14.0					
CL	L 14.0		L 4.0	N 15.0					
K	L 12.00		L 5.00	L 14.00					
BIL	N 23.0		L 6.0	N 18.0					
SK	H 43.		N 7.	H 24.					
PHO	L 23.		L 8.	L 21.					

Courtesy of Triple G Corporation, Markham, Ontario, Canada.

```
┌─────┬─────────┬──────────────┬────────────────┬─────┬─┬────┬─────────────┐
│ seq │ Request │ Name,Last    │ First Name     │ Age │S│Col │ Panel Codes │
│   1 │ 101945  │ COOPER       │ STAN           │ 0 Y │F│DAY │ PRL FOL     │
└─────┴─────────┴──────────────┴────────┬┬──────┴─────┴─┴────┴─────────────┘
                                        EE
┌──────┬────────────┬────┬────────────┬┬──────┬────────────┬────┬──────────┐
│ code │ parameter  │  . │ result     ││ code │ parameter  │    │ result   │
│ pL   │ PROLACT    │  N │      6.8   ││ ff   │ BIL        │  N │  23.0    │
│ fo   │ FOLATE     │  H │     75.0   ││ gg   │ SK         │  H │  43.     │
│ aa   │ DIG        │  H │      7.6   ││ hh   │ PHO        │  L │  23.     │
│ bb   │ GLU        │  L │      2.0   ││ ii   │ CAL        │  H │  12.     │
│ cc   │ NA         │  N │     13.0   ││ jj   │ P22        │  L │   2.00   │
│ dd   │ CL         │  L │     14.0   ││ kk   │ P23        │  L │  12.0    │
│ ee   │ K          │  L │     12.00  ││      │            │    │          │
└──────┴────────────┴────┴────────────┴┴──────┴────────────┴────┴──────────┘
                                       88
 TST SP-202747       record status : Scrutiny      Operator : P        114
 [L]oad [E]nq [R]edo [0-9,A]ccept [S]end [C]hange [X]del [T]ext [P]anic [D]il [N]
```

Courtesy of Triple G Corporation, Markham, Ontario, Canada.

In the upper screen, results from a group of nine patients are presented in nine vertical columns, and the user can approve or elect to flag for further review or flag for repeat any column of results.

In the lower screen the results from column 1 of the upper screen are displayed for review on their own.

Once approved, the results are released for reporting.

MANUAL

The LIS should allow tests performed by manual methods or on noninterfaced instruments to be reported out as a single test or to be placed on a user definable worklist for repetitive batch entry.

Test results should be entered by numeric values, predefined codes, canned comments, and/or free text depending on the type of test defined. If the value entered is defined as a ridiculous or nonsensical result, the system should not allow it to be entered.

When appropriate, some tests should have default results available and a means of entering these defaults for a batch of requests (see worklist result entry later).

As tests are being resulted, normal values should display, as well as any user defined flags, which may appear if the test is abnormal, if it is a critical value, or if it fails user defined delta checks.

In the form on the facing page, note that the chloride result is highlighted, indicating that this result is the one being entered. At the bottom of the entry screen there is a field called *Ranges,* which indicates the user defined reference range for the tests currently being entered, in this case 95 to 105 mmol/L.

The result of 110 is flagged to the right as *H,* indicating it is a high abnormal result. Also to the right is another flag, *DH,* indicating that this result failed the delta check on the high end, that is, it is significantly higher than the last chloride result on this patient.

Also of interest is the potassium, which indicates a *L* low abnormal result but *N,* no delta failure, and the sodium which is normal (no high or low flag) and shows *N,* no delta failure. The bicarbonate results have not yet been entered.

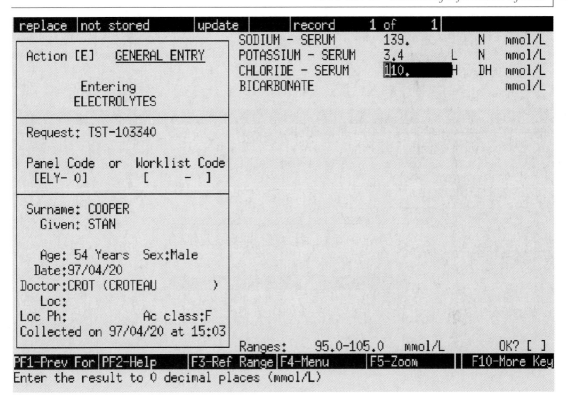

replace	not stored		update		record	1 of	1	

SODIUM - SERUM   139.   N   mmol/L
POTASSIUM - SERUM   3.4   L   N   mmol/L
CHLORIDE - SERUM   110.   H   DH   mmol/L
BICARBONATE   mmol/L

Action [E]   <u>GENERAL ENTRY</u>

Entering
ELECTROLYTES

Request: TST-103340

Panel Code or Worklist Code
[ELY- 0]   [-]

Surname: COOPER
  Given: STAN

  Age: 54 Years   Sex:Male
Date:97/04/20
Doctor:CROT (CROTEAU   )
  Loc:
Loc Ph: Ac class:F
Collected on 97/04/20 at 15:03

Ranges: 95.0-105.0   mmol/L   OK? [ ]

PF1-Prev For	PF2-Help		F3-Ref Range	F4-Menu		F5-Zoom			F10-More Key

Enter the result to 0 decimal places (mmol/L)

Courtesy of Triple G Corporation, Markham, Ontario, Canada.

Hot keys during result entry can be very useful to access additional information. In the example below a hot key has been used to access various user defined ranges for chloride. In addition, the high or low limits for delta checking based on the last previous result are shown.

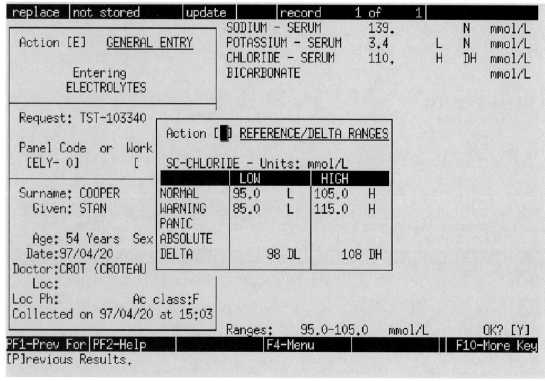

| replace | not stored | update | | record | 1 of | 1 | | |

Courtesy of Triple G Corporation, Markham, Ontario, Canada.

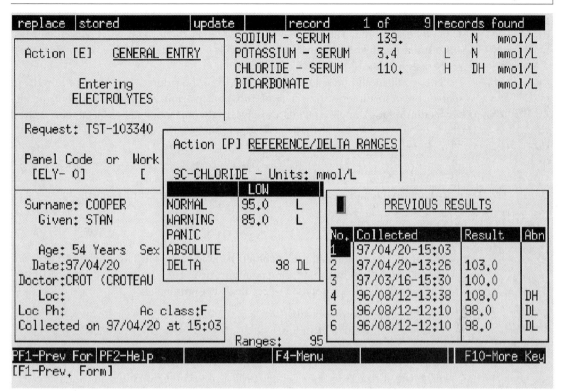

Courtesy of Triple G Corporation, Markham, Ontario, Canada.

Another hot key is used to access previous results for the test that is being entered.

The system should allow tests to be set up with user defined criteria that allow results to be autoreleased by the system.

If these criteria are exceeded in any way, the system should require the results to be reviewed and validated by a technologist, supervisor, or laboratory physician and should have some means of notifying appropriate personnel that results are waiting validation.

Such features should be available within an LIS and be used based on user or organizational preference or policy.

WORKLIST RESULT ENTRY

A worklist should define a specific batch of manual tests to be performed in either a user defined or a system defined order. The system usually defines the order of testing in ascending or descending numeric order. In these cases the user must sort the specimens into batch order.

For the user to define the order of testing, the user should be able t build a worklist batch by either wanding bar code labels (preferred) or keying numbers into the batch. In these cases the worklist order should be in the order of the specimens without sorting. Unless the number of specimens is very low (less than one or two dozen), scanning bar codes is far quicker, more efficient, and less prone to sample mix-up than sorting specimens.

Such lists can be hard copy printouts or, for those who are inclined to move toward a paperless environment, on-line and not printed.

Users should be able to enter results for tests in worklist batches by identifying only the batch number. The system should be able to then identify the patient and test result required and prompt for it. All the features available in the result entry process described above should be available here as well.

The result should be able to be entered from the printed worklist if required and available, but also directly from a noninterfaced instrument display, printout, or any other medium, for example, reading directly from a microbiology plate or slide, and so forth.

SPECIALIZED RESULT ENTRY SCREENS

See "Laboratory Departmental Modules or Compartmentalization," later.

INTERPRETATION AND EXPERT SYSTEMS

Once the results are entered the LIS should be able to perform as much or as little interpretation as required by the medical community it serves.

The first step in interpretation of results is the automatic:

■ Flagging of abnormal results
■ Flagging of delta check failures
■ Flagging of panic value results
■ Prevention of entry of absurd results
■ Routing of results by user defined criteria to a validation buffer or queue
■ Release of other results not blocked by the above criteria

All of these have been referred to previously. But this should be only the beginning. There many interpretive things an LIS should be able to do for the laboratory.

REFLEXING

The LIS should provide users with the ability to define reflex actions in response to certain results. Such user defined reflex functionality should include appropriate additional testing, billing, copies of reports, and diagnostic comments based on good laboratory practice and also based on standardized conditional orders from physicians. Doctors should be able to order some tests, with a requirement to order additional tests based on the outcome of the initial set.

 If this type of functionality is to be employed, the user should ensure that these actions do not contravene any local, state, or federal laws or regulations relating to medical laboratory testing and/or billing.

Reflexing should be available for numeric results based on set ranges of results. The user should be able to specify whether or not a delta check failure should be part of the criteria considered for a reflex to occur. For example if a complete blood count (CBC) is ordered and the white blood count (WBC) significantly increased, the user may wish to reflex a smear review or manual differential. However, this may not be required if the WBC had been previously elevated and a manual differential was done at that time. Such reflexes should automatically include any allowable billing codes.

Reflexing should also be available based on specific coded comment result entry. Based on a microbiology organism code or coded comment code, the user should be able to define the requirement to automatically send a copy of the report to the appropriate public health authority.

Another simple example would be a positive screening test such as an antinuclear factor (ANF) screen automatically reflexing addition of an antinuclear antibody (ANA) titer along with appropriate billing codes.

The user should be able to define multiple reflexes for any test result. This would allow the addition of more than one test or the addition of a test and additional reports, and so forth.

CALCULATED RESULTS

For any test results that are calculated, if a calculation formula can be defined by the user, then the user should be able to apply this formula to the definition of a test in the data tables.

This can be as simple as FTI = T3 * T4 (free thyroxine index = T3 result × T4 result) or as complex as CC = (Uc/(CR/1000)) * (((UV * 24)/cP)/864000) * (1.73/AA) where:

CC = creatinine clearance
Uc = urine creatinine
CR = serum creatinine
UV = urine volume collected
cP = time period of urine collection (usually but not necessarily 24 hours)
AA = body surface area

EXPERT SYSTEMS

When the calculation cannot be clearly written in a single line formula, the LIS should provide alternate means of achieving these results. This may require expert systems or artificial intelligence.

Many LISs provide expert system functionality, but in most cases the vendor is required to program the expert logic required by the user. This works very well provided the user can provide adequate specifications for the required routines and the vendor can provide the resource to perform the task at reasonable cost.

Ideally, an LIS should provide hooks from within the base software; this allows a "trained user" to write subroutines or algorithms that can be called by the system to analyze result information and provide the required actions. This may include complex reflex requirements, complex calculations, diagnostic interpretations, treatment advise, further testing recommendations, and so forth.

In Chapter 4 on p 68, there are flow charts for the assessment of lipids, the diagnosing of hypertriglyceridemia, and lipid interpretation for coronary heart disease.

These flow charts lend themselves very well to the use of expert systems. The programmer analyst should be capable of following the decision tree of the flow chart and creating a software algorithm to generate the required lipid testing based on provision of risk factors and secondary screening results and provide appropriate diagnostic interpretation and phenotyping if required. In addition, drug treatment, follow-up, and dietary recommendations could be provided as required in each of these complex situations.

The main requirement is a comprehensive specification, provided by the medical specialist, of the factors or conditions that need to be considered, which can be programmed into the expert system to provide the necessary analysis and information for each patient.

FEATURE	SINGLE SITE LAB	MULTISITE LAB
Result Entry—All	Whether single site or multisite organization, all result entry options should be available at all laboratory sites. Not all sites may require all options, e.g., perhaps not all sites perform microbiologic or anatomic pathologic analysis. However, users with appropriate security may need to access these functions from any site depending on their level of expertise and requirement to work at multiple sites. This is also true of the specialized departmental entry screens discussed later. Instrument interface functionality should be available at any site with instruments capable of being interfaced. Requirement is that appropriate connectivity be available for such sites, i.e. dial-up or dedicated communication lines depending on type of instrument, volume of work, and cost effectiveness of connection. Reflex functionality is of value to any lab that wants to and is able to take advantage of this type of powerful assistance from LIS.	

FEATURE	HOSPITAL LAB (HL)	INDEPENDENT LAB (IL)	REFERENCE LAB (RL)
Result Entry	Above comments on single site versus multisite laboratories also apply here for different types of laboratories. Each of result entry features, including reflex functionality, described in text may be equally important to users in any of these types of labs. Again, this is also true of specialized departmental entry screens discussed below.		

FEATURE	BENEFITS TO LAB MANAGEMENT	BENEFITS TO LAB STAFF	BENEFITS TO CLINICIAN
Result Entry—Automated	Highly accurate, cost effective method of entry of large volume of results with minimal operator intervention resulting in personnel savings. Elimination of transcription errors for these results. Much quicker turnaround time for these tests.	Elimination of large amount of tedious data entry.	More rapid response potentially resulting in better patient care. Fewer transcription errors provide better level of confidence in results.
Result Entry—Manual	LIS provides on-screen help for manual result entry, allowing users to concentrate on entry. User prompted when user defined criteria not met, providing safeguards that do not exist in manual non-LIS laboratory, including automatic delta checking, level of abnormality checking, and many other possible error checking routines.	User can concentrate on result entry with awareness and confidence that numerous error checking routines are in operation to assist in accuracy and quality assurance.	Can be more confident of reliability of manually performed test management.

Continued ▶

▶ Continued

FEATURE	BENEFITS TO LAB MANAGEMENT	BENEFITS TO LAB STAFF	BENEFITS TO CLINICIAN
Worklist Result Entry	Even without printing hard copies, computer worklists provide more efficient reliable entry of manually managed tests.	Easier to keep track of order of results being entered, less likely there will be patient result mix-up.	More reliable result entry should allow greater confidence in results.
Reflexing and Expert Systems	Protocols for *appropriate* additional testing, billing, and reporting can be set up and managed efficiently and automatically. No need to worry that conditional actions requiring human intervention may be missed.	Far fewer phone calls asking why test was not done. No need to remember that if "this cholesterol" is elevated, HDL is required. System will tell them. Or perhaps it will just recommend that physician order HDL as follow-up procedure.	Physicians have opportunity to receive expert advice, which hopefully they have had hand in defining in cooperation with the laboratory professionals. Also, less need to worry that their conditional testing may be missed.
Expert System Function Flexibility	Management needs to be aware that not all physicians want or appreciate diagnostic interpretations or treatment recommendations on their laboratory reports. These types of information should be optional and should be controlled by system according to user defined criteria, so that they can be switched off based on who physician is.	Should not need to be concerned about which physicians require additional information and which not.	Those who want it get it and appreciate it. Those who don't want it, don't get it.

Laboratory Departmental Modules or Compartmentalization

Historically some LISs have had separate modules and separate databases for disciplines like microbiology and anatomic pathology, not to mention accounting. With today's technology this type of compartmentalization should not be a system requirement.

Orders should not have to be entered either manually or by electronic transfer into multiple modules or databases unless the organization absolutely requires this approach. For example some LISs may not have a particular user requirement such as transfusion medicine. In such cases the user may elect to acquire one LIS for transfusion medicine and another for the rest of the laboratory. In such cases, the user should ensure that both systems are capable of communicating with each other.

If the laboratory requires compartmentalization for other reasons of workflow or confidentiality, this can be achieved using other configuration and security techniques. This is not to say that such disciplines as microbiology or anatomic pathology do not have specialized needs. They do, but these should be met by functions within the LIS software, not by structurally separate configurations.

Some examples are highlighted later.

LABORATORY WORKFLOW AND INFORMATION MANAGEMENT REQUIREMENTS

HEMATOLOGY RESULTS

With continuing improvements in hematology instrumentation technology, automated hematology interfaces should be pretty straightforward. However once a manual differential or review of the slide is required, the hematology technologist and/or physician should be able to access a single screen for the following functions:

- ▌ Hematology results entry and review
- ▌ On-line individualized cell counter for manual differential counting and reticulocyte counting
- ▌ Automatic correction of WBC for nucleated red blood cells (RBCs)
- ▌ Single key entry to grade RBC morphologic types
- ▌ Automatic correction of RBC indices if any related parameters are corrected
- ▌ Access to previous results with one keystroke

An example of such a screen is shown below.

```
replace |not stored    |update |       |record    1 of    1|

Action [E]  0          HAEMATOLOGY PANEL ENTRY    Cell Results
                           Prev   ICM,HPM,XDF,SED,ML,GT3,HP,GCH,CBC,RET,
Request: TST-103159    Panel: HPM 0  MASTER HPANEL-DO NOT ORD   progress
     Name: COOPER, STAN         DOB: 42/12/30  54 Years  Male    97/03/16
   Doctor: CROT  M. CROTEAU                                   905-305-0042
 Cells  1     WBC Differential 93.1  2       RBC Mrph  3    Platelets 4
 WBC    8.0   1 Neutrophils   43.3  3.7    Aniso          Estimate
 RBC    4.50  2 Lymphocytes   40.6  3.5    Macro
 HGB    175.  3 Monocytes      6.4  0.5    Micro          Fields
 HCT    0.455 0 Eosinophils    2.1  0.2    Hypo      ++   Count
 MCV    85.   . Basophils      0.7  0.1    Poly           Factor      20
 MCH    25.5  8 Metamyelocytes 0.0  0.0    Poik           Estimate
 MCHC   385.  5 Myelocytes     0.0  0.0    Target    +++  Other        5
 RDW    12.0  6 Promyelocytes  0.0  0.0    Stomato        ESR
 PLT    350.  + Blasts         0.0  0.0    Sphero    ++++ Malaria
 MPV    12.5  7 Atyp Lymphs    0.0  0.0    ICC            P.B.
 PDW          4              0.0  0.0    Schisto        Reticulocytes
 PLCR         9              0.0  0.0                   %
 N/LM   0.9   ^ Nuc Red Cells  0.0                      Abs.

PF1-Prev For|PF2-Help |       |F4-Menu   |      || F10-More Key
[E]nter/change results, [F]ree text, [N]otes, [T]racking...   [F2-Help]
```

Courtesy of Triple G Corporation, Markham, Ontario, Canada.

MICRORESULTS

The system should automatically generate bar coded plate labels. It should also be able to produce detailed user definable epidemiology reports and allow automatic recognition of reportable organisms and automatic generation of reports to the appropriate authority.

The microbiologists should be able to access a single screen for the following microbiology functions:

■ User definable worklists and workcards for paperless work-up and result entry

■ Result entry by default for cultures that usually do not have growth, e.g., urine, blood

■ Result entry by coded comment to allow rapid entry of paragraph style comments using simple codes

■ Automatic addition of biochemical and antibiotic panels for positive culture identification and sensitivities

■ User definable preliminary and final reporting

■ Automatic capture of billing for appropriate additional testing such as sensitivities

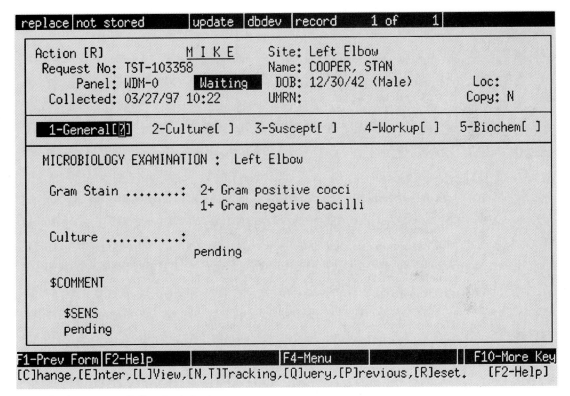

Courtesy of Triple G Corporation, Markham, Ontario, Canada.

The screen above is an example of such a screen for microbiology, showing five main entry functions with *General* highlighted as the section currently in use, i.e., Gram stain or microscopy. Notice that the lower portion of the form indicates work or results already complete. Gram stain results have been entered, and the culture results and sensitivity results are pending.

The foregoing screens are just some examples of the types of special treatment that can be provided for various disciplines such as hematology, microbiology, and anatomic pathology results, without going into detailed examples for all of them.

FEATURE	BENEFITS TO LAB MANAGEMENT	BENEFITS TO LAB STAFF	BENEFITS TO CLINICIAN
Specialized Departmental Result Entry Screens	Confidence that each discipline is using system that allows their special needs for workflow and data entry.	LIS work more accurately and efficiently when LIS functionality allows special needs of their department and in some case even individual users, e.g., user defined count keys for on-line manual differential counter.	Greater confidence in laboratory workflow, data entry, and therefore results.
Integrated System and Database	All data from all disciplines available for inquiry by users with appropriate security access, and for reporting to physicians on single integrated report, as well as cumulative reports if any of these are desired. Also available for integrated management reporting,	More efficient inquiry and reporting capabilities, depending on user security level.	More efficient inquiries and fewer reports.

The user should be able to request and view a list of requests for any test performed on the patient.

For any test request, the user should be able to view a list of any physicians associated with the request as well as any tracking information including demographic changes, test additions and/or deletions, result changes, reports printed and where, reports queued for future printing, and the status of all tests on the order (pending, resulted, or reported).

An important feature from within any inquiry function is to allow the user to print or fax a copy of the report to the physician without having to move to a special report printing screen while the physician may be waiting on the line. If user has to change screens when the physician asks for a copy, it is easy to say yes, hang up, get distracted, and forget.

It is also useful for the user to be able to inquire by physician and test, e.g., to view all orders for all patients from Dr. X with a CBC, within a given date range, or just all orders for Dr. X in the date range.

FEATURE	BENEFITS TO LAB MANAGEMENT	BENEFITS TO LAB STAFF	BENEFITS TO CLINICIAN
Hot Key Inquiry	More efficient and more manageable inquiry.	Users do not lose their current position and do not need to remember what they were doing; LIS remembers for them.	Quicker response to inquiries. Not on the line as long, waiting for user to navigate between functions.

Continued ▶

▶ Continued

FEATURE	BENEFITS TO LAB MANAGEMENT	BENEFITS TO LAB STAFF	BENEFITS TO CLINICIAN
Unique ID	User usually finds correct patient (may still key ID incorrectly but fewer mistakes). Better performance and productivity.	User usually finds correct patient (may still key ID incorrectly but fewer mistakes). Better performance and productivity.	Better reliability of information.
Flexible Search Criteria in Absence of Unique ID	More flexible criteria provide more chances to find incorrect patients but also better chance of finding correct patient.	More flexible criteria provide more chances to find incorrect patients but also better chance of finding correct patient.	If patient results are in system there is better chance of finding.
Print or Fax Report	Ability to print or fax a copy of the report to physician without having to move to special report printing screen while physician may be waiting on line provides more efficient service.	Ease of use, less time consuming, fewer problems.	Better, faster service.
Physician Specific Inquiries	Can review all orders by physician, or orders for specific tests by physician. Sometimes may be only way to find request if physician has forgotten patient's name (it happens). billing, and workload statistics.	Alternate search method sometimes useful.	Can obtain feedback about ordering patterns.

Inquiry on Results (and Other Information)

A user should be able to inquire about patient information and results without aborting and/or leaving whatever function the user is in when the inquiry becomes necessary. Use of one or more hot keys may allow this type of feature. In addition, once the inquiry is complete, a single keystroke should allow the user to return to the previous screen in the same field from which the user left it.

The inquiry function should allow the user to search by patient ID, such as medical record number, personal health number, social security number, or such means of unique patient record identification as might be available. Some reference and independent laboratories are implementing internal patient ID numbers similar to hospital medical record or numbers to allow such identification when they see a significant number of repeat visits from patients.

Failing the availability of a unique ID, the user should be able to search for patients using various other pieces of demographic information such as any part or all of the patient's last and first name, sex, date of birth, physician, and so forth.

Once the patient is found, the user should be able to view all visit and test request information including results and appropriate reference ranges and abnormal flags.

LABORATORY WORKFLOW AND INFORMATION MANAGEMENT REQUIREMENTS

Result Report Formatting

The user should have the ability to define the layout of the report with as much flexibility as possible. This should include the report page size, the layout and content of the header and footer information for each page, and the layout of test demographic, result, range, flag, and interpretive information for every test in the system.

This may sound like a painful amount of work and effort, but in the end the user has control of the laboratory's end product, the laboratory report. Without such functions the user must accept the vendor's standard report formatting capabilities or rely on the vendor to provide custom layouts.

Ideally the user should be able to define such layouts by laboratory client, doctor, ward, and so forth. The intensive care unit may require different information or a different sequence of information from long term care. One physician or group of physicians may have preferences for serial graphic reporting whereas others may not.

When such alternatives can be set up by the users, the system should then be able to select and report the appropriate format based on the provider or location of the patient.

FEATURE	HOSPITAL LAB (HL)	INDEPENDENT LAB (IL)	REFERENCE LAB (RL)
Flexible Report Formatting	Generally wants some flexibility but usually prefers to define select few formats to be used throughout institution. If told it could have or create as many different formats as it wishes, it often requests that its physicians not be informed of such capabilities. When hospital organization has outreach program or acts as reference laboratory for its community, reaction is more akin to that of IL and RL.	Here and at RL, both highly competitive and service oriented, this feature is highly desirable tool, particularly in eyes of sales and marketing departments.	Same as IL.

FEATURE	BENEFITS TO LAB MANAGEMENT	BENEFITS TO LAB STAFF	BENEFITS TO CLINICIAN
Flexible Report Formatting	Ability to meet varied requirements of different health care providers and services. More control of its end product and its impact on its clientele, and ability to respond to market demands quickly.	Ability to use different formatting within laboratory during performance of testing and result review provides user with better information and enhanced productivity, e.g., even if physician may not want serial reporting of various results, technologist may make use of such layouts in evaluating results for approval.	Physicians have availability of report layouts that in their experience provide them with better feedback and understanding of test results.

Result Report Delivery (Printing, Routing, Faxing, Phoning, Electronic Transfer—HL7)

PRINTING, DELIVERY, AND FAXING OF REPORTS

No matter how good the technical expertise of the laboratory staff, the excellence of the technology, equipment, and quality control employed in testing, i.e., no matter how good the test results may be or how quickly they are produced, they are useless until they are in the hands of the physician.

In its most primitive form, report delivery is accomplished by hand transport of the report from the laboratory to the ward or physician by porter, courier, or mail. In such situations the reports are generally printed at a central site (either in the laboratory or a mail room) and sorted and distributed for delivery. In such situations the LIS should be able to provide appropriate sorting of the reports by courier routes, delivery areas, specific locations, physicians, or other laboratory sort criteria.

The LIS should also be able to provide automatic or on-demand delivery of reports by remote printing to wards, clinics, and physicians' offices, and automatic faxing (provided that fax numbers are on-line in the database).

Ideally the system should have the capability to format output to any print device so that the user defined format can produce graphic page set quality reports on Post-Script laser printers and still be able alternatively to print a legible report on a dumb character or line printer or fax machine.

Faxing of reports is really only a specialized form of remote printing. In addition to the internal autofax capability that the LIS should have, there should also be inherent in the system the ability for on-demand fax reporting so that when a physician request that a copy be sent to an unidentified fax number, the user has the ability to request a copy report with the ability to supply a fax number, so that the system can then fax the report. In most cases there should not be a need to print a hard copy of the report and fax it manually.

ELECTRONIC TRANSFER OF REPORTS

In addition to electronic transfer of laboratory orders (O/E S2S interface) many hospitals, health maintenance organizations (HMOs), and even physicians' offices are moving more and more to a central result reporting repository. This requires that the LIS be able to transfer meaningful information to hospital information systems (HISs) and clinic management systems, preferably by using standardized communications file transfer protocols message structures such as Health Level Seven (HL7). For more detailed information on HL7, see the bibliography.

Although many one on one customized system to system (S2S) interfaces exist and can be created as required, the use of HL7 standard interfaces is becoming more and more widely required. S2S interfacing allows the LIS to transmit the data to the result repository and have it integrated into the repository database. The health care professionals then have a single source of information such as laboratory results, radiographic and other diagnostic imaging information, pharmacy, and so forth. However, even where this is the standard source of information, the ability to access the information from the LIS should always be available in an emergency.

DELIVERY AVAILABILITY

Whatever the mechanism of delivery of report information to the physician, it should always be available either on demand or in an automatic scheduler.

LABORATORY WORKFLOW AND INFORMATION MANAGEMENT REQUIREMENTS

The laboratory should be able to schedule print runs, fax runs, or electronic transfers as often or as infrequently as it wishes or requires. It should also be able to force an individual report or an entire print run or transfer manually as required.

REPORT TRACKING

The system should automatically create a tracking record in a permanent log every time a report is issued by any mechanism. Users should be able to inquire and see a record of any or all such events and know what or who initiated the report (scheduled or forced), the date and time it was initiated, the date and time it printed or transmitted, who it was printed for, and to what peripheral device it was sent.

FEATURE	SINGLE SITE LAB	MULTISITE LAB
Printing and Sorting	Single site laboratories need to be able to print and sort reports to go to any or all of their specimen collection areas or wards, as well as any individual physicians, group practices or other clients.	The multisite laboratory first of all should have ability to combine results of tests from same order onto single report even though testing may have been done by more than one testing facility.
Remote Printing, Auto Faxing, S2S, Interfacing, Scheduled Report Runs, and Report Tracking	Each of these other features would be equally as important to single site and multisite laboratories.	

FEATURE	BENEFITS TO LAB MANAGEMENT	BENEFITS TO LAB STAFF	BENEFITS TO CLINICIAN
Printing and Sorting	Even with hand or courier delivered reports, hours of costly manual labor can be saved and TAT improved by having LIS properly sort reports at time of printing.	Staff are freed up to concentrate on other tasks rather than something that is better done by automated technology.	Physicians receive reports earlier and more reliably.
Remote Printing	Elimination of costly delivery process provides additional cost savings and improved TAT. One negative factor here is that remote print devices can be management problem, especially if they are not under laboratory manager's control.	As above.	As above.
Autofaxing	Same advantages as remote printing. Better than manual faxing because controlled by computer and central hard copy is not required	As above.	As above.

Continued ▶

▶ Continued

FEATURE	BENEFITS TO LAB MANAGEMENT	BENEFITS TO LAB STAFF	BENEFITS TO CLINICIAN
S2S Interfacing	Less concern about report printing and delivery. Data repository provides single source of information such as laboratory results, radiographic and other diagnostic imaging information, pharmacy, and so forth. Direct access to LIS data can also be provided as apparently seamless access to laboratory data from HIS terminal.	Fewer phone calls from physicians looking for results. Whether available in central repository or direct access to LIS results, physicians may have direct inquiry access.	Physicians have direct access to inquiry either in data repository or online inquiry to LIS.
Scheduled Report Runs	Automatic scheduling of report runs allows lab to report as results are ready to be released without having to wait for human intervention to release reports.	Confidence that results are available to physician in quick reliable manner.	Confidence that they have results available quickly and reliably.
Report Tracking	Any and all reports printed or transmitted electronically by LIS are tracked and recorded.	Able to find and provide positive information regarding every report issued by LIS.	Confidence that reports are not lost or misdirected.

Quality Assurance and Quality Control

QUALITY ASSURANCE

In the last section it was stated that *no matter* how good the test results may be or how quickly they are produced, they are useless until they are reported. *However,* quickly and efficiently reporting an erroneous or invalid result is even more dangerous than not reporting a result at all.

The LIS may be very good at reporting results automatically, but it cannot maintain the quality of the laboratory. The first step in quality assurance (QA) in addition to an acceptable quality control (QC) system (see later) is the ability of the system to log as many relevant user and system activities as possible.

The second important step in the QA process is the reporting of this information in user defined management reports back to the appropriate managers or supervisors, either automatically for some frequently desired reports or on demand and possibly ad hoc for less frequently required information.

Some simple examples might be:

Lists of all changed results by original result entry user and changed result user
Lists of specimen integrity problems and originating collection locations, wards, and so forth
Lists of all late tests results
Lists of all critical value results and the date and time reported, by whom, and to whom

Relational database systems and SQL provide the most comprehensive and flexible capabilities for this type of reporting. Not only is it quicker and easier for LIS vendors to produce such reports, but laboratory staff or associated IS staff can learn to provide them very quickly.

LABORATORY WORKFLOW AND INFORMATION MANAGEMENT REQUIREMENTS

QUALITY CONTROL

QC is a major part of QA. The LIS should allow the laboratory to keep track of QC results on-line and perform all the required statistical analyses to ensure that the laboratory's testing accuracy and precision are maintained at acceptable levels.

Users should have the ability to define as many levels of QC material as they require and define what tests are performed on each material. In addition they should be able to assign what work areas are reported for each material down to individual analyzer by laboratory site if multiple site testing is performed.

Users should be able to enter results for any tests manually. The system should also be able to receive QC results automatically from any on-line instrument interface. The QC system should be able to recognize the source of any QC result, e.g., analyzer 1, analyser 2, even if they are the same make and model instrument.

Westgard rule application should be definable (i.e., which rules to use) for each test and should be applicable across single or multiple levels of control material by user definition.

When rule failures occur the use should be automatically prompted for error assessment or corrective action comments. The user should also have the ability to define whether acceptance of patient results can be blocked automatically by the QC system or whether this remains a technologist decision with appropriate security authority and logging.

At any time, a supervisor or manager should have the ability to review QC data on-line and comment on QC results and approve for internal audit and external inspection.

QUALITY CONTROL REPORTS AND GRAPHS

QC Reports and/or graphs should be able to be printed by the user at any time, or scheduled for printing at regular intervals if so desired. Users should have the option to print by test; by QC material; by level; by analyzer; by day, week, month, or any specified date range; and by any combination of these parameters.

Although graphics terminals and printers provide the most esthetic output for QC graphs, ideally the LIS should be able to send either graphics output to printers and terminals that can support them or character based outputs to any device that cannot support graphics. The latter may not be pretty, but they are visual and save the expense of the graphic displays for those who want to save money.

FEATURE	BENEFITS TO LAB MANAGEMENT	BENEFITS TO LAB STAFF	BENEFITS TO CLINICIAN
Automatic Logging of Activities and Problems	On-line tracking of compliance with defined QA protocols.	Built-in warnings and automatic reporting to help avoid errors or problems in system.	Better QA provides more reliable information from laboratory.
Reporting of Quality Information Logs	Routine reporting of QA information for supervisory review. May be helpful in determining weaknesses in workflow or staff requiring additional training.	Staff requiring remedial training can receive it quickly so that problems do not persist.	Improved quality of staff and service.

Continued ▶

▶ Continued

FEATURE	BENEFITS TO LAB MANAGEMENT	BENEFITS TO LAB STAFF	BENEFITS TO CLINICIAN
QC	On-line QC system saves hours of on-line entry of automated results and automatically performs all statistical analysis required. Staff are notified on-line when out of control errors occur.	On-line notification of rule failures, with automatic prompting for corrective actions or appropriate overrides, allows more rapid response, correction, and quicker acceptance of results	Confidence in quality of test performance.

Management Reporting

Most LISs have a battery of basic management reports that come as part of the system. Any additional reports or changes to layouts of existing reports are considered by most LIS vendors to be customizations.

The laboratory benefits if the LIS provides tools that allow users with appropriate security access to write their own ad hoc reports, rather than to have to request them of the LIS or IS department or the vendor.

Management reports whether canned, automatic, on demand, or ad hoc cover a wide range of laboratory areas and information such as (but certainly not limited to):

▎ Laboratory productivity

User data entry statistics

Workload statistics by area, location, client, facility (if multiple)

Turnaround time reports

Results waiting to be approved for release

Late test results

Missed pickups or deliveries

▎ Billing and Financial

Income by location or ward or clinic

Income by client or physician

Daily or weekly or monthly revenue for current month or year to date

▎ Client management

Referral statistics.

▎ Infection control reports

Organisms isolated by ward or service

Drug correlations (if drug information is available to the LIS)

▎ User definable

Special result surveys

Research and development

Specific test ordering patterns by physician.

Reference range studies

LABORATORY WORKFLOW AND INFORMATION MANAGEMENT REQUIREMENTS

The major limiting factors for management report availability should be only twofold:

1. Is the data you need to put in the report in the database?
2. Is the server powerful enough to do the job without degrading system performance?

Billing and Accounts Receivable

Ideally the LIS should have an integrated billing and accounts receivable (A/R) module. There should be no need to interface to a separate database and definitely no need to reenter orders into a separate system.

Order entry of data into the LIS the should automatically capture all the necessary billing information up front. The LIS should also be able to automatically generate legally and ethically acceptable additional billing as required. For example, when a request for culture yields positive results and sensitivity testing is indicated and additional billing is allowed, then the LIS should automatically add on the appropriate test and billing information.

If various test combinations result in application of different billing rules from when the tests are done separately, then this adjustment should be user definable and handled automatically by the LIS.

Beyond the special billing requirements of clinical laboratories, the A/R module should be fully functional and based on sound standard principles of accounting.

Regulatory and Standards Compliance

REGULATORY

Various agencies (CAP, CLIA, FDA (see later definitions), state health authorities, and so forth) monitor clinical laboratories for adherence to various sets of standards and/or regulations. Most of these standards or regulatory bodies do not specifically require laboratories to have LIS computers. However when the laboratory does have an LIS, most of these bodies have sections in their requirements specific to, or that can be interpreted to, apply to the LIS.

Many of the requirements differ from state to state. The LIS cannot define the compliance protocol that any laboratory wishes to follow. However the laboratory and LIS vendor should be able to ensure that as many of the standardized and regulated procedures as possible are monitored and any exception are logged by the LIS. Appropriate flags, warnings, or reports should be issued if compliance is violated. Some simple example are as follows:

- Certain tests may not be performed if specimen is older than a given time frame (the time may vary from state to state). The LIS should warn users if the time span from the time of collection to the time of entry exceeds the required time.
- If a result is changed, any subsequent report must display both the old and the new result. The LIS should be able to do this automatically.

AGENCIES THAT MAY REGULATE OR STANDARDIZE USE OF LABORATORY INFORMATION SYSTEMS

The following summary of external organizations is presented mainly to assist the reader in understanding *how and by whom the LIS may be affected,* which in fact is not that much different from how and by whom the laboratory may be affected.

Some of the agencies that need to be considered by laboratories are listed below. Additional information on how such agencies may expect to regulate LISs may be found in references in the bibliography.

DHHS. The Department of Health and Human Services, includes HCFA.

HCFA. Healthcare Finance Administration. HCFA is charged with the implementation and enforcement of CLIA (see later), including approval of proficiency testing programs, accreditation programs, and state exemption applications. On the financial side, HCFA also administers Medicare and Medicaid reimbursement for medical treatment, and in order to receive payments for covered services, a laboratory must meet the requirements of HCFA that are embodied by the CLIA regulations.

CLIA 88. Clinical Laboratory Improvement Amendments of 1988. CLIA was the result of congressional investigations after several media reports focused attention on deficiencies in the quality of service provided by some of the nation's clinical laboratories. The final regulations of CLIA 88, published in the February 28, 1992, Federal Register, are very comprehensive, set minimal standards for laboratory practice and quality, and specify requirements for proficiency testing, QC, patient test management, personnel, QA, certification, and inspections.

Proficiency Testing. Proficiency testing is central to the regulations' intent to ensure quality. This determines which laboratories comply and which fail. Failure to comply results in the application of sanctions, the penalty of which can range from loss of license to increased testing.

Inspection. Inspection is another key part of the regulations' tools to ensure quality. Several organizations have obtained status to perform inspections. Inspection is every 2 years.

Quality Control and Quality Assurance. Two areas of concern appear to be QC and QA. Key areas for inspection are appropriate QC and documentation as well as a QA program that monitors and evaluates the total laboratory.

CAP. College of American Pathologists. This nonprofit organization supports improvement of laboratory science and is a deemed proficiency testing organization. The CAP proficiency testing program may be utilized instead of the HCFA proficiency testing program.

JCAHO. Joint Commission for Accreditation of Healthcare Organizations. The JCAHO began evaluating laboratory services for hospitals in 1979 and in January 1995 was granted deeming authority under CLIA 88. Laboratories that are accredited by the JCAHO meet the most rigorous quality standards available today.

STATES. Each state has compliance regulations that are required of laboratories that wish to do business in that state. Some of the state programs are comprehensive enough to be deemed by the HCFA to meet their requirements.

UNITED STATES JUSTICE DEPARTMENT, OIG. Office of the Inspector General. The OIG ensures compliance to appropriate billing procedures by laboratories.

LABORATORY WORKFLOW AND INFORMATION MANAGEMENT REQUIREMENTS

STANDARDS

Clinical laboratories and health care institutions in general make strong efforts to standardize as many aspects of their work as possible. In addition the LIS should be produced using standardized procedures and should be able to help the laboratory monitor its own standard procedures in the same manner as for regulatory procedures previously described. Several of the standards being used in clinical Laboratories and in LISs are listed here. Again, additional information may be found in some of the references in the bibliography.

ISO 9000. International Standards Organization. ISO 9000 is a business management standard. The standard covers 20 main topics, including the way that the company trains its staff to do their job, the way that it ensures that the products or services are correct, how it handles mistakes and prevents them from happening in future, and many other considerations.

In 1988, the BS5750 standard of the British Standards Institute was adopted by the International Standards Organization, without changes, and was published internationally under the ISO 9000 name.

In 1994, ISO 9000 was revised and published internationally. There are a number of other standards and guidance documents that have been amended to reflect the requirements of ISO 9000. For example, The U.S. Food and Drug Administration (FDA) has revised its good manufacturing practice (GMP) regulations for medical devices to follow ISO 9001 with appropriate additional requirements.

Today, the term *ISO 9000* has become synonymous with quality, not just in English, but in most every language used to conduct trade and commerce.

FDA REQUIREMENTS. The FDA has been given jurisdiction by Congress to oversee the manufacture of medical devices and drugs in the United States. Any new device or drug must receive an Investigational Device Exemption before beginning its testing for certification. Then, when testing has been completed following "good science" rules for scientific evidence, a 510k must be filed complete with proofs of testing that meet the labeling claims for the device.

This has been the case for some time with in vivo devices and drugs, including blood bank laboratory systems, but the FDA at the time of this writing is now investigating extending the rules to software used in the medical field, particularly in laboratories.

ASTM. American Society for Testing Materials. A U.S. based nonprofit organization similar to ISO has created a body of standards and includes E31, the Committee for Clinical Information Systems that directly describes standards for the manufacture of computer software used in health care. ASTM has also produced a standard for analyzer interface communications that is rapidly being adopted by most instrument and LIS manufacturers.

LOINC. Logical Observation Identifier Names and Codes. This is a fairly new standard for clinical laboratory test nomenclature that is rapidly becoming popular internationally. It is a free database providing *unique* standard names and codes to identify tests and results in data transmissions and has recently been endorsed by the American Clinical Laboratory Association (ACLA).

HL7. Health Level Seven. HL7 is an organization of health care workers involved in the use of or production of health care informatics. Its ultimate goal is to produce a standard specification for communication of information or data interchange from one health care computer system to another.

System Acceptance, Validation

Every LIS should have a defined protocol for system acceptance or validation. This provides the vehicle for the laboratory to agree on acceptance of the system. Initially this will be the base unmodified system. The laboratory and the LIS vendor should then agree on a validation procedure for any required customizations.

These procedures together should also be the foundation for demonstrating first to the laboratory management and users and second to any of the regulating bodies that all their requirements have been met by the LIS.

The validation process for the LIS is as important as calibration and standardization of any clinical laboratory analyzer. It should be designed to validate:

▮ Existing data provided with the system (data definitions)
▮ New data entered into the system (new order, new test, or results entered, and so forth)
▮ Any and all processes in the LIS that manipulate and alter data (interfaced entry of orders, result reflexes, calculations, billing generation, and so forth)
▮ Any data so altered (calculated result, reflexed test added, and so forth)
▮ Production of user activity logs or tracking records (date, time, and user log for changed demographics, tests added or deleted, changed results, and so forth)

The LIS should provide the users with the tools to be able to set up and monitor any and all of these items. Such tools may include scripts for printing data sets, standard information reports, special validation reports, or patient result reports.

Each step in the process must be documented.

FEATURE	SINGLE SITE LAB	MULTISITE LAB
Regulatory Compliance and Voluntary Standards Utilization	Compliance, it should be obvious, is mandatory for all laboratories. Voluntary use of nonregulated standards is equally important to any laboratory. LIS should be useful in monitoring compliance for all laboratories whether small, large, single site, or multisite. As more and more laboratories implement them, the use of voluntary standards such as ASTM or HL7 provide laboratory with ability to communicate with other health care systems as required, with far less effort than with stand-alone proprietary interface requirements.	
System Validation	For any laboratory, LIS should provide users with tools to be able to set up and monitor any and all of these items. Such tools may include scripts for printing data sets, standard information reports, special validation reports, or patient result reports.	

FEATURE	HOSPITAL LAB (HL)	INDEPENDENT LAB (IL)	REFERENCE LAB (RL)
Regulatory Compliance and Voluntary Standards Utilization	As above, compliance, it should be obvious, is mandatory for all laboratories. Voluntary use of nonregulated standards is equally important to any laboratory. LIS should be useful in monitoring compliance for all laboratories whether HL, IL, or RL. As more and more laboratories implement them, use of voluntary standards such as ASTM or HL7 provide laboratory with ability to communicate with other health care systems as required, with far less effort than with stand-alone proprietary interface requirements.		
System Validation	As above, for any laboratory, LIS should provide users with tools to be able to set up and monitor any and all of these items. Such tools may include scripts for printing data sets, standard information reports, special validation reports, or patient result reports.		

LABORATORY WORKFLOW AND INFORMATION MANAGEMENT REQUIREMENTS

FEATURE	BENEFITS TO LAB MANAGEMENT	BENEFITS TO LAB STAFF	BENEFITS TO CLINICIAN
Regulatory Compliance	LIS should provide appropriate warnings if monitored compliance issues are not met. Less likelihood of inspection infractions.	LIS should provide appropriate warnings if monitored compliance issues are not met. Less likelihood of inspection infractions. Confidence that laboratory is following required or recommended procedures.	Confidence that laboratory is following required or recommended procedures.
Voluntary Standards Utilization	Use of voluntary standards such as ASTM or HL7 provide laboratory with ability to communicate with other health care systems as required, with far less effort than with stand-alone proprietary interface requirements. Viewed favorably by inspecting agencies.	Confidence that laboratory is following required or recommended procedures.	Confidence that laboratory is following required or recommended procedures.
System Validation	Confidence that LIS is working as intended and as required.	Confidence that LIS is working as intended and as required.	Confidence that LIS is working as intended and as required.

SUMMARY

Laboratory acquisitions, mergers, consolidation, and amalgamation, in addition to other causes of business growth, are putting tremendous pressures on LISs to be flexible and to play a key role in the integration of new business relationships while providing management and users with the tools necessary to ensure quality and cost effective lab services.

The interdependency between application design and the tools used cannot be overstated. One without the other results in an information tool that constrains an organization and its users, due to its inability to respond in a timely fashion to the ever changing reality of the laboratory business, be it public, private, profit, not for profit, commercial, hospital, or any or all of the above.

If one looks at LIS vendors and their origins in the market today, the bulk have been developed for and evolved from single hospital settings. In order to meet the demands imposed by the market over recent years to provide functions that deal with multiple sites, routing of specimens, external customer service, competition with reference labs, and unique specimen identification (one of the fundamental requirements of laboratory automation), the functional "retrofitting" of legacy software results in less than elegant solutions to fundamental business requirements.

This partially explains why small laboratory operations have upward of 50 to 60 LIS vendors that may offer acceptable LIS packages, whereas the larger, multisite operations have only four or five realistic options that would be considered viable solutions.

Today's vendor should offer an open system solution running on an industry standard RDBMS and proved in today's market in high volume multisite environments.

The American Society for Clinical Laboratory Sciences is offering complementary software developed by the Triple G Corporation that will complement this chapter. The software will enable individuals to access laboratory information system windows and makes the chapter interactive. To receive a free copy of these disks, write, FAX, or phone:

> The American Society for Clinical Laboratory Sciences
> 7910 Woodmont Avenue, Suite 530
> Bethesda, Maryland 20814
>
> Telephone (301) 657-2768 ext 3024
> FAX   (301) 657-2909

BIBLIOGRAPHY

Books, Journals, and Periodicals

Aller RD, Balis UJ: Informatics. In Henry JB: Clinical Diagnosis and Management by Laboratory Methods, 19th ed. Philadelphia, WB Saunders, 1996, Chapter 5.

Aller RD, Elvitch FR, eds: Laboratory and Hospital Information Systems. Philadelphia, WB Saunders, 1991.

Clinical Laboratory News: Various articles re LOINC—Standard for Electronic Reporting of Test Results. Clin Lab News 23(4), 1996.

Elvitch FR: Computers in the clinical laboratory. In Burtis CA, Ashwood ER, eds: Teitz Textbook of Clinical Chemistry, 2nd ed. Philadelphia, WB Saunders, 1994, Chapter 16.

Elvitch FR, Treling C, Spackman K, et al: A clinical laboratory automation system survey: challenge for the decade. Arch Pathol Lab Med, 117:12–21, 1993.

Kenny D, Solberg HE, eds: Special issue: computing in clinical laboratories. Clin Chim Acta 222:147–171, 1993.

McNeely MD, Smith BJ: An interactive expert system for the ordering and interpretation of laboratory tests to enhance diagnosis and control utilization. Can Med Informat 2(3):16–19, 1995. Also on Internet at http://vvv.com/ai/las/medinfo.html.

Ward K, Lehmann C, Leiken A: Clinical Laboratory Instrumentation and Automation. Philadelphia, WB Saunders, 1994.

Internet World Wide Web Sites

http://www.mcis.duke.edu/standards/termcode/loinc.htm—LOINC.

http://www.os.dhhs.gov—OIG.

http://www.jcaho.org—JCAHO.

http://nelle.mc.duke.edu/standards/HL7/hl7.htm—HL7.

http://www.hcfa.gov/oirm/hdplan1.htm—HCFA.

http://www.cap.org/html/lip/lap.html—CAP Laboratory Accreditation Program.

Chapter **47**

LABORATORY MATHEMATICS

Craig A. Lehmann, PhD, CC(NRCC)

Q U I C K   C O N T E N T S

INTRODUCTION

This chapter covers some of the more common mathematics problems encountered by laboratory personnel. Each problem is presented as if one were explaining the process to another individual. A step by step approach is taken, showing all the mathematics and explaining the logic for each step in the process.

METRICS

Metric Chart

PREFIX	MULTIPLE	GRAM	LITER
Kilo	1000	1000 milligrams	1000 milliliters
Deci	1/10	100 milligrams	100 milliliters
Centi	1/100	10 milligrams	10 milliliters
Milli	1/1000	1 milligram	1 milliliter
Micro	1/1,000,000	0.001 milligrams	0.001 milliliters
Nano	1/1,000,000,000	0.0000001 milligrams	0.0000001 milliliters
Pico	1/1,000,000,000,000	0.0000000000001 milligrams	0.0000000000001 milliliters
Femto	1/1,000,000,000,000,000	0.0000000000000001 milligrams	0.0000000000000001 milliliters

Converting One Metric Unit to Another

Example. Convert 0.036 g to milligrams.

Formula.

$$\frac{0.036 \text{ g}}{x \text{ mg}} = \frac{1 \text{ g}}{1000 \text{ mg}}$$

$$x = 0.036 \times 1000$$

$$\underline{x = 36 \text{ mg}}$$

Converting Fahrenheit and Celsius Temperatures

Formula. $\quad °F = \left(°C \times \dfrac{9}{5}\right) + 32 \quad$ or $\quad °F = (°C \times 1.8) + 32$

$$°C = (°F - 32) \times \frac{5}{9} \quad \text{or} \quad °C = (°F - 32) \times 0.556$$

Example. Convert 40°C to Fahrenheit.

$$°F = (40 \times 1.8) + 32$$

$$°F = 72 + 32$$

$$°F = 104$$

DILUTIONS

Example. Calculate the final concentration of serum in the dilution and calculate the dilution of each step.

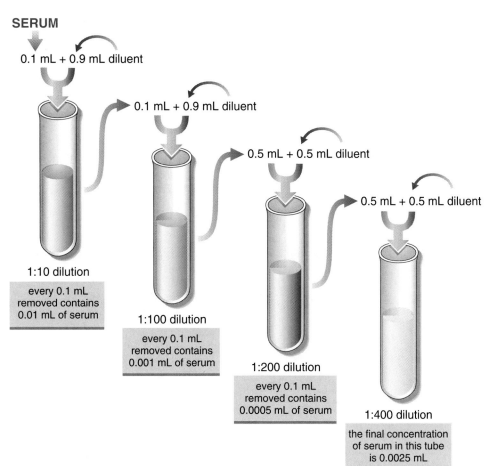

SERUM

0.1 mL + 0.9 mL diluent

0.1 mL + 0.9 mL diluent

0.5 mL + 0.5 mL diluent

0.5 mL + 0.5 mL diluent

1:10 dilution

every 0.1 mL removed contains 0.01 mL of serum

1:100 dilution

every 0.1 mL removed contains 0.001 mL of serum

1:200 dilution

every 0.1 mL removed contains 0.0005 mL of serum

1:400 dilution

the final concentration of serum in this tube is 0.0025 mL

DILUTIONS

SOLUTIONS

Weight/Weight

Example. Make 1800 mL of a 50% weight/weight, acetone/alcohol solution.

1. Since you are working with liquids, the first piece of information you need to know is the specific gravity of each:

   Specific gravity of acetone is 0.786.
   Specific gravity of alcohol is 0.810.

2. Since this is a percent (100) solution the next step is to find out how many milliliters of each you will need to get 50 g of each to make a total of 100 g:

$$\frac{50 \text{ g}}{0.786 \text{ specific gravity}} = 63.6 \quad \text{mL of acetone required to get 50 g}$$

$$\frac{50 \text{ g}}{0.810 \text{ specific gravity}} = 61.73 \quad \text{mL of alcohol required to get 50 g}$$

3. The second step is to add the milliliters of acetone and alcohol together. This tells you how many total milliliters are required to have 50 g of each substance:

$$
\begin{array}{ll}
63.6 & \text{mL of acetone} \\
+61.73 & \text{mL of alcohol} \\
\hline
125.33 & \text{total mL}
\end{array}
$$

4. Since the total volume needed is 1800, you need to find out how many 125.33s are in 1800 mL.
This is accomplished by dividing 125.33 into 1800:

$$1800 \div 125.33 = 14.36$$

5. The final step is to find the total volumes of acetone and alcohol needed to make 1800 mL of the 50% solution:

$$63.6 \text{ mL of acetone} \times 14.36 = \quad 913.296 \text{ mL} \qquad \text{total volume of acetone added to bottle}$$

$$61.73 \text{ mL of alcohol} \times 14.36 = \underline{+886.44} \quad \text{mL} \qquad \text{total volume of alcohol added to bottle}$$

$$\qquad\qquad\qquad\qquad\qquad\qquad 1799.74 \quad \text{mL} \qquad \text{total volume of solution}$$

Weight/Volume

Now make the same solution but a weight/volume. This means that you want 1800 mL of 50% acetone in alcohol.

1. The first step again because you are working with a liquid is to convert the weight to milliliters. Because the only weight in the calculation is acetone, you only need to convert acetone:

$$\frac{50 \text{ g}}{0.786} = 63.6 \quad \text{mL of acetone required to obtain 50 g of acetone}$$

Therefore, for every 100 mL of solution you need 63.6 mL of acetone.

2. The total volume needed is 1800 mL:

$$1800 \div 100 = 18$$

$$18 \times 63.6 = 1145.04 \qquad \text{total acetone required}$$

3. Subtract the amount of required acetone from the total volume. This shows you how much alcohol is needed:

$$\begin{array}{r} 1800 \\ -1145.04 \\ \hline 654.96 \end{array}$$

total volume
acetone required
mL of alcohol needed to be added to acetone to make final solution

Volume/Volume

Now take the same solution and make 1800 mL of 50% volume/volume. 1800 of a 50% volume/volume solution of acetone/alcohol is made as follows:

Since no weight is involved, there is no need to convert from grams to milliliters. Therefore:

$$50\% \text{ or } 0.50 \times 1800 = 900 \text{ mL}$$

$$\begin{array}{r} 900 \\ +900 \\ \hline 1800 \end{array}$$

mL of acetone
mL of alcohol
mL of solution = 50% volume/volume

Percent Solutions

Make a 10% solution of Na_2SO_4.

This is essentially a weight/volume solution. Therefore, 10 g of sodium sulfate is diluted to 100 mL with a liquid. However, if the only sodium sulfate that you have in stock is hydrated, you must account for the water molecules. Typically, hydrated sodium sulfate has 10 water molecules ($Na_2SO_4 \cdot 10H_2O$).

The gram molecular weight of sodium sulfate is 142.0396.
The gram molecular weight of sodium sulfate with 10 water molecules is 322.1896.

To demonstrate the effect of water, divide the molecular weight of the hydrated form into the needed anhydrous form:

$$322.1896\overline{)142.0396}^{\,0.44086}$$

Therefore, every gram of the hydrated form contains only 0.44086 of pure sodium sulfate.

The following formula accounts for the water:

$$\frac{142.0396}{322.1896} = \frac{10}{x}$$

$$142.0396x = 322.1896 \times 10$$

$$x = \frac{3221.896}{142.0396}$$

$$x = 22.684$$

g of $Na_2SO_4 \cdot 10\ H_2O$ diluted to 100 with water to make a 10% solution

MOLARITY

A molar solution is the gram molecular weight (GMW) of a substance dissolved and diluted to a final volume of 1 liter of solution.

Example. A 1 molar solution of sodium sulfate would be made by weighing out the GMW (142.0396 g) and diluting up to 1000 mL with a solute.
  More information is required if the chemical is a liquid and/or an acid.

Example. A 2 molar solution of phosphoric acid would be made by finding the correct volume of the acid needed to obtain the GMW (97.9938 g) of phosphoric acid. Since it is a liquid you need to account for the specific gravity. Also since it is an acid you need to account for its purity.

  The GMW of phosphoric acid = 97.9938 g
  The specific gravity = 1.5 g/mL
  The purity = 85.5%

Therefore, the formula should be written as follows:

$$\text{2 molar phosphoric acid} = \frac{97.9938 \text{ GMW}}{1.5 \text{ specific gravity} \times 0.855 \text{ purity}} \times 2$$
$$= 152.817 \text{ mL of acid diluted to } 1000 \text{ mL}$$

NORMALITY

A normal solution is the number of equivalent weights per 1000 mL of solvent or the GMW divided by the valence. Therefore, the previous 2 molar phosphoric acid solution would be a 6 normal solution because it has a valence of 3 (three replaceable hydrogens).
  The formula for making a 1 normal solution of phosphoric acid is as follows:

$$\text{1 normal phosphoric acid} = \frac{98 \text{ GMW}}{3 \text{ valence} \times 1.5 \text{ specific gravity} \times 0.855 \text{ purity}}$$

$$= 25.471 \quad \text{mL of acid needed}$$

Therefore, a 1 normal phosphoric acid solution requires 25.471 mL of acid to be diluted to 1000 mL with solvent.

MOLALITY

A molal solution is the GMW of a substance dissolved in 1000 g of a solvent.

Example. Make a 1 molal solution of sulfuric acid.

  The GMW of H_2SO_4 is 98.
  The specific gravity is 1.6.
  The purity is 98%.

Formula.

$$1 \text{ mole of } H_2SO_4 = \frac{98}{1.6 \text{ specific gravity} \times 0.98 \text{ purity}} = 62.42 \text{ mL}$$

Therefore 62.42 mL of sulfuric acid placed in 1000 g of solvent = 1 molal solution of H_2SO_4. The total volume of this solution is 1062.42 mL.

Milliequivalents

A milliequivalent is the equivalent weight expressed in milligrams.

Example. Typically the laboratory is required to convert milligrams per deciliter (mg/dL) to milliequivalents per liter (mEq/L). This can be accomplished by the following formula:

$$mEq/L = \frac{mg/dL \times 10 \times \text{valence}}{\text{molecular weight}}$$

In order to convert 3 mg/dL of magnesium to mEq/L:

$$mEq/L = \frac{3 \times 10 \times 2}{24.31} = 2.47 \qquad \begin{aligned} 3 &= mg/dL \\ 10 &= dl \text{ to L} \\ 2 &= \text{valence} \\ 24.31 &= mg \text{ molecular weight} \end{aligned}$$

MOLALITY

MILLIMOLES

Millimoles are the molecular weight expressed in milligrams. The following formula is used to calculate millimoles per liter:

$$mmol/L = \frac{mg/L}{mg \text{ molecular weight}}$$

Example. Convert a 3 mg/dL magnesium value to mmol/L.

$$mmol/L = \frac{3 \times 10}{24.31} = 1.23 \qquad \begin{aligned} 3 &= mg/dL \\ 10 &= dL \text{ to L} \\ 24.31 &= mg \text{ molecular weight} \end{aligned}$$

IONIC SOLUTIONS

Ionic compounds are present as either a base, an acid, or a salt.

The acid-base relationship is often expressed in the Henderson-Hasselbalch equation in determining pH in body fluids.

Example:

1. $pH = pK' + \log \dfrac{cHCO_3^-}{cdCO_2}$

Shows that an increase in [bicarbonations] increases pH

Shows that an increase in [dissolved CO_2] decreases pH

2. $pH = pK' + \log \dfrac{[salt]}{[acid]}$

3. $pH = pK' + \log \dfrac{total\ CO_2 - (a \times PCO_2)}{a \times PCO_2}$

4. $total\ CO_2\ (mmol/L) = 0.03\ PCO_2\ (antilog[pH - 6.1] + 1)$

5. $PCO_2\ (mm\ Hg) = \dfrac{total\ CO_2\ (mmol/L)}{0.03(antilog[pH - 6.1] + 1)}$

$c\ HCO_3^- = $ Total CO_2 ($ctCO_3$) $-$ the concentration of dissolved CO_2 ($cdCO_2$), which includes H_2CO_3

$cdCO_2 = $ concentration of dissolved CO_2, including undissociated H_2CO_3

$a = 0.03 = $ proportioning constant

$6.1 = $ pK of carbonic acid–bicarbonate buffer system

$PCO_2 = $ partial pressure of CO_2

Example:

1. Calculate the pH.

$$The\ PCO_2 = 57$$

$$The\ total\ CO_2 = 43$$

$$pH = 6.1 + \log \dfrac{43 - (0.03 \times 57)}{0.03 \times 57}$$

$$= 6.1 + \log \dfrac{41.29}{1.71}$$

$$= 6.1 + \log 24.15$$

$$pH = 7.48$$

2. Calculate the PCO_2.

$$The\ total\ CO_2 = 28$$

$$The\ pH = 7.43$$

$$PCO_2 = \frac{28}{0.03(\text{antilog}\,[7.43 - 6.1] + 1)}$$

$$= \frac{28}{0.3(21.38 + 1)}$$

$$PCO_2 = 41.79 \text{ mm Hg}$$

3. Prepare an acetate buffer with a concentration of 0.3 molar and a pH of 6.4.

$$6.4 = 4.76 + \log \frac{[\text{salt}]}{[\text{acid}]} \qquad \text{pK of acetic acid} = 4.76$$

$$\text{Antilog of } 1.64 = 43.65$$

$$\text{Ratio} - 43.65 \text{ mol/L salt} + 1 \text{ mol/L acid} = 44.65 \text{ mol/L buffer}$$

$$\frac{44.65}{1} = \frac{0.3}{x} = 0.0067 \text{ mol/L acid}$$

$$\text{mol/L acid} + \text{mol/L salt} = \text{mol/L total}$$

$$\text{mol/L salt} = 0.29$$

$$\text{MW} \times \text{M} = \text{g/L}$$

$$60 \times 0.0067 = 0.40 \text{ g/L acid}$$

$$82 \times 0.29 = 24.05 \text{ g/L salt}$$

$$\text{MW} = \text{molecular weight}$$

$$\text{M} = \text{moles}$$

ABSORBANCE

Beer's Law

Formula. $A = abc$

  A = absorbance
  a = absorptivity
  b = light path (cm)
  c = concentration

Formula. Concentration of an unknown =

$$\frac{\text{absorbance of unknown}}{\text{absorbance of standard}}$$

$\times$ mg of standard used

$$\times \frac{100}{\text{mL of sample used}}$$

Example. Calculate a patient's glucose concentration from the following information:

Methodology = glucose oxidase

Procedure is as follows:

- To prepare a filtrate place 0.5 mL of serum (patient), control, 100 mg/dL glucose standard, and water in their appropriate centrifuge tubes.

- To each tube add 7.5 mL of water and mix.

- To each tube add 1.0 mL of barium hydroxide, mix, and let stand for 1 minute.

- To each tube add 1.0 mL of zinc sulfate and let stand for 2 minutes.

- Centrifuge all tubes at 2000 rpm for 10 minutes.

- Pipet 0.2 mL of each filtrate (1:20 dilution) into a clean labeled tube.

- Add 1.0 mL of glucose oxidase reagent to each tube and incubate for 30 minutes in a 37°C bath.

- Add 5.0 mL of sulfuric acid to each tube, mix, and let stand at room temperature for 5 minutes.

- Read absorbances at 540 nm of all tubes against reagent blank.

Absorbance Readings:

Unknown = 0.225
Control = 0.105   Control value 100 mg/dL ± 5 mg/dL
Standard = 0.100

$$\text{Concentration of unknown} = \frac{0.225}{0.100} \times 0.01 \text{ mg} \times \frac{100}{0.01 \text{ mL}}$$

Unknown = 225 mg/dL of glucose   represents 0.2 mL of a 1:20 dilution

$$\text{Concentration of control} = \frac{0.105}{0.100} \times 0.01 \text{ mg} \times \frac{100}{0.01 \text{ mL}}$$

Control = 105 mg/dL of glucose.

BIBLIOGRAPHY

Burtis CA, Ashwood ER: Tietz, Fundamentals of Clinical Chemistry, 4th ed. Philadelphia, WB Saunders, 1996.

Campbell JM, Campbell JB: Laboratory Mathematics: Medical and Biological Applications, 4th ed. St Louis, CV Mosby, 1990.

Chapter **48**

LABORATORY STATISTICS

Thomas R. Sexton, PhD
Alan M. Leiken, PhD

Q U I C K   C O N T E N T S

INTRODUCTION

All laboratory measurements are subject to variation, which jeopardizes the clinical decisions they support. Laboratorians can improve the quality and effectiveness of health care by first recognizing and understanding variation and then taking steps to reduce it.

Statistics is the science of variation. This chapter is intended to convey certain essential statistical concepts that relate to the laboratorian's mission. Specifically, the goals of this chapter are as follows:

- To explain and illustrate commonly used statistical techniques for measuring and describing variation in laboratory settings
- To demonstrate the role of standard statistical computer software in applying these techniques.

TYPES OF VARIATION

Variation occurs when the measured value differs from the true value of the quantity of interest. For example, suppose that the true concentration of glucose in a particular sample is 101 mg/dL but that the measured value is 103 mg/dL. Our measurement variation, or measurement error, here is $103 - 101 = 2$ mg/dL. (Statistical convention is that measurement error is calculated by subtracting the true value from the measured value.) Had the measured value been 98 mg/dL, the measurement error would have been $98 - 101 = -3$ mg/dL.

We must come to terms with the fact that *we can never be absolutely certain of the true value of the quantity of interest.* We can measure the concentration with the most accurate equipment and techniques available, but we can never be sure that the resulting measured value exactly equals the true concentration. Even if the measured concentration happens exactly to equal the true concentration in a particular measurement, we will never *know* this to be the case. Thus, even when we (unknowingly) obtain the correct value, we must allow for the possibility of error.

In some situations, we can improve our estimate of the true value by obtaining several measurements and averaging the results. Suppose we split our sample into four subsamples, measured the glucose concentration in each subsample, and obtained the values:

$$103 \ 100 \ 102 \ 103.$$

The average measured value is:

$$\bar{x} = (103 + 100 + 102 + 103)/4 = 102 \text{ mg/dL}$$

which still differs from the true value of 101 mg/dL. Nonetheless, this procedure has the advantage that it can reduce one component of variation, called *random variation,* as we discuss later.

We find it useful to identify two distinct types of measurement variation—systematic and random. *Systematic variation* refers to methodic deviations of the measured value from the true value. An improperly calibrated analyzer, for example, will introduce systematic variation by consistently overestimating (or underestimating) the true value. *Random variation* refers to deviations of the measured value from the true value that follow no pattern. Unpredictable temperature changes, slight differences in reagents, and subtle changes in procedure, for example, may lead to random variation.

An important distinction between systematic and random variation is that systematic variation occurs primarily, if not always, in the same direction, whereas random variation occurs symmetrically in both directions. Consequently, we can often reduce the effects of random variation by repeating our measurements and averaging, but this is not so for systematic variation. In other words, random variations cancel eventually, whereas systematic variations accumulate.

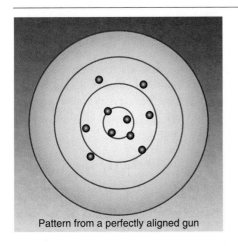

Pattern from a perfectly aligned gun

Let us consider an example. Suppose that we aim a gun at a bull's-eye target 100 m away by mounting it on a tripod and aligning it on the target's center using the sights on the gun (see left). Suppose, for now, that we have aligned the gun perfectly, meaning that a flawlessly designed bullet fired with precisely the proper charge and totally unaffected by atmospheric and other effects would hit the target at its exact center. If we fire 10 bullets at the target, we expect that the 10 hits will form a random pattern around the center of the target, as in the figure on the left. We should not expect that all 10 bullets will hit the exact center, because we realize that each bullet has microscopic flaws that will affect its flight, that the amount of gunpowder will vary slightly from round to round, causing the bullets to have different muzzle speeds, and that unpredictable wind shifts will influence each bullet's path differently.

All these factors result in random variation that generally cancels. If we compute the geometric center of the 10 hits, we will almost surely find that it lies very near the center of the target. If we repeat the experiment with 100 rounds rather than 10, we expect the center of the hits to be even closer to the center of the target. In other words, as we increase the number of repetitions (sample size) and average the results, we obtain a point increasingly close to the center of the target *provided the gun is perfectly aligned*.

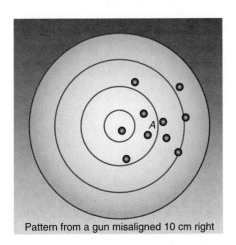

Pattern from a gun misaligned 10 cm right

Suppose, however, that the gun is misaligned such that a flawlessly designed bullet fired with precisely the proper charge and totally unaffected by atmospheric and other effects would hit the target 10 cm to the right of the center at a point called A (see left). The 10 (or 100) bullets will now form a random pattern centered at point A. Notice that increasing the sample size does not give us a midpoint closer to the center but rather it gives us a midpoint closer to point A, 10 cm away. In other words, we cannot affect the size of the systematic error by increasing the sample size, as we can affect the size of the random error. In fact, as the sample size increases, the systematic error—the distance from point A to the center—remains constant whereas the random error tends toward zero, making the systematic error much more prominent.

TYPES OF VARIATION

CALIBRATION AT A SINGLE POINT

Suppose we wish to calibrate a glucose analyzer at a specific level, say 102 mg/dL. Of course, we really need to calibrate the analyzer at several levels to ensure accuracy across a range of concentrations, but we focus on only one level for now. Using careful laboratory procedures, we prepare a sufficiently large volume of test material with a concentration of precisely 102 mg/dL. We then split the volume into 16 test samples and analyze each on the analyzer. We obtain the following 16 readings:

103 104 103 100 105 99 102 101 106 101 104 105 101 103 105 102

Can we conclude that the analyzer is properly calibrated at 102 mg/dL? The answer is yes if the average of these 16 observations is sufficiently close to 102 mg/dL for us to conclude that the difference is almost surely not the result of systematic error. That is, we need to conclude that the difference between the sample mean and 102 mg/dL falls well within the range we expect if the only variation present is random.

Compute the sample mean of these 16 observations:

$$\bar{x} = (103 + 104 + 103 + \ldots + 102) / 16 = 1644 / 16 = 102.75 \text{ mg/dL}$$

The sample mean does not exactly equal 102 mg/dL, but we should not expect that, just as we did not expect the center of the hits in the figure to be precisely the center of the bull's-eye. The relevant question is, Is the difference of 0.75 between the observed mean (102.75) and the target value (102) within the range of variation we expect if only random variation is present? To answer this question, we must turn to the measurement of random variation.

MEASUREMENT OF RANDOM VARIATION

Statisticians use many ways to measure random variation. We discuss *variance, standard deviation,* and *coefficient of variation* only, as these are by far the most important and most commonly used.

Variance

Variance measures random variation by computing the average squared distance of the observations from the sample mean. Thus it is sometimes called the *mean squared error* of the data. Conceptually, the computation is quite intuitive. It is based on the idea that if the data do not have much spread, then most of the observations will lie close to the sample mean. Conversely, if the data contain much spread, then many observations will lie far from the mean. Therefore, we begin by computing the difference between each observation and the sample mean, denoted symbolically as $x_i - \bar{x}$. In our calibration example, these 16 differences are as follows:

0.25, 1.25, 0.25, −2.75, 2.25, −3.75, −0.75, −1.75,

3.25, −1.75, 1.25, 2.25, −1.75, 0.25, 2.25, −0.75

Note that the sum of these differences is zero. This is no coincidence; it is a direct consequence of the definition of the sample mean. Thus, we cannot measure variation by simply averaging these differences because the positive deviations exactly cancel the negative deviations to produce an average deviation of zero.

We can avoid this cancellation in two ways: absolute value and squaring. We could replace each difference by its *absolute value,* that is, its magnitude (always positive or zero) without regard to its sign. This is a statistically proper approach and leads to a measure of variation known as the *mean absolute deviation from the mean* and related measures. However, it is not often used because the mathematical properties of absolute values create various difficulties when one attempts to derive or prove certain properties of this measure.

The other approach is to square each difference, since squared values are always either positive or zero, so that no cancellation can occur in the sum. In our calibration example, the squared differences are as follows:

$$0.0625, 1.5625, 0.0625, 7.5625, 5.0625, 14.0625, 0.5625, 3.0625,$$

$$10.5625, 3.0625, 1.5625, 5.0625, 3.0625, 0.0625, 5.0625, 0.5625$$

The sum of these 16 squared differences is 61, and the mean is 61/16 = 3.8125. However, for complex statistical reasons involving the concepts of *degrees of freedom* and *unbiased estimation,* we do not divide by 16, but by 15, 1 less than the sample size. Thus, the *variance* s^2 of this sample is the following:

$$s^2 = 61 / (16 - 1) = 61 / 15 = 4.0667 \ (mg/dL)^2$$

The variance is sometimes called the *mean squared deviation from the mean.*

Standard Deviation

The variance is often difficult to interpret. The differences have all been squared before summing, which implies that the units of measurement—mg/dL in the example—have also been squared. How does one interpret units like $(mg/dL)^2$?

For this reason, and others, it is common practice to compute the square root of the variance to produce the *standard deviation s.* In the calibration example, we obtain:

$$s = \sqrt{s^2} = \sqrt{4.0667} = 2.0166 \ mg/dL$$

as the value of the standard deviation. Note that by using the square root, we ensure that the units of the standard deviation are the same as those of the original observations. The standard deviation is sometimes called the *root mean squared deviation from the mean.*

Coefficient of Variation

The standard deviation expresses the spread in the data on the scale on which the data were measured. It may be viewed as a kind of average distance of the data from the mean in which the squaring and the square root roughly cancel one another. Sometimes, presenting the spread in the data as a percentage of the mean value is helpful. In our glucose concentration example, we may gain some insight into the precision of the analyzer by computing the *coefficient of variation,* CV, which is the standard deviation (2.0166 mg/dL) expressed as a percentage of the mean (102.75 mg/dL):

$$CV = \frac{s}{\bar{x}} \times 100\% = \frac{2.0166 \ mg/dL}{102.75 \ mg/dL} \times 100\% = 1.96\%$$

MEASUREMENT OF RANDOM VARIATION

Thus we learn that the standard deviation is approximately 2% of the mean, or that a "typical" measurement deviates from the mean by about 2%.

The coefficient of variation is also useful when we wish to compare the precisions of two analyzers that are measuring two entirely different quantities. For example, suppose we had $n = 12$ measurements of total cholesterol from a sample of known concentration equal to 200 mg/dL. Suppose further that the mean of these 12 measurements is 199 mg/dL with standard deviation equal to 3 mg/dL. Which measurement is more precise, that of the glucose concentration or that of the cholesterol concentration? The glucose measurements have the smaller standard deviation, so we might conclude that they were more precise. However, the coefficient of variation of the cholesterol measurements is:

$$CV = \frac{s}{\bar{x}} \times 100\% = \frac{3 \text{ mg/dL}}{199 \text{ mg/dL}} \times 100\% = 1.51\%$$

which is less than that of the glucose measurements. Therefore, in percentage terms, the cholesterol measurements are more precise.

The coefficient of variation may also be more useful than the standard deviation if we wish to compare the precision of an analyzer across its range of measurement. We often find that the standard deviation is larger when the mean is larger. For instance, we may find that the standard deviation of glucose concentration measurements is greater when the level is 106 mg/dL than when it is 99 mg/dL. However, the coefficient of variation may be the same at these levels, suggesting a constant percentage error.

NORMAL DISTRIBUTION

The standard deviation has some important mathematical properties that make it very useful. Most of these properties relate to a very important mathematical function called the *normal* (or *Gaussian*) *distribution*. The normal distribution is the familiar "bell-shaped" curve that is often used (and often misused!) to describe the manner in which observations are spread. The normal distribution is symmetric about its midpoint, where it attains its peak value. The height of the curve at any point represents the relative likelihood that a given observation will be found at that point. Thus, in normal distributions, the most likely location for an observation is in the center, which, by symmetry, is also the mean of the distribution. A frequency histogram of the glucose concentration data and the best fitting normal curve to the data is shown on the facing page:

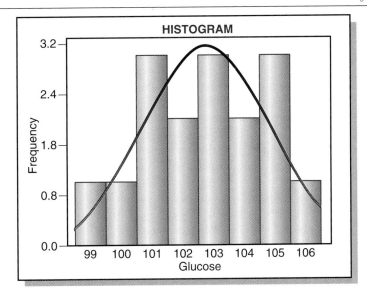

The normal distribution is characterized by two numbers: its location and its spread. Location is specified by the mean, which, as stated, is where the curve peaks. Spread is specified by its standard deviation. Normal curves with small standard deviations are tall and narrow and fall away quickly from the peak. Those with large standard deviations are short and wide and fall away slowly from the peak.

Whenever observations are normally distributed, we can use their mean and standard deviation to compute the percentage of observations expected to fall within any interval we specify. Most often we are interested in intervals centered at the mean and extending equally far in either direction. In any normal distribution, the interval that extends from 1 standard deviation below the mean to 1 standard deviation above the mean is expected to include 68.3% of the data. Similarly, the interval that extends from 2 standard deviations below the mean to 2 standard deviations above the mean is expected to include 95.4% of the data. An interval extending 3 standard deviations in either direction from the mean is expected to capture 99.7% of the observations.

These percentages can be used as rough approximations in data sets that are reasonably symmetric even if they deviate somewhat from the normal curve. Often, these percentages are rounded, and we say, "We expect about two thirds of the data to be within one standard deviation of the mean, about 95% to be within two standard deviations, and virtually all to be within three standard deviations." We commonly consider observations that are more than 3 standard deviations from the mean to be *outliers*, that is, very unusual and perhaps erroneous observations. However, we must use great caution and explore all possible explanations before we declare an observation to be an outlier.

SAMPLING DISTRIBUTIONS

Why is the normal distribution so important? The answer lies in understanding the concepts of a *sampling distribution* and the *Central Limit Theorem*. Consider again our example of glucose concentration measurements made on samples drawn at random from a specimen of known concentration equal to 102 mg/dL. Our sample of size $n = 16$ produced a sample mean of $\bar{x} = 102.75$ and a sample standard deviation of $s = 2.0166$. Suppose someone else had also collected a sample of $n = 16$ measurements from the same source. Their measurements would have differed from ours simply because of random variation, that is, the random conditions that would have affected their measurements in one way would have affected ours differently. Therefore, we would expect their sample mean (and their sample standard deviation) to be different from ours. Both would be legitimate estimates of the true concentration (102 mg/dL), but both would be subject to the effects of the random conditions.

Imagine, now, that thousands of people had each collected a sample of $n = 16$ measurements from the same source. Each would have generated a sample mean, and, taken together, these thousands of sample means could be graphed as a histogram to provide a picture of their distribution. If we imagine the number of people increasing without limit, the distribution portrayed by the histogram of sample means approaches a continuous curve called the *sampling distribution of $\bar{x}$*. In brief, the sampling distribution of $\bar{x}$ portrays the manner in which the sample mean varies, with higher points where the sample mean is more likely to occur and lower points where it is less likely to occur.

Much is known about the sampling distribution of the mean. One is that the average value of all the sample means exactly equals the true value of the quantity being measured. In the glucose example, some people would have obtained sample means less than 102 mg/dL and some would have obtained values larger than 102 mg/dL. However, the average of *all* their sample means would exactly equal 102 mg/dL. Therefore, we say that the sample mean is an *unbiased estimator* of the true value being measured. This has great practical significance. It tells us that although our particular sample mean is likely to be either too low or too high, on average we will be correct.

Recognizing that this property of the sample mean depends on the absence of any systematic error in our sampling process is important. If the technician performs the measurements improperly such that they overestimate the true glucose concentration, then the sample mean will also overestimate the true value. Recall the figures on p 1223. The geometric midpoint of the hits is at the center of the target only when the gun is perfectly aligned, that is, when systematic error is absent. Misalignment of the gun, or improper measurement procedure, causes the midpoint, or mean measurement, to be biased.

Another well known property of the sampling distribution is that its standard deviation, which we call the *standard error* (SE) *of the sample mean,* is equal to the standard deviation of the measurement process divided by the square root of the number of measurements included in the sample mean:

$$SE(\bar{x}) = \frac{\sigma}{\sqrt{n}}$$

In this formula, σ represents the standard deviation of the measurements that we would obtain if we performed an unlimited number of measurements. Of course, we can never know the value of σ because we only have a finite sample. However, we can estimate the value of σ to be approximately equal to that of the sample standard deviation s and therefore that the standard error of the sample mean is approximately:

$$SE(\bar{x}) \approx \frac{s}{\sqrt{n}}$$

In the glucose example, the estimated standard error of the sample mean would be:

$$\text{SE}(\bar{x}) \approx \frac{2.0166}{\sqrt{16}} = 0.5041$$

Two relevant observations can be gleaned from this formula. First, the spread in the sampling distribution of the sample mean is proportional to the spread in the measurement process. The greater the random effects are on the measurements, the greater will be their effects on the sample mean, and therefore the sample mean will be a less precise estimator of the true value. Second, the spread in the sampling distribution of the sample mean is inversely proportional to the square root of the number of measurements averaged into the sample mean. Clearly, this means that the standard error of the mean is lower when the sample size is greater, so that larger samples lead to more precise estimates of the true value. However, the square root causes the benefit of increasing the sample size to diminish as the sample size increases. For example, it requires four times as many observations to cut the standard error in half. In the glucose example, we would require $4 \times 16 = 64$ measurements to reduce the standard error from approximately 0.5041 to approximately $0.5041/2 = 0.2521$, assuming the estimated standard deviation remains constant.

CENTRAL LIMIT THEOREM

Thus, we know the mean and the standard deviation (standard error) of the sampling distribution of the sample mean. A remarkable theorem in mathematical statistics, known as the *Central Limit Theorem,* gives us another extremely valuable characteristic of the sampling distribution of the sample mean. The Central Limit Theorem tells us that if the sample size is sufficiently large, then the sampling distribution of the sample mean is very close to normal.

Why is this so valuable? Recall that the normal distribution is specified by two numbers: its mean and its standard deviation. Thus, to know that the sampling distribution of the sample mean is normal, combined with what we know about its mean and standard deviation (standard error), is to know everything about the distribution. Because we can now calculate the probability that the sample mean will fall in any interval we specify, we may construct *confidence intervals* for the population mean. These are intervals that capture its true value with prespecified likelihood. Also, we can conduct *hypothesis tests* involving the population mean. These are statistical tests that assess the evidence provided by the data relative to statements about the population mean. Confidence interval construction and hypothesis testing are important types of statistical analysis, and the Central Limit Theorem makes them possible.

The Central Limit Theorem is remarkable in its generality. The Central Limit Theorem applies whatever the distribution of the measurements themselves is. Whether the measurements tend roughly to resemble a normal distribution, as in the histogram on p 1227, or another, very differently shaped distribution, the Central Limit Theorem still applies. The shape of the measurement distribution has only one effect: the closer it is to normal, the smaller is the sample size required for the Central Limit Theorem to provide good approximations. Thus, if the measurement distribution is fairly symmetric with a single, centrally located peak, then the Central Limit Theorem will provide good approximations even if the sample size is small, even $n = 10$. If the measurement distribution is highly skewed to one side, or has multiple peaks, then a larger sample size will be required to obtain the same accuracy. Most often, sample sizes of $n = 30$ or more allow the Central Limit Theorem to provide a level of precision sufficiently great for practical purposes.

CONFIDENCE INTERVALS

In our glucose concentration example, we found that the sample mean was 102.75 mg/dL with a standard error of the mean of 0.5041 mg/dL based on a sample of size $n = 16$. We know in this example that the true value is 102 mg/dL because we produced the test specimens according to this criterion. However, suppose we did not know this value, as we would not if the measurements were being made on specimens of unknown (but equal) concentration. How might we estimate the true, unknown value of the glucose concentration?

The Central Limit Theorem tells us that the sample means in this situation are distributed roughly according to a normal distribution centered at the true value (102 mg/dL, although we do not know this value) and with a standard deviation approximately equal to 0.5041 mg/dL. If we were asked to make a *point estimate* of the true value based on our data, it would make sense to estimate it to be equal to our sample mean, 102.75 mg/dL. However, a point estimate gives us no sense of the precision in our estimate—how far off we are likely to be. A *confidence interval* is designed to convey that sense of precision.

Recall that we can easily calculate the probability of any interval when we know that the distribution is normal. This is true in particular for intervals centered at the mean. Thus, we can construct an interval centered at our best estimate of the mean (102.75 mg/dL) and extending an equal amount in each direction until we achieve a pre-specified probability that the interval contains the true but unknown value. How far out in either direction must we go?

We must first determine the *confidence* we wish to have that the interval will contain the true value. This is a matter of choice and should be selected based on two considerations: the importance of capturing the true value, and the importance of keeping the interval short. The higher we set the confidence, that is, the probability that the interval will contain the unknown true value, the longer will be our confidence interval. For example, 95% confidence intervals will capture the true value in 95% of the instances in which we construct such intervals but will be longer than 90% confidence intervals. Similarly, 99% confidence intervals will be longer still. Of course, the usefulness of long intervals is less than that of short intervals, so tradeoffs must be made between confidence level and interval length.

Suppose we select 95% confidence. We can then determine how many standard errors left and right of our estimated value (102.75 mg/dL) we must extend to construct our confidence interval. This number of standard errors is called the *critical t-value* and depends on the number of measurements used to compute the mean. The critical *t*-value is derived from a mathematical probability distribution called the *t-distribution*.

t—Distribution

The *t*-distribution is very similar to the normal distribution; it is symmetric (about zero) and bell shaped but slightly flatter than the standardized normal distribution, that is, the normal distribution with mean equal to zero and standard deviation equal to 1. Actually, there is an entire (infinite) family of t-distributions identified individually by a number called the *degrees of freedom* of the distribution. Recall that the concept of degrees of freedom was mentioned in the discussion of variance, where we divided the sum of squared deviations from the mean by $n - 1$ rather than by n. In the glucose concentration example, the appropriate degrees of freedom is 15.

The members of the t-distribution family that have large degrees of freedom (30 or more) look almost indistinguishable from the standardized normal distribution. In fact, as the degrees of freedom approaches infinity, the t-distribution approaches the standardized normal distribution exactly. However, because the t-distribution is flatter than the standardized normal distribution, we must extend further in each direction from the center to capture the same proportion of observations. The chart below shows the critical t-values for selected members of the t-distribution family and for the standardized normal distribution. These are the number of standard errors we must extend left and right from the estimated value to obtain the confidence levels shown.

CRITICAL VALUES OF THE *T*-DISTRIBUTION FOR SELECTED DEGREES OF FREEDOM AND CONFIDENCE LEVELS

DEGREES OF FREEDOM	CONFIDENCE LEVEL		
	90%	95%	99%
5	2.0150	2.5706	4.0322
15	1.7531	2.1315	2.9467
25	1.7081	2.0595	2.7874
50	1.6759	2.0086	2.6778
100	1.6602	1.9840	2.6259
Infinite (Normal)	1.6449	1.9600	2.5758

The chart above illustrates how the confidence intervals grow with the confidence level. In the glucose concentration example, with 15 degrees of freedom, the 90% confidence interval for the true value is:

$$102.75 \pm (1.7531)(0.5041) = 102.75 \pm 0.88 = (101.87, 103.63)$$

Nine times out of 10 in which we follow this procedure, the resulting interval will capture the true value. We can see that the true value (102 mg/dL) is indeed captured by this interval, but recall that in an actual situation, we would not know the true value so we would not know this to be the case.

The 95% confidence interval is:

$$102.75 \pm (2.1315)(0.5041) = 102.75 \pm 1.07 = (101.68, 103.82)$$

which we can see is longer than the 90% confidence interval. Similarly, the 99% confidence interval is:

$$102.75 \pm (2.9467)(0.5041) = 102.75 \pm 1.49 = (101.26, 104.24)$$

longer still.

The chart above also illustrates that the intervals computed with the t-distribution will become almost identical to those computed with the normal distribution as the degrees of freedom becomes very large. This occurs when the number of observations used to compute the mean becomes very large. Thus, in large samples, very little distinction exists between the normal and the t-distribution.

It may seem odd that we do not use the normal distribution to compute confidence intervals. After all, the Central Limit Theorem suggests that the normal distribution is appropriate for this situation. And the normal distribution would be appropriate *if we knew the value of the standard deviation σ exactly*. However, we do not, and we need to rely on the data itself to estimate σ by the sample standard deviation s. This step introduces additional uncertainty into our confidence interval calculation, and it is this uncertainty that causes the confidence intervals to be somewhat wider than they would be if σ were known and the normal distribution was used. As the number of observations increases, the sample standard deviation s becomes a better estimate of the true standard deviation σ, and the confidence interval expansion disappears.

We can now answer the question posed earlier: Is the difference of 0.75 between the observed mean (102.75) and the target value (102) within the range of variation we would expect if only random variation were present? We have observed that the target value (102) fell within the 90% confidence interval $102.75 \pm 0.88 = (101.87, 103.63)$. By the logic used to construct the confidence interval, we can say that there is a 90% chance that the difference between the observed mean and the target value would not exceed 0.88 mg/dL if only random variation were present. Since the actual difference, 0.75 mg/dL, is less than 0.88 mg/dL, we conclude that the actual difference is not unusual and that there is no evidence that systematic variation is present. Thus, we would conclude that the analyzer is properly calibrated at 102 mg/dL.

HYPOTHESIS TESTING

The statistical development that leads to confidence intervals can also be used to perform a *hypothesis test* that answers the same question. A *hypothesis* is simply a declarative statement that is either true or false. A hypothesis test involves two hypotheses: a *null hypothesis* (H_0) and an *alternative hypothesis* (H_A). The null hypothesis is a statement that we initially assume to be true, and the alternative hypothesis is its logical negation. Thus, either the null or the alternative hypothesis must be true and the other must be false.

Generally, the null hypothesis is taken to be the statement that describes the situation in which conditions are as expected. For example, in the glucose concentration example, the null hypothesis would be that the analyzer is properly calibrated at 102 mg/dL. This is the situation in which nothing is wrong, that is, no systematic variation is present, only random variation. We would express this as

$$H_0: \quad \mu = 102 \text{ mg/dL},$$

where μ is the mean measurement we would obtain from the analyzer if we tested an infinite number of samples. This is sometimes called the *population mean*. The alternative hypothesis is then the logical negation of the null hypothesis:

$$H_A: \quad \mu \neq 102 \text{ mg/dL}.$$

The test of these hypotheses proceeds as follows. We begin by assuming that the null hypothesis is true, that is, that the analyzer is properly calibrated at 102 mg/dL. This is a *tentative* assumption; the purpose of the hypothesis test is to decide if the evidence at hand (the 16 measurements) is sufficient for us to change our minds about the truth of the null hypothesis. From our previous development, we could show that, if H_0 is true, then:

$$t = \frac{\bar{x} - \mu_0}{s/\sqrt{n}}$$

follows a t-distribution with $n - 1$ degrees of freedom. In this expression, $\bar{x}$ is the mean of the n measurements, s is their standard deviation, and μ_0 is the mean under the null hypothesis. In the glucose concentration example, we compute:

$$t = \frac{102.75 - 102}{2.0166/\sqrt{16}} = \frac{0.75}{0.5042} = 1.49$$

with $n - 1 = 15$ degrees of freedom.

The question is, How unusual is a t-value of 1.49 or larger with 15 degrees of freedom? Here, the alternative hypothesis is *two-tailed*, that is, we would reject the null hypothesis if μ differed from 102 mg/dL in either direction. We should interpret this question to mean: 1.49 or larger in absolute value. This is because a mean of 101.25 mg/dL, with a deviation from μ_0 of 0.75 mg/dL in the other direction, would be just as much evidence to reject the null hypothesis as the data we actually obtained.

We can answer this question by determining how much confidence we would have if we extended 1.49 standard errors in either direction of the estimated value. The answer, which is obtainable from tables of the t-distribution and from standard statistical computer programs, is approximately 0.864. In the figure below, this confidence level is portrayed as the area under the *probability density function* of the t-distribution. From this it follows that the likelihood of obtaining a deviation from μ_0 as large as or larger than the one we obtained is roughly 0.136. This is called the *p-value* associated with the hypothesis test. As shown in the figure below, the p-value is the area under the probability density function in the two tails beyond -1.49 and 1.49. Because events with probability 0.136 (roughly 2 out 15) are not very unusual, we would not claim that the data provide evidence against the null hypothesis and we would not reject H_0. As before, we would conclude that the analyzer is properly calibrated at 102 mg/dL.

THE T-DISTRIBUTION WITH 15 DEGREES OF FREEDOM

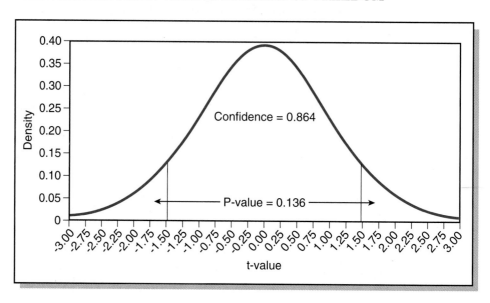

REGRESSION AND CORRELATION: CALIBRATION AT SEVERAL POINTS

At this point, we would be confident that the analyzer is properly calibrated at the given glucose concentration level, 102 mg/dL. Of course, we should be concerned about the calibration across a range of glucose concentration levels. In other words, we want to have confidence that the analyzer will provide accurate measurements whatever the actual glucose concentration within some defined range.

We can test the accuracy of the analyzer across a range of glucose concentrations by first preparing several batches with concentrations that range over the values of interest. Next, we obtain one or more measurements from each batch and compare the measured values to the known true values. This is analogous to the approach we took with one known concentration. However, in this situation we must take into account the variation in the true concentration value across batches.

Suppose that we analyze four batches at each of eight known concentrations and obtain the results shown in the chart below. We need to decide whether the measured values differ from the true values by amounts that are greater than those we would expect if only random variation were present. We can do this by constructing a *scatter plot* of the measured and true concentrations and fitting a straight line through the data points. This is shown in the scatter plot on the facing page.

MEASURED GLUCOSE CONCENTRATION LEVELS

BATCH	TRUE CONCENTRATION (mg/dL)							
	98	**99**	**100**	**101**	**102**	**103**	**104**	**105**
1	98	99	101	102	103	102	103	103
2	98	97	98	105	106	105	103	102
3	102	98	100	102	104	103	104	107
4	99	102	99	102	99	106	105	105

SCATTER PLOT

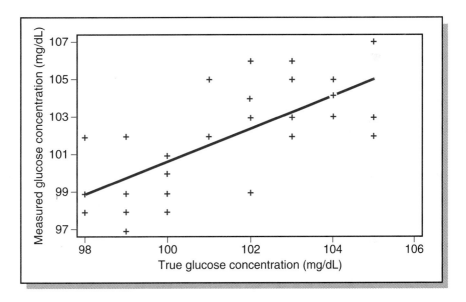

If the analyzer is properly calibrated, then we would expect that the straight line would almost match to the *identity line* $y = x$, where y is the measured concentration and x is the true concentration. The fitted straight line will have an equation of the form $y = b_0 + b_1x$, where b_1 is the slope of the line and b_0 is its y intercept. We can say that the analyzer is properly calibrated if b_1 is very close to 1 and b_0 is very close to zero. Thus, we need to test two sets of hypotheses:

$$\text{H}_0: \quad \beta_0 = 0 \qquad \text{vs} \qquad \text{H}_A: \quad \beta_0 \neq 0$$

and

$$\text{H}_0: \quad \beta_1 = 1 \qquad \text{vs} \qquad \text{H}_A: \quad \beta_1 \neq 1$$

where β_0 and β_1 are the *true* y intercept and slope. Of course, without an infinite amount of data, we can never *know* the values of β_0 and β_1, but we can test hypotheses about their values.

REGRESSION AND CORRELATION: CALIBRATION AT SEVERAL POINTS

Least Squares Regression

To test these hypotheses, we must first determine the equation of the fitted straight line, that is, the values of b_0 and b_1. The straight line we choose to fit the data should be the best possible according to some appropriate criterion. What criteria are appropriate?

If the line is to be a good fit to the data, requiring that it produce generally small residuals seems reasonable. The *residual* associated with a data point is simply the vertical distance between the data point and the fitted line. If the data point has coordinates (x_i, y_i) and the straight line has the equation $y = b_0 + b_1 x$, then the height of the straight line as it passes x_i is:

$$\hat{y}_i = b_0 + b_1 x_i$$

where $\hat{y}_i$ is called the *predicted value* of y_i. It follows that the residual associated with this point is:

$$e_i = y_i - \hat{y}_i$$

One criterion we might consider is to select the line that minimizes the sum of the residuals. Note, however, that some residuals are positive (if the data point is above the line) and others are negative (if the data point is below the line). Thus, the positive and negative residuals cancel one another in the sum. Indeed, we can construct many lines that produce a *zero* residual sum, some of which are clearly not good fits to the data. In fact, *any* line that passes through the point of means $(\bar{x}, \bar{y})$ produces a zero residual sum.

One way to avoid the cancellation is to select the line that minimizes the sum of the *absolute values* of the residuals. The absolute value of a residual is equal to the magnitude of the residual and is always taken as positive. Thus, the absolute value of 3 is 3, whereas the absolute value of -3 is also 3. Although this approach is sometimes used, its mathematical properties are difficult to establish.

The most commonly accepted method to avoid the cancellation is to select the line that minimizes the sum of the *squared* residuals. Since squaring a number always results in a non-negative value, no cancellation can occur in the sum. This approach is called *ordinary least squares* (OLS) *regression* and leads to well known and very useful mathematical results. Specifically, the slope and y intercept of the OLS regression line are:

$$b_1 = \frac{\sum_{i=1}^{n} x_i y_i - n\bar{x}\bar{y}}{\sum_{i=1}^{n} x_i^2 - n\bar{x}^2}$$

and

$$b_0 = \bar{y} - b_1 \bar{x}$$

The computer output for this data set is shown in the figure on p 1237. It was produced using Statistix for Windows, but many other standard statistical computer programs provide the same information. The values of b_0 and b_1 are shown in the "coefficient" column; they are $b_0 = 14.3333$ and $b_1 = 0.86310$. Recall that we want to decide whether $\beta_0 = 0$ and $\beta_1 = 1$. We need to decide whether the observed values of b_0 and b_1 differ significantly from zero and 1, respectively.

REGRESSION COMPUTER OUTPUT

```
UNWEIGHTED LEAST SQUARES LINEAR REGRESSION OF MEAS_CONC
Measured Glucose Concentration

PREDICTOR
VARIABLES        COEFFICIENT      STD ERROR      STUDENT'S T         P

CONSTANT           14.3333         15.0483          0.95          0.3485
TRUE_CONC          0.86310         0.14822          5.82          0.0000

R-SQUARED                 0.5306    RESID. MEAN SQUARE (MSE)    3.69087
ADJUSTED R-SQUARED        0.5149    STANDARD DEVIATION          1.92116

SOURCE            DF            SS           MS           F          P

REGRESSION         1        125.149      125.149      33.91      0.0000
RESIDUAL          30        110.726        3.69087
TOTAL             31        235.875

CASES INCLUDED    32    MISSING CASES    0
```

We can extract additional information from the computer output to help us make this choice. Recall that in our hypothesis test for μ, the population mean, we divided the difference between $\bar{x}$, the sample mean, and μ_0, the hypothesized population mean, by the standard error of $\bar{x}$ and used the t-distribution with $n - 1$ degrees of freedom. We will perform the hypothesis tests on β_0 and β_1 in analogous fashion. To test $H_0: \beta_0 = 0$ versus $H_A: \beta_0 \neq 0$, we compute:

$$t = \frac{b_0 - 0}{SE(\beta_0)}$$

and use the t-distribution with $n - 2$ degrees of freedom. To test $H_0: \beta_1 = 1$ versus $H_A: \beta_1 \neq 1$, we compute:

$$t = \frac{b_1 - 1}{SE(\beta_1)}$$

and, again, use the t-distribution with $n - 2$ degrees of freedom. The standard errors are available in the figure above in the column labeled "std error" as $SE(\beta_0) = 15.0483$ and $SE(\beta_1) = 0.14822$. Thus, the t-value for β_0 is $(14.3333 - 0)/15.0483 = 0.95$ (which is shown in the figure in the column labeled "student's t"), while that for β_1 is $(0.86310 - 1)/0.14822 = -0.92$. Both t-values have $n - 2 = 32 - 2 = 30$ degrees of freedom. The p-value for the test for β_0 is 0.3485 (which is shown in the figure in the column labeled "p"), while that for β_1 is 0.3649. This latter value is not shown in the figure, as the p-value there tests the hypotheses $H_0: \beta_1 = 0$ versus $H_A: \beta_1 \neq 0$. The p-value for our test was computed separately using the same software package. Neither p-value suggests that we should reject the null hypothesis. Therefore, we would conclude that the analyzer is properly calibrated over the range used.

Note the value of 0.5306 next to "r-squared" in the figure. We interpret this as the proportion of the total variation in y (measured glucose concentration) that is explained by variation in x (true glucose concentration). If the data points lie on or very close to the regression line, then most of the variation in y is accounted for by variation in x, and the r^2 value will be close to 1. If the points vary substantially around the line, then r^2 will be close to zero. In this example, we can say that approximately 53% of the variation in measured glucose concentration can be explained by variation in true glucose concentration. This is not a very high r^2 value, which is not surprising given the extent to which the data points in the scatter plot on p 1235 scatter about the regression line.

The *correlation coefficient* is another commonly used measure of the strength of a regression model. It is computed as the square root of r^2, choosing a positive or negative sign to match that of b_1, the slope coefficient. In this example, the slope is positive, so:

$$r = +\sqrt{r^2} = 0.7284$$

The correlation coefficient, by definition, varies between -1 and $+1$, with zero representing no linear relationship. As r approaches ± 1, the strength of the linear relationship is said to increase, with the sign showing the direction of the relationship.

Comparison with a "Gold Standard"

As people work to lower the cost of delivering health care, we regularly learn of newer methods of performing various tests. These methods are often attractive because they are faster, easier to perform, and less costly than the standard methods they are designed to replace. However, before we accept a new procedure as a replacement for a "gold standard," we need to ensure that it provides results that are consistent with the older and more reliable method.

An interesting example is described by V. Jones, who reported a statistical analysis of results from the hemodynamic monitor (HDM) and the blood urea nitrogen (BUN) recirculation tests. The BUN is considered the gold standard in hemodialysis, and the HDM is a newer noninvasive system that uses a small electromagnetic sensor and a hand held computer. The purpose of the analysis was to justify "substantial equivalence" between the two methods for submission to the Food and Drug Administration (FDA).

The analysis team collected 113 clinical observations, each consisting of an HDM measurement and a BUN measurement on the same patient. A regression analysis produced a slope of 0.976 and a y intercept of -1.69, with approximate standard errors of 0.0325 and 2.315, respectively. The t-values, each with 111 degrees of freedom, were -0.74 for the slope ($H_0: \beta_1 = 1$), and -0.73 for the y intercept ($H_0: \beta_0 = 0$). The corresponding p-values were 0.4609 for the slope and 0.4669 for the y intercept. Thus, the HDM measurements do not appear to differ from the BUN measurements. The correlation coefficient was $r = 0.94$, quite close to 1. Correspondingly, the value of r^2 was approximately 0.88, indicating that roughly 88% of the variation in the HDM measurements was associated with variation in the BUN measurements.

QUALITY CONTROL

Quality control is a critical component of every laboratory's operating procedure. The accuracy and precision of the results depend heavily on ensuring that the analyzers are properly calibrated. A standard technique is to analyze a control specimen simultaneously with a patient's specimen. If the control measurements show no systematic deviations from their mean, it is commonly assumed that the analyzer is reporting proper results. Statistical analysis is required to detect systematic deviations, and *control charts,* often called *Levey-Jennings charts,* are excellent tools for this purpose.

Many types of control charts are in use. They differ in that they use different measures to detect different types of systematic deviations, but they all use the same basic structure. We discuss one type, called an *x Chart* or an *i Chart,* which is used when the observations are individual measurements. Other charts are used when the observations are means of several measurements, counts or proportions of nonconforming units, measures of spread such as range or standard deviation, or any of several other possibilities.

The figure below shows a control chart for 30 individual cholesterol measurements.

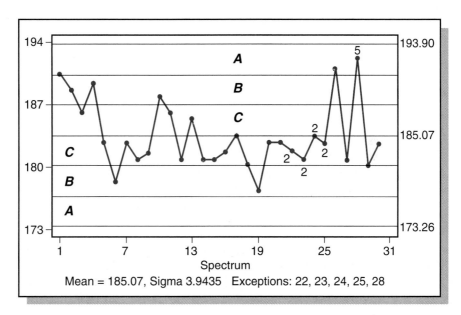

The center horizontal line is plotted at 185.07 mg/dL, the mean of the 30 measurements. Horizontal lines are also plotted at the mean plus and minus 1 standard deviation, and at the mean plus and minus 2 and 3 standard deviations. The standard deviation of the 30 measurements is 3.9435 mg/dL. We label as *A* the regions between the 2 and 3 standard deviation lines, as *B* those between the 1 and 2 standard deviation lines, and as *C* those between the mean and the 1 standard deviation lines. These labels are used with various rules we can use to decide if systematic deviations exist, as described later.

The control chart is useful because the probabilities associated with the labeled regions are known if the measurements follow a normal distribution. Specifically, if the data are normally distributed, then about 68.26% of the observations will lie in region C, 95.44% will lie in either region C or region B, and 99.73% will lie in either region C, region B, or region A. These percentages remain fairly stable even if the distribution is not normal provided that it is only moderately skewed about a single central peak.

We can use the control chart as a graphic representation of the measurements, and most general purpose statistical software packages can construct a variety of control charts with very little effort. The control chart like the one above can be produced using Statistix for Windows, which can produce 11 different types of graphs commonly used in quality assurance. Many of these packages are affordable to even the smallest laboratory. Thus, one of the commonly cited objections to the use of control charts—that they are cumbersome and time consuming to prepare—is no longer valid.

QUALITY CONTROL

Tests for Systematic Variations

Many quality assurance programs also apply several tests to the control chart data to detect if sufficient evidence exists to claim that the variations shown are systematic in nature rather than random. Variations exist, but the following is one set that typifies those in use:

Test 1: A point outside the mean ± 3 standard deviation limits
Rationale: The probability of this is about 0.27% for any measurement. We would expect this to occur only once in every 370 measurements due to randomness alone. Thus, there is a good chance that the measurement is inaccurate.

Test 2: Nine points in a row on one side of the mean line
Rationale: The probability of this is about 0.20% for any sequence of nine measurements. We would expect this to occur only once in every 512 such sequences due to randomness alone. Thus, there is a good chance that the mean has shifted.

Test 3: Six points in a row either all increasing or all decreasing
Rationale: The probability of this is about 0.28% for any sequence of six measurements. We would expect this to occur only once in every 360 such sequences due to randomness alone. Thus, there is a good chance that a trend has developed.

Test 4: Fourteen points in a row alternating up and down
Rationale: The probability of this is about 0.38% for any sequence of 14 measurements. We would expect this to occur only once in every 266 such sequences due to randomness alone. Thus, there is a good chance that a periodic source of variation has developed.

Test 5: Two out of three consecutive points in region A or beyond on the same side of the center line
Rationale: The probability of this is about 0.21% for any sequence of three measurements. We would expect this to occur only once in every 486 such sequences due to randomness alone. Thus, there is a good chance that a source of systematic variation has developed.

Test 6: Four out of five consecutive points in region B or beyond on the same side of the center line.
Rationale: The probability of this is about 0.55% for any sequence of five measurements. We would expect this to occur only once in every 181 such sequences due to randomness alone. Thus, there is a good chance that a source of systematic variation has developed.

Test 7: Fifteen consecutive points in region C on either side of the center line.
Rationale: The probability of this is about 0.32% for any sequence of 15 measurements. We would expect this to occur only once in every 314 such sequences due to randomness alone. Thus, there is a good chance that the process variance has become smaller.

Test 8: Five consecutive points on either side of the center line, but none in region C.
Rationale: The probability of this is about 0.33% for any sequence of five measurements. We would expect this to occur only once in every 306 such sequences due to randomness alone. Thus, there is a good chance that the process has become bimodal with one mode above the current mean and the other below.

Notice that measurements 22, 23, 24, and 25 in the control chart above have been marked by the computer program with the number 2. This indicates that those measurements violate the conditions of test 2. Measurement 22 was the ninth consecutive point to lie below the center line, and together there were 12 such points. This would normally be considered strong evidence that the process mean has shifted; the analyzer should be recalibrated and all patient's results starting with measurement 22 should not be reported and should be repeated.

Note also that measurement 28 has been marked by the computer with the number 5 to show a violation of the conditions of test 5. Measurements 26 and 28 are both in region A on the same side of the center line. This would suggest that a source of systematic variation has developed. Again, the analyzer should be recalibrated and patient's results should be discarded.

CONCLUSIONS

Statistics is the science of variation, and we have seen a small glimpse of its role in laboratory management. Many more techniques can be applied, and computer software has become readily available to help the laboratory manager in carrying out these methods. The central points to be taken from this discussion are the following:

- Variation is ubiquitous and must be understood for effective laboratory operation.
- The objective is to eliminate all sources of systematic variation and reduce as much as possible all sources of random variation. This will provide accurate and consistent patient results and better health care.
- Statistical methods may be employed to account for random variation so that the accuracy and precision of laboratory measurements are better understood and properly interpreted.
- New procedures may be scientifically evaluated using statistical methods so that real improvements can be properly identified and bogus innovations can be discarded.

BIBLIOGRAPHY

Jones V: My summer internship experience. Stats 17:24, 1996.
Statistix Version 4.1 User's Manual. Analytical Software; Tallahassee, Fla, 1994.

QUALITY CONTROL

Chapter *49*

SAFETY ISSUES FOR THE CLINICAL LABORATORY

Vincent Della Speranza, MS, HTL (ASCP), MT

Q U I C K   C O N T E N T S

INTRODUCTION

The safety of the clinical laboratory environment has come under great scrutiny by regulatory authorities in the past decade. The result has been a daunting morass of regulations that have a profound impact on laboratory practices with substantial penalties for facilities that fail to comply. The regulatory standards are often quite difficult to read and decipher and are voluminous. The purpose of this chapter is to make the reader familiar with significant aspects of the federal regulations pertaining to the clinical laboratory in easy to understand language. Space does not permit a more detailed examination of the regulatory standards, which could fill an entire volume. The reading list that has been provided at the end of this chapter should direct you to sources of specific information that you may require. It must be understood that safety regulations are constantly being created, reviewed, and revised, making it necessary to stay abreast of changes as they occur.

The responsibility for a safe, compliant work environment does not rest with your employer or supervisor but with each of us. The clinical laboratory professional must be familiar with the requirements of federal, state, and local authorities if we can hope to be successful in protecting the environment, ourselves, and those around us.

Brief History

It should come as no surprise that human interest in the hazards of the workplace has only come into focus during this century. In past civilizations, labor was performed by slaves, an expendable and readily available workforce. The practice of medicine in those times was available only to the ruling classes, so little attention was paid to the health consequences of labor practices. Reports of occupational injuries, including the hazards of grinding, gilding, marble cutting, and the smelting of mercury ore, however, can be found dating back to the Middle Ages, with some reports going as far back as the 1st century. In 1775, Percival Pott noted a trend of scrotal cancer (now referred to as Pott's disease) in young boys who were used to clean chimneys in England. It was the practice to lower these chimney sweeps by rope; they would clean the soot and creosote from the walls of the chimney with hand tools. Despite numerous documented observations of work associated illness or injury throughout history, organized efforts to identify and prevent their occurrence in the workforce did not begin until after the excesses of dangerous occupations of the American Industrial Revolution in the late 1800s.

It was only after a new social consciousness arose and industrialists began to appreciate that worker well-being was in their economic self-interest that the emphasis shifted from diagnosis and treatment of work related illness and injury to identification and prevention of hazards in the workplace. In the early 1900s, Alice Hamilton, MD, was credited as the first pathologist to study occupational health, systematically documenting lead poisoning in 35,000 workers that led to legislation known as the *lead laws.* In 1905, Massachusetts was the first state to employ health inspectors to investigate worker injuries. Twenty-one states had legislation in place to regulate industrial working conditions, including dust control, ventilation, and sanitation, by 1909. Worker compensation laws could be found in half of the states by 1913.

Few would argue that the most significant legislation for the American worker was the Occupational Health and Safety Act of 1970, which has had a dramatic and lasting impact on workplace practices. The passage of this act resulted in the establishment of a number of agencies involved with the examination of workplace safety and the creation of the safety standards that form the basis of regulatory agency enforcement today.

Agencies Regulating Laboratory Safety

Clinical laboratory safety receives significant emphasis from accrediting agencies such as the College of American Pathologists (CAP) and the Joint Commission of Accreditation of Healthcare Organizations (JCAHO), who promote the standards promulgated by the Occupational Safety and Health Administration (OSHA), an agency within the U.S. Department of Labor. OSHA was established to monitor and reduce the occurrence of occupational hazards, injuries, and illnesses. OSHA standards are federal law, and compliance is mandatory for all work environments.

OSHA standards are often based on the recommendations of a number of other agencies including the National Fire Protection Agency (NFPA), the Environmental Protection Agency (EPA), the Centers for Disease Control and Prevention (CDC), the National Institute for Occupational Safety and Health (NIOSH), and the U.S. Department of Transportation (DOT), which may offer specific expertise in various areas of concern. The DOT regulates the shipment of hazardous materials or biologics. NIOSH does not make laws but is involved with recommending permissible exposure levels for hazardous chemicals. One can begin to appreciate that an impressive array of resources is now devoted to limiting the risk of injury in the workplace.

AGENCIES ENGAGED IN THE CREATION AND ENFORCEMENT OF SAFETY STANDARDS	
Department	**Agencies**
U.S. Department of Labor	OSHA Bureau of Labor Statistics
U.S. Department of Health and Human Services	Centers for Disease Control and Prevention (CDC) National Institute for Occupational Health and Safety (NIOSH) Agency for Toxic Substances National Center for Health Statistics
U.S. Department of Transportation (DOT)	
Environmental Protection Agency (EPA)	

OCCUPATIONAL SAFETY AND HEALTH ADMINISTRATION

OSHA is the federal enforcement agency for safety compliance. It generally responds to an employee complaint or in some cases to an unusual rate of injury or illness. In such instances, the OSHA inspector will likely appear at your door without notice. Facilities find that it is generally less expensive to take the necessary steps to comply with OSHA standards. Citations for noncompliance can be quite costly. Violations categorized as "less than serious" may cost up to $7000 each in penalties, whereas findings of "willful neglect" result in fines up to $70,000 each. Fines in excess of $30,000 are not uncommon.

OSHA also offers programs for training and education, informational literature, and consultation services. On request, the agency will dispatch a consultant to survey your facility to make recommendations for compliance. When a laboratory has requested the agency's assistance, any deficiencies that are found by the consultant do not result in the assessment of penalties, so you should not be reluctant to use this resource.

Individual states may choose to establish their own programs for occupational safety; however, state programs must at least meet all federal requirements, although they may exceed federal standards, so it is important that you become knowledgeable with state and local regulations. OSHA inspectors monitor compliance in states not having such programs.

At present, there are a number of OSHA standards regulating aspects of laboratory operations that we must be familiar with. These include:

- The Hazard Communication Standard
- The Laboratory Standard
- The Bloodborne Pathogens Standard
- The Formaldehyde Standard

INTRODUCTION

❚ The Air Contaminants Standard
❚ The Respirator Standard
❚ The Personal Protective Equipment Standard

In addition, a tuberculosis (TB) standard is under development. These standards are examined more closely later in this chapter.

When standards are first enacted, they are initially published in the *Federal Register*. They are subsequently published in the Code of Federal Regulations (CFR), a multivolume set that is divided into titles. Title 29 contains all OSHA regulations such that each standard is referred to as *29 CFR* and the number of the specific document being referenced. For example, The Laboratory Standard is 29 CFR 1910.1450. It would be advisable for laboratories to have a copy of each standard, along with compliance guidelines, which may be obtained from OSHA. Your facility may also find it beneficial to obtain OSHA's Enforcement Procedures, the detailed instructions provided to OSHA inspectors that spells out exactly what will and will not pass a compliance inspection. Lastly, you may be interested in reading the preamble that accompanies each standard in the *Federal Register*, since this explains the data and rationale behind the standard.

One last note about OSHA. The best way to survive an OSHA inspection is to avoid having one. The repercussions of noncompliance are serious and expensive. The best way to avoid an OSHA inspection is to put your employees' fears to rest. Employees who feel secure that their employer is concerned about their personal safety are less apt to contact this agency. Facilities that appear to be cutting corners, perhaps by not having sufficient personal protective equipment on hand, or adequate ventilation, for example, will simply succeed in convincing employees that they may be at risk.

There is no question that a safe work environment is expensive to maintain. An unsafe work environment, however, will be more costly in the long run, not only because of penalties that could be levied for noncompliance but also because of the financial liabilities that may result if an employee becomes seriously injured as a result of noncompliance.

HAZARD COMMUNICATION STANDARD (29 CFR 1910.1200)

The Hazard Communication Standard, more commonly referred to as the "Right-to-Know" law, was directed to industrial facilities, including those involved with the manufacture of hazardous materials. In the clinical laboratory, this standard has been largely superseded by the Laboratory Standard. The intent of the Hazard Communication Standard is to ensure that workers know the hazards associated with the chemicals in their workplace to allow them to take appropriate precautions.

Facilities that must comply with the Hazard Communication Standard include:

❚ All manufacturing facilities
❚ Laboratories that are part of manufacturing facilities
❚ Nonmanufacturing facilities

Clinical laboratories must comply with certain aspects of the Hazard Communication Standard, especially if they prepare or distribute chemicals to clients or other facilities. For example, some laboratories commonly provide fixative or preservative solutions to physicians' offices and other clients as part of their outreach marketing program. Such activities would require full compliance with the standard.

The Hazard Communication Standard requires the following:

▮ Employers must have material safety data sheets (MSDSs) for any hazardous chemical used in the workplace. Since few of us are experts at what constitutes a "hazardous" chemical, it would be prudent to obtain an MSDS for each chemical used. The MSDS is readily obtainable from your chemical supplier.

▮ The MSDS must be accessible to employees at the location where the chemical is used.

▮ The employer must have a written hazard communication program. Clinical laboratories are exempt from this requirement because they are regulated by the Laboratory Standard, which requires a chemical hygiene plan.

▮ Each hazardous chemical must be labeled with the identity of its chemical constituents, and appropriate warnings for these compounds, including target organ effects, must be included. It is permissible to use symbols for hazard warnings.

▮ Employees must receive information and initial training on the proper handling of hazardous chemicals at hire and when new hazards are introduced into the work environment.

▮ Employees must receive annual training. Clinical laboratories covered by the Laboratory Standard are to follow the requirements of that standard. The employee education program must include instruction on the MSDS, significance and interpretation of labeling, interpretation of hazard information, procedures for safe use and storage, and appropriate disposal practices.

Labeling Requirements

The Hazard Communication Standard mandates that hazardous chemicals be labeled with appropriate warnings. Methods vary, incorporating the use of symbols or descriptives or a combination of the two. One well known symbol is the hazard rating diamond proposed by the National Fire Protection Agency. This diamond is divided into four compartments, each color coded to represent different hazards, red for flammability, blue for health hazards, yellow for reactivity warnings, and white for other descriptives. Numbers are placed into each of the category boxes within the diamond to reflect the severity of the hazard, ranging from "0" representing the least severe or normal to "4," which represents the greatest hazard. The drawback to this labeling system is that staff often forget what each color diamond is supposed to represent.

HAZARD COMMUNICATION STANDARD (29 CFR 1910.1200)

NATIONAL FIRE PROTECTION RATING SYSTEM

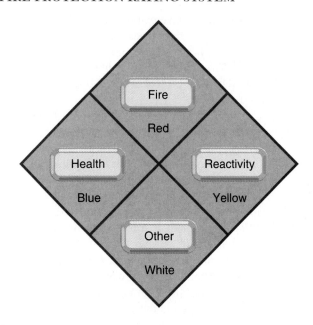

Health Hazards *(blue):*

0 = No hazard.
1 = Can cause irritation if left untreated.
2 = Can cause injury. Requires prompt treatment.
3 = Can cause serious injury despite medical treatment.
4 = Can cause death or major injury despite medical treatment.

Flammability *(red):*

0 = Will not burn.
1 = Ignites after considerable preheating.
2 = Ignites if moderately heated.
3 = Can be ignited at all normal temperatures.
4 = Very flammable gases or very volatile flammable liquid.

Reactivity *(yellow):*

0 = Normally stable. Not reactive with water.
1 = Normally stable. Unstable at high temperature and pressure. Reacts with water.
2 = Normally unstable but will not detonate.
3 = Can detonate or explode, but requires strong initiating force or heating.
4 = Readily detonates or explodes.

In the diamond designated *other* (**white**) one might use the following descriptions:

OX = Oxidizer.
ACID = Acid.
ALK = Alkali.
COR = Corrosive.
—W— = Use no water.

Hazard Definitions

COMBUSTIBLE. Flash point above 100°F. *Will not* ignite when exposed to ignition source below 100°F.

FLAMMABLE. Flash point below 100°F. Vapors *will ignite* when exposed to ignition source below 100°F.

EXPLOSIVE. Capable of causing an explosion when struck or shaken or when in contact with another chemical (i.e., picric acid).

OXIDIZER. A chemical that can initiate or promote combustion.

IRRITANT. A chemical that causes a reversible inflammatory effect on living tissue at the site of contact.

SENSITIZER. A chemical that causes an allergic reaction in normal tissue after repeated exposure.

CORROSIVE. Causes visible destruction to living tissue at the site of contact (i.e., mineral acids).

TARGET ORGAN EFFECTS. Chemically induced changes to liver, kidneys, reproductive organs, nervous system, respiratory system, blood, or fetus.

Material Safety Data Sheet

Most laboratory professionals are at least familiar with the MSDS, which has been in use now for about 10 years. The intent of the Hazard Communication Standard was that each of us would have the most critical information at our fingertips for those compounds in use in our laboratories. The standard requires the chemical supplier to provide an MSDS to its customers for any compound it sells. In addition, the standard requires that the MSDS contain the following data:

1. The product name as it appears on the label, as well as the chemical name and synonyms of each hazardous ingredient
2. Physical and chemical characteristics including flash point, boiling point, specific gravity, and so forth
3. Physical hazards: flammable, explosive, reactive
4. Health hazards to includes the signs and symptoms of exposure and any medical conditions that could be aggravated by exposure
5. Primary routes of entry to the body: inhalation, absorption, ingestion
6. Permissible exposure levels
7. Carcinogen rating
8. Handling precautions, including clean-up procedures
9. Recommended control measures to limit employee exposure, including appropriate engineering controls, work practices, and personal protective equipment.
10. Emergency first aid
11. Date of preparation and revisions
12. Name, address, and telephone number of manufacturer or distributor

In 1993, The American National Standards Institute (ANSI) recommended a new standard format for the MSDS to chemical manufacturers that would enhance the pre-

HAZARD COMMUNICATION STANDARD (29 CFR 1910.1200)

sentation, volume, and type of data provided on this document. Although conformance to this new format would be voluntary, it is likely that many firms will adopt it for use.

SAMPLE MATERIAL SAFETY DATA SHEET

MATERIAL SAFETY DATA SHEET

10% neutral buffered formalin

Date issued: 5-16-94

ACME Chemical Company
1000 Main Street
Omaha, Nebraska 91876

Replaces: 7-22-92

Telephone: (199) 123-4567

HAZARDOUS INGREDIENTS

	PEL 8 hr TWA	STEL	Agency
Formaldehyde*	0.75 ppm	2 ppm	OSHA, ACGIH
Methanol	200 ppm	250 ppm	OSHA, ACGIH

*Listed as probable carcinogen by NTP and IARC

PHYSICAL AND CHEMICAL DATA

Appearance and odor	Clear, colorless liquid, pungent odor
Boiling point	95.6°–99.4°C (204°–211°F)
Evaporation rate	0.43 (butyl acetate = 1)
Percent volatile by volume	98%
Solubility in water	Complete
Specific gravity	1.109 @ 21°C (water = 1)
Vapor density	1.1 (air = 1)
Vapor pressure	19 mm Hg

FIRE AND EXPLOSION HAZARD DATA

Flammability class (OSHA):	111A
Flash point	None observed below 82°C (180°F)
	Closed cup method 85°C (185°F)
Autoignition	430°C (806°F)
Flammable limits in air:	
% by volume	LOWER 7
	UPPER 73

Reactions: Reaction of formaldehyde with nitrogen dioxide, nitromethane, perchloric acid, and aniline or peroxyformic acid yields explosive compounds.

Extinguishing media: Alcohol foam, dry chemicals, carbon dioxide, water in flooding amounts as fog. Solid streams may not be effective. Cool fire-exposed containers with water from side until well after fire is out. Use of water spray to flush spills should also dilute the spill to produce nonflammable mixtures. Water run-off, however, should be contained for treatment.

Special firefighting procedures: Withdraw immediately in case of rising sound from venting safety device or any discoloration of storage tank due to fire.

REACTIVITY DATA

Stability: No known hazardous instability. May self-polymerize to form paraformaldehyde, which precipitates, and trioxane.

Incompatibility: Reaction with phenol, strong acids, or alkalis may be violent. Formaldehyde and hydrochloric acid may form the potent carcinogenic bischloromethylether. Formaldehyde reacts with nitrogen dioxide, nitromethane, and perchloric acid to yield explosive compounds. A violent reaction occurs when formaldehyde is mixed with strong oxidizers.

Hazardous decomposition: Occurs slowly at elevated temperatures, releasing formaldehyde gas.

HEALTH HAZARD DATA

Skin effects: Avoid contact. Solution is a severe skin irritant and a sensitizer. Contact with formaldehyde causes white discoloration, smarting, drying, cracking, and scaling. Previously exposed persons may react to future exposures with an allergic eczematous dermatitis or hives.

Eye effects: Solution sprayed in eye can cause injuries ranging from transient discomfort to severe, permanent corneal clouding and loss of vision. The severity of the effect depends on the concentration of the formaldehyde in the solution and whether or not the eyes were flushed with water immediately after the accident. Blindness may occur if the solution is swallowed. Vapors may cause discomfort and tearing of the eyes.

SYSTEMIC EFFECTS

Ingestion: Liquids containing formaldehyde may cause severe irritation to mucosal surfaces of the mouth, throat, and gastrointestinal tract, which may result in nausea and vomiting. Severe stomach pain may follow ingestion, with possible loss of consciousness and death.

Inhalation: Formaldehyde is highly irritating to the upper respiratory tract and eyes. Concentrations of 0.5–2.0 ppm may irritate the eyes, nose, and throat of some individuals. Concentrations of 3–5 ppm also cause tearing of the eyes and are intolerable in some people.

EMERGENCY AND FIRST AID PROCEDURES

Skin contact: Remove contaminated clothing immediately. Wash affected area with soap or mild detergent and large amounts of water until no evidence of the chemical remains—at least 15–20 minutes. If there are burns, get first aid to cover the area with sterile, dry dressings and bandages.

Eye contact: Immediately flush eye with plenty of water for at least 15 minutes, occasionally lifting upper and lower eyelid. Call a physician. If there is appreciable irritation, see an ophthalmologist.

Inhalation: If affected by vapors, move patient to fresh air immediately. Where formaldehyde concentration may be very high, rescuers must wear self-contained breathing apparatus before attempting to remove victim. If not breathing, give artificial respiration. Qualified medical personnel should administer oxygen, if available.

Ingestion: If victim is unconscious: dilute, inactivate, or absorb the ingested formaldehyde by giving milk, activated charcoal, or water. Keep affected person warm. Get medical attention immediately.

HAZARD COMMUNICATION STANDARD (29 CFR 1910.1200)

LABORATORY STANDARD (29 CFR 1910.1450)

Occupational Exposure to Hazardous Chemicals in Laboratories, otherwise referred to as the *Laboratory Standard,* was enacted by OSHA in 1990. This standard applies to all laboratories using hazardous chemicals in procedures that are not part of a production process where quantities small enough to be handled by one person are used.

Hazardous chemicals are defined as any compound that appears on the OSHA Z list (29 CFR 1910 Table Z-1-A) or that is found to be carcinogenic or potentially carcinogenic by the International Agency for Research on Cancer (IARC) or the National Toxicology Program (NTP). The standard targets individuals employed in a laboratory setting who may be exposed to hazardous chemicals in the performance of their duties.

This extends not only to laboratory technicians and technologists but also to maintenance and custodial staff who are called on to perform their duties in the laboratory setting.

Key Requirements of the Laboratory Standard

CHEMICAL HYGIENE PLAN

The standard requires employers to develop a chemical hygiene plan, which must outline procedures and policies to protect workers from hazardous chemicals. The plan must be readily available to employees in the lab, and it must specifically address all the hazardous materials in use. The plan must be reviewed annually and updated as new hazards are brought into the lab. More specifically, the chemical hygiene plan must include:

1. Standard operating procedures appropriate to the specific laboratory for any work that involves hazardous materials. This must include general safety precautions, response to accidents, general clean-up procedures, spill response, and disposal procedures.
2. Criteria that establish when specific exposure control measures must be undertaken. These might include the toxicity of a given compound, the likelihood and degree of exposure that can be anticipated with the procedures employed, and an assessment of the degree to which engineering controls (for example, the use of chemical fume hoods) are effective in limiting exposure. Measures to control exposure might include the use of personal protective equipment (PPE) or administrative controls. An example of an administrative control might be a policy that requires that employees rotate responsibility for the performance of a given procedure to limit any one individual's maximal exposure.
3. Verification that chemical fume hoods and other engineering controls are monitored on a regular basis to confirm that they are operating properly.
4. Provisions for employee training and a medical surveillance program to provide ongoing health assessment of individuals with exposure to hazardous compounds.
5. The name of someone (safety officer or committee) designated by the employer to be responsible for the administration of the chemical hygiene plan.

Laboratories using **select carcinogens** or other extremely hazardous substances, such as reproductive toxins and other highly toxic compounds, are required to have additional measures in the chemical hygiene plan. A *select carcinogen* is defined as a substance that:

▌ Is an OSHA regulated carcinogen *or*
▌ Is listed as a *known carcinogen* by the NTP *or*
▌ Is listed as *carcinogenic, probably carcinogenic,* or *possibly carcinogenic* to humans by the IARC

Facilities using select carcinogens, reproductive toxins, or highly toxic substances are required to:

1. Designate an area where the material is used and post appropriate signs that a hazardous compound is routinely used in the area. Employees who frequent the **designated** area must be aware that the substance is in use. It is important to stress that this requirement extends to all employees who may frequent the area, including housekeeping and maintenance personnel. Decontamination procedures must be available. An entire laboratory or a portion of a laboratory

may serve as a designated area. Since the designated area will likely have more than one hazardous substance in use, a list of hazardous substance(s) used in the designated area should be posted outside the immediate area to alert people before entering.

2. Provide engineering controls for procedures that create aerosols, or if volatile materials are in use or when there is anticipation of an uncontrollable release of the substance.

3. Provide a procedure for the collection and removal of hazardous waste.

EMPLOYEE TRAINING

The facility must be able to demonstrate that sufficient training is made available to staff for the complexity of procedures employed there. Training must include:

1. The physical and health hazards associated with the chemicals found in the work area.
2. Appropriate work practices, appropriate personal protective equipment, and emergency procedures to be used to limit or prevent employee exposure.
3. The permissible exposure limits (PELs) for OSHA regulated substances or exposure limits for other hazardous chemicals.
4. Signs and symptoms associated with exposure to hazardous chemicals in use.
5. The laboratory's chemical hygiene plan.
6. How to detect the presence of hazardous materials in the work area.

Training must be provided on initial hiring and before the assignment of any new procedures using hazardous chemicals.

MEDICAL CONSULTATIONS AND EXAMINATIONS

Employers must allow employees to receive appropriate medical attention if they demonstrate symptoms of hazardous chemical exposure. A medical consultation with a licensed physician must be provided without cost to the employee after a leak or spill or other event that may have caused a significant exposure to a hazardous chemical.

HAZARD IDENTIFICATION

Employees must be provided with hazard information for any substance produced in the laboratory for its own use. An MSDS must be available for each chemical that is purchased and used in the laboratory. Labels received on purchased chemicals must be maintained in a usable condition.

RESPIRATORS

If respirators are used to keep employee exposure below the PEL, their use must comply with the Respiratory Protection Standard (29 CFR 1910.134) This includes a written program for respirator use; criteria for the selection of appropriate respirators for the task performed and evidence of employee fit-testing; and training of proper use and maintenance of respirator equipment.

EMPLOYEE EXPOSURE

The employer is required to conduct a risk assessment, taking into account the frequency and duration of exposure to a hazardous chemical likely to occur for the procedures that are in use in that facility. Individual exposure must be within the OSHA PELs

LABORATORY STANDARD (29 CFR 1910.1450)

for OSHA regulated substances (29 CFR 1910 Table Z-1-A), time weighted average (TWA) over an 8 hour period, and the short term exposure limit (STEL).

A *PEL* is the maximal allowable airborne concentration to which an employee may be exposed. Airborne concentrations of vapors are measured in parts per million (ppm) and milligrams of substance per cubic meter of air (mg/m³) for particulates. It must be stressed that it is not sufficient for the employer to take air samplings of the work environment. The employee must be monitored to adequately assess exposure.

The *TWA* is the employee's average exposure over an 8 hour period. The TWA does not address brief high exposures. For a given substance, it may be possible for the employee to receive a significant exposure during the first hour and none for the remaining 7 hours, so that when averaged, the exposure falls below the PEL. For example, if the PEL for a substance is 1 ppm TWA, it is possible to be exposed to 1 ppm each hour for 8 hours. Conceivably, an individual might also be exposed to 8 ppm of the same substance for 1 hour and have no subsequent exposure for the next 7 hours; averaged over 8 hours (8 ppm/8 hr = 1 ppm TWA) this would not exceed the PEL for this substance.

STEL, short term exposure limit, is the employee's 15 minute time weighted average exposure. It represents the highest permissible exposure for any 15 minute period during a shift. The STEL is always higher than the TWA.

CL, the ceiling limit, is the maximal permissible exposure during any part of the shift.

Exposures are considered additive. If you are working with two regulated substances and have been exposed to 70% of the PEL for the first, you cannot be exposed to more than 30% of the PEL of the second.

The American Congress of Governmental Industrial Hygienists (ACGIH) has proposed biological exposure indices (BEIs) that reflect the amount of hazardous substance or its metabolite(s) in blood or urine. The BEI is the value expected to be found in a healthy worker who has been exposed to the PEL for a given regulated substance. No conclusions of the health effects of analyte levels exceeding the BEI have been determined.

OSHA Permissible Exposure Limits for Some Common Laboratory Substances

SUBSTANCE	PEL
Acetic acid	10 ppm TWA
Acetone	1000 ppm TWA
Ammonium hydroxide	25 ppm ammonia gas STEL
Chloroform	50 ppm ceiling limit
Dioxane	100 ppm TWA
Ethanol	1000 ppm TWA
Diethyl ether	400 ppm TWA.
Formaldehyde	0.75 ppm TWA
Hydrochloric acid	5 ppm CL hydrogen chloride gas
Iodine	0.1 ppm CL
Isopropanol	400 ppm TWA
Methanol	200 ppm TWA
Nitric acid	2 ppm TWA
Phenol	5 ppm TWA
Toluene	50 ppm TWA
Xylene	100 ppm TWA

FORMALDEHYDE STANDARD (29 CFR 1910.1048)

The Formaldehyde Standard has had a dramatic impact on the operation of laboratories that rely on this chemical for the preservation of tissues and organs. This standard has received significant emphasis by OSHA inspectors as well as those of the various laboratory accrediting agencies and so warrants an in-depth discussion here.

The Formaldehyde Standard applies to all histology and pathology laboratories as well as any laboratory using this compound in solutions containing formaldehyde in a concentration greater than 0.1%. Histology and pathology laboratories commonly use solutions of 3.7% to 4.0% formaldehyde called *formalin* to fix tissues and organs.

Before 1987, when this standard was enacted, the PEL for formaldehyde was 3 ppm. The standard reduced the PEL to 1.0 ppm and was subsequently revised in 1992 to further reduce the permissible exposure to its current level of 0.75 ppm. This reduction in permissible exposure has caused a hardship for some laboratories, so much so that a number of chemical suppliers have attempted to market so-called formalin substitutes to enable laboratories to avoid the burden of this stringent regulation.

The standard reflects a formal recognition by OSHA of the hazards associated with the use of formaldehyde in the workplace; this has been received by some with skepticism and controversy and has been discounted by many who have worked with this substance for many decades without any apparent deleterious effects.

Health Hazards Associated with Formaldehyde

IRRITANT. Formaldehyde is a strong skin and respiratory irritant. Many individuals cannot tolerate vapor levels above 3 ppm. Levels above 5 ppm may result in difficulty breathing. Fortunately, formaldehyde vapor is sufficiently unpleasant to be near that it is unlikely that individuals would be unaware of their exposure. However, with prolonged use, some individuals may become less able to detect formaldehyde odors. On contact with skin, formaldehyde may cause redness, blistering, and cracking of skin. Prolonged skin exposure may result in sensitization, causing an allergic dermatitis or hives.

SENSITIZER. Some individuals may become sensitized to formaldehyde after prolonged use, and this may result in an allergic reaction varying from allergic dermatitis to serious respiratory difficulties. Once sensitization has occurred, individuals may find themselves reacting to smaller and smaller exposures. Sensitization is often for life. Since formaldehyde is used in many consumer products, including hair products, wrinkle-free fabrics, plywood products, and several plastic resins including those used in houseware items, the sensitized individual's quality of life outside of work may be significantly affected.

CARCINOGEN. Studies have demonstrated that formaldehyde may be carcinogenic in humans, with squamous cell carcinomas arising in the nasal pharynx, oropharynx, and lung. It is believed that repeated exposures increase the risk of neoplasm.

Provisions of the Formaldehyde Standard

PERMISSIBLE EXPOSURE LIMIT

No employee may be exposed to more than *0.75 ppm TWA* (over 8 hours). The *STEL* is *2 ppm* averaged over 15 minutes. The STEL should represent the worst or highest anticipated exposure during the performance of one's duties. OSHA has also established an *action level* for formaldehyde at **0.5 ppm** TWA. The employer is required to additional steps to protect employees whose exposure, although not exceeding the PEL, has met or exceeded the action level of 0.5 ppm.

EMPLOYEE MONITORING

▌ The standard requires the employer to perform an initial monitoring of any employee who can be expected to experience exposure to formaldehyde, or a representative task sampling may be conducted. This means that the employer is not required to monitor the exposure of every employee but rather can monitor those performing tasks that are expected to provide formaldehyde exposure. This assumes that if employees rotate responsibilities for task performance in a laboratory, each individual's exposure would be expected to be comparable when performing the same task. Sampling the room air is *not* an acceptable measure of employee exposure. The employee must wear an exposure monitor near the breathing zone for either a full shift for the TWA measurement or for 15 minutes during the performance of high exposure tasks for the STEL measurement.

▌ Monitoring must be repeated if there should be a significant change in work practices or additional procedures are placed into use.

▌ In addition, individuals must be monitored immediately if any symptoms of formaldehyde exposure are reported.

▌ If the results of initial monitoring are at or above the action level, repeat monitoring must be performed annually. When results fall below the action level, no further testing is required.

▌ If the initial monitoring results exceed the STEL, repeat monitoring is required annually.

▌ If either the STEL or TWA were exceeded, the employer must develop a written plan to reduce employee exposure, using engineering and/or administrative controls and/or personal protective equipment.

▌ Employees must be notified of the monitoring results in writing. It is my practice to have employees sign a copy of the results, and I also post all monitoring results in a conspicuous area of the workstation.

Work areas demonstrated to have formaldehyde levels exceeding the PEL must be designated as a *regulated work area* (see the Laboratory Standard). Access to such areas must be restricted, and signs must be posted outside the area indicating that formaldehyde is in use.

OSHA Mandated Sign for Regulated Areas Where Formaldehyde Is Used

DANGER

FORMALDEHYDE
IRRITANT AND POTENTIAL CANCER HAZARD
AUTHORIZED PERSONNEL ONLY!

EXCESSIVE EXPOSURE

The employer must take steps to reduce the exposure of individuals exceeding the STEL or TWA. If administrative or engineering controls are not sufficient to bring the exposure into compliance, the employee must be provided with a respirator for use during procedures when exposure is excessive. The use of respirators is regulated by the Respiratory Protection Standard (29 CFR 1910.134). Respirator requirements as they apply to formaldehyde exposure include the following:

1. A full face respirator using approved cartridges for formaldehyde must be worn in situations in which exposure is likely to exceed acceptable limits.
2. A fit test must be performed to verify that the mask fits snugly against the face to prevent the leakage of formaldehyde vapors into the mask. Facial hair or eyeglasses may pose obstacles to proper respirator fit. Fit testing is often conducted using banana oil vapor or another harmless substance that is sprayed around the breathing zone. If the vapor cannot be detected by the wearer, the fit is suitable. After initial fit testing, the respirator fit must be checked annually.
3. Employee training must be conducted, covering the proper use and maintenance of the full face respirator. OSHA requires that formaldehyde cartridges be changed every 3 hours or at the end of the shift, *whichever is less.* Employees must also understand the limitations of the respirator, methods of checking the fit, and what to do in emergency situations.
4. Procedures must be established for inspecting, cleaning, and storing of respirators, which must be inspected before and immediately after each use.
5. A medical surveillance program must be conducted by a licensed physician, to include an annual health assessment of individuals required to wear respirators to perform their duties. The medical surveillance program is also required for any individual demonstrating symptoms of overexposure, whether or not the individual wears a respirator.
6. Employee exposure monitoring records must be kept on file for 30 years.
7. Employee medical surveillance records must be kept on file for 30 years.
8. Respirator fit test data must be retained until the next fit test is conducted.

PERSONAL PROTECTIVE EQUIPMENT (PPE)

Individuals working with formaldehyde solutions of a 1% or greater concentration must use gloves, a fluid impervious barrier such as a plastic apron, and chemical splash resistant goggles. Eye protection such as goggles or face shields must be rated to be chemical resistant (ANSI Z87.1-1989). Those often used as barrier protection under the Bloodborne Pathogens Standard are *not* adequate for use with chemicals. The laboratory is required to have eyewash facilities and an emergency shower.

REASSIGNMENT OF EMPLOYEES DEMONSTRATING SYMPTOMS OF OVEREXPOSURE

The 1992 revision of the Formaldehyde Standard requires employers to reassign employees who have signs of formaldehyde overexposure. The intent is to remove the individual from the offending environment. Symptoms of overexposure qualifying employees for reassignment include:

- Irritation of the eyes or mucosa of the upper respiratory tract
- Respiratory sensitization
- Irritation or sensitization of the skin

FORMALDEHYDE STANDARD (29 CFR 1910.1048)

Under such circumstances, the standard mandates that the employee be evaluated by a licensed physician selected by the employer. This may include the completion of a health assessment questionnaire. The employee has the option to seek a second opinion. If the physician recommends that the employee be removed from the work environment, the employee must be provided comparable work for which he or she is qualified or can be trained for in 6 months, with no loss of earnings or income, benefits, and seniority. If suitable work is not available, salary, benefits, and seniority must be maintained until one of the following, whichever comes first:

1. Work becomes available
2. The employee is determined to be unable to return to the exposure environment
3. The employee is determined to be able to return to work
4. Six months have passed

HAZARD COMMUNICATION REQUIREMENTS

The standard views formaldehyde solutions of 0.1% or greater to be hazardous and under such circumstances mandates strict labeling requirements for every container that holds this chemical. This includes any tissues that are being stored in the pathology laboratory containing as little as 1 mL of liquid. The OSHA required language for formaldehyde labeling is listed in the diagram below. The standard also requires all distributors of formaldehyde solutions to provide an MSDS to users. This requirement applies to laboratories that provide formalin solutions to clients. In a hospital setting, this would include clinics and other patient care areas such as the operating room where personnel use formaldehyde solutions.

OSHA Required Formaldehyde Warning Label

> ### CAUTION. CONTAINS FORMALDEHYDE.
> Toxic by inhalation and if swallowed. Irritating to the eyes, respiratory system, and skin. May cause sensitization by inhalation or skin contact. Risk of serious damage to eyes. May cause cancer; repeated exposure increases the risk.

TRAINING REQUIREMENTS

A training program that focuses on various aspects of formaldehyde usage and hazards must be provided to employees on initial hiring and annually thereafter. The program should include:

1. A thorough review of the MSDS for this chemical
2. Health hazards including an explanation of how to recognize signs of exposure
3. Correct procedures for working safely with formaldehyde, including labeling requirements of the standard
4. Use of PPE to limit exposure
5. Response to emergencies and spill containment
6. Engineering controls and work practices required by the standard

7. Discussion of the medical surveillance program
8. Disposal procedures

BLOODBORNE PATHOGENS STANDARD (29 CFR 1910.1030)

The intent of the Bloodborne Pathogens Standard, enacted in 1992, is to protect all individuals who could "reasonably be anticipated" as the result of performing their job duties to come into contact with blood and other potentially infectious material. The standard applies not only to laboratory personnel but to all workers in the health care environment who may come into contact with blood and body fluids, including housekeeping and maintenance personnel, security staff, sales representatives, firefighters, ambulance personnel, and so forth. The Bloodborne Pathogens Standard has been one of the most vigorously enforced laboratory regulations in history.

The standard applies to all occupational exposure to blood or other potentially infectious materials, including:

▌ Semen, vaginal secretions, cerebrospinal fluid, synovial fluid, pleural fluid, pericardial fluid, peritoneal fluid, amniotic fluid, saliva in dental procedures, any body fluid visibly contaminated with blood, and all body fluids in situations in which it is difficult or impossible to differentiate between body fluids.
▌ Unfixed tissues or organs (other than intact skin) from a human (living or dead)
▌ Human immunodeficiency virus (HIV) containing cell, tissue, or organ cultures and HIV or hepatitis B virus (HBV) containing culture media or other solutions and blood, organs, or other tissues from experimental animals infected with HIV or HBV as potentially infectious.

Blood borne pathogens are defined as pathogenic organisms that may be present in human blood and can cause disease in humans. These pathogens include, but are not limited to, HBV and HIV.

Epidemiology of Bloodborne Pathogens

OSHA estimates that about 75 to 110 of every 1000 workers who are frequently exposed to blood or other potentially infectious materials will become infected with HBV over the course of their working lifetime. Of those, 20 to 30 will suffer acute clinical illness, 4 to 6 will require hospitalization, and 2 to 3 will die of their disease. In addition, it is estimated that between 5% and 10% will become chronic carriers. Of those contracting hepatitis C, 50% will develop chronic disease, with 10% progressing to life threatening liver disease.

Symptoms of hepatitis infection resemble a flu-like illness. More severe clinical illness may be characterized by loss of appetite, jaundice, nausea, vomiting, abdominal pain, and diarrhea; 30% of those infected will pass HBV on to their sexual partner.

Acquired immunodeficiency syndrome (AIDS) is an almost invariably fatal illness resulting from infection with the HIV. The viral attack on the patient's immune system results in a spectrum of opportunistic infections that take an insurmountable toll. In its early stages, the patient experiences a retroviral syndrome not unlike mononucleosis. As it progresses, fever, fatigue, and diarrhea develop. Most individuals who are infected with HIV go on to develop AIDS, and although the symptoms can be treated somewhat, the immune deficiency appears irreversible.

THE BLOODBORNE PATHOGENS STANDARD (29 CFR 1910.1030)

Workplace Transmission

Although intact skin is thought to offer some protection against blood borne pathogens, they may be contracted by accidental skin puncture with contaminated needles, scalpels, capillary tubes, broken glass, or other "sharps." Broken skin, cuts, nicks, abrasions, and skin eruptions offer a portal of entry as well as splashes to the eyes and mucous membranes.

Universal Precautions

The concept of *universal precautions* is the cornerstone of efforts to prevent workplace transmission of blood borne pathogens. Under this concept, employees are trained to treat all patient specimens as though they are infectious. Therefore, precautions are taken in every instance, eliminating the need for judgments to be made that could otherwise be based on erroneous or incomplete information. This encourages employees to develop good work habits and to avoid having to remember which precautions are needed in each instance.

Requirements of the Bloodborne Pathogens Standard

EXPOSURE CONTROL PLAN

Employers are required to develop a written exposure control plan that is designed to eliminate or minimize exposure. The plan must identify, in writing, the tasks and procedures as well as job classifications *where occupational exposure to blood or other potentially infectious materials is likely to occur.* In addition, the plan must include recommendations for preventing exposure, using appropriate PPE, engineering controls, and work practice controls where feasible. A program must also be established to investigate all workplace exposure incidents. The exposure control plan must include the following:

- Exposure determination for each job category and task
- Methods for compliance with the standard
- Engineering and work practice controls, which include hand washing, and universal precautions
- Procedures for handling and disposal of infectious waste
- Proper handling and disposal of contaminated sharps
- The use and availability of PPE
- Emergency procedures
- Spill containment and clean-up
- Postexposure evaluation and follow-up to include a confidential medical evaluation and counseling
- Provision for HBV vaccine to be made available to each employee anticipated to experience exposure to blood borne pathogens during performance of routine duties
- Appropriate labeling of material believed to be potentially infectious
- Employee training on initial assignment and annually thereafter
- A plan to retain employee medical records for the duration of employment plus 30 years

HAZARD COMMUNICATION

The standard requires that warning labels including the orange biohazard symbol be affixed to containers of regulated waste, refrigerators and freezers, and other containers that are used to store or transport blood or other potentially infectious materials. An example of the required label is included below. Red bags or containers may be used in place of labeling. When a facility uses universal precautions, labeling is not required within the facility. Blood that has been tested and found to be free of HIV or HBV and regulated waste that has been decontaminated (i.e., autoclaved) need not be labeled. Signs must be posted to identify restricted areas in HIV and HBV research laboratories and production facilities.

OSHA Approved Biohazard Label

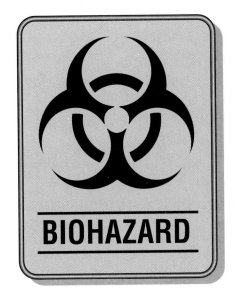

NOTE: The background of the biohazard symbol is usually orange

TRAINING

The standard mandates that training be provided to all employees who have a reasonable expectation of exposure to blood borne pathogens during the performance of their duties. Training must be conducted on initial work assignment and annually thereafter and must include making accessible a copy of the Bloodborne Pathogens Standard, an explanation of its contents, and a general discussion on blood borne diseases and their transmission, the facility's exposure control plan, engineering and work practice controls, personal protective equipment, HBV vaccine, response to emergencies involving blood, how to handle exposure incidents, the postexposure evaluation and follow-up program, signs, labels, and color coding. The trainer must be knowledgeable in the subject matter. Laboratory and production facility workers must receive additional specialized training.

PERSONAL PROTECTIVE EQUIPMENT

Employees who have a reasonable expectation of exposure to blood borne pathogens during the performance of their duties must be provided by the employer, at no cost to themselves, appropriate personal protective equipment such as, but not limited to, gloves, gowns, laboratory coats, face shields or masks, eye protection, mouthpieces, resuscitation bags, and pocket masks, or other ventilation devices. PPE will be considered

THE BLOODBORNE PATHOGENS STANDARD (29 CFR 1910.1030)

"appropriate" only if it does not permit blood or other potentially infectious materials to pass through to or reach the employee's work clothes, street clothes, undergarments, skin, eyes, and mouth or other mucous membranes under normal conditions of use and for the duration of time the device(s) are in use.

An entire industry has grown around the need for devices designed to protect the health care worker, offering facilities a selection of products that are useful for a wide range of activities. These range from devices to permit blood smears to be prepared without removing the Vacutainer stopper to whole blood analyzers utilizing direct tube sampling technologies that pierce the stopper to remove an aliquot of sample without exposing the technologist to the hazards of blood borne pathogens.

RECORD KEEPING REQUIREMENTS

The standard requires that the medical records of employees who have a reasonable expectation of exposure to blood borne pathogens during the performance of their duties be retained *for the duration of employment plus 30 years* and be kept confidential. Training records must be retained for 3 years and must include the dates, summary of the training content, trainer's name and qualifications, and names and job titles of all persons who attended the sessions.

TUBERCULOSIS EXPOSURE IN THE WORKPLACE

The recent resurgence of TB infections, especially drug resistant strains, in the general population has caused widespread alarm among the nation's health care providers. This problem is believed to have arisen among groups at risk for HIV infection, such as intravenous drug users, who often do not complete the lengthy therapeutic regimen for TB, leading to drug resistance. A depleted arsenal of pharmacologic agents to effectively deal with this organism sets the stage for a public health dilemma and significant challenges in the health care setting. Although there is no specific OSHA standard addressing this issue, laboratories are required to follow the 1994 CDC Guidelines for Preventing the Transmission of *Mycobacterium tuberculosis* in Health Care Facilities.

Transmission of *M. tuberculosis* is a recognized risk to patients and health care workers in the health care facilities. Transmission is most likely to occur from patients who have unrecognized pulmonary or laryngeal TB, are not on effective anti-TB therapy, and have not been placed in TB isolation. Several recent outbreaks in health care facilities, including outbreaks of multidrug resistant TB, have heightened concern about nosocomial transmission. Patients who develop multidrug resistant TB can remain infectious for prolonged periods, which increases the risk for nosocomial and/or occupational transmission.

Increases in the incidence of TB have been observed in some geographic areas; these increases are related partially to the high risk for TB among immunosuppressed persons, particularly those infected with HIV. Transmission of *m. tuberculosis* to HIV infected individuals is of particular concern because these persons are at high risk for developing active TB if they become infected with the bacterium. Thus, health care facilities should be particularly alert to the need for preventing transmission of *M. tuberculosis* in settings in which HIV infected persons work or receive care.

An effective TB infection control program requires early identification, isolation, and treatment of persons who have active TB. Implementation of a TB infection control program requires:

- Risk assessment and development of a TB infection control plan
- Early identification, treatment, and isolation of infectious TB patients
- Effective engineering controls
- An appropriate respiratory protection program
- Health care worker TB training, education, counseling, and screening

Although CDC guidelines are aimed primarily at individuals in the health care setting responsible for providing primary care to TB patients, some laboratory personnel can be expected to have direct exposure to infectious patients or infected material. These may include phlebotomists and technical staff performing bedside testing, microbiology technologists performing TB cultures, and personnel in the surgical pathology laboratory and autopsy room who may have exposure to infected lung tissue and other infected tissues in cases of extrapulmonary TB. The extent of an effective TB infection control program may vary from a simple program emphasizing administrative controls in settings where there is minimal risk for exposure to *M. tuberculosis* to a comprehensive program that includes administrative controls, engineering controls, and respiratory protection in settings where the risk for exposure is high. In all instances administrative measures must be used to limit the number of health care workers exposed.

Epidemiology

M. tuberculosis is carried in airborne particles or droplet nuclei that can be generated when persons who have pulmonary or laryngeal TB sneeze, cough, speak, or sing. The particles are an estimated 1 to 5 μm, and normal air currents can keep them airborne for prolonged periods of time and spread them throughout a room or building. Infection occurs when a susceptible person inhales droplet nuclei containing *M. tuberculosis* and these droplet nuclei make their way into the alveoli of the lung. Once in the alveoli, the organisms are taken up by the alveolar macrophages and spread throughout the body. Usually within 2 to 10 weeks after initial infection with *M. tuberculosis*, the immune response limits further multiplication and spread of the tubercle bacilli; however, some of the organisms remain dormant and viable for many years. This condition is referred to as *latent TB infection.* Individuals with latent TB will often test PPD positive, but they do not have symptoms of active TB and they are not infectious. Immunocompromised individuals have a greater risk for the progression of latent TB infection to active TB disease. HIV is the strongest known risk factor for this progression.

The probability that a person who is exposed to *M. tuberculosis* will become infected depends primarily on the concentration of infectious droplet nuclei in the air and the duration of exposure. Environmental factors that enhance the likelihood of transmission include:

- Exposure in a relatively small, enclosed space
- Inadequate local or general ventilation that results in insufficient dilution and/or removal of infectious droplet nuclei
- Recirculation of air containing infectious droplet nuclei

Fundamentals of Tuberculosis Infection Control

Specific measures to reduce the risk of transmission of *M. tuberculosis* include the following:

- Conducting a risk assessment to evaluate the risk of transmission of *M. tuberculosis* in all areas of the health care facility, developing a written TB infection

TUBERCULOSIS EXPOSURE IN THE WORKPLACE

control program based on risk assessment, and periodic reassessment of effectiveness of the program

▌ Developing, implementing, and enforcing policies and protocols to ensure early identification, diagnostic evaluation, and effective treatment of patients who may have infectious TB

▌ Promptly initiating and maintaining TB isolation for persons who may have infectious TB in the inpatient setting

▌ Developing, installing, maintaining, and evaluating ventilation and other engineering controls to reduce the potential for airborne exposure to *M. tuberculosis.*

▌ Developing, implementing, maintaining, and evaluating a respiratory protection program

▌ Educating and training health care workers about TB, effective methods for prevention of transmission, and the benefits of medical screening programs

▌ Developing a program for routine periodic screening of health care workers for active and latent TB infections

▌ Promptly evaluating possible episodes of *M. tuberculosis* transmission in health care facilities among health care workers, or patients and contacts of patients and health care workers

ENGINEERING CONTROLS

To prevent the escape of infectious droplet nuclei, TB isolation rooms, TB laboratories, and autopsy rooms should be kept under negative pressure relative to corridors and surrounding areas, which must be monitored daily. This is to prevent contaminated air from escaping into noncontaminated rooms and hallways. The American Society of Heating, Refrigerating and Air Conditioning Engineers (ASHRAE) further recommends a minimum of 6 air changes per hour for the areas previously listed. However, the effectiveness of this level of airflow in reducing the concentration of droplet nuclei the room, thus reducing the transmission of airborne pathogens, has not been evaluated directly or adequately. The CDC recommends that, where possible, the ventilation flow rate be increased to 12 air changes per hour, with air from TB rooms preferentially exhausted directly to the outside of the building. That is, air from these rooms should not be recirculated within the facility. In some cases, this may be unavoidable, in which instance HEPA (high efficiency particulate air) filters must be used with the ducting to prevent dissemination of tubercle bacilli.

RESPIRATORY PROTECTION

Personal respiratory protection should be used by persons entering rooms in which patients with known or suspected infectious TB are being isolated. Such protection should likewise be made available to those providing emergency surgical or dental care, autopsy personnel, and the surgical pathologist who may be exposed during the performance of frozen sections and tissue dissection.

Respiratory protection must meet the following criteria:

1. The respirator mask must be able to filter particles 1 μm or less. The HEPA respirator is designed to filter particulate matter less than one μm, which *should* successfully filter the tubercle bacillus

2. The facility must follow the provisions of the OSHA Respiratory Protection Standard, which includes the requirement for fit testing and employee education and training.

Surgical masks are designed to prevent the respiratory secretions of the person wearing the mask from entering the air and ***will offer no protection from TB exposure.*** TB patients who must be transported through the hospital will be required to wear a surgical mask to reduce the number of droplet nuclei entering the air. *A surgical mask should never be used by employees wishing to protect themselves from exposure.*

Education and Training

All health care workers, including physicians, should receive education regarding TB that is relevant to persons in their particular occupational group. Training should be conducted before initial assignment, and retraining should be conducted as needed. The level and detail of training will vary according to the individual's work responsibilities and the level of risk.

The program should include:

1. The basic concepts of TB transmission, pathogenesis, and diagnosis; signs and symptoms; and the difference between latent and active infection
2. The principles and practices of infection control that reduce the risk of transmission of *M. tuberculosis*
3. Infection control measures and the written policies and procedures specific to the various job titles identified to have exposure risk

BIBLIOGRAPHY

ACGIH: 1994–95 Threshold Limit Values for Chemical Substances and Physical Agents and Biological Exposure Indices. Cincinnati, Ohio, American Conference of Governmental Industrial Hygienists, 1994.

Dapson JC, Dapson R: Hazardous Chemicals in the Histopathology Laboratory. Battle Creek, Mich, Anatech, 1995.

Guidelines for Protecting the Safety and Health of Health Care Workers. Atlanta, Ga, U.S. Department of Health and Human Services, Centers for Disease Control Publication 88-119, 1988.

Guidelines for Preventing the Transmission of Tuberculosis in Healthcare Settings, with Special Focus on HIV-Related Issues. MMWR Morb Mortal Wkly Rep 39 (RR-17):1–29, 1990.

Guidelines for Preventing the Transmission of *Mycobacterium tuberculosis* in Healthcare Facilities, 1994. MMWR Morbid Mortal Wkly Rep 43 (RR-13):1–132, 1994.

NCCLS: Clinical Laboratory Safety: Tentative Guideline. Villanova, Pa, National Committee for Clinical Laboratory Standards, NCCLS Document GP-17T, 1994.

NCCLS: Clinical Laboratory Waste Management: Approved Guideline. Villanova, Pa, National Committee for Clinical Laboratory Standards, NCCLS Document GP-5A, 1993.

NCCLS: Protection of Laboratory Workers from Infectious Disease Transmitted by Blood, Body Fluids and Tissue, Tentative Guideline. Villanova, Pa, National Committee for Clinical Laboratory Standards, NCCLS Document M29-T2, 1991.

OSHA publications: CFR 1910.1030, The Bloodborne Pathogens Standard (1992); CFR 1910.1048, The Formaldehyde Standard (1987); CFR 1910.1200, The Hazard Communication Standard (1988); CFR 1910.1450, The Laboratory Standard (1990).

Rekus J: Bloodborne Pathogens. Occup Health Saf 12:31, 1991.

Sax NI: Dangerous Properties of Industrial Materials. New York, Van Nostrand Reinhold, 1991.

INDEX